Current Cancer Therapeutics
Fifth Edition

Academic Editors

David S. Ettinger, MD, FACP, FCCP
Alex Grass Professor of Oncology
Professor of Medicine
Professor of Radiation Oncology and Molecular Radiation Sciences
Johns Hopkins University School of Medicine
The Sidney Kimmel Comprehensive Cancer Center at Johns Hopkins
Baltimore, Maryland

Ross C. Donehower, MD, FACP
Virginia and DK Ludwig Professor in Clinical Investigation of Cancer
Professor of Oncology and Medicine
Director, Division of Medical Oncology
Johns Hopkins University School of Medicine
The Sidney Kimmel Comprehensive Cancer Center at Johns Hopkins
Baltimore, Maryland

Editors

Rowena N. Schwartz, PHARMD, BCOP
Director of Oncology Pharmacy
Johns Hopkins Hospital
Baltimore, Maryland

MiKaela Olsen, RN, MS, OCN
Oncology and BMT Clinical Nurse Specialist
The Sidney Kimmel Comprehensive Cancer Center at Johns Hopkins
Baltimore, Maryland

With 53 contributors

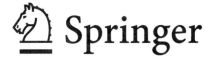

CURRENT MEDICINE GROUP LLC, PART OF SPRINGER SCIENCE+BUSINESS MEDIA LLC

400 Market Street, Suite 700 • Philadelphia, PA 19106

Developmental Editor	Jennifer Guimaraes
Editorial Assistant	Juleen Deaner
Design and Layout	Dan Britt
Illustrators	Heather Hoch, Wieslawa Langenfeld, Jacqueline Leonard, Maureen Looney
Production Coordinator	Carolyn Naylor
Indexer	Holly Lukens

ISBN 978-1-57340-285-9
ISSN 1074-2816

Although every effort has been made to ensure that drug doses and other information are presented accurately in this publication, the ultimate responsibility rests with the prescribing physician. Neither the publishers nor the authors can be held responsible for errors or for any consequences arising from the use of information contained herein. Products mentioned in this publication should be used in accordance with the prescribing information prepared by the manufacturers. No claims or endorsements are made for any drug or compound at present under clinical investigation.

www.springer.com

For more information, please call 1 (800) 777-4643
or email us at orders-ny@springer.com

10 9 8 7 6 5 4 3 2 1

Printed in the United States by IPC Print Services

This book was printed on acid-free paper

Preface

This is the fifth edition of Current Cancer Therapeutics, and 7 years since the last edition. During this time period, significant advances have been made in our understanding of cancer because of genetics and molecular biology. This understanding has led to the use of various target therapies to treat cancers either alone or in combination with other therapies, as well as improvement in the diagnosis, prevention, and early detection and treatment of these diseases. Cancer treatment has become more complex, in many situations involving a multimodality approach.

This edition is written by authors from the Sidney Kimmel Comprehensive Cancer Center at Johns Hopkins. Several authors have since moved to other academic positions. The information provided on specific chemotherapy, target therapy, combinations of therapy, and management of specific diseases and complications of disease and its treatment are concise, easily understandable, informative, and should aid the practicing oncologists, nurses, pharmacists, and other healthcare professionals in caring for their cancer patients.

The book is divided into five parts: Agents; Specific Neoplasms and Therapeutic Protocols; Supportive Care; Pharmacy-Specific Issues; and Nursing-Specific Issues. The latter two are new to this edition of the book. The part on clinical data collection was deleted.

The agent section is compendious but informative providing data on pharmacokinetics, indications, and toxicities of the specific therapies. Three new chapters were included: Targeted Therapies, Cancer Vaccines, and Radiation Therapy and Chemopotentiation.

The disease sections were updated and provide concise summaries of epidemiology, risk factors, screening, staging, and therapeutic options. The information for specific therapies is provided in either tabular or in a diagrammatic fashion.

The supportive care section contains information on the management of complications such as myelosuppression, renal and metabolic, pulmonary and cardiac, neurotoxicities, paraneoplastic syndromes, and cachexia. Also provided are information on palliative care, quality of life, and a new chapter on geriatric-specific issues.

As mentioned previously, new sections of the book include concise information on pharmacy as well as nursing-specific issues as they relate to the cancer patient.

We believe that the contributors to this volume provide the reader with an understandable, concise review of cancer and cancer therapeutics. It is hoped that this book will assist those healthcare providers interested in cancer to better understand and treat their patients.

David S. Ettinger
Ross C. Donehower
Editors

Contributors

Richard F. Ambinder, MD, PhD
James B. Murphy Professor of Oncology
Division Director, Hematologic Malignancies
Department of Oncology
The Sidney Kimmel Comprehensive
 Cancer Center at Johns Hopkins
Baltimore, Maryland

Deborah K. Armstrong, MD
Associate Professor of Oncology
Johns Hopkins Kimmel Cancer Center
Associate Professor of Gynecology
 and Obstetrics
Johns Hopkins University School of Medicine
Baltimore, Maryland

Douglas W. Ball, MD
Associate Professor
Departments of Medicine and Oncology
Johns Hopkins University School of Medicine
Baltimore, Maryland

Jaishri Blakeley, MD
Assistant Professor of Neurology,
 Neurosurgery, and Oncology
Department of Neurology
Johns Hopkins University School of Medicine
Baltimore, Maryland

Julie R. Brahmer, MD
Assistant Professor
Department of Oncology
Johns Hopkins University School of Medicine
The Sidney Kimmel Comprehensive Care
 Center at Johns Hopkins
Baltimore, Maryland

Johann C. Brandes, MD, PhD, FCCP
Assistant Professor of Hematology
 and Oncology
Emory University School of Medicine
Staff Physician, Atlanta VAMC
Atlanta, Georgia

Susanne Briest, MD
Head of Breast Cancer Center
University of Leipzig
Leipzig, Germany

Malcolm V. Brock, MD
Associate Professor
Department of Surgery
Department of Oncology
Johns Hopkins University School of Medicine
Baltimore, Maryland

Ilene Browner, MD
Instructor
Department of Medical Oncology
Johns Hopkins University School of Medicine
The Sidney Kimmel Comprehensive
 Cancer Center at Johns Hopkins
Baltimore, Maryland

Michael A. Carducci, MD, FACP
Professor of Oncology and Urology
Johns Hopkins University School of Medicine
The Sidney Kimmel Comprehensive
 Cancer Center at Johns Hopkins
Baltimore, Maryland

Hetty E. Carraway, MD, MBA
Instructor in Oncology
Department of Oncology/Cancer Biology
 Program and Division of Hematologic
 Malignancies
Johns Hopkins University School of Medicine
The Sidney Kimmel Comprehensive
 Cancer Center at Johns Hopkins
Baltimore, Maryland

Keri Culton, RD, LDN, CNSD
Clinical Dietitian Specialist
Department of Nutrition
Johns Hopkins Hospital
Baltimore, Maryland

Samuel R. Denmeade, MD
Associate Professor
Department of Oncology
Johns Hopkins University School of Medicine
The Sidney Kimmel Comprehensive
 Cancer Center at Johns Hopkins
Baltimore, Maryland

Luis A. Diaz, Jr, MD
Assistant Professor of Oncology
Director, Translational Medicine
Ludwig Center for Cancer Genetics
 and Therapeutics
Johns Hopkins University School of Medicine
The Sidney Kimmel Comprehensive Cancer
 Center at Johns Hopkins
Baltimore, Maryland

Erin M. Dunbar, MD
Assistant Professor
Department of Neurosurgery
University of Florida
Gainesville, Florida

Sydney Dy, MD
Assistant Professor of Health, Policy and
 Management
Johns Hopkins University
Baltimore, Maryland

Khaled El-Shami, MBBch, PhD
Postdoctoral Fellow
Department of Oncology
Johns Hopkins University School of Medicine
The Sidney Kimmel Comprehensive Cancer
 Center at Johns Hopkins
Baltimore, Maryland

David S. Ettinger, MD
Alex Grass Professor of Oncology
The Sidney Kimmel Comprehensive Cancer
 Center at Johns Hopkins
Baltimore, Maryland

Leslie A. Fecher, MD
Assistant Professor
Department of Medicine
Division of Hematology/Oncology
Abramson Cancer Center of the
 University of Pennsylvania
Philadelphia, Pennsylvania

Joanne Finley, MS, RN
Patient Education Coordinator
Johns Hopkins Hospital
The Sidney Kimmel Comprehensive
 Cancer Center at Johns Hopkins
Baltimore, Maryland

Arlene A. Forastiere, MD
Professor of Oncology
Johns Hopkins University School of Medicine
The Sidney Kimmel Comprehensive Cancer
 Center at Johns Hopkins
Baltimore, Maryland

Ignacio Garrido-Laguna, MD
Clinical Research Fellow, Gastrointestinal
 Oncology and Developmental
 Therapeutics Program
The Sidney Kimmel Comprehensive Cancer
 Center at Johns Hopkins
Baltimore, Maryland

Elizabeth A. Griffiths, MD
Senior Oncology Fellow
Department of Oncology
Johns Hopkins University School of Medicine
The Sidney Kimmel Comprehensive Cancer
 Center at Johns Hopkins
Baltimore, Maryland

Joseph Herman, MD, MSc
Assistant Professor
Department of Radiation Oncology and
 Molecular Radiation Sciences
Department of Urology
Department of Surgery
Johns Hopkins University School of Medicine
Baltimore, Maryland

Carol Ann Huff, MD
Assistant Professor of Oncology and Medicine
Director
Myeloma Program
Johns Hopkins University School of Medicine
The Sidney Kimmel Comprehensive
 Cancer Center at Johns Hopkins
Baltimore, Maryland

Salma Jabbour, MD
Assistant Professor
Department of Radiation Oncology
Robert Wood Johnson Medical School
University of Medicine and Dentistry of
 New Jersey
Piscataway, New Jersey

Elizabeth M. Jaffee, MD
Dana and Albert "Cubby" Broccoli Professor
 of Oncology
Department of Oncology
Johns Hopkins University School of Medicine
Baltimore, Maryland

Antonio Jimeno MD, PhD
Assistant Professor of Oncology
Director, Developmental
 Therapeutics/Pharmacodynamic Laboratory
University of Colorado Cancer Center
Aurora, Colorado

Yvette L. Kasamon, MD
Assistant Professor
Departments of Oncology and Medicine
Johns Hopkins University School of Medicine
Baltimore, Maryland

Peter S. Kim, PhD
Department of Oncology
Johns Hopkins University School of Medicine
Baltimore, Maryland

Daniel Laheru, MD
Associate Professor of Oncology
Clinical Director, Division of
 Gastrointestinal Oncology
Co-Director, The Skip Viragh Center for
 Pancreas Cancer Clinical Research and
 Patient Care
Johns Hopkins University School of Medicine
The Sol Goldman Pancreatic Cancer
 Research Center
The Sidney Kimmel Comprehensive
 Cancer Center at Johns Hopkins
Baltimore, Maryland

John Laterra, MD, PhD
Professor
Departments of Neurology, Oncology,
 and Neuroscience
Johns Hopkins University School of Medicine
Director of Neuro-oncology
Johns Hopkins Hospital
Director
Neuro-oncology Laboratory
The Kennedy Krieger Research Institute
Baltimore, Maryland

Dung Le, MD
Instructor
Department of Oncology
Johns Hopkins University School of Medicine
Baltimore, Maryland

Moshe Yair Levy, MD
Instructor
Department of Oncology
Johns Hopkins University
Baltimore, Maryland

David M. Loeb, MD, PhD
Assistant Professor, Oncology, and Pediatrics
Director
Musculoskeletal Tumor Program
The Sidney Kimmel Comprehensive Cancer
 Center at Johns Hopkins
Baltimore, Maryland

Wen Wee Ma, MD
Clinical and Research Fellow
Department of Oncology
Johns Hopkins University
Clinical Fellow
Department of Medical Oncology
The Sidney Kimmel Comprehensive
 Cancer Center at Johns Hopkins
Baltimore, Maryland

Wells A. Messersmith, MD
Director, GI Medical Oncology Program
Associate Professor, Division of
 Medical Oncology
Department of Medicine
University of Colorado School of Medicine
University of Colorado Cancer Center
Aurora, Colorado

MiKaela Olsen, RN, MS, OCN
Oncology and BMT Nurse Specialist
The Sidney Kimmel Comprehensive Cancer
 Center at Johns Hopkins
Baltimore, Maryland

Roberto Pili, MD
Associate Professor of Oncology and Urology
Department of Oncology
Johns Hopkins University
Baltimore, Maryland

**Rowena N. Schwartz,
 PharmD, BCOP**
Director of Oncology Pharmacy
Johns Hopkins Hospital
Baltimore, Maryland

Gary R. Shapiro, MD
Associate Professor of Oncology
Chairman, Department of Oncology
Johns Hopkins Bayview Medical Center
Director
Johns Hopkins Geriatric Oncology Program
The Sidney Kimmel Comprehensive Cancer
 Center at Johns Hopkins
Baltimore, Maryland

William H. Sharfman, MD
Associate Professor of Oncology
 and Dermatology
Director of Cutaneous Oncology
Clinical Co-Director
Melanoma Program
The Sidney Kimmel Comprehensive
 Cancer Center at Johns Hopkins
Johns Hopkins University
Baltimore, Maryland

Ori Shokek, MD
Division of Radiation Oncology
York Cancer Center
York, Pennsylvania

B. Douglas Smith, MD
Associate Professor,
Department of
 Oncology/Hematologic Malignancies
Johns Hopkins University School of Medicine
The Sidney Kimmel Comprehensive
 Cancer Center at Johns Hopkins
Baltimore, Maryland

Vered Stearns, MD
Associate Professor of Oncology
Johns Hopkins University School of Medicine
The Sidney Kimmel Comprehensive
 Cancer Center at Johns Hopkins
Baltimore, Maryland

Lode J. Swinnen, MD
Department of Oncology
Division of Hematologic Malignancies
Johns Hopkins University School of Medicine
Baltimore, Maryland

Katherine Thornton, MD
Assistant Professor
Johns Hopkins University School of Medicine
The Sidney Kimmel Comprehensive
 Cancer Center at Johns Hopkins
Baltimore, Maryland

Scott Wadler, MD (deceased)
Richard T. Silver Distinguished Professorship
 of Hematology and Medical Oncology
Weill Cornell Medical College
New York Presbyterian Hospital
New York, New York

Nina D. Wagner-Johnston, MD
Assistant Professor
Washington University School of Medicine
Saint Louis, Missouri

Janet R. Walczak, MSN, CRNP
Research Associate
Department of Oncology
Johns Hopkins University
Nurse Practitioner
The Sidney Kimmel Comprehensive
 Cancer Center at Johns Hopkins
Baltimore, Maryland

Erica D. Warlick, MD
Assistant Professor of Medicine
Division of Hematology, Oncology,
 and Transplantation
University of Minnesota
Minneapolis, Minnesota

Antonio C. Wolff, MD, FACP
Associate Professor of Oncology
Breast Cancer Program
The Sidney Kimmel Comprehensive
 Cancer Center at Johns Hopkins
Baltimore, Maryland

Rex C. Yung, MD
Assistant Professor of Medicine
Johns Hopkins University School
 of Medicine
The Sidney Kimmel Comprehensive
 Cancer Center at Johns Hopkins
Baltimore, Maryland

Contents

Chemotherapy

Rowena N. Schwartz

The pharmacologic approach to cancer therapy encompasses a wide variety of medications. Chemotherapy has historically referred to those cytotoxic agents that target rapidly dividing cancer cells. The strategy of drug therapy for treatment of cancer continues to evolve, yet chemotherapy remains an important pharmacotherapy approach for cancer treatment. This chapter provides a brief overview of some of the most common classes of chemotherapy. Additionally, the accompanying drug-specific pages provide information about individual agents, including proposed mechanism of anticancer activity, toxicities, therapeutic uses in cancer, and pharmacologic profile. The precise mechanism of the anticancer effect of many agents is not fully understood and the information provided is what is currently known about the pharmacologic mechanism of action. Additionally, doses and dose ranges for medications are not provided, as the dose and schedule of a specific agent is dependent on many aspects of the clinical situation (*eg*, combination, time in course of treatment, concurrent therapies, disease state). A review of pharmacologic aspects of individual agents may be found in many texts [1–3] and in published reviews. A quick reference list of toxicities for specific agents is available [4] and delineates between acute and delayed toxicities.

CLASSIFICATION OF AGENTS

Agents used as cancer therapy are commonly categorized by their mechanism of action (*eg*, antimetabolite or alkylating agents) or source (*eg*, vinca alkaloid). Within a specific class of agents, individual medications differ significantly with regard to their pharmacology, activity, toxicities, and clinical application. Certain toxicities may be unique to an individual agent within a class, while other side effects may be common among all drugs within a class. Importantly, the manifestation of a specific agent's side effect may vary significantly based on the drug dose, schedule, route, and duration of administration and drug therapy combination. The tolerability of most drugs used in the treatment of cancer depends upon patient-specific considerations such as disease, organ function (*eg*, renal function, liver function), comorbidities, and concomitant medications. Strategies and references for chemotherapy dose modifications is not discussed in this chapter, although information included in the agent-specific pages does provide some guidance for when practioners should consider dose modification. Modification of the dose of most drugs listed should be made with consideration to clinical situation (*eg*, goal of treatment), etiology for organ impairment (*eg*, renal dysfunction secondary to obstruction of lymphoma may respond to therapy and allow full dosing versus renal dysfunction secondary to comorbidities).

ALKYLATING AGENTS

Alkylating agents (Table 1-1) [5] are a diverse group of anticancer drugs that act through the covalent bonding of the alkyl group (one or more saturated carbon atoms) to cellular nucleophilic sites. This leads to DNA strand breaks and ultimately cell death. Alkylating agents differ in their pharmacokinetic profile, chemical properties, and cancer activity, although they share a common molecular mechanism of action. Cross-resistance is not complete between all alkylating agents, but may be seen between some agents. Bendamustine is a novel alkylator agent—actually a purine analogue–alkylator hybrid—that has been available in Germany for many years but was recently approved in the United States.

The usual dose-limiting toxicity of many alkylating agents is myelosuppression. The degree, duration, and manifestation of the myelosuppression vary among agents and are dependent on dose and/or schedule. Nausea and vomiting are often associated with drugs in this class; again, the degree and pattern vary depending upon the agent. The actions of alkylating agents are not selective for cancer cells, and damage to other tissues may result in a variety of acute and delayed organ toxicities. For example, cyclophosphamide and ifosfamide are associated with hemorrhagic cystitis secondary to

the effect of a toxic metabolite, acrolein, within the bladder wall. Busulfan, in addition to other alkylating agents, has been associated with interstitial pneumonitis and pulmonary fibrosis. Alopecia is a common effect seen with most of these agents. Long-term complications with alkylating agents include gonadal atrophy, infertility, and increased risk of secondary cancers.

Of note, many of these agents demonstrate a dose-response effect and are used at very high doses as part of the mobilization and/or preparative regimens preceding hematopoietic stem cell transplantation. The side effect profiles for agents such as cyclophosphamide are different when the dose is escalated in high-dose regimens.

NONCLASSICAL ALKYLATING AGENTS

A group of cytotoxic agents often referred to as nonclassical alkylating agents have diverse chemical structures and are able to covalently bind to biologic macromolecules in a manner similar to alkylating agents. The structure of nonclassical alkylating agents does not include the classic alkylating chloroethyl group seen with "classical" alkylating agents. The drugs within this classification of agents are diverse, ranging from platinum agents to the monoamine oxidase inhibitor procarbazine [5].

PLATINUM COMPOUNDS

A group of chemotherapeutic agents based on the inclusion of elemental platinum are among the most widely used antineoplastic agents (Table 1-2). The biologic actions of Pt(II) complexes are attributable to displacement reactions in which platinum binds to DNA, RNA, proteins, and other biomolecules. Through successive displacement, these agents form a complex, similar to alkylating agents, inducing cell damage and apoptosis.

Cisplatin, carboplatin, and oxaliplatin are the three commercially available platinum agents. The toxicity profile of each agent is unique, but there are some shared adverse effects. Cisplatin is associated with significant acute and delayed nausea and vomiting, which is at least partially prevented with aggressive prophylactic antiemetics. Renal toxicity, manifesting in

Table 1-1. Alkylating Agents and Nonclassical Alkylating Agents	
Drug class	**Drugs**
Nitrogen mustards	Cyclophosphamide
	Ifosfamide
	Mechlorethamine
	Melphalan
	Chlorambucil
Aziridines	Thiotepa
	Altretamine
Alkyl alkane sulfonates	Busulfan
Nitrosoureas	Carmustine
	Lomustine
	Streptozocin
Nonclassical alkylating agents	Procarbazine
	Dacarbazine
	Temozolomide
	Cisplatin
	Carboplatin
	Oxaliplatin
Alkylating agent hybrid	Bendamustine

tubular damage and associated electrolyte wasting, is dose limiting. Carbo-platin, developed with the intent of avoiding the problematic nephrotoxicity of cisplatin, is associated with hematologic toxicity. Oxaliplatin, the most recent agent widely used in the treatment of colorectal cancer, has signifi-cant neurotoxicity. The neurotoxicity may manifest as a chronic peripheral neuropathy, also seen with cisplatin and carboplatin, or a unique sensory neuropathy manifested by cold sensitivity (*eg*, a burning sensation when touching cold objects). In most patients, the neurotoxicity is reversible upon discontinuation of oxaliplatin [5].

ANTIMETABOLITES

The antimetabolites are drugs that are structurally related to naturally occur-ring compounds involved in cellular production (Table 1-3). Developed as drugs focused on causing disruption of cell division as "false" components of DNA, newer agents exert their cytotoxic effects through additional cel-lular mechanisms. Historically, these agents were most effective against rapidly dividing cells, as many of the individual agents are active during cell cycle. One of the advances of more recently developed antimetabolites is their impact on nondividing cells (*eg*, gemcitabine).

PYRIMIDINE ANALOGUES

FLUORINATED PYRIMIDINES
The fluoropyrimidines were originally synthesized based on the rationale that cancer cells used uracil more rapidly than nonmalignant cells. Fluo-rouracil (5-FU) is an analogue of uracil with a fluorine atom substituted for hydrogen at the carbon 5 position of the pyrimidine ring. The cytotoxic mechanism of action appears to be through inhibition of thymidylate syn-thetase, ultimately inhibiting both DNA and RNA synthesis. The presence of a reduced folate cofactor is required for tight binding of the active metabolite to thymidylate synthetase, and the addition of the reduced folate leucovorin has been incorporated into regimens with 5-FU to optimize cell kill.

The main toxicities of the fluoropyrimidines are based on the disruption of rapidly dividing cells; such toxicities primarily manifest as damage to the gastrointestinal (GI) tract (*eg*, mucositis and diarrhea) and bone mar-row suppression. The spectrum of toxicity associated with these agents is very dependent upon dose, schedule, and route of administration. Toxicities seen with chronic exposure, such as a daily dosing regimen used with oral capecitabine or a continuous infusion regimen, are often associated with damage to the GI tract. Regimens that include bolus dosing of antimetabo-lites are more commonly associated with bone marrow suppression.

CYTIDINE ANALOGUES

Nucleoside analogues compete with their physiologic counterpart for incor-poration into nucleic acids and eventually interfere with cell division. Cyta-rabine has long been considered a cornerstone of the treatment of acute myelogenous leukemia (AML), but its use may be limited secondary to development of drug resistance. The search for similarly effective alterna-tive agents has led to the development of a number of agents that have found their utility in leukemia and other cancers.

The toxicity profile of cytarabine, similar to other antimetabolites, is dependent upon dose and schedule. Lower doses administered as a con-tinuous infusion result in GI and hematologic toxicity. Higher doses given as intermittent bolus infusions are associated with additional toxicities such as neurotoxicity and ocular toxicity.

Gemcitabine is a difluorinated analogue of deoxycytidine. It was initially developed as an alternative for cytarabine for AML, but is now most com-monly used in a number of solid tumors (*eg*, pancreatic, lung, and breast cancer). The dose-limiting toxicity is hematologic. Of note, patients often

experience a mild but distressing flu-like syndrome following gemcitabine. Gemcitabine is also a powerful radiosensitizer.

PURINE ANTIMETABOLITES

GUANINE ANALOGUES
Some of the oldest anticancer agents are synthetic analogues to guanine. Mercaptopurine (6-MP) and thioguanine, the 2-amino analogue of 6-MP, are both rapidly converted to ribonucleotides that ultimately inhibit purine biosynthesis. Cross-resistance occurs between the two agents. Both agents are generally well tolerated. GI toxicity and bone marrow suppression are the most common toxicities.

ADENOSINE ANALOGUES
Many of the currently available analogues of adenosine were initially developed as an alternative to cytarabine. Fludarabine, unlike cytarabine, is incorporated into RNA, resulting in inhibition of transcription. Fludara-bine is used in the treatment of lymphoid malignancies, and has significant immunosuppressive effects. Toxicities include myelosuppression, immuno-suppression, and, at higher doses, cerebellar toxicities. Cladribine, another agent initially developed for acute leukemia, demonstrated activity in both dividing and resting cells and is associated with both myelosuppression and immunosuppression.

FOLATE ANTAGONISTS

Folate is an essential cofactor in many reactions for the synthesis of DNA; therefore, agents that inhibit the availability of cellular folate have been developed as cytotoxic agents. Dietary folates, dihydrofolates, are reduced to their biologically active tetrahydrofolate form to be utilized in the biosyn-thesis of DNA. Methotrexate is a folic acid analogue that inhibits dihydrofo-late reductase, the enzyme that reduces dietary folic acid to the biologically active folinic acid. Methotrexate is used in a variety of doses and schedules for both cancer and autoimmune disease [6].

Similar to other antimetabolites, toxicities of methotrexate include bone marrow suppression and GI toxicities. Methotrexate is also a good example of how the toxicities of an agent vary based on the strategy of use. High-dose methotrexate can precipitate in the renal tubule and result in renal dysfunction. Preventive strategies, including alkalinization of the urine and vigorous hydration, can help minimize precipitation of drug in the kidneys and subsequent nephrotoxicity. High-dose regimens (> 500 mg/m²) are followed within 24 hours with the reduced folate (folinic acid) leucovorin

Table 1-3. Antimetabolite Chemotherapeutic Agents

Drug class	Drug
Pyrimidine analogues	Fluorouracil
	Floxuridine
	Capecitabine
	Cytarabine
	Gemcitabine
Folate antagonists	Methotrexate
	Trimetrexate
	Pemetrexed
Purine analogues	Mercaptopurine
	Thioguanine
	Bendamustine*
	Cladribine
	Clofarabine
	Fludarabine
	Nelarabine
	Pentostatin

*Bendamustine is a purine analogue/alkylator hybrid.

Table 1-2. Platinum-Containing Compounds

Agent	Dose-limiting toxicity
Cisplatin	Nephrotoxicity, neurotoxicity
Carboplatin	Hematologic toxicity
Oxaliplatin	Neurotoxicity

as rescue to prevent lethal effects of myelosuppression and stomatitis. In fact, with appropriate leucovorin rescue strategies there is minimal bone marrow suppression or stomatitis with high-dose methotrexate regimens. On the other hand, hepatotoxicity with chronic administration of low-dose methotrexate may be a significant problem.

Pemetrexed is a multitargeted antifolate analogue that targets a number of enzymes involved in folate metabolism, including, but not limited to, thymidine synthetase and dihydrofolate reductase. The main toxicities include dose-limiting myelosuppression, mucositis, and rash. Toxicities are decreased with supplementation of folic acid and vitamin B_{12} [6].

ANTIMICROTUBULE AGENTS

A strategic cellular target for anticancer therapy is the microtubules, as they are known to play such an important role in mitosis as well in the maintenance of cell shape, scaffolding, and function. Antimicrotubule agents are often naturally occurring or semisynthetic compounds (Table 1-4) [7,8].

VINCA ALKALOIDS

Vinca alkaloids are naturally occurring or semisynthetic nitrogenous bases that interact with tubulin and disrupt microtubule assembly, ultimately inducing metaphase arrest in dividing cells. The principal toxicities of the vinca alkaloids differ despite structural and pharmacologic similarities. The primary toxicity of vincristine is peripheral neurotoxicity, which limits the dosing of the drug. Myelosuppression is the dose-limiting toxicity of vinblastine, although neurotoxicity can be seen. Dose-limiting toxicities for vindesine are hematologic and neurologic. Vinorelbine also has dose-limiting hematologic toxicity. Of note, all these agents can cause significant tissue damage if extravasation occurs.

TAXANES

Taxanes also exert their cytotoxic effect on microtubules, but through a different mechanism. By stabilizing microtubules against depolymerization, taxanes prevent disassembly and ultimately inhibit the dynamic reorganization of the microtubule network [9].

The primary toxicity of the agents in this class is myelosuppression. Paclitaxel has a high incidence of major hypersensivity reactions thought to be secondary to the diluent Cremophor EL (polyethoxylated castor oil, BASF Corp., Ludwigshafen, Germany), which is necessary for solubility. Paclitaxel requires premedication with histamine antagonists and corticosteroids. Docetaxel is formulated in polysorbate 80 and has significantly fewer infusion-related reactions. Unique to docetaxel is a cumulative fluid retention syndrome characterized by edema, weight gain, and pleural effusions. Premedication with dexamethasone (and continued posttherapy for 3 to 5 days) has helped ameliorate this toxicity. Docetaxel also has significant dermatologic effects, including rash and onychodystrophy. Alopecia is severe with these agents, and peripheral neuropathy can be dose limiting in some patients.

Nab-paclitaxel is a novel albumin-bound (nab) particle form of paclitaxel designed to circumvent the need for solvents and utilize the properties of albumin to increase intratumor concentrations of the paclitaxel [10]. Nab-paclitaxel is administered as a shorter infusion without the requirement for corticosteroid and antihistamine premedication.

EPOTHILONES

Epothilones are a novel class of cytotoxic agents that function similarly to taxanes, but have different binding to the microtubules and appear to be less susceptible to multidrug resistance. Ixabepilone, the first approved agent of this class, is a semisynthetic derivative of epothilone [11,12].

TOPOISOMERASE INHIBITORS

The DNA topoisomerases are key enzymes required for DNA replication, as they are responsible for relaxing the torsional stress that occurs during the unwinding of DNA double helix during cell division. Topoisomerase I and II can relax supercoiled DNA. Topoisomerase II enzymes can also decatenate intertwined DNA strands. Table 1-5 includes a list of various topoisomerase inhibitors.

CAMPTOTHECINS

The camptothecins are a group of anticancer agents that target the nuclear DNA topoisomerase I enzyme. Irinotecan and topotecan interface the topoisomerase I–DNA complex, reversibly trapping macromolecular complexes. Toxicities of these agents depend upon the agent. Irinotecan is associated with myelosuppression and diarrhea, whereas topotecan is predominantly associated with bone marrow suppression [13].

EPIPODOPHYLLOTOXIN DERIVATIVES

Podophyllotoxins have long been known to inhibit microtubule formation and block mitosis in rapidly dividing cells, but, more recently, their interaction with topoisomerase II enzymes has been postulated to be the mechanism of cytotoxicity. Etoposide and teniposide are large molecular weight podophyllotoxin derivatives that are poorly water soluble, requiring use of complex vehicles. The major dose-limiting toxicity is myelosuppression, but toxicities such as alopecia, mucositis, and hypersensitivity can also occur.

ANTHRACYLINE DERIVATIVES

The anthracycline antibiotics are natural products derived from actinobacteria. Traditionally, these agents have been thought to exert a cytotoxic effect via intercalation into the DNA, resulting in DNA strand breaks. More recently, the ability of these agents to complex topoisomerase II and to form free radical products with oxygen has indicated that there is likely more than one mechanism for cytotoxicity.

The toxicity of these agents includes myelosuppression, nausea and vomiting, and GI damage resulting in diarrhea and/or mucositis. Dose-limiting toxicity appears to be cardiotoxicity. Cardiotoxicity with anthracyclines may be seen with any administration, but the cardiomyopathy associated with tissue damage is thought to be based on damage to the tissue of the heart over time seen with cumulative doses greater than 400 mg/m^2.

Table 1-4. Antimicrotubule Chemotherapeutic Agents

Drug class	Drug
Vinca alkaloids	Vinblastine
	Vincristine
	Vinorelbine
Taxanes	Docetaxel
	Paclitaxel
	Paclitaxel, protein bound
Epothilones	Ixabepilone

Table 1-5. Topoisomerase Inhibitors

Drug class	Drug
Camptothecins	Irinotecan
	Topotecan
Anthracycline antibiotics	Daunorubicin
	Doxorubicin
	Liposomal doxorubicin
	Epirubicin
	Idarubicin
	Valrubicin
Anthracenedione	Mitoxantrone
Podophyllotoxin derivatives	Etoposide
	Teniposide

MISCELLANEOUS CYTOTOXIC AGENTS

A variety of agents or classes of drugs are used in the management of cancer. Although some of these agents are unique (*eg*, bleomycin) in mechanism of action, a number of groups of drugs (*eg*, histone deacetylase inhibitors) are emerging as entirely new methods of treating cancer. As the biology of cancer cell development and progression is further understood, it is anticipated that new targets and consequently new strategies of drug therapies will be identified. Of note with these new strategies is the introduction of new toxicities and the need to further evaluate the best way to optimize treatment without negatively impacting quality of life. Additionally, as new drugs are added to conventional treatment, there is a potential to broaden the scope of toxicities in an individual patient.

PROTEASOME INHIBITORS

Bortezomib is a reversible inhibitor of the 26S, a multicatalytic threonine protease responsible for intracellular protein turnover in eukaryotic cells. This includes the processing and degradation of several proteins involved in cell cycle control and the regulation of apoptosis. Inhibition of the 26S proteasome prevents this targeted proteolysis, thereby affecting multiple signaling cascades within the cell. This disruption of normal homeostatic mechanisms can lead to cell death. Preclinical trials demonstrate this agent has a wide range of biologic effects that result in decreased proliferation, induction of apoptosis, and sensitization of tumor cells to conventional che-motherapeutic agents and irradiation. Toxicities associated with bortezomib include fatigue, neuropathy, and thrombocytopenia. The side effect profile may differ depending on drug therapy combination and patient factors such as extent of pretreatment [14].

HISTONE DEACETYLASE INHIBITORS

Vorinostat is the first in the class of histone deacetylase inhibitors. Histone acetylation is a dynamic process of cellular gene regulation that is "epigenetic," that is, not heritable in the germline. Histones are DNA-binding proteins that allow for the compaction of large amounts of DNA, yet comprise a highly dynamic process that permits efficient transcriptional regulation. Histone deacetylase inhibitors modify gene expression in cancer cells without altering gene sequences, and cause expression of genes (often tumor suppressors) that have been inappropriately turned off during the oncogenic process.

DNA METHYLTRANSFERASE INHIBITORS

Aberrant DNA methylation patterns, including hypermethylation of tumor suppressor genes, have been described in many human cancers. These epigenetic mutations can be reversed by DNA methyltransferase inhibitors. Decitabine and azacitidine are two agents, used in the treatment of myelo-dysplastic syndrome, that are believed to exert a cytotoxic effect through this mechanism [15].

ARSENIC TRIOXIDE

MECHANISM OF ACTION

Cytotoxic action is not fully understood; DNA fragmentation; damage to fusion protein promyelocytic leukemia–retinoic acid receptor-α

PREPARATION

Dilute immediately after withdrawing from ampule; single-use vials

ADMINISTRATION

Intravenous (IV) infusion routinely administered over 1–2 hours, but rate may be increased

CONTRAINDICATIONS/PRECAUTIONS

Contraindicated in patients with known hypersensitivity to arsenic trioxide; precaution in patients with preexisting cardiac abnormalities including QT prolongation and atrioventricular block; teratogenic and may cause harm if administered to pregnant woman

TOXICITIES

Cardiovascular: QT prolongation, cardiac arrhythmias; **Dermatologic:** rash, alopecia; **GI:** nausea, vomiting, abdominal pain; **Hematologic:** leukocytosis, myelosuppression; **Metabolic:** hyperglycemia; **Neurologic:** headache, fatigue, peripheral neuropathy; **Respiratory:** dyspnea, cough; **Miscellaneous:** edema, cough, fatigue; **Acute promyelocytic leukemia (APL):** APL differentiation syndrome manifested by fever, weight gain, pulmonary edema, pleural effusions, pulmonary infiltrates with or without hyperleukocytosis

THERAPEUTIC USES

Indications: APL
Applications: AML; chronic myeloid leukemia; multiple myeloma; myelodysplastic syndrome

PHARMACOKINETICS

Absorption: not given orally; **Distribution:** arsenic is stored in the body in heart, liver, kidney, lung, hair, and nails; **Metabolism:** parent drug undergoes reduction and methylation; **Elimination:** trivalent form is excreted in the urine

DOSAGE ADJUSTMENTS

No clear guidelines for dose adjustment in organ dysfunction

AVAILABILITY

Supplied as Trisenox by Cephalon, Inc. (Frazer, PA)

ASPARAGINASE

MECHANISM OF ACTION

Enzyme that deaminates the amino acid asparagines to aspartic acid and ammonia, ultimately depleting tumor cells of asparagines required for protein synthesis

PREPARATION

Lyophilized powder should be reconstituted; only clear colorless solutions should be used

ADMINISTRATION

Intramuscularly (IM), deep IM injection into a large muscle; IV infusions over at least 30 minutes; an intradermal test dose is recommended prior to the initial administration of the drug and when more than one week has elapsed between doses, although false-negative skin tests greater than 75% have been reported

CONTRAINDICATIONS/PRECAUTIONS

Contraindicated in patients with hypersensitivity to asparaginase and in patients with pancreatitis or a history of pancreatitis; precaution in patients with hepatic dysfunction; pregnancy risk factor C

TOXICITIES

Many of the toxicities of asparaginase are a result of the drug's effect on protein synthesis, resulting in functional changes (*eg*, decreased insulin resulting in hyperglycemia); **Dermatologic:** rash, urticaria; **GI:** mild nausea, pancreatitis, hemorrhagic pancreatitis; **Hematologic:** coagulation defects, thrombosis; **Hepatic:** increased liver function test, hyperalbuminemia; **Metabolic:** hyperglycemia; **Musculoskeletal:** arthralgia; **Neurologic:** central nervous system (CNS) depression or excitability, fatigue, confusion, agitation, headache; **Renal:** renal insufficiency; **Respiratory:** bronchospasm from hypersensitivity reaction; **Miscellaneous:** hypersensitivity, coagulation defects secondary to protein inhibition of coagulation factors and procoagulation factors, fever, chills

THERAPEUTIC USES

Acute lymphocytic leukemia; acute nonlymphocytic leukemia (childhood AML); non-Hodgkin's lymphoma

PHARMACOKINETICS

Distribution: large volume of distribution (70%–80% of plasma volume); **Metabolism:** metabolic degradation; **Elimination:** trace amounts excreted in urine, hepatic

DOSAGE ADJUSTMENTS

No clear guidelines for dose adjustment in organ dysfunction

AVAILABILITY

Supplied as Elspar by Ovation Pharmaceuticals, Inc. (Deerfield, IL)

The information here is provided as guidance only. Prescribers should always consult the manufacturer's current prescribing information.

AZACITIDINE

MECHANISM OF ACTION
Hypomethylation of DNA

PREPARATION
Lyophilized powder that is prepared as a suspension (note: suspension is cloudy); reconstituted product may be refrigerated up to 8 hours prior to administration

ADMINISTRATION
Subcutaneous administration after suspension is resuspended immediately prior to use

CONTRAINDICATIONS/PRECAUTIONS
Contraindicated in patients who have demonstrated hypersensitivity to azacitidine or mannitol

TOXICITIES
Cardiovascular: congestive heart failure; **Dermatologic:** injection site reactions, alopecia; **GI:** anorexia, abdominal pain; **Hepatic:** increased liver function test; **Hematologic:** myelosuppression; **Musculoskeletal:** myalgia; **Neurologic:** anxiety, depression; **Respiratory:** cough, dyspnea; **Miscellaneous:** hypersensitivity

THERAPEUTIC USES
Myelodysplastic syndrome

PHARMACOKINETICS
Absorption: bioavailability is approximately 90% after subcutaneous injection; **Metabolism:** hepatic metabolism; **Elimination:** excreted in the urine

DOSAGE ADJUSTMENTS
Dose adjustments are based on hematologic parameters (white blood cell or platelet nadir as a percent decrease from baselines); dose adjustment may be required with renal impairment

AVAILABILITY
Supplied as Vidaza by Celgene Corp. (Summit, NJ)

BENDAMUSTINE

MECHANISM OF ACTION
Bifunctional mechlorethamine derivative; covalently bonds with nucleophilic moieties; purine analogue; activity against both quiescent and dividing cells

PREPARATION
Reconstitution with sterile water; dilute in normal saline within 30 minutes of reconstitution

ADMINISTRATION
IV administration over 30 minutes

CONTRAINDICATIONS/PRECAUTIONS
Contraindicated in patients with hypersensitivity to bendamustine or mannitol; use is not recommended in patients with hepatic dysfunction; pregnancy risk factor D

TOXICITIES
Cardiovascular: hypertensive crisis; **Dermatologic:** skin rash, bullous exanthema; **GI:** diarrhea, nausea and vomiting; **Hematologic:** bone marrow suppression; **Metabolic:** hyperuricemia associated with tumor lysis syndrome; **Miscellaneous:** fatigue, hypersensitivity reactions including anaphylaxis

THERAPEUTIC USES
Chronic lymphoid leukemia; non-Hodgkin's lymphoma

PHARMACOKINETICS
Distribution: highly protein bound; **Metabolism:** hepatic metabolism via hydrolysis and CYP1A2; **Elimination:** fecal excretion 90%

DOSAGE ADJUSTMENTS
Dose modifications required in patients with renal dysfunction and hepatic dysfunction

AVAILABILITY
Supplied as Treanda by Cephalon, Inc. (Frazer, PA)

BLEOMYCIN

MECHANISM OF ACTION
Oxidative cleavage of DNA

PREPARATION
Bleomycin should not be reconstituted with dextrose-containing solutions; dissolve in 50 to 100 mL normal saline for intrapleural administration

ADMINISTRATION
IV infusion at rate less than 1 unit/min; test dose is recommended for patients receiving bleomycin for lymphoma (2 units)

CONTRAINDICATIONS/PRECAUTIONS
Contraindicated in patients with hypersensitivity to bleomycin; precaution in patients with pulmonary disease; pregnancy risk factor D

TOXICITIES
Cardiovascular: Raynaud's phenomena; **Dermatologic:** erythema; induration and hyperkeratosis that predominantly affect digits, hands, joints, and areas of prior radiation; hyperpigmentation; alopecia; nail changes; phlebitis at injection site; **GI:** nausea and vomiting (mild), stomatitis; **Hematologic:** little myelosuppression; **Renal:** hemorrhagic cystitis; **Respiratory:** interstitial pneumonitis that may progress to interstitial fibrosis, patients at risk include those with underlying pulmonary disease, older than 70 years of age, prior chest irradiation, and/or oxygen therapy; **Miscellaneous:** hypersensitivity reactions (increased risk in patients with lymphoma); fevers and chills associated with administration; pain at site of cancer

THERAPEUTIC USES
Cervical cancer; esophageal cancer; head and neck cancer; Hodgkin's lymphoma; Kaposi's sarcoma; malignant pleural effusion; melanoma; non-Hodgkin's lymphoma; osteosarcoma; ovarian (germ cell) cancer; penis cancer; skin cancer; soft tissue sarcoma; squamous cell carcinomas of skin; testicular cancer; thyroid cancer; trophoblastic neoplasms; vulva cancer

PHARMACOKINETICS
Absorption: bioavailability is dependent on route; IM bioavailability 30%, intracavitary injection bioavailability 30%; **Distribution:** volume of distribution is 22 L/m^2; highest concentrations in skin, kidney, lung, and heart; drug does not cross the blood-brain barrier; **Metabolism:** activation by microsomal reduction, degradation by hydrolase found in tissues throughout the body including liver, gut, skin, lungs, kidneys, and serum; **Elimination:** renal elimination up to 70% in first 24 hours as active drug

DOSAGE ADJUSTMENTS
Dose reductions are recommended for patients with creatinine clearance (CrCl) < 60 mL/min

AVAILABILITY
Supplied as Blenoxane by Bristol-Myers Squibb (Princeton, NJ)

BORTEZOMIB

MECHANISM OF ACTION
Proteasome inhibitor; bortezomib reversibly inhibits the 26S proteasome, therefore preventing targeted proteolysis and disruption of normal cellular homeostatic mechanisms and leading to cell death

PREPARATION
Available as powder that requires reconstitution; reconstitution product should be used within 8 hours

ADMINISTRATION
IV over 3 to 5 seconds

CONTRAINDICATIONS/PRECAUTIONS
Contraindicated in patients with known hypersensitivity to bortezomib, boron, or mannitol; precaution in patients receiving hypotensive agents because the effect may be potentiated with concurrent bortezomib; precaution in patients with diabetes mellitus who are receiving hypoglycemic agents because the effect may be potentiated with concurrent bortezomib

TOXICITIES
Cardiovascular: congestive heart failure and decreased left ventricular ejection fraction, prolongation of QT interval, hypotension; **Dermatologic:** local skin irritation; **GI:** nausea, diarrhea, constipation, anorexia; **Hepatic:** increase in liver function test; **Hematologic:** myelosuppression (thrombocytopenia); **Neurologic:** peripheral neuropathy; **Respiratory:** pneumonitis, acute respiratory distress syndrome (rare); **Miscellaneous:** fevers

THERAPEUTIC USES
Multiple myeloma; non-Hodgkin's lymphoma

PHARMACOKINETICS
Distribution: highly protein bound (> 80%); **Metabolism:** metabolized by cytochrome P-450 systems to inactive metabolites (mainly 3A4, 2C19, 1A2); **Elimination:** hepatic and renal

DOSAGE ADJUSTMENTS
No clear guidelines for dose adjustment in organ dysfunction; dose modification may be considered for individuals with renal impairment or liver dysfunction

AVAILABILITY
Supplied as Velcade by Millenium Pharmaceuticals, Inc. (Cambridge, MA)

BUSULFAN

MECHANISM OF ACTION
Nitrogen mustard alkylating agent; alkylation of DNA through the formation of reactive intermediates that attack nucleophilic sites

PREPARATION
Final concentration of IV busulfan should be greater than 0.5 mg/mL

ADMINISTRATION
IV solutions should be administered via a central catheter over 2 hours; oral for high dose—doses of busulfan used in preparative regimens for stem cell transplantation require multiple 2-mg tablets; gelatin capsules may be used to package multiple tablets to minimize the number of oral dosing units required for patients at each dosing interval

CONTRAINDICATIONS/PRECAUTIONS
Contraindicated in patients with known hypersensitivity to busulfan; precaution in patients with history of seizure; pregnancy risk factor D

TOXICITIES
Dermatologic: skin hyperpigmentation, urticaria, erythema, alopecia; **Endocrine:** ovarian suppression, amenorrhea, infertility, sterility, gynecomastia; **GI:** nausea and vomiting, diarrhea, anorexia; **Hepatic:** hepatic veno-occlusive disease (high-dose regimen), hepatitis; **Hematologic:** myelosuppression, myeloablative (high-dose regimen); **Musculoskeletal:** weakness, fatigue; **Neurologic:** confusion, seizure (high-dose regimen); **Respiratory:** pulmonary fibrosis, pneumonitis; **Miscellaneous:** secondary malignancies, teratogenicity, cataracts

THERAPEUTIC USES
Acute nonlymphocytic leukemia; chronic myelocytic leukemia; preparative therapy in treatment of malignancies with bone marrow transplantation

PHARMACOKINETICS
Absorption: oral bioavailability $\geq$ 50%; **Metabolism:** enzymatic conjugation with glutathione; **Elimination:** renal

DOSAGE ADJUSTMENTS
No clear guidelines for dose adjustment in organ dysfunction

AVAILABILITY
Supplied as Myleran by GlaxoSmithKline (Research Triangle Park, NC) and Busulfex by Otsuka America Pharmaceuticals, Inc. (Rockville, MD)

CAPECITABINE

MECHANISM OF ACTION
Prodrug that is converted to 5-FU by enzymes that are expressed at higher concentrations in tumors; 5-FU is metabolized to 5-fluoro-2'-deoxyuridine 5'-monophosphate (FdUMP) and 5-fluorouridine triphosphate (FUTP). The cytotoxic activity is believed to be via binding of FdUMP and a folate cofactor to thymidylate synthetase, which ultimately interferes with DNA synthesis. In addition, FUTP can be incorporated into RNA and interfere with RNA processing and protein synthesis; leucovorin potentiates the antineoplastic activity and toxicity

PREPARATION
Oral tablets

ADMINISTRATION
Oral administration to be taken with water within 30 minutes after the end of a meal

CONTRAINDICATIONS/PRECAUTIONS
Contraindicated in patients with severe renal dysfunction (CrCl < 30 mL/min)

TOXICITIES
Cardiovascular: edema; other cardiovascular effects are rare but may include angina, cardiomyopathy, hypertension and hypotension; **Dermatologic:** palmar-plantar erythrodysesthesia (hand-foot syndrome), rash; **GI:** diarrhea (can be dose limiting); abdominal pain; mild nausea and vomiting that may be clinically problematic as the course of drug is 14 days; **Hepatic:** hyperbilirubinemia, hepatitis; **Hematologic:** myelo-suppression; **Musculoskeletal:** fatigue, myalgia; **Neurologic:** headache; **Ocular:** ocular irritation, corneal deposits; **Respiratory:** dyspnea; **Miscellaneous:** photosensitivity, radiation recall

THERAPEUTIC USES
Breast cancer; colorectal cancer; GI cancer

PHARMACOKINETICS
Absorption: oral bioavailability is approximately 70%, although there is interindividual variation; presence of food decreases the rate and extent of absorption of capecitabine; **Distribution:** distributed into tumors, intestinal mucosa, plasma, liver, and other tissues; plasma protein binding is less than 60% and not concentration dependent; **Metabolism:** capecitabine is metabolized in the liver and tumor; 5-FU is catabolized via dihydropyrimidine dehydrogenase; **Elimination:** capecitabine and metabolites excreted in urine (> 90%) and minimally in feces (< 5%)

DOSAGE ADJUSTMENTS
After initial course of capecitabine, subsequent doses are modified based on an individual response in terms of toxicity. Dose reductions are based on toxicity of diarrhea, nausea and vomiting, palmar-plantar erythrodysesthesia, and myelosuppression; dose adjustments are recommended in patients with renal dysfunction

AVAILABILITY
Supplied as Xeloda by Roche Laboratories (Nutley, NJ)

CARBOPLATIN

MECHANISM OF ACTION

Covalently binds to DNA bases and disrupts DNA function

PREPARATION

Dilution of reconstituted product is required for infusion

ADMINISTRATION

IV infusion over 15 minutes or longer; do not use aluminum needles for mixing or administration

CONTRAINDICATIONS/PRECAUTIONS

Contraindicated in patients with hypersensitivity to carboplatin, mannitol, or cisplatin; pregnancy risk factor D

TOXICITIES

Dermatologic: alopecia, skin rash, urticaria, pruritus; **GI:** nausea and vomiting, diarrhea; **Hepatic:** increased liver function test; **Hematologic:** bone marrow suppression including thrombocytopenia, hemolytic anemia; **Neurologic:** peripheral neuropathies, hearing loss, transient cortical blindness; **Renal:** nephrotoxicity associated with electrolyte wasting; **Respiratory:** bronchospasms; **Miscellaneous:** anaphylactic-like reactions have been reported and may occur within minutes of administration

THERAPEUTIC USES

Bladder cancer; brain cancer; breast cancer; carcinoma of unknown primary; cervix cancer; endometrial cancer; esophageal cancer; fallopian tube cancer; head and neck cancer; Hodgkin's lymphoma; lung cancer; melanoma; neuroblastoma; non-Hodgkin's lymphoma; ovarian cancer; peritoneal cancer; retinoblastoma; testicular cancer; Wilm's tumor

PHARMACOKINETICS

Metabolism: minimally to aquated and hydroxylated compounds; **Elimination:** approximately 90% is excreted in the urine within 24 hours

DOSAGE ADJUSTMENTS

Dose reductions are recommended for individuals with renal dysfunction; dose calculations using the Calvert formula incorporates the modification of renal function

AVAILABILITY

Supplied as Paraplatin by Bristol-Myers Squibb (Princeton, NJ)

CARMUSTINE (BCNU)

MECHANISM OF ACTION

Alkylating agent (nitrosourea); alkylates biologic molecules that ultimately result in DNA–DNA and DNA–protein cross-links, inhibition of enzymes such as DNA polymerase, DNA ligase, and RNA synthetic and processing enzymes, leading to inhibition of DNA and RNA synthesis

PREPARATION

Use supplied diluent and 27 mL of sterile water in 100-mg vial to get product that is 3.3 mg/mL; glass containers; protect from light. Note: diluent is alcohol, therefore high doses (*eg*, used as preparative regimen prior to stem cell transplantation) may contain significant alcohol

ADMINISTRATION

IV infusion given slowly over 1 to 2 hours (longer infusions used in high-dose regimens)

CONTRAINDICATIONS/PRECAUTIONS

Contraindicated in patients with hypersensitivity to carmustine or any component of the formulation (ethanol); pregnancy risk factor D

TOXICITIES

Cardiovascular: infusion-related hypotension (high-dose regimens); **Dermatologic:** alopecia, local phlebitis; **GI:** severe nausea and vomiting, stomatitis; **Hepatic:** increased liver function test (often reversible), veno-occlusive disease (high-dose regimen); **Hematologic:** myelosuppression (delayed, cumulative, and prolonged), refractory anemia; **Neurologic:** lethargy, ataxia, disorientation; seizures, ethanol intoxication with infusion secondary to diluent, perioral pain, fever (high-dose regimens); **Renal:** delayed renal damage; **Respiratory:** pulmonary toxicity following carmustine characterized as interstitial pneumonia and fibrosis; **Miscellaneous:** rapid infusions cause flushing and perioral pain, secondary malignancies; **Wafer:** toxicity of carmustine implant in polifeprosan 20 wafer—adverse events are seen postoperatively due to surgery or neurologic toxicities secondary to drug (including headache, somnolence, fever, seizure, aphasia, nausea/vomiting)

THERAPEUTIC USES

Brain cancer; colorectal cancer; cutaneous T-cell lymphoma; Hodgkin's lymphoma; melanoma; multiple myeloma; non-Hodgkin's lymphoma; stomach cancer; Waldenström macroglobulinemia

PHARMACOKINETICS

Distribution: crosses blood-brain barrier, enters breast milk, protein binding 80%; **Metabolism:** rapid hepatic; **Elimination:** urine excretion of 60%–70% in 96 hours, pulmonary 6%–10% as carbon dioxide

DOSAGE ADJUSTMENTS

No clear guidelines for dose adjustment in organ dysfunction

AVAILABILITY

Supplied as BiCNU by Bristol-Myers Squibb (Princeton, NJ) and Gliadel (wafer) by MGI Pharma, Inc. (Bloomington, MN)

The information here is provided as guidance only. Prescribers should always consult the manufacturer's current prescribing information.

CHLORAMBUCIL

MECHANISM OF ACTION
Alkylating agent; interferes with DNA replication and transcription of RNA

PREPARATION
2-mg tablets

ADMINISTRATION
Oral, may divide daily dose if nausea occurs; recommended to take 1 hour prior to meals or 2 hours after food

CONTRAINDICATIONS/PRECAUTIONS
Contraindicated in patients with hypersensitivity to chlorambucil; requires proper handling as a chemotherapeutic agent; pregnancy risk factor D

TOXICITIES
Dermatologic: rashes, alopecia; **GI:** infrequent nausea, vomiting, diarrhea, and stomatitis; **Hepatic:** infrequent hepatotoxicity; **Hematologic:** myelosuppression; **Metabolic:** menstrual irregularities; **Neurologic:** myoclonia, hallucinations; **Respiratory:** pulmonary infiltrates and fibrosis; **Miscellaneous:** secondary malignancy, infertility, sterility

THERAPEUTIC USES
Chronic lymphocytic leukemia; cutaneous T-cell lymphoma; hairy cell leukemia; Hodgkin's lymphoma; non-Hodgkin's lymphoma; ovarian (germ and nongerm cell) cancer; trophoblastic neoplasms; Waldenström macroglobulinemia

PHARMACOKINETICS
Absorption: oral bioavailability 50%–70% (decreases with food); **Distribution:** volume of distribution is 0.14 to 0.24 L/kg, protein binding > 90%; **Metabolism:** chemical decomposition to active phenyl acetic acid mustard and to inert dechlorination products (hepatic); **Elimination:** urine excretion as unchanged drug (< 1%) and metabolites (60%)

DOSAGE ADJUSTMENTS
Consider dose adjustment in patients receiving concurrent radiation; consider dose adjustment for individuals with bone marrow depression from disease, previous or current therapy

AVAILABILITY
Supplied as Leukeran by GlaxoSmithKline (Research Triangle Park, NC)

CISPLATIN

MECHANISM OF ACTION
Heavy metal compound (nonclassical alkylating agent); covalently binds to DNA bases and disrupts DNA function

PREPARATION
Available as powder or aqueous solution; prepare in saline solution, preparation stability is dependent on solution (most stable in normal saline); avoid aluminum IV sets and needles

ADMINISTRATION
IV infusions at maximum rate of 1 mg/min; intraperitoneal

CONTRAINDICATIONS/PRECAUTIONS
Contraindicated in patients with known hypersensitivity to platinum compounds; precaution in patients with renal impairment (CrCl < 60 mL/min) and/or patients on concurrent nephrotoxic medications; pregnancy risk factor D

TOXICITIES
Cardiovascular: Raynaud's phenomenon, postural hypotension, arrhythmias; **GI:** severe acute and delayed nausea and vomiting, anorexia, taste abnormalities, diarrhea; **Hematologic:** myelosuppression, specifically anemia; **Metabolic:** electrolyte wasting from renal toxicity including hypomagnesemia, hypokalemia, hypophosphatemia, hypocalcemia; **Neurologic:** peripheral neuropathy (motor and sensory), sensory loss including hearing loss; seizures, papilledema (rare); **Renal:** renal insuf-

ficiency associated with electrolyte (potassium, magnesium, calcium) wasting; **Respiratory:** pulmonary fibrosis; **Miscellaneous:** hypersensitivity reactions

THERAPEUTIC USES
Adrenal cortex cancer; anal cancer; bladder cancer; brain cancer; breast cancer; carcinoma of unknown primary; cervical cancer; endometrial cancer; esophageal cancer; fallopian tube cancer; head and neck cancer; Hodgkin's lymphoma; Kaposi's sarcoma; kidney (rhabdoid tumors) cancer; liver cancer; lung cancer; melanoma; mesothelioma; neuroblastoma; non-Hodgkin's lymphoma; osteosarcoma; ovarian (germ and nongerm cell) cancer; penis cancer; peritoneal cancer; prostate cancer; retinoblastoma; skin cancer; soft tissue sarcoma; stomach cancer; testicular cancer; thymoma; thyroid cancer; vulva cancer; Wilm's tumor

PHARMACOKINETICS
Distribution: long-term protein binding in many tissues; **Metabolism:** inactivated intracellularly and in the bloodstream by sulfhydryls on proteins; **Elimination:** unchanged in the urine

DOSAGE ADJUSTMENTS
Dose modifications are recommended for individuals with renal dysfunction

AVAILABILITY
Supplied as Platinol by Bristol-Myers Squibb (Princeton, NJ)

CLADRIBINE

MECHANISM OF ACTION
Purine nucleoside analogue antimetabolite; cladribine is a prodrug that requires intracellular phosphorylation to active metabolites; the 5'-triphosphaste metabolite results in DNA strand breaks and inhibition of DNA synthesis; high concentrations of the metabolite also inhibit DNA polymerases and ribonucleotide reductase, which causes an imbalance in deoxyribonucleotide triphosphate pools and inhibition of DNA synthesis and repair; the activity of cladribine is independent of cell division

PREPARATION
Although cladribine is given as a 7-day infusion, the drug does not contain a preservative and must be prepared in an appropriate environment (*eg*, clean room) if one preparation will be given for the full infusion

ADMINISTRATION
Continuous IV infusions; IV infusions

CONTRAINDICATIONS/PRECAUTIONS
Contraindicated in patients with a hypersensitivity to cladribine

TOXICITIES
Cardiovascular: tachycardia; **Dermatologic:** rash, pruritus, erythema; **GI:** mild nausea and vomiting, abdominal pain, constipation; **Hematologic:** myelosuppression, immunosuppression; **Musculoskeletal:** myalgia, arthralgia, fatigue; **Neurologic:** headache, insomnia, dizziness, peripheral neuropathy, paraparesis with high doses; **Renal:** nephrotoxicity at higher doses; **Respiratory:** shortness of breath; **Miscellaneous:** fevers (seen most commonly with treatment of hairy cell leukemia)

THERAPEUTIC USES
Chronic lymphocytic leukemia; cutaneous T-cell lymphoma; non-Hodgkin's lymphoma (refractory, low grade); hairy cell leukemia; Waldenström macroglobulinemia

PHARMACOKINETICS
Distribution: crosses the blood-brain barrier; **Metabolism:** activation to 2-CdATP within cells; **Elimination:** 50% urinary excretion

DOSAGE ADJUSTMENTS
No clear guidelines for dose adjustment in organ dysfunction, but may consider in individuals with renal dysfunction

AVAILABILITY
Supplied as Leustatin by Ortho Biotech Products (Raritan, NJ)

CLOFARABINE

MECHANISM OF ACTION
Purine nucleoside; converted intracellularly to clofarabine triphosphate, which inhibits DNA synthesis and ribonucleoside reductase, ultimately leading to inhibition of DNA synthesis

PREPARATION
Clofarabine should be diluted prior to administration; parenteral solutions should be inspected prior to administration for particulate matter and discoloration of product

ADMINISTRATION
IV infusion over 2 hours

CONTRAINDICATIONS/PRECAUTIONS
Contraindicated in patients with hypersensitivity to clofarabine; pregnancy risk factor D

TOXICITIES
Cardiovascular: tachycardia, pericardial effusions, edema, hypotension, hypertension; **Dermatologic:** dermatitis, pruritus, erythema, palmar-plantar erythrodysesthesia syndrome; **GI:** abdominal pain, diarrhea, nausea and vomiting; **Hepatic:** reversible hepatotoxicity; **Hematologic:** myelosuppression; **Musculoskeletal:** fatigue; **Neurologic:** headache, dizziness; **Miscellaneous:** tumor lysis syndrome

THERAPEUTIC USES
Acute lymphoblastic leukemia (pediatric)

PHARMACOKINETICS
Distribution: protein binding approximately 50% (predominantly albumin); **Metabolism:** limited hepatic metabolism, cellular phosphorylation to triphosphate; **Elimination:** renal elimination 50%–60% (unchanged drug)

DOSAGE ADJUSTMENTS
Recommendation for holding drug in individuals with hepatic dysfunction during therapy; if drug is restarted, recommendation to consider dose modification; consider dose modification for individuals with renal dysfunction

AVAILABILITY
Supplied as Clolar by Genzyme Corporation (Cambridge, MA)

CYCLOPHOSPHAMIDE

MECHANISM OF ACTION

Alkylating agent; interferes with DNA replication and transcription of RNA; cyclophosphamide requires biotransformation in the liver to active metabolite; immunosuppressive activity

PREPARATION

Use sterile paraben-preserved water to make 20-mg/mL concentration; oral tablets

ADMINISTRATION

Oral doses should be taken with food to minimize nausea; IV infusion, slow IV push, or short infusions (longer infusions may be used with high doses used for mobilization and/or preparative regimens associated with stem cell transplantation)

CONTRAINDICATIONS/PRECAUTIONS

Contraindicated in patients with hypersensitivity to cyclophosphamide; precaution in patients with impaired renal or hepatic function; pregnancy risk factor D

TOXICITIES

Cardiovascular: cardiomyopathy; **Dermatologic:** alopecia, rash, pruritus, facial flushing, toxic epidermal necrolysis; **GI:** severe acute and delayed nausea and vomiting, metallic taste with IV administration; **Hepatic:** increased liver function test; **Hematologic:** myelosuppression; **Metabolic:** hyponatremia (seen with high-dose infusions); **Neurologic:** headache, dizziness; **Renal:** renal tubular necrosis, acute hemorrhagic cystitis associated with infusion thought to be caused by the interaction of acrolein with the bladder; cystitis may be minimized with hydration and/or mesna; **Respiratory:** pneumonitis and pulmonary fibrosis, **Miscellaneous:** hypersensitivity reactions, sterility, infertility

THERAPEUTIC USES

Acute lymphocytic leukemia; acute nonlymphocytic leukemia; bladder cancer; brain cancer; breast cancer; cervical cancer; choriocarcinoma; chronic lymphocytic leukemia; chronic myelocytic leukemia; cryoglobulinemia; endometrial cancer; Ewing's sarcoma; head and neck cancer; Hodgkin's lymphoma; kidney cancer; lung cancer; multiple myeloma; neuroblastoma; non-Hodgkin's lymphoma; osteosarcoma; ovarian (germ and non-germ cell) cancer; pheochromocytoma; preparative regimen in treatment of malignancies with bone marrow transplantation; prostate cancer; retinoblastoma; soft tissue sarcoma; testicular cancer; thymoma cancer; trophoblastic neoplasms; Waldenström macroglobulinemia; Wilm's tumor

PHARMACOKINETICS

Absorption: well absorbed following oral administration; bioavailability > 75%; **Distribution:** widely distributed throughout the body; crosses the blood-brain barrier to reach the brain and cerebrospinal fluid (CSF); distributed into breast milk; **Metabolism:** metabolized in the liver via the mixed-function oxidase system to active metabolites; **Elimination:** cyclophosphamide and metabolites are excreted in urine

DOSAGE ADJUSTMENTS

No clear guidelines for dose adjustment in organ dysfunction for cyclophosphamide; dose modification may be considered for individuals with renal dysfunction receiving high-dose cyclophosphamide

AVAILABILITY

Supplied as Cytoxan by Bristol-Myers Squibb (Princeton, NJ)

The information here is provided as guidance only. Prescribers should always consult the manufacturer's current prescribing information.

CYTARABINE

MECHANISM OF ACTION

Nucleoside analogue; within the cell, cytarabine (Ara-C) is phosphorylated to triphosphate, which is a potent inhibitor of DNA polymerases that ultimately inhibits DNA synthesis and repair and DNA elongation

PREPARATION

Liposomal cytarabine should be prepared within 4 hours of administration

ADMINISTRATION

IM; subcutaneous; IV as continuous infusion or short infusion (high doses are given over 1–2 hours); cytarabine and liposomal cytarabine are available for intrathecal administration

CONTRAINDICATIONS/PRECAUTIONS

Contraindicated in patients with hypersensitivity to cytarabine; high-dose cytarabine should be used with caution in patients with renal dysfunction secondary to risk of cerebellar toxicity; pregnancy risk factor D

TOXICITIES

Note: toxicity profile is dependent on the dose and schedule of administration; **Dermatologic:** mucositis, rash, alopecia; **GI:** mild nausea and vomiting, mucositis, acute pancreatitis, anorexia; **Hepatic:** increased liver function test; **Hematologic:** bone marrow suppression; **Respiratory:** noncardiogenic pulmonary edema, acute respiratory distress; **Miscellaneous:** hypersensitivity; **High-dose therapy:** dermatologic—mucositis, hand-foot syndrome, rash, alopecia; GI—significant nausea and vomiting; hepatic—increased liver function test; hematologic—bone marrow suppression; neurologic—cerebellar toxicity presenting as dysarthria, dementia, and ataxia; respiratory—noncardiogenic pulmonary edema, acute respiratory distress; miscellaneous—conjunctivitis and photophobia, hypersensitivity; **Liposomal cytarabine:** chemical arachnoiditis that may present as neck pain, neck rigidity, headaches, fever, nausea, vomiting, and back pain; there is a decreased incidence of this toxicity with dexamethasone prophylaxis

THERAPEUTIC USES

Acute lymphocytic leukemia; acute nonlymphocytic leukemia; chronic myeloid leukemia; Hodgkin's lymphoma; lymphomatous meningitis; myelodysplastic syndromes; non-Hodgkin's lymphoma; lymphomatous meningitis (cytarabine liposomal)

PHARMACOKINETICS

Absorption: poor oral bioavailability; **Distribution:** widely distributed in total body water, crosses the blood-brain barrier; **Metabolism:** liver, plasma, and peripheral tissue; **Elimination:** within 24 hours up to 80% recovered in urine as inactive metabolite

DOSAGE ADJUSTMENTS

Dose modifications should be considered for individuals with renal dysfunction; caution about use of high-dose cytarabine in individuals with renal dysfunction

AVAILABILITY

Supplied as Cytosar by Teva Parenteral Medicine (Irving, CA) and Depo-Cyt (liposomal cytarabine) by Pacira Pharmaceuticals (Parsippany, NJ)

DACARBAZINE

MECHANISM OF ACTION

Exact mechanism of antitumor activity is not known; developed as a purine antimetabolite, although antitumor activity dose not result from interference with purine synthesis; metabolic activation to methylating species (MTIC) is necessary for antitumor activity; inhibition of DNA, RNA, and protein synthesis

PREPARATION

Dilute drug in 100 to 500 mL dextrose 5% in water or normal saline; protect preparation from light to decrease decomposition of drug

ADMINISTRATION

IV push over 1–2 minutes; IV infusion over 15–30 minutes

CONTRAINDICATIONS/PRECAUTIONS

Contraindicated in patients with history of hypersensitivity; pregnancy risk C

TOXICITIES

Dermatologic: local pain at infusion site, alopecia, facial flushing; **GI:** nausea and vomiting, anorexia, taste changes (metallic), diarrhea; **Hepatic:** increased liver function test, hepatic necrosis; **Hematologic:** myelosuppression; **Metabolic:** hypocalcemia; **Musculoskeletal:** paresthesia, myalgia, weakness; **Neurologic:** headache, blurred vision; **Respiratory:** sinus congestion; **Miscellaneous:** flu-like syndrome, photosensitivity, anaphylaxis

THERAPEUTIC USES

Indications: melanoma; Hodgkin's disease
Applications: sarcoma; neuroblastoma

PHARMACOKINETICS

Distribution: volume of distribution exceeds that of total body water suggesting some binding to tissue; **Metabolism:** activated by hepatic microsomal enzymes to cytotoxic metabolites; **Elimination:** hepatobiliary elimination, and renal (30%–50% unchanged in urine)

DOSAGE ADJUSTMENTS

No clear guideline for dose adjustment in organ dysfunction; may consider dose modifications in individuals with renal dysfunction

AVAILABILITY

Supplied as DTIC-Dome by Bayer Healthcare Pharmaceuticals (Wayne, NJ)

DACTINOMYCIN

MECHANISM OF ACTION

Intercalation into DNA between adjacent guanine–cytosine bases, ultimately poisoning topoisomerase II and leading to lethal double-strand DNA breaks

PREPARATION

Dilute with preservative-free sterile water for injection to final concentration (do not use preservative diluent because precipitation may occur); caution in dosing—doses are routinely written in micrograms, verify dose if written in milligrams

ADMINISTRATION

IV slow push and rapid infusion

CONTRAINDICATIONS/PRECAUTIONS

Contraindicated in individuals with concurrent or recent chickenpox or herpes zoster or in those with hypersensitivity to dactinomycin; precaution in children less than 6 months of age; pregnancy risk factor D

TOXICITIES

Dermatologic: tissue damage if extravasation occurs during administration; alopecia; skin eruptions; erythema; increased pigmentation at site of previous irradiated skin; **Endocrine:** hypocalcemia; **GI:** severe nausea and vomiting, stomatitis; **Hepatic:** hepatitis, increased liver function test; **Hematologic:** bone marrow suppression, aplastic anemia, agranulocytosis; **Metabolic:** hyperuricemia; **Musculoskeletal:** myalgia; **Neurologic:** malaise, fatigue, lethargy; **Miscellaneous:** radiation sensitization and recall reactions; anaphylactic reaction

THERAPEUTIC USES

Acute lymphocytic leukemia; Ewing's sarcoma; Kaposi's sarcoma; osteosarcoma; ovarian cancer; soft tissue sarcoma; testicular cancer; trophoblastic neoplasm; Wilm's tumor

PHARMACOKINETICS

Distribution: high concentration found in tissues including bone marrow, liver, kidney; crosses the placenta; poor penetration across blood-brain barrier; **Metabolism:** minimal; **Elimination:** urinary excretion varies by 5%–30%, and biliary excretion varies from 5%–10%; **Comments:** Distribution half-life is very short, but the plasma elimination half-life is > 30 hours

DOSAGE ADJUSTMENTS

Consider dose adjustment in patients with edema; consider dose adjustment in obese patients

AVAILABILITY

Supplied as Cosmegen by Ovation Pharmaceuticals, Inc. (Deerfield, IL)

DAUNORUBICIN

MECHANISM OF ACTION

Inhibition of DNA topoisomerase II catalytic activity resulting in DNA double-strand breaks; enhances the catalysis of oxidative-reduction reactions, resulting in generation of reactive oxygen intermediates; activation of signal transduction pathways; stimulation of apoptosis

PREPARATION

Lyophilized drug may be reconstituted with sterile water for injection or other IV solutions; IV push doses: recommended to reconstitute with dextrose 5% in water or normal saline to ensure isotonicity of preparation; protect from fluorescent light to decrease photo-inactivation; decomposed medication turns purple

ADMINISTRATION

IV push; IV short infusions

CONTRAINDICATIONS/PRECAUTIONS

Contraindicated in hypersensitivity to daunorubicin or any component of the formulation; use precaution in preexisting cardiomyopathy, with total cumulative doses of daunorubicin, with any preexisting treatment with anthracyclines, with treatment, and in history of or concurrent radiation; pregnancy risk factor D

TOXICITIES

Cardiovascular: electrocardiogram changes, arrhythmias, pericarditis–myocarditis (acute); cardiomyopathy (related to cumulative dose, concurrent therapy, preexisting cardiac status, method of administration) (delayed); **Dermatologic:** vesicant if extravasation occurs, alopecia, hyperpigmentation of nail beds, streaking of veins; **GI:** nausea, vomiting, mucositis, anorexia, diarrhea; **Hepatic:** hyperbilirubinemia and increased liver function test; **Hematologic:** myelosuppression; **Metabolic:** hyperuricemia; **Musculoskeletal:** fatigue, malaise; **Neurologic:** depression; **Respiratory:** shortness of breath and dyspnea on exertion secondary to congestive heart failure; **Miscellaneous:** discoloration of urine (red, orange), radiation recall, secondary malignancies, infertility and sterility

THERAPEUTIC USES

Acute lymphocytic leukemia; acute nonlymphocytic leukemia; chronic myelocytic leukemia; chronic myelomonocytic leukemia; Ewing's sarcoma; neuroblastoma; non-Hodgkin's lymphoma; Wilm's tumor

PHARMACOKINETICS

Absorption: poor oral absorption (< 50%); **Distribution:** distribution includes many body tissues including liver, spleen, kidney, lung, and heart; the CSF/plasma ratio is low, indicating that the drug does not cross the blood-brain barrier; protein binding is high; crosses the placenta and into human breast milk; **Metabolism:** primarily hepatic metabolism to active metabolite doxorubicinol, then to an inactive aglycone; there is significant patient variation in biotransformation; **Elimination:** a substantial fraction of parent drug is bound to DNA and cardiolipin in tissues and slowly dissociates; about 50%–60% of patient drug is accounted for by known routes of elimination

DOSAGE ADJUSTMENTS

Drug clearance is decreased in patients with hyperbilirubinemia and/or known liver disease (metastatic cancer, preexisting liver dysfunction); dose reductions are recommended for individuals with impaired hepatobiliary function; consider dose reduction for individuals with renal dysfunction

AVAILABILITY

Supplied as Cerubidine by Bedford Laboratories (Bedford, OH)

DOCETAXEL

MECHANISM OF ACTION

Docetaxel appears to shift the dynamic equilibrium between tubulin dimers and microtubules toward microtubule assembly and stabilize microtubules against depolymerization; this inhibits the reorganization of the microtubule network, and this inhibition is thought to impact the transmission of proliferative signals of cellular process

PREPARATION

Initial concentration is 10 mg/mL; diluted solutions should be stored in bottles or plastic bags

ADMINISTRATION

IV infusion over 1 hour

CONTRAINDICATIONS/PRECAUTIONS

Hypersensitivity and fluid retention have led to the recommendation of premedication with dexamethasone; pregnancy risk factor D

TOXICITIES

Cardiovascular: hypotension, arrhythmia; **Dermatologic:** nail changes, alopecia, hyperpigmentation; **GI:** mucositis, mild to moderate nausea and vomiting, diarrhea; **Hepatic:** increased liver function test; **Hematologic:** bone marrow suppression; **Musculoskeletal:** myalgia, arthralgia; **Neurologic:** peripheral neuropathies, asthenia; **Ocular:** conjunctivitis, lacrimation, lacrimal duct obstruction; **Respiratory:** dyspnea, pulmonary edema; **Miscellaneous:** fever, hypersensitivity reaction, fluid retention (generalized edema and effusions)

THERAPEUTIC USES

Bladder cancer; breast cancer; esophagus cancer; head and neck cancer; lung cancer; ovarian cancer; prostate cancer; stomach cancer

PHARMACOKINETICS

Distribution: extensive extravascular distribution and tissue binding; highly protein bound; **Metabolism:** hepatic metabolism by oxidation and CYP3A3/4; **Elimination:** majority via feces (< 10 % urine)

DOSAGE ADJUSTMENTS

Dose modifications are recommended for individuals with hepatic dysfunction

AVAILABILITY

Supplied as Taxotere by Sanofi-Aventis (Bridgewater, NJ)

The information here is provided as guidance only. Prescribers should always consult the manufacturer's current prescribing information.

DOXORUBICIN

MECHANISM OF ACTION

Inhibits DNA topoisomerase II catalytic activity, resulting in DNA double-strand breaks; enhances the catalysis of oxidative-reduction reactions, resulting in generation of reactive oxygen intermediates; activation of signal transduction pathways; stimulation of apoptosis

PREPARATION

Lyophilized drug may be reconstituted with sterile water for injection or other IV solutions; IV push doses—recommended to reconstitute with dextrose 5% in water or normal saline to ensure isotonicity of preparation

ADMINISTRATION

IV push; IV bolus; prolonged continuous infusion

CONTRAINDICATIONS/PRECAUTIONS

Contraindicated in hypersensitivity to doxorubicin or any component of the formulation; use precaution in preexisting cardiomyopathy, with total cumulative dose of doxorubicin, with any preexisting treatment with anthracyclines, with treatment, and with history or concurrent radiation; pregnancy risk factor D

TOXICITIES

Cardiovascular: electrocardiogram changes, arrhythmias, pericarditis–myocarditis (acute); cardiomyopathy (related to cumulative dose, concurrent therapy, preexisting cardiac status, method of administration) (delayed); **Dermatologic:** vesicant if extravasation occurs, alopecia, hyperpigmentation of nail beds, streaking of veins, stomatitis; **GI:** nausea, vomiting, mucositis, anorexia, diarrhea; **Hematologic:** myelosuppression; **Metabolic:** hyperuricemia; **Miscellaneous:** discoloration of urine (red, orange), radiation recall, secondary malignancies, fever

THERAPEUTIC USES

Acute lymphocytic leukemia; acute nonlymphocytic leukemia; adrenal cortex cancer; bladder cancer; breast cancer; carcinoid tumor; cervical cancer; chronic lymphocytic leukemia; endometrial cancer; esophageal cancer; Ewing's sarcoma; head and neck cancer; Hodgkin's lymphoma; Kaposi's sarcoma; liver cancer; lung cancer; multiple myeloma; non-Hodgkin's lymphoma; neuroblastoma; osteosarcoma; ovarian (germ and nongerm cell) cancer; pancreatic cancer; prostate cancer; retinoblastoma; soft tissue sarcoma; stomach cancer; testicular cancer; thyroid cancer; thymoma; trophoblastic neoplasms; Wilm's tumor

PHARMACOKINETICS

Absorption: poor oral absorption (< 50%); **Distribution:** distribution to many body tissues including liver, spleen, kidney, lung, and heart; the CSF/plasma ratio is low, indicating that the drug does not cross the blood-brain barrier; protein binding is high (60%–70%); doxorubicin does cross the placenta and into human breast milk; volume of distribution is 25 L/kg; **Metabolism:** primarily hepatic metabolism to active metabolite doxorubicinol, then to an inactive aglycone; there is significant interpatient variation in biotransformation; **Elimination:** a substantial fraction of parent drug is bound to DNA and cardiolipin in tissues and slowly dissociates; about 50%–60% of patient drug is accounted for by known routes of elimination

DOSAGE ADJUSTMENTS

Drug clearance is decreased in patients with hyperbilirubinemia and/or known liver disease (metastatic cancer, preexisting liver dysfunction); dose modifications are recommended in individuals with impaired hepatobiliary function

AVAILABILITY

Supplied as generic by various manufacturers; Adriamycin

DOXORUBICIN, LIPOSOMAL

MECHANISM OF ACTION

Liposomal doxorubicin incorporates a polyethylene glycol derivative around liposomal coated core of doxorubicin; inhibition of DNA topoisomerase II catalytic activity resulting in DNA double-strand breaks; enhances the catalysis of oxidative reduction reactions resulting in generation of reactive oxygen intermediates; activation of signal transduction pathways; stimulation of apoptosis

PREPARATION

Liposomal doxorubicin must be further diluted prior to administration

ADMINISTRATION

IV infusion over 30 minutes; do not administer as a bolus or as undiluted medication

CONTRAINDICATIONS/PRECAUTIONS

Contraindicated in hypersensitivity to doxorubicin or any component of the liposomal formulation; precaution in history or concurrent radiation; pregnancy risk factor D

TOXICITIES

Cardiovascular: electrocardiogram changes, arrhythmias, pericarditis–myocarditis (acute); cardiomyopathy (related to cumulative dose, concurrent therapy, preexisting cardiac status, method of administration) (delayed); **Dermatologic:** alopecia, hyperpigmentation of nail beds, stomatitis, palmar-plantar erythrodysesthesia and acral dysesthesia; **GI:** nausea, vomiting, mucositis, anorexia, diarrhea; **Hematologic:** myelosuppression; **Metabolic:** hyperuricemia; **Musculoskeletal:** back pain; **Neurologic:** dizziness, headache; **Respiratory:** dyspnea; **Miscellaneous:** discoloration of urine (red, orange), radiation recall , secondary malignancies, fever, allergic reaction

THERAPEUTIC USES

Breast cancer; Kaposi's sarcoma; multiple myeloma; ovarian cancer

PHARMACOKINETICS

Distribution: steady-state volume of distribution is confined to vascular fluid volume; bound to plasma proteins (70%); **Metabolism:** liver and plasma

DOSAGE ADJUSTMENTS

Drug clearance is decreased in patients with hyperbilirubinemia and/or known liver disease (metastatic cancer, preexisting liver dysfunction); dose modifications are recommended in individuals with impaired hepatobiliary function; dose modifications are recommended based on grade of dermatologic and/or hematologic toxicities

AVAILABILITY

Supplied as Doxil by Ortho Biotech Products (Raritan, NJ)

EPIRUBICIN

MECHANISM OF ACTION

Inhibition of DNA topoisomerase II catalytic activity resulting in DNA double-strand breaks; enhances the catalysis of oxidative reduction reactions resulting in generation of reactive oxygen intermediates; activation of signal transduction pathways; stimulation of apoptosis

PREPARATION

Available in a ready-to-use solution

ADMINISTRATION

IV push or short infusion through a free-flowing IV over 3–20 minutes
Etoposide phosphate: may be administered over short period without hypotension or anaphylactic reactions; doses used are equivalent to etoposide

CONTRAINDICATIONS/PRECAUTIONS

Contraindicated in hypersensitivity to epirubicin or any component of the formulation; precaution in preexisting cardiomyopathy, with total cumulative dose of epirubicin, with any preexisting treatment with anthracyclines, with treatment, and with history or concurrent radiation; pregnancy risk factor D

TOXICITIES

Cardiovascular: electrocardiogram changes, arrhythmias, pericarditis–myocarditis (acute); cardiomyopathy (related to cumulative dose, concurrent therapy, preexisting cardiac status, method of administration) (delayed); **Dermatologic:** vesicant if extravasation occurs, alopecia, hyperpigmentation of nail beds, streaking of veins; **GI:** nausea, vomiting, mucositis, anorexia; **Hepatic:** hyperbilirubinemia and liver function test; **Hematologic:** myelosuppression; **Metabolic:** hyperuricemia; **Respiratory:** shortness of breath and dyspnea on exertion secondary to congestive heart failure; **Miscellaneous:** discoloration of urine (red, orange), radiation recall, secondary malignancies, infertility and sterility

THERAPEUTIC USES

Breast cancer; esophageal cancer; Hodgkin's lymphoma; lung cancer; non-Hodgkin's lymphoma; ovarian cancer; soft tissue sarcoma; stomach cancer

PHARMACOKINETICS

Distribution: distribution to many body tissues including liver, spleen, kidney, lung, and heart; the CSF/plasma ratio is low, indicating that the drug does not cross the blood-brain barrier; protein binding is high; crosses the placenta and into human breast milk; **Metabolism:** extensive via hepatic and extrahepatic routes; **Elimination:** hepatic

DOSAGE ADJUSTMENTS

Dose modifications are recommended for individuals with impaired hepatobiliary function; dose modifications may be considered for individuals with renal dysfunction; clearance may be reduced in elderly women, monitor effect and consider dose reduction in subsequent cycles based on toxicity

AVAILABILITY

Supplied as Ellence by Pfizer (New York, NY)

ETOPOSIDE

MECHANISM OF ACTION

Topoisomerase II inhibitor leading to DNA strand break

PREPARATION

Stability of prepared drug is dependent on dilution; oral capsules (50 mg) must be refrigerated

ADMINISTRATION

IV infusion over 30–60 minutes minimum; IV infusion of high dose—rate dependent on dose; oral doses ≤ 400 mg are given as single daily dose and doses > 400 mg should be given as divided doses

CONTRAINDICATIONS/PRECAUTIONS

Contraindicated in hypersensitivity to etoposide, rapid bolus infusion, or intrathecal administration; pregnancy risk factor D

TOXICITIES

Cardiovascular: hypotension (associated with rapid infusion, thought to be secondary to the diluent of preparation); **Dermatologic:** alopecia, toxic epidermal necrolysis; **GI:** nausea, vomiting, mucositis (increased incidence and severity seen with higher doses); **Hepatic:** hepatitis (high-dose therapy); **Hematologic:** myelosuppression; **Miscellaneous:** secondary malignancies

THERAPEUTIC USES

Acute lymphocytic leukemia; acute nonlymphocytic leukemia; adrenal cortex cancer; bladder cancer; brain cancer; carcinoma of unknown primary; cutaneous T-cell lymphoma; endometrial cancer; Ewing's sarcoma; Hodgkin's lymphoma; Kaposi's sarcoma; liver cancer; lung cancer; multiple myeloma; neuroblastoma; non-Hodgkin's lymphoma; osteosarcoma; ovary (germ and nongerm cell) cancer; retinoblastoma; soft tissue sarcoma; stomach cancer; testes cancer; thymoma; trophoblastic neoplasms; Wilm's tumor

PHARMACOKINETICS

Absorption: significant patient to patient variability (bioavailability ranges 25%–75%); time to peak serum level between 1–2 hours; **Distribution:** high protein binding; poor penetration into CNS; **Metabolism:** hepatic metabolism to hydroxy acid and cis-lactone metabolites; **Elimination:** renal excretion (> 50%), feces (> 40%)

DOSAGE ADJUSTMENTS

Dose modifications are recommended for individuals with hepatic impairment; dose modifications are recommended for individuals with renal impairment; consider dose modifications for individuals with low albumin

AVAILABILITY

Supplied as VePesid and Etopophos (etoposide phosphate) by Bristol-Myers Squibb (Princeton, NJ)

FLOXURIDINE

MECHANISM OF ACTION

Pyrimidine analogue antimetabolite agent; inhibition of DNA and RNA synthesis

PREPARATION

Reconstituted lyophilized powder should be further diluted prior to infusion

ADMINISTRATION

IV infusion over 15 minutes; intra-arterially

CONTRAINDICATIONS/PRECAUTIONS

Contraindicated in known hypersensitivity to floxuridine; precaution in patients with myelosuppression; pregnancy risk factor D

TOXICITIES

Dermatologic: alopecia, dermatitis, rash; **GI:** nausea and vomiting, stomatitis; **Hepatic:** hepatotoxicity; **Hematologic:** myelosuppression; **Musculoskeletal:** weakness, lethargy; **Miscellaneous:** fever; **Regional arterial infusion:** toxicities related to procedure such as thrombosis, embolism, hepatic necrosis, and bleeding

THERAPEUTIC USES

Colorectal cancer; kidney cancer; liver cancer; ovarian cancer

PHARMACOKINETICS

Metabolism: metabolism in liver and tissue; **Elimination:** renal excretion is approximately 10%–13%, respiratory excretion 60% as carbon dioxide

DOSAGE ADJUSTMENTS

No clear guidelines for dose adjustment in organ dysfunction

AVAILABILITY

Supplied as generic by various manufacturers; FUDR

FLUDARABINE

MECHANISM OF ACTION
The active triphosphorylated metabolite F-ara-ATP incorporates into DNA and terminates chain formation, inhibits enzymes responsible in DNA replication and RNA function; active against dividing and nondividing cells

PREPARATION
Reconstitute vial with 2 mL of sterile water for injection for a concentration of 25 mg/mL (for further dilution)

ADMINISTRATION
IV short infusions; IV prolonged infusions (less common)

CONTRAINDICATIONS/PRECAUTIONS
Contraindication in patients with hypersensitivity to fludarabine; precaution in patients with renal impairment (not recommended in patients with CrCl < 30 mL/min); pregnancy risk factor D

TOXICITIES
Cardiovascular: edema; **Dermatologic:** rash, alopecia; **GI:** mild nausea, vomiting, diarrhea, stomatitis; **Hepatic:** transient increase in transaminase; **Hematologic:** myelosuppression, immunosuppression (T cells > B cells), hemolytic anemia; **Metabolic:** hyperglycemia; **Musculoskeletal:** arthralgia; **Neurologic:** at high doses CNS toxicity may occur and is dose limiting; complications include somnolence, blindness, and coma; **Respiratory:** interstitial pneumonitis

THERAPEUTIC USES
Acute nonlymphocytic leukemia; chronic lymphocytic leukemia; cutaneous T-cell lymphoma; hairy cell leukemia; non-Hodgkin's lymphoma; prolymphocytic leukemia; Waldenström macroglobulinemia

PHARMACOKINETICS
Distribution: widely distributed with extensive tissue binding; **Metabolism:** phosphorylation and dephosphorylation in serum and tissues; **Elimination:** urine

DOSAGE ADJUSTMENTS
Dosing modifications are recommended for individuals with renal impairment

AVAILABILITY
Supplied as Fludara by Bayer Healthcare Pharmaceuticals (Wayne, NJ)

5-FLUOROURACIL

MECHANISM OF ACTION
Fluorinated pyrimidine antimetabolite; 5-FU is metabolized to FdUMP and FUTP; the cytotoxic activity is believed to be via binding of FdUMP and a folate cofactor to thymidylate synthetase, which ultimately interferes with DNA synthesis. In addition, FUTP can be incorporated into RNA and myelosuppression with RNA processing and protein synthesis; leucovorin potentiates the antineoplastic activity and toxicity

PREPARATION
Preparation is dependent on the method of administration

ADMINISTRATION
IV administration including bolus, short infusion, and continuous infusion; topical

CONTRAINDICATIONS/PRECAUTIONS
Contraindication in patients with hypersensitivity to 5-FU and in patients with dihydropyrimidine dehydrogenase deficiency; pregnancy risk factor D

TOXICITIES
Cardiovascular: coronary vasospasm, edema, angina, cardiomyopathy, hypertension, hypotension; **Dermatologic:** hyperpigmentation, palmar-plantar erythrodysesthesia, rash; **GI:** diarrhea can be dose limiting; abdominal pain, mild nausea and vomiting, mucositis; increased GI side effects with prolonged continuous infusion regimens; **Hepatic:** hyperbilirubinemia, hepatitis; **Hematologic:** myelosuppression; **Musculoskeletal:** fatigue, myalgia; **Neurologic:** headache; **Ocular:** ocular irritation, photophobia, tearing; **Respiratory:** dyspnea; **Miscellaneous:** photosensitivity, radiation recall

THERAPEUTIC USES
Adrenal cortex cancer; anal cancer; bladder cancer; breast cancer; carcinoid tumor; cervix cancer; colorectal cancer; endometrial cancer; esophageal cancer; head and neck cancer; kidney cancer; liver cancer; lung cancer; ovarian cancer; pancreatic cancer; penis cancer; prostate cancer; skin (topical) cancer; stomach cancer; vulva cancer

PHARMACOKINETICS
Absorption: oral bioavailability is erratic; **Distribution:** 5-FU is distributed into tumors and many tissues; crosses the blood-brain barrier and distributes into CSF and into brain; there appears to be longer persistence of drug at tumor than in other tissues, which is thought to be due to impaired catabolism of uracil in tumor; **Metabolism:** parent drug is metabolized in the liver and tissue; following IV administration, the plasma elimination half-life is < 30 minutes; **Elimination:** metabolites are excreted as respiratory carbon dioxide and urea

DOSAGE ADJUSTMENTS
After initial course of 5-FU, subsequent doses are modified based on an individual response in terms of toxicity; dose reductions are based on toxicity of diarrhea and myelosuppression

AVAILABILITY
Supplied as Efudex by Valeant Pharmaceuticals (Costa Mesa, CA) and Fluoroplex by Allergan Inc. (Irvine, CA)

GEMCITABINE

MECHANISM OF ACTION

Intracellular conversion to gemcitabine diphosphate, which inhibits the synthesis of deoxynucleoside triphosphates required for DNA synthesis; intracellular conversion to gemcitabine triphosphate, which competes with deoxynucleosides triphosphates for incorporation into DNA with subsequent inhibition of DNA synthesis

PREPARATION

Reconstitute vials for further dilution prior to administration

ADMINISTRATION

IV infusion over 30 minutes (longer infusions may increase toxicity)

CONTRAINDICATIONS/PRECAUTIONS

Contraindicated in patients with known hypersensitivity to gemcitabine; precaution in patients receiving radiation therapy

TOXICITIES

Cardiovascular: edema; **Dermatologic:** rash, alopecia; **GI:** nausea and vomiting, diarrhea, constipation, stomatitis; **Hepatic:** increased trans- aminase; **Hematologic:** myelosuppression; **Renal:** proteinuria; **Respiratory:** dyspnea; **Miscellaneous:** flu-like syndrome seen following administration

THERAPEUTIC USES

Bladder cancer; breast cancer; gallbladder (and biliary tract) cancer; germ cell tumor; Hodgkin's lymphoma; lung (non-small cell) cancer; non-Hodgkin's lymphoma; ovarian cancer; pancreatic cancer; testicular cancer

PHARMACOKINETICS

Distribution: low protein binding; **Metabolism:** cellular metabolism; **Elimination:** urine

DOSAGE ADJUSTMENTS

Dose modifications are recommended for individuals with hepatic dysfunction; gemcitabine is a radiosensitizer and dose modifications are recommended for individuals receiving concurrent radiation therapy

AVAILABILITY

Supplied as Gemzar by Eli Lilly and Company (Indianapolis, IN)

HYDROXYUREA

MECHANISM OF ACTION

Interferes with synthesis of DNA during cell division; inhibits ribonucleoside diphosphate reductase, preventing deoxyribonucleotides; in sickle cell disease, mechanism is thought to be increased hemoglobin F levels in red blood cells, thereby increasing deformability of sickled cells and altering the adhesion of red blood cells to the endothelium

PREPARATION

Oral as tablets and capsules; oral capsules may be opened and suspended in water (does not go into solution)

ADMINISTRATION

Oral

CONTRAINDICATIONS/PRECAUTIONS

Contraindicated in patients with hypersensitivity to hydroxyurea; precaution in patients with severe anemia, thrombocytopenia, or neutropenia; pregnancy risk factor D

TOXICITIES

Cardiovascular: edema; **Dermatologic:** stomatitis, alopecia, erythema of hand and face, rash; **GI:** nausea and vomiting, anorexia, pancreatitis; **Hepatic:** increase in transaminases, increases in bilirubin, hepatotoxicity; **Hematologic:** bone marrow suppression; **Neurologic:** drowsiness, headache, dizziness; **Renal:** impairment of renal tubule; **Respiratory:** acute diffuse pulmonary infiltrates (rare), dyspnea; **Miscellaneous:** fevers

THERAPEUTIC USES

Cervical cancer; chronic myelocytic leukemia; head and neck cancer; melanoma; ovary cancer; polycythemia vera; thrombocytosis

PHARMACOKINETICS

Absorption: > 80% oral bioavailability (rapid); **Distribution:** volume of distribution equals total body water; crosses the blood-brain barrier and distributes into tissues including ascites; **Metabolism:** degradation by GI enzymes (50%); hepatic metabolism; **Elimination:** urine (50% as unchanged drug) and exhaled as carbon dioxide gas

DOSAGE ADJUSTMENTS

Dose modifications are recommended for individuals with renal dysfunction or with bone marrow depression

AVAILABILITY

Supplied as Hydrea by Bristol-Myers Squibb (Princeton, NJ)

IDARUBICIN

MECHANISM OF ACTION

Inhibition of DNA topoisomerase II catalytic activity; generation of reactive oxygen intermediates; activation of signal transduction pathways; stimulation of apoptosis

PREPARATION

Supplied as a preservative-free solution

ADMINISTRATION

IV slowly over 10 to 15 minutes

CONTRAINDICATIONS/PRECAUTIONS

Contraindicated in patients with a hypersensitivity to anthracyclines; precaution in patients with heart disease; pregnancy risk factor D

TOXICITIES

Cardiovascular: electrocardiogram changes, arrhythmias, pericarditis–myocarditis (acute); cardiomyopathy (related to cumulative dose, concurrent therapy, preexisting cardiac status, method of administration) (delayed); **Dermatologic:** vesicant if extravasation occurs, alopecia, hyperpigmentation of nail beds, palmar-plantar erythrodysesthesia; **GI:** nausea, vomiting, mucositis, anorexia, diarrhea; **Hepatic:** increase in liver function (rare); **Hematologic:** myelosuppression; **Metabolic:** hyperuricemia; **Miscellaneous:** discoloration of urine (red, orange), radiation recall, secondary malignancies

THERAPEUTIC USES

Acute lymphocytic leukemia; acute nonlymphocytic leukemia

PHARMACOKINETICS

Absorption: rapidly absorbed from GI tract following oral administration (unique from most other anthracyclines); **Distribution:** widely distributed in tissues; **Metabolism:** idarubicin is metabolized by aldoketoreductase to idarubicinol (active metabolite); extrahepatic metabolism; **Elimination:** idarubicin is excreted in bile; some renal elimination (primarily as metabolite idarubicinol)

DOSAGE ADJUSTMENTS

Dose modifications should be considered for individuals with hepatic dysfunction

AVAILABILITY

Supplied as Idamycin by Pfizer (New York, NY)

IFOSFAMIDE

MECHANISM OF ACTION

Alkylating agent; interferes with DNA replication and transcription of RNA; ifosfamide requires biotransformation in the liver to active metabolite

PREPARATION

Crystalline powder is reconstituted, and may be further diluted for administration; packaged with the uroprotectant mesna

ADMINISTRATION

IV infusion (minimum of 30 minutes); prolonged infusions (over 24 hours for multiple days)

CONTRAINDICATIONS/PRECAUTIONS

Contraindicated in patients with hypersensitivity to ifosfamide; pregnancy risk factor D

TOXICITIES

Cardiovascular: cardiomyopathy; **Dermatologic:** alopecia, skin hyperpigmentation, dermatitis; **GI:** severe acute and delayed nausea and vomiting, stomatitis, anorexia; **Hepatic:** increased liver function test; **Hematologic:** myelosuppression; **Metabolic:** syndrome of inappropriate antidiuretic hormone (SIADH), sterility; **Neurologic:** agitation, confusion, somnolence, hallucination; encephalopathy associated with higher-dose regimens, short infusions, patients with hypoalbuminemia, and/or renal dysfunction; **Renal:** nephrotoxicity associated with renal tubular damage; **Respiratory:** pneumonitis; **Miscellaneous:** hemorrhagic cystitis associated with infusion thought to be secondary to metabolite acrolein; management includes concurrent mesna and hydration to minimize effects of acrolein; infertility, sterility, secondary malignancy

THERAPEUTIC USES

Acute lymphocytic leukemia; bladder cancer; breast cancer; cervical cancer; endometrial cancer; Ewing's sarcoma; head and neck cancer; Hodgkin's lymphoma; lung cancer; neuroblastoma; non-Hodgkin's lymphoma; osteosarcoma; ovarian (germ and non-germ cells) cancer; pancreatic cancer; soft tissue sarcoma; testicular (germ cell) cancer; thymoma; uterus cancer; Wilm's tumor

PHARMACOKINETICS

Absorption: plasma concentrations of ifosfamide and its metabolites exhibit interindividual variation; **Distribution:** widely distributed throughout the body; crosses the blood-brain barrier into the CSF and brain; **Metabolism:** ifosfamide is metabolized in liver and lung by mixed-function oxidases; ifosfamide mustard is believed to be the primary alkylating metabolite; acrolein is the metabolite believed to be causative of hemorrhagic cystitis; **Elimination:** ifosfamide and its metabolites are excreted in urine

DOSAGE ADJUSTMENTS

Dose adjustments for renal impairment may be considered

AVAILABILITY

Supplied as Ifex by Bristol-Myers Squibb (Princeton, NJ)

IRINOTECAN

MECHANISM OF ACTION
Type I topoisomerase inhibitor; cytotoxic effect believed to occur through interaction with DNA–DNA topoisomerase cleavable complex, stabilizing the complex preventing topoisomerase for relegating single-strand breaks; the DNA damage results in apoptosis

PREPARATION
Irinotecan must be diluted prior to administration (final concentration of 0.12–2.8 mg/mL)

ADMINISTRATION
IV infusion

CONTRAINDICATIONS/PRECAUTIONS
Contraindicated in patients with hypersensitivity to irinotecan; precaution in patients with hyperbilirubinemia; pregnancy risk factor D

TOXICITIES
Cardiovascular: vasodilation, flushing, increase in venothrombosis events; **Dermatologic:** alopecia, rash; **GI:** acute diarrhea (within 24 hours of administration) as part of cholinergic response; management with atropine; later-onset diarrhea (> 24 hours after administration but often delayed up to 1 or 2 weeks) may be dose limiting; management with loperamide. Nausea and vomiting, anorexia, dyspepsia, stomatitis; **Hepatic:** transient elevation in liver function test; **Hematologic:** myelosuppression (increased in patients who are homozygous for UGT1A1*28 allele); **Metabolic:** electrolyte abnormalities associated with diarrhea; **Musculoskeletal:** weakness; **Neurologic:** dizziness; **Respiratory:** cough, rhinitis; **Miscellaneous:** insomnia, fever

THERAPEUTIC USES
Cervical cancer; colorectal cancer; lung (small cell) cancer; lung (non–small cell); ovarian (platinum-refractory, platinum-resistant) cancer

PHARMACOKINETICS
Distribution: protein binding for irinotecan (30%–70%) and for SN-38 (> 90%); **Metabolism:** irinotecan undergoes metabolic conversion to the active metabolite SN-38; **Elimination:** irinotecan is eliminated via conversion to SN-38, and through biliary and urinary excretion; SN-38 is eliminated via glucuronidation and biliary excretion; **Comments:** irinotecan and SN-38 undergo reversible conversion

DOSAGE ADJUSTMENTS
Following the initial course of irinotecan therapy, subsequent doses should be modified based on patient tolerance (*eg*, myelosuppression, diarrhea); dose modifications should be consideration for individuals with hepatic dysfunction

AVAILABILITY
Supplied as Camptosar by Pfizer (New York, NY)

IXABEPILONE

MECHANISM OF ACTION
Epothilone B analogue disrupting the activities of microtubules, therefore interfering with cell growth, proliferation, and signaling, which result in subsequent cell death

PREPARATION
Allow both ixabepilone powder and diluent vial to stand at room temperature for about 30 minute prior to reconstitution; prepare in DEHP-free containers to final concentration between 0.2 mg/mL and 0.6 mg/mL

ADMINISTRATION
IV infusion over 3 hours (must be complete within 6 hours of when drug is prepared)

CONTRAINDICATIONS/PRECAUTIONS
Pregnancy risk factor D

TOXICITIES
Cardiovascular: left ventricular dysfunction, myocardial ischemia, arrhythmia; **Dermatologic:** alopecia, hand-foot syndrome, nail changes; **GI:** abdominal pain, constipation, diarrhea, anorexia, nausea and vomiting, stomatitis; **Hematologic:** myelosuppression; **Musculoskeletal:** arthralgia, myalgia, musculoskeletal pain; **Neurologic:** sensory neuropathy, asthenia; **Miscellaneous:** fatigue, hypersensitivity reactions

THERAPEUTIC USES
Breast cancer; androgen-independent prostate cancer

PHARMACOKINETICS
Distribution: highly protein bound; **Metabolism:** extensive hepatic metabolism via CYP3A4; **Elimination:** renal elimination about 20%, fecal elimination about 65%

DOSAGE ADJUSTMENTS
Dose modification recommended for individuals with hepatic dysfunction

AVAILABILITY
Supplied as Ixempra by Bristol-Myers Squibb (Princeton, NJ)

LOMUSTINE (CCNU)

MECHANISM OF ACTION

Alkylating agent (nitrosourea); alkylates biologic molecules, which ultimately results in DNA–DNA and DNA–protein cross-links, inhibition of enzymes such as DNA polymerase, DNA ligase, and RNA synthetic and processing enzymes, leading to inhibition of DNA and RNA synthesis

PREPARATION

Supplied as capsules

ADMINISTRATION

Lomustine should be taken with fluid on an empty stomach; recommended that no food or fluid should be taken for 2 hours after administration to minimize nausea

CONTRAINDICATIONS/PRECAUTIONS

Contraindicated in patients with known hypersensitivity to lomustine; pregnancy risk factor D

TOXICITIES

Dermatologic: alopecia; **GI:** nausea, vomiting, stomatitis; **Hepatic:** increased liver function test (often reversible); **Hematologic:** myelosuppression (delayed, cumulative, and prolonged); refractory anemia; **Neurologic:** lethargy, ataxia, disorientation; **Respiratory:** pulmonary toxicity following lomustine characterized as interstitial pneumonia and fibrosis

THERAPEUTIC USES

Brain cancer; breast cancer; colorectal cancer; Hodgkin's lymphoma; lung cancer; melanoma; multiple myeloma

PHARMACOKINETICS

Absorption: oral bioavailability 60%–90%, rapidly absorbed after oral administration; **Distribution:** crosses blood-brain barrier (CSF concentrations approximately equal to plasma concentrations); **Metabolism:** metabolism in the liver via hydroxylation producing active metabolites; enterohepatically recycled; **Elimination:** renal excretion greater than feces (< 5%), which is greater than lung

DOSAGE ADJUSTMENTS

Lomustine is eliminated in the urine; therefore, some sources recommend reduction based on CrCl

AVAILABILITY

Supplied as CeeNU by Bristol-Myers Squibb (Princeton, NJ)

MECHLORETHAMINE

MECHANISM OF ACTION

Alkylating agent; cross-links strands of DNA, ultimately resulting in inhibition of DNA synthesis

PREPARATION

Crystalline powder is reconstituted, then further diluted for administration; solution is very unstable and should be used within 1 hour of reconstitution and dilution

ADMINISTRATION

Slow IV push through free-flowing IV fluid; topical; intracavitary; intrapericardial

CONTRAINDICATIONS/PRECAUTIONS

Contraindicated in patients with hypersensitivity to mechlorethamine; precaution in preexisting bone marrow depression; pregnancy risk factor D

TOXICITIES

Dermatologic: rash, alopecia; **GI:** nausea and vomiting, diarrhea, anorexia, taste changes (metallic), vesicant if extravasation occurs during administration (antidote: sodium thiosulfate); **Hepatic:** hepatotoxicity; **Hematologic:** myelosuppression, hemolytic anemia; **Metabolic:** hyperuricemia; **Musculoskeletal:** weakness; **Neurologic:** peripheral neuropathy, tinnitus; **Miscellaneous:** hypersensitivity, infertility and sterility

THERAPEUTIC USES

Chronic myelocytic leukemia; cutaneous T-cell lymphoma; Hodgkin's lymphoma; lung cancer; malignant pericardial effusion; malignant peritoneal effusion; malignant pleural effusion; non-Hodgkin's lymphoma

PHARMACOKINETICS

Metabolism: rapid hydrolysis and demethylation; **Elimination:** minimal as unchanged drug

DOSAGE ADJUSTMENTS

No clear guidelines for dose adjustment in organ dysfunction

AVAILABILITY

Supplied as Mustargen by Ovation Pharmaceuticals, Inc. (Deerfield, IL)

MELPHALAN

MECHANISM OF ACTION

Alkylating agent; bischloroethylamine; cytotoxicity secondary to cross-linking of DNA strands

PREPARATION

Dissolve powder with diluent, which is then further diluted for administration; the reconstituted and prepared medication is unstable and should be used within 60 minutes; do not refrigerate IV preparations; protect oral product from light and store and room temperature

ADMINISTRATION

IV infusion (rapid and short infusion); oral—take on an empty stomach, should be separated from food as food may decrease absorption

CONTRAINDICATIONS/PRECAUTIONS

Contraindicated in known hypersensitivity to melphalan; precaution with use of live virus vaccines; pregnancy risk factor D

TOXICITIES

GI: stomatitis, mild nausea; **Hepatic:** jaundice, elevation of liver function test; **Hematologic:** myelosuppression, hemolytic anemia, myeloproliferative disorder; **Respiratory:** pulmonary fibrosis, interstitial pneumonia; **Miscellaneous:** hypersensitivity and anaphylaxis (rare), sterility and infertility, secondary malignancies

THERAPEUTIC USES

Breast cancer; chronic myelocytic leukemia; endometrial cancer; Hodgkin's lymphoma; melanoma; multiple myeloma; osteosarcoma; ovarian cancer; prostrate cancer; soft tissue sarcoma; testes cancer; Waldenström macroglobulinemia

PHARMACOKINETICS

Absorption: poor bioavailability; **Distribution:** protein binding ranges from 60%–90%; **Metabolism:** extensive metabolism in the blood to inactive metabolites; **Elimination:** renal elimination is about 10%, fecal elimination from 20%–50%

DOSAGE ADJUSTMENTS

There are no clear dose modifications recommended; may consider dose reduction in patients receiving high-dose melphalan with renal dysfunction

AVAILABILITY

Supplied as Alkeran by GlaxoSmithKline (Research Triangle Park, NC)

MERCAPTOPURINE

MECHANISM OF ACTION

Purine antagonist that interferes with DNA and RNA synthesis

PREPARATION

Tablet (50 mg); can be made into an oral suspension (proper handling)

ADMINISTRATION

Do not administer with food

CONTRAINDICATIONS/PRECAUTIONS

Contraindicated in patients with known hypersensitivity to mercaptopurine; precaution in patients with liver impairment; precaution in patients receiving allopurinol because there is increased exposure of active drug; pregnancy risk factor D

TOXICITIES

Dermatologic: hyperpigmentation, rash; **GI:** nausea, vomiting, diarrhea, stomatitis, abdominal pain; **Hepatic:** intrahepatic cholestasis and focal centralobar necrosis presenting as increased liver function test and hyperbilirubinemia; **Hematologic:** myelosuppression; **Metabolic:** hyperuricemia; **Neurologic:** fever

THERAPEUTIC USES

Acute lymphocytic leukemia; acute nonlymphocytic leukemia; chronic myelocytic leukemia; Hodgkin's lymphoma; non-Hodgkin's lymphoma

PHARMACOKINETICS

Absorption: bioavailability is variable and ranges from 15%–50%; **Distribution:** volume of distribution approximates total body water; penetration into the CNS is poor; **Metabolism:** hepatic and GI metabolism; **Elimination:** renal elimination is seen at higher doses, but thought to be minor with lower doses

DOSAGE ADJUSTMENTS

Dose should be decreased by 75% in patients receiving concurrent allopurinol; dose reductions are recommended in patients with hepatic impairment or renal impairment

AVAILABILITY

Supplied as Purinethol by Teva Pharmaceuticals (Irvine, CA)

METHOTREXATE

MECHANISM OF ACTION

Antimetabolite; inhibition via irreversibly binding dihydrofolate reductase, which results in the inhibition of DNA, RNA, and protein synthesis; immune suppression, exact mechanism is not known

PREPARATION

IV lyophilized powder available to be reconstituted to either 25 mg/mL or 50 mg/mL; intrathecal—prepare with preservative-free solution; available as oral tablet

ADMINISTRATION

IV bolus or prolonged infusion; IM; intrathecal; oral

CONTRAINDICATIONS/PRECAUTIONS

Contraindicated in patients with known hypersensitivity to methotrexate; caution in patients with impaired renal and/or liver dysfunction; caution in patients with fluid accumulation (*eg*, pleural effusions, ascites); pregnancy risk factor D

TOXICITIES

The toxicity profile of methotrexate is dependent on dose, dose regimen, and the use of leucovorin posttherapy; **Cardiovascular:** vasculitis; **Dermatologic:** rash, urticaria; **GI:** nausea, vomiting, diarrhea, mucositis (note: mucositis can be minimized with appropriate leucovorin rescue after high-dose methotrexate therapy); **Hepatic:** increased liver function test; cirrhosis and portal fibrosis with chronic low-dose use; **Hematologic:** myelosuppression (may be minimized with leucovorin posttherapy); **Metabolic:** hyperuricemia; **Musculoskeletal:** arthralgia; **Neurologic:** CNS toxicity is seen with intrathecal administration ranging from arachnoiditis to demyelinating encephalopathy; **Ocular:** blurred vision; **Renal:** renal dysfunction may be caused by precipitation of the drug in the renal tubule resulting in decreased renal output and associated sequelae; **Respiratory:** pneumonitis; **Miscellaneous:** photosensitivity, radiation recall, infertility, sterility

THERAPEUTIC USES

Acute lymphocytic leukemia; acute nonlymphocytic leukemia; bladder cancer; brain cancer; breast cancer; carcinomatous meningitis; cervical cancer; colorectal cancer; esophageal cancer; head and neck cancer; Hodgkin's lymphoma; lung cancer; non-Hodgkin's lymphoma; osteosarcoma; ovarian cancer; pancreatic cancer; penis cancer; soft tissue sarcoma; stomach cancer; trophoblastic neoplasm

PHARMACOKINETICS

Absorption: methotrexate is absorbed from the GI tract by a saturable active transport system; therefore oral bioavailability is dose dependent and it is decreased by food and bile; **Distribution:** the volume of distribution of methotrexate approximates that of total body water; protein bound to plasma proteins (approximately 50%); third space retention of methotrexate is associated with prolongation of the terminal drug half-life; **Metabolism:** undergoes uptake, storage, and metabolism in the liver; in the hepatocytes methotrexate is converted to polyglutamate forms that persist for months after administration; **Elimination:** primarily excreted in the urine

DOSAGE ADJUSTMENTS

Dose adjustment is recommended for individuals with impaired renal dysfunction; dose adjustment may be warranted for individuals with hepatic dysfunction; caution should be used when administering methotrexate in patients with fluid accumulation (*eg*, pleural effusions, ascites); leucovorin rescue is recommended for methotrexate doses greater than 100 mg/m^2

AVAILABILITY

Supplied as Rheumatrex by Stada Pharmaceuticals (Cranbury, NJ) and Trexall by Barr Pharmaceuticals, Inc. (Montvale, NJ)

MITOMYCIN

MECHANISM OF ACTION

Classified as an antibiotic antineoplastic agent; cytotoxic action is thought to be secondary to alkylating; causes cross-linking of DNA and subsequent inhibition of DNA, RNA, and protein synthesis

PREPARATION

Powder for injection is reconstituted, and then further diluted for IV use

ADMINISTRATION

IV; intravesically (bladder cancer)

CONTRAINDICATIONS/PRECAUTIONS

Contraindicated in known hypersensitivity to mitomycin; precaution in coagulation disorders and with live viral vaccines; pregnancy risk factor D

TOXICITIES

Cardiovascular: cardiotoxicity; **Dermatologic:** vesicant if extravasation occurs, alopecia; **GI:** nausea and vomiting, stomatitis; **Hepatic:** increased liver enzymes; **Hematologic:** myelosuppression (cumulative and delayed); **Renal:** hemolytic uremic syndrome, nephrotoxicity; **Respiratory:** acute pulmonary toxicity, pulmonary fibrosis; **Miscellaneous:** bladder contracture with intravesical administration

THERAPEUTIC USES

Anal cancer; bladder cancer; breast cancer; cervical cancer; chronic myelocytic leukemia; colorectal cancer; esophageal cancer; gallbladder cancer; head and neck cancer; lung cancer; pancreas cancer

PHARMACOKINETICS

Metabolism: hepatic; **Elimination:** renal elimination of unchanged drug (10%)

DOSAGE ADJUSTMENTS

Consider dose reduction for those individuals with renal dysfunction

AVAILABILITY

Supplied as Mutamycin by Bristol-Myers Squibb (Princeton, NJ)

MITOXANTRONE

MECHANISM OF ACTION
Intercalates into DNA causing cross links and strand breaks in DNA; inhibition of topoisomerase II

PREPARATION
Dilute dose to at least 50 mL

ADMINISTRATION
IV infusion over at least 3 minutes

CONTRAINDICATIONS/PRECAUTIONS
Contraindicated in patients with hypersensitivity to mitoxantrone; precaution with hepatic dysfunction; pregnancy risk factor D

TOXICITIES
Cardiovascular: cardiomyopathy; **Dermatologic:** alopecia; **GI:** diarrhea, nausea and vomiting; **Hepatic:** increased liver function test, specifically bilirubin; **Hematologic:** myelosuppression; **Neurologic:** headache; **Miscellaneous:** secondary malignancies, sterility and infertility

THERAPEUTIC USES
Acute lymphocytic leukemia; acute nonlymphocytic leukemia; breast cancer; liver cancer; non-Hodgkin's lymphoma; prostate cancer; multiple sclerosis

PHARMACOKINETICS
Distribution: high protein binding; **Elimination:** fecal excretion about 25%

DOSAGE ADJUSTMENTS
Dose adjustment with myelosuppression when used in nonmalignant disease states (*eg*, multiple sclerosis); dose modifications should be considered for individuals with hepatic dysfunction

AVAILABILITY
Supplied as Novantrone by EMD Serono, Inc. (Rockland, MA)

NAB-PACLITAXEL (PACLITAXEL PROTEIN BOUND)

MECHANISM OF ACTION
Antimicrotubule agent; paclitaxel shifts the dynamic equilibrium between tubulin dimers and microtubules toward microtubule assembly and stabilizes microtubules against depolymerization; this inhibits the reorganization of the microtubule network and this inhibition is thought to impact the transmission of proliferative signals of cellular process

PREPARATION
IV powder for suspension reconstituted prior to use; inject dose into empty polyvinyl chloride–type IV bag; if suspension or clumps form during preparation, let stand until resolution; do not use in-line filter

ADMINISTRATION
IV infusion over 30 minutes

CONTRAINDICATIONS/PRECAUTIONS
Contraindicated in patients with hypersensitivity to paclitaxel or human albumin; pregnancy risk factor D

TOXICITIES
Dermatologic: alopecia; **GI:** diarrhea, nausea and vomiting; **Hepatic:** increased liver enzymes; **Hematologic:** myelosuppression; **Neurologic:** asthenia, sensory neuropathy; **Miscellaneous:** hypersensitivity reactions are rare (< 5%)

THERAPEUTIC USES
Breast cancer

PHARMACOKINETICS
Distribution: highly protein bound (90%–98%); **Metabolism:** hepatic metabolism via cytochrome P450 (CYP2C8, CYP3A4); **Elimination:** fecal elimination approximately 20%

DOSAGE ADJUSTMENTS
Dose modifications are recommended for individuals who experience sensory neuropathy while on therapy

AVAILABILITY
Supplied as Abraxane by Abraxis BioScience, Inc. (Los Angeles, CA)

NELARABINE

MECHANISM OF ACTION

Prodrug of deoxyguanosine analogue; after demethylation and triphosphorylation to ara-GTP accumulates in leukemia cells ultimately leading to inhibition of DNA synthesis and cell death

PREPARATION

Solution should not be further diluted prior to administration

ADMINISTRATION

IV infusion over 2 hours for adults, and 1 hour in children

CONTRAINDICATIONS/PRECAUTIONS

Contraindicated in patients with hypersensitivity to nelarabine; precaution in preexisting neurotoxicity; avoid live vaccines; pregnancy risk factor D

TOXICITIES

Cardiovascular: edema; **Dermatologic:** petechiae; **GI:** constipation, diarrhea, nausea, vomiting; **Hematologic:** myelosuppression; **Neurologic:** severe neurologic toxicity has occurred including altered mental states, somnolence, seizures, and peripheral neuropathy; there have been reports of demyelination and neuropathies similar to Guillain-Barré syndrome; **Miscellaneous:** tumor lysis syndrome

THERAPEUTIC USES

Acute lymphoblastic leukemia (T cell); lymphoblastic lymphoma (T cell)

PHARMACOKINETICS

Distribution: limited protein binding; **Metabolism:** primary route of metabolism is o-methylation by adenosine deaminase; **Elimination:** limited renal elimination of drug, although there is > 25% renal elimination of metabolite (ara-G)

DOSAGE ADJUSTMENTS

Dose modification may be required for individuals with neurologic toxicity; no clear guidelines for dose adjustment in organ dysfunction

AVAILABILITY

Supplied as Arranon by GlaxoSmithKline (Research Triangle Park, NC)

OXALIPLATIN

MECHANISM OF ACTION

DNA damage that ultimately inhibits DNA replication and transcription

PREPARATION

Lyophilized powder that requires reconstitution and further dilution; do not use chloride-containing solution for reconstitution or final dilution

ADMINISTRATION

IV infusion over 2 hours

CONTRAINDICATIONS/PRECAUTIONS

Contraindicated in patients with a history of known hypersensitivity to platinum compounds; use with caution in patients with renal dysfunction; pregnancy risk factor D

TOXICITIES

Dermatologic: rash, urticaria, erythema, pruritus; **GI:** nausea, vomiting, mucositis; **Hepatic:** hepatotoxicity; **Hematologic:** myelosuppression; **Musculoskeletal:** fatigue; **Neurologic:** severe peripheral sensory neuropathies may occur; an acute neuropathy that occurs with treatment and is exacerbated by cold may be seen during infusion to days following administration (pharyngolaryngeal dysesthesias); a more classic peripheral neuropathy associated with paresthesias and dysesthesias may be seen with chronic dosing, although it may exacerbate a preexisting toxicity; **Ocular:** decreased visual acuity; **Otic:** hearing loss; **Renal:** renal dysfunction; **Respiratory:** pulmonary fibrosis that may manifest as a nonproductive cough, dyspnea, pulmonary infiltrates; **Miscellaneous:** hypersensitivity reaction that may occur with any cycle

THERAPEUTIC USES

Colorectal cancer; stomach cancer

PHARMACOKINETICS

Distribution: rapid distribution into tissues; **Metabolism:** oxaliplatin undergoes rapid and extensive nonenzymatic biotransformation; **Elimination:** renal elimination

DOSAGE ADJUSTMENTS

Dose modifications should be considered for individuals who have treatment-related peripheral neuropathy, myelosuppression, mucositis; dose modifications should be considered for individuals who have renal dysfunction

AVAILABILITY

Supplied as Eloxatin by Sanofi Aventis (Bridgewater, NJ)

PACLITAXEL

MECHANISM OF ACTION

Antimicrotubule agent; paclitaxel shifts the dynamic equilibrium between tubulin dimers and microtubules toward microtubule assembly and stabilizes microtubules against depolymerization; this inhibits the reorganization of the microtubule network, and this inhibition is thought to impact the transmission of proliferative signals of cellular process

PREPARATION

Use non–polyvinyl chloride administration sets to prevent DEHP leaching

ADMINISTRATION

IV infusion, rate of infusion is determined by the dose regimen used; premedication with H2 blocker, antihistamine, corticosteroids, for most regimens, although corticosteroid may not be required for weekly regimen

CONTRAINDICATIONS/PRECAUTIONS

Contraindicated in patients with known hypersensitivity or reaction to paclitaxel; pregnancy risk factor D

TOXICITIES

Cardiovascular: arrhythmias, bradycardia, myocardial infarction; **Dermatologic:** alopecia, flushing, phlebitis; **GI:** mild nausea and vomiting, mucositis seen with prolonged infusion schedules; **Hepatic:** increased liver function test; **Hematologic:** myelosuppression that is dose and schedule dependent; **Musculoskeletal:** arthralgia, myalgia; **Neurologic:** peripheral neuropathies, ataxia; **Miscellaneous:** hypersensitivity reactions that may manifest as life-threatening anaphylaxis

THERAPEUTIC USES

Bladder cancer; breast cancer; carcinoma of unknown primary; cervical cancer; endometrial cancer; esophageal cancer; fallopian tube cancer; head and neck cancer; lung (non–small cell and small cell) cancer; Kaposi's sarcoma; ovarian cancer; peritoneal cancer; prostate cancer; stomach cancer; testicular cancer

PHARMACOKINETICS

Distribution: highly protein bound (> 95%); does not cross blood-brain barrier significantly; **Metabolism:** hepatic hydroxylation (P-450 enzymes); **Elimination:** elimination of metabolites via hepatobiliary system; less than 10% of dose eliminated as intact drug via urine

DOSAGE ADJUSTMENTS

Dose modifications are required in patients who experience peripheral neuropathy or severe neutropenia with treatment; dose modification are recommended for individuals with hepatic dysfunction

AVAILABILITY

Supplied as Taxol by Bristol-Myers Squibb (Princeton, NJ), Onxol by IVAX Pharmaceuticals (Miami, FL)

PEGASPARGASE

MECHANISM OF ACTION

Enzyme that deaminates the amino acid asparagines to aspartic acid and ammonia, ultimately depleting tumor cells of asparagines required for protein synthesis

PREPARATION

For IV preparation, dilute in 100 mL of normal saline or dextrose

ADMINISTRATION

IM; IV infusion over 1–2 hours through an infusion

CONTRAINDICATIONS/PRECAUTIONS

Contraindicated in hemorrhagic events and/or pancreatitis and/or thrombosis with prior asparaginase therapy; contraindicated in patients with hypersensitivity to pegaspargase; precaution in coagulopathy or thrombotic event; pregnancy risk factor C

TOXICITIES

Many of the toxicities of asparaginase are a result of the drug's effect on protein synthesis resulting in functional changes (*eg*, decreased insulin resulting in hyperglycemia); **Cardiovascular:** edema, hypotension, tachycardia; **Dermatologic:** rash, urticaria, local injection site hypersensitivity; **GI:** mild nausea, anorexia, constipation, diarrhea, flatulence, abdominal pain, pancreatitis; **Hematologic:** coagulation defects, thrombosis; **Hepatic:** increased liver function test, hyperalbuminemia; **Metabolic:** hyperglycemia; **Musculoskeletal:** arthralgia; **Neurologic:** depression, fatigue, confusion, agitation; **Renal:** renal insufficiency; **Respiratory:** bronchospasm from hypersensitivity reaction; **Miscellaneous:** hypersensitivity, coagulation defects secondary to protein inhibition of coagulation factors and procoagulation factors, fever, chills

THERAPEUTIC USES

Acute lymphoblastic leukemia

PHARMACOKINETICS

Distribution: 70%–80% of plasma volume, does not penetrate into the CSF; **Metabolism:** systematically degraded; **Elimination:** minimal renal excretion; **Comments:** asparaginase is measurable for up to 15 days following initial treatment

DOSAGE ADJUSTMENTS

No clear guidelines for dose adjustment in organ dysfunction

AVAILABILITY

Supplied as Oncaspar by Enzon Pharmaceuticals (Bridgewater, NJ)

PEMETREXED

MECHANISM OF ACTION

Folic acid antagonist that disrupts folate-dependent metabolic processes essential for cell replication; inhibits thymidylate synthetase, dihydrofolate reductase, and phosphoribosylglycinamide formyltransferase, which are involved in the biosynthesis of thymidine and purine nucleotides

PREPARATION

The reconstituted solution should be further diluted for administration

ADMINISTRATION

IV infusion over 10 minutes

CONTRAINDICATIONS/PRECAUTIONS

Contraindicated in patients with hypersensitivity to pemetrexed; patients should receive treatment with vitamin B_{12} and folic acid pretreatment to minimize hematologic and GI toxicity; pretreatment with corticosteroids reduces the incidence and severity of cutaneous toxicities; pemetrexed may accumulate in fluid, therefore large effusions should be drained prior to administration; pregnancy risk factor D

TOXICITIES

Cardiovascular: cardiac ischemia; **Dermatologic:** rash, desquamation (corticosteroids should be administered to minimize this toxicity); **GI:** stomatitis, nausea, vomiting; **Hepatic:** increased liver function test; **Hematologic:** myelosuppression; **Musculoskeletal:** myalgia; **Neurologic:** fever; **Respiratory:** dyspnea; **Miscellaneous:** anorexia

THERAPEUTIC USES

Lung cancer; mesothelioma

PHARMACOKINETICS

Elimination: renal; **Comments:** caution is recommended when using concurrently with nephrotoxic agents

DOSAGE ADJUSTMENTS

Dose modification should be considered for individuals with renal impairment

AVAILABILITY

Supplied as Alimta by Eli Lilly and Company (Indianapolis, IN)

PENTOSTATIN

MECHANISM OF ACTION

Inhibitor of enzyme (adenosine deaminase) involved in purine metabolism. The highest levels of this enzyme are found in lymphoid tissue and lymphocytes. The degree to which pentostatin inhibits adenosine deaminase varies among cell types; inhibition of RNA synthesis; DNA strand break; immunosuppressive

PREPARATION

Pentostatin powder is reconstituted with 5 mL of sterile water for final concentration of 2 mg/mL; this can be used for injection or further diluted

ADMINISTRATION

IV bolus or short infusion

CONTRAINDICATIONS/PRECAUTIONS

Contraindicated in patients with hypersensitivity to pentostatin; precaution in renal dysfunction; pregnancy risk factor D

TOXICITIES

Cardiovascular: chest pain, arrhythmia, peripheral edema; **Dermatologic:** rash; **GI:** mild nausea and/or vomiting, anorexia, diarrhea, stomatitis, abdominal pain; **Hepatic:** increases in transaminases; **Hematologic:** myelosuppression; **Neurologic:** dose-dependent neurotoxicity ranging from lethargy to coma; **Renal:** acute renal dysfunction (more commonly with high doses); **Respiratory:** pulmonary edema, dyspnea, bronchitis, sinusitis

THERAPEUTIC USES

Acute lymphocytic leukemia; chronic lymphocytic leukemia; cutaneous T-cell lymphoma; hairy cell leukemia; prolymphocytic leukemia

PHARMACOKINETICS

Distribution: distribution to all body tissues; enters erythrocytes; some penetration into the CSF; **Elimination:** 30%–90% of pentostatin is excreted in urine unchanged and/or as active metabolites

DOSAGE ADJUSTMENTS

Dose modifications are recommended in patients with CrCl < 60 mL/min

AVAILABILITY

Supplied as Nipent by Bedford Laboratories (Bedford, OH)

PROCARBAZINE

MECHANISM OF ACTION
Inhibition of transmethylation of methionine in RNA, ultimately resulting in cessation of protein, RNA, and DNA synthesis

PREPARATION
Oral capsules should be protected from light; oral capsules will decompose if exposed to moisture

ADMINISTRATION
Oral; because this agent has monoamine oxidase (MAO) inhibition activity, use caution with select concomitant foods; concomitant alcohol may cause a disulfiram-like reaction

CONTRAINDICATIONS/PRECAUTIONS
Contraindicated in patients with hypersensitivity to procarbazine; as a MAO inhibitor, procarbazine may cause reactions with certain foods (tyramine-containing) and/or medications; pregnancy risk factor D

TOXICITIES
Dermatologic: hyperpigmentation, alopecia; **GI:** nausea and vomiting, anorexia, abdominal pain, constipation and diarrhea; **Hepatic:** hepatotoxicity; **Hematologic:** myelosuppression, hemolysis; **Neurologic:** peripheral neuropathy, depression, hallucinations, headache, nervousness, insomnia, CNS stimulation; **Respiratory:** pleural effusions, cough, pneumonitis; **Miscellaneous:** nystagmus, disulfiram-like reaction with alcohol

THERAPEUTIC USES
Brain cancer; Hodgkin's lymphoma; lung cancer; multiple myeloma; non-Hodgkin's lymphoma

PHARMACOKINETICS
Absorption: rapid and complete, time to peak concentration approximately 60 minutes; **Distribution:** crosses blood-brain barrier; distribution into CSF; **Metabolism:** hepatic and renal auto-oxidation; **Elimination:** renal elimination (majority as metabolite as N-isopropylterephthalamic acid

DOSAGE ADJUSTMENTS
Consider dose modifications for individuals with severe hepatic dysfunction and/or renal dysfunction

AVAILABILITY
Supplied as Matulane by Sigma-Tau Pharmaceuticals (Gaithersburg, MD)

STREPTOZOCIN

MECHANISM OF ACTION
Alkylating agent (nitrosoureas); formation of DNA intrastrand crosslinks, ultimately resulting in inhibition of DNA synthesis; streptozocin has a diabetogenic or hyperglycemic effect; toxicity to the pancreatic islet β cells results in loss of insulin secretion

PREPARATION
Supplied as powder for injection, reconstitute prior to administration

ADMINISTRATION
Rapid IV administration (over 15 to 30 minutes); short or prolonged IV infusion (over 6 hours)

CONTRAINDICATIONS/PRECAUTIONS
Contraindicated in patients with known hypersensitivity to streptozocin; precaution with live viral vaccines; pregnancy risk factor D

TOXICITIES
Dermatologic: pain at injection site; **GI:** nausea and vomiting, diarrhea; **Hepatic:** increased liver function test, jaundice; **Hematologic:** myelosuppression (uncommon), eosinophilia; **Metabolic:** hypoglycemia, hyperglycemia; **Neurologic:** depression, confusion; **Renal:** renal dysfunction (dose related and cumulative), nephrogenic diabetes insipidus; **Miscellaneous:** fever, secondary malignancy

THERAPEUTIC USES
Carcinoid tumors; colorectal cancer; pancreatic cancer

PHARMACOKINETICS
Metabolism: liver; **Elimination:** renal elimination of metabolites

DOSAGE ADJUSTMENTS
No clear guidelines for dose adjustment in organ dysfunction; use with caution in individuals with severe renal and/or hepatic dysfunction

AVAILABILITY
Supplied as Zanosar by Teva Parenteral (Irvine, CA)

TEMOZOLOMIDE

MECHANISM OF ACTION
Temozolomide is converted to the active alkylating metabolite MTIC

PREPARATION
Oral

ADMINISTRATION
Recommended that the drug be taken on an empty stomach to decrease the incidence of nausea and vomiting

CONTRAINDICATIONS/PRECAUTIONS
Contraindicated in patients with hypersensitivity to temozolomide or dacarbazine; precaution in patients with severe renal impairment; pregnancy risk factor D

TOXICITIES
Cardiovascular: peripheral edema; **Dermatologic:** rash, pruritus; **GI:** nausea, vomiting, constipation, anorexia, mucositis; **Hematologic:** myelosuppression; **Musculoskeletal:** weakness; **Neurologic:** headache, fatigue, seizures, hemiparesis, dizziness, fever, insomnia (it is difficult to distinguish toxicity of drug from disease effects in cancers involving the CNS); **Miscellaneous:** vision abnormalities

THERAPEUTIC USES
Brain (refractory anaplastic astrocytoma, glioblastoma multiforme); melanoma

PHARMACOKINETICS
Absorption: bioavailability is 100%; **Distribution:** approximately 15% protein bound; **Metabolism:** temozolomide is a prodrug that is hydrolyzed to the active form MTIC; **Elimination:** small amount (5%–10%) in urine

DOSAGE ADJUSTMENTS
No clear dose adjustments are recommended for hepatic or renal impairment

AVAILABILITY
Supplied as Temodar by Schering Corporation (Kenilworth, NJ)

TENIPOSIDE

MECHANISM OF ACTION
Semisynthetic podophyllotoxin derivative that is structurally related to etoposide; topoisomerase II inhibitor leading to DNA strand breaks

PREPARATION
Teniposide concentrate must be diluted prior to infusions (usual concentration is 0.1, 0.2, 0.4, or 1 mg/mL)

ADMINISTRATION
Slow IV infusion (minimum of 30–60 minutes to minimize hypotensive reactions)

CONTRAINDICATIONS/PRECAUTIONS
Contraindicated in patients with hypersensitivity to teniposide or polyoxyl 35 castor oil; precaution in patients with Down syndrome because they may be sensitive to the myelosuppressive effects of teniposide; pregnancy risk factor D

TOXICITIES
Cardiovascular: transient hypotension; **Dermatologic:** alopecia, rash; **GI:** diarrhea, nausea and vomiting, mucositis; **Hepatic:** hepatic impairment; **Hematologic:** myelosuppression; **Neurologic:** acute CNS depression (high-dose regimen); **Renal:** renal impairment; **Miscellaneous:** hypersensitivity reactions (increased incidence in patients with neuroblastoma or brain tumors), secondary malignancies

THERAPEUTIC USES
Acute lymphocytic leukemia; neuroblastoma; non-Hodgkin's lymphoma

PHARMACOKINETICS
Metabolism: hepatically metabolized

DOSAGE ADJUSTMENTS
Dose adjustment of initial dose of teniposide for individuals with Down syndrome, as there has been evidence of increased myelosuppression; some sources recommend dose modifications for individuals with hepatic and/or renal insufficiency

AVAILABILITY
Supplied as Vumon by Bristol-Myers Squibb (Princeton, NJ)

THIOGUANINE

MECHANISM OF ACTION

Purine antimetabolite; thioguanine is converted to ribonucleotides, which ultimately results in the synthesis and utilization of purine nucleotides; immunosuppression

PREPARATION

Tablets 40 mg (scored)

ADMINISTRATION

Dose maybe given as single daily dose; give at consistent time daily in regard to meals

CONTRAINDICATIONS/PRECAUTIONS

Contraindicated in patients with hypersensitivity to thioguanine; precaution in resistance to thioguanine or mercaptopurine (there is usually complete cross resistance between the two agents); pregnancy risk factor D

TOXICITIES

Dermatologic: rash; **GI:** mild nausea and vomiting, anorexia, stomatitis, diarrhea; **Hepatic:** hepatotoxicity may manifest as veno-occlusive disease, jaundice; **Hematologic:** myelosuppression; **Metabolic:** hyperuricemia; **Neurologic:** unsteady gait

THERAPEUTIC USES

Acute lymphocytic leukemia; acute nonlymphocytic leukemia; chronic myelocytic leukemia

PHARMACOKINETICS

Absorption: bioavailability is variable and incomplete (approximately 30%); absorption may be increased if administered on an empty stomach; **Distribution:** incorporated into the DNA and RNA of bone marrow cells; does not appear to cross blood-brain barrier; crosses placenta; **Metabolism:** rapidly converted to active compound (2-amino-6-methylthioguanine) and to inactive metabolites in the liver and other tissues; **Elimination:** urine as metabolites; **Comments:** hemodialysis is unlikely to reduce toxicity of drug as it is converted rapidly into active metabolites

DOSAGE ADJUSTMENTS

Consider dose modifications for individuals with renal dysfunction or hepatic dysfunction

AVAILABILITY

Supplied as generic by various manufacturers

THIOTEPA

MECHANISM OF ACTION

Alkylating agent; interferes with DNA replication; immunosuppressive effects

PREPARATION

Preparation is dependent on route of administration

ADMINISTRATION

IV as rapid infusion; IM; intracavitary; intravesical (bladder instillation); intrathecal

CONTRAINDICATIONS/PRECAUTIONS

Contraindicated in patients with hypersensitivity to thiotepa; pregnancy risk factor D

TOXICITIES

Dermatologic: alopecia, rash, hyperpigmentation of skin; **GI:** anorexia; **Genitourinary:** hemorrhagic cystitis; **Hepatic:** increased transaminases with high-dose regimens; **Hematologic:** myelosuppression; **Metabolic:** hyperuricemia; **Neurologic:** dizziness, fever, headache; **Renal:** hematuria; **Miscellaneous:** allergic reactions

THERAPEUTIC USES

Bladder cancer; breast cancer; carcinomatous meningitis; Hodgkin's lymphoma; malignant pericardial effusion; malignant peritoneal effusion; malignant pleural effusion; ovarian cancer

PHARMACOKINETICS

Absorption: variable absorption through membranes; absorption through bladder mucosa ranges greatly depending on integrity of the bladder mucosa; **Distribution:** wide distribution of drug and active metabolite thiethylene phosphoramide (TEPA) and other metabolites; **Metabolism:** hepatic metabolism to active metabolite TEPA; **Elimination:** urine as metabolites; feces elimination is unknown; sweat when given at high doses; **Comments:** the pharmacokinetics of the agent varies based on the route of administration (*eg*, IV vs intrathecal)

DOSAGE ADJUSTMENTS

Some sources recommend dose reduction for individuals with hepatic and/or renal dysfunction

AVAILABILITY

Supplied as generic by various manufacturers

TOPOTECAN

MECHANISM OF ACTION

Semisynthetic derivative of camptothecin; type I DNA topoisomerase inhibitor, causing stabilization of DNA–DNA topoisomerase complex preventing relegating of single-strand breaks; this DNA damage is thought to lead to apoptosis

PREPARATION

IV administration over minimum of 30 minutes; oral—store capsules at room temperature and protect from light

ADMINISTRATION

IV administration over minimum of 30 minutes; oral—capsules should not be opened or crushed

CONTRAINDICATIONS/PRECAUTIONS

Contraindicated in patients with known hypersensitivity to topotecan; pregnancy risk factor D

TOXICITIES

Dermatologic: alopecia, rash; **GI:** nausea, vomiting, diarrhea; **Hepatic:** transient elevations in liver function tests; **Hematologic:** myelosuppression; **Neurologic:** headache, paresthesia; **Respiratory:** dyspnea, cough

THERAPEUTIC USES

Cervical cancer; chronic myelomonocytic leukemia; lung (small and non–small cell); myelodysplastic syndromes; ovarian cancer

PHARMACOKINETICS

Absorption: bioavailability is 30%; **Distribution:** approximately 35% is bound to plasma proteins; **Metabolism:** hepatic metabolism; **Elimination:** majority as unchanged drug; urine (55%), feces (20%); **Comments:** at pH $\leq$ 4 the lactone moiety of topotecan undergoes hydrolysis to the pharmacologically active form of drug

DOSAGE ADJUSTMENTS

Dose modification are recommended for individuals with renal impairment

AVAILABILITY

Supplied as Hycamtin by GlaxoSmithKline (Research Triangle Park, NC)

VINBLASTINE

MECHANISM OF ACTION

Binds to tubulin, therefore preventing the polymerization of the tubulin subunit into microtubules, resulting in inhibition of microtubule assembly and cellular metaphase arrest

PREPARATION

Use normal saline preserved with phenol or benzyl alcohol for final concentration of 1 mg/mL; protect from light

ADMINISTRATION

IV push or dilute IV infusion

CONTRAINDICATIONS/PRECAUTIONS

Contraindicated in intrathecal administration (may result in death) and known hypersensitivity to vincristine; pregnancy risk factor D

TOXICITIES

Cardiovascular: hypertension, Raynaud's phenomena; **Dermatologic:** alopecia, vesicant if extravasation occurs; **GI:** nausea, vomiting, constipation, anorexia, metallic taste; **Hematologic:** bone marrow suppression; **Musculoskeletal:** myalgia; **Neurologic:** constipation, peripheral neuropathy, depression, malaise; **Renal:** urinary retention; **Respiratory:** bronchospasm

THERAPEUTIC USES

Bladder cancer; breast cancer; cutaneous T-cell lymphoma; head and neck cancer; Hodgkin's lymphoma; immune or idiopathic thrombocytopenic purpura; Kaposi's sarcoma; kidney cancer; lung cancer; melanoma; neuroblastoma; non-Hodgkin's lymphoma; ovarian (germ cell) cancer; prostate cancer; testicular cancer; trophoblastic neoplasms

PHARMACOKINETICS

Distribution: binds to tissue, does not cross the blood-brain barrier; highly protein bound (> 99%); **Metabolism:** hepatic metabolism to inactive metabolite; **Elimination:** feces (95%); < 1% in urine as unchanged drug

DOSAGE ADJUSTMENTS

Dose modifications are recommended for individuals with hepatobiliary dysfunction

AVAILABILITY

Supplied as generic by various manufacturers; Velban

The information here is provided as guidance only. Prescribers should always consult the manufacturer's current prescribing information.

VINCRISTINE

MECHANISM OF ACTION

Vincristine binds to tubulin, therefore preventing the polymerization of the tubulin subunit into microtubules, resulting in inhibition of microtubule assembly and cellular metaphase arrest; immunosuppressive effects

PREPARATION

Recommendation to prepare in minibag to avoid inadvertent intrathecal administration

ADMINISTRATION

IV short infusion or IV push

CONTRAINDICATIONS/PRECAUTIONS

Contraindicated in patients with hypersensitivity to vincristine or in patients with demyelinating form of Charcot-Marie-Tooth syndrome; precaution in patients with underlying neuropathy

TOXICITIES

Cardiovascular: hypotension, hypertension; **Dermatologic:** tissue irritation and necrosis if extravasation occurs during administration (managed with warm compresses); alopecia; phlebitis; **Endocrine:** SIADH; **GI:** constipation secondary to peripheral neuropathy, anorexia, mild nausea and vomiting, metallic taste; **Hematologic:** mild myelosuppression; **Musculoskeletal:** myalgia; **Neurologic:** peripheral neuropathy that may be severe; **Otic:** eighth cranial nerve damage that may manifest by vestibular manifestation; **Respiratory:** bronchospasm, shortness of breath

THERAPEUTIC USES

Acute lymphocytic leukemia; acute nonlymphocytic leukemia; brain cancer; breast cancer; cervical cancer; chronic lymphocytic leukemia; chronic myelocytic leukemia; colorectal cancer; cutaneous T-cell lymphoma; Ewing's sarcoma; Hodgkin's lymphoma; Kaposi's sarcoma; immune or idiopathic thrombocytopenic purpura; kidney sarcoma; liver cancer; lung cancer; melanoma; multiple myeloma; neuroblastoma; non-Hodgkin's lymphoma; osteosarcoma; ovarian (germ cell) cancer; retinoblastoma; rhabdomyosarcoma; soft tissue sarcoma; trophoblastic neoplasms; Waldenström macroglobulinemia; Wilm's tumor

PHARMACOKINETICS

Distribution: rapidly and widely distributed throughout the body, does not appear to cross the blood-brain barrier; **Metabolism:** thought to be hepatically metabolized; **Elimination:** vincristine and metabolites excreted in feces via biliary eliminations

DOSAGE ADJUSTMENTS

Dose reduction is recommended for individuals with hepatic impairment

AVAILABILITY

Supplied as generic by various manufacturers; Oncovin

VINORELBINE

MECHANISM OF ACTION

Semisynthetic vinca alkaloid; binds to tubulin and inhibits microtubule formation; binds to microtubular protein of mitotic spindle causing metaphase arrest

PREPARATION

For syringe, concentration 1.5–3 mg/mL; for minibag, concentration 0.5–2 mg/mL

ADMINISTRATION

IV short infusion over minimum of 6–10 minutes, flush the vein with 75–125 mL of normal saline or dextrose 5% in water to reduce phlebitis and local irritation; IV infusion over 20–30 minutes, flush the vein with 75–125 mL of normal saline or dextrose 5% in water to reduce phlebitis and local irritation

CONTRAINDICATIONS/PRECAUTIONS

Contraindicated in hypersensitivity to vinorelbine; contraindicated in intrathecal administration; pregnancy risk factor D

TOXICITIES

Cardiovascular: chest pain (rare); **Dermatologic:** vesicant if extravasation occurs, injection site reactions including pain, alopecia; **GI:** nausea, vomiting, constipation; **Hepatic:** increased liver function test; **Hematologic:** myelosuppression; **Metabolic:** SIADH; **Musculoskeletal:** weakness; **Neurologic:** peripheral neuropathy; **Respiratory:** dyspnea; **Miscellaneous:** asthenia

THERAPEUTIC USES

Breast cancer; cervical cancer; lung (non–small cell) cancer; ovarian cancer

PHARMACOKINETICS

Absorption: unreliable; **Distribution:** binds extensively to platelets and lymphocytes; **Metabolism:** extensive hepatic metabolism; **Elimination:** feces (> 45%), urine (< 20%)

DOSAGE ADJUSTMENTS

Dose modification are recommended for individuals with hepatic impairment (manifested by hyperbilirubinemia)

AVAILABILITY

Supplied as Navelbine by Pierre Fabre Pharmaceuticals, Inc. (Parsippany, NJ)

REFERENCES

1. Abeloff MD, Armitage JO, Niederhuber JE, *et al.*: *Clinical Oncology*, edn 3. Philadelphia: Elsevier Churchill Livingstone; 2004.

2. DeVita VT, Lawrence TS, Rosenberg SA, eds.: *DeVita, Hellman, and Rosenberg's Cancer: Principles and Practices of Oncology*, edn 8. Philadelphia: Lippincott Williams & Wilkins; 2008.

3. Chabner BA, Longo DL, eds.: *Cancer Chemotherapy and Biotherapy: Principles and Practices*, edn 3. Philadelphia: Lippincott Williams & Wilkins; 2001.

4. Drugs of choice for cancer. *Treat Guidel Med Lett* 2003, 1: 41–52.

5. Tew KD: Alkylating agents. In *DeVita, Hellman, and Rosenberg's Cancer: Principles and Practices of Oncology*, edn 8. Edited by Devita VT, Lawrence TS, Rosenberg SA. Philadelphia: Lippincott Williams & Wilkins; 2008:407–419.

6. McGuire JJ: Anticancer antifolates: current status and future directions. *Curr Pharm Des* 2003, 9:2593–2613.

7. Nagle A, Hur W, Gray NS: Antimitotic agents of natural origin. *Curr Drug Targets* 2006, 7:305–326.

8. Kiselyov A, Balakin KV, Tkachenko SE, *et al.*: Recent progress in discovery and development of antimitotic agents. *Anticancer Agents Med Chem* 2007, 7:189–208.

9. Kingston DG, Newman DJ: Taxoids: cancer fighting compounds from nature. *Curr Opin Drug Discov Devel* 2007, 10:130–144.

10. Socinski M: Update on nanoparticle albumin-bound paclitaxel. *Clin Adv Hematol Oncol* 2006, 4:745–746.

11. Altmann KH: Epothilone B and its analogs: a new family of anticancer agents. *Min Rev Med Chem* 2003, 3:149–158.

12. Donovan D, Vahdat LT: Epothilones: clinical update and future directions. *Oncology* 2008, 22:408–416.

13. Pommier Y: Topoisomerase I inhibitors: camptothecins and beyond. *Nat Rev Cancer* 2006, 6:789–802.

14. Zavrski I, Jakob C, Kaiser M, *et al.*: Molecular and clinical aspects of proteosome inhibition in treatment of cancer. *Recent Results Cancer Res* 2007, 176:165–176.

15. Brueckner B, Kuck D, Lyko E: DNA methyltransferase inhibitors for cancer treatment. *Cancer J* 2007, 13:17–22.

16. Adams VR, Liewer S: Guide for the administration and use of cancer therapeutic agents 2008: solid tumors. *Clinical Oncology News Special Edition* 2008, 11:43–64.

17. Saif MW, Chu E: Antimetabolites. In *DeVita, Hellman, and Rosenberg's Cancer Principles & Practice of Oncology*, edn 8. Edited by DeVita VT, Lawrence TS, Rosenberg SA. Philadelphia: Lippincott Williams & Wilkins; 2008:427–436.

18. Rasheed ZA, Rubin EH: Topoisomerase-interacting agents. In *DeVita, Hellman, and Rosenberg's Cancer Principles & Practice of Oncology*, edn 8. Edited by DeVita VT, Lawrence TS, Rosenberg SA. Philadelphia: Lippincott Williams & Wilkins; 2008:437–446.

19. Lee JJ, Harris LN: Antimicrotubule agents. In *DeVita, Hellman, and Rosenberg's Cancer Principles & Practice of Oncology*, 8th ed. Edited by DeVita VT, Lawrence TS, Rosenberg SA. Philadelphia: Lippincott Williams & Wilkins; 2008:447–456.

20. Doroshow JH: Anthracyclines and anthracenediones. In *Cancer Chemotherapy & Biotherapy Principles and Practice*, edn 3. Edited by Chabner BA, Longo DL. Philadelphia: Lippincott Williams & Wilkins; 2001:500–538.

21. Superfin D, Iannucci AA, Davies AM: Commentary: oncologic drugs in patients with organ dysfunction: a summary. *Oncologist* 2007, 12:1070–1083.

Hormones play a pivotal role in regulating the growth and development of their target organs. Various hormonal agents have been used in the treatment of tumors originating from these target organs, namely the breast, uterus, ovary, and prostate.

MECHANISM OF ACTION

Estrogens, androgens, and progestins exert their function mainly through their respective receptors. After binding to the receptors in high affinity, the steroids alter the configuration of receptor molecules and make them capable of binding to a segment of DNA template called hormone response element, where they regulate gene transcription and control cellular growth and function [1].

COMPLEX CELLULAR REGULATION

A complex system governs the growth of normal and cancerous cells. Endocrine functions are under tight feedback loops of autoregulation within one type of hormone as well as under interregulation between hormones. The former can best be illustrated using the case of pharmacologic dosages of estrogen that downregulate expression of the estrogen receptors. Regarding interhormonal regulation, estrogens promote the production of progesterone receptor, and progestins, acting through their receptor, can then downregulate the estrogen receptors.

There is also a second level of fine tuning at the site of the local microenvironment, in which cellular functions are mediated through the paracrine effects of various growth factors [2]. Estrogen supports breast cancer growth through an enhanced autocrine production of transforming growth factor-α. Estrogen also increases cellular sensitivity to other mitogens such as the insulin-like growth factors.

Hormonal therapy aims to disrupt these regulatory pathways. Tamoxifen, progestins, and ovariectomy act to reverse the effects of estrogen on growth factor production. Various modalities of endocrine therapy can be classified arbitrarily as additive, ablative, competitive, and inhibitive (Table 2-1).

APOPTOSIS AS A MECHANISM OF ANTITUMOR EFFECTS

It is well documented that the antitumor effects of many endocrine therapies are mediated through the process of apoptosis (programmed cell death). Deprivation of hormones by orchiectomy or ovariectomy induces apoptosis of tumor cells in prostate and breast cancer, respectively [3]. Both antiestrogen and antiprogestin act through competitive mechanisms to achieve tumor regression through the apoptotic process [4].

TISSUE-SPECIFIC RESPONSE TO TAMOXIFEN

Although the action of tamoxifen in humans is mainly an antiestrogenic effect, tamoxifen also possesses an estrogenic effect depending on the type and condition of target tissues. We now understand that the ability of tamoxifen to influence estrogen receptors is cell context dependent [5]. In breast cancer, tamoxifen acts mainly to antagonize estrogen receptor function. In vaginal epithelium, endometrium, and skeletal bones, however,

tamoxifen acts like estrogen. This differential function explains why tamoxifen inhibits breast cancer growth while increasing the risk of endometrial cancer. It also explains why tamoxifen, instead of causing osteoporosis, promotes mineral bone formation as estrogens do. Thus, tamoxifen can be an agonist or antagonist of estrogen receptor-α function depending on the cell type. The term *selective estrogen receptor modulator* (SERM) is now used to describe such agents. When breast cancer progresses after an initial response to tamoxifen, a minority of patients can have a response to tamoxifen withdrawal. In this setting, either tamoxifen itself, or some of its metabolites, may have become agonists for the breast cancer cells.

Tamoxifen may affect cancer cell growth through mechanisms other than the steroid receptor pathway, such as through the protein kinase C system, by inhibiting ornithine decarboxylase and polyamine [6], by suppressing the plasma level of insulin-like growth factor [7], by modulating the multidrug resistance gene *MDR*, or through antiangiogenesis [8].

INDICATIONS FOR HORMONAL THERAPY

The types of cancers that have shown responses to hormonal agents are listed in Table 2-2. Because the major action of hormones is mediated through steroid receptors, theoretically only receptor-positive tumor cells will respond to this modality of therapy. Indeed, 60% of receptor-positive breast cancers responded to first-line hormonal therapy. Early reports suggested that 10% of estrogen receptor–negative breast cancer cells could respond to tamoxifen. However, newer methods used to detect estrogen receptors have shown that in the absence of estrogen receptor expression, the response to tamoxifen is nonexistent. Prostate cancer cells have a high level of androgen receptor expression and respond to androgen deprivation, either by orchiectomy or by a combination of antiandrogen (flutamide) and a luteinizing hormone–releasing hormone (LH-RH) analogue. The presence of steroid receptors in ovarian and endometrial cancers is less frequent than their presence in breast and prostate cancers. However, even in receptor-positive tumors, the response of ovarian and uterine cancers to hormonal agents is at best modest or rare.

There is no clear, rational basis for treating renal cell cancer or melanoma with hormonal therapy because no genuine steroid receptor has been found in these two types of cancer. Unlike hamster kidney cancer, human renal cell carcinoma is hormonally independent. The estrogen receptors previously reported in melanoma are actually tyrosinase. However, because tamoxifen may bind proteins other than the estrogen receptor, it is possible that tamoxifen could influence other growth-regulatory pathways. For example, in one uncontrolled study, the response rate of melanoma to combination chemotherapy was reported to be improved from 10% without tamoxifen to 51% with tamoxifen [9]. However, additional randomized trials have not shown a benefit for tamoxifen with chemotherapy [10].

FLARE FOLLOWING HORMONAL THERAPY

Tumor flare has been observed with every known hormonal therapy. The most frequent manifestations of a tumor flare are an abrupt increase of pain at sites of known metastases, erythema around skin lesions, and induced hypercalcemia. However, evidence of actual tumor growth increase

Table 2-1. Categories of Current Endocrine Therapy

Additive	Ablative
Estrogens	Ovariectomy
Progestins	Luteinizing hormone–releasing hormone analogues
Androgens	
Competitive	**Inhibitive**
Selective estrogen receptor modulators	Aromatase inhibitors
Antiandrogens	Luteinizing hormone–releasing hormone analogues
Antiprogestins	

Table 2-2. Type of Tumor Subjected to Hormonal Therapy

High probability of response (40%–80%)	Low probability of response (10%–30%)	Rare response (< 10%)
Steroid receptor–positive	Endometrial cancer	Steroid receptor–negative
Breast cancer		Prostate cancer
Prostate cancer		Ovarian cancer
Meningioma		Renal cell cancer

is lacking. Indeed, the flare may be a good prognostic sign that the tumor is hormonally responsive. Therefore, by an adequate control of pain or hypercalcemia, a continued use of the hormonal agent may result in tumor regression. This practice is especially important and prudent in the use of LH-RH analogues for prostate cancer, in which an initial increase of the blood androgen level and bone pain is frequently inevitable.

DURATION OF TREATMENT

Because of the cytostatic effects on tumor cells from most hormonal agents, a minimal period of 2 months of continuous treatment is needed to adequately determine the efficacy of these agents.

COMBINED OR SEQUENTIAL USE OF HORMONAL THERAPY

As described earlier, when cancer cell growth is dependent on hormones, there are many ways to interrupt such dependency: by removing or reducing the hormone source, blocking peripheral conversion of steroids into estrogens, or blocking hormonal action at the receptor site. Therefore, a combined hormone approach makes sense and has been used for treatment of advanced prostate cancer (LH-RH analogue plus flutamide) [11]. The results of such combination approaches in breast cancer are less convincing, although some data suggest that a combination of tamoxifen plus an LH-RH analogue is superior to tamoxifen alone [12] in the treatment of premenopausal patients with advanced disease. These early results suggest that improved survival may be obtained by combining hormone therapies in breast cancer; however, several issues remain unanswered regarding appropriate sequencing of these therapies [13]. Because an initial response to hormone therapy predicts response to a second- or third-line hormonal manipulation, it is recommended that hormone therapy in advanced breast cancer be used in sequence (Fig. 2-1).

COMBINED HORMONAL THERAPY AND CHEMOTHERAPY

A combination of hormonal therapy and chemotherapy is theoretically logical because these two modalities have different mechanisms of antitumor action and different types of side effects. However, clinical studies around the world have not shown benefit for such a combination, especially in terms of the duration of response or survival in patients with breast cancer [14]. Therefore, for palliative purposes in advanced breast cancer, sequential application of hormonal therapy and chemotherapy to achieve a prolonged control of the disease is advised (Fig. 2-2). It has also been suggested that "hormonal priming" with an estrogen or androgen could enhance subsequent chemotherapeutic responses by placing more cells in S-phase. However, this has not been shown to be clinically useful and may in fact be detrimental.

NEW DEVELOPMENTS

In the past decade, several new hormonal agents for the management of malignant diseases have been added. Most of the new agents belong to the category of antiestrogens (toremifene, raloxifene), antiandrogens (bicalutamide, nilutamide), aromatase inhibitors (anastrozole, letrozole), and aromatase inactivators (exemestane). In general, these agents do not seem to advance the therapeutic indexes; rather, a marked improvement is achieved in compliance (*eg*, once-daily dose) and in the reduction of untoward side effects.

In breast cancer, recent studies have shown that third-generation aromatase inhibitors (anastrozole, exemestane, letrozole) are superior to tamoxifen in previously untreated hormone receptor–positive advanced breast cancer [15]. In the adjuvant setting, several studies have demonstrated that 5-year treatment with an aromatase inhibitor instead of tamoxifen or a sequential therapy of tamoxifen followed by an aromatase inhibitor for a total of 5 or 10 years is superior to 5 years of tamoxifen alone [16]. Importantly, fewer thromboembolic effects and less vaginal bleeding were seen in patients receiving aromatase inhibitors.

These agents have also provided new options for patients with hormonally responsive disease. For example, patients who initially responded to tamoxifen may respond to an aromatase inhibitor. Given the favorable side effect profile of most hormonal agents, it is advisable to try a second hormonal manipulation in a patient who has previously had a good clinical response.

A major recent advancement is the development of new hormonal agents based on an improved understanding of steroid receptor function. As noted, hormonal agents have different effects on their target tissues in a cell context manner. Once SERMs bind the receptor complex, the receptor undergoes a conformational change that allows the binding of coregulatory proteins. Both coactivators and corepressors have been discovered that significantly influence steroid hormone receptor action. For example, the SERM tamoxifen acts as an estrogen in the uterus, whereas raloxifene does not share this property. Presumably, this differential effect of tamoxifen and raloxifene on the uterus is caused by their ability to induce conformational changes that alter the coregulatory protein binding. In the case of tamoxifen, coactivator proteins (or release of corepressor proteins) are favored and induce gene transcription. Fulvestrant, another SERM, can be used in women with hormone receptor–positive advanced breast cancer and is under investigation in the adjuvant setting. Initial clinical trials suggest that tamoxifen and fulvestrant are not cross-resistant. In animal models and human clinical trials, tamoxifen-resistant tumors may respond to these newer modulators [17,18]. Thus, development of new hormonal agents for cancer treatment has a promising future.

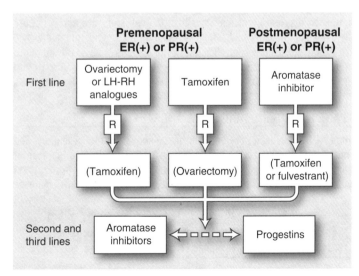

Figure 2-1. Sequential hormonal therapy in advanced breast cancer. ER(+)—estrogen receptor–positive; LH-RH—luteinizing hormone–releasing hormone; PR(+)—progesterone receptor–positive; R—responders.

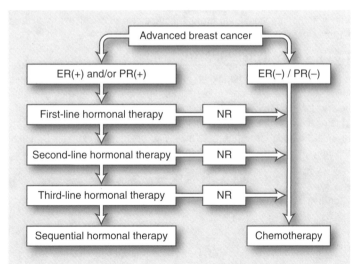

Figure 2-2. Treatment for advanced breast cancer. ER(+)—estrogen receptor–positive; ER(-)—estrogen receptor–negative; NR—nonresponder; PR(+)—progesterone receptor–positive; PR(-)—progesterone receptor–negative.

AMINOGLUTETHIMIDE

EFFICACY AND USAGE

Aminoglutethimide has been casually referred to as a medical adrenalectomy. The role of this agent in therapy for breast cancer is attributed to its action as an inhibitor of the enzyme aromatase. Aromatase catalyzes the conversion of testosterone to estradiol and the conversion of androstenedione to estrone. This enzyme is present in the adrenal cortex and extraglandular peripheral tissues, including adipose and breast cancer tissues.

DOSAGE AND ADMINISTRATION

250 mg two to four times daily with hydrocortisone 20-mg supplement. Mineralocorticoid replacement (*eg*, fludrocortisone) may be necessary.

SPECIAL PRECAUTIONS

Given its similarity to the sedative glutethimide, severe sedation may occur, especially in elderly patients.

TOXICITIES

Side effects are unpredictable and occur in 50% of patients; **Most common:** skin (morbilliform maculopapular) rashes (30%), lethargy, somnolence; **Hematologic:** thrombocytopenia, leukopenia; **Metabolic:** hypothyroidism; **Cardiovascular:** hypotension; **GI:** loss of appetite, nausea; **Other:** flu-like syndrome

INDICATIONS

Second- or third-line endocrine therapy for advanced breast cancer in postmenopausal patients. With development of third-generation aromatase inhibitors for breast cancer, aminoglutethimide has no advantages for the treatment of breast cancer. However, use as second-line therapy in prostate cancer is still warranted.

CONTRAINDICATIONS

History of hypersensitivity to glutethimide

PHARMACOKINETICS

Addition of hydrocortisone is necessary to suppress a reflex rise in adrenocorticotropic hormone (ACTH) levels, which could act to overcome the blockade in steroid synthesis caused by aminoglutethimide

DRUG INTERACTIONS

Binds to CYP-450 enzymes and may increase the clearance rate of warfarin, antipyrine, theophylline, digitoxin, and tamoxifen

RESPONSE RATES

Third-line therapy for breast cancer: ~ 30% in patients who previously responded to endocrine therapy

NURSING INTERVENTIONS

Carefully monitor for side effects, especially mental status

PATIENT INFORMATION

Patient should check for skin rashes and drowsiness

AVAILABILITY

Supplied as Cytadren by Novartis Pharmaceuticals, East Hanover, NJ; 250-mg tablets stored in light-protected container at room temperature

ANASTROZOLE

EFFICACY AND USAGE

Anastrozole is a newer nonsteroidal aromatase inhibitor for the treatment of postmenopausal breast cancer. It specifically suppresses the enzyme that converts androgens to estrogens, with no effect on corticosteroid or aldosterone synthesis.

DOSAGE AND ADMINISTRATION

1 mg daily orally

SPECIAL PRECAUTIONS

Should not be administered in pregnant woman and should be closely monitored for side effects in patients with impaired liver function

TOXICITIES

The drug is generally well tolerated; **Most common:** gastrointestinal disturbance, musculoskeletal discomfort, headache, hot flashes, and edema. Incidence of rashes and central nervous system symptoms (*eg*, lethargy) may occur but much less often than with the first-generation aromatase inhibitors

INDICATIONS

For adjuvant therapy in postmenopausal women with hormone receptor–positive tumors; first- or second-line therapy in advanced breast cancer in postmenopausal patients with hormone receptor–positive tumors; neoadjuvant treatment for hormone receptor–positive, operable or potentially operable, locally advanced disease in postmenopausal women for 3 months prior to surgery

CONTRAINDICATIONS

Prior history of hypersensitivity reaction to the drug

PHARMACOKINETICS

Well absorbed and bound to plasma proteins; it is metabolized in liver and excreted mainly through the biliary tract; reaches the steady-state level at ~ 7 d with a half-life of 50 h in postmenopausal women

DRUG INTERACTIONS

Although anastrozole inhibits reactions catalyzed by certain CYP-450 enzymes, it does not have known interactions with other drugs. It should not be used with tamoxifen

RESPONSE RATES

In patients having prior treatment with tamoxifen for advanced breast cancer, about one third had an objective response (10%) or stable disease (24%), with an overall median time to progression of 21 wk

NURSING INTERVENTIONS

In patients with poor liver function, closely monitor the side effects of anastrozole. Bone density should be monitored

PATIENT INFORMATION

May cause edema or bone or muscle pain

AVAILABILITY

Supplied as Arimidex by AstraZeneca Pharmaceuticals, Wilmington, DE; 1-mg tablets stored at room temperature between 20° to 25°C

BICALUTAMIDE

EFFICACY AND USAGE

Bicalutamide is a nonsteroidal "pure" antiandrogen used in the treatment of advanced prostate cancer. It competitively binds to androgen receptors and inhibits the action of androgens.

DOSAGE AND ADMINISTRATION

50 mg daily orally

SPECIAL PRECAUTIONS

Moderate to severe hepatic impairment

TOXICITIES

Most common: hot flashes, bone pain, hematuria, and gastrointestinal symptoms (diarrhea)

INDICATIONS

In combination with an LH-RH analogue for the treatment of advanced prostate cancer

CONTRAINDICATIONS

Prior history of a hypersensitivity reaction to this drug

PHARMACOKINETICS

Bicalutamide is well absorbed orally and not affected by food intake; the active component (R-enantiomer) is highly protein bound; it reaches its maximal plasma level by 19 h and a steady-state level by 1 mo. It is metabolized mainly in the liver by glucuronidation and excreted in feces and urine with a half-life of ~ 6–7 d

DRUG INTERACTIONS

May interact with warfarin at its protein-binding sites

RESPONSE RATES

The response and survival rates of patients with advanced prostate cancer treated with bicalutamide monotherapy are inferior to those treated with castration; tumors that progress from bicalutamide monotherapy have a high-level amplification of the androgen receptor gene; therefore, bicalutamide should be used in combination with an LH-RH analogue for total androgen blockade. For bicalutamide in combination with an LH-RH analogue, the median time to treatment failure in prostate cancer is 97 wk.

NURSING INTERVENTIONS

Closely monitor side effects in patients with impaired liver function; adjust warfarin dosages according to prothrombin time

PATIENT INFORMATION

Bicalutamide should be started simultaneously with an LH-RH analogue; it may cause gynecomastia and breast pain

AVAILABILITY

Supplied as Casodex by AstraZeneca Pharmaceuticals, Wilmington, DE; 50-mg tablets stored at room temperature

DIETHYLSTILBESTROL

EFFICACY AND USAGE

Diethylstilbestrol is a synthetic estrogen used for breast cancer and prostate cancer treatment. Because of its dichotomous effects on breast cancer—tumor flare at physiologic doses and regression at pharmacologic doses—the dosage for breast cancer should be in the pharmacologic range. On the contrary, the dosage used for prostate cancer should be low to prevent cardiovascular complications. The suppression of serum androgens may be measured to document the adequacy of dosage.

DOSAGE AND ADMINISTRATION

Breast cancer: 5 mg three times daily orally
Prostate cancer: 1–3 mg daily orally

SPECIAL PRECAUTIONS

Pregnant patients; patients with poor liver or renal function, congestive heart failure, gallbladder disease, endometrial problems, or history of thrombophlebitis or embolism

TOXICITIES

Tumor flare occurs in 5%–10%; **GI:** nausea and vomiting, cholestatic jaundice, increased gallbladder disease; **Cardiovascular:** exacerbation of congestive heart failure, thromboembolism; **GU:** vaginal bleeding, candidiasis, cystitis-like symptoms; **Metabolic:** hypercalcemia, fluid retention; **CNS:** headache, migraine, mental depression; **Skin:** pigmentation of nipple and axillae; **Breasts:** gynecomastia in men

INDICATIONS

Postmenopausal female patients or male patients with advanced breast cancer; patients with metastatic prostate cancer

CONTRAINDICATIONS

Pregnancy, active thrombophlebitis, known or suspected estrogen-dependent malignancy

PHARMACOKINETICS

Relatively completely absorbed; binding to serum hormone–binding globulin is 40%–50%; blood levels are 0.15–6.0 mg/mL after administration at 1 mg three times daily; hepatic biotransformation and biliary excretion

DRUG INTERACTIONS

None directly; however, estrogen decreases the prothrombin time, impairs glucose tolerance, and increases thyroid-binding globulin

RESPONSE RATES

Approximately 30% of postmenopausal breast cancers and 55%–60% of estrogen receptor–positive cancers will respond; the response rate in male breast cancer is similar to that in female breast cancer; the objective response rate in prostate cancer is ~ 65%; if patients with subjective pain relief are included as responders, the total response rate could be up to 85%

NURSING INTERVENTIONS

Carefully monitor and document signs and symptoms

PATIENT INFORMATION

Patient should be aware of increased risk of endometrial carcinoma, carcinogenic effects on fetus during pregnancy, and all the potential side effects listed above

AVAILABILITY

No longer available in the United States

EXEMESTANE

EFFICACY AND USAGE

Exemestane is a steroidal aromatase inactivator for the treatment of post-menopausal breast cancer. It specifically suppresses the enzyme that converts androgens to estrogens, with no effect on corticosteroid or aldosterone synthesis. Compared with anastrozole and letrozole, exemestane binds irreversibly to the aromatase substrate–binding site. This causes downregulation of aromatase. It is unclear if this mechanism of action correlates with enhanced clinical response.

DOSAGE AND ADMINISTRATION

25 mg daily orally

SPECIAL PRECAUTIONS

Should not be administered in pregnant woman and should be closely monitored for side effects in patients with impaired liver function

TOXICITIES

The drug is generally well tolerated; **Most common:** hot flashes, nausea, fatigue, musculoskeletal discomfort, increased sweating

INDICATIONS

As adjuvant therapy in postmenopausal women with hormone receptor–positive tumors; for advanced breast cancer in postmenopausal patients with hormone receptor–positive tumors who progressed on antiestrogen; also effective for patients who have progressed on anastrozole

PHARMACOKINETICS

Well absorbed and bound to plasma proteins; metabolized in liver and excreted mainly through the biliary tract. It has a half-life of ~ 24 h, thus once-daily dosing is appropriate. Steady-state levels are achieved in less than 1 wk

DRUG INTERACTIONS

Although exemestane inhibits reactions catalyzed by certain CYP-450 enzymes, it does not have known interactions with other drugs

RESPONSE RATES

Early results suggest that first-line treatment of estrogen receptor–positive breast cancer results in an objective response rate at least equivalent to, if not better than, tamoxifen. For patients who have progressed on tamoxifen therapy, the objective response rate is ~ 15% and stable disease is 22%. In this setting, median time to treatment failure is 16 wk

NURSING INTERVENTIONS

In patients with poor liver function, closely monitor the side effects of exemestane. Bone density should be monitored

AVAILABILITY

Supplied as Aromasin by Pharmacia & Upjohn, a division of Pfizer, Inc., New York, NY; 25-mg tablets stored at room temperature between 15° to 30°C

FLUOXYMESTERONE

EFFICACY AND USAGE

Fluoxymesterone is a synthetic steroid hormone used for the treatment of advanced breast cancer. The response rate is lower than that of tamoxifen. It has been used as a third-line therapy. The erythropoietic effects may provide a sense of well being in anemic patients.

DOSAGE AND ADMINISTRATION

10 mg twice daily orally

SPECIAL PRECAUTIONS

Masculinization effects and, occasionally, induced hypercalcemia

TOXICITIES

GU: virilization, amenorrhea, irregular menstrual periods; **GI:** nausea, cholestatic jaundice; **Hematologic:** suppression of clotting factors, polycythemia; **CNS:** increased libido, headache, anxiety, aggressiveness, depression; **Skin:** acne, hirsutism

INDICATIONS

Advanced breast cancer

CONTRAINDICATIONS

Known hypersensitivity to the drug, suspected prostate cancer, pregnancy, or serious cardiac, hepatic, or renal disease

PHARMACOKINETICS

Absorption is rapid; biotransformation occurs in liver; half-life is 9.2 h; 90% is excreted in urine after being glucuronidated

DRUG INTERACTIONS

Increases the sensitivity to anticoagulants, decreasing the requirement for insulin and interfering with laboratory testing for thyroid function

RESPONSE RATES

15%–25% in breast cancer

NURSING INTERVENTIONS

Monitor and document signs and symptoms

PATIENT INFORMATION

Causes masculinization, hoarseness, acne, and changes in menstrual periods

AVAILABILITY

Supplied as Halotestin by Pharmacia & Upjohn, a division of Pfizer, Inc., New York, NY; 2-, 5-, and 10-mg tablets stored at room temperature

---

The information here is provided as guidance only. Prescribers should always consult the manufacturer's current prescribing information.

FLUTAMIDE

EFFICACY AND USAGE

Flutamide is a nonsteroidal antiandrogen. It is used in combination with an LH-RH analogue for the treatment of metastatic prostate cancer. The drug blocks the androgenic action at its target site.

DOSAGE AND ADMINISTRATION

250 mg every 8 h orally

SPECIAL PRECAUTIONS

Patients with hepatic toxicity with elevation of hepatic transaminases and cholestatic jaundice

TOXICITIES

Most common: diarrhea, hot flashes, impotence, loss of libido; **GI:** anorexia, nausea, vomiting; **Cardiovascular:** hypertension, edema; **CNS:** drowsiness, depression, anxiety; **Hematologic:** anemia, leukopenia, thrombocytopenia (occasionally)

INDICATIONS

Advanced prostate cancer

CONTRAINDICATIONS

Liver function impairment

PHARMACOKINETICS

Rapidly orally absorbed; its biologic metabolites reach a maximal plasma level in 2 h and a steady-state level in 9.6 h; plasma half-life is ~ 8 h; mainly excreted in the urine

DRUG INTERACTIONS

Increased prothrombin time in patients on long-term warfarin

RESPONSE RATES

Flutamide is frequently used in combination with an LH-RH analogue, which suppresses the production of testicular androgens. The overall response rate for the combination therapy is about 70%, and the drug provides a significantly prolonged survival compared with LH-RH analogue alone (36 vs 28 mo)

NURSING INTERVENTIONS

Monitor signs and symptoms

PATIENT INFORMATION

May cause hepatic injury such as cholestatic jaundice; the patient may need more frequent monitoring of prothrombin time while on warfarin

AVAILABILITY

Available in generic form only; 125-mg capsules stored at room temperature and protected from heat and moisture

FULVESTRANT

EFFICACY AND USAGE

Fulvestrant is a pure steroidal antiestrogen. Unlike other SERMs, it is a pure antiestrogen in all tissues studied. Fulvestrant also causes degradation of the estrogen receptor, resulting in a decreased cellular concentration of the receptor. Early clinical trials suggest it is useful in patients who have progressive disease on tamoxifen.

DOSAGE AND ADMINISTRATION

250-mg monthly injection

SPECIAL PRECAUTIONS

Should not be administered in pregnant woman and should be closely monitored for side effects in patients with impaired liver function

TOXICITIES

Injection site reaction, pain, and inflammation; **GI:** abdominal pain, constipation, diarrhea, nausea, vomiting; **Musculoskeletal:** backache; **Neurologic:** headache; **Respiratory:** pharyngitis

INDICATIONS

Treatment of hormone receptor–positive metastatic breast cancer in postmenopausal women with disease progression following antiestrogen therapy

CONTRAINDICATIONS

Pregnant women; hypersensitivity to the drug or its components

RESPONSE RATES

Early results suggest that good responses can be obtained in patients who have progressed through tamoxifen, suggesting a lack of cross-resistance

AVAILABILITY

Supplied as Faslodex by AstraZeneca Pharmaceuticals, Wilmington, DE; 50 mg/mL solution for injection in prefilled syringes to be refrigerated at 2° to 6°C

GOSERELIN ACETATE

Goserelin is a synthetic decapeptide analogue of LH-RH with a much prolonged half-life and 100 times greater potency than that of the natural releasing hormone. Therefore, it downregulates the LH-RH receptors and reduces the release of gonadotropic hormones, which in turn results in a decrease in blood testosterone or estrogen levels. Thus, the functional result of LH-RH analogue therapy is equivalent to medical castration.

DOSAGE AND ADMINISTRATION

A depot dose of 3.6-mg implant given subcutaneously every 4 wk or a 10.8-mg implant given subcutaneously every 12 wk

SPECIAL PRECAUTIONS

Patients with hypersensitivity to LH-RH; initial exacerbation of symptoms from prostate cancer; pregnant nursing patients

TOXICITIES

GU: sexual dysfunction, gynecomastia, hot flashes, loss of libido; **Respiratory:** bronchitis; **Cardiovascular:** arrhythmias, hypertension; **CNS:** depression, anxiety, headache; **GI:** constipation, diarrhea, dyspepsia

INDICATIONS

Advanced breast cancer and endometriosis (the 4-wk dose has been studied in these settings); advanced prostate cancer; in combination with flutamide for locally confined stage B2-C prostate cancer (the 12-wk dose has been studied in this setting)

CONTRAINDICATIONS

Pregnant nursing patients; history of hypersensitivity to LH-RH

PHARMACOKINETICS

Absorption is very slow; peak blood level achieved in 12–15 d following a single-dose (3.6-mg) injection; following goserelin therapy, the mean serum estradiol or testosterone values fall into the range of castrated level within 2–3 wk; the drug is excreted through both urine and hepatic metabolism, and there is no drug accumulation on an every-28-d schedule

RESPONSE RATES

Advanced prostate cancer: in combination with flutamide, 70%
Pre- and perimenopausal receptor–positive breast cancer: 45%

NURSING INTERVENTIONS

Monitor signs and symptoms

PATIENT INFORMATION

Because of the initial, but transient, surge of blood testosterone level, patients may experience exacerbation of bone pain at metastatic sites of prostate cancer or urethral obstruction; patients may experience hot flushes and sexual dysfunction

AVAILABILITY

Supplied as Zoladex by AstraZeneca Pharmaceuticals, Wilmington, DE; 3.6-mg and 10.8-mg disposable syringe device to be stored at room temperature below 25°C

KETOCONAZOLE

EFFICACY AND USAGE

Ketoconazole is a synthetic imidazole with antifungal action. It inhibits the synthesis of ergosterol, a vital membranous component of fungal cells. Because of its inhibition of testosterone synthesis, ketoconazole is also used for the treatment of advanced prostate cancer.

DOSAGE AND ADMINISTRATION

400 mg every 8 h orally in order to sustain the androgen suppression with hydrocortisone 20 mg orally as a supplement

SPECIAL PRECAUTIONS

Hypersensitivity to the drug; at high dosage, decreases the ACTH-induced corticosteroid level

TOXICITIES

GI: nausea and vomiting can be prominent; **Skin:** pruritus; **Other:** hepatic toxicity, hypersensitivity; in patients treated with 1200 mg daily for prostate cancer, death within 2 wk from unknown mechanism was observed

INDICATIONS

Used for advanced prostate cancer but is not approved by the FDA for this indication

CONTRAINDICATIONS

Coadministration with terfenadine, astemizole, cisapride, and oral triazolam

PHARMACOKINETICS

Absorption is rapid; requires gastric acidity; peak blood level is reached within 1–2 h; half-life is biphasic, initially 2 h during the first 10 h then 8 h thereafter; plasma binding is 99% to albumin; converts into inactive metabolites; the major route of excretion is via bile; central nervous system penetration is poor

DRUG INTERACTIONS

Inhibits the metabolism of the drugs listed in the Contraindications section and increases their blood level, resulting in cardiac arrhythmia including ventricular tachycardia; may increase phenytoin serum concentrations; may enhance the anticoagulant effect of warfarin; should not be given concomitantly with rifampin or isoniazid; interacts with cyclosporine and methylprednisolone; coadministration with miconazole (another imidazole) may potentiate hypoglycemia episodes; antacids, anticholinergics, and H$_2$ blockers reduce the dissolution and absorption of ketoconazole

RESPONSE RATES

Difficult to assess the tumor response rate; most study series included pain relief as response

NURSING INTERVENTIONS

Closely monitor the signs and symptoms and determine the potential interaction with other medications; for overdose, use gastric lavage with sodium bicarbonate

PATIENT INFORMATION

Take the medication with a meal and avoid alcohol consumption

AVAILABILITY

Supplied as Nizoral by Janssen Pharmaceutica, Titusville, NJ; 200-mg tablets. Requires acidity for dissolution; store at room temperature

LETROZOLE

EFFICACY AND USAGE

Letrozole is a selective and potent aromatase inhibitor. The circulating estrogens decrease by more than 95% within 2 wk of daily doses of letrozole, with no change in aldosterone or clinically significant changes in cortisol levels.

DOSAGE AND ADMINISTRATION

2.5 mg daily orally

SPECIAL PRECAUTIONS

Should not be used in pregnant woman

TOXICITIES

Letrozole is well tolerated; **Hematologic:** transient thrombocytopenia; **GI:** nausea, vomiting; **CNS:** headache, depression; **Cardiovascular:** hypertension, dyspnea; **Other:** elevation of liver transaminases, musculoskeletal pain, fatigue, hot flashes

INDICATIONS

For adjuvant therapy in postmenopausal women with hormone receptor–positive breast cancer; extended adjuvant therapy of breast cancer in postmenopausal women, following 5 years of tamoxifen therapy; first- or second-line therapy in advanced breast cancer in postmenopausal patients with hormone receptor–positive or –unknown tumors

CONTRAINDICATIONS

Known hypersensitivity to this drug

PHARMACOKINETICS

Letrozole is rapidly and completely absorbed through the oral route and reaches a steady-state blood level by 2–6 wk; it is metabolized through the glucuronidation pathway and excreted (90%) in urine, with a elimination half-life of 2 d

DRUG INTERACTIONS

None recorded

RESPONSE RATES

Objective response to letrozole as a second- and third-line hormonal therapy in patients with advanced breast cancer are ~ 24% and ~ 22%, respectively

NURSING INTERVENTIONS

Monitor the liver function tests in patients with impaired liver function. Bone density should be monitored

PATIENT INFORMATION

Be aware of symptoms that may be derived from estrogen depletion or potential side effects

AVAILABILITY

Supplied as Femara by Novartis Pharmaceuticals, East Hanover, NJ; 2.5-mg tablets stored at room temperature

LEUPROLIDE

EFFICACY AND USAGE

Leuprolide acetate is a synthetic nonapeptide analogue of natural LH-RH. It desensitizes the LH-RH receptor and reduces the production of gonadotropic hormones. It acts as medical castration in reducing testosterone in males and estrogens in females. It has been used for the treatment of advanced prostate cancer and breast cancer.

DOSAGE AND ADMINISTRATION

7.5-mg depot administered intramuscularly every month or 22.5-mg depot every 3 mo. The optimal dosing and timing in women with breast cancer is not yet defined

SPECIAL PRECAUTIONS

Hypersensitivity to the agent and tumor flare may occur owing to an initial surge of blood testosterone or estrogen levels in the beginning of therapy

TOXICITIES

Endocrine: sexual dysfunction, gynecomastia, hot flashes, loss of libido; **Respiratory:** bronchitis; **Cardiovascular:** hot flushes, arrhythmias, hypertension; **CNS:** depression, anxiety, headache; **GI:** constipation, diarrhea, dyspepsia

INDICATIONS

Palliative treatment of advanced prostate cancer and of premenopausal advanced breast cancer

CONTRAINDICATIONS

History of hypersensitivity to the drug; pregnant nursing patients

PHARMACOKINETICS

Bioavailability is 90%; metabolism, distribution, and excretion have not been fully determined

DRUG INTERACTIONS

None reported

RESPONSE RATES

40%–45% response rates have been observed in premenopausal patients with estrogen receptor–positive advanced breast cancer. The response rates of prostate cancer to leuprolide versus leuprolide/flutamide are not significantly different; however, the median survival is in favor of the combination (36 vs 28 mo)

NURSING INTERVENTIONS

Monitor signs and symptoms

PATIENT INFORMATION

Hypersensitivity and sexual dysfunction may occur

AVAILABILITY

Supplied as Lupron Depot by TAP Pharmaceuticals, Lake Forest, IL; 3.75-mg, 7.5-mg, and 22.5-mg depot formulations for intramuscular injection. Store at room temperature and protect from freezing. Long-acting implantable forms (Viadur, Alza Pharmaceuticals, Mountain View, CA) are also approved

The information here is provided as guidance only. Prescribers should always consult the manufacturer's current prescribing information.

MEGESTROL ACETATE

EFFICACY AND USAGE

Megestrol acetate is a synthetic progestational drug used in the treatment of advanced breast cancer and endometrial cancer. It is also used to improve anorexia and cachexia in cancer and AIDS patients. Progestins have significant antiestrogenic effects through either the conversion of estradiol to a less active estrone or downregulation of estrogen receptors.

DOSAGE AND ADMINISTRATION

Breast and endometrial cancer: 40-mg tablet four times daily orally
Cachexia/anorexia: 400–800 mg orally daily

SPECIAL PRECAUTIONS

Weight gain in obese patients; patients with history of thromboembolic episodes

TOXICITIES

In general, the drug is well tolerated; **Endocrine:** breakthrough bleeding, change in menstrual flow; **Metabolic:** weight gain, hypercalcemia; **Cardiovascular:** edema; thromboembolic episodes, hypertension, dyspnea; **GI:** nausea, vomiting

INDICATIONS

Advanced breast cancer, endometrial cancer, and cancer-related cachexia

CONTRAINDICATIONS

Early stage of pregnancy

PHARMACOKINETICS

Oral bioavailability is 97%; peak plasma levels are reached in 2–3 h; half-life is biphasic, with a terminal half-life of 15–20 h; metabolized in liver; majority excreted in urine

DRUG INTERACTIONS

Decreases the clearance of warfarin

RESPONSE RATES

Approximately 60% of steroid receptor–positive breast cancers respond to megestrol; response rate is higher in tumors with positive progesterone receptors; the response rate in endometrial cancer is ~ 30%

NURSING INTERVENTIONS

Monitor signs and symptoms

PATIENT INFORMATION

Patient should be aware of the effects of weight gain and thromboembolic episodes and the need to avoid pregnancy. May cause photosensitivity

AVAILABILITY

Supplied as Megace from Bristol-Myers Squibb Co., Princeton, NJ; 20- and 40-mg tablets to be stored at room temperature. Also available in micronized megestrol acetate 40-mg/mL oral suspension with alcohol 0.06% to be stored below 25°C

MIFEPRISTONE

EFFICACY AND USAGE

Mifepristone is a synthetic derivative of progesterone. It acts as an antiprogestin and antiglucocorticoid. It has an antitumor effect on rat mammary tumors and human breast cancer and meningioma cell lines. Clinical trials in Europe have shown tumor regression from mifepristone in human breast cancers and unresectable meningioma. It should be noted that about 72% of meningiomas are progesterone receptor positive.

DOSAGE AND ADMINISTRATION

100–200 mg twice daily

SPECIAL PRECAUTIONS

Pregnant patients

TOXICITIES

In general, it is well tolerated; **Most common:** nausea, anorexia, hot flashes, dizziness, lethargy, gynecomastia in male patients

INDICATIONS

Medical termination of pregnancy through 49 days. Not FDA-approved for treatment of cancer or meningioma; however, clinical studies show modest activity in palliative treatment for advanced breast cancer and unresectable meningioma

CONTRAINDICATIONS

Pregnant patients

PHARMACOKINETICS

Half-life is 20 h

DRUG INTERACTIONS

None reported

RESPONSE RATES

Mifepristone showed minimal activity against breast cancer in two small European trials; preliminary results from a recent Canadian phase 2 study also showed a modest antitumor activity; partial responses observed in only 2 of 22 patients [11]; the response rate for meningioma was reported to be ~ 30%–40%

NURSING INTERVENTIONS

Monitor and document signs and symptoms

PATIENT INFORMATION

Should not be used in patients who are pregnant or planning for conception

AVAILABILITY

Supplied as Mifeprex by Danco Laboratories, New York, NY; 200-mg tablets

---

The information here is provided as guidance only. Prescribers should always consult the manufacturer's current prescribing information.

NILUTAMIDE

EFFICACY AND USAGE

Nilutamide is a nonsteroidal antiandrogen used in conjunction with surgical castration or an LH-RH analogue for advanced prostate cancer.

DOSAGE AND ADMINISTRATION

300 mg daily orally for the first month, then 150 mg daily orally

SPECIAL PRECAUTIONS

Be aware of the untoward side effects mentioned in the Toxicities section

TOXICITIES

GI: diarrhea; **Ophthalmologic:** visual disturbance (dark adaptation); **Respiratory:** interstitial pneumonitis (2% up to 17% in a small study); **Hepatic:** hepatitis (1%) with liver function abnormalities; **Other:** hot flashes; the inhibition of the mitochondrial respiratory chain and adenosine triphosphate formation by nilutamide may contribute to the aforementioned untoward, sometimes serious, toxicities

INDICATIONS

In combination with castration for metastatic prostate cancer; it should be started simultaneously with castration

CONTRAINDICATIONS

Severe impairment of liver function and respiratory insufficiency or history of hypersensitivity to this drug

PHARMACOKINETICS

Rapidly and completely absorbed through the oral route; ~ 84% of the drug is bound to plasma proteins; the steady-state plasma concentration is reached within 2–4 wk; the drug is extensively metabolized and mainly excreted through the kidneys; the plasma elimination half-life is ~ 50–60 h

DRUG INTERACTIONS

Intolerance to ethanol consumption (hot flashes, malaise, and hypotension); interaction with drugs (noticeably, vitamin K antagonists, phenytoin, theophylline, and others) that are metabolized via the CYP-450 system

RESPONSE RATES

Comparing nilutamide/orchiectomy combination therapy with orchiectomy alone, the response rates were 40%–50% versus 24%–33%; progression-free survival was 21 versus 15 mo, and overall survival was 37 versus 30 mo. The improvement of bone pain and prostate-specific antigen is also in favor of the combination; however, no data are currently available to compare nilutamide with other newer antiandrogens (*eg*, bicalutamide) in a combination modality with orchiectomy or with LH-RH analogues.

NURSING INTERVENTIONS

Patient should have a chest radiograph taken before initiation of nilutamide and have liver functions closely monitored; be aware of those drugs that may interact with nilutamide, and monitor the drug level closely

PATIENT INFORMATION

Patients should be aware of possible visual disturbance (delayed adaptation to dark) and should be cautious about driving at night; patients should also be informed about the symptoms of interstitial pneumonitis and potential deterioration of liver functions

AVAILABILITY

Supplied as Nilandron by Sanofi-Aventis, Bridgewater, NJ; 150-mg tablets stored at room temperature and protected from light

TAMOXIFEN

EFFICACY AND USAGE

Tamoxifen is a nonsteroidal antiestrogen that exerts its effect on breast cancer by competitively inhibiting the binding of estrogen to estrogen receptors. Tamoxifen has been used in combination with chemotherapeutic agents for cancers other than breast in origin.

DOSAGE AND ADMINISTRATION

20–40 mg daily orally

SPECIAL PRECAUTIONS

Barrier forms of contraception should be considered in premenopausal patients because tamoxifen may initially induce ovulation; close monitoring of endometrium is required in prolonged use of tamoxifen for early detection of endometrial cancer

TOXICITIES

Vascular: light-headedness, thromboembolism; **Gynecologic:** vaginal bleeding, altered menses, ovarian cyst, increased incidence of endometrial cancer; **GI:** nausea, vomiting, anorexia; **Metabolic:** hypercalcemia; **CNS:** hot flashes, emotional instability, depression; **Ophthalmologic:** at prolonged high dosage, visual disturbance (macular retinopathy and corneal opacity), cataracts

INDICATIONS

Hormone receptor–positive female and male advanced breast cancer; adjuvant therapy after surgical removal of primary breast cancer or intraductal carcinoma lesion for 5 years; breast cancer prevention; in combination with chemotherapy, tamoxifen has been used for other cancer, such as melanoma

CONTRAINDICATIONS

Known hypersensitivity to tamoxifen; pregnant patients

PHARMACOKINETICS

Well absorbed; plasma peak level is reached within 4–7 h; hydroxylation or N-oxidation to active metabolites; the half-life is biphasic, initially 9–12 h, then later 7 d; mainly excreted in the feces

DRUG INTERACTIONS

Tamoxifen is a cytostatic drug that blocks the cell cycle at the late G1 phase; therefore, it may attenuate cytotoxicity of many chemotherapeutic agents such as 5-fluorouracil and doxorubicin. Use of strong CYP-450 2D6 inhibitors such as paroxetine, fluoxetine, and bupropion should be avoided

RESPONSE RATES

When tamoxifen is used as first-line hormonal therapy in advanced breast cancer, ~ 60% of steroid receptor–positive female and male breast cancers respond

NURSING INTERVENTIONS

Monitor and document signs and symptoms

PATIENT INFORMATION

Barrier form of contraception in premenopausal patients, and frequent gynecologic examination for early detection of endometrial cancer

AVAILABILITY

Supplied as Nolvadex by AstraZeneca Pharmaceuticals, Wilmington, DE; 10 or 20 mg tablets; several generics are also available

TOREMIFENE

EFFICACY AND USAGE

Toremifene is a nonsteroidal antiestrogen used for the treatment of advanced breast cancer in patients with steroid receptor–positive tumors. It appears to be nearly identical to tamoxifen in action and side effects. However, it has fewer tumorigenic effects in a rodent hepatic model, although this may not be clinically relevant.

DOSAGE AND ADMINISTRATION

60 mg daily orally

SPECIAL PRECAUTIONS

Should be cautious in patients with severe renal and hepatic insufficiency; drug-related hypercalcemia may occur

TOXICITIES

Most common: hot flashes, nausea, vaginal discharge or bleeding, and dizziness. **Other (minor):** anorexia, headache, diarrhea, vaginitis, rash, pruritus, depression, and insomnia. Thromboembolic events (3%), elevated liver function tests (19%), and hypercalcemia (3%) have also been observed

INDICATIONS

Advanced breast cancer in postmenopausal patients with hormone receptor–positive tumors

CONTRAINDICATIONS

Pregnant patients

PHARMACOKINETICS

Toremifene is well absorbed after oral administration; the steady-state blood level could be reached in 4–6 wk; the drug is mainly metabolized through the CYP-450 system in liver and is excreted in feces; the elimination half-life is ~ 5 d

DRUG INTERACTIONS

May interact with warfarin and CYP-450 inducers (phenobarbital, phenytoin) or inhibitors (ketoconazole)

RESPONSE RATES

As first-line hormonal therapy for estrogen receptor–positive or unknown advanced breast cancer, the response rates (21%–31%) in various randomized trials are comparable with those of tamoxifen (19%–37%); the time to progression and overall survival are also comparable

NURSING INTERVENTIONS

Monitor prothrombin time and adjust warfarin dosage

PATIENT INFORMATION

Should not be used in pregnant woman

AVAILABILITY

Supplied as Fareston by GTx Inc., Memphis, TN; 60-mg tablets stored at room temperature and protected from heat and light

REFERENCES

1. Baxter JD, Funder JW: Hormone receptors. *N Engl J Med* 1979, 301:1149–1161.

2. Lippman ME, Dickson RB, Bates S, *et al.*: Autocrine and paracrine growth regulation of human breast cancer. *Breast Cancer Res Treat* 1986, 7:59–71.

3. Buttyan R: Genetic response of prostate cells to androgen deprivation: insights into the cellular mechanism of apoptosis. In *Apoptosis: The Molecular Basis of Death.* Edited by Tomei LD, Cope FO. Plainview, NY: Cold Spring Harbor Laboratory Press; 1991:157–173.

4. Bardon S, Vignon F, Montcourrier PH: Steroid receptor-mediated cytotoxicity of an antiestrogen and an antiprogestin in breast cancer cells. *Cancer Res* 1987, 47:1441–1448.

5. Osborne CK, Zhao H, Fuqua SA: Selective estrogen receptor modulators: structure, function, and clinical use. *J Clin Oncol* 2000, 18:3172–3186.

6. Thomas T, Trend B, Butterfield JR, *et al.*: Regulation of ornithine decarboxylase gene expression in MCF-7 breast cancer cells by antiestrogens. *Cancer Res* 1989, 49:5852–5857.

7. Winston R, Kao PC, Kiang DT: Regulation of insulin-like growth factors by antiestrogen. *Breast Cancer Res Treat* 1994, 31:107–115.

8. Gagliardi A, Collins DC: Inhibition of angiogenesis by antiestrogens. *Cancer Res* 1993, 53:533–535.

9. McClay EF, McClay ME: Tamoxifen: is it useful in the treatment of patients with metastatic melanoma? *J Clin Oncol* 1994, 12:617–626.

10. Creagan ET, Suman VJ, Dalton RJ, *et al.*: Phase III clinical trial of the combination of cisplatin, dacarbazine, and carmustine with or without tamoxifen in patients with advanced malignant melanoma. *J Clin Oncol* 1999, 17:1884–1890.

11. Crawford ED, Eisenberger MA, McLeod DG, *et al.*: A controlled trial of leuprolide with and without flutamide in prostatic carcinoma. *N Engl J Med* 1989, 321:419–424.

12. Klijn JG, Beex LV, Mauriac L, *et al.*: Combined treatment with buserelin and tamoxifen in premenopausal metastatic breast cancer: a randomized study. *J Natl Cancer Inst* 2000, 92:903–911.

13. Davidson NE: Combined endocrine therapy for breast cancer: new life for an old idea? *J Natl Cancer Inst* 2000, 92:859–860.

14. Rausch DJ, Kiang DT: Interaction between endocrine and cytotoxic therapy. In *Endocrine Therapy in Cancer.* Edited by Stoll BA. Basel, Switzerland: Karger; 1988:102–118.

15. Gibson LJ, Dawson CL, Lawrence DJ, Bliss JM: Aromatase inhibitors for treatment of advanced breast cancer in postmenopausal women. *Cochrane Database Syst Rev* 2007, 3:CD003370.

16. Winer EP, Hudis C, Burstein HJ, *et al.*: American Society of Clinical Oncology technology assessment on the use of aromatase inhibitors as adjuvant therapy for postmenopausal women with hormone receptor-positive breast cancer: status report 2004. *J Clin Oncol* 2005, 23:619–629.

17. Osborne CK, Coronado-Heinsohn EB, Hilsenbeck SG, *et al.*: Comparison of the effects of a pure steroidal antiestrogen with those of tamoxifen in a model of human breast cancer. *J Natl Cancer Inst* 1995, 87:746–750.

18. Robertson JF: Fulvestrant (Faslodex): how to make a good drug better. *Oncologist* 2007, 12:774–784.

Targeted Therapies
Ignacio Garrido-Laguna, Antonio Jimeno

3

TARGETED AGENTS

HER-DIRECTED THERAPIES

The ErbB receptor family is abnormally activated in many epithelial tumors. Members of this family are HER1/EGFR, HER2/ErbB2, HER3/ErbB3, and HER4/ErbB4. These receptors, with the exception of HER3, share the same molecular structure, with an extracellular, cysteine-rich ligand-binding domain, a single α-helix transmembrane domain, and an intracellular domain with tyrosine kinase activity in the carboxy-terminal tail.

Ligand binding induces epidermal growth factor receptor (EGFR) homodimerization, as well as heterodimerization with other types of HER proteins. HER2 does not bind to any known ligand, but it is the preferred heterodimerization partner for EGFR after ligand-induced activation [1].

EGFR dimerization induces tyrosine kinase catalytic activity, which leads to the autophosphorylation of the tyrosine residues in the carboxy-terminal tail, activating a downstream pathway that is ultimately involved in cell proliferation, transformation, decreased apoptosis, and metastasis development. Several mechanisms may lead to aberrant receptor activation, including receptor overexpression, gene amplification, activating mutations, overexpression of receptor ligands, and loss of negative regulatory mechanisms.

Two strategies have been more extensively explored in clinical trials targeting EGFR: 1) The use of monoclonal antibodies directed against the external domain of the receptor, and 2) the use of small molecules that compete with adenosine triphosphate (ATP) for binding to the receptor's kinase pocket, thus blocking receptor activation; these are also known as tyrosine kinase inhibitors (TKIs).

MONOCLONAL ANTIBODIES

TRASTUZUMAB

Trastuzumab (Herceptin, Genentech, San Francisco, CA), is a recombinant DNA-derived humanized monoclonal antibody that selectively binds with high affinity to the extracellular domain of the human EGFR-2 protein, HER2 [2]. The antibody is an IgG_1 κ that contains human framework regions with the complementarity-determining regions of a murine antibody (4D5) that binds to HER2 [3]. HER2 protein overexpression is observed in 25% to 30% of primary breast cancers. Patients whose tumors have overexpression of this receptor or amplification of its gene have decreased overall survival. HER2 status can be assessed by measuring the number of HER2 gene copies (using fluorescence in situ hybridization [FISH]), or by a complementary method in which the number of HER2 cell surface receptors is evaluated (immunohistochemistry [IHC]) [4].

Trastuzumab consists of two antigen-specific sites that bind to the extracellular domain of the HER2 receptor, thereby preventing the activation of its intracellular tyrosine kinase. Trastuzumab decreases signaling by prevention of HER2-receptor dimerization, increased endocytotic destruction of the receptor, inhibition of shedding of the extracellular domain, and immune activation [5]. Trastuzumab is a mediator of antibody-dependent cellular cytotoxicity in cells overexpressing HER2 [6].

As a single agent, trastuzumab is indicated for the treatment of patients with metastatic breast cancer whose tumors overexpress the HER2 protein and who have received one or more chemotherapy regimens for their metastatic disease. Trastuzumab in combination with paclitaxel is indicated for the treatment of patients with metastatic breast cancer whose tumors overexpress HER2 and who have not received chemotherapy for their metastatic disease. The pivotal randomized clinical trial that showed the activity of trastuzumab in combination with chemotherapy enrolled 469 patients with previously untreated HER2-positive metastatic breast cancer. Chemotherapy was administered either alone or in combination with trastuzumab. Trastuzumab treatment increased both progression-free survival (PFS; 7.4 vs 4.6 months) and overall survival (25 vs 20 months) [7]. Trastuzumab as part of a treatment regimen containing doxorubicin, cyclophosphamide, and paclitaxel is indicated for the adjuvant treatment of patients with HER2-overexpress-

ing node-positive breast cancer. Four large, multicenter randomized trials reported a significant benefit from the addition of trastuzumab in the adjuvant and neoadjuvant setting. Two North American studies with similar design, the North Central Cancer Treatment Group (NCCTG) N-9831 trial and the National Surgical Adjuvant Breast and Bowel Project (NSABP) B31, randomized 3752 patients with early-stage, HER2-positive breast cancer to adjuvant chemotherapy administered concurrent with trastuzumab or chemotherapy alone [8]. Data were pooled for efficacy analyses. The hazard ratio (HR) for disease-free survival was 0.48 ($P < 0.0001$), meaning that the rate of progression in patients not receiving trastuzumab nearly doubled that of trastuzumab-treated patients. In Europe, HERA (Herceptin Adjuvant Trial) included more than 5000 women with HER2-positive breast cancer who on completion of adjuvant chemotherapy were randomized to observation or 1 to 2 years of trastuzumab every third week. One year of trastuzumab treatment after adjuvant chemotherapy led to a 36% reduction in the risk of recurrence [9]. Although the optimal duration of adjuvant trastuzumab therapy is not known [10], the guidelines of the National Comprehensive Cancer Network suggest that trastuzumab treatment should consist of 1 year of trastuzumab therapy beginning after completion of adjuvant anthracycline therapy and administered either concurrently with a taxane or as a single agent [11].

Seventy to eighty percent of patients with HER2-overexpressing breast cancer will not respond to trastuzumab therapy given as single agent, due to either primary or acquired resistance. Potential explanations for this resistance are inactivation of PTEN [12] activation of other tyrosine kinase receptors (insulin-like growth factor receptor 1 [IGFR-1]) [13] and accumulation of truncated forms of the HER2 receptor (p95Her2) [14].

Trastuzumab may be administered on a weekly basis (4 mg/kg loading dose then 2 mg/kg weekly) or every 3 weeks (8 mg/kg loading dose followed by 6 mg/kg every 21 days). Half-life is approximately 21 days [15].

The most important secondary event was cardiac dysfunction, which is influenced by the extent of prior therapy with anthracyclines and preexisting cardiac dysfunction. Left ventricular function should be evaluated in all patients prior to and during treatment with trastuzumab. Trastuzumab dosing should be withheld in case of a greater than 16% absolute decrease in left ventricular ejection fraction (LVEF) from pretreatment values or LVEF below institutional limits of normal and greater than 10% absolute decrease in LVEF from pretreatment values. As opposed to anthracycline cardiac toxicity, patients will usually respond to treatment with angiotensin-converting enzyme (ACE) inhibitors. Trastuzumab may be resumed if, within 4 to 8 weeks, the LVEF returns to normal limits and the absolute decrease from baseline is less than 15%. Permanently discontinue trastuzumab for a persistent (> 8 weeks) LVEF decline or if trastuzumab dosing is suspended on more than three occasions for cardiomyopathy. An acute hypersensitivity-like reaction is seen in less than 10% of patients and is preventable when antihistamines, anti-inflammatory drugs, and corticosteroids are used.

CETUXIMAB

Cetuximab (Erbitux, ImClone Systems, New York, NY) is a chimeric mouse-human monoclonal antibody. It binds the EGFR in its extracellular domain, and blocks EGF-induced autophosphorylation of the EGFR cell lines in vitro [16], induces dimerization and downregulation of the EGFR [17], perturbs cell cycle progression by inducing a G1 arrest through an increase in the protein levels of the p27kip1 inhibitor of cyclin-dependent kinases [18], and inhibits tumor-induced angiogenesis [19]. Cetuximab has shown preclinical activity in vitro and in vivo, as a single agent and in combination with cytotoxic agents and radiotherapy in a wide range of human cancer cell lines, including colorectal, pancreatic, prostate, breast, head and neck, glioma, and ovarian cancer.

Cetuximab is indicated in locally or regionally advanced squamous cell carcinoma of the head and neck (SCCHN) in combination with radiation therapy. In a randomized phase 3 trial, patients with locoregionally advanced head and neck cancer were randomly assigned to treatment with high-dose radiotherapy alone (213 patients) or high-dose radiotherapy plus weekly cetuximab (211 patients) at an initial dose of 400 mg/m^2 of body surface area (BSA), followed by 250 mg/m^2 weekly for the duration of radiotherapy. The primary end point was duration of control of locoregional disease; a secondary end point was overall survival. The median duration of locoregional control was 24.4 months in the combined arm and 15 months in the radiotherapy alone arm (HR 0.68; $P = 0.005$). With a median follow-up of 54 months, overall survival in the combined arm was 49 months versus 29.3 in the radiotherapy-alone arm (HR for death 0.74; $P = 0.03$) [20].

Cetuximab is indicated as a single agent for the treatment of patients with recurrent or metastatic SCCHN progressing after platinum-based therapy. A phase 2 study included 103 patients with recurrent or metastatic SCCHN who had progressed within 30 days after two to six cycles of a platinum-based chemotherapy. Patients received a 20-mg test dose of cetuximab on day 1, followed by a 400 mg/m^2 initial dose and 250 mg/m^2 weekly until disease progression or unacceptable toxicity. Upon progression, patients were given the option of receiving cetuximab plus the platinum regimen that they failed prior to enrollment. The objective response rate on the monotherapy phase was 13% (95% CI, 7%–21%). Median time to progression was 70 days [21].

Cetuximab is indicated as a single agent in EGFR-expressing metastatic colorectal cancer after failure of both irinotecan- and oxaliplatin-based regimens or in patients who are intolerant to irinotecan-based regimens. These indications are based on the results of a phase 3 trial that randomized 572 patients with EGFR-expressing, previously treated, recurrent metastatic colorectal cancer who were randomized (1:1) to receive cetuximab plus best supportive care (BSC) or BSC alone. Cross-over was not permitted. The primary end point was overall survival. Median overall survival in the cetuximab group was 6.14 months (95% CI, 5.36–6.70) with an HR for survival of 0.77 (95% CI, 0.64–0.92), whereas in the BSC group median survival was 4.57 months (95% CI, 4.21–4.86) [22].

Cetuximab is indicated in combination with irinotecan in EGFR-expressing metastatic colorectal carcinoma in patients who are refractory to irinotecan-based chemotherapy. Approval was based on objective response rate; no data are available demonstrating an improvement in survival. Three hundred twenty nine patients whose disease had progressed during or within 3 months after treatment with an irinotecan-based regimen were randomly assigned to receive either cetuximab and irinotecan or cetuximab monotherapy. The primary end point was response rate. In case of disease progression, the addition of irinotecan to cetuximab monotherapy was permitted. The rate of response rate in the combination therapy group was doubled (22.9 vs 10.8; 95% CI, 5.7%–18.1%; $P = 0.007$). The median time to progression was greater in the combination arm (4.1 vs 1.5 months; $P < 0.001$). Median survival time was 8.6 months in the combination therapy group and 7 months in the monotherapy group; it did not reach statistical significance ($P = 0.48$) [23].

Recent evidence has shown that patients harboring a *KRAS* mutation (about 35%–40% of all metastatic cases) do not accrue benefit from the administration of cetuximab in the first-line [24,25] or second-line [26] settings. Therefore, it is expected that the indication will soon be modified to exclude those patients from treatment with cetuximab and only treat those with an intact *KRAS* gene.

Recent evidence has shown that patients harboring a KRAS mutation (about 35%–40%) of all metastatic cases) do not accrue benefit from the administration of cetuximab in the first-line [24,25] or second-line [26] settings. Therefore, it is expected that the indication will soon be modified to exclude those patients from treatment with cetuximab and only treat those with an intact KRAS gene.

Cetuximab should be premedicated with an H$_1$ antagonist. Administer 400 mg/m^2 initial dose as 120-minute intravenous (IV) infusion followed by 250 mg/m^2 weekly infused over 60 minutes. Initiate cetuximab 1 week prior to initiation of radiation therapy.

In phase 1 studies, doses ranking from 5 to 400 mg/m^2 were explored without reaching a maximum tolerated dose. Pharmacokinetics analyses showed a nonlinear behavior, with saturation of drug clearance at doses over 200 mg/m^2, and therefore the dose regimen selected for phase 2/3 trials was a loading dose of 400 mg/m^2 followed by a weekly maintenance

dose of 250 mg/m^2. Phase 1 trials revealed a favorable tolerability, with the most significant toxicity reported being an acneiform rash and folliculitis involving the face and upper chest, which occurs in 80% of patients [27–29] (for specific data about skin toxicity management, see Management of Toxicity section below). Hypersensitivity reactions have been reported (some of them occurring within minutes of the first infusion) but are uncommon and rarely life-threatening. Other adverse effects include asthenia, fever, and alteration in liver function tests.

PANITUMUMAB

Panitumumab (Vectibix, Amgen, Inc., Thousand Oaks, CA) is a recombinant, human IgG$_2$ κ monoclonal antibody that binds specifically to the human EGFR. It is produced in genetically engineered mammalian cells. Panitumumab binds specifically to EGFR on both normal and tumor cells and competitively inhibits the binding of ligands for EGFR. Nonclinical studies show that binding of panitumumab to the EGFR prevents ligand-induced receptor autophosphorylation and activation of receptor-associated kinases, resulting in inhibition of cell growth, induction of apoptosis, and internalization of the EGFR [30].

Panitumumab is indicated for the treatment of EGFR-expressing metastatic colorectal carcinoma with disease progression on or following fluoropyrimidine-, oxaliplatin-, and irinotecan-containing chemotherapy regimens. Currently, no data are available that demonstrate an improvement in disease-related symptoms or increased survival. Approval was based on PFS benefit shown during an open-label phase 3 trial that randomized 463 patients with 1% or more EGFR tumor cell membrane staining to panitumumab 6 mg/kg every 2 weeks plus BSC ($n = 231$) or BSC alone ($n = 232$) [31]. The primary end point was PFS. Panitumumab significantly prolonged PFS (HR 0.54; 95% CI, 0.44–0.66; $P < 0.0001$). Median PFS was 8 weeks for panitumumab versus 7.3 weeks for BSC. The overall response rate in the panitumumab arm was 8% (95% CI, 5%–12.6%). No patient in the control arm had an objective response. No difference was observed in overall survival between the study arms, but 76% of the patients in the BSC arm entered the cross-over study.

Evidence from mature clinical studies suggests that—as with cetuximab—panitumumab is only active in patients with an intact *KRAS* gene, and this drug has been formally approved in the European Union only for these patients [32].

Evidence from mature clinical studies suggests that—as with cetuximab—panitumumab is only active in patients with an intact *KRAS* gene, and this drug has been formally approved in the European Union only for these patients [32].

The recommended dose of panitumumab is 6 mg/kg administered over 60 minutes as an IV infusion every 14 days. Doses higher than 1000 mg should be administered over 90 minutes.

Ninety percent of patients displayed dermatologic toxicity, which was severe in 16%. Clinical manifestations included but were not limited to, dermatitis acneiform, pruritus, erythema, rash, skin exfoliation, paronychia, dry skin, and skin fissures (for specific data about skin toxicity management, see Management of Toxicity section below). Toxicity involving gastrointestinal mucosa, the eye, and nail was also reported. Four percent of patients experienced infusion reactions, and in 1% reactions were graded as severe (National Cancer Institute Common Toxicity Criteria [NCI-CTC] grade 3–4). Pulmonary fibrosis occurred in less than 1% of patients. Electrolyte depletion hypomagnesemia occurred in 2% of the patients. Patient electrolytes should be periodically monitored during and for 8 weeks after completion of treatment.

TYROSINE KINASE INHIBITORS

TKIs compete with ATP for binding to the receptor's kinase pocket, thus blocking receptor activation. A large number of TKIs are currently being evaluated. They can be classified according to their selectivity (specific agents with HER1-selective activity, as opposed to nonspecific agents that target several members of the HER family or other receptors) or according to the reversibility of their interaction with their target (reversible or irreversible inhibitors). Two TKIs have received regulatory approval for use in non–small cell lung cancer (NSCLC) patients, gefitinib and erlotinib. One has been approved for advanced metastatic breast cancer.

Gefitinib

Gefitinib (Iressa, ZD1839, AstraZeneca, Wilmington, DE) is an orally active, low molecular weight, synthetic quinazoline [33]. Gefitinib reversibly and selectively targets the EGFR and blocks signal transduction processes implicated in the proliferation and survival of cancer cells with minimal activity against other tyrosine kinases and serine/threonine kinases. Gefitinib prevents autophosphorylation of EGFR, resulting in the inhibition of downstream signaling pathways [34–36].

Gefitinib is indicated as monotherapy for the continued treatment of patients with locally advanced or metastatic NSCLC after failure of both platinum-based and docetaxel-based chemotherapies who are benefiting or have benefited from gefitinib. It was approved by the US Food and Drug Administration (FDA) based on the results of IDEAL-1 and -2 (Iressa Dose Evaluation in Advanced Lung Cancer), two phase 2 studies that evaluated the clinical activity of gefitinib at two dose levels (250 and 500 mg) in patients with NSCLC who had failed at least one previous chemotherapy regimen. Patient selection was not based on EGFR expression. Both studies found similar response rates for each dose level (18% vs 19% and 12% vs 9%) leading to approval of gefitinib 250 mg/d as the standard dose [37,38]. A phase 3 study (ISEL [Iressa Survival Evaluation in Lung Cancer]) in 1692 patients compared gefitinib with BSC. The primary end point was survival in the overall population and in those with adenocarcinomas. No differences were found. Preplanned subgroup analysis found statistically significant increased survival in two subgroups of gefitinib-treated patients: never-smokers (HR 0.67; 95% CI, 0.49–0.91; median survival 8.6 vs 5.1 months) and patients of Oriental origin (HR 0.66; 95% CI, 0.48–0.91; median survival 9.5 vs 5.5 months) [39]. Posterior biomarker analysis from ISEL showed that a high EGFR gene copy number was a predictive biomarker for a gefitinib effect versus placebo on overall survival [40]. Different groups have reported longer median time to progression and overall survival in patients with EGFR amplification [41], but whether amplified wild-type EGFR contributes to lung cancer oncogenesis and susceptibility to gefitinib remains to be established. Increased response rates based on the presence of EGFR mutations have been reported [42,43]. The addition of gefitinib to standard chemotherapy has failed to induce an improvement in response or survival in chemotherapy-naive NSCLC patients. Two placebo-controlled, double-blinded, phase 3 randomized trials evaluating chemotherapy (either gemcitabine plus cisplatin or paclitaxel plus cisplatin) plus either gefitinib (250–500 mg) or placebo have rendered negative results [44,45]. On the basis of these results, gefitinib was subsequently not granted full approval, but allowed to remain on the market for those patients who were still deriving benefit.

The recommended daily dose of gefitinib is one 250 mg tablet with or without food. For management of skin toxicity and diarrhea, read the specific section (Management of Toxicity) below.

Erlotinib

Erlotinib (Tarceva, OSI-774, OSI Pharmaceuticals, Melville, NY) is a quinazoline derivative. Erlotinib inhibits the kinase activity of EGFR. It has shown in vitro and in vivo activity in preclinical trials in multiple human cancer cell lines, including ovarian, head and neck, and NSCLC [46,47]. Erlotinib has been evaluated in several phase 1 studies using different doses and schedules, including weekly administration for 3 weeks every 4 weeks, and a continuous daily dosing [48,49]. The schedule that was ultimately chosen for further evaluation consists of the daily administration of 150 mg orally; higher doses have resulted in dose-limiting diarrhea and cutaneous acneiform rash [48].

Erlotinib monotherapy is indicated for the treatment of patients with locally advanced or metastatic NSCLC after failure of at least one prior chemotherapy regimen. The indication is based on the results of a trial that randomized pretreated NSCLC patients 2:1 to erlotinib:placebo. In this study, subjects receiving the study drug survived 6.7 months compared with 4.7 months in those taking placebo (*P* < 0.001). Erlotinib has been the first EGFR-targeted therapy to receive regulatory approval on the basis of prolongation of survival [50]. Data from two phase 3 clinical trials in patients with NSCLC comparing standard chemotherapy regimens (cisplatin plus gemcitabine [51], and carboplatin plus paclitaxel [52]) with or without erlotinib showed that this approach failed to demonstrate a response or survival advantage; thus erlotinib is not indicated in combination with che-

motherapy in this setting. In initial small clinical trials, erlotinib has shown significant antitumor activity in the first-line treatment of advanced NSCLC [53]. The discovery of activating mutations in the EGFR has prompted novel patient selection strategies. Preliminary results from a clinical trial that sequenced the EGFR gene in chemotherapy-naive patients with NSCLC and treated those who were positive with erlotinib showed that 37 of 297 subjects were found to harbor a mutation, and 19 of 21 treated patients presented a response to therapy [54].

Erlotinib in combination with gemcitabine is indicated for the first-line treatment of patients with locally advanced, unresectable or metastatic pancreatic cancer based on the results of a phase 3 trial that randomized 569 patients with advanced pancreatic cancer to standard gemcitabine plus placebo versus gemcitabine plus erlotinib. The primary end point was overall survival and the combined arm showed a modest increase in survival (6.24 vs 5.91 months; *P* = 0.038). One-year survival rate was also greater in the combined arm (23 vs 17%; *P* = 0.023) [55].

The recommended daily dose of erlotinib is 150 mg for NSCLC and 100 mg for pancreatic cancer, taken at least 1 hour before or 2 hours after the ingestion of food. Treatment should continue until disease progression or unacceptable toxicity occurs. There is no evidence that treatment beyond progression is beneficial. The most common adverse reactions in patients receiving single-agent erlotinib were rash and diarrhea. Grade 3 to 4 rash and diarrhea occurred in 9% and 6%, respectively. The cutaneous toxicity was dose dependent, affected the face and upper trunk areas, appeared at the end of the first week of dosing, and progressively recovered even in patients who continued taking the same dose of erlotinib (for specific data about skin toxicity management, see Management of Toxicity section below). When dose reduction is necessary, the erlotinib dose should be reduced in 50-mg decrements. Exceptionally, serious interstitial lung disease has been reported in less than 1% of patients, with symptoms starting as soon as 5 days after treatment initiation. In the event of acute-onset, new unexplained pulmonary symptoms such as dyspnea, cough, and fever, erlotinib should be interrupted pending diagnostic evaluation.

Lapatinib

Lapatinib (GW572016; GlaxoSmithKline, Research Triangle Park, NC) is an oral dual kinase inhibitor targeting both the HER1 and HER2 receptors. Increased expression and activation of HER1 and HER2 in breast cancer are associated with a high risk for recurrence after primary treatment and consequently a poor clinical outcome. HER1 or HER2 overexpression is seen respectively in 30% and 20% to 25% of breast cancers. Lapatinib inhibits HER-driven tumor growth in vitro and in various animal models [56].

Lapatinib is indicated in patients with HER2-overexpressing (IHC 3+ or IHC 2+ confirmed by FISH), locally advanced or metastatic breast cancer, progressing after prior treatment with anthracyclines, taxanes, and trastuzumab [57]. A phase 3 trial randomized 324 women to receive either combination therapy (lapatinib at a dose of 1250 mg/d continuously plus capecitabine at a dose of 2000 mg/m^2 of BSA on days 1–14 of a 21-day cycle) or monotherapy (capecitabine alone at a dose of 2500 mg/m^2 on days 1–14 of a 21-day cycle). The primary end point was time to progression. The median time to progression was 8.4 months in the combination therapy group as compared with 4.4 months in the monotherapy group. The HR for the independently assessed time to progression was 0.49 (95% CI, 0.34–0.71; *P* < 0.001). There was no increase in serious toxic effects or symptomatic cardiac events.

The recommended dose of lapatinib is 1250 mg (five tablets) given orally once daily on days 1 through 21 continuously in combination with capecitabine 2000 mg/m^2/d (administered orally in two doses ~ 12 hours apart) on days 1 through 14 in a repeating 21-day cycle. Lapatinib should be taken at least 1 hour before or 1 hour after a meal.

In the phase 3 trial, the most common adverse effects were diarrhea, hand-foot syndrome, nausea, vomiting, fatigue, and rash that was distinct from the hand-foot syndrome. Most adverse events were grade 1, 2, or 3. Grade 4 diarrhea occurred in two women in the combination therapy group (1%). Diarrhea, dyspepsia, and rash occurred more often in the group of women who received combination therapy (for specific data about skin toxicity management, see Management of Toxicity section below). There were no withdrawals from treatment due to declines in LVEF, no cases of congestive heart failure, and no decreases in the mean LVEF values in the group receiving lapatinib.

MANAGEMENT OF TOXICITY

RASH

Skin toxicities are uncommon with traditional cancer therapies; therefore, grading and categorization of these cutaneous toxicities have been fairly inconsistent. Rash is a common adverse effect of HER1/EGFR-targeted agents and it might be of great clinical value. Current data indicate that onset and intensity of rash is related to drug exposure, although rash etiology remains unclear. Rash does not affect all patients and there is a high level of interpatient variability. It is possible that some patients are genetically predisposed to developing rash and these same genetic features may modulate response to HER1/EGFR-targeted agents. Histologic data from skin biopsy specimens indicate that the rash is similar with erlotinib, cetuximab, and gefitinib, suggesting this is a class effect of HER1/EGFR-targeted agents. There are no controlled data to show that any topical applications are useful for managing rash; moreover rash often improves spontaneously, thus there are no evidence-based guidelines for managing rash [58]. Nonetheless, general measures frequently accepted include maximal hydration of the skin and use of bath oil instead of shower gel. Xerosis may be prevented with an emollient cream. Sun exposure should be avoided. For grade 1 acneiform eruptions, no treatment or treatment with topical antiacne or antirosacea agents with anti-inflammatory properties can be started (metronidazole gel or cream, clindamycin gel or lotion). When acneiform eruption is fading or becoming scaly, one should switch topical treatment to cream bases [59]. In cases in which rash becomes infected, short courses of oral tetracyclines, amoxicillin/clavulanic acid, or cephalosporins may be useful.

DIARRHEA

Diarrhea is a common untoward event of EGFR inhibition. The median time to onset of diarrhea was 12 days for erlotinib. Patients with severe diarrhea who are unresponsive to loperamide or who become dehydrated may require dose reduction or temporary interruption of therapy. Diarrhea can usually be managed with loperamide; patients may start taking two 2-mg loperamide tablets immediately, followed by one 2-mg tablet after every loose bowel movement, up to a maximum daily dose of 10 tablets (20 mg). If the diarrhea does not resolve with this regimen, the patient should stop treatment with EGFR inhibitors and contact a physician promptly [60].

MULTI-TYROSINE KINASE INHIBITORS

SUNITINIB

Sunitinib (Sutent, SU11248, Pfizer, Inc., New York, NY) is an oral multikinase inhibitor. Sunitinib is a small molecule that binds to the ATP-binding pocket of multiple receptor tyrosine kinases, some of which are implicated in tumor growth, pathologic angiogenesis, and metastatic progression of cancer. Sunitinib inhibited the phosphorylation of multiple receptor tyrosine kinases (platelet-derived growth factor receptor [PDGFR]-β, vascular endothelial growth factor receptor [VEGFR]-2, KIT) in tumor xenografts expressing receptor tyrosine kinase targets in vivo and demonstrated inhibition of tumor growth or tumor regression. Sunitinib inhibited PDGFR-β and VEGFR-2–dependent tumor angiogenesis in vivo [61,62].

Sunitinib is indicated for the treatment of gastrointestinal stromal tumors (GIST) after disease progression or intolerance to imatinib mesylate. The study that led to sunitinib approval in this setting was a two-arm, international, randomized, double-blind, placebo-controlled trial of sunitinib in patients with GIST who had disease progression during prior imatinib treatment or who were intolerant to imatinib. The main end point was time to tumor progression. Three hundred twelve patients were randomized (2:1) to receive either 50 mg of sunitinib or placebo once daily, 4 weeks on followed by 2 weeks off. A planned interim analysis showed a benefit in the sunitinib arm over placebo, with a 67% reduction in the risk of progression. The time to tumor progression increased from 6.4 weeks in the placebo arm to 27.3 weeks in the sunitinib arm ($P < 0.0001$) [63].

Sunitinib is also indicated for the treatment of advanced renal cell carcinoma (RCC) based on the results of a phase 3 trial that enrolled 750 patients with previously untreated metastatic RCC. Patients were randomized to receive either 6-week cycles of sunitinib, 50 mg given orally daily for 4 weeks followed by 2 weeks rest, or interferon-α, 9 MU subcutaneously three times weekly. The primary end point was PFS. PFS was significantly longer in the sunitinib group, 11 versus 5 months, with a HR of 0.42 (95% CI, 0.32–0.54). Response rates were also higher in the sunitinib arm (31% vs 6%; $P < 0.001$) [64].

The recommended dose of sunitinib for GIST and RCC is one 50-mg oral dose taken once daily, on a schedule of 4 weeks on treatment followed by 2 weeks off. It may be taken with or without food. A dose reduction for sunitinib to a minimum of 37.5 mg daily should be considered if it must be coadministered with a strong CYP3A4 inhibitor. A dose increase to a maximum of 87.5 mg daily should be considered if sunitinib must be administered with a CYP3A4 inducer.

In the phase 3 trial, the proportion of grade 3 or 4 adverse events with sunitinib ranged from 1% to 13% for all categories. Most were ameliorated by interruption or modification of the dose; a total of 38% of patients in the sunitinib arm had a dose interruption because of adverse events and 32% had a dose reduction, and less than 10% of patients needed treatment discontinuation because of adverse events. The incidence of grade 3 to 4 fatigue was 12%, diarrhea grade 3 was present in 5% and was managed in a similar way to another TKI (see Erlotinib section). Hypertension grade 4 developed in 8% of patients, thus patients should be monitored for hypertension and treated with standard antihypertensive therapies. In the GIST study, 11% of the patients had treatment-emergent LVEF below the normal limits, 50% of them recovered without intervention, 25% recovered after dose reduction or initiation of standard antihypertensive therapy, and 25% went off study without documented recovery. Hand-foot syndrome grade 3 to 4 developed in 5% of the patients. Thyroid function should be monitored and standard substitutive treatment should be started in case hypothyroidism develops. Thirty percent of the patients had bleeding events, most of which were grade 1 to 2, with epistaxis being the most common.

SORAFENIB

Sorafenib (Nexavar, BAY43-9006, Bayer Pharmaceuticals Corp., West Haven, CT and Onyx Pharmaceuticals Corp., Emeryville, CA) is a multikinase inhibitor. Sorafenib was shown to interact with multiple intracellular (*CRAF*, *BRAF*, and mutant *BRAF*) and cell surface kinases (KIT, FLT-3, VEGFR-2, VEGFR-3, and PDGFR-β). Several of these kinases are thought to be involved in angiogenesis. Sorafenib inhibits tumor growth of the murine RCC line, RENCA, and several other human tumor xenografts in athymic mice. A reduction in tumor angiogenesis was seen in some tumor xenograft models.

Sorafenib is indicated in the treatment of advanced RCC. A randomized, placebo-controlled, phase 3 trial called TARGET (Treatment Approaches in Renal Cancer Global Evaluation Trial) confirmed the efficacy of sorafenib in cytokine-refractory RCC. Nine hundred three patients with RCC were randomized to sorafenib versus placebo. Patients were required to have confirmed metastatic clear cell RCC that had progressed after one systemic treatment within the previous 8 months. The primary end point was overall survival. The first interim analysis of overall survival showed a reduction in the risk of death of 38% in the sorafenib arm (95% CI, 0.54–0.94; $P = 0.02$). The PFS analysis included 769 patients stratified by Memorial Sloan-Kettering Cancer Center prognostic risk category (low or intermediate) and country. The median PFS for patients randomized to sorafenib was 5.5 months compared with 2.8 months in the placebo arm. The HR was 0.44 (95% CI, 0.35–0.55). Tumor response was determined according to RECIST Response Evaluation Criteria in Solid Tumors). Overall, of the 672 patients who were evaluable for response, seven (2%) in the sorafenib arm had a confirmed partial response. Thus the gain in PFS in the sorafenib arm primarily reflects the stable disease population [65].

The recommended daily dose of sorafenib is 400 mg (two tablets of 200 mg) taken twice daily, without food (at least 1 hour before or 2 hours after eating). When dose reduction is necessary, sorafenib may be reduced to 400 mg once daily. If additional dose reduction is required, sorafenib may be reduced to a single 400 mg dose every other day.

In the TARGET study, the proportion of patients who discontinued the study drug due to adverse events was similar in both arms (10% in the sorafenib and 8% in the placebo group), discontinuation was mostly due to constitutional, gastrointestinal, dermatologic, or pulmonary upper respiratory tract symptoms. Dose interruptions were mostly due to dermatologic events (hand-foot skin reactions or rash) and gastrointestinal events. The most common events were diarrhea (43%), rash (40%), fatigue (37%), hand-foot skin reactions (30%), alopecia (27%), and nausea. Most adverse events occurring during treatment were grade 1 or 2. The most frequent drug-related serious adverse event was hypertension (1%); it usually occurred during the first treatment cycle and was managed with standard antihypertension drugs.

Dasatinib

Dasatinib (Sprycel, Bristol-Myers Squibb, Princeton, NJ) is an inhibitor of multiple tyrosine kinases. Dasatinib inhibits several critical oncogenic proteins, including BCR-ABL, SRC family (SRC, LCK, YES, FYN), c-KIT, PDGFR-α, and PDGFR-β. Dasatinib blocks G1/S transition and inhibits cell growth in normal and neoplastic cells [66]. Based on modeling studies, dasatinib is predicted to bind to multiple conformations of the ABL kinase. Dasatinib inhibited the growth of chronic myeloid leukemia (CML) and acute lymphoblastic leukemia (ALL) cell lines overexpressing BCR-ABL [67]. Under the conditions of the assays, dasatinib was able to overcome imatinib resistance resulting from BCR-ABL kinase domain mutations, activation of alternate signaling pathways involving the SRC family kinases (LYN, HCK), and multidrug resistance gene overexpression.

Dasatinib is indicated for the treatment of adults with chronic-, accelerated-, or myeloid or lymphoid blast-phase CML with resistance or intolerance to prior therapy including imatinib. The effectiveness of dasatinib is based on hematology and cytogenetic response rates. There are no controlled trials demonstrating a clinical benefit, such as improvement in disease-related symptoms or increased survival. It is also indicated for the treatment of adults with Philadelphia-positive acute lymphoblastic leukemia (Ph+ ALL) with resistance or intolerance to prior therapy. Four single-arm, multicenter studies were conducted to determine efficacy and safety of dasatinib in patients with CML or Ph+ ALL resistant to or intolerant of treatment with imatinib. The chronic-phase CML study enrolled 186 patients [68], the accelerated-phase CML study enrolled 107 patients [69], the myeloid blast-phase study enrolled 74 patients, and the lymphoid blast-phase CML/Ph+ ALL study enrolled 78 patients [70]. The studies are ongoing and the results are based on a minimum of 6 months' follow-up. The primary end point in chronic-phase CML was major cytogenetic response defined as elimination or substantial diminution (at least 65%) of Ph+ hematopoietic cells. The primary end point in the rest of phases was major hematologic response. Dasatinib treatment resulted in cytogenetic and hematologic response in patient with all phases of CML and with Ph+ ALL. In chronic-phase CML patients, the major cytogenetic response rate was 45%, with a complete response rate (0% Ph+ cells) of 33%. The major hematologic response rate was 59% in accelerated-phase patients, 32% in myeloid phase patients, 31% in lymphoid blast-phase patients, and 42% in Ph+ ALL patients. Most cytogenetic responses occurred after 12 weeks of treatment. Hematologic and cytogenetic responses were stable during the 6-month follow-up of patients with chronic-phase, accelerated-phase, and myeloid blast-phase CML. The median durations of major hematologic response were 3.7 months in lymphoid blast CML and 4.8 months in Ph+ ALL.

The recommended dose of dasatinib is 140 mg/d administered orally in two divided doses with or without meal. Tablets should not be crushed or cut and should be swallowed whole.

Anemia, thrombocytopenia, and neutropenia grade 3 to 4 developed in 50% to 80% of patients. Their occurrence is more frequent in patients with advanced CML or Ph+ ALL than in chronic-phase CML. Complete blood counts should be performed weekly for the first 2 months and then monthly. Myelosuppression was generally reversible and managed by withholding dasatinib temporarily or by dose reduction. Severe gastrointestinal hemorrhage occurred in 7% of patients and generally required treatment interruptions and transfusions. Other common adverse events were fluid retention, events such as pleural effusion, and gastrointestinal events (diarrhea, nausea, abdominal pain, and vomiting).

Imatinib

Imatinib mesylate (Gleevec, Novartis Pharmaceuticals, East Hanover, NJ) is an oral selective inhibitor of Abelson (c-ABL), PDGRFR-α and -β, and c-KIT tyrosine kinases. Imatinib inhibits the BCR-ABL tyrosine kinase, the constitutive abnormal tyrosine kinase created by the Philadelphia chromosome abnormality in CML. In vitro, imatinib inhibits proliferation and induces apoptosis in GIST cells, which express an activating c-kit mutation. In vivo, imatinib inhibits tumor growth of BCR-ABL–transfected murine myeloid cells as well as BCR-ABL–positive leukemia lines derived from CML patients in blast crisis. It is also an inhibitor of the receptor tyrosine kinases for PDGF, stem cell factor (SCF), and c-kit and inhibits PDGF- and SCF-mediated cellular events [71,72].

Imatinib is indicated in the treatment of newly diagnosed CML. An open-label, multicenter, international randomized phase 3 trial was conducted in patients recently diagnosed with Ph+ CML in chronic phase. One thousand one hundred six patients were randomized to either single-agent imatinib or a combination of interferon-α plus cytarabine (Ara-C). Cross-over was permitted if patients failed to reach a complete hematologic response at 6 months, a major cytogenetic response at 12 months, or if they lost a complete hematologic or major cytogenetic response. Patients in the imatinib arm were initially treated with 400 mg daily. Dose escalations were allowed up to 800 mg daily. In the interferon arm, patients received interferon 5 MIU/m² subcutaneously in combination with subcutaneous cytarabine 20 mg/m²/d for 10 days per month. Baseline characteristics were well balanced. The primary end point of the study was PFS, defined as any of the following events: progression to accelerated phase or blast crisis; death; loss of complete hematologic response or major cytogenetic response; or in patients not achieving a complete hematologic response, an increasing white blood cell count despite appropriate therapeutic management. The estimated rate of PFS at 60 months in the intent-to-treat population was 83% in the imatinib arm and 64% in the interferon arm (P < 0.0001, log-rank test). At 60 months, the estimated overall survival was 89.4% versus 85.6%, respectively [73].

Imatinib is also indicated in the treatment of late chronic-phase CML and advanced-stage CML. Three international, open-label, single-arm, phase 2 studies have shown that imatinib induces high response rates in patients with chronic-phase CML in whom previous interferon therapy has failed. In one of the studies, 532 patients with late chronic-phase CML in whom previous therapy with interferon had failed were treated with imatinib 400 mg daily. Imatinib induced major cytogenetic responses in 60% of the patients and complete hematologic response in 95% [74]. In the second study, which included 237 patients with Ph+ accelerated-phase CML who were treated with imatinib at two different doses (400 and 600 mg), rates of complete and partial responses were 80% and 10%. Responses rates were higher for the 600-mg group only in the univariate analysis (hematologic response 75% vs 64%; P < 0.01) [75]. The last trial included 260 patients with myeloid blast crisis. These patients had more than 30% blasts in peripheral blood or bone marrow and/or extramedullary involvement other than spleen or liver, and 37% of the patients had received prior chemotherapy for treatment of either accelerated phase or blast crisis. The primary end point was hematologic response. The hematologic response rate was 31% (25.2%–36.8%) [76].

Imatinib is indicated in patients with Kit-positive unresectable and/or metastatic malignant GIST. The effectiveness of imatinib in GIST is based on objective response rate. There are no controlled trials demonstrating a clinical benefit, such as improvement in disease-related symptoms or increased survival. An open-label, multicenter trial randomized 147 patients with unresectable or metastatic GIST to receive 400 or 600 mg of imatinib daily. The study was not powered to show a statistically significant difference in response rates between the two dose groups. The primary end point was response rate. Sixty-seven percent of the patients had a partial response; 28% had stable disease. No patient had a complete response to the treatment [77].

Other approved indications include pediatric patients with Ph+ CML in chronic phase who are newly diagnosed or whose disease has recurred after stem cell transplant or who are resistant to interferon therapy (there are no controlled trials in pediatric patients demonstrating a clinical benefit, such as improvement in disease-related symptoms or increased survival). Imatinib is also indicated in adult patients with myelodysplastic/myeloproliferative diseases associated with PDGFR gene rearrangements, and in adult patients with aggressive systemic mastocytosis without the D816V c-Kit mutation or with unknown c-Kit mutational status.

Doses of 400 or 600 mg should be administered once daily, whereas a dose of 800 mg should be administered as 400 mg twice a day. In children, imatinib can be given as a once-daily dose or alternatively the daily dose may be split into two—once in the morning and once in the evening. There is no experience with imatinib in children younger than 2 years of age.

Most adverse reactions were mild to moderate grade but the drug was discontinued for drug-related adverse reactions in 2.4% of newly diagnosed patients, 4% of patients in chronic phase after failure of interferon-α therapy, 4% in accelerated phase, and 5% in blast crisis. The most frequently reported drug-related adverse reactions were edema, nausea and vomiting, muscle cramps, musculoskeletal pain, diarrhea, and rash. A variety of adverse reactions represent local or general fluid retention including pleural effusion, ascites, pulmonary edema, and rapid weight gain with or without superficial edema. Edema was most frequently periorbital or in lower limbs and was managed with diuretics, other supportive measures, or by reducing the dose of imatinib.

MAMMALIAN TARGET OF RAPAMYCIN INHIBITORS

TEMSIROLIMUS

Temsirolimus (CCI-779) is an inhibitor of mammalian target of rapamycin (mTOR). Temsirolimus binds to an intracellular protein (FKBP-12), and the protein-drug complex inhibits the activity of mTOR that controls cell division [78]. Inhibition of mTOR activity results in a G1 growth arrest in treated tumor cells [79]. When mTOR is inhibited, its ability to phosphorylate p70S6k and S6 ribosomal protein, which are downstream of mTOR in the PI3 kinase/AKT pathway, is blocked. In vitro studies in RCC cell lines has shown that temsirolimus inhibits the activity of mTOR and results in reduced levels of the hypoxia-inducible factors HIF1 and HIF2-α as well as VEGF.

Temsirolimus is indicated for the treatment of advanced RCC based on the results of a phase 3, multicenter, three-arm, randomized, open-label study conducted in previously untreated patients with advanced RCC (clear cell and non–clear cell histologies) [80]. This study randomized 626 patients with previously untreated, poor-prognosis metastatic RCC to receive 25 mg of IV temsirolimus weekly, 3 MU of interferon-α subcutaneously three times weekly, or combination therapy with 15 mg of temsirolimus weekly plus 6 million U of interferon-α three times weekly. The primary end point was overall survival. Patients in the temsirolimus-alone arm had longer overall survival (HR for death, 0.73; 95% CI, 0.58–0.92; P = 0.008) and PFS (P < 0.001) than did patients who received interferon alone, while the addition of temsirolimus to interferon did not improve survival (P = 0.70). Patients in the temsirolimus group had a median overall survival benefit greater than 3 months as compared with interferon (10.9 vs 7.3 months).

The recommended dose of temsirolimus for advanced RCC is 25 mg infused over a 30- to 60-minute period once a week. As premedication, patients should receive prophylactic IV diphenhydramine, 25 to 50 mg, 30 minutes before the start of each dose of temsirolimus. Temsirolimus should be held for an absolute neutrophil count less than 1000/mm³, platelet count less than 75,000/mm³, or NCI-CTC adverse event grade 3 or greater adverse reactions. Once toxicities have resolved to grade 2 or less, temsirolimus may be restarted with the dose reduced by 5 mg/week to a dose no lower than 15 mg/week. If a patient develops a hypersensitivity reaction during temsirolimus infusion, stop the infusion and observe the patient for 30 to 60 minutes. Treatment may be resumed with the administration of an H₁ receptor antagonist (such as diphenhydramine), if not previously administered and/or an H₂ receptor antagonist (IV famotidine 20 mg or IV ranitidine 50 mg) approximately 30 minutes before restarting the temsirolimus infusion at a slower rate (up to 60 minutes). Hyperglycemia during temsirolimus treatment may result in the need for an increase in the dose of, or initiation of, insulin and/or oral hypoglycemic agent therapy.

The most common adverse effects related to temsirolimus (> 30%) are rash, asthenia, mucositis, nausea, and edema. The most common laboratory abnormalities are anemia, hyperglycemia, hyperlipemia, elevated serum creatinine, and leukopenia. The most common grade 3 to 4 adverse effect was anemia in 10% of patients. Five percent of patients had grade 3 to 4 hyperglycemia and 18 (9%) patients experienced hypersensitivity reactions. Eighty-nine percent of patients in the phase 3 trial had at least one elevated serum glucose while on treatment, and 26% of patients reported hyperglycemia as an adverse event. Interstitial lung disease occurred in five patients (2%) that required discontinuation of temsirolimus and treatment with corticosteroids and/or antibiotics. Twenty-seven percent of patients in the temsirolimus arm had at least one elevated serum triglyceride value. This may require initiation of, or increase in, the dose of lipid-lowering agents. One patient had fatal bowel perforation.

ANTI–VASCULAR ENDOTHELIAL GROWTH FACTOR

BEVACIZUMAB

Bevacizumab (Avastin, Genentech) is a recombinant humanized monoclonal IgG₁ antibody that binds VEGF. Bevacizumab prevents the interaction of VEGF to its receptors (Flt-1 and KDR) on the surface of endothelial cells. The interaction of VEGF with its receptors leads to endothelial cell proliferation and new blood vessel formation in in vitro models of angiogenesis.

Bevacizumab in combination with IV 5-fluorouracil–based chemotherapy is indicated for first- or second-line treatment of patients with metastatic carcinoma of the colon or rectum. Bevacizumab gained approval based on the results of an Eastern Cooperative Oncology Group (ECOG) open-label, multicenter, randomized, three-arm, active-controlled trial enrolling 829 adult patients. Patients had received a fluoropyrimidine and irinotecan-based regimen as initial therapy for metastatic disease, or they had received prior adjuvant irinotecan-based chemotherapy and had recurred within 6 months of completing therapy. Treatments included bevacizumab 10 mg/kg as a 90-minute IV infusion on day 1 every 2 weeks, either alone or in combination with FOLFOX4 (oxaliplatin, leucovorin, and 5-fluorouracil), or FOLFOX4 alone. The bevacizumab monotherapy arm was closed to accrual after an interim efficacy analysis showed shorter survival in that arm. The primary end point of the study was overall survival [81]. A survival benefit of nearly 5 months was observed in the bevacizumab arm (20.3 vs 15.6, corresponding to a HR for death of 0.66; P < 0.001).

Bevacizumab in combination with carboplatin and paclitaxel is indicated for first-line treatment of patients with unresectable, locally advanced, recurrent or metastatic nonsquamous NSCLC. The FDA granted approval for bevacizumab in this setting based on a significant improvement in overall survival. A randomized, open label, multicenter clinical trial, conducted by the ECOG, in chemotherapy-naive patients with stage IIIb/IV nonsquamous NSCLC, evaluated bevacizumab plus carboplatin and paclitaxel versus carboplatin and paclitaxel alone. Exclusion of patients with squamous or predominantly squamous histology was based on life-threatening or fatal hemoptysis occurring in 4 of 13 patients with squamous histology who received bevacizumab plus chemotherapy in a phase 2 trial. Eight hundred seventy eight patients were randomized; the median age was 63, 46% were female, 76% had stage IV disease, and 40% had an ECOG performance status score of 0. An overall survival benefit of 2 months was observed in the bevacizumab arm (12.3 vs 10.3; HR 0.80; P = 0.013) [82].

Bevacizumab should not be initiated until at least 28 days following major surgery. The surgical incision should be fully healed prior to initiation of bevacizumab. For colorectal cancer, the recommended dose of bevacizumab depends on the drugs used in the treatment combination. In combination with IV 5-fluorouracil–based chemotherapy, the recommended dose of bevacizumab is 5 or 10 mg/kg every 14 days. When combined with bolus IFL (irinotecan, 5-fluorouracil, leucovorin), the dose should be 5 mg/kg. The recommended dose of bevacizumab in combination with FOLFOX is 10 mg/kg. For lung cancer, the recommended dose of bevacizumab is 15 mg/kg as an IV infusion every 3 weeks. Bevacizumab should be permanently discontinued in patients who develop gastrointestinal perforation, fistula formation involving an internal organ, wound dehiscence requiring medical intervention, serious bleeding, hypertensive crisis, or nephrotic syndrome. Bevacizumab should be suspended at least several weeks prior to elective surgery.

The incidence of gastrointestinal perforation ranged from 0% to 3.7%. In patients with metastatic colorectal cancer, the incidence in the combined arm was 2.4% versus 0.3% in the chemotherapy-alone arm. The incidence of postoperative wound healing and/or bleeding complications occurred in 15% of patients receiving bolus IFL plus bevacizumab versus 4% of patients receiving bolus IFL alone. The incidence of severe of fatal hemorrhage, including hemoptysis, gastrointestinal bleeding, hematemesis, and central nervous system hemorrhage occurred up to five-fold more frequently in bevacizumab-treated patients compared with those treated with chemotherapy alone. These events were generally mild in severity (NCI-CTC grade 1) and resolved without medical intervention. The incidence of severe hypertension was increased in patients receiving bevacizumab. The incidence of NCI-CTC grade 3 or 4 hypertension ranged from 8% to 18%. Management of hypertension in this setting included ACE inhibitors, β-blockers, diuretics, and calcium channel blockers. Nephrotic syndrome occurred in 0.5% of patients receiving bevacizumab.

BIOLOGIC AGENTS

ALDESLEUKIN

Aldesleukin (rIL-2, Proleukin, Chiron Therapeutics, Everyville, CA) is nonglycosylated and is produced in *Escherichia coli*. This preparation differs from natural human interleukin (IL)-2 in that the N-terminal alanine is lacking and the cysteine residue at amino acid position 125 is replaced by serine. These alterations permit correct folding and maintain the biologic activity of this agent. An International Unit of rIL-2 is defined as the reciprocal of the dilution that produces 50% of the maximal proliferation of murine TH2 cells in a short-term tritiated thymidine incorporation assay.

IL-2 is indicated in the treatment of metastatic renal cell cancer. It produces responses in 20% of patients with a median duration of response of 54 months. The median survival of the 8% of patients who achieved a complete response has not been reached and 60% of these patients are alive at a median follow-up of more than 10 years. The treatment requires high dependency or intensive care support due to capillary leak syndrome.

The supraphysiologic doses of IL-2 that have been used for therapy are associated with myriad side effects, which are most likely mediated by other cytokines (tumor necrosis factor-α in particular). Hematologic toxicity, including anemia requiring transfusion and thrombocytopenia less than 20,000/mm^3, have been observed in 60% and about 15% of treatment courses, respectively. Effects on the kidney include oliguria and decreased fractional excretion of sodium associated with rising serum creatinine and blood urea nitrogen in most patients. These can be managed successfully in most patients with the IV administration of volume expanders and dopamine infusions (2–3 µg/kg/min). Renal toxicity resolves in nearly all instances within several days. Cardiovascular toxicity includes increased heart rate and myocardial depression manifested by decreased ejection fraction. Elevations of adrenocorticotropic hormone, endorphins, growth hormone, prolactin, and glucocorticoids have been observed in treated patients.

Some patients develop clinically overt hypothyroidism that requires long-term thyroid hormone replacement therapy. Nearly all patients develop a vascular leak syndrome that is associated with egress of intravascular fluid into the soft tissues, where it remains sequestered until therapy ends. This redistribution of fluid probably contributes to the hypotension observed in most treated patients and can be managed effectively with vigorous fluid resuscitation using volume as crystalloid [39]. The volume of administered fluid is limited in some patients by noncardiogenic pulmonary edema secondary to capillary leak. In these patients, phenylephrine can be used to support the blood pressure in lieu of volume expansion, often while the patient remains in a conventional ward.

INTERFERONS

The interferons are a family of naturally occurring small proteins and glycoproteins with molecular weights of approximately 15,000 to 27,600 daltons produced and secreted by cells in response to viral infections and to synthetic or biological inducers. Interferons exert their cellular activities by binding to specific membrane receptors on the cell surface, initiating a complex sequence of intracellular events, including induction of certain enzymes, suppression of cell proliferation, immunomodulating activities such as enhancement of phagocytic activity of macrophages, and augmentation of the specific cytotoxicity of lymphocytes for target cells.

Interferon alpha-2b is indicated as an adjuvant to surgical treatment in patients 18 years of age or older with malignant melanoma who are free of diseases but at high risk for systemic recurrence, within 56 days of surgery. In a randomized controlled trial, 280 patients with resected melanoma were randomized to adjuvant interferon alpha-2b at 20 million IU/m^2 IV five times per week for 4 weeks (induction phase) followed by 10 million IU/m^2 subcutaneously three times per week for 48 weeks (maintenance). There was a benefit in relapse-free and overall survival in the interferon arm (1.72 vs 0.98 years; $P < 0.01$). The estimated 5-year relapse-free survival rate was 37% for interferon versus 26% in the observation group [83]. Interferon alpha-2b is also indicated in the treatment of hairy cell leukemia and follicular lymphoma.

The recommended daily dose of interferon alpha-2b in induction is 20 million IU as an IV infusion over 20 minutes, 5 consecutive days per week for 4 weeks. The recommended dose of interferon alpha-2b for maintenance is 10 million IU/m^2 as a subcutaneous injection three times per week for 48 weeks.

In the previously mentioned study [83], interferon alpha-2b was modified because of adverse events in 65% of the patients. It was discontinued because of adverse events in 8% of the patients in the induction phase and 18% of the patients during maintenance. The most frequently reported adverse reaction was fatigue, which was observed in 96% of patients. Other adverse reactions recorded in more than 20% of interferon alpha-2b–treated patients included neutropenia (92%), fever (81%), and myalgia (75%). Severe adverse reactions recorded in more than 10% of interferon-treated patients included neutropenia/leukopenia (26%), fatigue (23%), and fever (18%).

REFERENCES

1. Arteaga CL: The epidermal growth factor receptor: from mutant oncogene in nonhuman cancers to therapeutic target in human neoplasia. *J Clin Oncol* 2001, 19:32S–40S.

2. Coussens L, Yang-Feng TL, Liao YC, *et al.*: Tyrosine kinase receptor with extensive homology to EGF receptor shares chromosomal location with neu oncogene. *Science* 1985, 230:1132–1139.

3. Slamon DJ, Godolphin W, Jones LA, *et al.*: Studies of the HER-2/neu proto-oncogene in human breast and ovarian cancer. *Science* 1989, 244:707–712.

4. Wang S, Saboorian MH, Frenkel E, *et al.*: Laboratory assessment of the status of Her-2/neu protein and oncogene in breast cancer specimens: comparison of immunohistochemistry assay with fluorescence in situ hybridisation assays. *J Clin Pathol* 2000, 53:374–381.

5. Valabrega G, Montemurro F, Aglietta M: Trastuzumab: mechanism of action, resistance and future perspectives in HER2-overexpressing breast cancer. *Ann Oncol* 2007, 18:977–984.

6. Barok M, Isola J, Palyi-Krekk Z, *et al.*: Trastuzumab causes antibody-dependent cellular cytotoxicity-mediated growth inhibition of submacroscopic JIMT-1 breast cancer xenografts despite intrinsic drug resistance. *Mol Cancer Ther* 2007, 6:2065–2072.

7. Slamon DJ, Leyland-Jones B, Shak S, *et al.*: Use of chemotherapy plus a monoclonal antibody against HER2 for metastatic breast cancer that overexpresses HER2. *N Engl J Med* 2001, 344:783-92.

8. Romond EH, Perez EA, Bryant J, *et al.*: Trastuzumab plus adjuvant chemotherapy for operable HER2-positive breast cancer. *N Engl J Med* 2005, 353:1673–1684.

9. Smith I, Procter M, Gelber RD, *et al.*: 2-year follow-up of trastuzumab after adjuvant chemotherapy in HER2-positive breast cancer: a randomised controlled trial. *Lancet* 2007, 369:29–36.

10. Joensuu H, Kellokumpu-Lehtinen PL, Bono P, *et al.*: Adjuvant docetaxel or vinorelbine with or without trastuzumab for breast cancer. *N Engl J Med* 2006, 354:809–820.

11. Carlson RW, Moench SJ, Hammond ME, *et al.*: HER2 testing in breast cancer: NCCN Task Force report and recommendations. *J Natl Compr Canc Netw* 2006, 4(Suppl 3):S1–S22; quiz S23–S24.

12. Nagata Y, Lan KH, Zhou X, *et al.*: PTEN activation contributes to tumor inhibition by trastuzumab, and loss of PTEN predicts trastuzumab resistance in patients. *Cancer Cell* 2004, 6:117–127.

13. Lu Y, Zi X, Zhao Y, *et al.*: Insulin-like growth factor-I receptor signaling and resistance to trastuzumab (Herceptin). *J Natl Cancer Inst* 2001, 93:1852–1857.

14. Scaltriti M, Rojo F, Ocana A, *et al.*: Expression of p95HER2, a truncated form of the HER2 receptor, and response to anti-HER2 therapies in breast cancer. *J Natl Cancer Inst* 2007, 99:628–638.

15. Lin A, Rugo HS: The role of trastuzumab in early stage breast cancer: current data and treatment recommendations. *Curr Treat Options Oncol* 2007, 8:47–60.

16. Goldstein NI, Prewett M, Zuklys K, *et al.*: Biological efficacy of a chimeric antibody to the epidermal growth factor receptor in a human tumor xenograft model. *Clin Cancer Res* 1995, 1:1311–1318.

17. Fan Z, Lu Y, Wu X, *et al.*: Antibody-induced epidermal growth factor receptor dimerization mediates inhibition of autocrine proliferation of A431 squamous carcinoma cells. *J Biol Chem* 1994, 269:27595–27602.

18. Wu X, Rubin M, Fan Z, *et al.*: Involvement of p27KIP1 in G1 arrest mediated by an anti-epidermal growth factor receptor monoclonal antibody. *Oncogene* 1996, 12:1397–1403.

19. Ciardiello F, Bianco R, Damiano V, *et al.*: Antiangiogenic and antitumor activity of anti-epidermal growth factor receptor C225 monoclonal antibody in combination with vascular endothelial growth factor antisense oligonucleotide in human GEO colon cancer cells. *Clin Cancer Res* 2000, 6:3739–3747.

20. Bonner JA, Harari PM, Giralt J, *et al.*: Radiotherapy plus cetuximab for squamous-cell carcinoma of the head and neck. *N Engl J Med* 2006, 354:567–578.

21. Vermorken JB, Trigo J, Hitt R, *et al.*: Open-label, uncontrolled, multicenter phase II study to evaluate the efficacy and toxicity of cetuximab as a single agent in patients with recurrent and/or metastatic squamous cell carcinoma of the head and neck who failed to respond to platinum-based therapy. *J Clin Oncol* 2007, 25:2171–2177.

22. Jonker DJ, O'Callaghan CJ, Karapetis CS, *et al.*: Cetuximab for the treatment of colorectal cancer. *N Engl J Med* 2007, 357:2040–2048.

23. Cunningham D, Humblet Y, Siena S, *et al.*: Cetuximab monotherapy and cetuximab plus irinotecan in irinotecan-refractory metastatic colorectal cancer. *N Engl J Med* 2004, 351:337–345.

24. Van Cutsem E, Lanf I, D'haens G, *et al.*: KRAS status and efficacy in the first-line treatment of patients with metastatic colorectal cancer (mCRC) treated with FOLFIRI with or without cetuximab: the CRYSTAL experience [abstract]. *J Clin Oncol* 2008, 26(Suppl): abstract 2.

25. Bokemeyer C, Bondarenko I, Hartmann JT, *et al.*: KRAS status and efficacy of first-line treatment of patients with metastatic colorectal cancer (mCRC) with FOLFOX with or without cetuximab: the OPUS experience [abstract]. *J Clin Oncol* 2008, 26(Suppl): abstract 4000.

26. Tejpar S, Peeters M, Humblet Y, *et al.*: Relationship of efficacy with KRAS status (wild type versus mutant) in patients with irinotecan-refractory metastatic colorectal cancer (mCRC) treated with irinotecan (q2W) and escalating doses of cetuximab (q1W): the EVEREST experience (preliminary data) [abstract]. *J Clin Oncol* 2008, 26(Suppl): abstract 4001.

27. Robert F, Ezekiel MP, Spencer SA, *et al.*: Phase I study of anti-epidermal growth factor receptor antibody cetuximab in combination with radiation therapy in patients with advanced head and neck cancer. *J Clin Oncol* 2001, 19:3234–3243.

28. Baselga J, Pfister D, Cooper MR, *et al.*: Phase I studies of anti-epidermal growth factor receptor chimeric antibody C225 alone and in combination with cisplatin. *J Clin Oncol* 2000, 18:904–914.

29. Shin DM, Donato NJ, Perez-Soler R, *et al.*: Epidermal growth factor receptor-targeted therapy with C225 and cisplatin in patients with head and neck cancer. *Clin Cancer Res* 2001, 7:1204–1213.

30. Yang XD, Jia XC, Corvalan JR, *et al.*: Development of ABX-EGF, a fully human anti-EGF receptor monoclonal antibody, for cancer therapy. *Crit Rev Oncol Hematol* 2001, 38:17–23.

31. Van Cutsem E, Peeters M, Siena S, *et al.*: Open-label phase III trial of panitumumab plus best supportive care compared with best supportive care alone in patients with chemotherapy-refractory metastatic colorectal cancer. *J Clin Oncol* 2007, 25:1658–1664.

32. Amado RG, Wolf M, Peeters M, *et al.*: Wild-type KRAS is required for panitumumab efficacy in patients with metastatic colorectal cancer. *J Clin Oncol* 2008, 26:1624–1634.

23. Wakeling AE, Guy SP, Woodburn JR, *et al.*: ZD1839 (Iressa): an orally active inhibitor of epidermal growth factor signaling with potential for cancer therapy. *Cancer Res* 2002, 62:5749–5754.

34. Barker AJ, Gibson KH, Grundy W, *et al.*: Studies leading to the identification of ZD1839 (IRESSA): an orally active, selective epidermal growth factor receptor tyrosine kinase inhibitor targeted to the treatment of cancer. *Bioorg Med Chem Lett* 2001, 11:1911–1914.

35. Anderson NG, Ahmad T, Chan K, *et al.*: ZD1839 (Iressa), a novel epidermal growth factor receptor (EGFR) tyrosine kinase inhibitor, potently inhibits the growth of EGFR-positive cancer cell lines with or without erbB2 overexpression. *Int J Cancer* 2001, 94:774–782.

36. Ciardiello F, Caputo R, Bianco R, *et al.*: Inhibition of growth factor production and angiogenesis in human cancer cells by ZD1839 (Iressa), a selective epidermal growth factor receptor tyrosine kinase inhibitor. *Clin Cancer Res* 2001, 7:1459–1465.

37. Fukuoka M, Yano S, Giaccone G, *et al.*: Multi-institutional randomized phase II trial of gefitinib for previously treated patients with advanced non-small-cell lung cancer. *J Clin Oncol* 2003, 21:2237–2246.

38. Kris MG, Natale RB, Herbst RS, *et al.*: Efficacy of gefitinib, an inhibitor of the epidermal growth factor receptor tyrosine kinase, in symptomatic patients with non-small cell lung cancer: a randomized trial. *JAMA* 2003, 290:2149–2158.

39. Thatcher N, Chang A, Parikh P, *et al.*: Gefitinib plus best supportive care in previously treated patients with refractory advanced non-small-cell lung cancer: results from a randomised, placebo-controlled, multicentre study (Iressa Survival Evaluation in Lung Cancer). *Lancet* 2005, 366:1527–1537.

40. Hirsch FR, Varella-Garcia M, Bunn PA Jr, *et al.*: Molecular predictors of outcome with gefitinib in a phase III placebo-controlled study in advanced non-small-cell lung cancer. *J Clin Oncol* 2006, 24:5034–5042.

41. Cappuzzo F, Hirsch FR, Rossi E, *et al.*: Epidermal growth factor receptor gene and protein and gefitinib sensitivity in non-small-cell lung cancer. *J Natl Cancer Inst* 2005, 97:643–655.

42. Lynch TJ, Bell DW, Sordella R, *et al.*: Activating mutations in the epidermal growth factor receptor underlying responsiveness of non-small-cell lung cancer to gefitinib. *N Engl J Med* 2004, 350:2129–2139.

43. Paez JG, Janne PA, Lee JC, *et al.*: EGFR mutations in lung cancer: correlation with clinical response to gefitinib therapy. *Science* 2004, 304:1497–1500.

44. Giaccone G, Herbst RS, Manegold C, *et al.*: Gefitinib in combination with gemcitabine and cisplatin in advanced non-small-cell lung cancer: a phase III trial—INTACT 1. *J Clin Oncol* 2004, 22:777–784.

45. Herbst RS, Giaccone G, Schiller JH, *et al.*: Gefitinib in combination with paclitaxel and carboplatin in advanced non-small-cell lung cancer: a phase III trial—INTACT 2. *J Clin Oncol* 2004, 22:785–794.

46. Pollack VA, Savage DM, Baker DA, *et al.*: Inhibition of epidermal growth factor receptor-associated tyrosine phosphorylation in human carcinomas with CP-358,774: dynamics of receptor inhibition in situ and antitumor effects in athymic mice. *J Pharmacol Exp Ther* 1999, 291:739–748.

47. Moyer JD, Barbacci EG, Iwata KK, *et al.*: Induction of apoptosis and cell cycle arrest by CP-358,774, an inhibitor of epidermal growth factor receptor tyrosine kinase. *Cancer Res* 1997, 57:4838–4848.

48. Hidalgo M, Siu LL, Nemunaitis J, *et al.*: Phase I and pharmacologic study of OSI-774, an epidermal growth factor receptor tyrosine kinase inhibitor, in patients with advanced solid malignancies. *J Clin Oncol* 2001, 19:3267–3279.

49. Karp D, Ferrante D, Tensfeldt TG, *et al.*: A phase I dose escalation study of epidermal growth factor receptor (EGFR) tyrosine kinase (TK) inhibitor CP-358,774 in patients (pts) with advanced solid tumors [abstract]. *Lung Cancer* 2000, 29:72.

50. Shepherd FA, Rodrigues Pereira J, Ciuleanu T, *et al.*: Erlotinib in previously treated non-small-cell lung cancer. *N Engl J Med* 2005, 353:123–132.

51. Gatzemeier U, Pluzanska A, Szczesna A, *et al.*: Results of a phase III trial of erlotinib (OSI-774) combined with cisplatin and gemcitabine (GC) chemotherapy in advanced non-small cell lung cancer (NSCLC) [abstract]. *J Clin Oncol* 2004, 22(14S):abstract 7010.

52. Herbst RS, Prager D, Hermann R, *et al.*: TRIBUTE: a phase III trial of erlotinib hydrochloride (OSI-774) combined with carboplatin and paclitaxel chemotherapy in advanced non-small-cell lung cancer. *J Clin Oncol* 2005, 23:5892–5899.

53. Giaccone G, Gallegos Ruiz M, Le Chevalier T, *et al.*: Erlotinib for frontline treatment of advanced non-small cell lung cancer: a phase II study. *Clin Cancer Res* 2006, 12:6049–6055.

54. Paz-Ares L, Sanchez J, García-Velasco A, *et al.*: A prospective phase II trial of erlotinib in advanced non-small cell lung cancer (NSCLC) patients (p) with mutations in the tyrosine kinase (TK) domain of the epidermal growth factor receptor (EGFR) [abstract]. *J Clin Oncol* 2006, 24(18S):abstract 7020.

55. Moore MJ, Goldstein D, Hamm J, *et al.*: Erlotinib plus gemcitabine compared with gemcitabine alone in patients with advanced pancreatic cancer: a phase III trial of the National Cancer Institute of Canada Clinical Trials Group. *J Clin Oncol* 2007, 25:1960–1966.

56. Rusnak DW, Lackey K, Affleck K, *et al.*: The effects of the novel, reversible epidermal growth factor receptor/ErbB-2 tyrosine kinase inhibitor, GW2016, on the growth of human normal and tumor-derived cell lines in vitro and in vivo. *Mol Cancer Ther* 2001, 1:85–94.

57. Geyer CE, Forster J, Lindquist D, *et al.*: Lapatinib plus capecitabine for HER2-positive advanced breast cancer. *N Engl J Med* 2006, 355:2733–2743.

58. Perez-Soler R, Saltz L: Cutaneous adverse effects with HER1/EGFR-targeted agents: is there a silver lining? *J Clin Oncol* 2005, 23:5235–5246.

59. Segaert S, Van Cutsem E: Clinical signs, pathophysiology and management of skin toxicity during therapy with epidermal growth factor receptor inhibitors. *Ann Oncol* 2005, 16:1425–1433.

60. Shah NT, Kris MG, Pao W, *et al.*: Practical management of patients with non-small-cell lung cancer treated with gefitinib. *J Clin Oncol* 2005, 23:165–174.

61. Wilhelm SM, Carter C, Tang L, *et al.*: BAY 43-9006 exhibits broad spectrum oral antitumor activity and targets the RAF/MEK/ERK pathway and receptor tyrosine kinases involved in tumor progression and angiogenesis. *Cancer Res* 2004, 64:7099–7109.

62. Wan PT, Garnett MJ, Roe SM, *et al.*: Mechanism of activation of the RAF-ERK signaling pathway by oncogenic mutations of B-RAF. *Cell* 2004, 116:855–867.

63. Demetri GD, van Oosterom AT, Garrett CR, *et al.*: Efficacy and safety of sunitinib in patients with advanced gastrointestinal stromal tumour after failure of imatinib: a randomised controlled trial. *Lancet* 2006, 368:1329–1338.

64. Motzer RJ, Hutson TE, Tomczak P, *et al.*: Sunitinib versus interferon alfa in metastatic renal-cell carcinoma. *N Engl J Med* 2007, 356:115–124.

65. Escudier B, Eisen T, Stadler WM, *et al.*: Sorafenib in advanced clear-cell renal-cell carcinoma. *N Engl J Med* 2007, 356:125–134.

66. Fabarius A, Giehl M, Frank O, *et al.*: Centrosome aberrations after nilotinib and imatinib treatment in vitro are associated with mitotic spindle defects and genetic instability. *Br J Haematol* 2007, 138:369–373.

67. Tokarski JS, Newitt JA, Chang CY, *et al.*: The structure of dasatinib (BMS-354825) bound to activated ABL kinase domain elucidates its inhibitory activity against imatinib-resistant ABL mutants. *Cancer Res* 2006, 66:5790–5797.

68. Hochhaus A, Kantarjian HM, Baccarani M, *et al.*: Dasatinib induces notable hematologic and cytogenetic responses in chronic-phase chronic myeloid leukemia after failure of imatinib therapy. *Blood* 2007, 109:2303–2309.

69. Guilhot F, Apperley J, Kim DW, *et al.*: Dasatinib induces significant hematologic and cytogenetic responses in patients with imatinib-resistant or -intolerant chronic myeloid leukemia in accelerated phase. *Blood* 2007, 109:4143–4150.

70. Cortes J, Rousselot P, Kim DW, *et al.*: Dasatinib induces complete hematologic and cytogenetic responses in patients with imatinib-resistant or -intolerant chronic myeloid leukemia in blast crisis. *Blood* 2007, 109:3207–3213.

71. Heinrich MC, Griffith DJ, Druker BJ, *et al.*: Inhibition of c-kit receptor tyrosine kinase activity by STI 571, a selective tyrosine kinase inhibitor. *Blood* 2000, 96:925–932.

72. Heinrich MC, Corless CL, Duensing A, *et al.*: PDGFRA activating mutations in gastrointestinal stromal tumors. *Science* 2003, 299:708–710.

73. O'Brien SG, Guilhot F, Larson RA, *et al.*: Imatinib compared with interferon and low-dose cytarabine for newly diagnosed chronic-phase chronic myeloid leukemia. *N Engl J Med* 2003, 348:994–1004.

74. Kantarjian H, Sawyers C, Hochhaus A, *et al.*: Hematologic and cytogenetic responses to imatinib mesylate in chronic myelogenous leukemia. *N Engl J Med* 2002, 346:645–652.

75. Kantarjian HM, O'Brien S, Cortes JE, *et al.*: Treatment of Philadelphia chromosome-positive, accelerated-phase chronic myelogenous leukemia with imatinib mesylate. *Clin Cancer Res* 2002, 8:2167–2176.

76. Sawyers CL, Hochhaus A, Feldman E, *et al.*: Imatinib induces hematologic and cytogenetic responses in patients with chronic myelogenous leukemia in myeloid blast crisis: results of a phase II study. *Blood* 2002, 99:3530–3539.

77. Demetri GD, von Mehren M, Blanke CD, *et al.*: Efficacy and safety of imatinib mesylate in advanced gastrointestinal stromal tumors. *N Engl J Med* 2002, 347:472–480.

78. Sabatini DM, Erdjument-Bromage H, Lui M, *et al.*: RAFT1: a mammalian protein that binds to FKBP12 in a rapamycin-dependent fashion and is homologous to yeast TORs. *Cell* 1994, 78:35–43.

79. Schmelzle T, Hall MN: TOR, a central controller of cell growth. *Cell* 2000, 103:253–262.

80. Hudes G, Carducci M, Tomczak P, *et al.*: Temsirolimus, interferon alfa, or both for advanced renal-cell carcinoma. *N Engl J Med* 2007, 356:2271–2281.

81. Hurwitz H, Fehrenbacher L, Novotny W, *et al.*: Bevacizumab plus irinotecan, fluorouracil, and leucovorin for metastatic colorectal cancer. *N Engl J Med* 2004, 350:2335–2342.

82. Sandler A, Gray R, Perry MC, *et al.*: Paclitaxel-carboplatin alone or with bevacizumab for non-small-cell lung cancer. *N Engl J Med* 2006, 355:2542–2550.

83. Kirkwood JM, Strawderman MH, Ernstoff MS, *et al.*: Interferon alfa-2b adjuvant therapy of high-risk resected cutaneous melanoma: the Eastern Cooperative Oncology Group Trial EST 1684. *J Clin Oncol* 1996, 14:7–17.

Cancer vaccines aim to target protein antigens that are differentially expressed by cancer cells relative to the normal cells from which they are derived. The adaptive immune system has an immense capacity to recognize an infinite number of antigens. Through its network of specialized antigen-presenting and effector cells, the immune system can become activated to recognize and lyse cancer cells while sparing normal tissue. Recent advances in understanding how to effectively activate an immune response against cancer-specific antigens has led to the approval of two vaccines for the prevention of virus-associated cancers. The administration of a hepatitis B vaccine has reduced the risk of hepatoma worldwide, and prophylaxis with the human papillomavirus (HPV) vaccine offers protection against the development of cervical cancer precursor lesions [1–3]. Such results would not have occurred without molecular technology advances during the past 10 years that have led to an exponential understanding of how the immune system is regulated in the setting of many diseases, including autoimmunity, infection, and cancer. Animal models and early-phase clinical trials have shown that combinations of agents that modulate these immune system regulatory signaling pathways as well as vaccines that efficiently activate multiple components of the immune system will be required to effectively treat and prevent cancer.

HISTORICAL PERSPECTIVE

Vaccines that target infectious agents are one of modern medicine's greatest contributions to preventing morbidity and mortality worldwide in the 20th century. Therefore, it is important to point out that the first vaccine, the smallpox vaccine, was introduced by Edward Jenner in the late 1700s [4]. It took another 150 years to implement this vaccine into general practice. In fact, many of the same controversies and challenges that surrounded this vaccine now exist for cancer vaccines. For example, public debate existed about whether the smallpox vaccine could really eradicate this deadly disease or was responsible for additional medical problems. Once the principles of how to safely and effectively produce this vaccine were perfected, however, smallpox became eradicated worldwide.

Similarly, cancer vaccines had their start about 100 years ago. In the late 1800s, Dr. William Coley noted that some patients developed tumor regressions after experiencing immune activation from a bacterial infection [5]. Over the next 50 years, a number of investigators attempted to treat cancers with a mixture of tumor lysates or whole tumor cells and bacterial extracts. These were crude attempts to activate a cancer-specific immune response at a time when the adaptive arms of the immune system were not yet identified. However, this observation was subsequently postulated to be the result of endotoxin-mediated production of cytokines such as tumor necrosis factor (TNF) and interleukin-12 (IL-12) [6]. In the 1960s, Thomas and Burnet introduced the concept of immune surveillance and proposed that the immune system had the ability to recognize tumor antigens, resulting in elimination of microscopic malignant cells [7,8].

B and T cells are the key effector cells mediating responses to infections and cancer, yet these cellular components of the immune response were not defined until the 1970s and 1980s. Furthermore, the integrated innate and adaptive immune system pathways were not well understood until the development of the newer genetic technologies in the 1990s. The past decade and a half of immunology research has led to an exponential understanding of how T cells are generated, matured, and activated (Fig. 4-1). It has also led to the understanding that the immune system has natural mechanisms or signaling pathways in place that provide a fine balance or checkpoints for regulating the vast number of potential responses to infection and cancer. These checkpoints must be considered when designing vaccines for cancer treatment as well as for cancer prevention (Fig. 4-2).

This chapter focuses primarily on the host immune system and tumor interactions as well as vaccine strategies aimed at activating endogenous T cells that are under the control of multiple mechanisms of host and tumor regulation.

MECHANISMS OF IMMUNE TOLERANCE

SYSTEMIC MECHANISMS

A cancer vaccine's ultimate goal is to train the immune system to recognize tumors as foreign, ultimately resulting in tumor cell death. The inherent difficulty in such an approach is that tumors emerge from normal host cell precursors. Precursor cells slowly acquire genetic mutations that promote survival and proliferation in such a manner that the antigens presented on their surfaces are perceived as self-antigens. The immune system has naturally evolved to integrate immune tolerance mechanisms to protect the host from autoimmunity, thus making the process of generating antitumor immunity complex. Tumors come to clinical attention after they have already escaped the process of immune surveillance or more likely, immune editing. This dynamic process shapes the T-cell repertoire available in the host so that the tumor is no longer recognized by these cells. Therefore, clinically apparent cancers have survived the pressures of immune selection, resulting in the establishment of nonimmunogenic tumors in the immune editing process [9].

Tolerance to self-antigens can occur by multiple mechanisms, including thymic deletion of autoreactive T cells, peripheral deletion, peripheral ignorance, immune modulation, and peripheral suppression by signals provided by T regulatory cells (T_{regs}) or other cellular signals. The premise of active immunotherapy is that tumor-specific T cells have not been deleted and, under the appropriate circumstances, can be recruited and activated. Evidence that tumor-specific T cells have not been deleted in tolerant conditions has been supported in preclinical and clinical systems. As an example, latent high-avidity tumor-specific T cells can be uncovered in a tolerant mouse model after administration of T_{reg} modifying doses of cyclophospha-

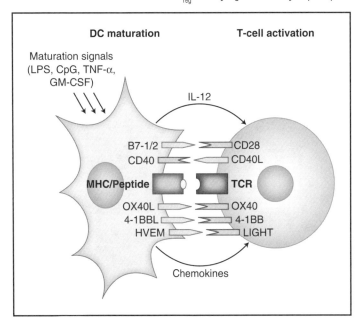

Figure 4-1. T-cell activation requires the proper signals from mature antigen-presenting cells. T cells recognize antigens in the context of major histocompatibility complex (MHC) molecules (signal 1) and receive costimulation via cell surface receptors such as CD28 (signal 2). Mature dendritic cells (DC) also secrete cytokines and express other stimulatory cell surface proteins. GM-CSF—granulocyte-macrophage colony-stimulating factor; IL—interleukin; LPS—lipopolysaccharide; TCR—T-cell receptor; TNF—tumor necrosis factor.

mide together with a vaccine targeting the same antigen [10]. Furthermore, human melanoma–specific tumor-infiltrating lymphocytes, activated by exposure to cytokines ex vivo, have been reinfused into patients, resulting in objective tumor regressions [11]. Effective vaccine strategies must not only recruit these endogenous T cells but also overcome the systemic and local barriers to their function.

Tumors and tumor-infiltrating immune cells can also secrete a variety of immune-suppressive cytokines that promote not only local tumor growth but generalized immune suppression. IL-6, IL-10, and transforming growth factor-β (TGF-β) are among the most commonly implicated cytokines [12–14]. In addition, T cells from patients with pancreatic and renal cell carcinomas and melanoma have been shown to have reduced expression of the T-cell receptor (TCR) zeta chain. This reduction in expression has been correlated with decreased T-cell activation and survival [15–17]. These findings further support the concept that cancer patients have specific immune regulatory defects that provide formidable barriers to effective immunization.

More recently, there has been increasing interest in the ability of $CD4^+CD25^+$ T_{regs} to suppress tumor-specific T cells. This suppression not only contributes to malignant pathogenesis but also inhibits vaccine-induced responses. The concept of suppressor T cells was introduced in the 1970s, but it was not until the 1990s that Sakaguchi *et al.* [18] identified thymically derived $CD4^+CD25^+$ T cells as important in the control of autoreactive T cells. Subsequently, FOXP3, a member of the forkhead/winged-helix family of transcriptional regulators, was found to be crucial in the development and function of T_{regs} [18–20]. An increase of T_{regs} has been demonstrated in the peripheral blood of cancer patients and in the tumor microenvironment of a number of cancers, including breast, ovarian, and pancreatic cancers [21–24]. More recent studies of tumor immune infiltrates have correlated an increased frequency of T_{regs} with poor prognosis [25,26]. Interestingly, there appears to be an increasing number of T_{regs} in precursor lesions, suggesting that these cells may need to be modulated prior to immunization even in the setting of primary prevention [27].

LOCAL MECHANISMS IN THE TUMOR

Researchers have identified a multitude of mechanisms employed by tumors to escape immune surveillance (Table 4-1). For T cells to recognize their targets, tumor antigens must be presented in the context of major histocompatibility complexes (MHC). Tumors have altered antigen presentation pathways to downregulate this prerequisite for recognition. Examples include the downregulation of genes involved in antigen presentation, including transporter associated with antigen presentation (TAP), subunits of the proteasome, and MHC class I molecules [28,29]. Additionally, during the evolution of a cancer, tumor antigens themselves may be lost [30]. T cells receive signals not only through their TCRs but through other surface receptors. Tumor manipulation of these signals can result in suppression of T-cell responses. For example, B7-H1 (PDL-1) is expressed on a variety of cancers. B7-H1 interacts with PD-1 on T cells, resulting in apoptosis of activated T cells. Adding to the complexity of tumor-induced immune regulation is the discovery that *STAT-3* is activated in many tumors. *STAT-3* not only induces antiapoptotic genes such as *CYCLIN D1* and *BCL-X$_L$* within the malignant cells but also promotes the release of factors such as vascular endothelial growth factor (VEGF) and IL-10, resulting in immune inhibitory effects. Moreover, tumor-secreted factors promote *STAT-3* activation in dendritic cells, natural killer cells, and neutrophils, leading to inhibition of their function [31–34].

Impaired function of infiltrating immune cells is not only mediated by immune-suppressive cytokines and tumor cell surface–associated molecules but a myriad of other secreted factors and suppressor populations that have been described and that contribute to the tolerant microenvironment. Tumor secretion of cyclooxygenase-2 has been postulated to inhibit dendritic cell function [35]. Furthermore, other suppressive cell types such as immature myeloid cells and myeloid suppressor cells generate reactive oxygen and nitrogen species that are inhibitory to T cells [36–40]. Additionally, indoleamine 2,3-dioxygenase (IDO)-producing plasmacytoid dendritic cells contribute to tolerance by several mechanisms. IDO initiates the degradation of tryptophan via the kynurenine pathway, which results in the depletion of tryptophan required by T cells to function. It also leads to the production of T-cell and natural killer cell–suppressive tryptophan metabolites [41,42]. Thus, it is becoming clear that an optimal vaccine approach would require multiple components, including a T-cell–activating vaccine and agents that modulate the mechanisms of T-cell inhibition.

SCIENTIFIC TOOLS FOR VACCINE DEVELOPMENT

At a minimum, three requirements must be met for the successful development of the most effective vaccine approaches. The first is the identification of antigens expressed by tumors that are the targets of immunized T cells. The second is the identification of methods to most efficiently deliver these antigens to the immune system for activation of T cells. The third requirement is the identification of the critical T-cell checkpoint targets and

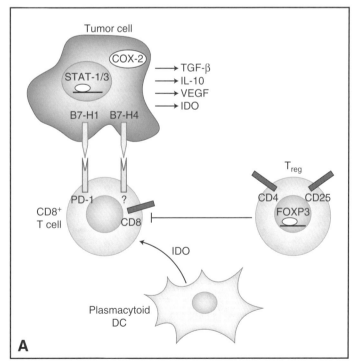

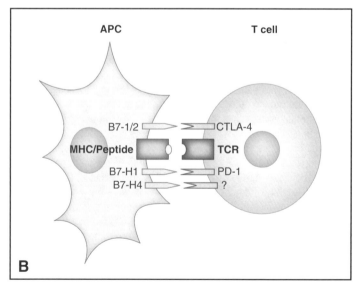

Figure 4-2. Downregulation of tumor-specific T cells results both from direct interaction with the tumor microenvironment (**A**) and as a consequence of immune checkpoints (**B**) that naturally regulate immune responses to infection and cancer. APC—antigen-presenting cell; COX— cyclooxygenase; CTLA—cytotoxic T-lymphocyte antigen; DC—dendritic cell; IDO—indoleamine 2,3-dioxygenase; IL—interleukin; MHC—major histocompatibility complex; TCR—T-cell receptor; TGF—transforming growth factor; T_{reg}—regulatory T cell; VEGF—vascular endothelial growth factor.

the development of agents that can bypass these checkpoints, which regulate T-cell function. Emerging technologies are facilitating the discovery of immunogenic antigens that are targets of T cells and signaling proteins involved in regulating T-cell responses.

Ideally, tumor antigens should be unique to and overexpressed in cancer cells, presented on the surface by human leukocyte antigen (HLA) molecules, essential for tumor survival, and immunogenic or capable of being recognized by T cells. These antigen characteristics provide specificity and may retard the capacity for immune escape. One method being used to identify antigens is the serological analysis of recombinant tumor cDNA expression libraries (SEREX). This method uses patient serum to screen libraries prepared from autologous or allogeneic tumors. In the initial application of this method, the use of autologous antibodies identified MAGE and tyrosinase, which were originally defined as melanoma T-cell antigens [43]. This finding led to the discovery that humoral immunity analysis could lead to the identification of T-cell antigens. Subsequently, these methods were used to identify coactosin-like protein found in pancreatic cancer and NY-ESO-1, which is widely expressed by many cancers [44,45].

A second method involves the use of T cells from cancer patients to screen autologous tumor cDNA libraries. This method has identified the majority of melanoma-specific T-cell antigens [46,47]. However, because this method requires pairs of autologous tumors and T-cell clones, it has been difficult to adapt this approach for the identification of antigens expressed by tumors other than melanoma. A newer method of antigen discovery involves the use of patient lymphocytes after whole cell vaccination to evaluate responses to proteins found to be differentially expressed on tumors. The candidate antigens are identified by serial analysis of gene expression (SAGE), which uses differential gene-display technology to identify genes that are more strongly expressed by tumor cells relative to normal cells [48,49]. Using enzyme-linked immunosorbent spot (ELISPOT) analysis, these antigens are then evaluated as T-cell targets using lymphocytes from vaccinated patients [50]. This method has identified mesothelin as a candidate T-cell target. Mesothelin is expressed at low levels in mesothelial cells, but is highly expressed by 56% of lung cancers and by the majority of mesotheliomas and ovarian and pancreatic adenocarcinomas [51–53].

While examination at the RNA level provides great insight into gene expression, it does not entirely reflect the final repertoire of the protein end products. This problem is further driving the development of proteomic-based techniques for tumor antigen discovery [54]. The "proteome" of a cell is the set of proteins it produces under a particular stimulus. Protein diversity is complex given that RNA transcripts can undergo alternative splicing and most proteins undergo posttranslational modifications. Proteins isolated from tumor cells can be separated by a series of techniques that often requires isoelectric-focusing two-dimensional gel electrophoresis. These proteins can then be quantified and isolated by blotting with sera from untreated patients or those treated with a vaccine. Individual spots representing the protein can then be identified by mass spectrometry. These techniques are being used to isolate disease biomarkers and to identify drug and immune targets. For immunotherapy, this strategy allows for the identification of targets that actually elicit a vaccine-mediated antibody response, resulting in the elucidation of targets for immune monitoring and eventually for immune targeting.

These and other technologic advances are also facilitating the actual translation of new immune targets into effective therapeutics. For example, new recombinant DNA technology and engineered mice are being used to generate humanized antibodies at a rapid pace. This, in turn, has resulted in the emergence of an entirely new class of monoclonal antibody therapeutics, the immune checkpoint modulators. Cytotoxic T-lymphocyte antigen-4 (CTLA-4) antibody is the prototype of this class, and is currently under evaluation in a variety of tumor types for its ability to block a negative regulatory checkpoint on activated T cells (Fig. 4-2). This molecule has been shown to have antitumor activity as a single agent in melanoma patients in particular [55,56]; however, it has also been shown to enhance the development of antigen-specific T cells when given in sequence with a vaccine in both preclinical and phase 1 clinical studies [57–60]. Combinatorial therapy is already being tested in prostate cancer patients who are receiving a granulocyte-macrophage colony-stimulating factor (GM-CSF)–secreting tumor vaccine concurrently with ipilimumab. In an early phase 1 study, evidence of clinical responses has been observed in the majority of patients treated [60].

TARGETING THE DENDRITIC CELL

A review of every vaccine approach currently being pursued is beyond the scope of this chapter. However, the underlying principles of most vaccine approaches can be unified by a single goal: antigen delivery to the most potent antigen-presenting cell (APC), the dendritic cell. In addition to signaling through its TCR, a T cell requires costimulatory signals to promote T-cell activation rather than T-cell anergy. Dendritic cells have the natural capacity to provide the necessary costimulation and are also able to process and present antigen for optimal T-cell activation. In addition, dendritic cells can present antigen peptides to both CD8+ and CD4+ T cells in the context of the MHC class I and II molecules, respectively. MHC class I antigen presentation was previously thought to be restricted to antigens generated in the cytosol. More recently, dendritic cells have been found to be capable of cross-priming, which involves the uptake of extracellular antigens into the endosomes (for processing and presentation on MHC class II molecules) and subsequently transferring these proteins to the cytosol (cross-priming) for processing and presentation on MHC class I molecules [50,61,62]. Dendritic cell maturation can be stimulated through a variety of receptors, including Toll-like receptors (TLRs), which bind to chemical moieties from pathogens and receptors from the TNF receptor family. After maturation, a dendritic cell is able to provide costimulation to T cells in the form of released cytokines such as IL-12 and the expression of cell surface molecules such as B7.1/B7.2, which interacts with CD28 on the T cell. In addition, activated dendritic cells also express the TNF receptor family members 4-1BBL and OX40-L, which also provide costimulatory signals to T cells [63–68]. While vaccine approaches are diverse, the universal goal of cancer vaccines is to enhance the presentation of antigens to tumor-specific T cells in the context of costimulation by mature dendritic cells.

Table 4-1. Mechanisms of Tumor Immune Evasion

Alterations to immune response	Local factors	Systemic factors
Antigen processing and presentation molecules	Human leukocyte antigen class I, TAP, β_2-microglobulin	—
Immune cell inhibitory molecules	IL-10, TGF-β, COX-2, vascular endothelial growth factor, B7-H1, B7-H4, STAT-1/3, IDO	IL-1, IL-6, IL-10, TGF-β
Immune checkpoint dysregulation	B7-H1, B7-H4	Signaling by dendritic cells (B7.1/B7.2:CTLA-4, B.7-DC/B7-H1:PD-1)
Suppressor populations	T regulatory cells and immature dendritic cells at the tumor site	T regulatory cells prominent in peripheral blood
Loss of costimulation	—	B7 molecules, OX40, CD40

COX—cyclooxygenase; CTLA—cytotoxic T-lymphocyte antigen; IDO—indoleamine 2,3-dioxygenase; IL—interleukin; TAP—transporter associated with antigen presentation; TGF—transforming growth factor.

TUMOR ANTIGENS ADMINISTERED WITH ADJUVANTS

A simple strategy for improving antigen presentation is to provide dendritic cells with an exogenous source of antigens together with an adjuvant to provide an activating signal. Tumor antigens may be administered in the form of cell lysates, DNA, or peptides. Several strategies have been used to improve the quality of antigen presentation by dendritic cells. First, CD4 T-helper epitopes have been combined with cytotoxic CD8 T-cell epitopes to promote activation of both T-cell populations [69]. Additionally, incorporation of costimulatory agents such as GM-CSF and CpG oligonucleotides as adjuvants can enhance a vaccine response [70]. Another technique used is the modification of peptides to generate agonist peptides. CAP1-6D is a modified CAP1, an immunodominant epitope of carcinoembryonic antigen (CEA) that has been shown to enhance T-cell activation and is currently being combined with two adjuvants, Montanide (Seppic, Paris, France) and GM-CSF, for the treatment of pancreatic cancer [71]. This method of epitope enhancement has also been applied to gp100, a melanoma antigen [72]. Another method used is the complexing of antigens to heat shock proteins designed to promote the targeting of antigens to dendritic cell MHC processing pathways. As an example, a DNA vaccine in which DNA encoding for the HPV E7 protein is fused to a heat shock protein is being studied in HPV-positive cervical and head and neck cancers [73]. Similar approaches with other adjuvants are being used to target a range of tumor antigens in various cancer types.

DENDRITIC CELL VACCINES

As discussed above, the most potent vaccines target the dendritic cells. Ex vivo expansion and antigen loading of dendritic cells is attractive for several reasons. First, direct loading of dendritic cells ensures that the peptides reach their targets. Second, conditions can be altered to promote dendritic cell maturation. Ex vivo dendritic cell maturation is complex and likely requires a combination of both cytokines and ligands to pathogen-sensing receptors such as TLRs. However, there are a number of technical hurdles that require solutions before this approach will become feasible. First, it is difficult to obtain an unlimited source of autologous dendritic cells because these cells are only available in small numbers in peripheral blood and bone marrow. Second, the optimal number and route of administration have been difficult to study in patients due to the difficulty of obtaining adequate numbers and the lack of standardized methods for evaluating treatment efficacy. Third, it is unclear whether these cells—if prepared as a batch prior to initiating therapy—can be stored and still maintain adequate function weeks or months later.

One trial in which 35 patients with relapsed stage IV follicular lymphoma were immunized with dendritic cells loaded with tumor-specific idiotype protein showed interesting responses. Twenty-three of 35 patients had a T-cell response (14 patients), an antibody response (six patients), or both (three patients). Among 28 patients with residual tumor mass, eight had an objective response [74]. While the results of a phase 3 trial of a dendritic cell–based vaccine in melanoma were disappointing, a dendritic cell–based vaccine in prostate cancer is currently under evaluation for approval by the US Food and Drug Administration [75,76]. Sipuleucel-T is composed of autologous APCs cultured with a fusion protein, PA2024, which consists of prostatic acid phosphatase linked to colony-stimulating factor. A phase 3 trial in hormone-refractory prostate cancer did not meet its primary end point of improvement in time to progression; however, sipuleucel-T did show a survival advantage.

WHOLE TUMOR CELL VACCINES

A number of whole tumor vaccine approaches have been studied in preclinical models and in patients. The best studied whole tumor vaccine in patients has been the GM-CSF modified tumor cell approach. Whole cell vaccine approaches are appealing because a multiantigen platform negates the need for identification of specific tumor antigens and may overcome the problem of antigen loss variants. Both autologous and allogeneic tumor cells have been modified to secrete GM-CSF. GM-CSF is an important growth and differentiation factor for dendritic cells and this method of delivery provides local and sustained levels of GM-CSF needed for recruitment and adequate

priming of dendritic cells. Although autologous tumor cells would appear to be the best source of tumor antigens, this approach was found to lack feasibility for most cancer types. Several lines of evidence support the rationale of using a more practical allogeneic approach. First, characterization of tumor-associated antigens expressed by human melanomas revealed that at least 50% of tumors share common antigens regardless of HLA type [77,78]. Furthermore, a process called cross-presentation occurs in which the patient's own APCs are able to take up non–HLA-matched vaccine–expressing whole proteins and process them into antigenic peptides through the class I pathway that then primes host CD8+ T cells [50].

A number of allogeneic vaccine studies of this GM-CSF approach have been tested in phase 1 to 3 trials. In a phase 1 study of 14 patients with resected pancreatic adenocarcinoma, an allogeneic vaccine was combined with chemoradiation in the adjuvant setting. This study reported that three long-term survivors in the two highest dose cohorts were the only subjects who developed postvaccination delayed-type hypersensitivity responses and mesothelin-specific T-cell responses. Furthermore, these T-cell responses were not dependent on having the same HLA restriction as the vaccine cells; rather, they correlated with the patient's HLA type, thereby supporting the concept of cross-presentation by dendritic cells [50,79]. A subsequent phase 2 pancreatic cancer adjuvant trial of 60 patients reported a 1-year survival rate of 88% and a 2-year survival rate of 76%, which compares favorably with previously reported survival data [80].

This GM-CSF vaccine approach is being evaluated in two multicenter phase 3 trials in hormone-refractory metastatic prostate cancer [81]. It is also being combined with the most active immune-modulating agent currently being tested as a single agent in clinical trials, the CTLA-4 antagonist antibody, ipilimumab [60]. Of the six patients in the two highest-dose cohorts (three patients receiving 3 mg/kg and three receiving 5 mg/kg), one patient had stable disease and five had a least a 50% reduction in prostate-specific antigen, with three of the five showing improvement on imaging. These results are beyond the expectations of either agent's potency as single agents. Presumably, GVAX (Cell Genesys, San Francisco, CA) is important in priming a prostate-specific immune response, and the CTLA-4 antagonist antibody enhances the prostate antigen–specific response by blocking inhibitory signals on the activated T cells. These studies are the prototype of what to expect from immune-based clinical trials during the next 10 years.

RECOMBINANT MICROORGANISM-BASED VACCINES

While whole tumor cell vaccines have the advantage of providing a range of tumor antigens for priming, their delivery efficiency may not be sufficient to induce the most potent immune responses. New platforms that modify bacterial and viral vectors to express antigens and costimulatory molecules are forming a new group of immune-based targeted agents that are undergoing clinical testing. Recombinant viral and bacterial vector systems take advantage of the capability of immunogenic infectious vectors to stimulate both adaptive and innate immune responses. The virulence of these agents can be modified to prevent clinical infections without reducing their capacity to present artificially introduced tumor antigens. These agents typically have natural mechanisms for engaging and activating immune cells including dendritic cells.

The poxviruses have received a significant amount of attention since the use of vaccinia to eradicate smallpox worldwide. To overcome the natural consequence of the memory response to clear subsequent boost vaccinations, investigators have employed a "prime and boost" strategy using sequential fowlpox and vaccinia vaccines [82]. While this approach has resulted in induction of tumor antigen–specific responses, a phase 3 study of PANVAC (Therion Biologics, Corp., Cambridge, MA), which targets CEA and Muc-1, failed to demonstrate a survival benefit.

The manipulation of *Listeria monocytogenes* is another interesting strategy for active immunization [83,84]. *Listeria* is an intracellular bacterium that not only induces both innate and adaptive immunity but specifically has access to both class I and II antigen-processing pathways. A *Listeria* platform currently undergoing early clinical development uses a strain that has been engineered without the capacity for cell-to-cell transfer. Thus, this modified strain prevents the possibility of propagation of infection. Additionally, this strain is able to infect APCs, including dendritic cells, without the capacity to infect other normal cells. Clinical protocols utilizing the platform to target mesothelin-expressing tumors are currently under development.

FUTURE DIRECTIONS

Combinatorial strategies that provide signals to induce the most vigorous T-cell responses while temporarily turning off checkpoint signals that prevent T-cell activation will be needed to produce clinically meaningful outcomes. These strategies will focus not only on adequate dendritic cell maturation and antigen delivery but will likely have to counter multiple immune checkpoints. Much will be learned from the currently ongoing clinical trials testing anti-CTLA-4 blockade in combination with vaccines (specific information about many such trials can be accessed at http://www.clinicaltrials.gov).

Antibodies directed at other B7 family members such as B7-H1 (PDL-1) and B7-H4 are also under development. B7-H1 and B7-H4 are expressed on various tumor types and may play a role in T-cell suppression [85–87]. PD-1 is expressed on T cells and is thought to play a role in negative regulation. An anti–PD-1 antagonist monoclonal antibody is currently being tested in phase 1 trials in a number of cancer types. Agonist antibodies are also entering clinical trials. These include anti–4-1BB, which binds to a TNF family receptor on T cells, resulting in enhanced activation [66].

Clinical grade immunostimulatory cytokines, such as IL-7, IL-15, and IL-21, are also becoming available [88]. When given in the right sequence with vaccines, these agents may have important antitumor immune activity.

Immune modulation is not limited to the effects of these specific checkpoint inhibitors. Chemotherapeutic agents such as gemcitabine and paclitaxel are thought to have immunostimulatory capacity and are being combined with vaccine approaches [89,90]. Strategies combining vaccines with agents that target the microenvironment (*eg*, VEGF-targeted agents) further enhance antitumor immunity and are effective in preclinical models [91]. Additionally, tumor antigen–targeted monoclonal antibodies, such as trastuzumab (anti-HER-2/neu) in breast cancer and cetuximab (anti–epidermal growth factor receptor) in pancreatic cancer, are being combined with vaccines because of their ability to enhance apoptosis and antigen presentation [92].

Other agents that combine with vaccines and target dendritic cell activation or maturation are also being evaluated. Soluble CD40L, which binds CD40 on dendritic cells, is being tested in early phase trials [93]. Of the TLR agonists, CpG oligodeoxynucleotide promotes the most potent induction of antigen-specific Th1 responses and is currently being studied as a peptide adjuvant in both melanoma and breast cancer vaccine studies [94].

CONCLUSIONS

The increasing understanding of the complex immune regulatory networks allows for the incorporation of immunostimulatory chemotherapeutic agents and more novel immune-modulating agents into vaccine strategies. Strategies that consider both the importance of immune priming and local and systemic tolerance mechanisms may ultimately promote the synergy required to harness the potential of immunotherapy.

REFERENCES

1. Chien YC, Jan CF, Kuo HS, Chen CJ: Nationwide hepatitis B vaccination program in Taiwan: effectiveness in the 20 years after it was launched. *Epidemiol Rev* 2006, 28:126–135.

2. Shepard CW, Simard EP, Finelli L, *et al.*: Hepatitis B virus infection: epidemiology and vaccination. *Epidemiol Rev* 2006, 28:112–125.

3. Rambout L, Hopkins L, Hutton B, Fergusson D: Prophylactic vaccination against human papillomavirus infection and disease in women: a systematic review of randomized controlled trials. *CMAJ* 2007, 177:469–479.

4. Stewart AJ, Devlin PM: The history of the smallpox vaccine. *J Infect* 2006, 52:329–334.

5. Coley WB: The treatment of malignant tumors by repeated inoculations of erysipelas with a report of ten original cases: 1893. *Clin Orthop Relat Res* 1991, 262:3–11.

6. Tsung K, Norton JA: Lessons from Coley's toxin. *Surg Oncol* 2006, 15:25–28.

7. Lawrence HS: *Discussion of Cellular and Humoral Aspects of the Hypersensitive States.* New York: Hoeber-Harper; 1959.

8. Burnet FM: The concept of immunological surveillance. *Prog Exp Tumor Res* 1970, 13:1–27.

9. Dunn GP, Old LJ, Schreiber RD: The immunobiology of cancer immunosurveillance and immunoediting. *Immunity* 2004, 21:137–148.

10. Ercolini AM, Ladle BH, Manning EA, *et al.*: Recruitment of latent pools of high-avidity CD8(+) T cells to the antitumor immune response. *J Exp Med* 2005, 201:1591–1602.

11. Dudley ME, Wunderlich JR, Yang JC, *et al.*: Adoptive cell transfer therapy following non-myeloablative but lymphodepleting chemotherapy for the treatment of patients with refractory metastatic melanoma. *J Clin Oncol* 2005, 23:2346–2357.

12. Martignoni ME, Kunze P, Hildebrandt W, *et al.*: Role of mononuclear cells and inflammatory cytokines in pancreatic cancer-related cachexia. *Clin Cancer Res* 2005, 11:5802–5808.

13. Shibata M, Nezu T, Kanou H, *et al.*: Decreased production of interleukin-12 and type 2 immune responses are marked in cachectic patients with colorectal and gastric cancer. *J Clin Gastroenterol* 2002, 34:416–420.

14. von Bernstorff W, Voss M, Freichel S, *et al.*: Systemic and local immunosuppression in pancreatic cancer patients. *Clin Cancer Res* 2001, 7(Suppl):925s–932s.

15. Schmielau J, Nalesnik MA, Finn OJ: Suppressed T-cell receptor zeta chain expression and cytokine production in pancreatic cancer patients. *Clin Cancer Res* 2001, 7(Suppl):933s–939s.

16. Dworacki G, Meidenbauer N, Kuss I, *et al.*: Decreased zeta chain expression and apoptosis in CD3+ peripheral blood T lymphocytes of patients with melanoma. *Clin Cancer Res* 2001, 7(Suppl):947s–957s.

17. Cardi G, Heaney JA, Schned AR, *et al.*: T-cell receptor zeta-chain expression on tumor-infiltrating lymphocytes from renal cell carcinoma. *Cancer Res* 1997, 57:3517–3519.

18. Sakaguchi S, Sakaguchi N, Shimizu J, *et al.*: Immunologic tolerance maintained by CD25+ CD4+ regulatory T cells: their common role in controlling autoimmunity, tumor immunity, and transplantation tolerance. *Immunol Rev* 2001, 182:18–32.

19. Hori S, Nomura T, Sakaguchi S: Control of regulatory T cell development by the transcription factor Foxp3. *Science* 2003, 299:1057–1061.

20. Fontenot JD, Gavin MA, Rudensky AY: Foxp3 programs the development and function of CD4+CD25+ regulatory T cells. *Nat Immunol* 2003, 4:330–336.

21. Wolf AM, Wolf D, Steurer M, *et al.*: Increase of regulatory T cells in the peripheral blood of cancer patients. *Clin Cancer Res* 2003, 9:606–612.

22. Curiel TJ, Coukos G, Zou L, *et al.*: Specific recruitment of regulatory T cells in ovarian carcinoma fosters immune privilege and predicts reduced survival. *Nat Med* 2004, 10:942–949.

23. Liyanage UK, Moore TT, Joo HG, *et al.*: Prevalence of regulatory T cells is increased in peripheral blood and tumor microenvironment of patients with pancreas or breast adenocarcinoma. *J Immunol* 2002, 169:2756–2761.

24. Liyanage UK, Goedegebuure PS, Moore TT, *et al.*: Increased prevalence of regulatory T cells (Treg) is induced by pancreas adenocarcinoma. *J Immunother* 2006, 29:416–424.

25. Bates GJ, Fox SB, Han C, *et al.*: Quantification of regulatory T cells enables the identification of high-risk breast cancer patients and those at risk of late relapse. *J Clin Oncol* 2006, 24:5373–5380.

26. Gao Q, Qiu SJ, Fan J, *et al.*: Intratumoral balance of regulatory and cytotoxic T cells is associated with prognosis of hepatocellular carcinoma after resection. *J Clin Oncol* 2007, 25:2586–2593.

27. Hiraoka N, Onozato K, Kosuge T, Hirohashi S: Prevalence of FOXP3+ regulatory T cells increases during the progression of pancreatic ductal adenocarcinoma and its premalignant lesions. *Clin Cancer Res* 2006, 12:5423–5434.

28. Alpan RS, Zhang M, Pardee AB: Cell cycle-dependent expression of TAP1, TAP2, and HLA-B27 messenger RNAs in a human breast cancer cell line. *Cancer Res* 1996, 56:4358–4361.

29. Seliger B, Hohne A, Knuth A, *et al.*: Reduced membrane major histocompatibility complex class I density and stability in a subset of human renal cell carcinomas with low TAP and LMP expression. *Clin Cancer Res* 1996, 2:1427–1433.

30. Uyttenhove C, Maryanski J, Boon T: Escape of mouse mastocytoma P815 after nearly complete rejection is due to antigen-loss variants rather than immunosuppression. *J Exp Med* 1983, 157:1040–1052.

31. Bromberg JF, Wrzeszczynska MH, Devgan G, *et al.*: Stat3 as an oncogene. *Cell* 1999, 98:295–303.

32. Kortylewski M, Kujawski M, Wang T, *et al.*: Inhibiting Stat3 signaling in the hematopoietic system elicits multicomponent antitumor immunity. *Nat Med* 2005, 11:1314–1321.

33. Wang T, Niu G, Kortylewski M, *et al.*: Regulation of the innate and adaptive immune responses by stat-3 signaling in tumor cells. *Nat Med* 2004, 10:48–54.

34. Cheng F, Wang HW, Cuenca A, *et al.*: A critical role for Stat3 signaling in immune tolerance. *Immunity* 2003, 19:425–436.

35. Sharma S, Stolina M, Yang SC, *et al.*: Tumor cyclooxygenase 2-dependent suppression of dendritic cell function. *Clin Cancer Res* 2003, 9:961–968.

36. Drake CG, Jaffee E, Pardoll DM: Mechanisms of immune evasion by tumors. *Adv Immunol* 2006, 90:51–81.

37. Apolloni E, Bronte V, Mazzoni A, *et al.*: Immortalized myeloid suppressor cells trigger apoptosis in antigen-activated T lymphocytes. *J Immunol* 2000, 165:6723–6730.

38. Bronte V, Apolloni E, Cabrelle A, *et al.*: Identification of a CD11b(+)/Gr-1(+)/CD31(+) myeloid progenitor capable of activating or suppressing CD8(+) T cells. *Blood* 2000, 96:3838–3846.

39. Kusmartsev S, Nefedova Y, Yoder D, Gabrilovich DI: Antigen-specific inhibition of CD8+ T cell response by immature myeloid cells in cancer is mediated by reactive oxygen species. *J Immunol* 2004, 172:989–999.

40. Kusmartsev S, Gabrilovich DI: Role of immature myeloid cells in mechanisms of immune evasion in cancer. *Cancer Immunol Immunother* 2006, 55:237–245.

41. Muller AJ, DuHadaway JB, Donover PS, *et al.*: Inhibition of indoleamine 2,3-dioxygenase, an immunoregulatory target of the cancer suppression gene Bin1, potentiates cancer chemotherapy. *Nat Med* 2005, 11:312–319.

42. Munn DH, Mellor AL: Indoleamine 2,3-dioxygenase and tumor-induced tolerance. *J Clin Invest* 2007, 117:1147–1154.

43. Sahin U, Tureci O, Schmitt H, *et al.*: Human neoplasms elicit multiple specific immune responses in the autologous host. *Proc Natl Acad Sci U S A* 1995, 92:11810–11813.

44. Nakatsura T, Senju S, Ito M, *et al.*: Cellular and humoral immune responses to a human pancreatic cancer antigen, coactosin-like protein, originally defined by the SEREX method. *Eur J Immunol* 2002, 32:826–836.

45. Chen YT, Scanlan MJ, Sahin U, *et al.*: A testicular antigen aberrantly expressed in human cancers detected by autologous antibody screening. *Proc Natl Acad Sci U S A* 1997, 94:1914–1918.

46. Rosenberg SA: Progress in human tumour immunology and immunotherapy. *Nature* 2001, 411:380–384.

47. Boon T, Cerottini JC, Van den Eynde B, *et al.*: Tumor antigens recognized by T lymphocytes. *Annu Rev Immunol* 1994, 12:337–365.

48. Argani P, Iacobuzio-Donahue C, Ryu B, *et al.*: Mesothelin is overexpressed in the vast majority of ductal adenocarcinomas of the pancreas: identification of a new pancreatic cancer marker by serial analysis of gene expression (SAGE). *Clin Cancer Res* 2001, 7:3862–3868.

49. Argani P, Rosty C, Reiter RE, *et al.*: Discovery of new markers of cancer through serial analysis of gene expression: prostate stem cell antigen is overexpressed in pancreatic adenocarcinoma. *Cancer Res* 2001; 61:4320–4324.

50. Thomas AM, Santarsiero LM, Lutz ER, *et al.*: Mesothelin-specific CD8(+) T cell responses provide evidence of in vivo cross-priming by antigen-presenting cells in vaccinated pancreatic cancer patients. *J Exp Med* 2004, 200:297–306.

51. Hassan R, Remaley AT, Sampson ML, *et al.*: Detection and quantitation of serum mesothelin, a tumor marker for patients with mesothelioma and ovarian cancer. *Clin Cancer Res* 2006, 12:447–453.

52. Hassan R, Bera T, Pastan I: Mesothelin: a new target for immunotherapy. *Clin Cancer Res* 2004, 10(12 Pt 1):3937–3942.

53. Ho M, Bera TK, Willingham MC, *et al.*: Mesothelin expression in human lung cancer. *Clin Cancer Res* 2007, 13:1571–1575.

54. Shoshan SH, Admon A: Novel technologies for cancer biomarker discovery: humoral proteomics. *Cancer Biomark* 2007, 3:141–152.

55. Attia P, Phan GQ, Maker AV, *et al.*: Autoimmunity correlates with tumor regression in patients with metastatic melanoma treated with anti-cytotoxic T-lymphocyte antigen-4. *J Clin Oncol* 2005, 23:6043–6053.

56. Hodi FS, Mihm MC, Soiffer RJ, *et al.*: Biologic activity of cytotoxic T lymphocyte-associated antigen 4 antibody blockade in previously vaccinated metastatic melanoma and ovarian carcinoma patients. *Proc Natl Acad Sci U S A* 2003, 100:4712–4717.

57. Hurwitz AA, Foster BA, Kwon ED, *et al.*: Combination immunotherapy of primary prostate cancer in a transgenic mouse model using CTLA-4 blockade. *Cancer Res* 2000, 60:2444–2448.

58. van Elsas A, Hurwitz AA, Allison JP: Combination immunotherapy of B16 melanoma using anti-cytotoxic T lymphocyte-associated antigen 4 (CTLA-4) and granulocyte/macrophage colony-stimulating factor (GM-CSF)-producing vaccines induces rejection of subcutaneous and metastatic tumors accompanied by autoimmune depigmentation. *J Exp Med* 1999, 190:355–366.

59. Hurwitz AA, Yu TF, Leach DR, Allison JP: CTLA-4 blockade synergizes with tumor-derived granulocyte-macrophage colony-stimulating factor for treatment of an experimental mammary carcinoma. *Proc Natl Acad Sci U S A* 1998, 95:10067–10071.

60. Gerritsen W, Van Den Eertwegh A, De Gruijl T, *et al.*: A dose-escalation trial of GM-CSF-gene transduced allogeneic prostate cancer cellular immunotherapy in patients with hormone-refractory prostate cancer [abstract]. *J Clin Oncol* 2006, 24(18S):2500.

61. Huang AY, Bruce AT, Pardoll DM, Levitsky HI: In vivo cross-priming of MHC class I-restricted antigens requires the TAP transporter. *Immunity* 1996, 4:349–355.

62. Huang AY, Golumbek P, Ahmadzadeh M, *et al.*: Role of bone marrow-derived cells in presenting MHC class I-restricted tumor antigens. *Science* 1994, 264:961–965.

63. Sallusto F, Lanzavecchia A: Efficient presentation of soluble antigen by cultured human dendritic cells is maintained by granulocyte/macrophage colony-stimulating factor plus interleukin 4 and downregulated by tumor necrosis factor alpha. *J Exp Med* 1994, 179:1109–1118.

64. Caux C, Massacrier C, Vanbervliet B, *et al.*: Activation of human dendritic cells through CD40 cross-linking. *J Exp Med* 1994, 180:1263–1272.

65. Cella M, Scheidegger D, Palmer-Lehmann K, *et al.*: Ligation of CD40 on dendritic cells triggers production of high levels of interleukin-12 and enhances T cell stimulatory capacity: T-T help via APC activation. *J Exp Med* 1996, 184:747–752.

66. Melero I, Shuford WW, Newby SA, *et al.*: Monoclonal antibodies against the 4-1BB T-cell activation molecule eradicate established tumors. *Nat Med* 1997, 3:682–685.

67. Weinberg AD, Rivera MM, Prell R, *et al.*: Engagement of the OX-40 receptor in vivo enhances antitumor immunity. *J Immunol* 2000, 164:2160–2169.

68. Bansal-Pakala P, Jember AG, Croft M: Signaling through OX40 (CD134) breaks peripheral T-cell tolerance. *Nat Med* 2001, 7:907–912.

69. Zarour HM, Maillere B, Brusic V, *et al*.: NY-ESO-1 119-143 is a promiscuous major histocompatibility complex class II T-helper epitope recognized by Th1- and Th2-type tumor-reactive CD4+ T cells. *Cancer Res* 2002, 62:213–218.

70. Valmori D, Souleimanian NE, Tosello V, *et al*.: Vaccination with NY-ESO-1 protein and CpG in Montanide induces integrated antibody/Th1 responses and CD8 T cells through cross-priming. *Proc Natl Acad Sci U S A* 2007, 104:8947–8952.

71. Zaremba S, Barzaga E, Zhu M, *et al*.: Identification of an enhancer agonist cytotoxic T lymphocyte peptide from human carcinoembryonic antigen. *Cancer Res* 1997, 57:4570–4577.

72. Walker EB, Haley D, Miller W, *et al*.: gp100(209-2M) peptide immunization of human lymphocyte antigen-A2+ stage I-III melanoma patients induces significant increase in antigen-specific effector and long-term memory CD8+ T cells. *Clin Cancer Res* 2004, 10:668–680.

73. Peng S, Trimble C, Ji H, *et al*.: Characterization of HPV-16 E6 DNA vaccines employing intracellular targeting and intercellular spreading strategies. *J Biomed Sci* 2005, 12:689–700.

74. Timmerman JM, Czerwinski DK, Davis TA, *et al*.: Idiotype-pulsed dendritic cell vaccination for B-cell lymphoma: clinical and immune responses in 35 patients. *Blood* 2002, 99:1517–1526.

75. Schadendorf D, Ugurel S, Schuler-Thurner B, *et al*.: Dacarbazine (DTIC) versus vaccination with autologous peptide-pulsed dendritic cells (DC) in first-line treatment of patients with metastatic melanoma: a randomized phase III trial of the DC study group of the DeCOG. *Ann Oncol* 2006, 17:563–570.

76. Small EJ, Schellhammer PF, Higano CS, *et al*.: Placebo-controlled phase III trial of immunologic therapy with sipuleucel-T (APC8015) in patients with metastatic, asymptomatic hormone refractory prostate cancer. *J Clin Oncol* 2006, 24:3089–3094.

77. Cox AL, Skipper J, Chen Y, *et al*.: Identification of a peptide recognized by five melanoma-specific human cytotoxic T cell lines. *Science* 1994, 264:716–719.

78. Kawakami Y, Eliyahu S, Delgado CH, *et al*.: Cloning of the gene coding for a shared human melanoma antigen recognized by autologous T cells infiltrating into tumor. *Proc Natl Acad Sci U S A* 1994, 91:3515–3519.

79. Jaffee EM, Hruban RH, Biedrzycki B, *et al*.: Novel allogeneic granulo-cyte-macrophage colony-stimulating factor-secreting tumor vaccine for pancreatic cancer: a phase I trial of safety and immune activation. *J Clin Oncol* 2001, 19:145–156.

80. Laheru DA, Yeo C, Biedrzycki B, *et al*.: A safety and efficacy trial of lethally irradiated allogeneic pancreatic tumor cells transfected with the GM-CSF gene in combination with adjuvant chemoradiotherapy for the treatment of adenocarcinoma of the pancreas [abstract]. *J Clin Oncol* 2007, 25(18S):3010.

81. Small EJ, Sacks N, Nemunaitis J, *et al*.: Granulocyte macrophage colony-stimulating factor–secreting allogeneic cellular immunotherapy for hormone-refractory prostate cancer. *Clin Cancer Res* 2007, 13:3883–3891.

82. Petrulio CA, Kaufman HL: Development of the PANVAC-VF vaccine for pancreatic cancer. *Expert Rev Vaccines* 2006, 5:9–19.

83. Brockstedt DG, Giedlin MA, Leong ML, *et al*.: Listeria-based cancer vaccines that segregate immunogenicity from toxicity. *Proc Natl Acad Sci U S A* 2004, 101:13832–13837.

84. Brockstedt DG, Leong ML, Luckett W, *et al*.: Recombinant Listeria mono-cytogenes-based immunotherapy targeting mesothelin for the treatment of pancreatic and ovarian cancer [abstract]. *Proc Am Assoc Cancer Res* 2005, 46:abstract 6028.

85. Dong H, Strome SE, Salomao DR, *et al*.: Tumor-associated B7-H1 promotes T-cell apoptosis: a potential mechanism of immune evasion. *Nat Med* 2002, 8:793–800.

86. Hirano F, Kaneko K, Tamura H, *et al*.: Blockade of B7-H1 and PD-1 by monoclonal antibodies potentiates cancer therapeutic immunity. *Cancer Res* 2005, 65:1089–1096.

87. Sadun RE, Sachsman SM, Chen X, *et al*.: Immune signatures of murine and human cancers reveal unique mechanisms of tumor escape and new targets for cancer immunotherapy. *Clin Cancer Res* 2007, 13:4016–4025.

88. Lin WW, Karin M: A cytokine-mediated link between innate immunity, inflammation, and cancer. *J Clin Invest* 2007, 117:1175–1183.

89. Yanagimoto H, Mine T, Yamamoto K, *et al*.: Immunological evaluation of personalized peptide vaccination with gemcitabine for pancreatic cancer. *Cancer Sci* 2007, 98:605–611.

90. Machiels JP, Reilly RT, Emens LA, *et al*.: Cyclophosphamide, doxorubicin, and paclitaxel enhance the antitumor immune response of granulocyte/macrophage-colony stimulating factor-secreting whole-cell vaccines in HER-2/neu tolerized mice. *Cancer Res* 2001, 61:3689–3697.

91. Manning EA, Ullman JG, Leatherman JM, *et al*.: A vascular endothelial growth factor receptor-2 inhibitor enhances antitumor immunity through an immune-based mechanism. *Clin Cancer Res* 2007, 13:3951–3959.

92. Wolpoe ME, Lutz ER, Ercolini AM, *et al*.: HER-2/neu-specific monoclonal antibodies collaborate with HER-2/neu-targeted granulocyte macrophage colony-stimulating factor secreting whole cell vaccination to augment CD8+ T cell effector function and tumor-free survival in her-2/neu-transgenic mice. *J Immunol* 2003, 171:2161–2169.

93. Vonderheide RH, Flaherty KT, Khalil M, *et al*.: Clinical activity and immune modulation in cancer patients treated with CP-870,893, a novel CD40 agonist monoclonal antibody. *J Clin Oncol* 2007, 25:876–883.

94. Krieg AM: Development of TLR9 agonists for cancer therapy. *J Clin Invest* 2007, 117:1184–1194.

Since the development of the Nigro regimen for the definitive treatment of anal cancer in the 1970s, combined modality chemotherapy and radiation has emerged as the primary management of multiple solid malignancies. Concurrent chemoradiotherapy (CRT) is now used for cancers of the central nervous system (CNS), head and neck, lung, esophagus, stomach, pancreas, rectum, cervix, anus, and bladder. Reduced-dose chemotherapy is used in combination with full-dose radiotherapy (RT) to achieve a synergistic effect. Advances on the forefront of chemotherapy have led to improved clinical outcomes. Noncytotoxic (targeted) agents also have become available and have allowed for new combinations of treatments.

When combined with chemotherapy, radiation is responsible for improved tumor cell kill through increased DNA double-strand breaks, which lead to mitosis-associated cell death, decreased DNA repair, and apoptosis [1]. Radiation also disrupts the blood-brain barrier and causes vascular leaks, which can permit better drug delivery to CNS tumors [2]. In addition, radiation can potentiate the cytotoxic effects of chemotherapy by permitting prolonged tumor retention of 5-fluorouracil (5-FU) [3]. Still, the mechanisms of radiosensitization continue to be delineated.

A radiosensitizer can be defined as a chemical or pharmacologic agent that increases the lethal effects of radiation if administered in conjunction with it. These agents must show a differential effect between tumor and normal tissues, so as to increase the tumor's sensitivity to a greater extent than normal cells [4]. When combined with RT, chemotherapy doses may be reduced to allow the toxicity profile to become safer. This chapter discusses the mechanisms by which chemotherapeutic and newer targeted agents achieve cell death in combination with radiation and the clinical trials using CRT therapies to potentiate tumor killing.

CHEMOTHERAPEUTIC AGENTS

5-FLUOROURACIL

Combined 5-FU and RT has been studied extensively. 5-FU shows DNA-directed effects by inhibiting thymidylate synthase; it also shows RNA-directed effects through incorporation into RNA [5]. Although damage to DNA or RNA can result in cell death, it is postulated that radiosensitization occurs primarily through the inhibition of thymidylate synthase. Combined radiation and 5-FU–based regimens have led to landmark clinical trials in treatments for cancers of the esophagus [6], stomach [7], pancreas [8], rectum [9], and head and neck [10] (Table 5-1).

Evidence has suggested comparable outcomes between intravenous 5-FU and capecitabine, an orally administered prodrug. A phase 3 trial from Spain compared oxaliplatin with either capecitabine or continuous infusional 5-FU as first-line therapy in metastatic colorectal cancer and found no significant differences in efficacy between the arms. There were also no significant differences between time to progression, median overall survival, or response rate, although there was a trend for slightly lower survival in the capecitabine group [11]. Capecitabine offers the advantage of oral administration, whereas 5-FU is often given in continuous infusion and thus requires an indwelling catheter or infusional pump. Capecitabine is a fluoropyrimidine carbamate selectively activated to 5-FU at the tumor. Specifically, it passes through the intestinal mucosal membrane intact and is subsequently activated by a cascade of three enzymes that results in the preferential release of 5-FU at the tumor site. Dose-limiting toxicities include diarrhea with hypotension, abdominal pain, and leukopenia. Palmar-plantar erythrodysesthesia can also occur at higher dose levels after prolonged treatment [12]. 5-FU and capecitabine remain important chemotherapies used in combination with RT.

PLATINUM

The platinum analogues, including cisplatin, carboplatin, and oxaliplatin, are used frequently in the treatment of multiple solid tumors. Carboplatin causes increased single- and double-strand breaks via intercalation in the presence of RT [13]. In irradiated cells, RT causes increased cellular uptake of carboplatin and can inhibit DNA repair pathways [14,15]. Oxaliplatin is a third-generation cisplatin analogue that reacts with DNA, forming DNA adducts through guanine/guanine and adenosine/guanine cross-links [16]. Oxaliplatin has a different spectrum of activity and low cross-resistance to cisplatin and can therefore be used in cisplatin-refractory patients [17]. Oxaliplatin is more efficient than cisplatin in inhibiting DNA chain elongation; however, it produces fewer DNA and protein cross-links than cisplatin [18].

Table 5-1. Studies of Combined Radiotherapy and 5-FU–Based Chemotherapy Regimens

Study	Population	Study arms	CRT regimen	Median survival/outcome
Herskovic *et al.* [6]	SCC or ACA of thoracic esophagus	Arm 1: CRT Arm 2: RT only	RT + 5-FU + cisplatin	12.5 vs 8.9 mo*
Macdonald [7]	Resected gastric ACA	Arm 1: Surgery + postoperative CRT → chemotherapy Arm 2: Surgery only	LV + 5-FU → LV + 5-FU + RT → LV + 5-FU	36 vs 27 mo*
Kalser and Ellenberg [8]	Resected pancreatic ACA	Arm 1: CRT → maintenance 5-FU Arm 2: Surgery only	5-FU + RT	20 vs 11 mo*
Sauer *et al.* [9]	T3/T4 or node-positive rectal ACA	Arm 1: Preoperative CRT → adjuvant 5-FU Arm 2: Postoperative CRT → adjuvant 5-FU	5-FU + RT	Reduced acute and long-term toxicity in preoperative arm*; local recurrence 6% (preoperative) vs 13% (postoperative)*
Brizel *et al.* [10]	T3/T4 or N1/N2 M0 head and neck SCC	Arm 1: Hyperfractionated RT Arm 2: Hyperfractionated CRT → chemotherapy	5-FU + cisplatin	3-y OS 55% vs 34%; RFS 61% vs 41%; local control 70% vs 44%*

*Significant difference between treatment groups.
5-FU—fluorouracil; ACA—adenocarcinoma; CRT—chemoradiotherapy; LV—leucovorin; OS—overall survival; RFS—recurrence-free survival; RT—radiotherapy; SCC—squamous cell carcinoma.

Clinical results support the administration of concurrent cisplatin with RT for head and neck cancers [19,20], non–small cell lung cancer (NSCLC) [21], small cell lung cancer [22], and cervical cancer [23] (Table 5-2). Bladder conservation has been successful with the combination of cisplatin and RT in carefully selected patients [24].

Oxaliplatin has been used most commonly with RT in rectal cancer, based on the successful use of oxaliplatin, 5-FU, and leucovorin (FOLFOX) for advanced colorectal cancer [25]. Preoperative RT, oxaliplatin, and 5-FU for rectal cancer have been used without increased toxicity [26]. Oxaliplatin is also currently used in combination with gemcitabine and radiation for pancreatic cancer; however, long-term follow-up is necessary to determine its efficacy in this setting [27].

GEMCITABINE

Gemcitabine radiosensitization is thought to be due to nucleotide misincorporations in the presence of deoxyadenosine triphosphate (dATP) imbalances. If these imbalances are not repaired, cell death is augmented after RT. The activity of gemcitabine has also been correlated with the inhibition of ribonucleotide reductase [5]; radiosensitization has been correlated with dATP depletion and S-phase accumulation. Gemcitabine radiosensitization occurs through mismatched nucleotides, suggesting a role for deficiency in mismatch repair contributing to radiosensitization [28]. Treatment of cells with gemcitabine immediately before irradiation significantly reduces the variation in radiosensitivity by reversal of S-phase radioresistance [29], and implies that gemcitabine interferes with mismatch repair [30] and homologous recombination in the setting of RT [31].

Multiple clinical trials have evaluated various dosing regimens of gemcitabine with radiation in an attempt to determine the most effective regimen for each disease site. Trials have included full-dose gemcitabine (1000 mg/m^2 weekly for 3 weeks) with an abbreviated course of 36-Gy RT over 3 weeks in the neoadjuvant setting to the primary tumor [32,33], or low-dose weekly [34] or biweekly gemcitabine (40 mg/m^2 twice weekly) with full-dose RT in the adjuvant setting after a Whipple procedure [35]. Other studies have reported increased toxicity with large-field RT, including regional lymphatics delivered as 30 to 33 Gy in 10 to 11 fractions with 250 to 500 mg/m^2 of weekly gemcitabine [36]. It appears that RT with gemcitabine may be feasible and safe when attenuated gemcitabine doses are given with smaller radiation fields.

Gemcitabine has also been combined with radiation in head and neck cancers, showing efficacy but also increased mucositis rates [37]. In bladder cancer, the combination has shown safety at doses of gemcitabine 27 mg/m^2 weekly with 60-Gy RT [38]. Gemcitabine and RT have also been combined for use in chest wall recurrences in breast cancer [39], and the combination is in phase 2 testing in NSCLC [40]. Overall, early results with gemcitabine and RT are encouraging.

TAXANES

Taxanes enhance the stability of microtubules, promoting microtubule formation and inhibiting disassembly, thereby preventing the separation of chromosomes during mitosis [41]. Taxanes lead to tumor radio-enhancement through reoxygenation of radioresistant hypoxic cells and G2/M arrest [42]. Despite inducing G2/M block in vitro, it is thought that G2/M block is not a sufficient condition for paclitaxel radiosensitization [43]. On a molecular level, it appears that the effects of taxanes are mainly p53 independent and primarily involve phosphorylation of the *Bcl-2* gene [42].

Paclitaxel has been combined with radiation in various clinical settings. One example is the definitive management of head and neck cancers with carboplatin, paclitaxel, and daily RT [44].

IRINOTECAN

Irinotecan is an inhibitor of topoisomerase I, which unwinds double-stranded DNA, permitting repair and replication. When combined with radiation, irinotecan can lead to dose-dependent delay of cells in S phase, followed by a dose-dependent trapping in G2/M phase [45]. Irinotecan with RT has shown comparable response rates in NSCLC to traditional platinum doublets with RT, while maintaining acceptable toxicity [46]. However, when evaluated in esophageal cancer, neither irinotecan/cisplatin/RT nor cisplatin/paclitaxel/RT improved outcomes compared with standard cisplatin/5-FU/RT [47].

TIRAPAZAMINE

Tirapazamine, a hypoxia-selective cytotoxin, has demonstrated activity in cancer clinical trials. Under hypoxic conditions, tirapazamine is reduced to a radical that leads to DNA double-strand breaks, single-strand breaks, and base damage. Conversion of DNA radicals to cytotoxic DNA double strand-breaks usually requires molecular oxygen, but tirapazamine allows for full cytotoxicity to hypoxic cells [48]. Tirapazamine is also a topoisomerase II inhibitor [49].

Phase 2 testing has been completed for concurrent tirapazamine and RT in glioblastoma multiforme, advanced head and neck cancer, and cervical cancer. Tirapazamine did not reveal a survival benefit in glioblastoma multiforme [50], but did show acceptable toxicity and disease control in head and neck cancer, although it was not combined with cisplatin chemotherapy [51]. When combined with cisplatin and RT for locally advanced cervical cancer, tirapazamine appeared to have acceptable toxicity levels [52]. Further study is warranted in the CRT setting.

Table 5-2. Studies of Combined Radiotherapy and Cisplatin-Based Chemotherapy Regimens

Study	Population	Study arms	Median survival/outcome, %
Forastiere *et al.* [19]	Locally advanced laryngeal cancer	Arm 1: Cisplatin + RT Arm 2: Cisplatin + 5-FU → RT Arm 3: RT only	Laryngeal preservation/local control: 88/78* (arm 1); 75/61 (arm 2); 70/56 (arm 3)
Cooper *et al.* [20]	Postoperative high-risk head and neck cancer	Arm 1: RT Arm 2: Cisplatin + RT	2-y local control: 72 (arm 1); 82* (arm 2); significant DFS improvement overall
Furuse *et al.* [21]	Unresectable non–small cell lung cancer	Arm 1: MVP → RT Arm 2: MVP + RT	Response rate/5-y survival: 66/9 (arm 1); 84/16* (arm 2)
Turrisi *et al.* [22]	Limited-stage small cell lung cancer	Arm 1: Daily RT + cisplatin/etoposide Arm 2: Hyperfractionated RT + cisplatin/etoposide	2-y/5-y survival: 41/16 (arm 1); 47/26 (arm 2)
Rose *et al.* [23]	Stage IIB, III, IVa cervical cancer without para-aortic lymph nodes	Arm 1: Cisplatin + RT Arm 2: Cisplatin + hydroxyurea + RT Arm 3: Hydroxyurea + RT	2-y survival: 74 (arm 1); 74 (arm 2); 60 (arm 3)

*Significant difference between treatment groups.
5-FU—fluorouracil; DFS—disease-free survival; MVP—mitomycin, vindesine, platinum; RT—radiotherapy.

TEMOZOLOMIDE

Temozolomide, an oral alkylating agent, has shown activity in the treatment of glioblastoma multiforme, both as a single agent and in combination with RT. The DNA-repair enzyme, O^6-methylguanine-DNA methyltransferase (MGMT) inhibits the killing of tumor cells by alkylating agents. Promoter methylation leads to epigenetic silencing of MGMT, preventing its activity. Methylation of the MGMT promoter results in an improved response to carmustine (BCNU) and therefore improved overall and disease-free survival [53]. MGMT methylation status was confirmed to be an independent predictor for glioblastoma multiforme patients in other studies [54].

The European Organisation for Research and Treatment of Cancer (EORTC) 26981/22981 study compared RT with and without temozolomide in glioblastoma multiforme patients. The addition of temozolomide during and after RT resulted in a significant survival benefit (14.6 vs 12.1 months). The 2-year survival rate was 26.5% with RT and temozolomide compared with 10.4% for RT alone. Concomitant RT and temozolomide resulted in grade 3 or 4 hematologic toxicities in 7% of patients [55]. The methylation status of the MGMT DNA-repair gene was assessed in this cohort of patients; 45% of assessable patients had a methylated MGMT promoter. This subgroup benefited most from temozolomide [56].

MOTEXAFIN GADOLINIUM

Motexafin gadolinium, formerly gadolinium texaphyrin, was developed as a radiosensitizer for the preferential sensitization of cancers but not their surrounding tissues via a mechanism that allows uptake in both oxic and hypoxic tumor cells. It also allows tumor visualization by magnetic resonance imaging (MRI) because of the paramagnetism of gadolinium, thereby allowing for a means of localization and response to treatment.

The mechanism by which motexafin gadolinium is postulated to work is a biological redox reaction, a defense system that may play a role in protecting cells from damage caused by ionizing radiation and reactive oxygen species. Motexafin gadolinium catalytically reacts with various intracellular reducing metabolites, such as ascorbate and NADPH, to produce hydrogen peroxide and other reactive oxygen species. Changes in the intracellular redox state affect the signaling pathways controlling apoptosis and replication. Therefore, motexafin gadolinium has been shown to improve the effects of RT by a mechanism known as "futile" redox cycling, which is encountered as a property of electron-affinic molecules [57].

Phase 3 testing in patients with brain metastases from solid tumors (251 with NSCLC and 75 with other cancers), receiving whole-brain radiation therapy (WBRT) with or without motexafin gadolinium showed no difference in median survival between the two groups (5.2 months for motexafin gadolinium and WBRT group vs 4.9 months for WBRT alone group). There was also no difference in time to neurologic progression. However, in the cohort with NSCLC, there was an improvement in time to neurologic progression (median not reached for motexafin gadolinium and WBRT group vs 7.4 months for WBRT alone group) and neurocognitive function [58]. The most frequent adverse effects seen with motexafin gadolinium were dose-dependent, transient, greenish skin, urine, and scleral discoloration due to the dark-green color of motexafin gadolinium itself [59]. In another study in which motexafin gadolinium was given during the course of WBRT [60], patients with brain metastases due to lung cancer appeared to benefit the most from the perspective of improved memory and executive and neurologic function.

TARGETED AGENTS

EPIDERMAL GROWTH FACTOR RECEPTOR INHIBITORS

The epidermal growth factor receptor (EGFR) family of receptors regulates mesenchymal-epithelial interactions during growth and development. Four known receptors: EGFR, HER2 (ERBB2), HER3 (ERBB3), and HER4 (ERBB4) contain an extracellular ligand-binding domain, transmembrane domain, and an intracellular tyrosine kinase domain [61,62]. Ligand binding activates dimerization, which results in phosphorylation and activation of various signaling cascades (Fig. 5-1). Receptor activation can initiate multiple downstream signal transduction pathways including protein kinase C (PKC), PI3K-AKT, and STAT pathways [63].

CETUXIMAB

Cetuximab (Erbitux, ImClone Systems, Inc., New York, NY, and Bristol-Myers Squibb, Princeton, NJ) is an anti-EGFR monoclonal antibody that binds to the extracellular domain of EGFR and interferes with ligand binding and dimerization. Studies have demonstrated that upregulation of EGFR family receptors leads to radioresistance in many cancers, including breast [64], brain [65], and head and neck cancer [66]. In some patients, EGFR upregulation results in decreased local control [67]. In vitro combination of radiation and EGFR inhibitors results in modest radiosensitization. In some cases, radiosensitization is more pronounced in vivo than in vitro and with fractionated- as opposed to single-dose irradiation [68]. EGFR or HER2 inhibitors arrest cells in the G1 phase with a subsequent decrease in the S phase, leading to decreased proliferation. Some models suggest that when EGFR inhibitors are combined with radiation, there is an increase in apoptosis and interference with repair of radiation-induced DNA damage [69]. Feng *et al.* [70] recently reported on the effects of cetuximab and gefitinib with or without gemcitabine in a head and neck cancer animal model. The researchers found EGFR inhibition delayed tumor doubling time from 40 days with gemcitabine and radiation to 106 and 66 days if cetuximab or gefitinib were added respectively (both $P <$ 0.005). Cetuximab caused prolonged suppression of EGFR, STAT3, and Bcl-X$_1$; these may be candidates for treatment response biomarkers in future clinical trials.

The primary toxicity of cetuximab is an acneiform skin rash secondary to known EGFR inhibition in the epidermis of hair follicles. As a single agent, cetuximab has modest activity, but is enhanced when combined with cytotoxic therapy. In a phase 3 trial, patients with stage III/IV squamous cell carcinoma of the oropharynx, hypopharynx, or larynx were treated with standard RT (three different fractionation schedules) with or without cetuximab [71]. Concurrent chemotherapy was not given. Three-year and median survival rates were significantly improved with RT plus cetuximab compared with RT alone (57% vs 44% and 54 vs 28 months, respectively; $P =$ 0.02). There was an increase in skin toxicity but not mucosal toxicity. Phase 2 studies have evaluated the role of adding cetuximab to CRT for patients with esophageal and stomach cancer [72]. When cetuximab was combined with paclitaxel, carboplatin, and radiation, there was an increased incidence of rash but no increase in mucositis or esophagitis.

TRASTUZUMAB

Overexpression of HER2/neu in cancer cells results in homodimerization and activation of the tyrosine kinase receptor and survival pathways [73]. Trastuzumab is a monoclonal antibody that inhibits uncontrolled HER2/neu amplification by binding to the extracellular domain, blocking heterodimerization, and resulting in receptor internalization with subsequent degradation [74]. Koukourakis *et al.* [75] reported on the efficacy of concurrent trastuzumab, amifostine, liposomal doxorubicin, and docetaxel with hypofractionated radiation for the treatment of c-erbB-2–positive breast cancer. Inclusion of trastuzumab with CRT did not increase radiation or systemic toxicity. Coadministration of aggressive RT with docetaxel and liposomal doxorubicin and trastuzumab was feasible when supported with amifostine. In a phase 1 study of esophageal adenocarcinoma, trastuzumab has been combined with RT (50.4 Gy), paclitaxel, and cisplatin [76]. HER-2/neu was overexpressed in approximately one third of the 12 patients with esophageal adenocarcinoma. The researchers concluded that trastuzumab can be safely added to cisplatin, paclitaxel, and radiation.

PANITUMUMAB

Panitumumab (Vectibix, Amgen Inc., Thousand Oaks, CA) is a fully humanized anti-EGFR antibody generated using the transgenic Xeno-Mouse technology (Amgen Inc.) [77]. It is an IgG$_2$ subclass monoclonal antibody and does not mediate a significant level of antibody-dependent cellular cytotoxicity on EGFR-expressing tumor cells. Patients with refractory colorectal cancer had an improved response with panitumumab, but there was no significant benefit seen in disease-free or overall survival. Panitumumab is being evaluated in other sites such as head and neck cancer [78], but at this time, there have not been any studies combining panitumumab with radiation.

SMALL MOLECULE TYROSINE KINASE INHIBITORS

Gefitinib (Iressa, AstraZeneca, Wilmington, DE) and erlotinib (Tarceva, OSI Pharmaceuticals/Genentech, San Francisco, CA) are two small molecule tyrosine kinase inhibitors of EGFR. The primary toxicities of gefitinib and erlotinib are skin effects (similar to Erbitux) and diarrhea; there are also rare reports of life-threatening interstitial lung disease for both agents.

GEFITINIB

When combined with full-dose chemotherapy and radiation, gefitinib can result in additional toxicity. One study combined capecitabine, gefitinib (250 mg daily), and RT (50.4 Gy to tumor and lymph nodes) for locally advanced pancreatic cancer. The study was closed due to 6 of 10 patients developing a dose-limiting toxicity (diarrhea) [79].

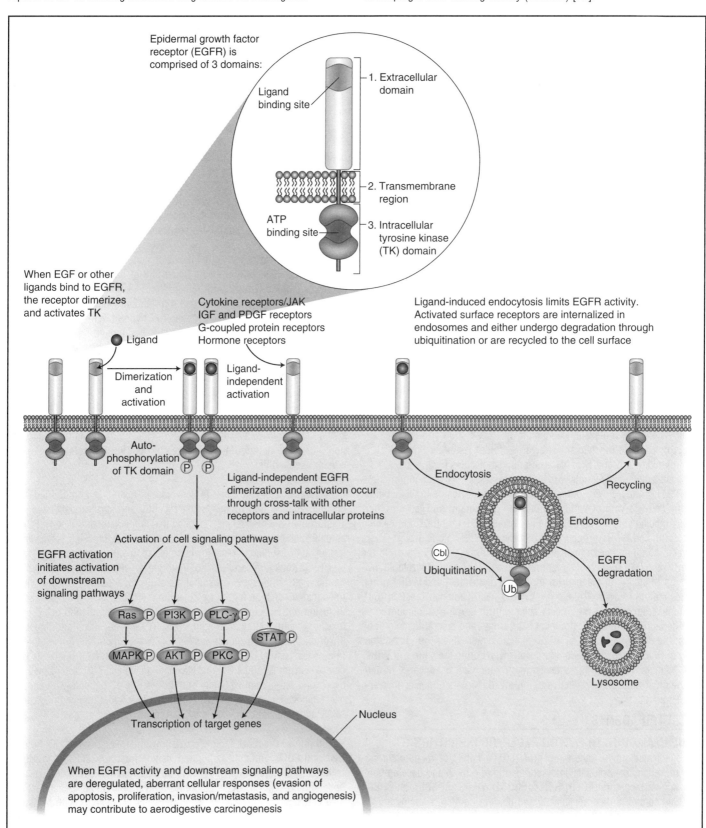

Figure 5-1. Epidermal growth factor receptor activation, processing, and signaling. ATP—adenosine triphosphate; IGF—insulin-like growth factor; PDGF—platelet-derived growth factor. (*Adapted from* Karamouzis *et al.* [106].)

Another study by Maurel *et al.* [80] combined gefitinib with concurrent RT and gemcitabine in patients with locally advanced pancreatic cancer. Gemcitabine was administered at 100, 150, and 200 mg/m²/d in a 2-hour infusion weekly with gefitinib (250 mg/d). The targeted irradiated volume included the tumor plus a 2-cm margin. Patients with a tumor volume greater than 500 cm³ were excluded. There were no dose-limiting toxicities; common toxicities were mild neutropenia, asthenia, diarrhea, cutaneous rash, and nausea/vomiting. The median progression-free survival was 3.7 months, and the median overall survival was 7.5 months (95% CI, 5.2–9.9). No significant reduction of vascular endothelial growth factor (VEGF) and interleukin-8 was observed after treatment. Combined gefitinib, RT, and gemcitabine had an acceptable toxicity profile but minimal activity in locally advanced pancreatic cancer. These studies suggest that small fields should be used when adding gefitinib to CRT in patients with locally advanced pancreatic cancer.

A recent phase 1 trial combined gefitinib with radiation for patients with locally advanced squamous cell head and neck cancer [81]. Patients with intermediate-stage disease were treated with concomitant boost RT with escalating doses of gefitinib (250 or 500 mg; cohort I). Patients with high-risk disease were treated with daily gefitinib (250 or 500 mg), weekly cisplatin (30 mg/m²), and once-daily RT (cohort II). Patients also received post-RT gefitinib at 250 mg daily for a period of up to 2 years. Gefitinib (250 or 500 mg daily) was well tolerated with concomitant boost RT or concurrent CRT with weekly cisplatin. Protracted administration of gefitinib for up to 2 years at 250 mg daily was also well tolerated.

ERLOTINIB

Erlotinib has been evaluated in several clinical trials. The combination of gemcitabine and erlotinib was found to be superior to gemcitabine alone in patients with locally advanced or metastatic pancreatic cancer, with a significant improvement in survival (1-year survival 17% vs 24%) [82]. This led to the integration of erlotinib into various treatment paradigms for pancreatic cancer. Erlotinib has been shown to be a radiosensitizer in vivo [83]. In a study by Duffy *et al.* [84], patients with unresectable pancreatic cancer received RT (50.4 Gy) with a fixed dose of gemcitabine at 40 mg/m² (over 30 minutes) twice weekly and erlotinib (maximum tolerated dose, 100 mg/d). Seventeen patients were assessable for response. The partial response rate was 35%, and 53% had stable disease. The median survival for all patients was an encouraging 18.7 months.

Iannitti *et al.* [85] recently reported another phase 1 study combining erlotinib (50–150 mg/d), paclitaxel, and RT (50.4 Gy to tumor and lymph nodes) followed by maintenance erlotinib (150 mg/d) for patients with unresectable or incompletely resected pancreatic cancer. The maximum tolerated dose of erlotinib was 50 mg when combined with paclitaxel and concurrent RT. Reported toxicities included diarrhea, dehydration, rash, myelosuppression, and small bowel stricture. In this study, the median survival of 13 patients with locally advanced pancreatic cancer was 14 months, and 46% had a partial response. Ma *et al.* [86] recently reported on a phase 1 trial in which patients with resected pancreatic cancer received combined capecitabine, erlotinib, and RT (50.4 Gy). Their preliminary analysis suggests that this regimen is safe; efficacy results are pending.

Krishnan *et al.* [87] reported on a phase 1 trial of erlotinib with RT in patients with glioblastoma multiforme. Patients received 1 week of erlotinib followed by erlotinib with RT (60 Gy). Median time to progression was 26 weeks, and median survival was 55 weeks. Toxicity was tolerable. Temozolomide has now been added to erlotinib in glioblastoma multiforme patients, and accrual is in progress.

Dobelbower *et al.* [88] combined RT (50.4 Gy), 5-FU, cisplatin, and erlotinib in patients with esophageal carcinoma. Eleven patients with squamous or adenocarcinoma of the esophagus were enrolled. The phase 1 study demonstrates the safety and tolerability of erlotinib delivered at 150 mg/d with concurrent 5-FU, cisplatin, and thoracic RT. The major toxicities encountered were grade 1 to 2 diarrhea, grade 1 skin rash, grade 1 to 3 nausea, and grade 3 dehydration. Additional studies are needed to determine how to safely combine targeted EGFR inhibitors with chemotherapy and radiation.

ANGIOGENESIS INHIBITORS

BEVACIZUMAB

Angiogenesis is necessary for tumor growth and is partially mediated by VEGF receptors (VEGFR). Bevacizumab is a humanized mouse monoclonal antibody that binds VEGFR. In a phase 3 trial of metastatic colorectal patients, bevacizumab was combined with continuous infusion 5-FU, leucovorin, and irinotecan and showed prolonged overall survival and DFS compared with chemotherapy alone [89]. Czito *et al.* [90] recently reported a phase 1 trial evaluating the combination of bevacizumab, capecitabine, oxaliplatin, and RT (50.4 Gy) in patients with rectal cancer. All patients (*N* = 11) were evaluable for toxicity and efficacy. The recommended phase 2 dose was bevacizumab 15 mg/kg on day 1 plus 10 mg/kg on days 8 and 22, oxaliplatin 50 mg/m² weekly, and capecitabine 625 mg/m² twice daily on Monday through Friday. Six patients had clinical responses, two had a pathologic complete response, and three had microscopic disease only. This regimen appears tolerable, with encouraging response rates. For a thorough summary of bevacizumab, readers should refer to the review by Willett *et al.* [91].

NUCLEAR FACTOR KAPPA B INHIBITORS

BORTEZOMIB

Nuclear factor kappa B (NF-κB) is a transcription factor thought to be a potentially important inhibitor of apoptosis when initiated by chemotherapy and/or RT. NF-κB is a collection of homodimers and heterodimers comprising a family of five subunits. Specific heterodimers result in the inhibition of apoptosis [92]. NF-κB is bound by a repressor protein known as I-κB. When I-κB is phosphorylated by I-κB kinase (IKK), NF-κB dimers translocate from the cytoplasm into the nucleus where they bind to a large number of promoter elements that influence apoptosis. Nonspecific inhibition of NF-κB can be achieved by proteasome inhibitors, which prevent degradation of I-κB thus inhibiting NF-κB upregulation. The proteasome inhibitor bortezomib (Velcade, Millenium Pharmaceuticals, Cambridge, MA) resulted in enhanced radiosensitization of LoVo colorectal cancer cells in a xenograft model [93]. Van Waes *et al.* [94] evaluated bortezomib and reirradiation in patients with recurrent head and neck squamous cell carcinoma and found that the maximally tolerated dose of bortezomib was exceeded at a dose of 0.6 mg/m². Bortezomib induced detectable differences in NF-κB localization, apoptosis, and NF-κB–modulated genes and cytokines in tumor and serum, resulting in tumor reduction. Therefore, other schedules of bortezomib combined with primary RT or reirradiation may merit future investigation. However, a combination of bortezomib with radiation may inhibit normal tissue repair, resulting in additional toxicity. More studies are needed to determine the efficacy of bortezomib with RT in various malignancies.

HISTONE DEACETYLASE INHIBITORS

The packaging and compaction of DNA into chromatin is necessary for transcription, replication, and repair [95]. Chromatin comprises nucleosomes that are made up of four core histones (H2A, H2B, H3, and H4) [96]. Chromatin structure can be altered by posttranslational acetylation. The acetylation status of histones is balanced by two actions: histone acetyltransferase (HAT) and histone deacetylase (HDAC). Alteration of these actions can induce differentiation, cell cycle arrest, apoptosis, growth inhibition, and cell death. HDAC inhibitors have been found to act as radiosensitizers to tumor cells and concurrently protect normal structures from radiation damage. Multiple studies have shown that HDAC inhibitors such as sodium butyrate, phenylbutyrate [97], valproic acid [98], benzamides (MS-275) [99], and suberoylanilide hydroxamic acid (SAHA) [100] can enhance the sensitivity of various cancer cell lines to radiation. Treatment of cells with HDAC inhibitors prior to irradiation results in increased levels of γH2AX, suggesting an increase in double-strand breaks with combination therapy compared with radiation alone [101]. These studies suggest a change in chromatin conformation results in increased double-strand breaks [102]. HDAC inhibitors also appear to decrease the expression of DNA repair proteins Ku70 and Ku86 [103]. The exact mechanisms that lead to the enhanced radiosensitivity and paradoxical radioprotection of HDAC inhibitors for each malignancy are unknown and require additional study.

CONCLUSIONS

This chapter outlines some of the common chemotherapeutic and targeted therapies that have been evaluated for their ability to sensitize cancer cells to irradiation. Early radiation studies relied heavily on in vitro clonogenic survival curves to determine the optimal dose of drug and radiation necessary to impose a therapeutic benefit. Historically, lower doses of chemotherapy were combined with full-dose RT to obtain an optimal sensitizing effect. As outlined in this chapter, unique combinations of chemotherapy and targeted agents are being evaluated to further enhance the therapeutic benefit of combined modality therapy. Some targeted therapies cannot be adequately evaluated in vitro. These limitations have paved the way for sophisticated in vivo experiments attempting to closely simulate combined modality therapy that mimics treatment in the clinical setting. New orthotopic and transgenic animal models [104] combined with small animal imaging closely approximate treatment conditions that can potentially be translated into phase 1 clinical trials. These models should lead to a deeper understanding of the mechanisms underlying radiation sensitization prior to being tested in the clinic.

It has become increasingly difficult to determine the optimal combinations of chemotherapeutic and targeted agents with radiation. As we gain a greater understanding of the complicated and unique mechanisms of tumor growth and development it is clear that one combined modality regimen will not be equally effective for all patients with a specific tumor type. Therefore, patient selection becomes paramount and stresses the need to better determine which patients are more likely to respond to a specific regimen based on genetic mutations or tumor markers [105]. It is imperative that future clinical trials include collection of serum and tumor samples to better select patients for specific therapies. Future combinations of chemotherapy, targeted therapy, immunotherapy, and radiation should lead to improved outcomes and less treatment-related toxicity.

REFERENCES

1. Kolesnick R, Fuks Z: Radiation and ceramide-induced apoptosis. *Oncogene* 2003, 22:5897–5906.

2. Deeken JF, Loscher W: The blood-brain barrier and cancer: transporters, treatment, and Trojan horses. *Clin Cancer Res* 2007, 13:1663–1674.

3. Blackstock AW, Kwock L, Branch C, *et al.*: Tumor retention of 5-fluorouracil following irradiation observed using 19F nuclear magnetic resonance spectroscopy. *Int J Radiat Oncol Biol Phys* 1996, 36:641–648.

4. Hall EJ: *Radiobiology for the Radiologist*, edn 5. Philadelphia: Lippincott Williams & Wilkins; 2000.

5. Shewach DS, Lawrence TS: Antimetabolite radiosensitizers. *J Clin Oncol* 2007, 25:4043–4050.

6. Herskovic A, Martz K, al-Sarraf M, *et al.*: Combined chemotherapy and radiotherapy compared with radiotherapy alone in patients with cancer of the esophagus. *N Engl J Med* 1992, 326:1593–1598.

7. Macdonald JS: Clinical overview: adjuvant therapy of gastrointestinal cancer. *Cancer Chemother Pharmacol* 2004, 54(Suppl 1):S4–S11.

8. Kalser MH, Ellenberg SS: Pancreatic cancer: adjuvant combined radiation and chemotherapy following curative resection. *Arch Surg* 1985, 120:899–903.

9. Sauer R, Becker H, Hohenberger W, *et al.*: German Rectal Cancer Study Group: Preoperative versus postoperative chemoradiotherapy for rectal cancer. *N Engl J Med* 2004, 351:1731–1740.

10. Brizel DM, Albers ME, Fisher SR, *et al.*: Hyperfractionated irradiation with or without concurrent chemotherapy for locally advanced head and neck cancer. *N Engl J Med* 1998, 338:1798–1804.

11. Diaz-Rubio E, Tabernero J, Gomez-Espana A, *et al.*: Spanish Cooperative Group for the Treatment of Digestive Tumors Trial: Phase III study of capecitabine plus oxaliplatin compared with continuous-infusion fluorouracil plus oxaliplatin as first-line therapy in metastatic colorectal cancer: final report of the Spanish Cooperative Group for the Treatment of Digestive Tumors Trial. *J Clin Oncol* 2007, 25:4224–4230.

12. Mackean M, Planting A, Twelves C, *et al.*: Phase I and pharmacologic study of intermittent twice-daily oral therapy with capecitabine in patients with advanced and/or metastatic cancer. *J Clin Oncol* 1998, 16:2977–2985.

13. Yang LX, Double EB, O'Hara JA, Wang HJ: Production of DNA double-strand breaks by interactions between carboplatin and radiation: a potential mechanism for radiopotentiation. *Radiat Res* 1995, 143:309–315.

14. Yang LX, Double EB, Wang HJ: Irradiation enhances cellular uptake of carboplatin. *Int J Radiat Oncol Biol Phys* 1995, 33:641–646.

15. Amorino GP, Freeman ML, Carbone DP, *et al.*: Radiopotentiation by the oral platinum agent, JM216: role of repair inhibition. *Int J Radiat Oncol Biol Phys* 1999, 44:399–405.

16. Saris CP, van de Vaart PJ, Rietbroek RC, Blommaert FA: In vitro formation of DNA adducts by cisplatin, lobaplatin and oxaliplatin in calf thymus DNA in solution and in cultured human cells. *Carcinogenesis* 1996, 17:2763–2769.

17. Rixe O, Ortuzar W, Alvarez M, *et al.*: Oxaliplatin, tetraplatin, cisplatin, and carboplatin: spectrum of activity in drug-resistant cell lines and in the cell lines of the National Cancer Institute's Anticancer Drug Screen Panel. *Biochem Pharmacol* 1996, 52:1855–1865.

18. Woynarowski JM, Faivre S, Herzig MC, *et al.*: Oxaliplatin-induced damage of cellular DNA. *Mol Pharmacol* 2000, 58:920–927.

19. Forastiere AA, Goepfert H, Maor M, *et al.*: Concurrent chemotherapy and radiotherapy for organ preservation in advanced laryngeal cancer. *N Engl J Med* 2003, 349:2091–2098.

20. Cooper JS, Pajak TF, Forastiere AA, *et al.*: Radiation Therapy Oncology Group 9501/Intergroup: Postoperative concurrent radiotherapy and chemotherapy for high-risk squamous-cell carcinoma of the head and neck. *N Engl J Med* 2004, 350:1937–1944.

21. Furuse K, Fukuoka M, Kawahara M, *et al.*: Phase III study of concurrent versus sequential thoracic radiotherapy in combination with mitomycin, vindesine, and cisplatin in unresectable stage III non-small-cell lung cancer. *J Clin Oncol* 1999, 17:2692–2699.

22. Turrisi AT III, Kim K, Blum R, *et al.*: Twice-daily compared with once-daily thoracic radiotherapy in limited small-cell lung cancer treated concurrently with cisplatin and etoposide. *N Engl J Med* 1999, 340:265–271.

23. Rose PG, Bundy BN, Watkins EB, *et al.*: Concurrent cisplatin-based radiotherapy and chemotherapy for locally advanced cervical cancer. *N Engl J Med* 1999, 340:1144–1153.

24. Shipley WU, Kaufman DS, Zehr E, *et al.*: Selective bladder preservation by combined modality protocol treatment: long-term outcomes of 190 patients with invasive bladder cancer. *Urology* 2002, 60:62–67; discussion 67–68.

25. de Gramont A, Vignoud J, Tournigand C, *et al.*: Oxaliplatin with high-dose leucovorin and 5-fluorouracil 48-hour continuous infusion in pretreated metastatic colorectal cancer. *Eur J Cancer* 1997, 33:214–219.

26. Gerard JP, Chapet O, Nemoz C, *et al.*: Preoperative concurrent chemoradiotherapy in locally advanced rectal cancer with high-dose radiation and oxaliplatin-containing regimen: the Lyon R0-04 phase II trial. *J Clin Oncol* 2003, 21:1119–1124.

27. Desai SP, Ben-Josef E, Normolle DP, *et al.*: Phase I study of oxaliplatin, full-dose gemcitabine, and concurrent radiation therapy in pancreatic cancer. *J Clin Oncol* 2007, 25:4587–4592.

28. Flanagan SA, Robinson BW, Krokosky CM, Shewach DS: Mismatched nucleotides as the lesions responsible for radiosensitization with gemcitabine: a new paradigm for antimetabolite radiosensitizers. *Mol Cancer Ther* 2007, 6:1858–1868.

29. Latz D, Fleckenstein K, Eble M, *et al.*: Radiosensitizing potential of gemcitabine (2',2'-difluoro-2'-deoxycytidine) within the cell cycle in vitro. *Int J Radiat Oncol Biol Phys* 1998, 41:875–882.

30. Robinson BW, Im MM, Ljungman M, *et al.*: Enhanced radiosensitization with gemcitabine in mismatch repair-deficient HCT116 cells. *Cancer Res* 2003, 63:6935–6941.

31. Wachters FM, van Putten JW, Maring JG, *et al.*: Selective targeting of homologous DNA recombination repair by gemcitabine. *Int J Radiat Oncol Biol Phys* 2003, 57:553–562.

32. McGinn CJ, Zalupski MM, Shureiqi I, *et al.*: Phase I trial of radiation dose escalation with concurrent weekly full-dose gemcitabine in patients with advanced pancreatic cancer. *J Clin Oncol* 2001, 19:4202–4208.

33. Talamonti MS, Small W Jr, Mulcahy MF, *et al.*: A multi-institutional phase II trial of preoperative full-dose gemcitabine and concurrent radiation for patients with potentially resectable pancreatic carcinoma. *Ann Surg Oncol* 2006, 13:150–158.

34. Demols A, Peeters M, Polus M, *et al.*: Adjuvant gemcitabine and concurrent continuous radiation (45 Gy) for resected pancreatic head carcinoma: a multicenter Belgian phase II study. *Int J Radiat Oncol Biol Phys* 2005, 62:1351–1356.

35. Blackstock AW, Mornex F, Partensky C, *et al.*: Adjuvant gemcitabine and concurrent radiation for patients with resected pancreatic cancer: a phase II study. *Br J Cancer* 2006, 95:260–265.

36. Crane CH, Varadhachary G, Wolff RA, *et al.*: The argument for pre-operative chemoradiation for localized, radiographically resectable pancreatic cancer. *Best Pract Res Clin Gastroenterol* 2006, 20:365–382.

37. Aguilar-Ponce J, Granados-Garcia M, Villavicencio V, *et al.*: Phase II trial of gemcitabine concurrent with radiation for locally advanced squamous cell carcinoma of the head and neck. *Ann Oncol* 2004, 15:301–306.

38. Kent E, Sandler H, Montie J, *et al.*: Combined-modality therapy with gemcitabine and radiotherapy as a bladder preservation strategy: results of a phase I trial. *J Clin Oncol* 2004, 22:2540–2545.

39. Suh WW, Schott AF, Hayman JA, *et al.*: A phase I dose escalation trial of gemcitabine with radiotherapy for breast cancer in the treatment of unresectable chest wall recurrences. *Breast J* 2004, 10:204–210.

40. Hirsh V, Soulieres D, Duclos M, *et al.*: Phase II multicenter trial with carboplatin and gemcitabine induction chemotherapy followed by radiotherapy concomitantly with low-dose paclitaxel and gemcitabine for stage IIIA and IIIB non-small cell lung cancer. *J Thorac Oncol* 2007, 2:927–932.

41. Nabell L, Spencer S: Docetaxel with concurrent radiotherapy in head and neck cancer. *Semin Oncol* 2003, 30(Suppl 18):89–93.

42. Milas L, Milas MM, Mason KA: Combination of taxanes with radiation: preclinical studies. *Semin Radiat Oncol* 1999, 9(Suppl 1):12–26.

43. Liebmann J, Cook JA, Fisher J, *et al.*: In vitro studies of Taxol as a radiation sensitizer in human tumor cells. *J Natl Cancer Inst* 1994, 86:441–446.

44. Suntharalingam M, Haas ML, Conley BA, *et al.*: The use of carboplatin and paclitaxel with daily radiotherapy in patients with locally advanced squamous cell carcinomas of the head and neck. *Int J Radiat Oncol Biol Phys* 2000, 47:49–56.

45. Falk SJ, Smith PJ: DNA damaging and cell cycle effects of the topoisomerase I poison camptothecin in irradiated human cells. *Int J Radiat Biol* 1992, 61:749–757.

46. Takeda K, Negoro S, Kudoh S, *et al.*: Phase I/II study of weekly irinotecan and concurrent radiation therapy for locally advanced non-small cell lung cancer. *Br J Cancer* 1999, 79:1462–1467.

47. Kleinberg L, Powell ME, Forastiere A, *et al.*: E1201: an Eastern Cooperative Oncology Group (ECOG) randomized phase II trial of neoadjuvant preoperative paclitaxel/cisplatin/RT or irinotecan/cisplatin/RT in endoscopy with ultrasound (EUS) staged adenocarcinoma of the esophagus [ASCO abstract]. *J Clin Oncol* 2007, 25(18S):4533.

48. Denny WA: The role of hypoxia-activated prodrugs in cancer therapy. *Lancet Oncol* 2000, 1:25–29.

49. Peters KB, Brown JM: Tirapazamine: a hypoxia-activated topoisomerase II poison. *Cancer Res* 2002, 62:5248–5253.

50. Del Rowe J, Scott C, Werner-Wasik M, *et al.*: Single-arm, open-label phase II study of intravenously administered tirapazamine and radiation therapy for glioblastoma multiforme. *J Clin Oncol* 2000, 18:1254–1259.

51. Lee DJ, Trotti A, Spencer S, *et al.*: Concurrent tirapazamine and radiotherapy for advanced head and neck carcinomas: a phase II study. *Int J Radiat Oncol Biol Phys* 1998, 42:811–815.

52. Craighead PS, Pearcey R, Stuart G: A phase I/II evaluation of tirapazamine administered intravenously concurrent with cisplatin and radiotherapy in women with locally advanced cervical cancer. *Int J Radiat Oncol Biol Phys* 2000, 48:791–795.

53. Esteller M, Garcia-Foncillas J, Andion E, *et al.*: Inactivation of the DNA-repair gene MGMT and the clinical response of gliomas to alkylating agents. *N Engl J Med* 2000, 343:1350–1354.

54. Hegi ME, Diserens AC, Godard S, *et al.*: Clinical trial substantiates the predictive value of O-6-methylguanine-DNA methyltransferase promoter methylation in glioblastoma patients treated with temozolomide. *Clin Cancer Res* 2004, 10:1871–1874.

55. Stupp R, Mason WP, van den Bent MJ, *et al.*: European Organisation for Research and Treatment of Cancer Brain Tumor and Radiotherapy Groups, National Cancer Institute of Canada Clinical Trials Group: Radiotherapy plus concomitant and adjuvant temozolomide for glioblastoma. *N Engl J Med* 2005, 352:987–996.

56. Hegi ME, Diserens AC, Gorlia T, *et al.*: MGMT gene silencing and benefit from temozolomide in glioblastoma. *N Engl J Med* 2005, 352:997–1003.

57. Magda D, Lepp C, Gerasimchuk N, *et al.*: Redox cycling by motexafin gadolinium enhances cellular response to ionizing radiation by forming reactive oxygen species. *Int J Radiat Oncol Biol Phys* 2001, 51:1025–1036.

58. Mehta MP, Rodrigus P, Terhaard CH, *et al.*: Survival and neurologic outcomes in a randomized trial of motexafin gadolinium and whole-brain radiation therapy in brain metastases. *J Clin Oncol* 2003, 21:2529–2536.

59. Carde P, Timmerman R, Mehta MP, *et al.*: Multicenter phase Ib/II trial of the radiation enhancer motexafin gadolinium in patients with brain metastases. *J Clin Oncol* 2001, 19:2074–2083.

60. Meyers CA, Smith JA, Bezjak A, *et al.*: Neurocognitive function and progression in patients with brain metastases treated with whole-brain radiation and motexafin gadolinium: results of a randomized phase III trial. *J Clin Oncol* 2004, 22:157–165.

61. Yarden Y: The EGFR family and its ligands in human cancer: signalling mechanisms and therapeutic opportunities. *Eur J Cancer* 2001, 37(Suppl 4):S3–S8.

62. Ullrich A, Schlessinger J: Signal transduction by receptors with tyrosine kinase activity. *Cell* 1990, 61:203–212.

63. Schlessinger J: Cell signaling by receptor tyrosine kinases. *Cell* 2000, 103:211–225.

64. Pietras RJ, Poen JC, Gallardo D, *et al.*: Monoclonal antibody to HER-2/neureceptor modulates repair of radiation-induced DNA damage and enhances radiosensitivity of human breast cancer cells overexpressing this oncogene. *Cancer Res* 1999, 59:1347–1355.

65. Barker FG II, Simmons ML, Chang SM, *et al.*: EGFR overexpression and radiation response in glioblastoma multiforme. *Int J Radiat Oncol Biol Phys* 2001, 51:410–418.

66. Miyaguchi M, Takeuchi T, Morimoto K, Kubo T: Correlation of epidermal growth factor receptor and radiosensitivity in human maxillary carcinoma cell lines. *Acta Otolaryngol* 1998, 118:428–431.

67. Gupta AK, McKenna WG, Weber CN, *et al.*: Local recurrence in head and neck cancer: relationship to radiation resistance and signal transduction. *Clin Cancer Res* 2002, 8:885–892.

68. Raben D, Helfrich B, Bunn PA Jr: Targeted therapies for non-small-cell lung cancer: biology, rationale, and preclinical results from a radiation oncology perspective. *Int J Radiat Oncol Biol Phys* 2004, 59(Suppl):27–38.

69. Hidalgo M: Erlotinib: preclinical investigations. *Oncology (Williston Park)* 2003, 17(Suppl 12):11–16.

70. Feng FY, Lopez CA, Normolle DP, *et al.*: Effect of epidermal growth factor receptor inhibitor class in the treatment of head and neck cancer with concurrent radiochemotherapy in vivo. *Clin Cancer Res* 2007, 13:2512–2518.

71. Bonner JA, Harari PM, Giralt J, *et al.*: Radiotherapy plus cetuximab for squamous-cell carcinoma of the head and neck. *N Engl J Med* 2006, 354:567–578.

72. Mukogawa T, Koyama F, Tachibana M, *et al.*: Adenovirus-mediated gene transduction of truncated I kappa B alpha enhances radiosensitivity in human colon cancer cells. *Cancer Sci* 2003, 94:745–750.

73. Di Fiore PP, Pierce JH, Kraus MH, *et al.*: erbB-2 is a potent oncogene when overexpressed in NIH/3T3 cells. *Science* 1987, 237:178–182.

74. Pegram MD, Konecny G, Slamon DJ: The molecular and cellular biology of HER2/neu gene amplification/overexpression and the clinical development of Herceptin (trastuzumab) therapy for breast cancer. *Cancer Treat Res* 2000, 103:57–75.

75. Koukourakis MI, Manavis J, Simopoulos C, *et al.*: Hypofractionated accelerated radiotherapy with cytoprotection combined with trastuzumab, liposomal doxorubicin, and docetaxel in c-erbB-2-positive breast cancer. *Am J Clin Oncol* 2005, 28:495–500.

76. Safran H, DiPetrillo T, Nadeem A, *et al.*: Trastuzumab, paclitaxel, cisplatin, and radiation for adenocarcinoma of the esophagus: a phase I study. *Cancer Invest* 2004, 22:670–677.

77. Zhu Z: Targeted cancer therapies based on antibodies directed against epidermal growth factor receptor: status and perspectives. *Acta Pharmacol Sin* 2007, 28:1476–1493.

78. Harari PM: Stepwise progress in epidermal growth factor receptor/radiation studies for head and neck cancer. *Int J Radiat Oncol Biol Phys* 2007, 69(Suppl):S25–S27.

79. Czito BG, Willett CG, Bendell JC, *et al.*: Increased toxicity with gefitinib, capecitabine, and radiation therapy in pancreatic and rectal cancer: phase I trial results. *J Clin Oncol* 2006, 24:656–662.

80. Maurel J, Martin-Richard M, Conill C, *et al.*: Phase I trial of gefitinib with concurrent radiotherapy and fixed 2-h gemcitabine infusion, in locally advanced pancreatic cancer. *Int J Radiat Oncol Biol Phys* 2006, 66:1391–1398.

81. Chen C, Kane M, Song J, *et al.*: Phase I trial of gefitinib in combination with radiation or chemoradiation for patients with locally advanced squamous cell head and neck cancer. *J Clin Oncol* 2007, 25:4880–4886.

82. Dragovich T, Huberman M, Von Hoff DD, *et al.*: Erlotinib plus gemcitabine in patients with unresectable pancreatic cancer and other solid tumors: phase IB trial. *Cancer Chemother Pharmacol* 2007, 60:295–303.

83. Chinnaiyan P, Huang S, Vallabhaneni G, *et al.*: Mechanisms of enhanced radiation response following epidermal growth factor receptor signaling inhibition by erlotinib (Tarceva). *Cancer Res* 2005, 65:3328–3335.

84. Duffy A, Kortmansky J, Schwartz GK, *et al.*: A phase I study of erlotinib in combination with gemcitabine and radiation in locally advanced, non-operable pancreatic adenocarcinoma. *Ann Oncol* 2008, 19:86–91.

85. Iannitti D, Dipetrillo T, Akerman P, *et al.*: Erlotinib and chemoradiation followed by maintenance erlotinib for locally advanced pancreatic cancer: a phase I study. *Am J Clin Oncol* 2005, 28:570–575.

86. Ma W, Herman JM, Jimeno A, *et al.*: A phase I tolerability and pharmacokinetic study of adjuvant erlotinib and capecitabine with concurrent radiation in resected pancreatic cancer [abstract]. *Presented at the 2007 ASCO/ASTRO Gastrointestinal Cancers Symposium*; January 19–21, 2007; Orlando, FL.

87. Krishnan S, Brown PD, Ballman KV, *et al.*: North Central Cancer Treatment Group: Phase I trial of erlotinib with radiation therapy in patients with glioblastoma multiforme: results of North Central Cancer Treatment Group protocol N0177. *Int J Radiat Oncol Biol Phys* 2006, 65:1192–1199.

88. Dobelbower MC, Russo SM, Raisch KP, *et al.*: Epidermal growth factor receptor tyrosine kinase inhibitor, erlotinib, and concurrent 5-fluorouracil, cisplatin and radiotherapy for patients with esophageal cancer: a phase I study. *Anticancer Drugs* 2006, 17:95–102.

89. Hurwitz H, Fehrenbacher L, Novotny W, *et al.*: Bevacizumab plus irinotecan, fluorouracil, and leucovorin for metastatic colorectal cancer. *N Engl J Med* 2004, 350:2335–2342.

90. Czito BG, Bendell JC, Willett CG, *et al.*: Bevacizumab, oxaliplatin, and capecitabine with radiation therapy in rectal cancer: phase I trial results. *Int J Radiat Oncol Biol Phys* 2007, 68:472–478.

91. Willett CG, Kozin SV, Duda DG, *et al.*: Combined vascular endothelial growth factor-targeted therapy and radiotherapy for rectal cancer: theory and clinical practice. *Semin Oncol* 2006, 33(Suppl 10):S35–S40.

92. Roccaro AM, Vacca A, Ribatti D: Bortezomib in the treatment of cancer. *Recent Patents Anticancer Drug Discov* 2006, 1:397–403.

93. Russo SM, Tepper JE, Baldwin AS Jr, *et al.*: Enhancement of radiosensitivity by proteasome inhibition: implications for a role of NF-kappa B. *Int J Radiat Oncol Biol Phys* 2001, 50:183–193.

94. Van Waes C, Chang AA, Lebowitz PF, *et al.*: Inhibition of nuclear factor-kappa B and target genes during combined therapy with proteasome inhibitor bortezomib and reirradiation in patients with recurrent head-and-neck squamous cell carcinoma. *Int J Radiat Oncol Biol Phys* 2005, 63:1400–1412.

95. Karagiannis TC, El-Osta A: Clinical potential of histone deacetylase inhibitors as stand alone therapeutics and in combination with other chemotherapeutics or radiotherapy for cancer. *Epigenetics* 2006, 1:121–126.

96. Horn PJ, Peterson CL: Heterochromatin assembly: a new twist on an old model. *Chromosome Res* 2006, 14:83–94.

97. Lopez CA, Feng FY, Herman JM, *et al.*: Phenylbutyrate sensitizes human glioblastoma cells lacking wild-type p53 function to ionizing radiation. *Int J Radiat Oncol Biol Phys* 2007, 69:214–220.

98. Duenas-Gonzalez A, Candelaria M, Perez-Plascencia C, *et al.*: Valproic acid as epigenetic cancer drug: preclinical, clinical and transcriptional effects on solid tumors. *Cancer Treat Rev* 2008 [ePub ahead of print].

99. Camphausen K, Scott T, Sproull M, Tofilon PJ: Enhancement of xenograft tumor radiosensitivity by the histone deacetylase inhibitor MS-275 and correlation with histone hyperacetylation. *Clin Cancer Res* 2004, 10(Pt 1):6066–6071.

100. Kodym E, Kodym R, Choy H, Saha D: Sustained metaphase arrest in response to ionizing radiation in a non-small cell lung cancer cell line. *Radiat Res* 2008, 169:46–58.

101. Camphausen K, Burgan W, Cerra M, *et al.*: Enhanced radiation-induced cell killing and prolongation of gammaH2AX foci expression by the histone deacetylase inhibitor MS-275. *Cancer Res* 2004, 64:316–321.

102. Furuta T, Takemura H, Liao ZY, *et al.*: Phosphorylation of histone H2AX and activation of Mre11, Rad50, and Nbs1 in response to replication-dependent DNA double-strand breaks induced by mammalian DNA topoisomerase I cleavage complexes. *J Biol Chem* 2003, 278:20303–20312.

103. Munshi A, Kurland JF, Nishikawa T, *et al.*: Histone deacetylase inhibitors radiosensitize human melanoma cells by suppressing DNA repair activity. *Clin Cancer Res* 2005, 11:4912–4922.

104. Tuveson DA, Hingorani SR: Ductal pancreatic cancer in humans and mice. *Cold Spring Harb Symp Quant Biol* 2005, 70:65–72.

105. Spalding AC, Lawrence TS: New and emerging radiosensitizers and radioprotectors. *Cancer Invest* 2006, 24:444–456.

106. Karamouzis MV, Grandis JR, Argiris A: Therapies directed against epidermal growth factor receptor in aerodigestive carcinomas. *JAMA* 2007, 298:70–82.

Breast Cancer

Susanne Briest, Antonio C. Wolff

6

EPIDEMIOLOGY

In 2005, cancers accounted for 13% of deaths worldwide, most of them (70%) occurring in low and middle income countries. Deaths from cancer worldwide are projected to continue rising, with an estimated 9 million people dying from cancer in 2015 and 11.4 million dying in 2030 [1]. Although people living in industrialized countries are twice as likely to be diagnosed with cancer as those in developing countries, fewer people are dying in affluent countries (50% vs 80%, respectively). Breast cancer is the number one cause of cancer death in women worldwide (502,000 deaths/year). The United States has the highest overall cancer rate among industrialized countries; there were approximately 178,480 new breast cancer cases in 2007 and 40,460 deaths (26% of all cancer deaths) [2].

A reduction in the number of new cases has been observed recently, likely due to a decrease in the use of menopausal hormonal therapy [3]. Breast cancer mortality has also declined over time due to the increased use of mammography and improvements of adjuvant systemic therapy [4]. There is a strong relation between stage at diagnosis and prognosis, with 5-year survival rates of 98% for localized disease, 83% for regional disease, and 26% for metastatic disease [2]. However, in the United States, there are observed differences in incidence and survival across various groups. For instance, the age-adjusted mortality from breast cancer in African American women is 36.4 deaths per 100,000 compared with 28.3 deaths per 100,000 in white women [5]; this is likely a combination of biologic and socioeconomic factors. Premenopausal African American women have a particularly unfavorable situation. As an example, these women are more likely to present with a basal-like breast cancer subtype. Furthermore, breast cancers in African American women often have higher tumor grade and stage at diagnosis, which may explain an observed worse outcome even after adjusting for stage.

RISK FACTORS

Age and gender are the most important risk factors, and only 1% of breast cancers occur in men. There is a bimodal breast cancer age-at-onset distribution with a dominant peak near age 50 and a smaller peak near age 70. The median age of diagnosis in the United States is 61 [6].

These observations may not apply for women with a strong family history of breast cancer. Mutations of the breast cancer–related genes *BRCA1* and *BRCA2* are a main factor associated with inherited breast cancer phenotypes. Ovarian cancer is also frequently observed, and the risk of being a carrier is highest in families with many cases of breast cancer (both breast and ovarian cancer), one or more family members with bilateral cancer, or an Ashkenazi (Eastern European) Jewish background. Women with a proven mutation of *BRCA1* or *BRCA2* have an expected three- to sevenfold increase in their lifetime risk of developing breast cancer. Other risk factors include prior histologic-proven atypical hyperplasia, in situ or invasive cancer in the breast, prolonged exposure to estrogen, obesity, and reproductive factors (Table 6-1).

DIAGNOSTIC METHODS

IMAGING

Monthly breast self-examination (BSE) is recommended, preferably around day 5 to 12 of the menstrual cycle, although evidence of its effectiveness (beyond raising awareness) is lacking [7]. Changes in size and shape of breast and the nipple/areola (including discharge), visible and/or palpable abnormality, and signs of inflammation require further evaluation.

Various imaging modalities are available; however, only annual mammography (film-based or digital) should be considered standard for screening the average-risk woman. Suspicious findings like asymmetry, architectural distortions, spiculated or poorly circumscribed mass, or suspicious or new micro-calcifications require additional imaging. Mammography is less sensitive in young patients with dense breast tissue, and ultrasound may be considered to further distinguish suspicious areas in all age groups and to guide any

diagnostic biopsy intervention in the breast or axilla [8]. Magnetic resonance imaging (MRI) of the breast or magnetic resonance mammography with contrast agents like gadolinium diethylenetriamine penta-acetic acid (Gd-DTPA) is another imaging method, but should not be used for routine screening of the average-risk woman. Its potential uses include the exclusion of multicentricity before planned breast conservation or after surgery to distinguish scars from a new abnormality, to potentially identify occult contralateral lesions not seen with conventional imaging, and in patients with high-risk lesions like atypical hyperplasia or a known diagnosis of invasive breast cancer [9]. All these techniques require dedicated equipment (including MRI coils) able to guide any biopsies and expert radiologists able to integrate the data obtained with all imaging techniques used. Other breast imaging techniques assessing vascular flow, electrical activity, glucose metabolism, and mitochondrial activity are under development and should be considered investigational [10,11].

Needle biopsies should be considered the standard method for the evaluation of most palpable and nonpalpable abnormalities, often performed under imaging guidance. Excisional biopsies should be reserved for situations in which a needle biopsy is not possible (*eg*, location of the tumor or nondiagnostic and/or discordant imaging and needle biopsy findings). Core biopsy is the preferred method in the breast or chest wall to properly assess architecture, presence of invasion, and perform immunohistologic assays. Fine-needle aspiration (FNA) should be reserved primarily for the assessment of suspicious lymph nodes. Experienced cytopathologists are needed for the interpretation of FNA findings.

TYPE OF BREAST CANCER

Breast cancer is increasingly understood as a collection of different tumor phenotypes with various prognostic and therapeutic implications. Several subtypes can be distinguished, based on histopathologic features, biologic patterns, and gene expression profiles. The designation into a specific tumor subtype may become an important factor for determination of prognosis and for treatment decision-making.

The tumor, node, metastasis (TNM) staging system reflects the anatomic features of breast cancer. The American Joint Committee on Cancer (AJCC) published a revised (sixth) edition in 2002 to take new data and current treatment standards into account (Table 6-2 and Table 6-3).

Table 6-1. Risk Factors for Breast Cancer
Female gender
Advanced age
Prior history of atypical ductal hyperplasia or in situ carcinoma
Prior history of invasive carcinoma of the breast
Strong family history of breast cancer
Proven mutation of *BRCA1* and/or *BRCA2*
Mutations in p53 and phosphatase and tensin homologue (PTEN)
Obesity
Dense breast tissue on mammography
Radiation of breast/chest, particularly at young age
Prolonged exposure to estrogen
Early menarche
Late onset of menopause
Nulliparity
Higher age at first pregnancy
Prolonged use of menopausal hormonal therapy

PATHOLOGIC CLASSIFICATION

There are two major categories of invasive breast cancer, invasive ductal and invasive lobular [12]. Seventy-five percent of the invasive ductal carcinomas are not otherwise specified, and the Nottingham modification of the Bloom-Richardson system of grade 1, 2, and 3 (well-differentiated, moderately differentiated, and poorly differentiated, respectively) is frequently used. The special types of invasive ductal carcinoma are described according to various criteria, such as cell type (*ie*, apocrine carcinoma), type of secretion (*ie*, mucinous carcinoma), architectural patterns (*ie*, papillary or cribriform carcinoma), and patterns of spread (*ie*, inflammatory carcinoma) [13]. Mucinous, tubular, medullary, invasive papillary apocrine, metaplastic, and secretory carcinomas are included in this group. Many of these various subtypes have a better prognosis. Invasive lobular carcinomas constitute 10% to 14%

of invasive breast cancer. Whereas the prognosis does not differ from invasive ductal carcinoma when stratified by stage, invasive lobular subtypes have a higher incidence of bilaterality and multicentricity. Other rare types are tubulolobular, signet-ring cell carcinoma, and unusual malignant primary tumors like cystosarcoma phyllodes and angiosarcoma [14].

TRADITIONAL BIOLOGIC MARKERS

Besides the histologic classification of breast cancer, various biologic markers may influence the choice of therapy. The steroid receptors are a strong predictive factor of endocrine therapy. The estrogen receptor (ER) was first described by Toft and Gorski [15]. Immunohistochemical (IHC) assays can distinguish ER-α and -β, although this distinction in clinical practice is of unclear significance [16], and 75% of tumors are ER α-positive [17]. Tumors expressing ER-α are usually smaller than the ER-negative tumors and more often found

Table 6-2. TNM Classification of Breast Cancer	
Class	**Description**
Primary tumor (T)	
TX	Primary tumor cannot be assessed
T0	No evidence of primary tumor
Tis	Intraductal carcinoma (DCIS), LCIS, or Paget disease of the nipple with no associated invasion of normal breast tissue
T1	Tumor not > 2.0 cm in greatest dimension
T1mic	Microinvasion not > 0.1 cm in greatest dimension
T1a	Tumor > 0.1 cm but not > 0.5 cm in greatest dimension
T1b	Tumor > 0.5 cm but not > 1.0 cm in greatest dimension
T1c	Tumor > 1.0 cm but not > 2.0 cm in greatest dimension
T2	Tumor > 2.0 cm but not > 5.0 cm in greatest dimension
T3	Tumor > 5.0 cm in greatest dimension
T4	Tumor of any size with direct extension to (a) chest wall or (b) skin, only as described below
T4a	Extension to chest wall, not including pectoralis muscle
T4b	Edema (including peau d'orange) or ulceration of the skin of the breast, or satellite skin nodules confined to the same breast
T4c	Both T4a and T4b
T4d	Inflammatory carcinoma
Regional lymph nodes (N)	
NX	Regional lymph nodes cannot be assessed (*eg*, previously removed)
N0	No regional lymph node metastasis
N1	Metastasis to movable ipsilateral axillary lymph node(s)
N2	Metastasis to ipsilateral axillary lymph node(s), fixed or matted, or in clinically apparent* ipsilateral internal mammary nodes in the absence of clinically evident lymph node metastasis
N2a	Metastasis in ipsilateral axillary lymph nodes fixed to one another (matted) or to other structures
N2b	Metastasis only in clinically apparent* ipsilateral internal mammary nodes and in the absence of clinically evident axillary lymph node metastasis
N3	Metastasis in ipsilateral infraclavicular lymph node(s) with or without axillary lymph node involvement, or in clinically apparent* ipsilateral internal mammary lymph node(s) and in the presence of clinically evident axillary lymph node metastasis; or metastasis in ipsilateral supraclavicular lymph node(s) with or without axillary or internal mammary lymph node involvement
N3a	Metastasis in ipsilateral infraclavicular lymph node(s)
N3b	Metastasis in ipsilateral internal mammary lymph node(s) and axillary lymph node(s)
N3c	Metastasis in ipsilateral supraclavicular lymph node(s)

*Clinically apparent is defined as detected by imaging studies (excluding lymphoscintigraphy) or by clinical examination or grossly visible pathologically.
†Classification is based on axillary lymph node dissection with or without SLN dissection. Classification based solely on SLN dissection without subsequent axillary lymph node dissection is designated (sn) for sentinal node, *eg*, pN0(I+) (sn).
‡ITCs are defined as single tumor cells or small cell clusters not > 0.2 mm usually detected only by IHC or molecular methods but that may be verified on hematoxylin and eosin stains. ITCs do not usually show evidence of malignant activity (*eg*, proliferation of stromal reaction).
§Not clinically apparent is defined as not detected by imaging studies (excluding lymphoscintigraphy) or by clinical examination.
¶Clinically apparent is defined as detected by imaging studies (excluding lymphoscintigraphy) or by clinical examination.
DCIS—ductal carcinoma in situ; IHC—immunohistochemical; ITC—isolated tumor cells; LCIS—lobular carcinoma in situ; RT-PCR—reverse transcriptase polymerase chain reaction; SLN—sentinel lymph node.
(*From* Singletary *et al.* [30].)

in older patients. ER-negative tumors also correlate with high grade and lymph node involvement, and are more commonly seen in African American women.

The epidermal growth factor receptor (EGFR) 2 (also known as HER2) is another important predictive and prognostic marker in breast cancer. It is overexpressed in about 20% of patients with invasive breast cancer and almost all cases of comedo-type intraductal carcinoma, although its significance in ductal carcinoma in situ (DCIS) is unclear [18]. This 185-kilodalton transmembrane glycoprotein with tyrosine kinase activity was first described in the mid-1980s [19]. Four different EGFRs have since been described, of which HER2 has special importance as a therapeutic target. Overexpression of HER2 is also associated with worse prognosis [20], even in lymph node–negative disease [21]. HER2 is a predictive factor for benefit from trastuzumab, a humanized monoclonal anti-HER2 antibody against the extracellular domain number IV of the receptor [22].

Other promising predictive factors include markers like urokinase-type plasminogen activator (uPA) and plasminogen activator inhibitor 1 (PAI-1). A strong relation between high uPA levels and/or high PAI-1 in fresh frozen tumor extracts and poor disease-free survival (DFS) and overall survival have been described in a pooled analysis of 17 data sets [23]. The prognostic impact of uPA and PAI-1 has further been demonstrated in a large clinical trial [24].

GENE EXPRESSION PROFILES

Breast cancer can be classified according to the expression of a certain gene profile. Perou *et al.* [25] described different molecular portraits of human breast tumors on the basis of gene expression patterns using complementary DNA (cDNA) microarrays. They identified several subtypes, such as luminal A and B, basal-like, HER2 positive, and normal-like. The basal-like tumors show a high expression of proliferation-associated genes and the overexpression

---

Table 6-2. TNM Classification of Breast Cancer *(Continued)*

Class	Description
Pathologic classification (pN)†	
pNX	Regional lymph nodes cannot be assessed (*eg*, not removed for pathologic study or previously removed)
pN0	No regional lymph node metastasis histologically, and no additional examination for ITC‡
pN0(I-)	No regional lymph node metastasis histologically, negative IHC
pN0(I+)	No regional lymph node metastasis histologically, positive IHC, and no IHC cluster > 0.2 mm
pN0(mol-)	No regional lymph node metastasis histologically, and negative molecular findings (RT-PCR)
pN0(mol+)	No regional lymph node metastasis histologically and positive molecular findings (RT-PCR)
pN1	Metastasis in 1–3 axillary lymph nodes, and/or in internal mammary nodes with microscopic disease detected by SLN dissection but not clinically apparent§
pN1mi	Micrometastasis (> 0.2 mm but not > 2.0 mm)
pN1a	Metastasis in 1–3 axillary lymph nodes
pN1b	Metastasis in internal mammary nodes with microscopic disease detected by SLN dissection but not clinically apparent§
pN1c	Metastasis in 1–3 axillary lymph nodes and in internal mammary lymph nodes with microscopic disease detected by SLN dissection but not clinically apparent§ (if associated with > 3 positive axillary lymph nodes, the internal mammary nodes are classified as pN3b to reflect increased tumor burden)
pN2	Metastasis in 4–9 axillary lymph nodes, or in clinically apparent¶ internal mammary lymph nodes in the absence of axillary lymph node metastasis to ipsilateral axillary lymph node(s) fixed to each other or to other structures
pN2a	Metastasis in 4–9 axillary lymph nodes (at least 1 tumor deposit > 2.0 mm)
pN2b	Metastasis in clinically apparent¶ internal mammary lymph nodes in the absence of axillary lymph node metastasis
pN3	Metastasis in ≥ 10 axillary lymph nodes, or in infraclavicular lymph nodes, or in clinically apparent¶ ipsilateral internal mammary lymph node(s) in the presence of ≥ 1 positive axillary lymph node(s); or in > 3 axillary lymph nodes with clinically negative microscopic metastasis in internal mammary lymph nodes; or in ipsilateral supraclavicular lymph nodes
pN3a	Metastasis in ≥ 10 axillary lymph nodes (at least 1 tumor deposit > 2.0 mm); or metastasis to the infraclavicular lymph nodes
pN3b	Metastasis in clinically apparent¶ ipsilateral internal mammary lymph nodes in the presence of ≥ 1 positive axillary lymph node(s); or in > 3 axillary lymph nodes and in internal mammary lymph nodes with microscopic disease detected by SLN dissection but not clinically apparent§
pN3c	Metastasis in ipsilateral supraclavicular lymph nodes
Distant metastasis (M)	
MX	Presence of distant metastasis cannot be assessed
M0	No distant metastasis
M1	Distant metastasis

*Clinically apparent is defined as detected by imaging studies (excluding lymphoscintigraphy) or by clinical examination or grossly visible pathologically.
†Classification is based on axillary lymph node dissection with or without SLN dissection. Classification based solely on SLN dissection without subsequent axillary lymph node dissection is designated (sn) for sentinel node, *eg*, pN0(I+) (sn).
‡ITCs are defined as single tumor cells or small cell clusters not > 0.2 mm usually detected only by IHC or molecular methods but that may be verified on hematoxylin and eosin stains. ITCs do not usually show evidence of malignant activity (*eg*, proliferation of stromal reaction).
§Not clinically apparent is defined as not detected by imaging studies (excluding lymphoscintigraphy) or by clinical examination.
¶Clinically apparent is defined as detected by imaging studies (excluding lymphoscintigraphy) or by clinical examination.
DCIS—ductal carcinoma in situ; IHC—immunohistochemical; ITC—isolated tumor cells; LCIS—lobular carcinoma in situ; RT-PCR—reverse transcriptase polymerase chain reaction; SLN—sentinel lymph node.
(*From* Singletary *et al.* [30].)

of genes that are normally expressed in myoepithelial or basal cells in normal breast tissue, such as basal keratins 5 and 17 and laminin [26]. The luminal A subtype highly expresses the ER-α gene, and tumors classified as luminal A subtypes overexpress genes involved in biologic processes like fatty acid metabolism and steroid-mediated signaling [27]. In contrast, the typical basal-like pattern shows a list of genes that are important for cancer development, including those involved in cell cycle, cell proliferation and differentiation, protein phosphorylation, and B-cell– and antibody-mediated immunity.

Tumors characterized as basal-like by gene expression profiling often show IHC patterns of so-called "triple-negative tumors," lacking ER, progesterone receptor (PR), and HER2 expression, and have an unfavorable prognosis. They are frequently observed in young women and often seen in *BRCA1* carriers [26]. Ninety percent of the tumors in women with *BRCA1* mutations are triple negative, and approximately 80% to 90% of the triple-negative breast cancer are basal-like [28,29]. Most of these tools remain investigational and ongoing studies are directly testing their predictive and prognostic utility in clinical practice.

PREDICTIVE AND PROGNOSTIC FACTORS

Predictive factors (*eg*, hormone receptor status) reflect the resistance or sensitivity of a given tumor to a specific therapy, while prognostic factors predict outcome independently of therapy, and thus reflect the natural history of the cancer and its risk. Classical prognostic factors include axillary lymph node status, tumor size, histopathologic subtype, and nuclear grade. Many factors like HER2 and ER are both prognostic and predictive.

Prognosis can be estimated based on stage of the tumor using the AJCC criteria (Table 6-2 and Table 6-3) [30]. It currently includes only anatomic information and an update is planned in the near future.

TREATMENT

IN SITU DISEASE

Lobular carcinoma in situ (LCIS) and DCIS are premalignant lesions that have the potential to relapse locally as in situ or invasive disease. However, there are some considerable differences between these two.

LCIS is an uncommon pathologic finding (< 5% in the general female population) usually detected by chance and reflects the elevated risk for an invasive breast cancer, ipsilateral and contralateral [31]. In contrast, atypical lobular hyperplasia (ALH) appears to be a risk factor for the ipsilateral breast cancer [32]. When LCIS or ALH are found in a core biopsy, an excisional biopsy is frequently recommended to rule out existing DCIS (17%) or invasive disease (27%) [33]. LCIS is regarded as a risk marker and clear margins do not appear to be needed. The pathologic distinction between ALH and LCIS is often not clear [34]. The presence of hyperplasia with atypia as compared with no atypia significantly increases the subsequent risk of developing cancer [35,36].

Widespread use of screening mammography has resulted in a remarkable increase in the diagnosis of DCIS, which comprises a heterogeneous group of lesions with different histopathologic features and prognoses. More than 62,030 (~ 25% of all cases) newly diagnosed DCIS occurred in 2007 [2], three times as many as in 1993 [37]. While a simple mastectomy leads to a nearly 100% cure rate, the adoption of breast conservation for invasive cancer also questioned the need for more radical surgery for preinvasive disease. It is sometimes difficult to image the extent of the disease, and the pathologic evaluation can also pose problems. The goal of the treatment is the complete removal of the lesion with clear margins. Excision alone may be used in selected patients as it may be associated with a higher risk of local recurrence in otherwise unselected patients [38]. The definition of adequate margins remains unsettled. Radiation after breast-conserving therapy decreases the recurrence rate by approximately 50% without a survival benefit. Large, randomized trials of lumpectomy with or without radiation have been conducted [39–41]. When subgroups were analyzed according to margin status (less than or greater than 10 mm), the differences for recurrence nearly vanished [42]. Other limitations included the quality of critical data like tumor size and nuclear grade [43]. Therefore, it may be possible to treat some patients with DCIS with adequate excision alone. Prognostic markers, such as the Van Nuys Prognostic Index [44], are an example of tools used to identify patients who might potentially be treated with just wide local excision (Table 6-4). Adjuvant tamoxifen following lumpectomy and radiotherapy has been evaluated. The National Surgical Adjuvant Breast and Bowel Project (NSABP) B24 study randomized patients to radiation plus placebo or radiation plus 5 years of tamoxifen (20 mg) after local excision. Neither adequacy of margin nor steroid receptor status was examined upfront. The addition of tamoxifen showed a reduction of the ipsilateral tumor recurrence from 11% to 7.7% ($P = 0.02$), mainly due to the reduction of invasive recurrences (5.3% to 2.6%; $P = 0.01$), but no difference was seen for DCIS [45]. In the United Kingdom, patients with DCIS were randomized to tamoxifen or nothing after excision only without a beneficial effect on recurrence [41]. The value of tamoxifen may be limited to the reduction of invasive recurrences in patients with ER-positive DCIS treated with wide excision and radiation, but prospective validation is needed. Ongoing trials, like NSABP B35 and the International Breast Cancer Intervention Study (IBIS) 2 are testing the value of aromatase inhibitors (AIs) for the risk reduction after DCIS.

OPERABLE INVASIVE DISEASE

LOCAL THERAPY

Breast cancer was at first considered a local disease with regional spread, which influenced the work of surgeons like Halsted [46] in the United States who favored a radical local approach to attempt cure (Halsted hypothesis). The radical mastectomy involves the removal of the breast, the pectoralis

Table 6-3. Staging of Breast Cancer According to the American Joint Committee on Cancer Staging System

Stage 0	Tis, N0, M0
Stage I	T1*, N0, M0
Stage IIA	T0, N1, M0
	T1*, N1, M0
	T2, N0, M0
Stage IIB	T2, N1, M0
	T3, N0, M0
Stage IIIA	T0, N2, M0
	T1*, N2, M0
	T2, N2, M0
	T3, N1, M0
	T3, N2, M0
Stage IIIB	T4, N0, M0
	T4, N1, M0
	T4, N2, M0
Stage IIIC†	Any T, N3, M0
Stage IV	Any T, any N, M1

*T1 includes T1mic.
†Stage IIIC breast cancer includes patients with any T stage who have pN3 disease. Patients with pN3a and pN3b disease are considered operable. Patients with pN3c disease are considered inoperable.
(*From* Woodward *et al.* [182].)

Table 6-4. The Van Nuys Prognostic Index Scoring System*

Score	Tumor size, *mm*	Margin width, *mm*	Pathologic classification
1	≤ 15	≥ 10	Nonhigh grade without necrosis
2	16–40	1–9	Nonhigh grade with necrosis
3	≥ 40	< 1	High grade with or without necrosis

*Van Nuys Prognostic Index (VNPI) 3 or 4—wide excision; VNPI 5, 6, or 7—wide excision plus radiation; VNPI 8 or 9—mastectomy.
(*Adapted from* Silverstein *et al.* [44].)

major and minor muscles, and all locoregional axillary nodes. The switch to less radical surgery including breast conservation was due to improved understanding of the systemic nature of breast cancer. This hypothesis was successfully tested in the NSABP B04 trial, which recruited patients with clinically node-negative disease to radical mastectomy, simple mastectomy and radiation, or simple mastectomy with observation and delayed dissection when positive nodes developed. After 25 years, the results for the distant DFS are the same [47]. This landmark study opened the way for a new understanding of local therapy. The change in paradigm was pushed forward by Fisher, who proposed that breast cancer is a systemic disease at presentation and would best be treated with conservative local treatment plus systemic chemotherapy (Fisher hypothesis). Breast conservation became the favorable locoregional treatment. It could be shown that radiotherapy after breast conservation reduced an otherwise high risk of local recurrence without compromising overall survival after 20 years of follow-up [48,49]. The decision to pursue mastectomy or breast conservation with radiotherapy should take into account specific contraindications (Table 6-5) and patient's choice. Immediate reconstruction with an implant or an autologous flap should always be considered by those treated with mastectomy.

The surgical evaluation of the axilla is considered gold standard. The number of involved nodes is an important predictor of prognosis and guides the choice of adjuvant radiation and systemic treatment. A positive impact on the rate of distant metastases and survival has been suggested [50]. Recently, sentinel lymph node biopsy has evolved as a new approach for the evaluation of the axilla in patients with early breast cancer. This operation avoids the known side effects of the complete axillary dissection while maintaining the accuracy of staging, and is now considered a standard procedure [51].

Postmastectomy radiation to the chest wall and regional lymph nodes has been shown to improve DFS and overall survival in patients with node-positive disease [52]. An American Society of Clinical Oncology (ASCO) guideline suggested the use of radiotherapy for patients with more than four involved lymph nodes, tumors larger than 5 cm, and locally advanced cancer [53]. However, the irradiation of patients with one to three involved lymph nodes has been controversial when the tumor is smaller than 5 cm. A 15-year survival benefit and reduced rate of locoregional failure after postmastectomy radiation of patients with one to three positive lymph nodes has recently been shown [54]. There is considerable disagreement concerning the radiation of the internal mammary nodes, and decisions should be individualized [55]. For patients with negative axillary nodes, chest wall radiation is recommended for those with a high risk of recurrence, which is defined as positive or close margin (< 1 mm) or tumors larger than 5 cm. There are also unresolved issues about the need to radiate the ipsilateral internal mammary and the supraclavicular lymph nodes.

SYSTEMIC THERAPY

The risk for recurrence and death from breast cancer can be high with local therapy alone, even in patients with node-negative disease. However, the degree of benefit from systemic therapy varies among patients depending on their tumor biology, stage, and age. Therefore, the therapeutic index should be defined for every individual patient as part of the decision to use systemic therapy.

ADJUVANT ENDOCRINE TREATMENT

Although Sir George Beatson showed a relationship between the removal of the ovaries and breast cancer response early on [56], the concept of systemic treatment was not further pursued until the mid-20th century [57]. First attempts of endocrine therapy were evaluated in patients with advanced disease using ovarian function suppression (OFS) achieved with adrenalectomy [58] or radiation of the ovaries [57]. Following the characterization of the estrogen receptor, the use of tamoxifen as a selective estrogen receptor modulator (SERM) was described. In 2000, the Early Breast Cancer Trialist's Collaborative Group (EBCTCG) reported that adjuvant tamoxifen reduces breast cancer recurrences in women whose tumors are ER-positive by more than 40%, and their annual breast cancer death rate by 31%. The benefits from tamoxifen are independent of the use of chemotherapy, age, PR status, or other tumor characteristics [59]. Endocrine therapy with tamoxifen is an affordable and effective therapy option

for women of all ages, and therefore access to accurate and reliable ER testing is key.

It was not until 1995 that 5-year tamoxifen therapy was shown to improve survival of premenopausal women [60]. The 2000 update of the Oxford overview showed that 5 years of tamoxifen reduced annual odds of recurrence by 34% and death by 24% in women younger than 50 years of age [59].

When considering endocrine therapy for premenopausal women, several factors may affect outcome. Breast cancer in younger premenopausal women (< 35 years) is more likely to be ER/PR-negative, larger than 2 cm in size, poorly differentiated, and to have high Ki-67 [61]. Their 10-year DFS and overall survival is shorter and, paradoxically, premenopausal women with ER-positive disease treated with chemotherapy alone have a worse outcome when compared with those with ER-negative disease [62].

OFS decreases the risk of recurrence and death when compared with no therapy [59], and ongoing studies are evaluating the role of OFS in women who may also be receiving tamoxifen and chemotherapy. Oophorectomy is a useful alternative to cytotoxic therapy in less affluent countries [63]. In the United States, OFS is mostly done with oophorectomy or luteinizing hormone–releasing hormone (LH-RH) agonists for 2 to 5 years as ovarian irradiation is technically challenging and frequently unreliable.

OFS in ER-positive disease offers similar DFS when compared with chemotherapy alone [64–67]. Similar results were observed with the combination of LH-RH agonists and tamoxifen versus chemotherapy [68–71], although the Austrian Breast and Colorectal Study Group trial (ABCSG 5) showed improved outcome in women treated with endocrine therapy [68]. The use of OFS after anthracycline and nonanthracycline chemotherapy [72,73] may offer a survival benefit that appears limited to women younger than 40 years, which again highlights the importance of adequate endocrine therapy in patients most likely to regain ovarian function after chemotherapy [74]. Overall, the Intergroup trial (INT) 0101 in node-positive patients revealed no difference in terms of survival after a median follow-up of 9.6 years, but the addition of tamoxifen to CAF (cyclophosphamide, doxorubicin, and 5-fluorouracil) followed by 5 years of monthly goserelin improved time to recurrence and DFS [73].

The data on OFS with LH-RH agonists were the subject of a recent overview [75]. However, they are limited by the primary use of CMF (cyclophosphamide, methotrexate, and fluorouracil) as standard chemotherapy as opposed to more contemporary regimens that include a taxane or an anthracycline. Another limitation of the existing data is that many trials did not use tamoxifen optimally. Tamoxifen remains the standard of care for premenopausal women with functioning ovaries, and ongoing clinical trials are examining the role of AIs and OFS in this setting [76]. However, concerns about the long-term effects of AIs on bone and cardiovascular health and quality of life exist and must be further characterized.

The endocrine treatment of postmenopausal women has been subject to important changes over the past years. The tissue-specific agonist/antagonist effect of tamoxifen is associated with potential adverse events like endometrial cancer and thromboembolic disease, and the identification of the aromatase enzyme [77] led to the development of a new class of drugs with a different safety profile. The third generation of more potent and

Table 6-5. Contraindications to Breast-Conserving Therapy

Absolute contraindications

Multicentric disease

Widespread malignant-appearing microcalcifications in separate quadrants

Prior radiation of the breast region

Pregnancy (use of radiation contraindicated)

Persistent positive margins after several surgical attempts to remove the tumor

Relative contraindications

Collagen vascular disease, like scleroderma

Tumor/breast volume relation

selective AIs includes letrozole, anastrozole, and exemestane. These agents directly target the aromatase enzyme (CYP19 enzyme complex) and can be divided into different classes regarding their chemical structure and mode of action. Since 2001, a large body of data has been released in the adjuvant setting testing various AI approaches as compared with tamoxifen (upfront, sequential, and extended) [78–85]. The first approach compared 5 years of an AI upfront instead of tamoxifen; trials included the ATAC (Arimidex, Tamoxifen, Alone or in Combination) trial [86], the Breast International Group trial 1-98 (BIG 1-98) [87], and the TEAM (Tamoxifen and Exemestane Adjuvant Multicenter) trial (data not published). Both ATAC and BIG 1-98 showed improvements in DFS favoring the upfront use of AI.

The sequential approach compared 5 years of tamoxifen with tamoxifen followed by an AI for a total of 5 years of endocrine therapy as studied in the Intergroup Exemestane Study (IES) [88]. The pooled analysis of the Italian Tamoxifen Anastrozole (ITA) trial [89,90] and an earlier trial of 3 years of tamoxifen followed by 2 years of the first-generation AI aminoglutethimide versus 5 years of tamoxifen showed a decreased all-cause mortality and breast cancer–specific mortality favoring a sequential approach [91]. A combined analysis of the Arimidex/Nolvadex (ARNO 95) and the ABCSG 8 trials [80,92] and a meta-analysis that included the ITA and IES [93] studies also favored the sequential approach.

Finally, the National Cancer Institute of Canada Clinical Trials Group (NCIC CTG) MA.17 [94], the ABCSG 6a [84], and the NSABP B-33 [85] trials evaluated the role for the AI in the extended adjuvant treatment. The MA.17 study showed an overall survival benefit, especially in women with node-positive disease. Furthermore, the initiation of the treatment with an AI seems to be beneficial even when started a few years after finishing 5 years of tamoxifen therapy [94]. Studies testing tamoxifen after an AI and upfront AI versus AI after a few years of tamoxifen have not been completed yet. Based on these data, ASCO and National Comprehensive Cancer Network (NCCN) guidelines recommend that, at some point, AIs be considered a part of the adjuvant treatment for postmenopausal women with hormone receptor–positive breast cancer [95,96].

At this time, available data do not identify patients who are more likely to benefit from AIs as compared with tamoxifen (*eg*, patients with HER2-positive breast cancer or patients with certain ER/PR patterns) [97,98].

For a summary of available agents for the endocrine treatment of breast cancer, see Table 6-6.

Adjuvant chemotherapy

The EBCTCG overview also evaluated prospective clinical trials of adjuvant chemotherapy. Compared with none, chemotherapy of any type reduced the risk of breast cancer recurrence and mortality by 22% and 15%, respectively, and all-cause mortality by 13%. Women who received anthracycline-based regimens had a greater reduction in annual odds of breast cancer recurrence by 11% and any death by 15% compared with those who received CMF-like regimens. Chemotherapy is associated with a larger benefit in younger women. In patients younger than 50 years of age, polychemotherapy was associated with a 12% reduction in absolute risk of breast cancer recurrence at 15 years and a 10% decrease in disease-related mortality compared with no chemotherapy. The results were more modest in women 50 to 59 years of age (4.1% and 3.0%, respectively) [59]. The magnitude of benefit was inversely correlated with age. Indeed, women aged 65 or older had substantially less gain. Because age under 50 has been often used as an indicator for menopause, it is not possible to determine whether it is indeed young age or premenopausal status that is associated with an improved benefit from chemotherapy in the younger age group. Premenopausal women with ER-positive disease may gain additional benefit from chemotherapy-induced ovarian suppression. In addition, cancer in younger women is more likely to lack hormone receptors and display high grade, factors that may predict relative chemosensitivity [99]. Older women may also gain less benefit from chemotherapy due to competing comorbidities and remaining lower life expectancy.

Recently, researchers compared differences in benefits from adjuvant chemotherapy in patients with ER-negative and ER-positive tumors. Data from three major adjuvant studies conducted by the US-American Breast Cancer Intergroup (Cancer and Acute Leukemia Group B [CALGB] 9741, CALGB 9344, and CALGB 8541) were included [100–102]. The addition of chemotherapy was associated with a statistically significantly higher benefit in patients with ER-negative tumors, compared with the benefits observed with the same therapy in patients with ER-positive disease who had also received tamoxifen. In patients with ER-negative and ER-positive tumors, chemotherapy overall reduced mortality by 55% and 23%, respectively [103]. The most beneficial regimen in this analysis was the biweekly, or dose dense, regimen of doxorubicin and cyclophosphamide (AC) followed by paclitaxel with growth factor support.

Whether there is an optimal adjuvant chemotherapy regimen for breast cancer treatment is not known. Choice of specific agents or combinations, dose, schedule, sequence, and duration are still debated [99]. Polychemotherapy, sequential or in combination, is better than single-agent therapy [59]. Other questions include the role of individual anthracyclines, whether to add a taxane, and if so, which one. The choice and the dose of the anthracycline have been mostly dictated by cost and geographical preferences (doxorubicin in the United States and epirubicin in Europe and Canada). Head-to-head comparisons of the different regimens are not available.

Based on encouraging experiences in metastatic breast cancer, several prospective trials evaluated the role of taxanes in addition to or instead of anthracycline therapy. The first study, CALBG 9344, reported that the addition of four cycles of paclitaxel to standard four cycles of AC improved DSF and resulted in the US Food and Drug Administration (FDA) approval of taxanes in the adjuvant therapy [101]. The NSABP B-28 study has also investigated the use of paclitaxel following four cycles of standard AC, and supported the results from the CALBG 9344 study, although the benefit appeared to be less likely due to enrollment of a lower-risk population and concomitant use of chemotherapy and tamoxifen [104]. However, in both the CALGB 9344 and NSABP B-28 comparisons, a confounding factor was the number of cycles: four in the standard AC arm compared with eight in the AC followed by paclitaxel investigational arm. Another study addressing the question was the Breast Cancer International Research Group (BCIRG) 001 study, which compared TAC (docetaxel, doxorubicin, and cyclophosphamide) versus FAC (5-fluorouracil, doxorubicin, and cyclophosphamide). With a median follow-up of 55 months, TAC, compared with FAC, was associated with a reduction in the risk of relapse by 28% (*P* = 0.001) and of death by 30% (*P* = 0.008), respectively [105]. Another trial compared four cycles of AC versus four cycles of TC (docetaxel and cyclophosphamide). Improved DFS was seen in the TC-treated patients (hazard ratio [HR] 0.67; *P* = 0.015), but the study was underpowered to assess overall survival [106]. In contrast, the Eastern Cooperative Oncology Group (ECOG)/INT 2197 trial had a much larger sample size and compared four cycles of AC

Table 6-6. Agents for the Endocrine Treatment of Breast Cancer

Agent	Dosage
Selective estrogen receptor modulator	
Tamoxifen	20 mg orally daily
Raloxifene	60 mg orally daily
Toremifene	60 mg orally daily*
Selective estrogen receptor downregulator*	
Fulvestrant	250 mg intramuscularly monthly
Aromatase inhibitors	
Anastrozole	1 mg orally daily
Letrozole	2.5 mg orally daily
Exemestane	25 mg orally daily
Luteinizing hormone–releasing hormone agonists	
Goserelin	3.6 mg subcutaneously monthly
Triptorelin	3.75 mg intramuscularly monthly
Leuprolide	11.25 mg subcutaneously every 3 mo

*Use in the metastatic setting.

with four cycles of AT (the combination of doxorubicin and paclitaxel). DFS and overall survival were equivalent in the treatment groups [107]. Finally, the first results of a head-to-head comparison of the two taxanes following adjuvant AC were reported. In ECOG 1199, women received four cycles of AC followed by paclitaxel or docetaxel administered every 3 weeks or weekly for a total of 12 weeks. With a median follow-up of 46.5 months, DFS and overall survival did not differ among the groups; however, a trend favoring weekly paclitaxel was seen in ER-negative women [108].

The Intergroup CALGB 40101 trial is randomizing patients with zero to three positive lymph nodes to AC or paclitaxel given every 2 weeks for four or six cycles. Results from the NSABP B-30, in which 4000 lymph node–positive patients were randomly assigned to AC followed by docetaxel versus a combination of doxorubicin and docetaxel versus all three drugs given concurrently should be available soon. Accrual to NSABP B-38 comparing TAC versus dose-dense AC followed by paclitaxel with or without gemcitabine concluded in 2007.

LOCALLY ADVANCED AND METASTATIC DISEASE

Systemic treatment is usually the first and main treatment modality for locally advanced or metastatic disease. The goals of therapy in metastatic breast cancer include improvement in overall response rate (ORR), time to progression, quality of life, and overall survival. Control of disease-related symptoms and the prevention of serious complications should ideally be achieved with minimal toxicities. Therefore, the therapeutic index of any therapy should be carefully considered.

ENDOCRINE TREATMENT

Women with ER/PR-positive disease and minimal symptoms (even if they have visceral involvement) should be considered candidates for endocrine therapy as a first step.

Tamoxifen is an effective therapy. Anastrozole, letrozole, and exemestane have been found to be as effective as megestrol acetate in postmenopausal women and better tolerated, and are also commonly used in postmenopausal women with ER-positive disease [109]. AIs were then examined in large, randomized trials as first-line treatment in postmenopausal women with ER-positive or ER-unknown breast cancer [110]. The selective estrogen receptor downregulator fulvestrant has been shown to be active in tamoxifen-resistant patients and as effective as AIs in the second-line setting [111]. Additionally, fulvestrant is an option in the first-line treatment of tamoxifen-resistant metastatic breast cancer or after progression on an AI [112].

OFS plays a major role in the treatment of premenopausal women with advanced breast cancer in combination with tamoxifen [113]. There are limited data concerning the combination of AIs and LH-RH agonists in the treatment of premenopausal women with metastatic breast cancer, and AIs alone are contraindicated in premenopausal women.

CHEMOTHERAPY

Chemotherapy is the only treatment option for women with endocrine nonresponsive breast cancer (*ie*, tumors that are ER/PR-negative and ER/PR-positive tumors that are refractory to endocrine therapy). Other indications are rapidly progressing visceral metastasis regardless of hormonal receptor status and a short disease-free interval following adjuvant treatment. There is a broad spectrum of classes of agents to consider: anthracyclines, taxanes, alkylating agents, antimetabolites, and vinca alkaloids as single agents or in combination with varied rates of response [114].

Although combination regimens may have an improved response rate and/or time to progression, their impact on overall survival is limited [115]. Combination chemotherapy is also accompanied by an increased risk of toxicity. Therefore, a sequential single-agent strategy is frequently favored.

Cyclophosphamide is the most extensively studied of the alkylating substances, and was among the first agents introduced in the nonendocrine treatment of breast cancer [116]. The introduction of doxorubicin in the 1970s led to improved outcomes in comparison with nonanthracycline regimens [117], and a meta-analysis published in 1993 revealed that anthracycline-containing regimens were superior to CMF [118].

Liposomal formulations of doxorubicin have been developed. Pegylated liposomal doxorubicin given at a dose of 50 mg/m^2 every 4 weeks was found to be equally effective to doxorubicin 60 mg/m^2 every 3 weeks with apparently less cardiotoxicity [119–122]. Other studies revealed that pegylated liposomal doxorubicin may be associated not only with decreased cardiotoxicity but an improved response and a longer median time to treatment failure [123].

Paclitaxel and docetaxel are commonly used in patients with metastatic disease who are anthracycline naive or after minimal anthracycline treatment, as well as after anthracycline failure. Taxanes were used as single agents or in combination with different classes of drugs. A meta-analysis investigating the effects of taxanes alone or in combination with anthracyclines revealed a HR of 1.19 ($P = 0.01$) for progression-free survival (PFS) and 1.01 ($P = 0.90$) for overall survival favoring taxanes compared with anthracyclines as a single agent [124].

Newer developments include the nanoparticle albumin-bound paclitaxel (nab-paclitaxel) which was shown in a randomized phase 3 study to have higher response rates in metastatic breast cancer when compared with 3-times-weekly paclitaxel (33% vs 19%, respectively; $P = 0.001$) and a longer time to progression (23.0 vs 16.9 weeks, respectively; HR = 0.75; $P = 0.006$) [125].

Capecitabine, an oral fluoropyrimidine, has a high single-agent efficacy in metastatic breast cancer [126]. Given its efficacy, safety, and ease of administration, it became an attractive agent for combination strategies [127]. Other agents with activity include vinorelbine, a third-generation semisynthetic vinca alkaloid with activity as first-line therapy alone [128,129] or in combination with doxorubicin [130] and as second-line treatment [129], and the pyrimidine antimetabolite gemcitabine, which was tested as a single agent in the first- and second-line setting, and associated with a high response rate in phase 2 trials [131].

PREOPERATIVE SYSTEMIC THERAPY

Neoadjuvant, preoperative, or primary systemic chemotherapy was first used for the treatment of patients with locally advanced disease. Nowadays, the main goals of preoperative chemotherapy in women with operable disease are to enhance breast conservation and to improve surgical options [132]. Another important goal is to use preoperative therapy as an "in vivo" sensitivity marker of the tumor response, as pathologic response to preoperative chemotherapy can be used as a window into the treatment of systemic micrometastasis and correlates with improved DFS and overall survival [133]. Others have hypothesized that drug resistance could be minimized with early exposure to systemic therapy [134]. The preoperative approach has also become an important vehicle for the evaluation of new agents and the introduction and testing of surrogate markers for the prediction of tumor response and clinical outcome [135–137].

PREOPERATIVE ENDOCRINE THERAPY

The idea of preoperative treatment was first introduced many decades ago to avoid surgery in elderly women [138]. Three phase 3 trials compared 3 to 4 months of treatment with AIs to tamoxifen in this setting. The IMPACT (Immediate Preoperative Anastrozole, Tamoxifen, or Combined with Tamoxifen) trial was designed to mirror the large adjuvant ATAC trial [139]. The investigators did not observe significant differences in the objective response between the three treatment groups. In contrast to the IMPACT trial, the PROACT (Preoperative Arimidex Compared to Tamoxifen) trial compared objective responses to anastrozole or tamoxifen in the preoperative setting with or without chemotherapy [140]. The authors demonstrated that preoperative treatment with anastrozole was at least as effective as tamoxifen in all patients and was perhaps more effective than tamoxifen in certain subgroups. In a third trial that compared letrozole and tamoxifen, the overall objective response was statistically significantly higher in the letrozole group (55% vs 36%; $P < 0.001$) [141]. Interestingly, tumors that overexpressed EGFR or HER2 were associated with response rates of 88% versus 21% ($P = 0.0004$) for letrozole and tamoxifen, respectively [142].

At the moment, preoperative endocrine therapy is most frequently used in patients with ER- or PR-positive disease who are not likely to be offered adjuvant chemotherapy.

PREOPERATIVE CHEMOTHERAPY

More than a dozen studies have compared chemotherapy in the neoadjuvant setting versus the same regimen in the adjuvant setting. Although a difference in survival could not be found, the trials established that preoperative chemotherapy is equivalent to the postoperative therapy in terms of survival [132,143]. Newer studies have evaluated the addition of taxanes. The first trial comparing the efficacy of docetaxel with an anthracycline-based regimen in the neoadjuvant setting was the Aberdeen trial [144]. An impressive survival benefit was demonstrated in this study after 65 months of follow-up for women who received docetaxel in addition to anthracycline-based regimen [145]. The largest neoadjuvant trial was NSABP B-27, which demonstrated an increase in pathologic complete response with the addition of four cycles of docetaxel to AC in comparison with AC alone [146]. While large differences in survival could not be demonstrated among the treatment arms, women with a pathologic complete response in the breast had improved OFS and overall survival [147].

TARGETED THERAPY AND NEW AGENTS

TRASTUZUMAB

TRASTUZUMAB IN THE METASTATIC SETTING

Trastuzumab was introduced into breast cancer treatment first as monotherapy, with an overall response of approximately 20% in patients with metastatic breast cancer [148,149]. When given in combination with doxorubicin (or epirubicin) and cyclophosphamide or with single-agent paclitaxel if there has been prior anthracycline exposure, the addition of trastuzumab was associated with longer time to disease progression, higher rate of objective response, longer duration of response, and improved survival [150]. Meanwhile, trastuzumab has been combined with different chemotherapeutic agents as a single agent or in combination with drugs like docetaxel [151] or vinorelbine [152]. Another combination regimen with trastuzumab is with paclitaxel and carboplatin in a weekly [153] or 3-times-weekly [154] schedule. Whereas the latter study demonstrated an improved ORR (57% vs 36%; P = 0.04) and PFS (13.8 vs 7.6 months) for paclitaxel, carboplatin, and trastuzumab compared with paclitaxel and trastuzumab, these results could not be confirmed when paclitaxel was replaced with docetaxel [155].

TRASTUZUMAB IN THE ADJUVANT SETTING

Since 2005, results of five pivotal trials that investigated the role of the addition of trastuzumab to adjuvant chemotherapy in patients with HER2-positive tumors have been published. All trials revealed improvement in disease or recurrence-free survival. An improvement in overall survival was seen in the North American studies (when combining the data from the NSABP B31 and the North Central Cancer Treatment Group [NCCTG]/INT 9831 trials) [156] and in the HERA (HERceptin Adjuvant) trial [157]. The BCIRG 006 trial was the only one containing an anthracycline-free regimen, thus demonstrating new possibilities to reduce the cardiac toxicity for high-risk patients [158]. Additional follow-up is required to assess whether trastuzumab benefit is equal in women who received the agent in combination with chemotherapy or following the completion of all chemotherapy.

The optimal duration of trastuzumab is not yet determined. Recently, the 2-year follow-up data of the HERA study were released, showing that 1 year of treatment with trastuzumab is associated with a significant overall survival benefit with a short median follow-up of 23.5 months. The unadjusted HR for the risk of death with trastuzumab compared with observation alone was 0.66 (P = 0.0115) [157]. Interestingly, the FinHer trial [159] has demonstrated improved outcomes for the addition of 9 weeks of trastuzumab to chemotherapy. Comparison data between 1 versus 2 years of trastuzumab in the HERA trial had not been released as of August 2008.

TRASTUZUMAB IN THE PREOPERATIVE SETTING

Trastuzumab was evaluated in small studies in the preoperative setting. M.D. Anderson Cancer Center investigators conducted a study that compared paclitaxel followed by FEC (5-fluorouracil, epirubicin, cyclophosphamide) with or without trastuzumab. The authors noted a high proportion of pathologic complete response (66.7%) in women who received combination trastuzumab and chemotherapy as compared with 25% of women who received chemotherapy alone, which led to premature closure of the trial [160]. A recently published update revealed that the pathologic complete response among a larger cohort treated with chemotherapy plus trastuzumab was 60% [161].

BEVACIZUMAB

Tumor growth is dependent on angiogenesis. A major stimulator for this process is the vascular endothelial growth factor (VEGF), and it has been shown that the humanized monoclonal antibody bevacizumab directed against VEGF is able to inhibit the growth of human tumors in animal models [162]. A large phase 3 trial was initiated to compare capecitabine monotherapy with the combination of capecitabine and bevacizumab in the treatment of patients after therapy with both an anthracycline and a taxane [163]. The primary end point of PFS was not statistically different between the combination and the monotherapy arm (4.86 vs 4.17 months, respectively; HR 0.98) and overall survival was similar (15.1 vs 14.5 months). However, the combination of capecitabine and bevacizumab increased the response rate significantly (19.8% vs 9.1%; P = 0.001). The most important side effect due to the addition of bevacizumab was hypertension, requiring therapy in 17.9% versus 0.5%. Capecitabine-related toxicities were not significantly increased. In contrast, the E2100 trial randomized 722 patients with no prior treatment for metastatic breast cancer to receive either paclitaxel monotherapy or the combination of paclitaxel and bevacizumab [164]. A first analysis demonstrated that the combination of the taxane with the VEGF antibody improved the response rates in all patients (28.2% vs 14.2%; P < 0.0001) and improved PFS (10.97 vs 6.11 months; HR 0.498; P < 0.0001). However, no improvement in overall survival was observed in this trial, and the data are now mature. Adjuvant trials have since started testing the role of bevacizumab in lymph node–positive patients in various duration schedules.

TYROSINE KINASE INHIBITORS

Tyrosine kinase inhibitors are small molecules that compete with adenosine triphosphate (ATP) for the binding site of ATP in the receptor, thus disrupting its phosphorylation and downstream effects in cells [165]. The best studied tyrosine kinase inhibitor in breast cancer is lapatinib, which is an orally active selective inhibitor of the EGFR as well as the HER2 tyrosine kinase [166]. In contrast to the antibody trastuzumab, lapatinib as a small molecule is able to penetrate the blood-brain barrier. Thus, tyrosine kinase inhibitors may prove useful in patients with HER2-positive disease and central nervous system (CNS) progression. The high incidence of brain metastases (28%–43%) in the group of patients with HER2-positive breast cancer [167] indicates a need for improved treatment strategies. In 2006, Geyer et al. [168] published the results of a phase 3 study randomizing patients with HER2-positive locally advanced or metastatic breast cancer that progressed after therapy with anthracycline, a taxane, and trastuzumab to either capecitabine in combination with lapatinib or capecitabine alone [168]. A longer median time to progression for the combination (8.4 vs 4.4 months; HR 0.49; P < 0.001) led to the approval of lapatinib by the FDA in March 2007. Other tyrosine kinase inhibitors target the VEGF receptor. As an example, the addition of axitinib twice daily to docetaxel showed a significant increase in objective response and a potential advantage in the prior chemotherapy subgroup [169].

OTHER NEW AGENTS

The humanized monoclonal antibody pertuzumab also binds to the extracellular domain of HER2 but in a different site than trastuzumab [170]. This prevents HER2/HER3 heterodimerization and thus inhibits cell signaling. This HER2 antibody has been combined with trastuzumab and shows preliminary evidence of activity in patients who have progressed on trastuzumab [171]. Other agents under investigation are summarized in Table 6-7.

Breast cancer is the most common cancer for women in the United States and second leading cause for cancer-related death. Over the past few decades, advances in adjuvant treatment have improved outcomes dramatically. A large body of data has been collected to individualize treatment and new exciting approaches are undergoing clinical testing. In addition, special attention must be paid to issues related to screening, chemoprevention, long-term follow-up, and survivorship.

RECOMMENDATIONS FOR SCREENING

Screening mammography has been found to reduce breast cancer mortality by 23% [172] to 32% [173] and has therefore been recommended in the United States for women starting in their 40s. Whereas the National Cancer Institute suggests the screening in 1- to 2-year intervals, the American Cancer Society and the American College of Radiology specify annual screening. According to the NCCN guidelines, periodic breast self-examination should be added. There is no upper age limit, but the screening should take into account life expectancy and comorbidities. These recommendations apply for women at a normal risk; those for women at higher risk are described in Table 6-8.

CHEMOPREVENTION

Endocrine agents like the SERMs tamoxifen and raloxifene as well as AIs have been considered as possible agents to reduce the risk of invasive breast cancer for women with an increased risk for the disease. Tamoxifen was first approved by the FDA for breast cancer prevention in 1998. Raloxifene received approval in 2007, offering a second choice for postmenopausal women seeking nonsurgical risk reduction. Clinical trials

with AIs are ongoing. Current recommendations are based on the results of various trials that have been conducted in the United States (NSABP P-1 [174], NSABP P-2 [175]) and Europe (Royal Marsden trial [176], Italian Chemoprevention trial [177]). After 48 months of follow-up, NSABP P-1 showed that the risk for predominantly ER-positive breast cancer could be decreased by 50%, and women with LCIS and atypical ductal hyperplasia had the greatest benefit. Recently, the results of the STAR (Study of Tamoxifen and Raloxifene) and NSABP P-2 trials were released and showed the equivalence of tamoxifen and raloxifene in reducing the risk of invasive breast cancer. The European trials randomized patients with either a positive family history for breast cancer (Royal Marsden) or women without an increased risk for breast cancer but after removal of the uterus (Italian trial). The Italian trial failed to demonstrate the risk-reducing effect. The high rate of noncompliance and the relatively low number of events were discussed to explain this inconsistency. Today, tamoxifen is recommended for premenopausal women and tamoxifen and raloxifene are recommended for postmenopausal patients at increased risk for the development of breast cancer as chemoprevention (for risk assessment, see Table 6-8).

LONG-TERM FOLLOW-UP

The follow-up of patients after adjuvant treatment should be done by physicians experienced in breast examination and surveillance. According to the ASCO guidelines [178], visits are recommended every 3 to 6 months during the first 3 years, every 6 to 12 months for years 4 and 5, and annually thereafter. During the follow-up visits, a careful taking of history and physical examination should be done with special regard for symptoms of recurrence and those caused by therapy. Further mammography on an annual basis (with the exception of a mammogram 6 months after definitive radiation therapy for women with breast-conserving therapy) and BSE are recommended. Stress is laid on patient education and genetic counseling for those at high risk for familiar breast cancer. No routine laboratory or radiologic testing beyond mammography is recommended for asymptomatic patients in the absence of clinical abnormalities [179].

SURVIVORSHIP AND LONG-TERM NEEDS OF PATIENTS WITH EARLY-STAGE BREAST CANCER

Issues of survivorship—the period of health and well being experienced by survivors following diagnosis and active cancer treatment—are closely related with follow-up [180]. Whereas the follow-up is more focused on the detection of recurrence, specific needs of patients after a cancer have to be addressed by caregivers. Besides the screening for breast cancer, the possible development of rare cancers that are caused by treatment, such as angiosarcoma, myeloid leukemia, and endometrial cancer, should be taken into consideration, even though their frequency is less than 1% [181]. Additional problems may be derived from endocrine treatment, like

Table 6-7. New Targeted Agents Under Investigation

Multitargeted tyrosine kinase inhibitors

Sorafenib

Sunitinib

Pazopanib

Vandetanib

Axitinib

New chemotherapeutics

Vinfluvine

Ixabepilone

Inhibitors of p53-mediated signal transduction

Farnesyl protein transferase inhibitors (tipifarnib, lonafarnib)

Epidermal growth factor inhibitors

Gefitinib

Erlotinib

Cetuximab

Selective inhibitor of the 26S proteasome

Bortezomib

Mammalian target of rapamycin inhibitors

Temsirolimus

Everolimus

Table 6-8. NCCN Breast Screening Recommendations for Women at Increased Risk

Population	Recommendations
Women with prior thoracic radiation	
< 25 y	Yearly clinical breast exam; periodic breast self-exam
25 y	6–12 monthly clinical breast exam; periodic breast self-exam; annual mammogram starting 8–10 y after exposure or with 40 y
5-y risk of invasive breast cancer ≥ 1.7 at age 35 or older	6–12 monthly clinical breast exam; periodic breast self-exam; annual mammogram; surgical or nonsurgical risk-reduction strategies
Women with a strong family history of genetic predisposition*	6–12 monthly clinical breast exam; periodic breast self-exam; annual mammogram starting 5–10 y prior to the youngest breast cancer case in the family (strong family history) or with age 25 (genetic predisposition); annual MRI; surgical or nonsurgical risk-reduction strategies
Women with ductal carcinoma in situ or atypical ductal hyperplasia	6–12 monthly clinical breast exam; periodic breast self-exam; annual mammogram; consider surgical or nonsurgical risk-reduction strategies

*According to the American Society of Clinical Oncology [184], defined as individuals with the following: 1) two breast cancer and ≥ 1 ovarian cancer in the family; 2) > 3 breast cancer diagnosed before the age of 50; 3) sisters diagnosed before the age of 50 with 2 breast cancer, 2 ovarian cancer, or 1 breast and 1 ovarian cancer. (*From the* National Cancer Comprehensive Network [183].)

hot flashes, sexual dysfunction, and arthralgia. Only recently problems like cognitive dysfunction, fatigue, and depression were acknowledged as related to cancer therapy. A trained mental health expert should be part of this multidisciplinary modality. Other long-term issues affecting breast cancer survivors include osteoporosis and cardiovascular disease. At pres-

ent, there are no specific recommendations regarding surveillance for these specific potential late complications. Surveillance should be mostly done by patients' primary care physicians during routine health maintenance evaluations that include screening for other tumors like colon and cervical cancer, immunizations, cholesterol screening, and bone health surveillance.

REFERENCES

1. Pan American Health Organization. Available at http://www.paho.org/Project.asp?SEL=TP&LNG=ENG&ID=538. Accessed July 28, 2008.

2. Jemal A, Siegel R, Ward E, *et al.*: Cancer statistics, 2007. *CA Cancer J Clin* 2007, 57:43–66.

3. Ravdin PM, Cronin KA, Howlader N, *et al.*: The decrease in breast-cancer incidence in 2003 in the United States. *N Engl J Med* 2007, 356:1670–1674.

4. Berry DA, Cronin KA, Plevritis SK, *et al.*: Effect of screening and adjuvant therapy on mortality from breast cancer. *N Engl J Med* 2005, 353:1784–1792.

5. Carey LA, Perou CM, Livasy CA, *et al.*: Race, breast cancer subtypes, and survival in the Carolina Breast Cancer Study. *JAMA* 2006, 295:2492–2502.

6. Anderson WF, Reiner AS, Matsuno RK, *et al.*: Shifting breast cancer trends in the United States. *J Clin Oncol* 2007, 25:3923–3929.

7. Thomas DB, Gao DL, Ray RM, *et al.*: Randomized trial of breast self-examination in Shanghai: final results. *J Natl Cancer Inst* 2002, 94:1445–1457.

8. Chagpar AB, Middleton LP, Sahin AA, *et al.*: Accuracy of physical examination, ultrasonography, and mammography in predicting residual pathologic tumor size in patients treated with neoadjuvant chemotherapy. *Ann Surg* 2006, 243:257–264.

9. Pediconi F, Catalano C, Roselli A, *et al.*: Contrast-enhanced MR mammography for evaluation of the contralateral breast in patients with diagnosed unilateral breast cancer or high-risk lesions. *Radiology* 2007, 243:670–680.

10. Freedman M: Imaging: new techniques. In *Diseases of the Breast*. Edited by Harris JR, Lippman ME, Morrow M, *et al.* Philadelphia: Lippincott Williams & Wilkins; 2004:181–198.

11. Chance B, Nioka S, Zhang J, *et al.*: Breast cancer detection based on incremental biochemical and physiological properties of breast cancers: a six-year, two-site study. *Acad Radiol* 2005, 12:925–933.

12. Elston CW, Ellis IO: Pathological prognostic factors in breast cancer. I. The value of histological grade in breast cancer: experience from a large study with long-term follow-up. *Histopathology* 1991, 19:403–410.

13. Berg JW, Hutter RV: Breast cancer. *Cancer* 1995, 75:257–269.

14. McCormick BM, Hudis C, Heerdt A, *et al.*: Breast cancer. In *Principles and Practice of Gynecologic Oncology*. Edited by Hoskins WJ, Perez CA, Young RC. Philadelphia: Lippincott Williams & Wilkins; 2000:1134–1239.

15. Toft D, Gorski J: A receptor molecule for estrogens: isolation from the rat uterus and preliminary characterization. *Proc Natl Acad Sci U S A* 1966, 55:1574–1581.

16. Speirs V: Oestrogen receptor beta in breast cancer: good, bad or still too early to tell? *J Pathol* 2002, 197:143–147.

17. Anderson WF, Chatterjee N, Ershler WB, *et al.*: Estrogen receptor breast cancer phenotypes in the Surveillance, Epidemiology, and End Results Database. *Breast Cancer Res Treat* 2002, 76:27–36.

18. Wolff AC, Hammond ME, Schwartz JN, *et al.*: American Society of Clinical Oncology/College of American Pathologists guideline recommendations for human epidermal growth factor receptor 2 testing in breast cancer. *J Clin Oncol* 2007, 25:118–145.

19. Coussens L, Yang-Feng TL, Liao YC, *et al.*: Tyrosine kinase receptor with extensive homology to EGF receptor shares chromosomal location with neu oncogene. *Science* 1985, 230:1132–1139.

20. Slamon DJ, Clark GM, Wong SG, *et al.*: Human breast cancer: correlation of relapse and survival with amplification of the HER-2/neu oncogene. *Science* 1987, 235:177–182.

21. Norris B CS, Cheang M, Gilks B, *et al.*: Poor 10 yr breast cancer specific survival and relapse free survival for HER2 positive T1N0 tumors [abstract]. *Breast Cancer Res Treat* 2006, 100:abstract 2031.

22. Cho HS, Mason K, Ramyar KX, *et al.*: Structure of the extracellular region of HER2 alone and in complex with the Herceptin Fab. *Nature* 2003, 421:756–760.

23. Look MP, van Putten WL, Duffy MJ, *et al.*: Pooled analysis of prognostic impact of urokinase-type plasminogen activator and its inhibitor PAI-1 in 8377 breast cancer patients. *J Natl Cancer Inst* 2002, 94:116–128.

24. Harbeck N, Kates RE, Schmitt M, *et al.*: Urokinase-type plasminogen activator and its inhibitor type 1 predict disease outcome and therapy response in primary breast cancer. *Clin Breast Cancer* 2004, 5:348–352.

25. Perou CM, Sorlie T, Eisen MB, *et al.*: Molecular portraits of human breast tumours. *Nature* 2000, 406:747–752.

26. Sorlie T, Perou CM, Tibshirani R, *et al.*: Gene expression patterns of breast carcinomas distinguish tumor subclasses with clinical implications. *Proc Natl Acad Sci U S A* 2001, 98:10869–10874.

27. Sorlie T, Wang Y, Xiao C, *et al.*: Distinct molecular mechanisms underlying clinically relevant subtypes of breast cancer: gene expression analyses across three different platforms. *BMC Genomics* 2006, 7:1–15.

28. Kandel MJ, Stadler Z, Masciari S, *et al.*: Prevalence of BRCA1 mutations in triple negative breast cancer (BC) [abstract]. *J Clin Oncol* 2006, 24(18S):508.

29. Carey LA, Dees EC, Sawyer L, *et al.*: The triple negative paradox: primary tumor chemosensitivity of breast cancer subtypes. *Clin Cancer Res* 2007, 13:2329–2334.

30. Singletary SE, Allred C, Ashley P, *et al.*: Revision of the American Joint Committee on Cancer staging system for breast cancer. *J Clin Oncol* 2002, 20:3628–3636.

31. McDivitt RW, Hutter RV, Foote FW Jr, *et al.*: In situ lobular carcinoma. A prospective follow-up study indicating cumulative patient risks. *JAMA* 1967, 201:82–86.

32. Page DL, Schuyler PA, Dupont WD, *et al.*: Atypical lobular hyperplasia as a unilateral predictor of breast cancer risk: a retrospective cohort study. *Lancet* 2003, 361:125–129.

33. Foster MC, Helvie MA, Gregory NE, *et al.*: Lobular carcinoma in situ or atypical lobular hyperplasia at core-needle biopsy: is excisional biopsy necessary? *Radiology* 2004, 231:813–819.

34. Newman LA: Lobular carcinoma in situ: clinical management. In *Diseases of the Breast*. Edited by Harris JR, Lippman ME, Morrow M, *et al.* Philadelphia: Lippincott Williams & Wilkins; 2004:497–505.

35. Dupont WD, Page DL: Risk factors for breast cancer in women with proliferative breast disease. *N Engl J Med* 1985, 312:146–151.

36. Page DL, Dupont WD, Rogers LW, *et al.*: Atypical hyperplastic lesions of the female breast. A long-term follow-up study. *Cancer* 1985, 55:2698–2708.

37. Ernster VL, Barclay J: Increases in ductal carcinoma in situ (DCIS) of the breast in relation to mammography: a dilemma. *J Natl Cancer Inst Monogr* 1997, 151–156.

38. Morrow M, Harris JR: Ductal carcinoma in situ and microinvasive carcinoma. In *Diseases of the Breast*. Edited by Harris JR, Lippman ME, Morrow M, *et al.* Philadelphia: Lippincott Williams & Wilkins; 2004:521–537.

39. Fisher B, Dignam J, Wolmark N, *et al.*: Lumpectomy and radiation therapy for the treatment of intraductal breast cancer: findings from National Surgical Adjuvant Breast and Bowel Project B-17. *J Clin Oncol* 1998, 16:441–452.

40. Julien JP, Bijker N, Fentiman IS, *et al.*: Radiotherapy in breast-conserving treatment for ductal carcinoma in situ: first results of the EORTC randomised phase III trial 10853. EORTC Breast Cancer Cooperative Group and EORTC Radiotherapy Group. *Lancet* 2000, 355:528–533.

41. Houghton J, George WD, Cuzick J, *et al.*: Radiotherapy and tamoxifen in women with completely excised ductal carcinoma in situ of the breast in the UK, Australia, and New Zealand: randomised controlled trial. *Lancet* 2003, 362:95–102.

42. Cutuli B: Is radiotherapy needed after adequate local excision of localized DCIS? *Int J Fertil Womens Med* 2004, 49:231–236.

43. Silverstein MJ, Lagios MD: Should all patients undergoing breast conserving therapy for DCIS receive radiation therapy? No. One size does not fit all: an argument against the routine use of radiation therapy for all patients with ductal carcinoma in situ of the breast who elect breast conservation. *J Surg Oncol* 2007, 95:605–609.

44. Silverstein MJ, Lagios MD, Craig PH, *et al.*: A prognostic index for ductal carcinoma in situ of the breast. *Cancer* 1996, 77:2267–2274.

45. Fisher B, Land S, Mamounas E, *et al.*: Prevention of invasive breast cancer in women with ductal carcinoma in situ: an update of the National Surgical Adjuvant Breast and Bowel Project experience. *Semin Oncol* 2001, 28:400–418.

46. Halsted WS: The results of radical operation for the cure of carcinoma of the breast. *Ann Surg* 1907, 46:1–19.

47. Fisher B, Jeong JH, Anderson S, *et al.*: Twenty-five-year follow-up of a randomized trial comparing radical mastectomy, total mastectomy, and total mastectomy followed by irradiation. *N Engl J Med* 2002, 347:567–575.

48. Fisher B, Anderson S, Bryant J, *et al.*: Twenty-year follow-up of a randomized trial comparing total mastectomy, lumpectomy, and lumpectomy plus irradiation for the treatment of invasive breast cancer. *N Engl J Med* 2002, 347:1233–1241.

49. Veronesi U, Cascinelli N, Mariani L, *et al.*: Twenty-year follow-up of a randomized study comparing breast-conserving surgery with radical mastectomy for early breast cancer. *N Engl J Med* 2002, 347:1227–1232.

50. Blichert-Toft M: Axillary surgery in breast cancer management—background, incidence and extent of nodal spread, extent of surgery and accurate axillary staging, surgical procedures. *Acta Oncol* 2000, 39:269–275.

51. Lyman GH, Giuliano AE, Somerfield MR, *et al.*: American Society of Clinical Oncology guideline recommendations for sentinel lymph node biopsy in early-stage breast cancer. *J Clin Oncol* 2005, 23:7703–7720.

52. Clarke M, Collins R, Darby S, *et al.*: Effects of radiotherapy and of differences in the extent of surgery for early breast cancer on local recurrence and 15-year survival: an overview of the randomised trials. *Lancet* 2005, 366:2087–2106.

53. Recht A, Edge SB, Solin LJ, *et al.*: Postmastectomy radiotherapy: clinical practice guidelines of the American Society of Clinical Oncology. *J Clin Oncol* 2001, 19:1539–1569.

54. Overgaard M, Nielsen HM, Overgaard J: Is the benefit of postmastectomy irradiation limited to patients with four or more positive nodes, as recommended in international consensus reports? A subgroup analysis of the DBCG 82 b&c randomized trials. *Radiother Oncol* 2007, 82:247–253.

55. National Comprehensive Cancer Network: Breast cancer (V.2.2008). Available at http://www.nccn.org/professionals/physician_gls/PDF/breast.pdf. Accessed June 28, 2008.

56. Beatson G: On the treatment of inoperable cases of carcinoma of the mamma: suggestions for a new method of treatment with illustrative cases. *Lancet* 1896, 2:104–107.

57. Cole MP: The place of radiotherapy in the management of early breast cancer. A report of two clinical trials. *Br J Surg* 1964, 51:216–220.

58. Fracchia AA, Holleb AI, Farrow JH, *et al.*: Results of bilateral adrenalectomy in the management of incurable breast cancer; report of 155 cases. *Cancer* 1959, 12:58–68.

59. Effects of chemotherapy and hormonal therapy for early breast cancer on recurrence and 15-year survival: an overview of the randomised trials. *Lancet* 2005, 365:1687–1717.

60. Tamoxifen for early breast cancer: an overview of the randomised trials. Early Breast Cancer Trialists' Collaborative Group. *Lancet* 1998, 351:1451–1467.

61. Colleoni M, Rotmensz N, Peruzzotti G, *et al.*: Role of endocrine responsiveness and adjuvant therapy in very young women (below 35 years) with operable breast cancer and node negative disease. *Ann Oncol* 2006, 17:1497–1503.

62. Aebi S, Gelber S, Castiglione-Gertsch M, *et al.*: Is chemotherapy alone adequate for young women with oestrogen-receptor-positive breast cancer? *Lancet* 2000, 355:1869–1874.

63. Love RR, Duc NB, Allred DC, *et al.*: Oophorectomy and tamoxifen adjuvant therapy in premenopausal Vietnamese and Chinese women with operable breast cancer. *J Clin Oncol* 2002, 20:2559–2566.

64. Jonat W, Kaufmann M, Sauerbrei W, *et al.*: Goserelin versus cyclophosphamide, methotrexate, and fluorouracil as adjuvant therapy in premenopausal patients with node-positive breast cancer: the Zoladex Early Breast Cancer Research Association study. *J Clin Oncol* 2002, 20:4628–4635.

65. Schmid P, Untch M, Wallwiener D, *et al.*: Cyclophosphamide, methotrexate and fluorouracil (CMF) versus hormonal ablation with leuprorelin acetate as adjuvant treatment of node-positive, premenopausal breast cancer patients: preliminary results of the TABLE-study (Takeda Adjuvant Breast cancer study with Leuprorelin Acetate). *Anticancer Res* 2002, 22:2325–2332.

66. von Minckwitz G, Graf E, Geberth M, *et al.*: CMF versus goserelin as adjuvant therapy for node-negative, hormone-receptor-positive breast cancer in premenopausal patients: a randomised trial (GABG trial IV-A-93). *Eur J Cancer* 2006, 42:1780–1788.

67. Castiglione-Gertsch M, O'Neill A, Price KN, *et al.*: Adjuvant chemotherapy followed by goserelin versus either modality alone for premenopausal lymph node-negative breast cancer: a randomized trial. *J Natl Cancer Inst* 2003, 95:1833–1846.

68. Jakesz R, Hausmaninger H, Kubista E, *et al.*: Randomized adjuvant trial of tamoxifen and goserelin versus cyclophosphamide, methotrexate, and fluorouracil: evidence for the superiority of treatment with endocrine blockade in premenopausal patients with hormone-responsive breast cancer—Austrian Breast and Colorectal Cancer Study Group Trial 5. *J Clin Oncol* 2002, 20:4621–4627.

69. Boccardo F, Rubagotti A, Amoroso D, *et al.*: Cyclophosphamide, methotrexate, and fluorouracil versus tamoxifen plus ovarian suppression as adjuvant treatment of estrogen receptor-positive pre-/perimenopausal breast cancer patients: results of the Italian Breast Cancer Adjuvant Study Group 02 randomized trial. *J Clin Oncol* 2000, 18:2718–2727.

70. Roche H, Fumoleau P, Spielmann M, *et al.*: Sequential adjuvant epirubicin-based and docetaxel chemotherapy for node-positive breast cancer patients: the FNCLCC PACS 01 trial. *J Clin Oncol* 2006, 24:5664–5671.

71. Roche H, Kerbrat P, Bonneterre J, *et al.*: Complete hormonal blockade versus epirubicin-based chemotherapy in premenopausal, one to three node-positive, and hormone-receptor positive, early breast cancer patients: 7-year follow-up results of French Adjuvant Study Group 06 randomised trial. *Ann Oncol* 2006, 17:1221–1227.

72. Arriagada R, Le MG, Spielmann M, *et al.*: Randomized trial of adjuvant ovarian suppression in 926 premenopausal patients with early breast cancer treated with adjuvant chemotherapy. *Ann Oncol* 2005, 16:389–396.

73. Davidson NE, O'Neill AM, Vukov AM, *et al.*: Chemoendocrine therapy for premenopausal women with axillary lymph node-positive, steroid hormone receptor-positive breast cancer: results from INT 0101 (E5188). *J Clin Oncol* 2005, 23:5973–5982.

74. De Placido S, De Laurentiis M, De Lena M, *et al.*: A randomised factorial trial of sequential doxorubicin and CMF vs CMF and chemotherapy alone vs chemotherapy followed by goserelin plus tamoxifen as adjuvant treatment of node-positive breast cancer. *Br J Cancer* 2005, 92:467–474.

75. Cuzick J, Ambroisine L, Davidson N, *et al.*: Use of luteinising-hormone-releasing hormone agonists as adjuvant treatment in premenopausal patients with hormone-receptor-positive breast cancer: a meta-analysis of individual patient data from randomised adjuvant trials. *Lancet* 2007, 369:1711–1723.

76. Jonat W, Pritchard KI, Sainsbury R, *et al.*: Trends in endocrine therapy and chemotherapy for early breast cancer: a focus on the premenopausal patient. *J Cancer Res Clin Oncol* 2006, 132:275–286.

77. Thompson EA Jr, Siiteri PK: The involvement of human placental microsomal cytochrome P-450 in aromatization. *J Biol Chem* 1974, 249:5373–5378.

78. Baum M, Budzar AU, Cuzick J, *et al.*: Anastrozole alone or in combination with tamoxifen versus tamoxifen alone for adjuvant treatment of postmenopausal women with early breast cancer: first results of the ATAC randomised trial. *Lancet* 2002, 359:2131–2139.

79. Boccardo F, Rubagotti A, Puntoni M, *et al.*: Switching to anastrozole versus continued tamoxifen treatment of early breast cancer: preliminary results of the Italian Tamoxifen Anastrozole Trial. *J Clin Oncol* 2005, 23:5138–5147.

80. Jakesz R, Jonat W, Gnant M, *et al.*: Switching of postmenopausal women with endocrine-responsive early breast cancer to anastrozole after 2 years' adjuvant tamoxifen: combined results of ABCSG trial 8 and ARNO 95 trial. *Lancet* 2005, 366:455–462.

81. Goss PE, Ingle JN, Martino S, *et al.*: A randomized trial of letrozole in postmenopausal women after five years of tamoxifen therapy for early-stage breast cancer. *N Engl J Med* 2003, 349:1793–1802.

82. Thurlimann B, Keshaviah A, Coates AS, *et al.*: A comparison of letrozole and tamoxifen in postmenopausal women with early breast cancer. *N Engl J Med* 2005, 353:2747–2757.

83. Coombes RC, Hall E, Gibson LJ, *et al.*: A randomized trial of exemestane after two to three years of tamoxifen therapy in postmenopausal women with primary breast cancer. *N Engl J Med* 2004, 350:1081–1092.

84. Jakesz R, Samonigg H, Greil R, *et al.*: Extended adjuvant treatment with anastrozole: results from the Austrian Breast and Colorectal Cancer Study Group Trial 6a (ABCSG-6a) [abstract]. *J Clin Oncol* 2005, 23(16S):527.

85. Mamounas E, Jeong JH, Wickerham L, *et al.*: Benefit from exemestane (EXE) as extended adjuvant therapy after 5 years of tamoxifen (TAM): intent-to treat analysis of NSABP B-33 [abstract]. *Breast Cancer Res Treat* 2006, 100:abstract 49.

86. Buzdar AU, Guastalla JP, Nabholtz JM, *et al.*: Impact of chemotherapy regimens prior to endocrine therapy: results from the ATAC (Anastrozole and Tamoxifen, Alone or in Combination) trial. *Cancer* 2006, 107:472–480.

87. Coates AS, Keshaviah A, Thurlimann B, *et al.*: Five years of letrozole compared with tamoxifen as initial adjuvant therapy for postmenopausal women with endocrine-responsive early breast cancer: update of study BIG 1-98. *J Clin Oncol* 2007, 25:486–492.

88. Coombes RC, Kilburn LS, Snowdon CF, *et al.*: Survival and safety of exemestane versus tamoxifen after 2-3 years' tamoxifen treatment (Intergroup Exemestane Study): a randomised controlled trial. *Lancet* 2007, 369:559–570.

89. Boccardo F, Rubagotti A, Guglielmini P, *et al.*: Switching to anastrozole versus continued tamoxifen treatment of early breast cancer. Updated results of the Italian Tamoxifen Anastrozole (ITA) trial. *Ann Oncol* 2006, 17(Suppl 7):vii10–vii14.

90. Boccardo F, Rubagotti A, Amoroso D, *et al.*: Sequential tamoxifen and aminoglutethimide versus tamoxifen alone in the adjuvant treatment of postmenopausal breast cancer patients: results of an Italian cooperative study. *J Clin Oncol* 2001, 19:4209–4215.

91. Boccardo F, Rubagotti A, Aldrighetti D, *et al.*: Switching to an aromatase inhibitor provides mortality benefit in early breast carcinoma: pooled analysis of 2 consecutive trials. *Cancer* 2007, 109:1060–1067.

92. Kaufmann M, Jonat W, Hilfrich J, *et al.*: Survival benefit of switching to anastrozole after 2 years' treatment with tamoxifen versus continued tamoxifen therapy: the ARNO 95 study [abstract]. *J Clin Oncol* 2006, 24(18S):abstract 547.

93. Jonat W, Gnant M, Boccardo F, *et al.*: Effectiveness of switching from adjuvant tamoxifen to anastrozole in postmenopausal women with hormone-sensitive early-stage breast cancer: a meta-analysis. *Lancet Oncol* 2006, 7:991–996.

94. Ingle JN, Tu D, Pater JL, *et al.*: Duration of letrozole treatment and outcomes in the placebo-controlled NCIC CTG MA.17 extended adjuvant therapy trial. *Breast Cancer Res Treat* 2006, 99:295–300.

95. Winer EP, Hudis C, Burstein HJ, *et al.*: American Society of Clinical Oncology technology assessment on the use of aromatase inhibitors as adjuvant therapy for postmenopausal women with hormone receptor-positive breast cancer: status report 2004. *J Clin Oncol* 2005, 23:619–629.

96. Carlson RW, Brown E, Burstein HJ, *et al.*: NCCN Task Force Report: adjuvant therapy for breast cancer. *J Natl Compr Canc Netw* 2006, 4(Suppl 1):S1–26.

97. Dowsett M, Allred DC: Relationship between quantitative ER and PgR expression and HER2 status with recurrence in the ATAC trial [abstract]. *Breast Cancer Res Treat* 2006, 100:abstract 48.

98. Viale G, Regan MM, Maiorano E, *et al.*: Prognostic and predictive value of centrally reviewed expression of estrogen and progesterone receptors in a randomized trial comparing letrozole and tamoxifen adjuvant therapy for postmenopausal women with early breast cancer: results from the BIG 1-98 collaborative groups. *J Clin Oncol* 2007, 25:3846–3852.

99. Stearns V, Davidson NE: Adjuvant chemotherapy or chemoendocrine therapy for primary breast cancer. In *Diseases of the Breast.* Edited by Harris JR, Lippman ME, Morrow M, *et al.* Philadelphia: Lippincott Williams & Wilkins; 2004:893.

100. Citron ML, Berry DA, Cirrincione C, *et al.*: Randomized trial of dose-dense versus conventionally scheduled and sequential versus concurrent combination chemotherapy as postoperative adjuvant treatment of node-positive primary breast cancer: first report of Intergroup Trial C9741/Cancer and Leukemia Group B Trial 9741. *J Clin Oncol* 2003, 21:1431–1439.

101. Henderson IC, Berry DA, Demetri GD, *et al.*: Improved outcomes from adding sequential paclitaxel but not from escalating doxorubicin dose in an adjuvant chemotherapy regimen for patients with node-positive primary breast cancer. *J Clin Oncol* 2003, 21:976–983.

102. Budman DR, Berry DA, Cirrincione CT, *et al.*: Dose and dose intensity as determinants of outcome in the adjuvant treatment of breast cancer. The Cancer and Leukemia Group B. *J Natl Cancer Inst* 1998, 90:1205–1211.

103. Berry DA, Cirrincione C, Henderson IC, *et al.*: Estrogen-receptor status and outcomes of modern chemotherapy for patients with node-positive breast cancer. *JAMA* 2006, 295:1658–1667.

104. Mamounas EP, Bryant J, Lembersky B, *et al.*: Paclitaxel after doxorubicin plus cyclophosphamide as adjuvant chemotherapy for node-positive breast cancer: results from NSABP B-28. *J Clin Oncol* 2005, 23:3686–3696.

105. Martin M, Pienkowski T, Mackey J, *et al.*: Adjuvant docetaxel for node-positive breast cancer. *N Engl J Med* 2005, 352:2302–2313.

106. Jones SE, Savin MA, Holmes FA, *et al.*: Phase III trial comparing doxorubicin plus cyclophosphamide with docetaxel plus cyclophosphamide as adjuvant therapy for operable breast cancer. *J Clin Oncol* 2006, 24:5381–5387.

107. Goldstein LJ, O'Neill A, Sparano J, *et al.*: E2197: Phase III AT (doxorubicin/docetaxel) vs AC (doxorubicin/cyclophosphamide) in the adjuvant treatment of node positive and high risk node negative breast cancer [abstract]. *J Clin Oncol* 2005, 23(16S):512.

108. Sparano JA, Wang M, Martino S, *et al.*: Phase III study of doxorubicin-cyclophosphamide followed by paclitaxel or docetaxel given every 3 weeks or weekly in patients with axillary node-positive or high-risk node-negative breast cancer: results of North American Breast Cancer Intergroup Trial E1199 [abstract]. *Breast Cancer Res Treat* 2006, 88:abstract 48.

109. Briest S, Davidson NE: Aromatase inhibitors for breast cancer. *Rev Endocr Metab Disord* 2007, 8:215–228.

110. Mauri D, Pavlidis N, Polyzos NP, *et al.*: Survival with aromatase inhibitors and inactivators versus standard hormonal therapy in advanced breast cancer: meta-analysis. *J Natl Cancer Inst* 2006, 98:1285–1291.

111. Robertson JF, Osborne CK, Howell A, *et al.*: Fulvestrant versus anastrozole for the treatment of advanced breast carcinoma in postmenopausal women: a prospective combined analysis of two multicenter trials. *Cancer* 2003, 98:229–238.

112. Ingle JN, Suman VJ, Rowland KM, *et al.*: Fulvestrant in women with advanced breast cancer after progression on prior aromatase inhibitor therapy: North Central Cancer Treatment Group Trial N0032. *J Clin Oncol* 2006, 24:1052–1056.

113. Klijn JG, Blamey RW, Boccardo F, *et al.*: Combined tamoxifen and luteinizing hormone-releasing hormone (LHRH) agonist versus LHRH agonist alone in premenopausal advanced breast cancer: a meta-analysis of four randomized trials. *J Clin Oncol* 2001, 19:343–353.

114. Ellis M, Hayes DF, Lippman ME: Treatment of metastatic breast cancer. In *Diseases of the Breast.* Edited by Harris JR, Lippman ME, Morrow M, *et al.* Philadelphia: Lippincott Williams & Wilkins; 2004.

115. Colozza M, de Azambuja E, Personeni N, *et al.*: Achievements in systemic therapies in the pregenomic era in metastatic breast cancer. *Oncologist* 2007, 12:253–270.

116. Carter SK: Single and combination nonhormonal chemotherapy in breast cancer. *Cancer* 1972, 30:1543–1555.

117. Smalley RV, Carpenter J, Bartolucci A, *et al.*: A comparison of cyclo-phosphamide, Adriamycin, 5-fluorouracil (CAF) and cyclophosphamide, methotrexate, 5-fluorouracil, vincristine, prednisone (CMFVP) in patients with metastatic breast cancer: a Southeastern Cancer Study Group project. *Cancer* 1977, 40:625–632.

118. A'Hern RP, Smith IE, Ebbs SR: Chemotherapy and survival in advanced breast cancer: the inclusion of doxorubicin in Cooper type regimens. *Br J Cancer* 1993, 67:801–805.

119. O'Brien ME, Wigler N, Inbar M, *et al.*: Reduced cardiotoxicity and compa-rable efficacy in a phase III trial of pegylated liposomal doxorubicin HCl (CAELYX/Doxil) versus conventional doxorubicin for first-line treatment of metastatic breast cancer. *Ann Oncol* 2004, 15:440–449.

120. Biganzoli L, Coleman R, Minisini A, *et al.*: A joined analysis of two Euro-pean Organization for the Research and Treatment of Cancer (EORTC) studies to evaluate the role of pegylated liposomal doxorubicin (Caelyx) in the treatment of elderly patients with metastatic breast cancer. *Crit Rev Oncol Hematol* 2007, 61:84–89.

121. Batist G, Ramakrishnan G, Rao CS, *et al.*: Reduced cardiotoxicity and preserved antitumor efficacy of liposome-encapsulated doxorubicin and cyclophosphamide compared with conventional doxorubicin and cyclophosphamide in a randomized, multicenter trial of metastatic breast cancer. *J Clin Oncol* 2001, 19:1444–1454.

122. Harris L, Batist G, Belt R, *et al.*: Liposome-encapsulated doxorubicin com-pared with conventional doxorubicin in a randomized multicenter trial as first-line therapy of metastatic breast carcinoma. *Cancer* 2002, 94:25–36.

123. Batist G, Harris L, Azarnia N, *et al.*: Improved anti-tumor response rate with decreased cardiotoxicity of non-pegylated liposomal doxorubicin com-pared with conventional doxorubicin in first-line treatment of metastatic breast cancer in patients who had received prior adjuvant doxorubicin: results of a retrospective analysis. *Anticancer Drugs* 2006, 17:587–595.

124. Piccart MJ, Burzykowski T, Sledge G, *et al.*: Effects of taxanes alone or in combination with anthracyclines on tumor response, progression-free survival and overall survival in first-line chemotherapy of patients with metastatic breast cancer: an analysis of 4,256 patients randomized in 12 trials [abstract]. *Breast Cancer Res Treat* 2005, 94:S278.

125. Gradishar WJ, Tjulandin S, Davidson N, *et al.*: Phase III trial of nanoparticle albumin-bound paclitaxel compared with polyethylated castor oil-based paclitaxel in women with breast cancer. *J Clin Oncol* 2005, 23:7794–7803.

126. Blum JL, Dieras V, Lo Russo PM, *et al.*: Multicenter, phase II study of capecitabine in taxane-pretreated metastatic breast carcinoma patients. *Cancer* 2001, 92:1759–1768.

127. O'Shaughnessy J, Miles D, Vukelja S, *et al.*: Superior survival with capecitabine plus docetaxel combination therapy in anthracycline-pre-treated patients with advanced breast cancer: phase III trial results. *J Clin Oncol* 2002, 20:2812–2823.

128. Zelek L, Barthier S, Riofrio M, *et al.*: Weekly vinorelbine is an effective palliative regimen after failure with anthracyclines and taxanes in meta-static breast carcinoma. *Cancer* 2001, 92:2267–2272.

129. Weber BL, Vogel C, Jones S, *et al.*: Intravenous vinorelbine as first-line and second-line therapy in advanced breast cancer. *J Clin Oncol* 1995, 13:2722–2730.

130. Spielmann M, Dorval T, Turpin F, *et al.*: Phase II trial of vinorelbine/doxo-rubicin as first-line therapy of advanced breast cancer. *J Clin Oncol* 1994, 12:1764–1770.

131. Seidman AD: Gemcitabine as single-agent therapy in the management of advanced breast cancer. *Oncology (Williston Park)* 2001, 15:11–14.

132. Kaufmann M, Hortobagyi GN, Goldhirsch A, *et al.*: Recommendations from an international expert panel on the use of neoadjuvant (primary) systemic treatment of operable breast cancer: an update. *J Clin Oncol* 2006, 24:1940–1949.

133. Symmans WF, Peintingerw F, Hatzis C, *et al.*: Measurement of residual breast cancer burden to predict survival after neoadjuvant chemotherapy. *J Clin Oncol* 2007, 25:4414–4422.

134. Wolmark N, Wang J, Mamounas E, *et al.*: Preoperative chemotherapy in patients with operable breast cancer: nine-year results from National Surgical Adjuvant Breast and Bowel Project B-18. *J Natl Cancer Inst Monogr* 2001, 96–102.

135. Wolff AC, Davidson NE: Primary systemic therapy in operable breast cancer. *J Clin Oncol* 2000, 18:1558–1569.

136. National Cancer Institute: Preoperative therapy in invasive breast cancer: reviewing the state of the science and exploring new research directions. Available at http://ctep.cancer.gov/bcmeeting/index.html. Accessed June 28, 2008.

137. Carey LA, Metzger R, Dees EC, *et al.*: American Joint Committee on Cancer Tumor-Node-Metastasis stage after neoadjuvant chemotherapy and breast cancer outcome. *J Natl Cancer Inst* 2005, 97:1137–1142.

138. Preece PE, Wood RA, Mackie CR, *et al.*: Tamoxifen as initial sole treat-ment of localised breast cancer in elderly women: a pilot study. *Br Med J (Clin Res Ed)* 1982, 284:869–870.

139. Smith IE, Dowsett M, Ebbs SR, *et al.*: Neoadjuvant treatment of post-menopausal breast cancer with anastrozole, tamoxifen, or both in combi-nation: the Immediate Preoperative Anastrozole, Tamoxifen, or Combined with Tamoxifen (IMPACT) multicenter double-blind randomized trial. *J Clin Oncol* 2005, 23:5108–5116.

140. Cataliotti L, Buzdar AU, Noguchi S, *et al.*: Comparison of anastrozole ver-sus tamoxifen as preoperative therapy in postmenopausal women with hormone receptor-positive breast cancer: the Pre-Operative "Arimidex" Compared to Tamoxifen (PROACT) trial. *Cancer* 2006, 106:2095–2103.

141. Eiermann W, Paepke S, Appfelstaedt J, *et al.*: Preoperative treatment of postmenopausal breast cancer patients with letrozole: a randomized double-blind multicenter study. *Ann Oncol* 2001, 12:1527–1532.

142. Ellis MJ, Coop A, Singh B, *et al.*: Letrozole is more effective neoadjuvant endocrine therapy than tamoxifen for ErbB-1- and/or ErbB-2-positive, estrogen receptor-positive primary breast cancer: evidence from a phase III randomized trial. *J Clin Oncol* 2001, 19:3808–3816.

143. Wolff AC, Davidson NE: Preoperative therapy in breast cancer: lessons from the treatment of locally advanced disease. *Oncologist* 2002, 7:239–245.

144. Smith IC, Heys SD, Hutcheon AW, *et al.*: Neoadjuvant chemotherapy in breast cancer: significantly enhanced response with docetaxel. *J Clin Oncol* 2002, 20:1456–1466.

145. Heys SD, Sarkar T, Hutcheon AW: Primary docetaxel chemotherapy in patients with breast cancer: impact on response and survival. *Breast Cancer Res Treat* 2005, 90:169–185.

146. Bear HD, Anderson S, Brown A, *et al.*: The effect on tumor response of adding sequential preoperative docetaxel to preoperative doxorubicin and cyclophosphamide: preliminary results from National Surgical Adjuvant Breast and Bowel Project Protocol B-27. *J Clin Oncol* 2003, 21:4165–4174.

147. Bear HD, Anderson S, Smith RE, *et al.*: Sequential preoperative or post-operative docetaxel added to preoperative doxorubicin plus cyclophos-phamide for operable breast cancer: National Surgical Adjuvant Breast and Bowel Project Protocol B-27. *J Clin Oncol* 2006, 24:2019–2027.

148. Cobleigh MA, Vogel CL, Tripathy D, *et al.*: Multinational study of the efficacy and safety of humanized anti-HER2 monoclonal antibody in women who have HER2-overexpressing metastatic breast cancer that has progressed after chemotherapy for metastatic disease. *J Clin Oncol* 1999, 17:2639–2648.

149. Vogel CL, Cobleigh MA, Tripathy D, *et al.*: Efficacy and safety of trastu-zumab as a single agent in first-line treatment of HER2-overexpressing metastatic breast cancer. *J Clin Oncol* 2002, 20:719–726.

150. Slamon DJ, Leyland-Jones B, Shak S, *et al.*: Use of chemotherapy plus a monoclonal antibody against HER2 for metastatic breast cancer that overexpresses HER2. *N Engl J Med* 2001, 344:783–792.

151. Esteva FJ, Valero V, Booser D, *et al.*: Phase II study of weekly docetaxel and trastuzumab for patients with HER-2-overexpressing metastatic breast cancer. *J Clin Oncol* 2002, 20:1800–1808.

152. Burstein HJ, Keshaviah A, Baron AD, *et al.*: Trastuzumab plus vinorelbine or taxane chemotherapy for HER2-overexpressing metastatic breast cancer: The trastuzumab and vinorelbine or taxane study. *Cancer* 2007, 110:965–972.

153. Perez EA: Carboplatin in combination therapy for metastatic breast cancer. *Oncologist* 2004, 9:518–527.

154. Robert N, Leyland-Jones B, Asmar L, *et al.*: Randomized phase III study of trastuzumab, paclitaxel, and carboplatin compared with trastuzumab and paclitaxel in women with HER-2-overexpressing metastatic breast cancer. *J Clin Oncol* 2006, 24:2786–2792.

155. Pegram M, Forbes J, Pienkowski T, *et al.*: BCIRG 007: first overall survival analysis of randomized phase III trial of trastuzumab plus docetaxel with or without carboplatin as first line therapy in HER2 amplified metastatic breast cancer (MBC) [abstract]. *J Clin Oncol* 2007, 25(18S):LBA1008.

156. Romond EH, Perez EA, Bryant J, *et al.*: Trastuzumab plus adjuvant chemotherapy for operable HER2-positive breast cancer. *N Engl J Med* 2005, 353:1673–1684.

157. Smith I, Procter M, Gelber RD, *et al.*: 2-year follow-up of trastuzumab after adjuvant chemotherapy in HER2-positive breast cancer: a randomised controlled trial. *Lancet* 2007, 369:29–36.

158. Slamon D, Eiermann W, Robert N, *et al.*: BCIRG 006: 2nd interim analysis phase III randomized trial comparing doxorubicin and cyclophosphamide followed by docetaxel (AC-T) with doxorubicin and cyclophosphamide followed by docetaxel and trastuzumab (AC-TH) with docetaxel, carboplatin and trastuzumab (TCH) in Her2neu positive early breast cancer patients [abstract]. *Breast Cancer Res Treat* 2006, 100:abstract 52.

159. Joensuu H, Kellokumpu-Lehtinen PL, Bono P, *et al.*: Adjuvant docetaxel or vinorelbine with or without trastuzumab for breast cancer. *N Engl J Med* 2006, 354:809–820.

160. Buzdar AU, Ibrahim NK, Francis D, *et al.*: Significantly higher pathologic complete remission rate after neoadjuvant therapy with trastuzumab, paclitaxel, and epirubicin chemotherapy: results of a randomized trial in human epidermal growth factor receptor 2-positive operable breast cancer. *J Clin Oncol* 2005, 23:3676–3685.

161. Buzdar AU, Valero V, Ibrahim NK, *et al.*: Neoadjuvant therapy with paclitaxel followed by 5-fluorouracil, epirubicin, and cyclophosphamide chemotherapy and concurrent trastuzumab in human epidermal growth factor receptor 2-positive operable breast cancer: an update of the initial randomized study population and data of additional patients treated with the same regimen. *Clin Cancer Res* 2007, 13:228–233.

162. Kim KJ, Li B, Winer J, *et al.*: Inhibition of vascular endothelial growth factor-induced angiogenesis suppresses tumour growth in vivo. *Nature* 1993, 362:841–844.

163. Miller KD, Chap LI, Holmes FA, *et al.*: Randomized phase III trial of capecitabine compared with bevacizumab plus capecitabine in patients with previously treated metastatic breast cancer. *J Clin Oncol* 2005, 23:792–799.

164. Miller KD, Wang M, Gralow J, *et al.*: A randomized phase III trial of paclitaxel versus paclitaxel plus bevacizumab as first-line therapy for locally recurrent or metastatic breast cancer: a trial coordinated by the Eastern Cooperative Oncology Group (E2100). *Breast Cancer Res Treat* 2005, 89:187–197.

165. Xia W, Mullin RJ, Keith BR, *et al.*: Anti-tumor activity of GW572016: a dual tyrosine kinase inhibitor blocks EGF activation of EGFR/erbB2 and downstream Erk1/2 and AKT pathways. *Oncogene* 2002, 21:6255–6263.

166. Konecny GE, Pegram MD, Venkatesan N, *et al.*: Activity of the dual kinase inhibitor lapatinib (GW572016) against HER-2-overexpressing and trastuzumab-treated breast cancer cells. *Cancer Res* 2006, 66:1630–1639.

167. Lin NU, Dieras V, Paul D, *et al.*: EGF105084, a phase II study of lapatinib for brain metastases in patients (pts) with HER2+ breast cancer following trastuzumab (H) based systemic therapy and cranial radiotherapy (RT) [abstract]. *J Clin Oncol* 2007, 25(18S):1012.

168. Geyer CE, Forster J, Lindquist D, *et al.*: Lapatinib plus capecitabine for HER2-positive advanced breast cancer. *N Engl J Med* 2006, 355:2733–2743.

169. Rugo HS, Stopeck A, Joy AA, *et al.*: A randomized, double-blind phase II study of the oral tyrosine kinase inhibitor (TKI) axitinib (AG-013736) in combination with docetaxel (DOC) compared to DOC plus placebo (PL) in metastatic breast cancer (MBC) [abstract]. *J Clin Oncol* 2007, 25(18S):1003.

170. Franklin MC, Carey KD, Vajdos FF, *et al.*: Insights into ErbB signaling from the structure of the ErbB2-pertuzumab complex. *Cancer Cell* 2004, 5:317–328.

171. Baselga J, Cameron D, Miles D, *et al.*: Objective response rate in a phase II multicenter trial of pertuzumab (P), a HER2 dimerization inhibiting monoclonal antibody, in combination with trastuzumab (T) in patients (pts) with HER2-positive metastatic breast cancer (MBC) which has progressed during treatment with T [abstract]. *J Clin Oncol* 2007, 25(18S):1004.

172. Shapiro S: Periodic screening for breast cancer: the HIP Randomized Controlled Trial. Health Insurance Plan. *J Natl Cancer Inst Monogr* 1997, 27–30.

173. Tabar L, Vitak B, Chen HH, *et al.*: The Swedish Two-County Trial twenty years later. Updated mortality results and new insights from long-term follow-up. *Radiol Clin North Am* 2000, 38:625–651.

174. Fisher B, Costantino JP, Wickerham DL, *et al.*: Tamoxifen for prevention of breast cancer: report of the National Surgical Adjuvant Breast and Bowel Project P-1 Study. *J Natl Cancer Inst* 1998, 90:1371–1388.

175. Vogel VG, Costantino JP, Wickerham DL, *et al.*: Effects of tamoxifen vs raloxifene on the risk of developing invasive breast cancer and other disease outcomes: the NSABP Study of Tamoxifen and Raloxifene (STAR) P-2 trial. *JAMA* 2006, 295:2727–2741.

176. Powles TJ, Ashley S, Tidy VA, *et al.*: 20 year follow-up of the Royal Marsden tamoxifen breast cancer prevention trial [abstract]. *Breast Cancer Res Treat* 2006, 88:abstract 51.

177. Veronesi U, Maisonneuve P, Costa A, *et al.*: Prevention of breast cancer with tamoxifen: preliminary findings from the Italian randomised trial among hysterectomised women. Italian Tamoxifen Prevention Study. *Lancet* 1998, 352:93–97.

178. Khatcheressian JL, Wolff AC, Smith TJ, *et al.*: American Society of Clinical Oncology 2006 update of the breast cancer follow-up and management guidelines in the adjuvant setting. *J Clin Oncol* 2006, 24:5091–5097.

179. Rojas MP, Telaro E, Russo A, *et al.*: Follow-up strategies for women treated for early breast cancer. *Cochrane Database Syst Rev* 2005, CD001768.

180. Rowland JH, Hewitt M, Ganz PA: Cancer survivorship: a new challenge in delivering quality cancer care. *J Clin Oncol* 2006, 24:5101–5104.

181. Hayes DF: Clinical practice. Follow-up of patients with early breast cancer. *N Engl J Med* 2007, 356:2505–2513.

182. Woodward WA, Strom EA, Tucker SL, *et al.*: Changes in the 2003 American Joint Committee on Cancer staging for breast cancer dramatically affect stage-specific survival. *J Clin Oncol* 2003, 21:3244–3248.

183. National Comprehensive Cancer Network: Breast cancer screening and diagnosis guidelines (V.1.2008). Available at http://www.nccn.org/professionals/physician_gls/PDF/breast-screening.pdf. Accessed June 28, 2008.

184. American Society of Clinical Oncology policy statement update: genetic testing for cancer susceptibility. *J Clin Oncol* 2003, 21:2397–2406.

7

Upper Gastrointestinal Cancer
Daniel Laheru

Malignancies of the upper gastrointestinal (GI) tract pose substantial challenges for therapy (Tables 7-1 and 7-2). Surgery remains the only known therapeutic method for this group of diseases; however, 5-year survival rates continue to be low even after definitive resection. Such results have stimulated interest in alternate and combined forms of management for these malignancies. Experience with chemotherapy and radiation therapy is growing. This chapter compares various therapeutic approaches within each disease group and highlights selected chemotherapy regimens that are in common use or have unique applications in upper GI tract cancer.

ESOPHAGEAL CANCER

In 2008, 16,470 new cases of esophageal carcinoma are expected in the United States; men will have more than a fourfold increase in risk compared with women. For unknown reasons, incidence of adenocarcinoma of the esophagus is increasing at a rate faster than that of nearly any other cancer.

Table 7-1. Risk Factors for Cancers of the Upper Gastrointestinal Tract

Esophagus

Exposure to nitrosomines

Cigarette smoking

Excessive alcohol use

Lye ingestion

Achalasia

Barrett's mucosa

Tylosis

Infection with transforming viruses (HPV, HSV, CMV, EBV)

Plummer-Vinson syndrome

Mycotoxin

Stomach

Achlorhydria

Helicobacter pylori infection

Previous gastrectomy, Billroth II procedures

Family history

Pancreas

Cigarette smoking

Exposure to β-naphthylamine, benzidine

Chronic pancreatitis

Family history

Liver

Hepatitis B carrier state

Chronic liver disease (chronic active hepatitis, cirrhosis)

Exposure to mycotoxin, ionizing radiation, steroid hormones, arsenic

Bile ducts

Sclerosing cholangitis

Parasitic infections

Use of steroid hormones

CMV—cytomegalovirus; EBV—Epstein-Barr virus; HPV—human papillomavirus; HSV—herpes simplex virus.

Overall 5-year survival rates have never exceeded 12% [1]. Locoregional or systemic spread of disease is often attributed to the lack of anatomic barriers to dissemination. The esophagus does not have a serosa to provide a natural defense for local invasion and is rich in submucosal lymphatics, which probably allow longitudinal spread from the primary site. Autopsy findings from patients who have recently undergone surgery for squamous cell carcinoma of the esophagus have demonstrated a high incidence of unsuspected early metastatic disease.

Patients with esophageal cancer usually present with dysphagia. Diagnosis is made with a contrast study alone or combined with endoscopy. Staging evaluation consists of a computed tomography (CT) scan of the chest and abdomen in addition to endoscopic ultrasound. Fine-needle aspirates should be performed on suspicious cervical or periumbilical adenopathy, and a bone scan should be done if symptoms of bone pain are present. Bronchoscopy should also be performed on patients with proximal lesions who are at risk of tracheobronchial fistula. Based on the staging evaluation and the patient's general state of health, a treatment protocol is designed (Table 7-3, Fig. 7-1). Patients with dysphagia whose disease is deemed unresectable often benefit from a percutaneous gastrostomy tube for alimentation during further therapy. This is not recommended for the surgical candidate because the stomach is the primary conduit used to replace the esophagus. Patients who are surgical candidates can be staged further with laparoscopy, and a feeding jejunostomy may be placed at that time for alimentation during neoadjuvant therapy prior to surgery [2].

THERAPY FOR ADVANCED DISEASE

Single-agent chemotherapy is now rarely used for advanced disease. Paclitaxel as a single agent has been reported to produce response rates of 34% and 28% in patients with adenocarcinoma and squamous cell carcinoma, respectively [3]. However, the best response rates are achieved with a combination of chemotherapeutic agents. The most commonly used combination chemotherapy regimen is 5-fluorouracil (5-FU) and cisplatin, which can produce an objective response rate as high as 42%. Other agents in cisplatin-containing combinations have included docetaxel, oxaliplatin, epirubicin, and protracted infusion 5-FU. These combinations have shown encouraging response rates of up to 65%. A phase 3 first-line study of docetaxel, cisplatin, and 5-FU compared with cisplatin and 5-FU demonstrated an improvement in time to progression (5.6 vs 3.7 months) as well as overall survival (9.2 vs 8.6 months) [4]. Another phase 3 first-line study demonstrated an improvement in overall survival when oxaliplatin/epirubicin was paired with capecitabine

Table 7-2. Guidelines for Prevention and Early Detection of Cancers of the Upper GI Tract

Prevention

Avoid cigarette smoking

Use alcohol in moderation

Eat a low-fat diet rich in fresh fruit and vegetables

Avoid exposure to occupational toxins

Immunize against infectious hepatitis

Avoid unnecessary use of steroid hormones

Early detection

Esophagus: annual upper GI endoscopy in patients with known Barrett's mucosa, tylosis, or history of caustic esophageal injury

Hepatoma: periodic α-fetoprotein measurement and liver ultrasound for patients with chronic liver disease

GI—gastrointestinal.

Table 7-3. TNM Staging Criteria for Esophageal Cancer

Staging	Criteria
T (Tumor)	
TX	Primary tumor cannot be assessed
T0	No evidence of primary tumor
Tis	Carcinoma in situ
T1	Tumor invades lamina propria or submucosa
T2	Tumor invades muscularis propria
T3	Tumor invades adventitia
T4	Tumor invades adjacent structures
N (Node)	
NX	Regional lymph nodes cannot be assessed
N0	No regional lymph node metastasis
N1	Regional lymph node metastasis
M (Metastasis)	
MX	Distant metastasis cannot be assessed
M0	No distant metastasis
M1	Distant metastasis
Tumors of the lower thoracic esophagus:	
M1a	Metastasis in celiac lymph nodes
M1b	Other distant metastasis
Tumors of the midthoracic esophagus:	
M1a	Not applicable
M1b	Nonregional lymph nodes and/or other distant metastasis
Tumors of the upper thoracic esophagus:	
M1a	Metastasis in cervical nodes
M1b	Other distant metastasis
Stage	**TNM Groupings**
Stage 0	Tis, N0, M0
Stage I	T1, N0, M0
Stage IIA	T2, N0, M0
	T3, N0, M0
Stage IIB	T1, N1, M0
	T2, N1, M0
Stage III	T3, N1, M0
	T4, any N, M0
Stage IV	Any T, any N, M1
Stage IVA	Any T, any N, M1a
Stage IVB	Any T, any N, M1b

(11.2 months) versus oxaliplatin, epirubicin, and 5-FU (9.3 months) or versus epirubicin with cisplatin and 5-FU (9.9 months) or capecitabine (9.9 months) [5]. Cisplatin and irinotecan have recently been used in conjunction to produce objective responses of 57%, and have been associated with a median survival of 14.6 months and diminished dysphagia in 90% of treated patients [6]. More recently, cisplatin and irinotecan have been safely combined with small molecule drugs like bevacizumab; encouraging clinical outcomes have been demonstrated by a response rate of 65%, time to progression of 8.3 months, and overall survival of 12.3 months [7].

THERAPY FOR LOCALLY UNRESECTABLE DISEASE

Perhaps the most vigorously tested role of combination chemotherapy in esophageal cancer has been in the multimodal management of local or regional disease. In the past, radiation therapy had been the mainstay of therapy as palliation for patients who were believed to have disease that could not be resected with reasonable chance for cure (T4, M1 disease) (Table 7-3). Relief of dysphagia in these patients is excellent, with reported palliative responses of up to 80%. However, even a small change in tumor size can lead to marked improvement in swallowing function, which results from decreased resistance to flow; this may explain why the high palliative rate observed with radiation therapy alone has not resulted in significant changes in median survival. Various studies have assessed the safety, feasibility, and regression rates of combination chemotherapy and radiation for patients with locally unresectable disease. The mainstay of drug therapy in this setting has been 5-FU combined with other radiation-sensitizing drugs, such as cisplatin or mitomycin. Pilot experiences with this approach showed encouragingly high 2-year survival rates and, in some cases, durable complete responses were observed. One such approach in the treatment of patients with adenocarcinoma of the esophagus and gastroesophageal junction involved a combination of 5-FU and mitomycin in addition to radiation therapy as definitive treatment. Complete response in seven of eight patients with T1 and T2 disease and a median relapse-free survival of 10 months were observed. Studies such as these led the Radiation Therapy Oncology Group (RTOG), the Southwest Oncology Group (SWOG), and the North Central Cancer Treatment Group (NCCTG) to conduct a randomized trial [8] comparing a combination of 5-FU (1000 mg/m² by continuous infusion daily for 4 days) and cisplatin (75 mg/m² on day 1) plus 50 Gy of radiation therapy to 64-Gy radiation therapy alone in patients with epidermoid carcinoma or adenocarcinoma of the thoracic esophagus. As might be expected, severe and life-threatening side effects (predominantly mucositis and myelosuppression) were seen more frequently in patients treated with combined-modality therapy. One patient in the combined-modality group died from complications of renal and bone marrow failure and many were not able to complete the full chemotherapeutic course. A 5-year follow-up for all patients showed a median survival of 14 months and an overall survival of 26% in the combined treatment group, whereas the median survival was 9.3 months with no patient alive at 5 years in the group tested with radiation alone [9]. Actuarial incidence of local failure as the first site of failure was also significantly decreased in the combined-modality group (45% vs 68%; *P* = 0.0123). The randomizing protocol was closed early due to these posi-

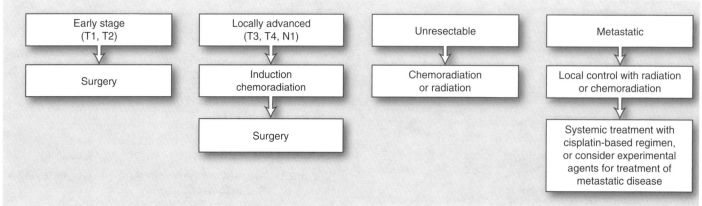

Figure 7-1. Treatment strategies for esophageal and esophagogastric cancer.

tive results; after this, an additional 50 patients were treated with combined therapy. The 5-year mortality for this group was 14% [10]. These survival results were also suggested by another broad-based practice survey [11].

Another approach has been to integrate irinotecan and cisplatin and radiation therapy or small molecule biologic drugs like cetuximab with radiation [12,13].

NEOADJUVANT THERAPY

Numerous randomized clinical trials have shown that neither radiation nor chemotherapy is of benefit when used alone prior to surgery [14,15]; however, the combination of the two has shown promising results. Early studies used 5-FU as a common denominator in induction chemotherapy as a single agent [16], in combination with cisplatin or mitomycin C, or as a multiagent regimen [17]. Although these trials varied in their study populations with respect to the proportion of epidermoid carcinomas to adenocarcinomas and with respect to presenting stage of disease, these reports were notable for the documentation of complete responses with eradication of pathologic evidence of disease. Naunheim *et al.* [18] reported an overall median survival of 23 months; in the report by Forastiere *et al.* [17], the median survival time was 29 months, and 34% of the patients were alive at 5 years. In both studies, the complete histologic response rate was more than 20%. These encouraging results led to several phase 3 investigations. Urba *et al.* [19] randomized 100 patients—75% with adenocarcinoma, 25% with squamous carcinoma—to surgery alone versus cisplatin, 5-FU, vinblastine, and 45-Gy radiation followed by surgery. The group receiving neoadjuvant therapy had a 3-year survival of 32% compared with 15% survival in the control group. This result was of borderline statistical significance ($P = 0.07$); a subsequent report updating this trial found no statistically significant survival difference [20]. In patients with esophageal adenocarcinoma, a prospective, randomized trial performed by Walsh *et al.* [21] clearly showed the superiority of combined-modality therapy (two courses of 5-FU and cisplatin with 40 Gy of radiotherapy followed by surgery) compared with surgery alone. The overall survival rates at 3 years were 32% and 6%, respectively. However, this study was criticized because the survival rate of those receiving surgery alone seemed unusually low. Randomized trials with squamous cell cancer have not shown a clear-cut benefit. In one multicenter, randomized trial, Bossett *et al.* [22] found improved disease-free survival and survival free of local disease, but no overall survival benefit between the groups receiving multimodal therapy and those receiving surgery alone. Notably, however, cisplatin was the only chemotherapeutic agent used in the combined treatment arm in the latter study. Law *et al.* [23] reported no survival benefit using cisplatin, 5-FU, and 40 Gy in addition to surgery for squamous cell cancer. Many had hoped that the present controversy would be clarified by Cancer and Leukemia Group B (CALGB) C9781, a phase 3 trial comparing neoadjuvant therapy to surgery alone, but unfortunately this trial has recently closed because of lack of accrual. There was a suggestion that combined modality chemoradiotherapy and surgery had a survival advantage over surgery alone, although the study was underpowered [24].

Preoperative strategies can be associated with a high toxicity profile, primarily from myelosuppression and esophagitis. For instance, Adelstein *et al.* [25] studied 5-FU and cisplatin chemotherapy in combination with accelerated fractionation radiation and found a perioperative mortality of 18%. Because of the toxicity of preoperative chemoradiotherapy and its unproven efficacy in phase 3 trials, both physicians and patients should weigh the benefits and side effects when electing treatment. Despite this, some well-designed phase 2 trials demonstrated 2-year survival as high as 60% and minimal morbidity with multimodal therapy [26]. Many physicians believe combined preoperative chemoradiotherapy should be considered in patients with clinical evidence of stage III disease (Fig. 7-1).

PALLIATIVE THERAPY

As already mentioned, combined chemoradiation is very effective at relieving the symptoms of obstruction. Unfortunately this usually takes 4 to 6 weeks to occur. Patients with severe obstruction who are at risk for aspiration can benefit from physical methods of maintaining esophageal patency while awaiting the benefits of chemoradiation. A 1998 study indicated that dilatation alone provided adequate palliation in this group compared with dilatation and neo-

dymium-yttrium-aluminum-garnet (Nd-YAG) laser therapy [27]. Endoscopic laser therapy and endoluminal radiation can be employed in patients whose dysphagia has not been lessened with chemoradiation. Expansile metal stents are particularly good for refractory obstruction or tracheoesophageal fistulas with an overall success rate of 90% [28]. These stents result in fewer complications compared with older plastic prostheses [29].

STOMACH CANCER

In 2008, approximately 21,500 new cases of stomach cancer will be diagnosed in the United States, and an estimated 10,800 people will die of this

Table 7-4. TNM Staging Criteria for Gastric Cancer

Staging	Criteria
T (Tumor)	
TX	Primary tumor cannot be assessed
T0	No evidence of primary tumor
Tis	Carcinoma in situ: intraepithelial tumor without invasion of the lamina propria
T1	Tumor invades lamina propria or submucosa
T2	Tumor invades muscularis propria or subserosa
T3	Tumor penetrates serosa (visceral peritoneum) without invasion of adjacent structures
T4	Tumor invades adjacent structures
N (Nodes)	
NX	Regional lymph node(s) cannot be assessed
N0	No regional lymph node metastasis
N1	Metastasis in 1–6 regional lymph nodes
N2	Metastasis in 7–15 regional lymph nodes
N3	Metastasis in > 15 regional lymph nodes
M (Metastasis)	
MX	Distant metastasis cannot be assessed
M0	No distant metastasis
M1	Distant metastasis
Stage	**TNM Groupings**
Stage 0	Tis, N0, M0
Stage IA	T1, N0, M0
Stage IB	T1, N1, M0
	T2, N0, M0
Stage II	T1, N2, M0
	T2, N1, M0
	T3, N0, M0
Stage IIIA	T2, N2, M0
	T3, N1, M0
	T4, N0, M0
Stage IIIB	T3, N2, M0
Stage IV	T4, N1, M0
	T1, N3, M0
	T2, N3, M0
	T3, N3, M0
	T4, N2, M0
	T4, N3, M9
	Any T, any N, M1

disease [1]. Cancer of the stomach appears to be decreasing in incidence. The explanation for this perplexing change in incidence is not known; however, some have attributed the decrease to the common practice of adding ascorbic acid as a food preservative, which decreases gastric pH and limits endogenous nitrosamine production by bacteria in the upper GI tract. A link between gastric cancer and *Helicobacter pylori* infections as a risk factor has been described [30,31]. The overall 5-year survival rate for affected patients remains low at approximately 21% [1]. Because the presenting symptoms of stomach cancer tend to be extremely vague, most patients are diagnosed with extensive local involvement or regional lymph node metastases. This explains in part the poor 5-year survival rate following surgery (Table 7-4). The staging work-up is similar to that used in esophageal cancer including endoscopy, endoscopic ultrasound, and abdominal CT.

THERAPY FOR LOCOREGIONAL DISEASE

Perhaps no topic in gastric cancer has received as much focus as the role of the extended lymphadenectomy. This aggressive surgical technique is embraced in Japan, where stage-specific survival is significantly higher than that reported in Western series. Three randomized trials compared D1 (removal of local draining lymph nodes) and D2 (removal of the next level of draining nodes) dissections in Western countries; increased morbidity was shown with the larger dissection but not increased survival [32–35]. For these reasons, D1 rather than D2 lymph node dissections have been accepted as standard cancer operations in the West.

The SWOG reviewed findings in 453 patients who underwent resection for gastric adenocarcinoma and demonstrated that a D0 dissection (an inadequate cancer operation) is what was performed in more than half of the cases [36]. This group went on to demonstrate that postoperative combined radiation and chemotherapy improved disease-free survival and overall survival in patients who had undergone resection of gastric adenocarcinoma [37]. The 557 patients who had undergone resection with curative intent and demonstrated no sign of metastasis were randomized to either treatment (with 5-FU, leucovorin, and 45 Gy of radiation) or observation. Nodal metastases were present in 85% of pathologic specimens. Therapy resulted in mortality in 1%, grade 3 toxicity in 32%, and grade 4 toxicity in 41% of patients treated. At a median of 3.3 years of follow-up, 3-year disease-free survival was 49% in treated patients compared with 32% in the control group ($P = 0.001$). Overall survival was 49% and 32%, respectively ($P = 0.003$). Although these were powerful results, some criticized the study [38], stating that perhaps the effect of the adjuvant therapy was to increase the survival from that obtained with an inadequate D0 dissection to that documented for D1 resections in the past [33].

Before the appearance of this analysis, results for adjuvant therapy in the United States had been poor. A meta-analysis involving 11 randomized trials had concluded that postoperative adjuvant therapy did not appear to be useful [39].

Previous disappointing results with postoperative adjuvant chemotherapy spawned attempts at improving surgical outcome with preoperative chemotherapy. Several studies are noteworthy in this regard. EAP (etoposide, doxorubicin, and cisplatin) has been tested preoperatively in patients with advanced locoregional disease (eg, those with positive lymph nodes, T3 or T4 primary lesions) [40,41]. EAP therapy was continued until patients achieved a maximum response to therapy, at which point resection was attempted. The objective response rate to preoperative EAP was 70%, including a 21% complete response rate. Twenty patients subsequently underwent resection. At a median follow-up of 20 months, the relapse rate was 60% at a median survival time of 18 months. The high complete remission rate with the EAP regimen could not be confirmed in another multi-institutional trial reported by Ajani *et al.* [42] involving early-stage gastric cancers. Ajani *et al.* [43] also evaluated the preoperative response rate and resectability following administration of etoposide, 5-FU, and cisplatin. In that study, 24% of the patients had major preoperative responses to chemotherapy, including two complete responses. The resection rate was 72%, and with a median follow-up of 25 months the median survival was 15 months. Safran *et al.* [44,45] evaluated the combination of paclitaxel with concurrent radiation therapy for locally advanced gastric cancer and determined a response rate of 70% in patients with evaluable disease. Of these patients, 30% subsequently underwent resection. Another approach incorporated postoperative intraperitoneal therapy with 5-FU and cisplatin in addition to preoperative FAMTX (5-FU, doxorubicin, methotrexate, and leucovorin). For patients who underwent curative resection in this study, the median survival was 31 months; peritoneal failure was seen in 16% of the patients, with acceptable levels of toxicity [44,45]. Ajani *et al.* [46] administered 5-FU, interferon, and cisplatin to 30 patients before scheduled surgery. Only half these patients could tolerate the planned five cycles. Clinical response was seen in 34% and complete response in 7%. Complete R0 resection was performed in 83%, producing a median survival of 30 months. These reports require confirmation in larger randomized trials before these approaches can be accepted as standard management for gastric cancer (Fig. 7-2).

THERAPY FOR ADVANCED DISEASE

Both single-agent and combination chemotherapy have been widely tested in advanced metastatic gastric cancer. More active agents in the past have included 5-FU, trimetrexate, mitomycin C, hydroxyurea, epirubicin, and carmustine, the partial response rates of which vary from 18% to 30%. Combination chemotherapy with these and other marginally active agents appears to produce higher objective response rates than those seen with single agents. Promising results have been seen with newer drug combinations involving the taxanes [47] and irinotecan; single-institution trials have reported objective response rates as high as 53% [48]. In a study by Buku *et al.* [49], irinotecan in combination with cisplatin showed objective responses in 42% to 57% of patients with acceptable toxicity and complete remission in 2%. Docetaxel has been used in a multicenter trial in conjunction with cisplatin inducing complete responses in 4%, partial responses in 52%, and a median survival of 9 months. Hematologic toxicities were the most severe, but 78% of patients were able to receive treatment as planned [50]. Murad *et al.* [51] treated 29 patients with paclitaxel and 5-FU to achieve objective responses in 65%, including complete responses in 24%. Of these patients, three had pathologic complete response confirmed at laparotomy. Toxicity was low and easily managed. Median survival was 12 months with a 2-year survival rate of 20%. In 45 patients, paclitaxel in combination with 5-FU and cisplatin produced complete responses in 11%, partial responses in 40%, and a median survival of 9 months. Treatment was reasonably well tolerated and had to be modified in only 17%

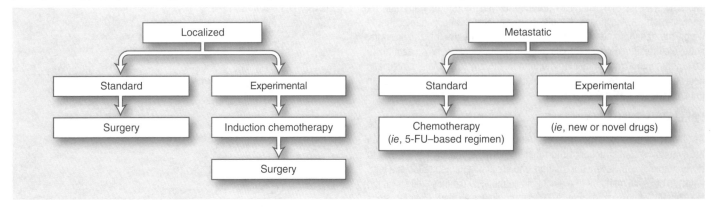

Figure 7-2. Treatment strategies for gastric cancer.

[52]. Another study used paclitaxel, etoposide, and cisplatin in 25 patients with advanced disease. Three of these patients had complete pathologic responses documented by laparotomy; 19 had partial responses [53].

Higher objective response rates did not hold up in phase 3 trials with past regimens, and to date, no single combination chemotherapy program tested in prospective randomized trials has shown a statistically significant improvement in median survival compared with those found in other regimens. Various multiagent regimens with activity against gastric cancer are available. Unfortunately, it is not yet clear whether any specific regimen can improve median survival compared with results accruing from the best single-agent or other combination regimens. Further phase 3 trials are needed to clarify the role of combination chemotherapy in advanced metastatic gastric cancer.

PANCREATIC CANCER

ADENOCARCINOMA

Adenocarcinoma of the pancreas represents the fourth most common cause of cancer-related death in US men. An estimated 37,680 cases may be expected to occur in 2008 [1]. Incidence of the disease approximately equals the age-adjusted mortality rate, which underscores the aggressive nature of this malignancy [1] (Table 7-5). In large studies, only 5% to 22% of presenting patients have resectable tumors. Unfortunately, even successful resection is associated with a low 5-year survival rate, ranging from 3.5% to 19%. Lesions in the body and tail of the pancreas present at an advanced stage with nonspecific symptoms. Lesions of the head and neck of the pancreas present at an earlier stage typically with painless jaundice. A spiral CT scan demonstrating a resectable mass in the absence of distant metastasis is the only staging necessary before surgery. A diagnosis based on tissue samples is only necessary to plan medical therapy for unresectable lesions. Patients with unresectable adenocarcinomas of the pancreas confined to the pancreas often undergo palliative surgery or biliary stent placement for relief of jaundice in addition to prophylactic duodenal bypass procedures to prevent obstruction (observed in 10% of patients). Chemotherapy can add to both quantity and quality of life in advanced pancreatic cancer, although the benefit could be limited to selected patients [54].

THERAPY FOR LOCOREGIONAL DISEASE

The role of chemotherapy in the management of pancreatic carcinoma is best understood in the context of combined-modality treatment for the adjuvant therapy of pancreatic carcinoma after resection or in the management of locally unresectable lesions. The Gastrointestinal Tumor Study Group (GITSG) reported a better than twofold increase in the 2-year actuarial survival (46% and 43% vs 18%) for patients treated with a combination of 5-FU and split-course radiation therapy following resection, compared with resection alone. In addition, the GITSG demonstrated an almost twofold increase in median survival in patients with unresectable disease treated with 5-FU plus split-course radiation, compared with high-dose radiation therapy alone. Intraoperative radiotherapy and interstitial brachytherapy have been employed rather than external-beam radiotherapy but neither technique has demonstrated improved survival. Bolus 5-FU has also been studied in combination with intraoperative radiation therapy and with brachytherapy, although randomized trials are not available to determine the role of 5-FU in this clinical setting. Protracted-infusion 5-FU combined with radiation has shown similar activity to bolus 5-FU and radiotherapy but with less toxicity [55]. Paclitaxel in combination with radiotherapy showed some promise in preliminary trials [56]. In their phase 2 trial using 5-FU, leucovorin, and cisplatin in conjunction with radiotherapy in 38 patients with locally unresectable disease, Kornek *et al.* [57] achieved 1- and 2-year survivals of 53% and 18%, respectively, without surgery. RTOG 97-04, a large randomized phase 3 trial, addressed the efficacy of postoperative infusional 5-FU and radiation coupled with repeating cycles of either infusional 5-FU or gemcitabine [58]. The addition of gemcitabine to adjuvant fluorouracil-based chemoradiation was associated with a survival benefit for patients with resected pancreatic cancer, although this improvement was not statistically significant [59]. RTOG 98-12 coupled radiation (50 Gy) with weekly paclitaxel (50 mg/m^2) in the treatment of unresectable disease

[57]. The median survival for patients with locally advanced unresectable disease was 11.2 months [60].

NEOADJUVANT THERAPY

Early reports of neoadjuvant therapy used standard fractionation radiation therapy 5000 cGy over 5.5 weeks with concomitant 5-FU, and one third of patients treated required hospital admission for GI toxicity [61]. Many newer approaches employ rapid fractionation delivering therapy over 2 weeks totaling 30 Gy with 300 cGy per fraction being delivered 5 days a week. Preliminary results suggest that neoadjuvant regimens can be delivered at this point without increasing the morbidity and mortality of subsequent surgical resections [62,63], and may in fact decrease the rate of pancreatic fistula [64]. Spitz *et al.* [65] reviewed the outcome of preoperative or postoperative chemoradiation and showed that preoperative chemoradiation could be delivered over a shorter time period without causing a delay in surgery. Planned postoperative therapy resulted in one quarter of eligible patients who remained untreated because of prolonged recovery or perioperative complications following surgery. Unfortunately, no survival benefit has yet been shown with this approach.

Table 7-5. TNM Staging Criteria for Pancreatic Cancer

Staging	Criteria
T (Tumor)	
TX	Primary tumor cannot be assessed
T0	No evidence of primary tumor
Tis	In situ carcinoma
T1	Tumor limited to the pancreas ≤ 2 cm or less in greatest dimension
T2	Tumor limited to the pancreas > 2 cm in greatest dimension
T3	Tumor extends directly into any of the following: duodenum, bile duct, peripancreatic tissues
T4	Tumor extends directly into any of the following: stomach, spleen, colon, adjacent large vessels
N (Node)	
NX	Regional lymph nodes cannot be assessed
N0	No regional lymph node metastasis
N1	Regional lymph node metastasis
pN1a	Metastasis in a single regional lymph node
pN1b	Metastasis in multiple regional lymph nodes
M (Metastasis)	
MX	Distant metastasis cannot be assessed
M0	No distant metastasis
M1	Distant metastasis
Stage	**TNM Grouping**
Stage 0	Tis, N0, M0
Stage I	T1, N0, M0
	T2, N0, M0
Stage II	T3, N0, M0
Stage III	T1, N1, M0
	T2, N1, M0
	T3, N1, M0
Stage IVA	T4, any N, M0
Stage IVB	Any T, any N, M1

Prophylactic preoperative irradiation of the liver has been advocated as this is a common site of metastasis, but this can be related with life-threatening toxicities [66].

Currently, an active area of investigation involves the use of preoperative chemotherapy and radiation to improve the opportunities for complete resection. Hoffman *et al.* [67] have reported on the preoperative regimen of 5-FU, mitomycin C, and local radiation; they observed a resection rate of 32%. Staley *et al.* [68] reported a resection rate of 61% after preoperative chemoradiation with a median survival of 19 months and 4-year actuarial survival rate of 19%. Subsequent efforts attempted to downstage disease that was deemed unresectable by radiologic evaluation or previous surgery. Brunner *et al.* [69] treated 27 unresectable patients with conformal radiation (50.4 Gy), 5-FU, and gemcitabine; after restaging, 60% were explored and a standard Whipple procedure was performed with negative margins on 37%. Resected patients had a 2-year survival of 50% as opposed to 6% in the unresected group.

BORDERLINE RESECTABLE DISEASE

There has been much recent discussion regarding a distinct classification that describes patients who are borderline resectable. The characteristics that would define this category of disease are still being formalized, but in general this is suggested to involve tumors that abut the superior mesenteric artery or celiac axis for less than half the circumference of the vessel, tumors that involve at most a short segment of the common hepatic artery, short-segment occlusion of the superior mesenteric vein (SMV) with patent proximal SMV–portal vein confluence, or a patient who has a marginal performance status. For this category of patient, the M.D. Anderson Cancer Center [70] recently reported retrospective results on 160 borderline resectable patients who were treated with combined chemorads (50.4 or 30 Gy) with or without gemcitabine-based chemotherapy. The majority of patients (78%) were able to complete therapy and 41% of patients were able to undergo resection (with 97% R0 resection). The median survival of patients in this selected group of patients was 40 months compared with 13 months for patients who were subsequently determined to be unresectable.

THERAPY FOR ADVANCED DISEASE

Use of chemotherapy for patients with widespread metastatic disease has been disappointing. The median survival of patients with advanced disease treated with best supportive care is approximately 2 to 4 months. There appears to be no highly active single agent and virtually all approved chemotherapy drugs have now been tested. 5-FU may have activity as a single agent; for instance, a phase 2 trial using 5-FU and more optimal biochemical modulation with leucovorin demonstrated a modest response rate of 7% and a median survival of 6.2 months [71]. Gemcitabine has been compared with 5-FU in a phase 3 trial. This study demonstrated a superior median survival of 5.7 months for gemcitabine compared with 4.4 months for 5-FU and also demonstrated improved relief of symptoms with gemcitabine. Due to its palliative potential, gemcitabine as a single agent should be considered for unresectable pancreatic adenocarcinoma [72,73]. In one study, fixed-dose rate gemcitabine (using a dose-intense regimen) was shown to have a better median survival than high-dose gemcitabine using a standard infusing schedule [74].

However, an Eastern Cooperative Oncology Group (ECOG)-sponsored phase 3 study of gemcitabine at standard dose and infusion versus fixed-dose rate infusion gemcitabine versus standard dose-infusion gemcitabine and oxaliplatin did not show survival benefit over gemcitabine alone [75]. There has been interest in gemcitabine combinations with statistically significant albeit modest improvement in survival over gemcitabine alone for gemcitabine plus the oral epidermal growth factor receptor (EGFR) tyrosine kinase inhibitor erlotinib [76] and gemcitabine plus capecitabine, respectively [77]. It seems clear that either new drugs or novel therapeutic approaches for pancreatic adenocarcinoma are desperately needed (Fig. 7-3) [78,79].

ISLET CELL CARCINOMA

Another important subgroup of pancreatic tumors includes islet cell tumors. These include malignant insulinoma, gastrinoma, vasoactive intestinal polypeptide-secreting tumor (VIPoma), glucagonoma, and somatostatinoma. It is important to recognize these lesions histologically because the natural history and management of these pancreatic tumors are different.

Many islet cell tumors produce fascinating and distinctive syndromes related to secretory hormones. These tumors are often indolent in their growth; management is often directed at palliation of the associated symptoms. Treatment may include surgical reduction of tumor bulk, up to and including total orthotopic liver transplantation, hepatic artery occlusion for symptomatic metastatic disease, and specific end-organ blockade of the hormonal system. Examples of the latter would include omeprazole, an inhibitor of the parietal cell hydrogen pump, which is more effective than H-2 blockers in the management of symptomatic gastrinomas. Octreotide, a somatostatin analogue now available in a long-acting preparation, has shown beneficial effect on tumor growth with stabilization of the disease as the most favorable response [80]. Octreotide is also helpful in palliating symptoms in patients with islet cell carcinomas depending upon the cell type.

In the past, chemotherapy was reserved as a therapy of last resort in patients with these indolent tumors. Active drugs have included streptozocin, doxorubicin, chlorozotocin, and dacarbazine. A randomized trial was conducted showing superiority of streptozocin and doxorubicin over streptozocin plus 5-FU or single-agent chlorozotocin [81]. In this trial, the combination of streptozocin and doxorubicin produced an improved response rate over the other two arms (69% vs 45% and 30%, respectively) and a significant survival advantage (median survival, 2.2 years vs 1.4 years and 1.4 years, respectively). These results may justify the use of this therapy as an initial approach in some patients. Chemoembolization also appears to be an effective alternative for patients with liver metastases of neuroendocrine origin. In various studies, Ruszniewski *et al.* [82–85] have reported that hepatic artery chemoembolization with iodized oil and doxorubicin can provide symptom control and tumor regression or stabilization in up to 80% of carcinoid tumors and gastrinomas. Recently, sunitinib, an oral small molecule tyrosine kinase inhibitor of vascular endothelial growth factor receptor (VEGFR), platelet-derived growth factor receptors, stem cell factor receptors, and glial cell line–derived neurotropic factors has been tested in advanced carcinoid and neuroendocrine tumors with a response rate of 16.7% for neuroendocrine cancers versus 2% for carcinoid tumors [86].

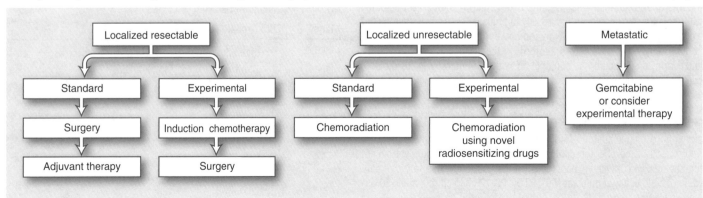

Figure 7-3. Treatment strategies for pancreatic cancer.

HEPATIC CANCER

Hepatocellular carcinoma (HCC) is the most prevalent cancer in the world. About 21,370 new cases are anticipated to occur in the United States in 2008 [1]. Any form of chronic liver injury and cirrhosis predisposes to the development of this malignancy. Worldwide, the most common risk factor is chronic viral hepatitis; in the United States, other causes of chronic liver disease, such as cirrhosis related to alcoholism, are also important risk factors. Regardless of the etiology, the only known curative modality for hepatoma is surgical resection.

Patients with liver disease should be monitored for the development of hepatoma with serum α-fetoprotein (AFP) levels and ultrasound examinations. When suspicions are raised, dynamic CT and magnetic resonance imaging (MRI) should be performed. Without elevated serum AFP levels, fine-needle aspiration may be required to diagnose radiologically indistinct lesions.

THERAPY FOR LOCOREGIONAL DISEASE

The patient's degree of cirrhosis and the anatomic location of tumor determine if partial hepatectomy can be performed. Even at high-volume centers specializing in the procedure, operative mortality has been shown to increase from 1% to 14% in the presence of cirrhosis [87]. For this reason, resection is reserved for patients with Child-Pugh A liver function. Multiple lesions do not preclude resection. Intraductal tumors causing obstructive jaundice can be successfully resected. In this situation, it is important to distinguish obstruction from underlying liver disease as the cause of the patient's jaundice. Patients with unresectable disease due to severe underlying liver disease, anatomic location of tumor, or the presence of distant metastases have an extremely poor prognosis (Tables 7-6 and 7-7).

Total hepatectomy followed by orthotopic liver transplantation is a sensible strategy to treat patients with cirrhosis and cancer, and experience is growing with this approach. As expected, the best results have been recorded in patients who had small HCC discovered incidentally at transplantation performed for liver failure [88]. Lesions smaller than 5 cm treated by transplantation have a significantly better prognosis, and, because organs are scarce, transplantation for HCC is usually limited to this setting. Mazzaferro *et al.* [89] have reported liver transplantation as an effective treatment for small, unresectable HCC in patients with cirrhosis, with 4-year recurrence-free survival of 83%.

Table 7-6. TNM Staging for Biliary Cancer

Staging	Criteria
T (Tumor)	
TX	Primary tumor cannot be assessed
T0	No evidence of primary tumor
Tis	Carcinoma in situ
T1	Tumor invades subepithelial connective tissue or fibromuscular layer
T1a	Tumor invades subepithelial connective tissue
T1b	Tumor invades fibromuscular layer
T2	Tumor invades perifibromuscular connective tissue
T3	Tumor invades adjacent structures: liver, pancreas, duodenum, gallbladder, colon, stomach
N (Node)	
NX	Regional lymph nodes cannot be assessed
N0	No regional lymph node metastasis
N1	Metastasis in cystic duct, pericholedochal and/or hilar lymph nodes (*ie*, in the hepatoduodenal ligament)
N2	Metastasis in peripancreatic (head only), periduodenal, periportal, celiac, and/or superior mesenteric and/or posterior pancreaticoduodenal lymph nodes
M (Metastasis)	
MX	Distant metastasis cannot be assessed
M0	No distant metastasis
M1	Distant metastasis
Stage	**TNM Grouping**
Stage 0	Tis, N0, M0
Stage I	T1, N0, M0
Stage II	T2, N0, M0
Stage III	T1, N1, M0
	T1, N2, M0
	T2, N1, M0
	T2, N2, M0
Stage IVA	T3, any N, M0
Stage IVB	Any T, any N, M1

Table 7-7. TNM Staging Criteria for Hepatocellular Carcinoma

Staging	Criteria
T (Tumor)	
TX	Primary tumor cannot be assessed
T0	No evidence of primary tumor
T1	Solitary tumor ≤ 2 cm in greatest dimension without vascular invasion
T2	Solitary tumor ≤ 2 cm in greatest dimension with vascular invasion, or multiple tumors limited to 1 lobe, none > 2 cm in greatest dimension without vascular invasion, or a solitary tumor > 2 cm in greatest dimension without vascular invasion
T3	Solitary tumor > 2 cm in greatest dimension with vascular invasion, or multiple tumors limited to 1 lobe, none > 2 cm in greatest dimension with vascular invasion, or multiple tumors limited to 1 lobe, any > 2 cm in greatest dimension with or without vascular invasion
T4	Multiple tumors in > 1 lobe or tumor(s) involve(s) a major branch of the portal or hepatic vein(s) or invasion of adjacent organs other than the gallbladder or perforation of the visceral peritoneum
N (Node)	
NX	Regional lymph nodes cannot be assessed
N0	No regional lymph node metastasis
N1	Regional lymph node metastasis
M (Metastasis)	
MX	Distant metastasis cannot be assessed
M0	No distant metastasis
M1	Distant metastasis
Stage	**TNM Grouping**
Stage I	T1, N0, M0
Stage II	T2, N0, M0
Stage IIIA	T3, N0, M0
Stage IIIB	T1, N1, M0
	T2, N1, M0
	T3, N1, M0
Stage IVA	T4, any N, M0
Stage IVB	Any T, any N, M1

Administration of an acyclic retinoid, polyprenoic acid, has been shown to reduce the incidence of recurrence of new hepatomas after surgical resection or percutaneous injection of ethanol [90–92]. Aggressive adjuvant chemotherapy protocols aimed at improving outcome following transplantation have been designed for hepatoma [93,94] (Figs. 7-4 and 7-5).

Chemotherapy that is directed through the hepatic artery has also been used to treat disease isolated to the liver. This can be done by percutaneous approach with chemoembolization, or with catheter placement at laparotomy. Using catheter-directed fluorodeoxyuridine (FUDR), mitomycin, and subcutaneous interferon-α, therapeutic responses in six of 10 patients with HCC have been reported [95].

Ablative techniques include ethanol injection, cryotherapy, and radiofrequency therapy. Percutaneous ethanol injection is a very effective technique for treating small hepatomas [96–98]. Cryoablation has been shown to be a safe and effective technique for destroying large HCCs by freezing. It is performed during laparotomy for lesions not amenable to surgical resection [99]. Radiofrequency ablation destroys tumor by heat; it can be performed on large or small tumors through percutaneous, laparoscopic, or open approaches [100].

THERAPY FOR ADVANCED DISEASE

Use of systemic chemotherapy in the management of unresectable or metastatic hepatoma has been extremely disappointing. Cisplatin, 5-FU, and mitomycin have all been used with little success [101,102]. Although doxorubicin is often considered to be an active single agent in hepatoma, the objective response rate to this agent is low and therapy with doxorubicin probably does not influence group survival when compared with no antitumor therapy.

Recently sorafenib, an oral small molecule inhibitor of the serine-threonine kinases Raf-1 and B-Raf and the receptor tyrosine kinase inhibitors of VEGFR-1, -2 and -3 and platelet-derived growth factor receptor, was compared to placebo in a multicenter, double-blinded clinical trial. Although there was no significant difference between the two groups with respect to median time to symptomatic progression (4.1 months for sorafenib vs 4.9 months for placebo), there was an improvement with respect to median

radiographic progression (5.5 vs 2.8 months in favor of sorafenib) and overall survival (10.7 vs 7.9 months in favor of sorafenib) [103].

BILIARY CANCER

Carcinoma of the gallbladder is often discovered as an incidental finding at surgery. If the disease is confined to the mucosa, cholecystectomy is curative. Unfortunately, advanced local and regional disease is usually present and the overall 5-year survival rate is less than 5%. The prognosis for patients with carcinoma of the distal bile duct is more optimistic, with an average 5-year survival after radical pancreaticoduodenectomy of approximately 40%. However, proximal bile duct carcinomas and hilar cholangiocarcinomas are much more difficult to treat surgically. In bile duct carcinomas, a favorable outcome is mainly determined by curative resection in the absence of lymph nodes metastases [104]. To achieve this, a major liver resection with extensive nodal dissection is often required. The operative mortality with this aggressive approach has now fallen below 10% in experienced centers, and median survival rates at 24 months (as opposed to those at 6 months) are being achieved [105].

THERAPY FOR LOCOREGIONAL DISEASE

Many researchers have examined the use of external-beam radiation in unresectable biliary cancer; no clear benefit has yet been demonstrated. Slightly more encouraging results have been achieved with intraoperative radiation and biliary bypass. In some cases, palliation and disease control can be achieved with brachytherapy using iridium 192 placed through a biliary drainage catheter.

THERAPY FOR ADVANCED DISEASE

The role of systemic chemotherapy in unresectable metastatic biliary tract cancers has also not been well defined. Because of the low incidence of these diseases, associated medical complications, and poor performance status of affected patients, few patients are referred for clinical trials. A recent review of the use of chemotherapy in the treatment of bile duct cancer suggests that possible active agents include 5-FU and mitomycin C either as single agents or in combination therapy with doxorubicin (FAM) or a combination of 5-FU and interferon [106]. Phase 2 studies with docetaxel have been disappointing [107]. Paclitaxel as a single agent appears to be ineffective. Combination of taxanes and other agents waits future testing [108]. In addition, hepatic artery infusion chemotherapy with agents such as 5-FU, FUDR, and doxorubicin has been studied in small numbers in patients, and objective partial responses have been reported.

Newer techniques, such as conformal radiation (which spares uninvolved liver), have permitted studies of combined chemotherapy and radiation in hepatobiliary cancers. Robertson *et al.* [109] studied hepatic artery infusion of FUDR and concurrent conformal radiation in localized hepatobiliary cancer and observed a high response to treatment, with a median survival of 19 months. Although modest progress is being made in hepatobiliary cancer, a concerted effort to better understand the role of chemotherapy in these diseases is needed.

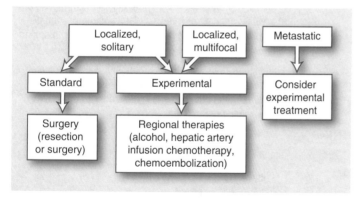

Figure 7-4. Treatment strategies for hepatoma.

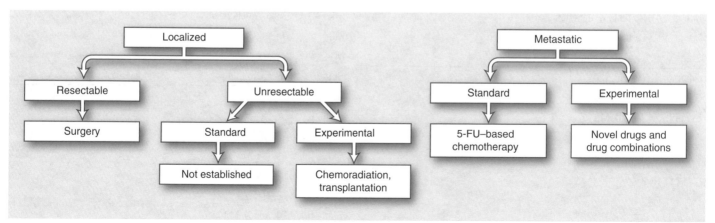

Figure 7-5. Treatment strategies for gallbladder and cholangiocarcinoma.

STREPTOZOCIN AND DOXORUBICIN

Streptozocin is a methyl nitrosourea produced by the fermentation of *Streptomyces achromogenes*. It decomposes spontaneously to generate alkylating and carbamoylating moieties, and alkylation is thought to be its principal mechanism of antitumor activity. Streptozocin is capable of transferring methyl groups to DNA but cannot form cross-links.

Doxorubicin is an antitumor antibiotic agent with an extremely wide spectrum of activity. It does not have a single mechanism of cytotoxicity but can produce cellular dysfunction and death by multiple means. Two of its most important mechanisms of cytotoxicity include intercalation among DNA base pairs and generation of toxic intracellular free radicals. These actions can cause single- and double-stranded DNA breaks, which in turn lead to inhibition of RNA and protein synthesis and defective mitoses.

CANDIDATES FOR TREATMENT

Patients with metastatic islet cell tumors

SPECIAL PRECAUTIONS

Patients with preexisting renal or heart disease

ALTERNATIVE THERAPIES

Chlorozotocin, dacarbazine

TOXICITIES

Streptozocin: renal toxicity (azotemia, anuria, hypophosphatemia, glycosuria, renal tubular acidosis), severe nausea and vomiting possible, mild to moderate abnormalities of glucose tolerance (hypoglycemia), hepatic toxicity and myelosuppression possible (usually mild); **Doxorubicin:** bone marrow suppression, anorexia, nausea and vomiting, alopecia, possible cardiotoxicity

DRUG INTERACTIONS

Streptozocin: none known; **Doxorubicin:** digoxin (suspected)

NURSING INTERVENTIONS

Monitor blood counts, liver function, pulmonary function, cardiac function; administer appropriate antiemetics to avoid severe nausea and vomiting; avoid extravasation; can cause severe necrosis

PATIENT INFORMATION

Myelosuppression may occur; call physician if signs and symptoms of infection develop; call physician if injection site becomes painful, red, or swollen; possible red-colored urine for 1–2 d after treatment; nausea and vomiting may occur; hair loss likely

Dosage and Scheduling
Streptozocin 500 mg/m^2 IV on d 1–5
Doxorubicin 50 mg/m^2 IV on d 1 and 22
• Repeat cycle every 6 wk
• Prior to therapy, complete blood count and platelets, liver chemistry, blood urea nitrogen, creatinine; baseline estimates of cardiac ejection fraction

Experiences and Response Rates				
Study	Evaluable patients, *n*	Dosage and Scheduling	Any regression/complete regression, %	Regression duration (median), *mo*
Moertel et al. [81]	36	Streptozocin 500 mg/m^2/d for 5 d Doxorubicin 50 mg/m^2/d on d 1 and 22	69/14	22
	33	Chlorozotocin 150 mg/m^2 every 7 wk	30/6	21
	33	Streptozocin 500 mg/m^2/d for 5 d 5-Fluorouracil 400 mg/m^2/d for 5 d (repeat every 6 wk)	45/4	13

EAP (ETOPOSIDE, DOXORUBICIN, AND CISPLATIN)

Etoposide is a semisynthetic derivative of podophyllotoxin. Its mechanism of cytotoxic action involves the inhibition of the nuclear enzyme topoisomerase II. This enzyme has the ability to disentangle topologically intertwined DNA helices, cleave double-stranded DNA, and then covalently bond to DNA to form DNA–topoisomerase II complexes. The cleaved DNA is then reunited after a second duplex DNA has passed through. Etoposide is believed to stabilize the DNA–topoisomerase II complex and prevent rejoining of the double-stranded DNA.

Doxorubicin is an antitumor antibiotic agent with an extremely wide spectrum of activity. It does not have a single mechanism of cytotoxicity but can produce cellular dysfunction and death by multiple means. Two of its most important mechanisms of cytotoxicity include intercalation among DNA base pairs and generation of toxic intracellular free radicals. These actions can cause single- and double-stranded DNA breaks, which in turn lead to inhibition of RNA and protein synthesis and defective mitoses.

Cisplatin is activated intracellularly to generate a positively charged aquated complex. This complex functions similarly to a bifunctional alkylating agent by interacting with the nucleophilic sites on DNA, RNA, and protein, producing intrastrand links and cross-links. These reactions alter the DNA template and inhibit DNA synthesis. Cisplatin lacks cell cycle specificity. Combination therapy with these drugs is based on in vitro and in vivo experimental data that have suggested synergistic cytotoxicity.

CANDIDATES FOR TREATMENT

Patients with advanced locoregional or metastatic gastric cancer prior to surgery

SPECIAL PRECAUTIONS

Patients with cardiac dysfunction or renal dysfunction

ALTERNATIVE THERAPIES

ELF or 5-FU, cisplatin, and etoposide for neoadjuvant therapy; FAM, FAM-TX, or ELF for metastatic disease

TOXICITIES

Drug combination: severe myelosuppression (leukopenia, anemia, thrombocytopenia); **Cisplatin:** renal toxicity, alopecia

DRUG INTERACTIONS

Etoposide: synergistic in vitro with cytarabine, cyclophosphamide, carmustine, vincristine, cisplatin, hydroxyurea, 5-FU, methotrexate, verapamil; **Doxorubicin:** digoxin (suspected)

NURSING INTERVENTIONS

Monitor blood counts, liver function, cardiac function, renal function, electrolytes; administer doxorubicin with caution (an extravasant); give adequate antiemetics and maintain adequate hydration; hypotension may occur with rapid administration of etoposide

PATIENT INFORMATION

Myelosuppression common; call physician if signs and symptoms of infection develop; call physician if injection site becomes painful, red, or swollen; possible red-colored urine for 1–2 d after treatment; nausea and vomiting may occur; hair loss likely

Dosage and Scheduling

Etoposide 120 mg/m^2 IV on d 4, 5, and 6

Doxorubicin 20 mg/m^2 IV on d 1 and 7

Cisplatin 40 mg/m^2 IV on d 2 and 8

- Repeat cycle every 3–4 wk

- Prior to therapy, complete blood count and platelets, liver chemistries, blood urea nitrogen, creatinine, electrolytes; baseline estimates of cardiac ejection fraction using a gated pool scan may be useful in some patients

Experiences and Response Rates

Study	Evaluable patients, *n*	Dosage and scheduling	CR/PR (%)	Median survival duration, *mo*
Lerner *et al.* [110]	36	Etoposide 120 mg/m^2/d on d 4, 5, and 6	3/9 (33)	7.5
		Doxorubicin 20 mg/m^2/d on d 1 and 7		
		Cisplatin 40 mg/m^2/d on d 2 and 8		
Kelsen *et al.* [111]	30	Etoposide 120 mg/m^2/d on d 4, 5, and 6	0/6 (20)	6.1
		Doxorubicin 20 mg/m^2/d on d 1 and 7		
		Cisplatin 40 mg/m^2/d on d 2 and 8		
Preusser *et al.* [112]	67	Etoposide 120 mg/m^2/d on d 4, 5, and 6	14/29 (64)	9.0
		Doxorubicin 20 mg/m^2/d on d 1 and 7		
		Cisplatin 40 mg/m^2/d on d 2 and 8		
Wilke *et al.* [113]	145	Etoposide 120 mg/m^2/d on d 4, 5, and 6	22/61 (57)	–
		Doxorubicin 20 mg/m^2/d on d 1 and 7		
		Cisplatin 40 mg/m^2/d on d 2 and 8		

CR—complete response; PR—partial response.

FAMTX (5-FLUOROURACIL, DOXORUBICIN, METHOTREXATE, AND LEUCOVORIN)

5-FU is a fluorinated uracil analogue that is metabolized intracellularly to its active forms, fluorouridine triphosphate (FUTP) and fluorodeoxyuridine monophosphate (FdUMP). FdUMP inhibits the enzyme, thymidylate synthetase, which is necessary for DNA synthesis. Another mechanism of cytotoxicity involves the false incorporation of 5-FUTP into RNA, causing transcription errors.

Doxorubicin is an antitumor antibiotic agent with an extremely wide spectrum of activity. It does not have a single mechanism of cytotoxicity, but can produce cellular dysfunction and death by multiple means. Two of its most important mechanisms of cytotoxicity include intercalation among DNA base pairs and generation of toxic intracellular free radicals. These actions can cause single- and double-stranded DNA breaks, which in turn lead to inhibition of RNA and protein synthesis and defective mitoses.

Methotrexate is an antifolate antimetabolite that exerts its primary cytotoxic effect during the S phase. Methotrexate is actively transported across the cell membrane where it binds to its target enzyme, dihydrofolate reductase (DHFR). This enzyme is essential for regenerating the oxidized folates produced during thymidine synthesis to their active forms. In the absence of unbound DHFR, thymidylate and purine biosynthesis can no longer occur.

Leucovorin, also known as folinic acid, is the active, chemically reduced derivative of folic acid, which is involved as a cofactor for one-carbon transfer reactions in the biosynthesis of purines and pyrimidines. It is a potent antidote for the hematopoietic and reticuloendothelial effects of folic acid antagonists because it is easily converted to tetrahydrofolic acid derivatives. Leucovorin also acts as a biochemical modulator of 5-FU by enhancing the ability of 5-FU to bind and then block the action of thymidylate synthetase.

CANDIDATES FOR TREATMENT

Patients with metastatic gastric cancer

SPECIAL PRECAUTIONS

Patients with cardiac dysfunction, renal dysfunction, any third-space fluid collection or ascites, pleural effusion, seroma

ALTERNATIVE THERAPIES

EAP, FAM, ELF, 5-FU (with or without leucovorin)

Continued on the next page

Dosage and Scheduling

5-Fluorouracil 500 mg/m^2 IV on d 1

Doxorubicin 30 mg/m^2 IV on d 15

Methotrexate 1500 mg/m^2 IV on d 1

Leucovorin 15 mg/m^2 orally every 6 h on d 2 and 3

• Repeat cycle every 4 wk

• Prior to therapy, complete blood count and platelets, liver chemistries, blood urea nitrogen, creatine; baseline estimates of cardiac ejection fraction using a gated pool scan may be useful in some patients

FAMTX (5-FLUOROURACIL, DOXORUBICIN, METHOTREXATE, AND LEUCOVORIN) (*CONTINUED*)

TOXICITIES

Drug combination: myelosuppression, mucositis, alopecia; **5-FU:** diarrhea; **Methotrexate:** renal toxicity, pulmonary fibrosis

DRUG INTERACTIONS

5-FU: leucovorin, methotrexate, interferon-α, dipyridamole, allopurinol, thymidine; **Doxorubicin:** digoxin (suspected); **Methotrexate:** salicylates, sulfonamides, tetracycline, phenylbutazone, chloramphenicol, phenytoin, probenecid, nonsteroidal anti-inflammatory drugs (NSAIDs), L-asparaginase, vincristine, etoposide, 5-FU

NURSING INTERVENTIONS

Monitor blood counts, renal function; patient must have normal renal function, adequate hydration, and urine alkalinization prior to high-dose methotrexate administration; monitor use of all NSAIDs (can enhance methotrexate toxicity); investigate and report pulmonary symptoms (such as dry, nonproductive cough); monitor for ascites or other third-space fluid collection (can enhance methotrexate toxicity); give antiemetics as necessary; monitor hepatic function; administer doxorubicin with caution (an extravasant); monitor methotrexate levels

PATIENT INFORMATION

Myelosuppression can occur; call physician if signs and symptoms of infection develop (fever, chills, flu-like symptoms); oral mucositis and diarrhea possible; hair loss likely; call physician if injection site becomes painful, red, or swollen; possible red-colored urine for 1–2 d after treatment; maintain adequate hydration

Experiences and Response Rates				
Study	Evaluable patients, *n*	Dosage and scheduling	CR/PR (%)	Median survival duration, *mo*
Kelsen *et al.* [111]	30	5-FU 1.5 g/m²/d on d 1	3/7 (33)	7.3
		Doxorubicin 30 mg/m²/d on d 15		
		Methotrexate 1.5 g/m²/d on d 1		
		Leucovorin 15 mg/m² orally every 6 h for 3 d starting on d 2		
Wils *et al.* [114]	81	5-FU 1.5 g/m2/d on d 1	5/28 (41)	10.5
		Doxorubicin 30 mg/m²/d on d 15		
		Methotrexate 1.5 g/m²/d on d 1		
		Leucovorin 15 mg/m² orally every 6 h for 48 h starting on d 2		
Wils *et al.* [115]	67	5-FU 1.5 g/m²/d on d 1	9/13 (33)	6.0
		Doxorubicin 30 mg/m²/d on d 15		
		Methotrexate 1.5 g/m²/d on d 1		
		Leucovorin 15 mg/m² orally every 6 h for 48 h starting on d 2		

CR—complete response; 5-FU—5-fluorouracil; PR—partial response.

ELF (ETOPOSIDE, LEUCOVORIN, AND 5-FLUOROURACIL)

Etoposide is a semisynthetic derivative of podophyllotoxin. Its mechanism of cytotoxic action involves the inhibition of the nuclear enzyme topoisomerase II. This enzyme has the ability to disentangle topologically intertwined DNA helices, cleave double-stranded DNA, and then covalently bond to DNA to form DNA–topoisomerase II complexes. The cleaved DNA is then reunited after a second duplex DNA has passed through. Etoposide is believed to stabilize the DNA–topoisomerase II complex and prevent rejoining of the double-stranded DNA.

Leucovorin, also known as folinic acid, is an active, chemically reduced derivative of folic acid. Reduction by the enzyme dihydrofolate reductase is not required for leucovorin to participate in reactions that use folates as a source of one-carbon moieties. Leucovorin also acts as a biochemical modulator of 5-FU by enhancing the ability of 5-FU to bind and then block the action of thymidylate synthetase.

5-FU is a fluorinated uracil analogue that is metabolized intracellularly to its active forms, FUTP and FdUMP. FdUMP inhibits the enzyme, thymidylate synthetase, which is necessary for DNA synthesis. Another mechanism of cytotoxicity involves the false incorporation of 5-FUTP into RNA, causing transcription errors.

Etoposide and 5-FU are both active agents in gastric carcinoma. In combination, they act synergistically and are not cross-resistant in vitro or in vivo. Leucovorin contributes to the synergism of this regimen by enhancing the cytotoxicity of 5-FU by increasing its ability to bind and then block the action of thymidylate synthetase.

CANDIDATES FOR TREATMENT

Patients with metastatic or advanced locoregional gastric cancer, especially for elderly or high-risk patients

SPECIAL PRECAUTIONS

None noteworthy

ALTERNATIVE THERAPIES

EAP, FAMTX, FAM, 5-FU (with or without leucovorin)

TOXICITIES

Myelosuppression, possible mucositis, diarrhea

DRUG INTERACTIONS

Etoposide: synergistic in vitro with cytarabine, cyclophosphamide, carmustine, vincristine, cisplatin, hydroxyurea, 5-FU, methotrexate, verapamil; **Leucovorin:** 5-FU; **5-FU:** leucovorin, methotrexate, interferon-α, dipyridamole, allopurinol, thymidine

NURSING INTERVENTIONS

Monitor blood counts; administer etoposide slowly over 45 to 60 minutes or longer (hypotension can occur if given too rapidly)

PATIENT INFORMATION

Oral mucositis may occur; skin reactions possible; call physician if diarrhea develops.

Dosage and Scheduling

Etoposide 120 mg/m² IV on d 1, 2, and 3

Leucovorin 300 mg/m² IV on d 1, 2, and 3

5-Fluorouracil 500 mg/m² IV on d 1, 2, and 3

• Prior to therapy, complete blood count and platelets

Experiences and Response Rates				
Study	Evaluable patients, n	Dosage and scheduling	CR/PR (%)	Median survival duration, *mo*
Wilke *et al.* [113]	51	Etoposide 120 mg/m²/d on d 1, 2, and 3	8/16 (53)	11
		Leucovorin 300 mg/m²/d on d 1, 2, and 3		
		5-FU 500 mg/m²/d on d 1, 2, and 3		
Wilke *et al.* [116]	33	Etoposide 120 mg/m²/d on d 1, 2, and 3	4/12 (48)	10.5
		Leucovorin 300 mg/m²/d on d 1, 2, and 3		
		5-FU 500 mg/m²/d on d 1, 2, and 3		

CR—complete response; 5-FU—5-fluorouracil; PR—partial response.

FAM (5-FLUOROURACIL, DOXORUBICIN, AND MITOMYCIN C)

5-FU is a fluorinated uracil analogue that is metabolized intracellularly to its active forms, FUTP and FdUMP. FdUMP inhibits the enzyme, thymidylate synthetase, which is necessary for DNA synthesis. Another mechanism of cytotoxicity involves the false incorporation of 5-FUTP into RNA, causing transcription errors.

Doxorubicin is an antitumor antibiotic agent with an extremely wide spectrum of activity. It does not have a single mechanism of cytotoxicity but can produce cellular dysfunction and death by multiple means. Its two most important mechanisms of cytotoxicity include intercalation among DNA base pairs and generation of toxic intracellular free radicals. These actions can cause single- and double-stranded DNA breaks, which in turn lead to inhibition of RNA and protein synthesis and defective mitoses.

Mitomycin C contains both quinoline and aziridine ring structures, allowing it to exert antitumor activity by two different mechanisms. Reduction of the quinoline ring by one electron transfer allows for free radical reactions similar to those seen with the anthracyclines. The aziridine ring functions as an alkylator producing DNA cross-links.

CANDIDATES FOR TREATMENT

Patients with metastatic gastric cancer

SPECIAL PRECAUTIONS

Patients with preexisting heart disease or pulmonary dysfunction

ALTERNATIVE THERAPIES

EAP, FAMTX, ELF, 5-FU (with or without leucovorin)

TOXICITIES

Drug combination: cumulative bone marrow suppression, including enhanced leukopenia and thrombocytopenia, alopecia, anorexia, nausea and vomiting; **Doxorubicin:** congestive cardiomyopathy, **Mitomycin C:** hemolytic anemia-like syndrome, pulmonary fibrosis

DRUG INTERACTIONS

5-FU: leucovorin, methotrexate, interferon-α, dipyridamole, allopurinol, thymidine; **Doxorubicin:** digoxin (suspected); **Mitomycin C:** none

NURSING INTERVENTIONS

Monitor blood counts, liver function, pulmonary function, cardiac function; administer doxorubicin and mitomycin C with great caution because extravasation injury can be extremely severe

PATIENT INFORMATION

Myelosuppression common; call physician if signs and symptoms of infection develop; call physician if area around site of injection becomes painful, red, or swollen; oral mucositis and diarrhea may occur; call physician if diarrhea persists; skin reactions possible; possible red-colored urine for 1–2 d after treatment.

Dosage and Scheduling
5-Fluorouracil 600 mg/m^2 IV on d 1 of wk 1, 2, 5, and 6
Doxorubicin 30 mg/m^2 IV on d 1 of wk 1 and 5
Mitomycin C 10 mg/m^2 IV on d 1 of wk 1
• Repeat cycle every 6 wk
• Prior to therapy, complete blood count and platelets, liver chemistries; baseline estimates of cardiac ejection fraction using a gated pool scan or pulmonary function tests may be useful in some patients

Experiences and Response Rates				
Study	Evaluable patients, *n*	Dosage and scheduling	CR/PR (%)	Median response duration, *mo*
MacDonald *et al.* [117]	62	5-FU 600 mg/m2/d on d 1, 8, 29, and 36	0/26 (42)	9
		Doxorubicin 30 mg/m2/d on d 1 and 29		
		Mitomycin C 10 mg/m2/d on d 1		
Biran H *et al.* [118]	43	5-FU 600 mg/m2/d on d 1, 8, 29, and 36	0/18 (42)	7
		Doxorubicin 30 mg/m2/d on d 1 and 29		
		Mitomycin C 10 mg/m2/d on d 1		
Arbuck *et al.* [119]	26	Leucovorin 500 mg/m2/d IV over 2 h on d 1, 8, 29 and 36	1/9 (38)	6
		5-FU 600 mg/m2/d as IV push 1 h after leucovorin on d 1, 8, 29, and 36		
		Doxorubicin 30 mg/m2/d on d 1 and 29		
		Mitomycin C 10 mg/m2/d on d 1		

CR—complete response; 5-FU—5-fluorouracil; PR—partial response.

5-FLUOROURACIL AND RADIATION THERAPY

5-FU is a fluorinated uracil analogue that is metabolized intracellularly to its active forms, FUTP and FdUMP. FdUMP inhibits the enzyme, thymidylate synthetase, which is necessary for DNA synthesis. Another mechanism of cytotoxicity involves the false incorporation of 5-FUTP into RNA, causing transcription errors.

When 5-FU is combined with radiation, enhancement of radiation effects is observed. It is known that 5-FU can significantly affect the slope of the radiation therapy survival curve when present in cytotoxic concentrations. The mechanism of this effect is unknown but may involve incorporation into DNA or RNA and cell cycle effects. Inhibition of sublethal damage repair does not seem to play a role.

CANDIDATES FOR TREATMENT

Patients with locally unresectable pancreatic cancer or with pancreatic cancer causing severe back pain from retroperitoneal extension of disease

SPECIAL PRECAUTIONS

None noteworthy

ALTERNATIVE THERAPIES

Radiation therapy alone, chemotherapy

TOXICITIES

Mucositis, diarrhea, myelosuppression, anorexia, nausea, vomiting, diarrhea, skin irritation

DRUG INTERACTIONS

5-FU: leucovorin, methotrexate, interferon-α, dipyridamole, allopurinol, thymidine

NURSING INTERVENTIONS

Monitor blood counts; inform patients of possible skin reactions, diarrhea, mucositis

PATIENT INFORMATION

Possible nausea, vomiting, anorexia, oral mucositis, skin reactions, diarrhea

Dosage and Scheduling

5-Fluorouracil 500 mg/m^2/d for 3 d every 2 wk for 2 cycles, then 500 mg/m^2 every wk* for a total of 2 y

Radiation 2000 cGy over 5 d for 2 courses; 2-wk separation period between doses

*Weekly doses of 5-fluorouracil begin 1 mo after radiation therapy is complete.

Experiences and Response Rates

Study	Evaluable patients, n	Dosage and scheduling*	Median survival duration, mo	2-y actuarial survival, %
Kalser and Ellenberg [120]	21	5-FU 500 mg/m^2/d for 3 d every 2 wk for 2 cycles, then 500 mg/m^2/wk starting 1 mo after radiation therapy is complete	21.0	43
		Radiation 2000 rads over 5 d for 2 courses (2-wk separation between doses)		
	22	No treatment (control group)	10.9	18
Gastrointestinal Tumor Study Group [121]	30	5-FU 500 mg/m^2/d for 3 d every 2 wk for 2 cycles, then 500 mg/m^2/wk starting 1 mo after radiation therapy is complete	18.0	46
		Radiation 2000 rads over 5 d for 2 courses (2-wk separation between doses)		

*Chemotherapy was continued on a weekly schedule for 2 y of therapy.
5-FU—5-fluorouracil.

CISPLATIN, 5-FLUOROURACIL, AND RADIATION THERAPY

Cisplatin is activated intracellularly to generate a positively charged aquated complex. This complex functions similarly to a bifunctional alkylating agent by interacting with the nucleophilic sites on DNA, RNA, and protein, producing intrastrand links and cross-links. These reactions alter the DNA template and inhibit DNA synthesis. Cisplatin lacks cell cycle specificity.

5-FU is a fluorinated uracil analogue that is metabolized intracellularly to its active forms, FUTP and FdUMP. FdUMP inhibits the enzyme, thymidylate synthetase, which is necessary for DNA synthesis. Another mechanism of cytotoxicity involves the false incorporation of 5-FUTP into RNA, causing transcription errors.

Both cisplatin and 5-FU, as single agents, are moderately active against esophageal carcinoma. When used in combination with radiation therapy, a radiation-enhancing effect is seen. Ideally, this multimodality approach would enhance the effects of radiation on local tumors and the systemic drug therapy would reduce the chance of distant micrometastases.

CANDIDATES FOR TREATMENT

Patients with esophageal carcinoma

SPECIAL PRECAUTIONS

Patients with renal dysfunction

ALTERNATIVE THERAPIES

Preoperative: 5-FU and mitomycin C; 5-FU, vinblastine, and cisplatin plus radiation; cisplatin and bleomycin with or without vindesine; cisplatin and 5-FU; etoposide, cisplatin, and 5-FU; etoposide, doxorubicin, and cisplatin; **Inoperable or metastatic disease:** cisplatin and bleomycin with or without vindesine; cisplatin, methotrexate, and bleomycin

TOXICITIES

Cisplatin: myelosuppression, nausea, vomiting, renal dysfunction, possible ototoxicity, possible neurotoxicity; **5-FU:** myelosuppression, mucositis, diarrhea; **Chemotherapy plus radiation therapy:** enhanced myelosuppression, severe esophagitis or stomatitis, nausea, vomiting, anorexia, diarrhea, possible ototoxicity, possible neurotoxicity

DRUG INTERACTIONS

5-FU: leucovorin, methotrexate, interferon-α, dipyridamole, allopurinol, thymidine; **Cisplatin:** none

NURSING INTERVENTIONS

Monitor blood counts, renal function, electrolytes; inform patients of possible skin reactions; give adequate amounts of antiemetics before and after cisplatin therapy; maintain adequate hydration; use diuretics as indicated

PATIENT INFORMATION

Oral mucositis and severe esophagitis may occur; myelosuppression is likely; call physician if signs of infection or diarrhea develop; call physician if hearing loss occurs; nausea and vomiting possible (possibly protracted); skin reactions possible, taste changes (metallic) possible.

Dosage and Scheduling

5-Fluorouracil 1000 mg/m^2/d as daily continuous infusion for 5 d

Cisplatin 70–100 mg/m^2 on d 1 only

• Prior to therapy, complete blood count and platelets, electrolytes, blood urea nitrogen, creatinine

Experiences and Response Rates

Study	Evaluable patients, *n*	Dosage and scheduling	Median survival duration, *mo*	Survival rates, %	
				12 mo	24 mo
Localized disease					
Herskovic *et al.* [8]	121	5-FU 1000 mg/m2/d for 4 d as CI + cisplatin 75 mg/m2 on d 1 only + radiation 5000 cGy over 5 wk	12.5	50	38
		Radiation alone (6400 cGy over 6.4 wk)	8.9	33	10
Seitz *et al.* [122]	35	5-FU 1000 mg/m2/d for 5 d as CI + cisplatin 70 mg/m2 on d 2 only + radiation 20 cGy over 5 d	17.0	–	41
Presurgical chemotherapy regimen					
Walsh *et al.* [21]	48	5-FU 15 mg/kg/d IV over 16 h daily for 5 d, wk 1 and 6 + cisplatin 75 mg/m2 IV over 8 h (1 dose) on d 7, wk 1 and 6 + radiation 40 cGy in 15 fractions (d 1–5, 8–12, 15–19)	16.0	52	37
Metastatic disease and control of primary tumor					
De Besi *et al.* [123]	37	5-FU 1000 mg/m2/d for 5 d as CI + cisplatin 100 mg/m2 on d 1 only + allopurinol 600 mg daily on d -2 to +5	3/10*		35†
Kies *et al.* [124]	26	5-FU 1000 mg/m2/d for 5 d as CI + cisplatin 100 mg/m2 on d 1 only	3/8*		42†

*Value indicates number of complete responses/partial reponses.
†Value indicates an overall response rate.
CI—continuous infusion; 5-FU—5-fluorouracil.

5-FLUOROURACIL, RECOMBINANT INTERFERON-α-2B, AND CISPLATIN

Cisplatin is activated intracellularly to generate a positively charged aquated complex. This complex functions similarly to a bifunctional alkylating agent by interacting with the nucleophilic sites on DNA, RNA, and protein, producing intrastrand links and cross-links. These reactions alter the DNA template and inhibit DNA synthesis. Cisplatin lacks cell cycle specificity.

5-FU is a fluorinated uracil analogue that is metabolized intracellularly to its active forms, FUTP and FdUMP. FdUMP inhibits the enzyme thymidylate synthetase, which is necessary for DNA synthesis. Another mechanism of cytotoxicity involves the false incorporation of 5-FUTP into RNA, causing transcription errors.

Biochemical modulation with recombinant interferon-α has been shown to augment the cytotoxicity of both 5-FU and cisplatin in vitro and may be a viable strategy in the treatment of esophageal carcinoma.

CANDIDATES FOR TREATMENT

Patients with regionally advanced or metastatic esophageal carcinoma

SPECIAL PRECAUTIONS

Patients with renal dysfunction

ALTERNATIVE THERAPIES

Cisplatin and bleomycin with or without vindesine, cisplatin and 5-FU, cisplatin and etoposide, methotrexate, and bleomycin

TOXICITIES

Myelosuppression, primarily thrombocytopenia, fatigue, neurologic toxicities, mucositis, diarrhea

DRUG INTERACTIONS

5-FU: leucovorin, methotrexate, dipyridamole, allopurinol, thymidine; **Interferon:** cisplatin, and 5-FU (augments cytotoxicity)

NURSING INTERVENTIONS

Monitor blood counts, renal function, electrolytes; inform patients of possible skin reactions; give adequate antiemetics and maintain adequate hydration during cisplatin administration

PATIENT INFORMATION

Possible nausea, vomiting, anorexia, oral mucositis, diarrhea; call physician if signs of infection or diarrhea develop. Possible neurologic toxicities include dizziness and gait disturbances.

Dosage and Scheduling

Interferon α-2b 10 MU subcutaneously weekly on d 1 (immediately before cisplatin) then on d 3 and 5

Cisplatin 100 mg/m^2 IV over 2 h on d 1, then at 25 mg/m^2 every wk (immediately before 5-fluorouracil bolus) beginning on d 15

5-Fluorouracil 750 mg/m^2/d IV for 5 d beginning on d 1, then at 750 mg/m^2 every wk beginning on d 15

Granulocyte-macrophage colony-stimulating factor 5 μ/kg subcutaneously on d 7–13, then on d 2–5 each wk beginning the day after chemotherapy

• Prior to therapy, complete blood count and platelets, electrolytes, blood urea nitrogen, creatinine, liver function

Experiences and Response Rates

Study	Evaluable patients, *n*	Dosage and scheduling	CR/PR	Response rate, %
Wadler *et al.* [125]	23	5-FU 750 mg/m^2/d for 5 d, then 750 mg/m^2 every wk beginning on d 15	1/14	65
		Cisplatin 100 mg/m^2 IV on d 1, then 25 mg/m^2 weekly beginning on d 15		
		IFN-α (Intron) 10 MU subcutaneously on d 1, 3, and 5		
Kelsen *et al.* [126]	37	5-FU 750 mg/m^2/d IV for 5 d as CI, then 750 mg/m^2 once weekly as IV push beginning on d 12	1/9	27
		IFN-α (Roferon-A) 9 MU subcutaneously 3 times/wk		
Wadler *et al.* [127]	20	5-FU 750 mg/m^2/d IV for 5 d as CI, then 750 mg/m^2 once weekly as IV push	2/3	25
		IFN-α (Roferon-A) 9 MU subcutaneously 3 times/wk		
Ilson *et al.* [128]	26	5-FU 750 mg/m^2/d IV for 5 d as CI (repeated every 28 d)	2/13	50
		Cisplatin 100 mg/m^2 IV on d 1 every 28 d for 3 cycles, then every 56 d		
		IFN-α (Roferon-A) 3 MU subcutaneously daily on d 1–28		

CI—continuous infusion; 5-FU—5-fluorouracil; IFN—interferon; IV—intravenous.

HIGH-DOSE CISPLATIN AND ETOPOSIDE

Etoposide is a semisynthetic derivative of podophyllotoxin. Its mechanism of cytotoxic action involves the inhibition of the nuclear enzyme topoisomerase II. This enzyme has the ability to disentangle topologically intertwined DNA helices, cleave double-stranded DNA, and then covalently bond to DNA to form DNA–topoisomerase II complexes. The cleaved DNA is then reunited after a second duplex DNA has passed through. Etoposide is believed to stabilize the DNA–topoisomerase II complex and prevent rejoining of the double-stranded DNA.

Cisplatin is activated intracellularly to generate a positively charged aquated complex. This complex functions similarly to a bifunctional alkylating agent by interacting with the nucleophilic sites on DNA, RNA, and protein, producing intrastrand links and cross-links. These reactions alter the DNA template and inhibit DNA synthesis. Cisplatin lacks cell cycle specificity.

Combination therapy with these drugs is based on in vitro and in vivo experimental data that have suggested synergistic cytotoxicity.

DOSAGE MODIFICATIONS

Patients older than 70 years of age are given reduced doses of cisplatin and etoposide. Patients with responding metastatic disease were given one additional cycle of chemotherapy. Patients with locoregional disease received radiation 1.8 Gy daily for 5 days/week for a total of 41.4 Gy. 5-FU is administered by continuous infusion at 300 mg/m^2/d for the duration of the radiation.

CANDIDATES FOR TREATMENT

Patients with unresectable or metastatic esophageal adenocarcinoma

SPECIAL PRECAUTIONS

Patients with renal dysfunction and patients with both renal and hepatic dysfunction

ALTERNATIVE THERAPIES

5-FU and interferon; 5-FU, interferon, and cisplatin

TOXICITIES

Neutropenia, thrombocytopenia, nausea and vomiting, peripheral sensory neuropathy, renal dysfunction, ototoxicity

DRUG INTERACTIONS

Cisplatin: interferon; **Etoposide:** synergistic in vitro with cytarabine, cyclophosphamide, carmustine, vincristine, cisplatin, hydroxyurea, 5-FU, methotrexate, verapamil

NURSING INTERVENTIONS

Monitor blood counts, renal function, electrolytes; give adequate amounts of antiemetics; maintain adequate hydration; use diuretics as indicated

PATIENT INFORMATION

Myelosuppression is likely; call physician if signs of infection develop. Nausea and vomiting (possibly protracted) and taste changes (metallic) may occur; inform physician if hearing loss occurs.

Dosage and Scheduling

Cisplatin 30 mg/m^2/d on d 1–5

Etoposide 60 mg/m^2/d on d 1–5

• Repeat cycle every 21 d for a total of 3 cycles

• Prior to therapy, complete blood count and platelets, blood urea nitrogen, creatinine, electrolytes, liver chemistries

Experiences and Response Rates

Study	Evaluable patients, *n*	Dosage and scheduling	CR/PR	Response rate, %
Spiridonidis *et al.* [129]	24	Cisplatin 30 mg/m2/d IV over 1 h for 5 d	5/8	54
		Etoposide 60 mg/m2/d IV over 2 h for 5 d		
		(3 cycles of cisplatin/etoposide followed by 5-FU and radiation in patients with locoregional disease)		

CR—complete response; 5-FU—5-fluorouracil; PR—partial response.

REFERENCES

1. Jemal A, Siegel R, Ward E, *et al.*: Cancer Statistics 2008. *CA Cancer J Clin* 2008, 58:71–96.

2. Heath EI, Kaufman HS, Talamini MA, *et al.*: The role of laparoscopy in pre-operative staging of esophageal cancer. *Surg Endosc* 2000, 14:495–499.

3. Kelsen D, Ajani J, Ilson D, *et al.*: A phase II trial of paclitaxel (Taxol) in advanced esophageal cancer: preliminary report. *Semin Oncol* 1994, 21(Suppl 8):44–48.

4. Van Cutsem E, Moseyenko VM, Tjulandin S, *et al.*: Phase III study of docetaxel and cisplatin plus fluorouracil compared with cisplatin and fluorouracil as first-line therapy for advanced gastric cancer: a report of the V324 study group. *J Clin Oncol* 2006, 24:4991–4997.

5. Cunningham D, Starling N, Rao S, *et al.*: Capecitabine and oxaliplatin for advanced esophagogastric cancer. *N Engl J Med* 2008, 358:36–46.

6. Ilson DH, Saltz L, Enzinger P, *et al.*: Phase II trial of weekly irinotecan plus cisplatin in advanced esophageal cancer. *J Clin Oncol* 1999, 17:3270–3275.

7. Shah M, Ramanathan RK, Ilson D, *et al.*: Multicenter phase II study of irinotecan, cisplatin and bevacizumab in patients with metastatic gastric or gastro-esophageal junction adenocarcinoma *J Clin Oncol* 2006, 24:5201–5206.

8. Herskovic A, Martz K, al-Sarraf M, *et al.*: Combined chemotherapy and radiotherapy compared with radiotherapy alone in patients with cancer of the esophagus. *N Engl J Med* 1992, 326:1593–1598.

9. al-Sarraf M, Herskovic A, Leichman L, *et al.*: Progress report of combined chemoradiotherapy versus radiotherapy alone in patients with esophageal cancer: an intergroup study. *J Clin Oncol* 1997, 15:277–284.

10. Cooper JS, Guo MD, Herskovic A, *et al.*: Chemoradiotherapy of locally advanced esophageal cancer: long-term follow-up of a prospective randomized trial (RTOG 85-01). Radiation Therapy Oncology Group. *JAMA* 1999, 281:1623–1627.

11. Coia LR, Minsky BD, Berkey BA, *et al.*: Outcome of patients receiving radiation for cancer of the esophagus: results of the 1992–1994 Patterns of Care Study. *J Clin Oncol* 2000, 18:455–462.

12. Ilson DH, Bains M, Kelsen DP, *et al.*: Phase I trial of escalating dose irinotecan given weekly with cisplatin and concurrent radiotherapy in locally advanced esophageal cancer. *J Clin Oncol* 2003, 21:2926–2932.

13. Safran H, Suntharalingam M, Dipetrillo T, *et al.*: Cetuximab with concurrent chemoradiation for esophagogastric cancer: assessment of toxicity. *Int J Radiat Oncol Biol Phys* 2008, 70:391–395.

14. Arnott SJ, Duncan W, Gignoux M, *et al.*: Preoperative radiotherapy in esophageal carcinoma: a meta-analysis using individual patient data (Oesophageal Cancer Collaborative Group). *Int J Radiat Oncol Biol Phys* 1998, 41:579–583.

15. Kelsen DP, Ginsberg R, Pajak TF, *et al.*: Chemotherapy followed by surgery compared with surgery alone for localized esophageal cancer. *N Engl J Med* 1998, 339:1979–1984.

16. Urba SG, Orringer MB, Perez-Tamayo C, *et al.*: Concurrent preoperative chemotherapy and radiation therapy in localized esophageal adenocarcinoma. *Cancer* 1992, 69:285–291.

17. Forastiere AA, Orringer MB, Perez-Tamayo C, *et al.*: Preoperative chemoradiation followed by transhiatal esophagectomy for carcinoma of the esophagus: final report. *J Clin Oncol* 1993, 11:1118–1123.

18. Naunheim KS, Petruska P, Roy TS, *et al.*: Preoperative chemotherapy and radiotherapy for esophageal carcinoma [with discussion]. *J Thorac Cardiovasc Surg* 1992, 103:887–895.

19. Urba S, Orringer MB, Turrisi A, *et al.*: A randomized trial comparing surgery to preoperative concomitant chemoradiation plus surgery in patients with resectable esophageal cancer: updated analysis [abstract]. *Proc Am Soc Clin Oncol* 1997, 16:277.

20. Urba S, Orringer MB, Turrisi A, *et al.*: Randomized trial of preoperative chemoradiation versus surgery alone in patients with locoregional esophageal carcinoma. *J Clin Oncol* 2001, 19:305–313.

21. Walsh TN, Noonan N, Hollywood D, *et al.*: A comparison of multimodal therapy and surgery for esophageal adenocarcinoma. *N Engl J Med* 1996, 335:462–467.

22. Bosset JF, Gignoux M, Triboulet JP, *et al.*: Chemoradiotherapy followed by surgery compared with surgery alone in squamous-cell cancer of the esophagus. *N Engl J Med* 1997, 337:161–167.

23. Law S, Kwong D, Tung H, *et al.*: Preoperative chemoradiation for squamous cell esophageal cancer: a prospective randomized trial [abstract]. *Can J Gastroenterol* 1998, 12:56B.

24. Tepper J, Krasna MJ, Niedzwiecki D, *et al.*: Phase III trial of trimodality therapy with cisplatin, fluorouracil, radiotherapy, and surgery compared with surgery alone for esophageal cancer: CALGB 9781. *J Clin Oncol* 2008, 26:1086–1092.

25. Adelstein DJ, Rice TW, Becker M, *et al.*: Use of concurrent chemotherapy, accelerated fractionation radiation, and surgery for patients with esophageal carcinoma. *Cancer* 1997, 80:1011–1020.

26. Heath EI, Burtness BA, Heitmiller RF, *et al.*: Phase II evaluation of preoperative chemoradiation and postoperative adjuvant chemotherapy for squamous cell and adenocarcinoma of the esophagus. *J Clin Oncol* 2000, 18:868–876.

27. Anand BS, Saeed ZA, Michaletz PA, *et al.*: A randomized comparison of dilatation alone versus dilatation plus laser in patients receiving chemotherapy and external beam radiation for esophageal carcinoma. *Dig Dis Sci* 1998, 43:2255–2260.

28. Reed CE: Endoscopic palliation of esophageal carcinoma. *Chest Surg Clin North Am* 1994, 4:155–172.

29. Knyrim K, Wagner HJ, Bethge N, *et al.*: A controlled trial of an expansile metal stent for palliation of esophageal obstruction due to inoperable cancer. *N Engl J Med* 1993, 329:1302–1307.

30. Parsonnet J, Friedman GD, Vandersteen DP, *et al.*: Helicobacter pylori infection and the risk of gastric carcinoma. *N Engl J Med* 1991, 325:1127–1131.

31. Parsonnet J, Friedman GD, Orentreich N, Vogelman H: Risk for gastric cancer in people with CagA positive or CagA negative Helicobacter pylori infection. *Gut* 1997, 40:297–301.

32. Bonenkamp JJ, Songun I, Hermans J, *et al.*: Randomised comparison of morbidity after D1 and D2 dissection for gastric cancer in 996 Dutch patients. *Lancet* 1995, 345:745–748.

33. Bonenkamp JJ, Hermans J, Sasako M, *et al.*: Extended lymph-node dissection for gastric cancer. Dutch Gastric Cancer Group. *N Engl J Med* 1999, 340:908–914.

34. Cuschieri A, Weeden S, Fielding J, *et al.*: Patient survival after D1 and D2 resections for gastric cancer: long- term results of the MRC randomized surgical trial. Surgical Co-operative Group. *Br J Cancer* 1999, 79:1522–1530.

35. Cuschieri A, Fayers P, Fielding J, *et al.*: Postoperative morbidity and mortality after D1 and D2 resections for gastric cancer: Preliminary results of the MRC randomised controlled surgical trial. The Surgical Cooperative Group. *Lancet* 1996, 347:995–999.

36. Estes NC, MacDonald JS, Touijer K, *et al.*: Inadequate documentation and resection for gastric cancer in the United States: a preliminary report. *Am Surg* 1998, 64:680–685.

37. Macdonald JS, Smalley S, Benedetti J, *et al.*: Postoperative combined radiation and chemotherapy improves disease-free survival (DFS) and overall survival (OS) in resected adenocarcinoma of the stomach and gastroesophageal junction [abstract]. *Proc Am Soc Clin Oncol* 2000, 19:6.

38. Kelsen DP: Postoperative adjuvant chemoradiation therapy for patients with resected gastric cancer: Intergroup 116. *J Clin Oncol* 2000, 18(Suppl):32S–34S.

39. Hermans J, Bonenkamp JJ, Boon MC, *et al.*: Adjuvant therapy after curative resection for gastric cancer: Meta- analysis of randomized trials. *J Clin Oncol* 1993, 11:1441–1447.

40. Wilke H, Stahl M, Fink U, *et al.*: Preoperative chemotherapy for unresectable gastric cancer. *World J Surg* 1995, 19:210–215.

41. Wilke H, Meyer HJ, Fink U: Preoperative chemotherapy in gastric cancer. *Recent Results Cancer Res* 1996, 142:237–248.

42. Ajani JA, Mayer RJ, Ota DM, *et al.*: Preoperative and postoperative combination chemotherapy for potentially resectable gastric carcinoma. *J Natl Cancer Inst* 1993, 85:1839–1844.

43. Ajani JA, Ota DM, Jessup JM, *et al.*: Resectable gastric carcinoma. An evaluation of preoperative and postoperative chemotherapy. *Cancer* 1991, 68:1501–1506.

44. Safran H, King TP, Choy H, *et al.*: Paclitaxel and concurrent radiation for locally advanced pancreatic carcinoma. *Front Biosci* 1998, 3:E204–E206.

45. Safran H, King TP, Choy H, *et al.*: Paclitaxel and concurrent radiation for locally advanced pancreatic and gastric cancer: a phase I study. *J Clin Oncol* 1997, 15:901–907.

46. Ajani JA, Mansfield PF, Lynch PM, *et al.*: Enhanced staging and all chemotherapy preoperatively in patients with potentially resectable gastric carcinoma. *J Clin Oncol* 1999, 17:2403–2411.

47. Choy H: Taxanes in combined-modality therapy for solid tumors. *Oncology (Williston Park)* 1999, 13(Suppl 5):23–38.

48. Karpeh MS, Brennan MF: Gastric carcinoma [review]. *Ann Surg Oncol* 1998, 5:650–656.

49. Buku N, Ohtsu A, Shimada Y, *et al.*: Phase II study of a combination of irinotecan and cisplatin against metastatic gastric cancer. *J Clin Oncol* 1999, 17:319–323.

50. Roth AD, Maibach R, Martinelli G, *et al.*: Docetaxel (Taxotere)-cisplatin (TC): an effective drug combination in gastric carcinoma. Swiss Group for Clinical Cancer Research (SAKK), and the European Institute of Oncology (EIO). *Ann Oncol* 2000, 11:301–306.

51. Murad AM, Petroianu A, Guimaraes RC, *et al.*: Phase II trial of the combination of paclitaxel and 5-fluorouracil in the treatment of advanced gastric cancer: a novel, safe, and effective regimen. *Am J Clin Oncol* 1999, 22:580–586.

52. Kollmannsberger C, Quietzsch D, Haag C, *et al.*: A phase II study of paclitaxel, weekly, 24-hour continuous infusion 5- fluorouracil, folinic acid and cisplatin in patients with advanced gastric cancer. *Br J Cancer* 2000, 83:458–462.

53. Lokich JJ, Sonneborn H, Anderson NR, *et al.*: Combined paclitaxel, cisplatin, and etoposide for patients with previously untreated esophageal and gastroesophageal carcinomas. *Cancer* 1999, 85:2347–2351.

54. Glimelius B, Hoffman K, Sjoden PO, *et al.*: Chemotherapy improves survival and quality of life in advanced pancreatic and biliary cancer. *Ann Oncol* 1996, 7:593–600.

55. Ishii H, Okada S, Tokuuye K, *et al.*: Protracted 5-fluorouracil infusion with concurrent radiotherapy as a treatment for locally advanced pancreatic carcinoma. *Cancer* 1997, 79:1516–1520.

56. Safran H, Akerman P, Cioffi W, *et al.*: Paclitaxel and concurrent radiation therapy for locally advanced adenocarcinomas of the pancreas, stomach, and gastroesophageal junction. *Semin Radiat Oncol* 1999, 9(Suppl 1):53–57.

57. Kornek GV, Schratter-Sehn A, Marczell A, *et al.*: Treatment of unresectable, locally advanced pancreatic adenocarcinoma with combined radiochemotherapy with 5-fluorouracil, leucovorin and cisplatin. *Br J Cancer* 2000, 82:98–103.

58. Rich TA: Chemoradiation for pancreatic and biliary cancer: current status of RTOG studies [review]. *Ann Oncol* 1999, 10(Suppl 4):231–233.

59. Regine WF, Winter KA, Abrams RA, *et al.*: Fluorouracil vs gemcitabine chemotherapy before and after fluorouracil-based chemoradiation following resection of pancreatic adenocarcinoma: a randomized controlled trial. *JAMA* 2008, 299:1019–1026.

60. Rich T, Harris J, Abrams RA, *et al.*: Phase II study of external irradiation and weekly paclitaxel for nonmetastatic unresectable pancreatic cancer: RTOG-98-12. *Am J Clin Oncol* 2004, 27:51–60.

61. Evans DB, Rich TA, Byrd DR, *et al.*: Preoperative chemoradiation and pancreaticoduodenectomy for adenocarcinoma of the pancreas. *Arch Surg* 1992, 127:1335–1339.

62. Miller AR, Robinson EK, Lee JE, *et al.*: Neoadjuvant chemoradiation for adenocarcinoma of the pancreas. *Surg Oncol Clin North Am* 1998, 7:183–197.

63. Breslin TM, Janjan NA, Lee JE, *et al.*: Neoadjuvant chemoradiation for adenocarcinoma of the pancreas. *Front Biosci* 1998, 3:E193–E203.

64. Evans DB, Pisters PW, Lee JE, *et al.*: Preoperative chemoradiation strategies for localized adenocarcinoma of the pancreas. *J Hepatobiliary Pancreat Surg* 1998, 5:242–250.

65. Spitz FR, Abbruzzese JL, Lee JE, *et al.*: Preoperative and postoperative chemoradiation strategies in patients treated with pancreaticoduodenectomy for adenocarcinoma of the pancreas. *J Clin Oncol* 1997, 15:928–937.

66. Evans DB, Abbruzzese JL, Cleary KR, *et al.*: Preoperative chemoradiation for adenocarcinoma of the pancreas: excessive toxicity of prophylactic hepatic irradiation. *Int J Radiat Oncol Biol Phys* 1995, 33:913–918.

67. Hoffman JP, Weese JL, Solin LJ, *et al.*: A pilot study of preoperative chemoradiation for patients with localized adenocarcinoma of the pancreas [with discussion]. *Am J Surg* 1995, 169:71–78.

68. Staley CA, Lee JE, Cleary KR, *et al.*: Preoperative chemoradiation, pancreaticoduodenectomy, and intraoperative radiation therapy for adenocarcinoma of the pancreatic head [with discussion]. *Am J Surg* 1996, 171:118–125.

69. Brunner TB, Grabenbauer GG, Kastl S, *et al.*: Preoperative chemoradiation in locally advanced pancreatic carcinoma: a phase II study. *Onkologie* 2000, 23:436–442.

70. Katz MH, Pisters PW, Evans DB, *et al.*: Borderline resectable pancreatic cancer: the importance of this emerging state of disease. *J Am Coll Surg* 2008, 206:833–846.

71. DeCaprio JA, Mayer RJ, Gonin R, Arbuck SG: Fluorouracil and high-dose leucovorin in previously untreated patients with advanced adenocarcinoma of the pancreas: results of a phase II trial. *J Clin Oncol* 1991, 9:2128–2133.

72. Burris HA, Moore MJ, Andersen J, *et al.*: Improvements in survival and clinical benefit with gemcitabine as first-line therapy for patients with advanced pancreas cancer: a randomized trial. *J Clin Oncol* 1997, 15:2403–2413.

73. Au E: Clinical update of gemcitabine in pancreas cancer. *Gan To Kagaku Ryoho* 2000, 27(Suppl 2):469–473.

74. Tempero M, Plunkett W: Randomized phase II trial of dose intense gemcitabine by standard infusion vs. fixed dose rate in metastatic pancreatic adenocarcinoma [abstract]. *Proc Am Soc Clin Oncol* 1999, 18:273.

75. Poplin E, Levy D, Berlin J, *et al.*: Phase III trial of gemcitabine (30 minute infusion) versus gemcitabine (fixed dose infusion) versus gemcitabine + oxaliplatin (GEMOX) in patients with advanced pancreas cancer (ECOG 6201) [abstract]. *J Clin Oncol* 2006, 24(18S):LBA 4004.

76. Moore MJ, Goldstein D, Hamm J, *et al.*: Erlotinib plus gemcitabine compared with gemcitabine alone in patients with advanced pancreatic cancer: a phase III trial of the National Cancer Institute of Canada Clinical Trial Group. *J Clin Oncol* 2007, 25:1960–1966.

77. Cunningham D, Chau I, Stocken C, *et al.*: Phase III randomized comparison of gemcitabine versus gemcitabine plus capecitabine in patients with advanced pancreatic cancer [abstract]. *Eur J Cancer* 2005, 3(Suppl 4): abstract PS11.

78. van der Schelling GP, Jeekel J: Palliative chemotherapy and radiotherapy for pancreatic cancer: is it worthwhile? *World J Surg* 1999, 23:950–953.

79. Cascinu S, Graziano F, Catalano G: Chemotherapy for advanced pancreatic cancer: it may no longer be ignored. *Ann Oncol* 1999, 10:105–109.

80. Arnold R, Frank M, Kajdan U: Management of gastroenteropancreatic endocrine tumors: the place of somatostatin analogues. *Digestion* 1994, 55(Suppl 3):107–113.

81. Moertel CG, Lefkopoulo M, Lipsitz S, *et al.*: Streptozocin-doxorubicin, streptozocin-fluorouracil or chlorozotocin in the treatment of advanced islet-cell carcinoma. *N Engl J Med* 1992, 326:519–523.

82. Ruszniewski P, Rougier P, Roche A, *et al.*: Hepatic arterial chemoembolization in patients with liver metastases of endocrine tumors: a prospective phase II study in 24 patients. *Cancer* 1993, 71:2624–2630.

83. Dominguez S, Denys A, Madeira I, *et al.*: Hepatic arterial chemoembolization in the management of advanced digestive endocrine tumours. *Ital J Gastroenterol Hepatol* 1999, 31(Suppl 2):S213–S215.

84. Dominguez S, Denys A, Madeira I, *et al.*: Hepatic arterial chemoembolization with streptozotocin in patients with metastatic digestive endocrine tumours. *Eur J Gastroenterol Hepatol* 2000, 12:151–157.

85. Ruszniewski P, Malka D: Hepatic arterial chemoembolization in the management of advanced digestive endocrine tumors. *Digestion* 2000, 62(Suppl 1):79–83.

86. Kulke M, Lenz HJ, Meropol NJ, *et al.*: Activity of sunitinib in patients with advanced neuroendocrine tumors. *J Clin Oncol* 2008, 26:3403–3410.

87. Vauthey JN, Klimstra D, Franceschi D, *et al.*: Factors affecting long-term outcome after hepatic resection for hepatocellular carcinoma [with discussion]. *Am J Surg* 1995, 169:28–35.

88. Haug CE, Jenkins RL, Rohrer RJ, *et al.*: Liver transplantation for primary hepatic cancer. *Transplantation* 1992, 53:376–382.

89. Mazzaferro V, Regalia E, Doci R, *et al.*: Liver transplantation for the treatment of small hepatocellular carcinomas in patients with cirrhosis [see comments]. *N Engl J Med* 1996, 334:693–699.

90. Muto Y, Moriwaki H, Saito A: Prevention of second primary tumors by an acyclic retinoid in patients with hepatocellular carcinoma. *N Engl J Med* 1999, 340:1046–1047.

91. Muto Y, Moriwaki H, Ninomiya M, *et al.*: Prevention of second primary tumors by an acyclic retinoid, polyprenoic acid, in patients with hepatocellular carcinoma. *Digestion* 1998, 59(Suppl 2):89–91.

92. Muto Y, Moriwaki H, Ninomiya M, *et al.*: Prevention of second primary tumors by an acyclic retinoid, polyprenoic acid, in patients with hepatocellular carcinoma. Hepatoma Prevention Study Group. *N Engl J Med* 1996, 334:1561–1567.

93. Holman M, Harrison D, Stewart A, *et al.*: Neoadjuvant chemotherapy and orthotopic liver transplantation for hepatocellular carcinoma. *N J Med* 1995, 92:519–522.

94. Stone MJ, Klintmalm GB, Polter D, *et al.*: Neoadjuvant chemotherapy and liver transplantation for hepatocellular carcinoma: a pilot study in 20 patients. *Gastroenterology* 1993, 104:196–202.

95. Atiq OT, Kemeny N, Niedzwiecki D, Botet J: Treatment of unresectable primary liver cancer with intrahepatic fluorodeoxyuridine and mitomycin C through an implantable pump. *Cancer* 1992, 69:920–924.

96. Orlando A, D'Antoni A, Camma C, *et al.*: Treatment of small hepatocellular carcinoma with percutaneous ethanol injection: a validated prognostic model. *Am J Gastroenterol* 2000, 95:2921–2927.

97. Bartolozzi C, Lencioni R: Ethanol injection for the treatment of hepatic tumours. *Eur Radiol* 1996, 6:682–696.

98. Livraghi T, Giorgio A, Marin G, *et al.*: Hepatocellular carcinoma and cirrhosis in 746 patients: long-term results of percutaneous ethanol injection. *Radiology* 1995, 197:101–108.

99. Onik GM, Atkinson D, Zemel R, Weaver ML: Cryosurgery of liver cancer. *Semin Surg Oncol* 1993, 9:309–317.

100. McGhana JP, Dodd GD Jr: Radiofrequency ablation of the liver: current status. *AJR Am J Roentgenol* 2001, 176:3–16.

101. Farmer DG, Busuttil RW: The role of multimodal therapy in the treatment of hepatocellular carcinoma. *Cancer* 1994, 73:2669–2670.

102. Farmer DG, Rosove MH, Shaked A, Busuttil RW: Current treatment modalities for hepatocellular carcinoma. *Ann Surg* 1994, 219:236–247.

103. Llovet J, Ricci S, Mazzaferro V, *et al.*: Sorafenib in advanced hepatocellular carcinoma. *N Engl J Med* 2008, 359:378–390.

104. Klempnauer J, Ridder GJ, von Wasielewski R, *et al.*: Resectional surgery of hilar cholangiocarcinoma: a multivariate analysis of prognostic factors. *J Clin Oncol* 1997, 15:947–954.

105. Baer HU, Stain SC, Dennison AR, *et al.*: Improvements in survival by aggressive resections of hilar cholangiocarcinoma. *Ann Surg* 1993, 217:20–207.

106. Patt YZ, Jones DV, Hoque A, *et al.*: Phase II trial of intravenous fluorouracil and subcutaneous interferon alfa-2b for biliary tract cancer. *J Clin Oncol* 1996, 14:2311–2315.

107. Pazdur R, Royce ME, Rodriguez GI, *et al.*: Phase II trial of docetaxel for cholangiocarcinoma. *Am J Clin Oncol* 1999, 22:78–81.

108. Jones DV, Lozano R, Hoque A, *et al.*: Phase II study of paclitaxel therapy for unresectable biliary tree carcinomas. *J Clin Oncol* 1996, 14:2306–2310.

109. Robertson JM, Lawrence TS, Dworzanin LM, *et al.*: Treatment of primary hepatobiliary cancers with conformal radiation therapy and regional chemotherapy. *J Clin Oncol* 1993, 11:1286–1293.

110. Lerner A, Gonin R, Steele GD Jr, Mayer RJ: Etoposide, doxorubicin, and cisplatin chemotherapy for advanced gastric adenocarcinoma: results of a phase II trial. *J Clin Oncol* 1992, 10:536–540.

111. Kelsen D, Atiq OT, Saltz L, *et al.*: FAMTX versus etoposide, doxorubicin, and cisplatin: a randomized assignment trial in gastric cancer. *J Clin Oncol* 1992, 10:541–548.

112. Preusser P, Wilke H, Achterrath W, *et al.*: Phase II study with the combination etoposide, doxorubicin, and cisplatin in advanced measurable gastric cancer. *J Clin Oncol* 1989, 7:1310–1317.

113. Wilke H, Preusser P, Fink U, *et al.*: New developments in the treatment of gastric carcinoma. *Semin Oncol* 1990, 17(Suppl 2):61–70.

114. Wils JA, Klein HO, Wagener DJ, *et al.*: Sequential high-dose methotrexate and fluorouracil combined with doxorubicin: a step ahead in the treatment of advanced gastric cancer: a trial of the European Organization for Research and Treatment of Cancer Gastrointestinal Tract Cooperative Group. *J Clin Oncol* 1991, 9:827–831.

115. Wils JA, Bleiberg H, Dalesio O, *et al.*: An EORTC Gastrointestinal Group evaluation of the combination of sequential methotrexate and 5-fluorouracil combined with Adriamycin in advanced measurable gastric cancer. *J Clin Oncol* 1986, 4:1799–1803.

116. Wilke JA, Preusser P, Fink U, *et al.*: High dose folinic acid/etoposide/5-fluorouracil in advanced gastric cancer: a phase II study in elderly patients or patients with cardiac risk. *Invest New Drugs* 1990, 8:65–70.

117. MacDonald JS, Schein PS, Woolley PV, *et al.*: 5-Fluorouracil, doxorbicin, and mitomycin (FAM) combination chemotherapy for advanced gastric cancer. *Ann Intern Med* 1980, 93:533–536.

118. Biran H, Sulkes A, Biran S: 5-Fluorouracil, doxorubicin (Adriamyin), and mitomycin C (FAM) in advanced gastric cancer: observations on response, patient characteristics, myelosuppression and delivered dosage. *Oncology* 1989, 46:83–87.

119. Arbuck SG, Silk Y, Douglass HO Jr, *et al.*: A phase II trial of 5-fluorouracil, doxorubicin, mitomycin C, and leucovorin in advanced gastric carcinoma. *Cancer* 1990, 65:2442–2445.

120. Kalser MH, Ellenberg SS: Pancreatic cancer. Adjuvant combined radiation and chemotherapy following curative resection. *Arch Surg* 1985, 120:899–903.

121. Further evidence of effective adjuvant combined radiation and chemotherapy following curative resection of pancreatic cancer. Gastrointestinal Tumor Study Group. *Cancer* 1987, 59:2006–2010.

122. Seitz JF, Giovannini M, Padaut-Cesana J, *et al.*: Inoperable nonmetastatic squamous cell carcinoma of the esophagus managed by concomitant chemotherapy (5-fluorouracil and cisplatin) and radiation therapy. *Cancer* 1990, 66:214–219.

123. De Besi P, Sileni VP, Salvagno L, *et al.*: Phase II study of cisplatin, 5-FU, and allopurinol in advanced esophageal cancer. *Cancer Treat Rep* 1986, 70:909–910.

124. Kies MS, Rosen ST, Tsang TK, *et al.*: Cisplatin and 5-fluorouracil in the primary management of squamous esophageal cancer. *Cancer* 1987, 60:2156–2160.

125. Wadler S, Haynes H, Beitler JJ, *et al.*: Phase II clinical trial with 5-fluorouracil, recombinant interferon-alpha-2b, and cisplatin for patients with metastatic or regionally advanced carcinoma of the esophagus. *Cancer* 1996, 78:30–34.

126. Kelsen D, Lovett D, Wong J, *et al.*: Interferon alfa-2a and fluorouracil in the treatment of patients with advanced esophageal cancer. *J Clin Oncol* 1992, 10:269–274.

127. Wadler S, Fell S, Haynes H, *et al.*: Treatment of carcinoma of the esophagus with 5-fluorouracil and recombinant alpha-2a interferon. *Cancer* 1993, 71:1726–1730.

128. Ilson DH, Sirott M, Saltz L, *et al.*: A phase II trial of interferon alpha-2A 5-fluorouracil, and cisplatin in patients with advanced esophageal carcinoma. *Cancer* 1995, 75:2197–2202.

129. Spiridonidis CH, Laufman LR, Jones JJ, *et al.*: A phase II evaluation of high dose cisplatin and etoposide in patients with advanced esophageal adenocarcinoma. *Cancer* 1996, 77:2070–2077.

Lower Gastrointestinal Cancer
Wen Wee Ma, Wells A. Messersmith

8

COLORECTAL CANCER

Cancers arising in the large bowel are the third most common type of cancer in men and women in the United States. Approximately 153,760 new cases were diagnosed in the year 2007, with approximately 52,180 cancer deaths [1]. The incidence of colorectal cancer has been decreasing over the past two decades, from 66.3 cases per 100,000 persons in 1985 to 49.5 in 2003. The incidence declined significantly from 1998 to 2003 by 2.1%, partly from increased screening and removal of colorectal polyps that would have transformed to invasive cancer.

The survival of patients with resectable colorectal cancer is improving, most likely due to earlier diagnosis, improvements in surgical technique, and the use of adjuvant therapy. The prognosis of patients with metastatic colorectal cancer is also improving due to increasing availability of more effective cytotoxics, such as oxaliplatin and irinotecan, and biologics, such as bevacizumab, cetuximab, and panitumumab. As more active chemotherapeutic agents and surgical techniques become available, patients with metastatic disease confined to a single organ, such as lung or liver, can expect better survival—or even cure in a subset of patients—when managed in a multidisciplinary fashion.

About 73% of new colorectal cancer cases originate in the colon (defined as the segment of the large bowel proximal to the peritoneal reflection), with the remaining new cases in the rectum. During the past 25 years, a shift in tumor location has been observed, with a decrease in the percentage of tumors arising in the rectum and descending colon, and an increasing incidence of tumors arising in the proximal colon. Adenocarcinomas account for the vast majority (> 90%) of large bowel cancers, whereas carcinoid tumors account for most of the remaining malignant neoplasms. Rarely, primary lymphomas, melanomas, and sarcomas of the large bowel are reported.

ETIOLOGY AND RISK FACTORS

Most colorectal cancer cases are sporadic (ie, no obvious excess risk factors), whereas about 5% to 10% are hereditary [2]. The other 1% to 2% of colorectal cancer cases are associated with chronic inflammation, as seen in inflammatory bowel disease (IBD). In sporadic cases, both genetic and environmental factors play important roles (Table 8-1). The risk for colorectal cancer increases with older age, with more than 90% of the disease diagnosed in patients older than 50 years of age [1]. In the United States, the incidence of colorectal cancer increases from less than 10 per 100,000 patients at risk among the 40-year-old group, to 125 per 100,000 at 60 years, 250 per 100,000 at 70 years, and 400 per 100,000 for those 85 years of age and older [3]. The disease is more likely to be diagnosed in male than female individuals.

About 20% of sporadic cases have some component of familial risk, although not adequate to fulfill the strict criteria of hereditary colorectal cancer syndromes [4]. For this group, the patients have two or more first- or second-degree relatives with colorectal cancer.

The progression of adenomatous polyps to colorectal adenocarcinoma is well described and is often an accumulation of multiple molecular genetic events [5]. Data from the National Polyp Study Workgroup indicates that it takes about 10 years for the smallest polyp and 5.5 years for a large polyp (> 1 cm) to transform into cancer [6]. Genetic and epigenetic abnormalities commonly seen in sporadic colorectal cancer involve either activation of certain oncogenes, such as K-ras, or inactivation/loss of functional tumor suppressor genes, such as APC, DCC (deleted in colon cancer, found on 18q), and p53 (found on 17p) [5,7–9]. About 10% to 13% of sporadic colorectal cancers exhibit the phenotype of microsatellite instability.

The two main forms of hereditary cancer syndromes are familial adenomatous polyposis (FAP) and hereditary nonpolyposis colorectal cancer (HNPCC; Lynch syndromes I and II) [4]. FAP and its variants, including Gardner's syndrome, attenuated adenomatous polyposis, and hereditary flat adenoma syndrome, are associated with mutations in the APC gene (chromosome 5q) that result in a truncated protein product. Patients with FAP develop multiple colonic adenomas at an early age, often in distal colon, with malignant transformation in most patients by the fifth decade. Families with HNPCC almost always harbor microsatellite instability and mismatch-repair gene mutations. Mutations in at least five different mismatch-repair genes have been found, including MSH2 (2p), MSH6 (2p), MLH1 (3p), PMS1 (2q), and PMS2 (7p).

Other rare hamartomatous polyposis syndromes are also associated with increased colorectal cancer risk. The genetic mutations underlying these syndromes include PTEN in Cowden's disease and Bannayan-Ruvalcaba syndrome [10,11], LKB1(STK11) in Peutz-Jeghers syndrome [12], and Smad4(DPC4) in familial juvenile polyposis [13].

In patients with IBD, cancers arise in areas of chronically inflamed epithelium, and the duration and extent of involvement are two independent risk factors [14]. For patients with extensive ulcerative and Crohn's colitis, the risk of developing colon cancer begins to increase above age-matched controls after 7 to 10 years of disease. Cancers associated with IBD do not arise from adenomatous polyps, but rather from dysplastic epithelium that is generally indistinguishable from nondysplastic adjacent epithelium. Therefore, multiple, random biopsies are needed for surveillance, with the risk for sampling error. APC mutations are infrequent and occur late, whereas p53 mutations occur early in malignant transformation.

Diets high in total fat, protein, and calories and low in calcium and folate are associated with an increased risk of colorectal cancer [15]. However,

Table 8-1. Etiology and Risk Factors for Colorectal Cancer

General

Age

Male gender

Cholecystectomy

Ureterocolic anastomosis

Hormonal factors

Environmental factors

Diet rich in meat and fat and poor in fiber, folate, and calcium

Sedentary lifestyle

Obesity

Diabetes mellitus

Smoking

Previous radiation

High alcohol intake

Asbestos exposure

Personal factors

History of colorectal polyps

History of colorectal cancer

History of small intestine, endometrial, breast, or ovarian cancer

History of inflammatory bowel disease

Family history of colorectal disease in first or second relatives

Hereditary colorectal cancer

Familial adenomatous polyposis

Hereditary nonpolyposis colorectal cancer

Hamartomatous polyposis syndrome

(Adapted from Weitz et al. [2].)

dietary supplementation with cereal fiber, or diets high in fiber, fruits, and vegetables and low in fat, have not reduced the rate of adenoma recurrence over a 3- to 4-year period. Cigarette smoking has been associated with an increased tendency to form adenomas and develop colorectal cancer. There has been much interest in the role of nonsteroidal anti-inflammatory drugs (NSAIDs) in chemoprevention for colorectal cancer following the observation that NSAIDs prevent formation or cause regression of adenomatous polyps in FAP individuals. Case-control studies in normal-risk populations also suggest a lower risk of colorectal cancer with regular use of aspirin or other NSAIDs. However, recent evidence showed unacceptable cardiovascular and gastrointestinal adverse effects of NSAIDs and cyclooxygenase-2 inhibitors to justify their use in colorectal cancer prevention [16].

SCREENING RECOMMENDATIONS

In 2003, the US Multisociety Task Force on Colorectal Cancer recommended a risk-based approach to screening [17]. For risk stratification, individuals should be evaluated for personal history, presence of predisposing illness (*eg*, IBD), and family history of colorectal cancer or adenomatous polyps. Positive response to any of the above factors should prompt further investigation into the condition associated with the increased risk. For individuals with average risk, screening with one of the following methods should be offered beginning at age 50:

- Fecal occult blood test (FOBT) or fecal immunochemical test (FIT) – yearly
- Flexible sigmoidoscopy – every 5 years
- FOBT or FIT, plus flexible sigmoidoscopy – every 5 years
- Double-contrast barium enema – every 5 years
- Colonoscopy – every 10 years

All positive results should be followed up with a colonoscopy. It is important to note that double-contrast barium enema has not been shown to reduce the incidence of mortality from colorectal cancer in individuals with average risk. Similarly, colonoscopy alone has not been shown to reduce incidence or mortality, although when evaluated together with FOBT in clinical trials, the combined approach did reduce colorectal cancer mortality [18–21].

All polyps should be removed when detected and examined pathologically because removal of adenomatous polyps may reduce the risk of subsequent colorectal cancer. Colonoscopy should be repeated in 3 years for individuals with advanced or more than three adenomas, and in 5 years for those with one or two small (< 1 cm) tubular adenomas. For individuals who had a curative resection for colorectal cancer, colonoscopy should be performed 6 months after surgery if the lesion was obstructive preoperatively; baseline colonoscopy should be performed at the time of initial diagnosis for synchronous lesions. If the result is normal, colonoscopy should be offered after 3 years, and if again normal, every 5 years.

No randomized trials are available to guide colorectal cancer screening in individuals with IBD, although it is common practice to perform surveillance colonoscopy with extensive biopsy protocol beginning at 8 to 10 years of disease. Prophylactic colectomy may be offered to a subset of IBD patients with severe disease. Individuals with or at risk of FAP should have annual sigmoidoscopy beginning at 10 to 12 years of age, whereas those at risk of or with HNPCC should have a colonoscopy every 1 to 2 years beginning at age 20 to 25 years or 10 years earlier than the youngest age of colon cancer diagnosis in the family (whichever comes first).

STAGING AND PROGNOSIS

The most reproducible prognostic indicator for large bowel cancers is operative staging. Tables 8-2 and 8-3 briefly summarize the staging definition and survival rates of the 2002 American Joint Commission on Cancer (AJCC) tumor, node, metastasis (TNM) system for colorectal cancer [22]. It is recommended that clinical decisions be made with reference to TNM classification instead of the older Dukes' or modified Astler-Coller classification schema. At least 12 lymph nodes should be examined to confirm the absence of involvement [23,24].

Stage 0 tumors are carcinoma in situ with intraepithelial or lamina propria invasion. Stage I tumors invade through to muscularis propria but without lymph node involvement or distant metastasis. Stage II tumors invade through the muscularis propria and may extend to adjacent structures, but show no further tumor involvement. Lymph node involvement without metastatic disease defines stage III; stage IIIA to IIIC differ in the local extent of disease and number of lymph nodes involved. The presence of distant metastases (commonly in the liver or lungs) is described as stage IV.

Prognosis for respective stages was analyzed based on 119,363 patients with colon adenocarcinoma in the Surveillance, Epidemiology and End Results (SEER) national cancer registry from 1991 to 2000 [25]. The 5-year survival is 93.2% for stage I, 72% to 85% for stage II, 44% to 84% for stage III, and 8% for stage IV. Interestingly, stage IIIA had a better survival than stage IIB based on the historical data, which clinicians may have to take into consideration when recommending treatment.

SURGICAL CONSIDERATIONS

En bloc surgical resection of primary colorectal cancer, including the adjacent mesentery and regional lymph nodes, remains the primary therapy for colorectal cancer and provides the optimal opportunity for cure and

Table 8-2. TNM Staging Definition for Colorectal Cancer

Primary tumor (T)

TX: Primary tumor cannot be assessed

T0: No evidence of primary tumor

Tis: Carcinoma in situ (intraepithelial or invasion of the lamina propria)

T1: Tumor invades submucosa

T2: Tumor invades muscularis propria

T3: Tumor invades through the muscularis propria into the subserosa or into nonperitonealized pericolic or perirectal tissues

T4: Tumor directly invades other organs or structures and/or perforates visceral peritoneum

Regional lymph nodes (N)

NX: Regional nodes cannot be assessed

N0: No regional lymph node metastasis

N1: Metastasis in 1–3 regional lymph nodes

N2: Metastasis in ≥ 4 regional lymph nodes

Distant metastasis (M)

MX: Distant metastasis cannot be assessed

M0: No distant metastasis

M1: Distant metastasis

Table 8-3. AJCC TNM Survival Rates in Colorectal Cancer

AJCC stage	Staging groupings	5-y stage-specific survival, %
Stage 0	Tis, N0, M0	—
Stage I	T1, N0, M0	93.2
	T2, N0, M0	
Stage IIA	T3, N0, M0	84.7
Stage IIB	T4, N0, M0	72.2
Stage IIIA	T1, N1, M0	83.4
	T2, N1, M0	
Stage IIIB	T3, N1, M0	64.1
	T4, N1, M0	
Stage IIIC	Any T, N2, M0	44.3
Stage IV	Any T, any N, M1	8.1

AJCC—American Joint Commission on Cancer; TNM—tumor, node, metastasis. (*Adapted from* O'Connell *et al.* [25].)

risk stratification. With increasingly active chemotherapy agents, surgical resection of both primary and metastatic lesions offers a potentially curative option in eligible patients with organ-confined metastases, often following preoperative (neoadjuvant) chemotherapy [26]. Adjuvant (postoperative) chemotherapy with fluoropyrimidine-based regimens decreases the risk of recurrence and improves survival in stage III colon cancer patients [27–31]. The role of adjuvant chemotherapy in stage II patients remains controversial given the small benefit in disease-free survival (DFS) and possibly overall survival [32]. Bowel obstruction or perforation, direct extension of tumor to adjacent structure (T4), and genetic/molecular features such as aneuploid DNA content, high S-phase fraction, or deletion of 18q are retrospectively associated with a higher risk of recurrence in stage II disease. The routine use of such tests for risk stratification is not recommended given the lack of prospective studies.

In rectal cancer, total mesorectal excision offers the best local control [33–35]). Neoadjuvant and adjuvant chemoradiotherapy or chemotherapy have been shown to benefit rectal cancer patients, although neoadjuvant chemotherapy may provide better local control and reduced toxicity [36–38]. Finally, laparoscopic versus open colorectal cancer resections have been found to have similar oncologic outcomes [39].

ADJUVANT THERAPY FOR RESECTED COLON CANCER

Adjuvant chemotherapy with fluorouracil (5-FU)–based regimens is considered standard of care for stage III patients but not routinely recommended for stage II patients after resection of the primary tumor [32,40]. However, stage II patients with poor prognostic features can reasonably be offered adjuvant therapy. Such features include an inadequate number of lymph nodes sampled (< 13 lymph nodes examined), T4 lesion, perforation, obstruction, and poorly differentiated histology. Stratification of stage II patients based on tumor molecular markers remains experimental. Eligible patients should receive 6 months of adjuvant chemotherapy [41].

Oxaliplatin-based combinations (FOLFOX, FLOX) are the standard regimens for adjuvant therapy. FOLFOX consists of infusional 5-FU, leucovorin (LV), and oxaliplatin, whereas FLOX uses bolus rather than infusional 5-FU. In the Multicenter International Study of Oxaliplatin/5-FU-LV in the Adjuvant Treatment of Colon Cancer (MOSAIC) trial, 2246 patients with completely resected stage II and III colon cancer were randomized to receive FOLFOX4 or infusional 5-FU/LV [42]. For stage III patients, the DFS at 6 years was 72.9% in the FOLFOX4 arm and 68.3% in the 5-FU/LV arm. For stage II patients, 6-year DFS was equivalent between both arms (86.8% vs 86.8%; hazard ratio [HR] 1.00). More patients (12.4%) in the FOLFOX4 arm developed grade 3 sensory neuropathy during therapy, which decreased to 1.1% after 1 year. In the National Surgical Adjuvant Breast and Bowel Project (NSABP) C-07 trial, 2407 patients with stage II (28.6%) or III colon cancer were randomized to receive FLOX or bolus 5-FU/LV [43]. Four-year DFS was 73.1% and 67.0% for FLOX and 5-FU/LV, respectively (HR 0.8; $P = 0.0034$). Side effects such as neurosensory toxicity, diarrhea, or dehydration associated with bowel wall thickening were more frequent in the FLOX arm [44].

Alternative regimens in the adjuvant setting include single-agent oral capecitabine and 5-FU/LV. Capecitabine was shown to be at least equivalent to bolus 5-FU/LV (Mayo regimen) with respect to DFS and overall survival for stage III patients [45]. Furthermore, capecitabine plus oxaliplatin (CapeOx) has a manageable toxicity profile in stage III colon cancer patients, although the comparative efficacy remains unknown [46]. Unlike in advanced or metastatic colon cancer, irinotecan-based regimens (IFL [irinotecan plus bolus 5-FU/LV] and FOLFIRI [irinotecan plus infusional 5-FU/LV]) failed to improve DFS and overall survival in multiple trials, and cannot be recommended in the adjuvant setting [47–49]. The role of biologic agents, such as cetuximab and bevacizumab, is under investigation.

THERAPY FOR EARLY-STAGE RECTAL CANCER

The management of early-stage rectal cancer (stage I–III) differs from similarly staged colon cancer in regard to the role of radiation and surgery. In addition to computed tomography (CT) scans, endorectal ultrasound or endorectal or pelvis magnetic resonance imaging (MRI) should be used to stage rectal cancer, when available, to determine the extent of

mucosal invasion and nodal status [50]. Local excision, such as transanal excision, achieves comparable results to anteroposterior resection in T1 tumors with favorable features (negative margins, no lymphovascular or perineural invasion, < 3 cm, well to moderately differentiated histology) [51,52]. However, the benefit of local excision in T2 tumors is controversial; therefore, an approach using neoadjuvant chemoradiation followed by local excision is being examined (American College of Surgeons Oncology Group [ACOSOG] Z6041 trial) [53]. Currently, transabdominal resection should be performed if the pathology of the excision reveals greater than T2 lesion or T1 or T2 lesions with poor risk features, such as positive margin, lymphovascular invasion, and poorly differentiated histology. Patients with invasive rectal cancer not amenable to local excision should undergo sharp mesorectal excision, with the removal of mesentery distal to the tumor as an intact unit [54]. Such an approach reduces local recurrence and perioperative morbidity.

As in colon cancer, adjuvant therapy is not indicated in stage I rectal cancer [55]. Adjuvant therapy is recommended for stage II and III rectal cancers and radiation is important in reducing locoregional recurrence. The NSABP R-02 trial showed that addition of pelvic radiation to adjuvant systemic chemotherapy reduced locoregional relapse in Duke's B and C rectal cancer patients from 13% to 8% at 5-year follow-up compared with a chemotherapy-only group [56]. In addition, infusional 5-FU during pelvic radiation was found to be more effective than bolus 5-FU [57]. As such, patients with stage II/III rectal cancer should receive adjuvant 5-FU–containing chemotherapy (bolus/infusional 5-FU, FOLFOX, or capecitabine) followed by concurrent 5-FU (bolus or infusional) and pelvic radiation, then another course of 5-FU–containing chemotherapy. Because the initial chemotherapy was often included in clinical trials to permit central review of planned radiation fields, in practice, many oncologists simply start with chemoradiation followed by chemotherapy. The use of FOLFOX or capecitabine in the adjuvant setting for rectal cancer is a reasonable extrapolation from colon cancer, and it is important to recall that most patients relapse with metastatic rather then localized disease. For concurrent chemoradiation, bolus 5-FU can be administered at an intravenous (IV) dose of 500 mg/m^2 for 3 days during weeks 1 and 5 of radiation; however, infusional 5-FU at 225 mg/m^2/d throughout radiation appears to be preferable. The roles of capecitabine, cetuximab, and bevacizumab in adjuvant chemoradiation of rectal cancer are being investigated.

Preoperative (or neoadjuvant) rectal cancer therapy has the advantages of debulking the primary tumor, preserving sphincter function, improving local control, rendering initially unresectable lesions resectable, and theoretically enhancing the radiosensitizing effects of chemotherapy by preserving the vascular integrity of the tumor tissues [38,58]. Sauer *et al.* [38] compared neoadjuvant against adjuvant chemoradiotherapy in a randomized trial and reported superior local control and reduced toxicity with preoperative chemoradiotherapy in patients with greater than T3 rectal cancer with nodal involvement. However, overall survival was not significantly different between both approaches. Interestingly, posttreatment staging had significant prognostic importance with regard to DFS. The European Organisation for Research and Treatment of Cancer (EORTC) 22921 phase 3 trial demonstrated the benefit of adding 5-FU to radiation compared with radiation alone. There was a significant reduction in tumor size, nodal involvement, and lymphovascular/perineural invasion [59]. Currently, the recommendation for resectable stage II to III rectal cancer is preoperative infusional 5-FU with radiation [55]. Following resection of the primary tumor, patents should then receive postoperative adjuvant 5-FU–containing chemotherapy (bolus/infusional 5-FU, capecitabine, or FOLFOX). Patients with locally unresectable rectal cancer should be considered for preoperative 5-FU/LV (infusional/bolus) or capecitabine with radiation followed by evaluation for possible surgical resection. The addition of other cytotoxics (*eg*, oxaliplatin) and biologics is being actively explored.

There is currently a lack of rigorous outcome data on patients who achieved pathologic downstaging with neoadjuvant therapy and underwent subsequent surgical resection. As such, postoperative chemotherapy should be administered for all patients who received preoperative chemotherapy regardless of the surgical pathology results [55].

SURVEILLANCE GUIDELINES FOR DETECTION OF RECURRENT COLORECTAL CANCER

The risk of recurrence remains high after primary therapy for resectable colorectal cancer. According to the American Society of Clinical Oncology's 2005 practice guidelines, patients with high risk for recurrence who are candidates for salvage surgery should be offered annual CT of the chest and abdomen for 3 years after primary therapy [60]. The National Comprehensive Cancer Center Network's surveillance algorithms are similar [41,55]. Pelvic CT scan is recommended for rectal cancer surveillance, especially for individuals with poor prognostic factors. Colonoscopy should be performed at 1 year after surgery (6 months if a full colonoscopy was not possible due to an obstructing lesion at diagnosis) and every 3 to 5 years thereafter if the result is normal. Rectal cancer patients without previous pelvic radiation should have flexible proctosigmoidoscopy every 6 months for 5 years. These patients should also have history and physical examination every 3 to 6 months for the first 3 years, every 6 months during years 4 and 5, and subsequently at the discretion of the treating physician. Carcinoembryonic antigen (CEA) every 3 months postoperatively for at least 3 to 5 years after diagnosis is recommended in patients who are candidates for surgery or systemic therapy. Elevation of CEA should be further investigated.

MANAGEMENT OF ADVANCED COLORECTAL CANCER

The goal for management of advanced or metastatic (stage IV) colorectal cancer depends upon the extent of metastases. Most patients have widespread disease, and the goal of therapy is palliation and incremental prolongation of life. However, there is a small subset of patients with organ-confined and limited metastases in whom cure is possible, generally with a combination of surgery and chemotherapy. Moreover, modern colorectal cancer chemotherapy is highly active and can render some initially unresectable metastases resectable. A retrospective analysis reported higher 5-year survival (> 30%) in patients with initially unresectable colorectal metastases who underwent metastectomy after receiving neoadjuvant chemotherapy [61]. As such, the subset of patients with potentially resectable liver- or lung-confined metastases should be identified early, treated aggressively, and referred for curative-intent surgery accordingly.

Palliative chemotherapy should be initiated in symptomatic patients with unresectable or metastatic colorectal cancer, provided they have reasonable performance status and are able to tolerate intensive therapy. Local symptoms in rectal cancer should be treated with appropriate regional or localized therapy. Chemotherapy treatments for advanced rectal cancer are otherwise similar to advanced colon cancer.

5-FU–BASED REGIMENS

The evidence for the benefit of systemic chemotherapy in advanced colorectal cancer became apparent following a meta-analysis of 13 randomized trials [62]. 5-FU forms the backbone of contemporary colorectal cancer chemotherapy, and combination regimens are superior to single-agent regimens [63]. In addition, infusional 5-FU appears superior to bolus 5-FU regimens, although they differ in their side effect profiles. The bolus regimens are associated with increased bone marrow suppression, mucostomatitis, and diarrhea, whereas palmar-plantar erythrodysesthesia (or hand-foot syndrome) is more common in the infusional regimens [64–66].

In previously untreated colorectal cancer patients (first-line setting), contemporary chemotherapy options include regimens combining infusional 5-FU with either oxaliplatin or irinotecan (FOLFOX/FOLFIRI), often with bevacizumab. Intravenous 5-FU may be substituted by oral capecitabine with similar safety and efficacy profiles in oxaliplatin combinations (CapeOx with or without bevacizumab) [67,68]. For patients less able to tolerate intensive therapy, 5-FU/LV alone or with bevacizumab are appropriate options [69]. Patients who have exhausted the above regimens are candidates (third-line or more) for irinotecan plus cetuximab, single-agent cetuximab, or panitumumab therapies.

CAPECITABINE

Capecitabine, a fluoropyrimidine carbamate, is an oral prodrug that undergoes enzymatic conversion in the liver to 5-FU [70]. Capecitabine is superior to daily bolus 5-FU (Mayo regimen) in response rate, although there is no

significant difference in metastatic disease survival [71–73]. Capecitabine can be used to replace the less convenient IV 5-FU in combination regimens [67,68]. The toxicity profile is comparable to infusional 5-FU regimens; hand-foot syndrome predominates. Other side effects include stomatitis, nausea, vomiting, bone marrow suppression, and diarrhea.

Due to the dependence on hepatic activation, caution is advised when administering capecitabine together with cytochrome-P450–interacting medications such as warfarin because unpredictable international normalized ratio prolongation can occur [74].

OXALIPLATIN

Oxaliplatin is a third-generation platinum compound that forms bulky DNA adducts and induces cellular apoptosis [75]. The agent can be administered with 5-FU and LV in different dosages and methods; such regimens are generally referred to as FOLFOX (infusional 5-FU) or FLOX (bolus 5-FU). In FOLFOX6, oxaliplatin is combined with bolus 5-FU/LV on day 1 followed by 46 hours of continuous infusion 5-FU. In FOLFOX4, oxaliplatin is administered with bolus 5-FU/LV followed by 22-hour infusional 5-FU for 2 consecutive days. Both combinations are repeated every 2 weeks.

FOLFOX has an established track record in both the first- and second-line setting. Giacchetti et al. [76] reported the superior median progression-free survival (PFS) of 8.7 months in previously untreated patients receiving oxaliplatin with chronomodulated 5-FU/LV, compared with 6.1 months in those receiving only 5-FU/LV ($P < 0.05$). In the first-line setting, de Gramont et al. [77] also reported significantly longer median PFS (9.0 vs 6.2 months; $P = 0.0003$) and response rate (50.7% vs 22.3%; $P = 0.0001$) in patients receiving FOLFOX4 compared with infusional 5-FU/LV alone. There was a trend toward longer survival (16.2 vs 14.7 months; $P = 0.12$) in the FOLFOX4 arm. In the second-line setting, metastatic colorectal cancer patients who failed IFL achieved longer median time to progression (4.6 vs 2.7 months; $P < 0.0001$) and response rate (12% vs 0%; $P < 0.0001$) with FOLFOX4 than those receiving bolus 5-FU/LV [78]. More patients who received FOLFOX4 achieved relief from tumor-related symptoms than those treated with 5-FU/LV (33% vs 12%; $P < 0.01$).

Neuropathy is a common side effect in patients receiving oxaliplatin-based regimens, with approximately 15% experiencing interference with activities of daily living [79]. The unique neuropathy includes an acute form that is reversible and transient, and is described as cold-induced paresthesia of hands, feet, or oral or pharyngeal regions during or for a short period of time after infusion. The cumulative form is dose dependent and longer lasting, and is described as peripheral dysesthesia that develops following months of treatment. The cumulative form is usually reversible with interruption of therapy. Fortunately, the neuropathy is reversible to a tolerable level in more than 99% of patients within 18 months after stopping oxaliplatin. Neutropenia and diarrhea are also more frequent with oxaliplatin-containing regimens [31].

Oxaliplatin-related neuropathy causes significant morbidity and limits the amount of therapy patients can receive. Oxaliplatin "stop-and-go" strategies have been developed to deal with this troublesome side effect; the Optimized 5-FU/Oxaliplatin Strategy (OPTIMOX-1) trial was the first such study [80]. In this trial, 620 patients with advanced colorectal cancer were randomized to receive FOLFOX4 until progression or a "stop-and-go" approach with six cycles of FOLFOX7 (using slightly higher oxaliplatin doses), followed by 5-FU/LV maintenance for 12 cycles, and then reintroduction of FOLFOX7. There was no decrement in PFS or overall survival, but the decrease in toxicity was disappointingly small. The OPTIMOX-2 trial, which examined a complete stoppage of chemotherapy, was stopped early due to the need to include bevacizumab in the chemotherapy arms. As a result, definitive conclusions cannot be drawn.

IRINOTECAN

Irinotecan is a topoisomerase I inhibitor derived from the natural alkaloid camptothecin that is hydrolyzed to SN38, the active metabolite [81]. Irinotecan can be administered with bolus 5-FU (IFL) or infusional 5-FU (FOLFIRI). The FOLFIRI regimen is recommended due to its superior efficacy and decreased toxicity. When compared with bolus 5-FU/LV (Mayo regimen), patients with advanced colorectal cancer receiving IFL achieved a longer median survival (14.8 vs 12.6 months; $P = 0.04$) and higher response rate

(39% vs 21%; $P < 0.001$) in a randomized trial sponsored by the Irinotecan Study Group in North America [82]. In Europe, patients receiving irinotecan with FOLFIRI also achieved longer median survival (6.7 vs 4.4 months; $P < 0.001$) and response rate (35% vs 22%; $P < 0.01$) compared with those receiving infusional 5-FU/LV [83].

The toxicity of irinotecan includes nausea, vomiting, diarrhea, and bone marrow suppression. Interestingly, irinotecan-related side effects have been retrospectively found to correlate with the polymorphism of uridine diphosphate glucuronosyltransferase isoform 1A1 (UGT1A1), an enzyme needed to clear SN38. Patients with reduced UGT1A1 activity have increased SN38 levels, probably leading to increased gastrointestinal toxicities and bone marrow suppression [84,85]. A US Food and Drug Administration (FDA)–approved UGT1A1 polymorphism test is currently available for use in patients who are to receive irinotecan. However, there are no prospective data validating clinical use of the test, and optimal dose adjustments remain largely unknown [86].

OXALIPLATIN OR IRINOTECAN FIRST?

As described in previous sections, both oxaliplatin- and irinotecan-containing infusional 5-FU regimens achieve superior efficacy compared with bolus 5-FU/LV regimens. The North Central Cancer Treatment Group N9741 trial showed that administering oxaliplatin with infusional 5-FU (FOLFOX) achieved superior response rate, time to progression, and median survival compared with IFL or irinotecan plus oxaliplatin (IROX) in previously untreated metastatic colorectal cancer patients [87]. When evaluated in a head-to-head randomized trial, FOLFOX and FOLFIRI demonstrated similar efficacy in terms of response rate, time to progression, and survival in the first-line treatment of advanced colorectal cancer [88].

Given their comparable efficacy, which regimen should a newly diagnosed metastatic colorectal cancer patient receive first? Tournigand *et al.* [89] randomized previously untreated advanced colorectal cancer patients to two sequences: FOLFIRI followed by FOLFOX6 (arm A) or FOLFOX6 followed by FOLFIRI (arm B). The trial reported similar efficacy in both sequences, although toxicity profiles were different. Neutropenia and neurosensory toxicity were more frequent with FOLFOX6, whereas mucositis, nausea, vomiting, and alopecia were more common in FOLFIRI. Analysis of seven phase 3 trials in advanced colorectal cancer showed that patients who received all three agents (5-FU, irinotecan, and oxaliplatin) during a treatment course achieved longer survival than those who did not, indicating that overall exposure to the agents, rather than any particular order, was more important [90]. As such, the choice of first-line regimen (FOLFOX vs FOLFIRI) in advanced colorectal cancer is often guided by toxicity profiles and institutional practice. To maximize outcomes, patients should be offered all three agents during their treatment course.

BEVACIZUMAB

At the beginning of this century, a new class of chemotherapy agents became available for clinical care of metastatic colorectal cancer. Unlike conventional cytotoxic agents, this class of drugs tends to be cytostatic and disrupts cellular signaling pathways important for cancer growth, survival, differentiation, and metastasis.

Angiogenesis is important in the delivery of essential nutrients and oxygen to tumors and is regulated by pro- and antiangiogenic factors [91]. The rationale of targeting tumor vasculature in cancer therapy was first raised in the 1940s and rehypothesized by Folkman in the 1970s [92]. Interaction between vascular endothelial growth factor (VEGF)-A and VEGF receptor (VEGFR)-2 is thought to be the main mediator of angiogenesis seen in tumors [93,94].

Bevacizumab is a humanized VEGF-binding monoclonal antibody and was approved by the FDA for use with IV 5-FU–based regimens in patients with metastatic colorectal cancer [95]. In a pivotal randomized trial, 813 previously untreated metastatic colorectal cancer patients were randomized to receive IFL with or without bevacizumab (5mg/kg every 2 weeks) [96]. Patients receiving the bevacizumab-containing arm achieved a longer median survival (20.3 vs 15.6 months; $P < 0.001$), better response rate (44.8% vs 34%; $P = 0.004$), and median duration of response (10.4 vs 7.1 months; $P = 0.001$) than those without. The side effects reported to be bevacizumab-related include reversible hypertension and proteinuria. Other rarer events include gastrointestinal perforation, thrombotic events, and

wound dehiscence. As the chemotherapy standards have been a moving target, FOLFIRI has largely replaced IFL when combined with bevacizumab in clinical practice. In the randomized NO16966 trial, preliminary analysis also supported slightly superior efficacy of adding bevacizumab to oxaliplatin-based regimens (FOLFOX4, CapeOx) [68].

The benefit of bevacizumab with FOLFOX as second-line therapy was demonstrated in a phase 3 randomized trial (Eastern Cooperative Oncology Group [ECOG] E3200) [97]. In this trial, 829 metastatic colorectal cancer patients refractory to irinotecan/fluoropyrimidine combination were randomized to receive FOLFOX4 with or without bevacizumab (10 mg/kg every 2 weeks). Patients in the bevacizumab plus FOLFOX4 arm achieved superior response rate (22.7% vs 8.6%; $P < 0.0001$) and median survival (12.9 vs 10.8 months; HR for death = 0.75; $P = 0.0011$) compared with those receiving FOLFOX4 only. More than 50% of the patients treated with FOLFOX4 plus bevacizumab needed bevacizumab dose reduction to 5 mg/kg every 2 weeks for hypertension, bleeding, thrombosis, liver dysfunction, and proteinuria. Secondary analysis revealed that the overall survival and PFS were not compromised in this patient group, indicating that the 5-mg/kg dose is as efficacious as the 10-mg/kg dose, albeit with less toxicity [98].

It remains unclear if bevacizumab should be continued into second-line therapy in patients who failed a first-line regimen containing bevacizumab. At present there are no prospective clinical data to support such a practice. The efficacy of administering both bevacizumab and cetuximab (see below) with first-line combination therapy is under investigation in a large intergroup trial (Cancer and Leukemia Group B/Southwest Oncology Group [CALGB/SWOG] C80405).

CETUXIMAB AND PANITUMUMAB

Epidermal growth factor receptor (EGFR) became a target of interest in colorectal cancer therapy upon recognition of its role in carcinogenesis. Cetuximab is a chimeric murine/human monoclonal antibody that targets the extracellular domain and inhibits ligand-dependent activation of EGFR. The drug was approved by the FDA for treatment of colorectal cancer patients who failed previous irinotecan-based chemotherapy. In a multicenter phase 3 trial, 329 metastatic colorectal cancer patients who progressed on irinotecan-based therapy were randomized to receive cetuximab plus irinotecan versus cetuximab monotherapy [99]. The patients receiving cetuximab/irinotecan achieved a better response rate (22.9% vs 10.8%; $P = 0.007$) and median time to progression (4.1 vs 1.5 months; $P < 0.001$) compared with cetuximab monotherapy. Similar results were reported in two other smaller studies [100,101]. Cetuximab monotherapy may be an option for patients intolerant of irinotecan. The benefits of adding cetuximab to FOLFOX in a second-line setting and FOLFIRI in first-line settings are being investigated [102,103].

In these trials, only patients with EGFR-expressing tumors were eligible to receive cetuximab, leading to FDA approval for use in patients with EGFR-expressing tumors. This was based on preclinical evidence suggestive a predictive value of EGFR expression for cetuximab efficacy and clinical experience with drugs such as trastuzumab for HER2/neu–expressing breast cancers. However, further analysis showed that cetuximab benefit was not related to the degree of EGFR expression, and patients with EGFR-negative colorectal cancers also responded to cetuximab therapy [104,105]. The side effects of cetuximab were fairly well tolerated. About 75% of patients develop mild acneiform-like rash; about 12% of these were grade 3. About 3% of patients developed hypersensitivity infusional reactions. Secondary analysis seems to correlate rash development with cetuximab response, a phenomenon that is seen across the entire class of EGFR inhibitors [106].

Panitumumab is a fully humanized anti-EGFR antibody that has the advantage of a biweekly schedule and fewer hypersensitivity reactions. In a multicenter phase 3 trial, 463 patients with refractory metastatic EGFR-expressing colorectal cancer were randomized to receive panitumumab plus best supportive care or best supportive care alone [107]. Panitumumab was administered at 6 mg/kg every 2 weeks. Patients receiving panitumumab had significantly prolonged PFS (HR 0.54; $P < 0.0001$) compared with the best supportive care arm. Crossover was allowed in the trial, which may explain why there was no difference in overall survival. Skin rash, hypomagnesemia, paronychia, and diarrhea were the most common toxicities. The agent is approved by the FDA for use in patients with EGFR-expressing metastatic colorectal cancer refractory to fluoropyrimidine-, oxaliplatin-, and irinotecan-containing regimens [108]. The role of panitumumab in combination regimens is under investigation. The Panitumumab Advanced Colorectal Cancer Evaluation (PACCE) trial, which compared FOLFOX/bevacizumab with or without panitumumab, was discontinued early due to increased mortality in the panitumumab arm. This surprising result calls into question the benefit of adding panitumumab to conventional cytotoxic chemotherapy.

SUPPORTIVE CARE

Mucostomatitis and diarrhea are common toxicities of patients receiving 5-FU–containing chemotherapy, especially with the bolus schedule. Diarrhea is more pronounced with the addition of irinotecan. Such gastrointestinal toxicities can lead to pain, discomfort, poor caloric intake, and dehydration if not managed promptly and can affect the completion of therapy.

To decrease the risk of mucostomatitis during colorectal cancer therapy, patients should be advised to adopt a proper oral care regimen, such as the use of a soft toothbrush that is replaced regularly, and have regular dental follow-up [109]. Oral cryotherapy, such as holding ice chips or an iced slurry in the mouth, before, during, and for 30 minutes after bolus 5-FU therapy can lessen the severity of stomatitis. Appropriate patient-controlled analgesics, including the use of opioids, are important in alleviating associated pain. Chlorhexidine is not recommended to treat established oral mucositis.

Chemotherapy-induced diarrhea also causes significant morbidity. Diarrhea-related deaths attributed to irinotecan plus a high-dose 5-FU/LV regimen (IFL) further highlighted the need for vigilant monitoring and aggressive treatment of chemotherapy-induced diarrhea in colorectal cancer patients [110]. Patients should be evaluated regularly and details such as symptom duration and severity, associated symptoms, and hydration status should be noted. Risk factors for complications should be monitored, which include grade 2 or higher nausea and vomiting, fever, sepsis, neutropenia, bleeding, dehydration, abdominal pain or cramping, and deteriorating performance status.

Patients experiencing grade 1 or 2 diarrhea with no complicating features may be classified as "uncomplicated" and managed conservatively (Table 8-4) [110]. Patients with grade 3 or higher diarrhea, or with any of the risk factors described above, should be managed as "complicated" cases. Complicated cases should be managed aggressively with IV fluids and octreotide at a starting dose of 100 to 150 µg subcutaneously 3 times a day (or IV at 25–50 µg/h), with titration up to 500 µg/h until diarrhea is controlled. Antibiotics (*eg*, fluoroquinolones) should be instituted with

Table 8-4. Classification of Chemotherapy-Induced Diarrhea

Uncomplicated

NCI CTC grade 1–2 diarrhea

No complicating features

Complicated

NCI CTC grade 3 or 4 diarrhea

Grade 1 or 2 diarrhea with one or more of the following:

  Nausea/vomiting ($\geq$ grade 2)

  Cramping

  Deteriorating performance status

  Fever

  Sepsis

  Neutropenia

  Frank bleeding

  Dehydration

NCI CTC—National Cancer Institute's Common Toxicity Criteria.
(*Adapted from* Benson *et al.* [110].)

neutropenia or in cases with a high suspicion of infectious complication. For uncomplicated cases, initial management should include dietary modifications, such as avoiding lactose-containing products and high-osmolar dietary supplements. Loperamide should be started and titrated regularly until formed stool is produced (not to exceed 16 mg/d). If symptoms persist beyond 24 hours, oral antibiotics should be considered as prophylaxis for infection. If the diarrhea persists for more than 48 hours on high-dose loperamide, the loperamide should be replaced by second-line agents (octreotide, oral budesonide, or tincture of opium) and appropriate stool and blood work-up should be performed.

As discussed above, about 15% of patients receiving oxaliplatin-containing regimens develop neuropathy interfering with daily activities. It has been reported that supplementation with 1 g of calcium gluconate and 1 g of magnesium chloride before and after oxaliplatin infusion can prevent or ameliorate symptoms associated with acute neuropathy [79]. However, this strategy has been called into question after an unplanned interim analysis of the Combined Oxaliplatin Neurotoxicity Prevention trial (CONCEPT), a "stop-and-go" study, showed a reduced response rate (17% vs 33%) in patients who had received calcium and magnesium infusions compared with patients who did not (unpublished data, Sanofi-Aventis, Bridgewater, NJ) [111].

Xaliproden is an oral nonpeptide neurotrophic agent with promising neuroprotective properties against oxaliplatin-induced neuropathy [112]. In a randomized, double-blind, placebo-controlled trial, 640 patients with untreated metastatic colorectal cancer were randomized to receive FOLFOX4 with xaliproden or placebo. The xaliproden-receiving arm achieved a significant risk reduction of 39% in the development of grade 3/4 peripheral sensory neuropathy. Equally important, xaliproden administration did not affect FOLFOX4 antitumor efficacy. Other neuromodulatory agents reported to have some activity in the prevention and treatment of oxaliplatin-related neuropathy include glutamine, glutathione, carbamazepine, gabapentin, venlafaxine, amifostine, and α-lipoic acid, although none had proven efficacy in definitive randomized trials [113].

The common side effects of bevacizumab are hypertension and proteinuria. Less common but potentially catastrophic side effects include arterial (not venous) thrombosis, impaired wound healing/dehiscence, and gastrointestinal perforation. These issues require vigilant monitoring by oncologists [114]. Bevacizumab-related hypertension is generally grade 3 or lower and can be managed with standard oral antihypertensive medications. It is recommended that bevacizumab not be used in cases of uncontrolled hypertension. Blood pressure should be measured at least every 2 to 3 weeks during bevacizumab therapy, and more frequently with development or exacerbation of hypertension. Although angiotensin-converting enzyme inhibitors were suggested as more appropriate antihypertensives, standard guidelines for the selection of antihypertensive medications are appropriate. Bevacizumab-related proteinuria is usually grade 1 or 2; less than 2% of patients develop grade 3 proteinuria. Spot urine protein-to-creatinine ratio is the preferred way to monitor for proteinuria, although dipstick urine assays may be substituted when the former is not readily available. The testing should be performed every 2 to 8 weeks and dipstick values of 2+ or higher should be confirmed by urine protein-creatinine ratio or 24-hour urine collection. Bevacizumab therapy should be interrupted in patients with proteinuria greater than or equal to 2 g per 24 hours.

Arterial thrombosis is not an absolute contraindication to bevacizumab and oncologists should discuss with patients the risk-benefit ratio of continuing bevacizumab. Pooled analysis of five randomized trials reported an incidence of 5.5 events per 100 person-years in the bevacizumab group versus 3.4 in those without (odds ratio 1.8; 95% CI, 0.94–3.33; $P = 0.076$) [115]. Thirty-day mortality from arterial thrombosis in the bevacizumab group was 0.6% versus 0.4% [116]. Patients taking aspirin while receiving bevacizumab therapy have a slightly increased risk (1.3-fold) of grade 3 or greater bleeding than those without. Patients with metastatic colorectal cancer who started full-dose anticoagulation therapy after the development of thromboembolism during bevacizumab therapy did not seem to be at higher risk of serious bleeding [96]. Bevacizumab-associated delayed wound healing is statistically nonsignificant but clinically significant. The risk is not considered large enough to postpone emergent or urgent surgery, but elective surgery should be postponed for 6 to 8 weeks after the last bevacizumab dose [117]. Patients on bevacizumab should be monitored closely for gastrointestinal perforation and the agent should be discontinued permanently in patients who developed perforations [118].

Acneiform rash is the most frequent side effect of EGFR inhibitors such as cetuximab and panitumumab, occurring in more than 50% of patients receiving such therapy [119]. Fortunately, only a small portion (5%–18%) experience a grade 3 reaction and the rash seems to be dose dependent. Other cutaneous toxicities include xerosis, eczema, fissures, telangiectasia, hyperpigmentation, hair changes, and paronychia. The side effects can cause itching, pain, and cosmetic discomfort that may affect therapy compliance if inappropriately treated. General recommended measures include keeping the skin well hydrated and avoiding sun. For mild acneiform rash, oral or topical clindamycin, metronidazole, or erythromycin can be considered. Topical or systemic steroids and anticomedonal topicals should be avoided. Topical menthol cream or an oral antihistamine may be considered for itching. Oral tetracyclines (minocycline 100 mg/d, lymecycline 300 mg/d, or doxycycline 100 mg/d) can be considered for more severe rash. A delay in EGFR inhibitor therapy should be considered in grade 3 or higher rash, and grade 4 rash should be managed in specialized unit.

ANAL CANCER

Anal cancer is defined as cancer arising in the anal canal from the anorectal ring to the anal verge. The lining of the proximal anal canal is columnar epithelium, whereas the distal anal canal comprises stratified squamous epithelium. The dentate line is the transition zone between the proximal and distal anal canal.

Anal cancer is a rare tumor with increasing incidence, and is often associated with sexually transmitted disease [120]. Keratinizing squamous cell carcinomas are the predominant histology; typically they occur distal to the dentate line. Nonkeratinizing tumors (also referred to as transitional cell tumors) occur proximal to the dentate line. The natural history and prognosis of keratinizing and nonkeratinizing tumors is similar. Adenocarcinomas arising from anal glands or fistulae formation are rare, but appear to behave like rectal adenocarcinomas. Most of the tumor morbidity and mortality is

associated with uncontrolled locoregional disease. Regional lymph node involvement generally occurs prior to spread to distant organs, and the pattern of lymphatic drainage depends on the primary tumor location. For tumors below the dentate line, the arterial supply is provided by the inferior and middle rectal arteries, venous drainage is systemic through the inferior rectal vein, and lymphatic drainage occurs most commonly through the inguinal nodes. For tumors above the dentate line, the superior and middle rectal arteries provide the arterial supply, venous drainage is through the superior rectal vein to the portal vein, and lymphatic drainage predominantly flows to pelvic and periaortic nodes.

Anal cancer is best managed by a multimodality approach. Chemoradiation is the standard in managing localized anal cancer and surgery is reserved for chemoradiation failure, inability to tolerate radiation, or incontinence due to irreversible sphincter damage or vaginal fistula [121].

ETIOLOGY AND RISK FACTORS

In the United States, about 4650 cases of anal cancer occurred in 2007 [1]. The average age at diagnosis is above 60 years. The etiology for anal cancer is multifactorial. Human papillomavirus infection and chronic immunodeficient states, such as HIV/AIDS and solid organ transplant immunosuppression, are significant risk factors for anal cancer [122–124]. HIV-positive men are twice as likely to develop anal cancer compared with HIV-negative men [125]. Other risk factors include more than 10 sexual partners in a lifetime, receptive anal intercourse before the age of 30, age older than 50 years, and active tobacco use [120,126].

STAGING AND PROGNOSIS

Initial diagnostic evaluation includes anorectal digital examination and palpation of inguinal nodes as well as direct visualization with anoscopy and proctoscopy. Suspicious lesions and enlarged lymph nodes should be biopsied, but an inguinal node dissection is not useful. Concurrent benign anal pathology, such as fissures or fistulas, is common. A malignant process should be pursued if a clinically benign lesion fails to improve after a 2-week trial of appropriate analgesics and topical therapy. The lesion must be biopsied or evaluated under anesthesia. HIV testing is recommended and gynecologic examination, including cervical cancer screening, is suggested in female patients [127].

The prognosis depends on the tumor size and the likelihood of lymphatic spread, and is reflected in the AJCC TNM staging system (Table 8-5 and Table 8-6). In the TNM staging system, stage 0 comprises carcinoma in situ, stage I includes tumors up to 2 cm in diameter with negative nodes, and stage II includes tumors larger than 2 cm but not invading adjacent organ(s) (T2 to T3) with negative nodes [22]. Tumors of any size that extend into adjacent pelvic or peritoneal structures are classified as T4. Stage III

Table 8-5. TNM Staging Definition for Anal Cancer

Primary tumor (T)

TX: Primary tumor cannot be assessed

T0: No evidence of primary tumor

Tis: Carcinoma in situ (intraepithelial or invasion of the lamina propria)

T1: Tumor ≤ 2 cm in greatest dimension

T2: Tumor < 2 cm but not > 5 cm in greatest dimension

T3: Tumor > 5 cm in greatest dimension

T4: Tumor of any size invades adjacent organ(s) (eg, vagina, urethra, bladder)

Regional lymph nodes (N)

NX: Regional nodes cannot be assessed

N0: No regional lymph node metastasis

N1: Metastasis in perirectal lymph node(s)

N2: Metastasis in unilateral internal iliac and/or inguinal lymph node(s)

N3: Metastasis in perirectal and inguinal lymph nodes and/or bilateral internal iliac and/or inguinal lymph nodes

Distant metastasis (M)

MX: Distant metastasis cannot be assessed

M0: No distant metastasis

M1: Distant metastasis

Table 8-6. AJCC TNM Staging Groupings for Anal Cancer

AJCC stage	Staging groupings
Stage 0	Tis, N0, M0
Stage I	T1, N0, M0
Stage II	T2, N0, M0
	T3, N0, M0
Stage IIIA	T1, N1, M0
	T2, N1, M0
	T3, N1, M0
	T4, N0, M0
Stage IIIB	T4, N1, M0
	Any T, N2, M0
	Any T, N3, M0
Stage IV	Any T, any N, M1

AJCC—American Joint Committee on Cancer; TNM—tumor, node, metastasis.

describes the involvement of regional nodes or a T4 tumor, and is subdivided into IIIA and IIIB. Stage IV comprises metastatic disease. Tumors less than 2 cm in diameter are cured in 80% of cases, whereas less than 50% of patients with tumors that are 5 cm or larger are cured.

The 5-year survival rate is about 78% for patients with localized disease, 56% for those with regional disease, and 18% for those with distant disease [125]. The median survival for locally invasive tumors, distant metastatic disease, and recurrent cancers is in the range of 7 to 12 months.

THERAPY FOR PRIMARY DISEASE

Chemoradiation has superseded abdominoperineal resection in the management of anal cancers. However, very early-stage lesions (Tis and T1) are exceedingly rare (~ 10% of all anal cancers) and are often diagnosed in excisions of benign anal lesions [127]. These lesions can be treated with local excision with adequate margins, and reexcision if the margins of the initial specimen were inadequate. Local radiation with or without 5-FU–based chemotherapy can be considered as an alternate option [128].

Historically, abdominoperineal resection was the standard treatment for invasive anal carcinoma; however, it resulted in considerable morbidity with a permanent colostomy and achieved a moderate 5-year survival of 40% to 75% [129]. Over the past two decades, the use of combined-modality radiation plus chemotherapy with 5-FU and mitomycin C in anal cancers has resulted in a lower colostomy rate, longer DFS, and has shown an advantage in delaying salvage surgery for relapse [130,131]. In the randomized Radiation Therapy Oncology Group (RTOG_/ECOG phase 3 trial, patients who received radiation along with 5-FU and mitomycin C achieved a higher pathologic response (7.7% positive posttreatment biopsies vs 15% in the radiation/5-FU group), lower colostomy rate (9% vs 22%), and higher DFS (73% vs 51%) [132]. Patients with relapsed disease underwent salvage surgery, likely explaining the nonsignificant difference in 4-year survival between the two groups. There was a higher toxicity in patients receiving mitomycin C. Mitomycin C can be given at 10 mg/m^2/dose for two doses (on days 1 and 29), 5-FU at 1000 mg/m^2/d for 4 days every 4 weeks (on days 1–4 and 29–32), and pelvic radiation at the dose of 45 to 50 Gy. A radiation boost (9 Gy) was delivered with 5-FU and cisplatin (100 mg/m^2) if posttreatment biopsies showed residual disease.

The combined regimen of radiotherapy (45–59 Gy, starting on day 57) with cisplatin (75 mg/m^2 on days 1, 29, 57, and 85) and 5-FU (1000 mg/m^2 on days 1–4, 29–32, 57–60, and 85–88) offers an alternative to the mito-mycin C–containing regimen. However, the colostomy rate was higher in the randomized phase 3 RTOG 98-11 trial [133] and, thus, 5-FU/mitomycin remains the standard of care. Five-year survival was similar between the two arms, and the hematologic toxicity was significantly lower in the 5-FU/cisplatin/radiotherapy arm than 5-FU/mitomycin C/radiotherapy arm. Of note, 5-FU and cisplatin were given as induction followed by the addition of radiation.

The randomized trials evaluating primary chemoradiation in anal cancer have not included HIV-positive patients. The available data suggest that HIV-positive patients can be treated with the same regimen as non-HIV patients. However, patients with active HIV/AIDS with associated complications may not tolerate a full-dose regimen and require dose adjustment [134,135].

FOLLOW-UP AND SURVEILLANCE AFTER PRIMARY THERAPY

Patients should be reevaluated about 8 to 12 weeks after primary therapy for anal cancer. Biopsies should be obtained if there is suspicion of residual or progressive disease so that salvage therapy can be instituted early [136]. Due to postchemoradiation changes, patients may be followed for up to 16 weeks posttreatment prior to performing a tissue biopsy. Multiple biopsies under general anesthesia may be required for complete evaluation.

Once residual disease has been excluded, patients should be evaluated every 3 to 6 months for 5 years with digital rectal examination, anoscopy, inguinal palpation, and CT scan for recurrences [127]. It is important to note that the optimal strategy to detect anal cancer relapse has not been studied in randomized trials. About 10% to 17% of patients who underwent chemoradiation developed distant metastases, most commonly in the liver, while the rest developed locoregional recurrence [130,131]. As such, symptom-driven investigation may be the optimal approach, instead of routine imaging, to detect distant metastases.

THERAPY FOR ADVANCED DISEASE

There are a lack of definitive trials to guide therapy in metastatic anal cancer due to its rarity. Experiences from the management of other squamous cell carcinomas have been extrapolated to anal cancer and various agents have been studied, including platinum analogues, 5-FU, mitomycin C, porfiromycin, bleomycin, vincristine, vinblastine, doxorubicin, and methotrexate [121]. The current recommended combination is 5-FU with cisplatin. 5-FU can be administered as a 96-hour or 120-hour continuous infusion at 750 to 1000 mg/m^2/d together with a bolus infusion of cisplatin 100 mg/m^2 on day 1 or 2, repeated every 4 weeks [121,127].

5-FU AND LEUCOVORIN, BOLUS REGIMEN

CANDIDATES FOR TREATMENT
Patients with colorectal cancer

SPECIAL PRECAUTIONS
Pregnant and nursing patients

ALTERNATIVE THERAPY
Other 5-FU–based regimens

TOXICITIES
Myelosuppression, mucositis, diarrhea

DRUG INTERACTIONS
5-FU: allopurinol, cimetidine, folinic acid, methotrexate, thymidine

PATIENT INFORMATION
Patient should report diarrhea of > 4 bowel movements per day or less severe diarrhea lasting > 3 d, soreness in mouth, difficulty swallowing, rash, fever; patient should be informed of possible skin reactions. Use of oral cryotherapy may reduce severity of mucositis

DOSAGE AND SCHEDULING

Roswell Park regimen (weekly bolus):

Leucovorin 500 mg/m^2 IV over 2 h, repeated weekly

5-FU 500 mg/m^2 IV bolus 1 h after leucovorin, repeated weekly for 6 wk followed by 2 wk of rest

• Repeat cycle every 8 wk

• Adjuvant therapy: repeat for 4 cycles

Mayo regimen (daily bolus):

Leucovorin 20 mg/m^2 IV followed by

 5-FU 425 mg/m^2/d for 5 consecutive days

• Repeat cycle every 4 wk

• Adjuvant therapy: repeat for 6 cycles

(*From* Petrelli *et al.* [137] and Poon *et al.* [138].)

5-FU AND LEUCOVORIN, CONTINUOUS INFUSION REGIMEN

5-FU is a fluorine-substituted uracil that blocks the methylation reaction of deoxyuridylic acid to thymidylic acid, interfering with DNA synthesis. Direct incorporation of fluoropyrimidine nucleotide into DNA and RNA also occurs. With continuous daily infusion, the activity and toxicity profiles are different than those seen with bolus therapy. The mechanism responsible for these differences is not completely understood.

CANDIDATES FOR TREATMENT
Patients with colorectal cancer

SPECIAL PRECAUTIONS
Pregnant and nursing patients

ALTERNATIVE THERAPY
Other 5-FU–based regimens

TOXICITIES
Myelosuppression and mucositis are less severe, palmar-plantar erythro-dysesthesia (possibly dose-limiting); loss of appetite, diarrhea, abdominal cramps, difficulty with coordination, mouth sores, dry skin or nose, splitting fingernails, metallic taste, watery eyes, nausea, vomiting, temporary alopecia, leukopenia leading to anemia, photosensitivity, skin rash, hyperpigmentation, local tissue irritation if drug extravasation occurs

DRUG INTERACTIONS
5-FU: allopurinol, cimetidine, folinic acid, methotrexate, thymidine

NURSING INTERVENTIONS
Instruct patients in care of semipermanent IV access and ambulatory pump; assess patient performance and mental status; monitor weight, encourage adequate fluid, caloric, and protein intake; give antiemetics, antidiarrheals, and food supplements as necessary; monitor blood counts and liver function

PATIENT INFORMATION
Patient should report diarrhea of > 4 bowel movements per day or less severe diarrhea lasting > 3 d, soreness in mouth, difficulty swallowing, rash, fever; patient should be informed of possible skin reactions

DOSAGE AND SCHEDULING

de Gramont regimen:

Leucovorin 200 mg/m^2 over 2 h on d 1

5-FU 400 mg/m^2 bolus followed by 22-h infusion of
 5-FU 600 mg/m^2 on d 1 and 2

• Repeat cycle every 2 wk

(*From de* Gramont *et al.* [139].)

FOLFOX (INFUSIONAL 5-FU, LEUCOVORIN, AND OXALIPLATIN)

CANDIDATES FOR TREATMENT

Patients with metastatic colorectal cancer in first- and second-line settings; stage III colorectal cancer

SPECIAL PRECAUTIONS

Pregnant and nursing patients, impaired renal and bone marrow function, preexisting neuropathy. Oxaliplatin product information contains an FDA black box warning regarding anaphylactic-like reactions that may occur within minutes of administration. Epinephrine, corticosteroids, and antihistamines have been used to alleviate symptoms.

ALTERNATIVE THERAPY

Other 5-FU–based regimens

TOXICITIES

Oxaliplatin: peripheral neuropathy, cold dysesthesia, myelosuppression, colitis, increased liver enzymes, anaphylaxis

DRUG INTERACTIONS

Oxaliplatin: rotavirus vaccine, Bacillus Calmette-Guérin vaccine, live vaccines for mumps, measles, poliovirus, rubella, smallpox, typhoid, varicella virus, yellow fever virus

NURSING INTERVENTIONS

Oxaliplatin: Wash skin exposed to oxaliplatin immediately and thoroughly with soap and water and flush exposed mucous membranes thoroughly with water

PATIENT INFORMATION

Oxaliplatin: Avoid cold temperature during oxaliplatin infusion. Wear gloves. Report worsening pain and/or numbness, diarrhea, or problems with writing, buttoning, swallowing, and walking

DOSAGE AND SCHEDULING

FOLFOX4:

Oxaliplatin 85 mg/m^2 IV over 2 h on d 1

Leucovorin 200 mg/m^2 IV over 2 h on d 1 and 2

5-FU 400 mg/m^2 IV bolus after leucovorin, followed by 5-FU 600 mg/m^2 over 22-h continuous infusion

• Repeat cycle every 2 wk

• Adjuvant therapy: administer a total of 6 mo

Modified FOLFOX6:

Oxaliplatin 85 mg/m^2 IV over 2 h on d 1

Leucovorin 400 mg/m^2 IV over 2 h on d 1

5-FU 400 mg/m^2 IV bolus on d 1 after leucovorin, followed by 5-FU 1200 mg/m^2/d continuous infusion for 2 d (total 2400 mg/m^2 over 46–48 h)

• Repeat cycle every 2 wk

• Adjuvant therapy: administer a total of 6 mo

(*From* Goldberg *et al.* [87] and Tournigand *et al.* [89].)

IRINOTECAN

CANDIDATES FOR TREATMENT

Patients with colorectal cancer whose disease has progressed on 5-FU therapy

FDA BLACK BOX WARNING

Irinotecan can induce early and late forms of diarrhea that appear to be mediated by different mechanisms. Both forms may be severe. Early diarrhea (occurring during or shortly after irinotecan infusion) may be accompanied by cholinergic symptoms of rhinitis, increased salivation, miosis, lacrimation, diaphoresis, flushing, and intestinal hyperperistalsis that can cause abdominal cramping. Early diarrhea and other cholinergic symptoms may be prevented or ameliorated by atropine. Late diarrhea (generally occurring > 24 h after irinotecan administration) can be life-threatening because it may be prolonged and lead to dehydration, electrolyte imbalance, or sepsis. Late diarrhea should be treated promptly with loperamide.

SPECIAL PRECAUTIONS

Pregnant and nursing patients; impaired hepatic function. The active form of irinotecan, SN-38, is metabolized by the polymorphic enzyme UGT1A1. UGT1A1 activity is reduced in individuals with genetic polymorphisms that lead to reduced enzyme activity such as UGT1A1*28 polymorphism (~ 10% of the North American population is homozygous for the UGT1A1*28 allele). Patients with reduced UGT1A1 activity are at increased risk of experiencing neutropenia and/or diarrhea when treated with irinotecan. When coadministered with other agents or as a single agent, a reduction in the starting dose by at least one level of irinotecan should be considered for patients known to be homozygous for the UGT1A1*28 allele. However, the precise dose reduction in this patient population is not known and subsequent dose modifications should be considered based on individual patient tolerance to treatment.

ALTERNATIVE THERAPIES

Infusional 5-FU regimens in patients with prior bolus 5-FU regimens

TOXICITIES

Early diarrhea, delayed diarrhea, myelosuppression, nausea and vomiting

DRUG INTERACTIONS

Prior pelvic/abdominal irradiation increases risk of myelosuppression

NURSING INTERVENTIONS

Atropine can relieve early diarrhea; patients with diarrhea should be carefully monitored and given fluid and electrolyte replacement if they become dehydrated or antibiotic therapy if they develop ileus, fever, or severe neutropenia

PATIENT INFORMATION

Loperamide 4 mg orally at the first onset of delayed diarrhea, then 2 mg every 2 h until the patient is diarrhea free for at least 12 h. During the night, the patient can take 4 mg every 4 h

DOSAGE AND SCHEDULING

Irinotecan 300–350 mg/m^2 over 30–90 min on d 1

• Repeat cycle every 3 wk

or

Irinotecan 125 mg/m^2 over 30–90 min weekly for 4 wk followed by 2 wk of rest (total of 6 wk)

• Repeat cycle every 6 wk

(*From* Rougier *et al.* [140] and Saltz *et al.* [82].)

IFL (IRINOTECAN, BOLUS 5-FU, AND LEUCOVORIN)

CANDIDATES FOR TREATMENT

Patients with metastatic colorectal cancer who failed oxaliplatin-containing regimen or who were unable to tolerate FOLFIRI regimen

SPECIAL PRECAUTIONS

Pregnant and nursing patients; impaired hepatic function

ALTERNATIVE THERAPIES

Other 5-FU–based regimens

TOXICITIES

Early and late diarrhea, myelosuppression, nausea and vomiting, mucositis

DRUG INTERACTIONS

Prior pelvic/abdominal irradiation may increase risk of myelosuppression with irinotecan; **5-FU:** allopurinol, cimetidine, folinic acid, methotrexate, thymidine

PATIENT INFORMATION

Loperamide 4 mg orally at the first onset of delayed diarrhea, then 2 mg every 2 h until the patient is diarrhea free for at least 12 h

DOSAGE AND SCHEDULING

Irinotecan 125 mg/m^2 IV over 90 min

Leucovorin 20 mg/m^2 IV bolus

5-FU 500 mg/m^2 IV bolus repeated weekly for 4 wk followed by 2 wk of rest (total of 6 wk)

FOLFIRI (INFUSIONAL 5-FU, LEUCOVORIN, AND IRINOTECAN)

CANDIDATES FOR TREATMENT

Patients with new diagnosis of metastatic colorectal cancer or who failed oxaliplatin-containing regimen

SPECIAL PRECAUTIONS

Pregnant and nursing patients; impaired hepatic function; also refer to the irinotecan FDA black box warning regarding diarrhea

ALTERNATIVE THERAPIES

Other 5-FU–based regimens

TOXICITIES

Early and late diarrhea, myelosuppression, nausea and vomiting, mucositis

DRUG INTERACTIONS

Prior pelvic/abdominal irradiation may increase risk of myelosuppression with irinotecan; **5-FU:** allopurinol, cimetidine, folinic acid, methotrexate, thymidine

PATIENT INFORMATION

Patient should report diarrhea of > 4 bowel movements per day or less severe diarrhea lasting > 3 d, soreness in mouth, difficulty swallowing, rash, and fever; patient should be informed of possible skin reactions. Loperamide 4 mg orally at the first onset of delayed diarrhea, then 2 mg every 2 h until the patient is diarrhea free for at least 12 h

DOSAGE AND SCHEDULING

Irinotecan 180 mg/m^2 IV over 90 min on d 1

Leucovorin 400 mg/m^2 IV over 2 h during irinotecan infusion

5-FU 400 mg/m^2 bolus after leucovorin followed by 5-FU 2400–3000 mg/m^2 over 46-h continuous infusion

• Repeat cycle every 3 wk

• Adjuvant therapy: not for use in adjuvant therapy*

or

Irinotecan 180 mg/m^2 IV over 30–120 min on d 1

Leucovorin 200 mg/m^2 IV infusion during irinotecan infusion on d 1 and 2

5-FU 400 mg/m^2 IV bolus after leucovorin followed by 5-FU 600 mg/m^2 over 22-h continuous infusion

• Repeat cycle every 2 wk

• Adjuvant therapy: not for use in adjuvant therapy*

*FOLFIRI should not be used in adjuvant therapy due to lack of efficacy in randomized trials [48,49].)
(*From* Andre *et al.* [141] and Douillard *et al.* [83].)

CETUXIMAB WITH OR WITHOUT IRINOTECAN

CANDIDATES FOR TREATMENT

Patients with metastatic EGFR-expressing colorectal cancer who failed 5-FU– and irinotecan-containing regimens

FDA BLACK BOX WARNING

Severe infusion reactions occurred with administration of cetuximab in ~ 3% of patients, rarely with fatal outcome (< 1 in 1000). About 90% of severe infusion reactions were associated with first cetuximab infusion. Such reactions are characterized by rapid onset of airway obstruction (bronchospasm, stridor, hoarseness), urticaria, and hypotension. Severe infusion reactions require immediate interruption of cetuximab infusion and permanent discontinuation from further treatment.

SPECIAL PRECAUTIONS

Pregnant and nursing patients

ALTERNATIVE THERAPIES

Single-agent EGFR inhibitors

TOXICITIES

Rash, acne, dry skin, diarrhea, dyspnea, infusion reaction

NURSING INTERVENTIONS

Use antihistamine premedication before each infusion or at least during the first infusion. Monitor for anaphylactic reactions

PATIENT INFORMATION

Avoid sun and tanning beds; use sunscreen. Patients should report diarrhea of > 4 bowel movements per day or less severe diarrhea lasting > 3 d. Report worsening rash, dyspnea, and eye problems

DOSAGE AND SCHEDULING

Single-agent regimen:

Cetuximab 400 mg/m^2 during first infusion, then 250 mg/m^2 weekly

• Repeat cycle every 6 wk

Combination regimen:

Cetuximab 400 mg/m^2 during first infusion, then 250 mg/m^2 weekly

with

Irinotecan 300–350 mg/m^2 IV every 3 wk

or

Irinotecan 125 mg/m^2 weekly for 4 wk followed by 2 wk of rest

or

Irinotecan 180 mg/m^2 every 2 wk

• Repeat cycle every 6 wk

(*From* Cunningham *et al.* [99].)

PANITUMUMAB

CANDIDATES FOR TREATMENT

Patients with refractory metastatic EGFR-expressing colorectal cancer

FDA BLACK BOX WARNING

Dermatologic toxicities related to panitumumab blockade of EGF binding and subsequent inhibition of EGFR-mediated signaling pathways were reported in 89% of patients and were severe in 12% receiving panitumumab monotherapy. The clinical manifestations included, but were not limited to, dermatitis acneiform, pruritus, erythema, rash, skin exfoliation, paronychia, dry skin, and skin fissures. Severe dermatologic toxicities were complicated by infection including sepsis, septic death, and abscesses requiring incisions and drainage. Withhold or discontinue panitumumab and monitor for inflammatory or infection sequelae in these patients. Severe infusion reactions also occurred with panitumumab administration (~ 1%). Such reactions were identified by reports of anaphylactic reaction, bronchospasm, fever, chills, and hypotension. Stop infusion if a severe reaction occurs; depending on the severity and/or persistence of the reaction, permanently discontinue panitumumab.

SPECIAL PRECAUTIONS

Pregnant and nursing patients; impaired hepatic function

ALTERNATIVE THERAPIES

Supportive care

TOXICITIES

Cutaneous toxicities, infusion reaction, diarrhea, hypomagnesemia, conjunctivitis, eye irritation

NURSING INTERVENTIONS

Monitor for infusion reactions, including fever, chills, rash, hypotension, and dyspnea

PATIENT INFORMATION

Avoid sun and tanning beds; use sunscreen. Patients should report diarrhea of > 4 bowel movements per day or less severe diarrhea lasting > 3 d. Report worsening rash, dyspnea, and eye problems

DOSAGE AND SCHEDULING

Panitumumab 6 mg/kg IV over 60 min every 2 wk

(*From* Van Cutsem *et al.* [107].)

BEVACIZUMAB

CANDIDATES FOR TREATMENT

Patients with metastatic colorectal cancer in first- or second-line settings

FDA BLACK BOX WARNING

Bevacizumab administration can result in GI perforation development, in some instances resulting in fatality. GI perforation, sometimes associated with intra-abdominal abscess, occurred throughout bevacizumab treatment (*ie*, was not correlated with duration of exposure). The incidence of GI perforation was 2.4%. The typical presentation was reported as abdominal pain associated with symptoms such as constipation and vomiting. GI perforation should be included in the differential diagnosis of patients presenting with abdominal pain on bevacizumab. Permanently discontinue therapy in patients with GI perforation. Bevacizumab administration can result in development of wound dehiscence, in some instances resulting in fatality. Permanently discontinue therapy in patients with wound dehiscence requiring medical intervention. The appropriate interval between termination of bevacizumab and subsequent elective surgery required to avoid risk of impaired wound healing/wound dehiscence has not been determined.

SPECIAL PRECAUTIONS

Pregnant and nursing patients. Bevacizumab may delay wound healing and increase bleeding risk within 28 days of major surgery

ALTERNATIVE THERAPIES

Other 5-FU–based regimens

TOXICITIES

Proteinuria, hypertension, arterial thromboembolism, impaired wound healing, wound dehiscence, hemorrhage, gastrointestinal perforation, increased bleeding risk, hypersensitivity reaction, reversible posterior leukoencephalopathy syndrome

NURSING INTERVENTIONS

Monitor blood pressure and urinary protein

PATIENT INFORMATION

Avoid sun and tanning beds; use sunscreen. Patients should report diarrhea of > 4 bowel movements per day or less severe diarrhea lasting > 3 d. Report worsening rash, dyspnea, and eye problems

DOSAGE AND SCHEDULING

With 5-FU–containing regimens:

With 5-FU/LV, FOLFOX, FLOX: Bevacizumab 5 mg/kg IV every 2 wk

With CapeOx: Bevacizumab 7.5 mg/kg IV every 3 wk

(*From* Kabbinavar *et al.* [69], Hurwitz *et al.* [96], and Giantonio *et al.* [142].)

MITOMYCIN C, 5-FU, AND RADIOTHERAPY

CANDIDATES FOR TREATMENT
Patients with primary anal cancer

SPECIAL PRECAUTIONS
Immunocompromised patients; pregnant and nursing patients; avoid in patients with preexisting cytopenias

ALTERNATIVE THERAPIES
Radiation therapy alone or radiation with 5-FU plus cisplatin

TOXICITIES
Diarrhea, cutaneous toxicities, myelosuppression

DRUG INTERACTIONS
5-FU: allopurinol, cimetidine, folinic acid, methotrexate, thymidine

NURSING INTERVENTIONS
Mitomycin is a vesicant and should be given through a free-flowing IV

PATIENT INFORMATION
Severe local skin reactions may occur

DOSAGE AND SCHEDULING

Primary therapy:

5-FU 1000 mg/m^2/24 h continuous for 96 h (d 1–4 and 29–32)

Mitomycin C 10 mg/m^2 IV on d 1 and 28 (maximum 20 mg per cycle)

Radiotherapy 45 Gy delivered 5 times per wk for 5 wk

Salvage therapy:

5-FU 1000 mg/m^2/24 h continuous for 96 h

Cisplatin 100 mg/m^2 IV over 6 h on d 2

Radiotherapy 9 Gy delivered from d 1–5

(*From* Flam *et al.* [132].)

CISPLATIN, 5-FU, AND RADIOTHERAPY

CANDIDATES FOR TREATMENT
Patients with primary anal cancer

SPECIAL PRECAUTIONS
Immunocompromised patients; pregnant and nursing patients; avoid in patients with preexisting cytopenias, hearing impairment, renal dysfunction, and neuropathy

ALTERNATIVE THERAPIES
Radiation therapy alone or with 5-FU plus mitomycin C

TOXICITIES
Diarrhea, cutaneous toxicities, myelosuppression, renal dysfunction, neuropathy, ototoxicity

DRUG INTERACTIONS
5-FU: allopurinol, cimetidine, folinic acid, methotrexate, thymidine

PATIENT INFORMATION
Severe local skin reactions, hearing problems, and numbness may occur

DOSAGE AND SCHEDULING

5-FU 1000 mg/m^2/24 h continuous for 96 h
 (d 1–4, 29–32, 57–60, and 85–88)

Cisplatin 75 mg/m^2 on d 1, 29, 57, and 85

Radiotherapy 45–59 Gy starting on d 57

(*From* Ajani *et al.* [133].)

The information here is provided as guidance only. Prescribers should always consult the manufacturer's current prescribing information.

REFERENCES

1. American Cancer Society: *Cancer Facts & Figures 2007*. Atlanta: American Cancer Society; 2007.

2. Weitz J, Koch M, Debus J, *et al.*: Colorectal cancer. *Lancet* 2005, 365:153–165.

3. Surveillance, Epidemiology, and End Results (SEER) Program: SEER*Stat Database: Incidence – SEER 17 Regs Limited-Use, Nov 2006 Sub (2000–2004). National Cancer Institute, DCCPS, Surveillance Research Program, Cancer Statistics Branch. http:www.seer.cancer.gov. Released April 2007, based on the November 2006 submission.

4. Lynch HT, de la Chapelle A: Hereditary colorectal cancer. *N Engl J Med* 2003, 348:919–932.

5. Kinzler KW, Vogelstein B: Lessons from hereditary colorectal cancer. *Cell* 1996, 87:159–170.

6. Winawer SJ, Zauber AG, Ho MN, *et al.*: Prevention of colorectal cancer by colonoscopic polypectomy. The National Polyp Study Workgroup. *N Engl J Med* 1993, 329:1977–1981.

7. Midgley R, Kerr D: Colorectal cancer. *Lancet* 1999, 353:391–399.

8. Aaltonen LA: Hereditary intestinal cancer. *Semin Cancer Biol* 2000, 10:289–298.

9. Kennedy EP, Hamilton SR: Genetics of colorectal cancer. *Semin Surg Oncol* 1998, 15:126–130.

10. Liaw D, Marsh DJ, Li J, *et al.*: Germline mutations of the PTEN gene in Cowden disease, an inherited breast and thyroid cancer syndrome. *Nat Genet* 1997, 16:64–67.

11. Marsh DJ, Coulon V, Lunetta KL, *et al.*: Mutation spectrum and genotype-phenotype analyses in Cowden disease and Bannayan-Zonana syndrome, two hamartoma syndromes with germline PTEN mutation. *Hum Mol Genet* 1998, 7:507–515.

12. Hemminki A, Markie D, Tomlinson I, *et al.*: A serine/threonine kinase gene defective in Peutz-Jeghers syndrome. *Nature* 1998, 391:184–187.

13. Howe JR, Roth S, Ringold JC, *et al.*: Mutations in the SMAD4/DPC4 gene in juvenile polyposis. *Science* 1998, 280:1086–1088.

14. Risques RA, Rabinovitch PS, Brentnall TA: Cancer surveillance in inflammatory bowel disease: new molecular approaches. *Curr Opin Gastroenterol* 2006, 22:382–390.

15. Janne PA, Mayer RJ: Chemoprevention of colorectal cancer. *N Engl J Med* 2000, 342:1960–1968.

16. Rostom A, Dube C, Lewin G, *et al.*: Nonsteroidal anti-inflammatory drugs and cyclooxygenase-2 inhibitors for primary prevention of colorectal cancer: a systematic review prepared for the U.S. Preventive Services Task Force. *Ann Intern Med* 2007, 146:376–389.

17. Winawer S, Fletcher R, Rex D, *et al.*: Colorectal cancer screening and surveillance: clinical guidelines and rationale—update based on new evidence. *Gastroenterology* 2003, 124:544–560.

18. Mandel JS, Bond JH, Church TR, *et al.*: Reducing mortality from colorectal cancer by screening for fecal occult blood. Minnesota Colon Cancer Control study. *N Engl J Med* 1993, 328:1365–1371.

19. Hardcastle JD, Chamberlain JO, Robinson MH, *et al.*: Randomised controlled trial of faecal-occult-blood screening for colorectal cancer. *Lancet* 1996, 348:1472–1477.

20. Kronborg O, Fenger C, Olsen J, *et al.*: Randomised study of screening for colorectal cancer with faecal-occult-blood test. *Lancet* 1996, 348:1467–1471.

21. Mandel JS, Church TR, Ederer F, Bond JH: Colorectal cancer mortality: effectiveness of biennial screening for fecal occult blood. *J Natl Cancer Inst* 1999, 91:434–437.

22. American Joint Committee on Cancer: *AJCC Cancer Staging Manual*. New York, NY: Springer; 2002.

23. Nelson H, Petrelli N, Carlin A, *et al.*: Guidelines 2000 for colon and rectal cancer surgery. *J Natl Cancer Inst* 2001, 93:583–596.

24. Compton CC, Greene FL: The staging of colorectal cancer: 2004 and beyond. *CA Cancer J Clin* 2004, 54:295–308.

25. O'Connell JB, Maggard MA, Ko CY: Colon cancer survival rates with the new American Joint Committee on Cancer sixth edition staging. *J Natl Cancer Inst* 2004, 96:1420–1425.

26. Adam R: Chemotherapy and surgery: new perspectives on the treatment of unresectable liver metastases. *Ann Oncol* 2003, 14(Suppl 2):13–16.

27. Andre T, Boni C, Mounedji-Boudiaf L, *et al.*: Oxaliplatin, fluorouracil, and leucovorin as adjuvant treatment for colon cancer. *N Engl J Med* 2004, 350:2343–2351.

28. Chau I, Norman AR, Cunningham D, *et al.*: A randomised comparison between 6 months of bolus fluorouracil/leucovorin and 12 weeks of protracted venous infusion fluorouracil as adjuvant treatment in colorectal cancer. *Ann Oncol* 2005, 16:549–557.

29. Poplin EA, Benedetti JK, Estes NC, *et al.*: Phase III Southwest Oncology Group 9415/Intergroup 0153 randomized trial of fluorouracil, leucovorin, and levamisole versus fluorouracil continuous infusion and levamisole for adjuvant treatment of stage III and high-risk stage II colon cancer. *J Clin Oncol* 2005, 23:1819–1825.

30. Wolmark N, Wieand HS, Kuebler JP, *et al.*: A phase III trial comparing FULV to FULV + oxaliplatin in stage II or III carcinoma of the colon: results of NSABP Protocol C-07 [ASCO abstract]. *J Clin Oncol* 2005, 23(16S):3500.

31. de Gramont A, Boni C, Navarro M, *et al.*: Oxaliplatin/5FU/LV in the adjuvant treatment of stage II and stage III colon cancer: efficacy results with a median follow-up of 4 years [ASCO abstract]. *J Clin Oncol* 2005, 23(16S):3501.

32. Figueredo A, Charette ML, Maroun J, *et al.*: Adjuvant therapy for stage II colon cancer: a systematic review from the Cancer Care Ontario Program in evidence-based care's gastrointestinal cancer disease site group. *J Clin Oncol* 2004, 22:3395–3407.

33. MacFarlane JK, Ryall RD, Heald RJ: Mesorectal excision for rectal cancer. *Lancet* 1993, 341:457–460.

34. Heald RJ: Total mesorectal excision is optimal surgery for rectal cancer: a Scandinavian consensus. *Br J Surg* 1995, 82:1297–1299.

35. Enker WE, Thaler HT, Cranor ML, Polyak T: Total mesorectal excision in the operative treatment of carcinoma of the rectum. *J Am Coll Surg* 1995, 181:335–346.

36. Prolongation of the disease-free interval in surgically treated rectal carcinoma. Gastrointestinal Tumor Study Group. *N Engl J Med* 1985, 312:1465–1472.

37. Kapiteijn E, Marijnen CA, Nagtegaal ID, *et al.*: Preoperative radiotherapy combined with total mesorectal excision for resectable rectal cancer. *N Engl J Med* 2001, 345:638–646.

38. Sauer R, Becker H, Hohenberger W, *et al.*: Preoperative versus postoperative chemoradiotherapy for rectal cancer. *N Engl J Med* 2004, 351:1731–1740.

39. Jayne DG, Guillou PJ, Thorpe H, *et al.*: Randomized trial of laparoscopic-assisted resection of colorectal carcinoma: 3-year results of the UK MRC CLASICC Trial Group. *J Clin Oncol* 2007, 25:3061–3068.

40. Benson AB III, Schrag D, Somerfield MR, *et al.*: American Society of Clinical Oncology recommendations on adjuvant chemotherapy for stage II colon cancer. *J Clin Oncol* 2004, 22:3408–3419.

41. National Comprehensive Cancer Network, Inc.: Colon cancer. NCCN Clinical Practice Guidelines in Oncology (Version 2.2007). Available at http://www.nccn.org. Accessed August 2, 2007.

42. de Gramont A, Boni C, Navarro M, *et al.*: Oxaliplatin/5FU/LV in adjuvant colon cancer: updated efficacy results of the MOSAIC trial, including survival, with a median follow-up of six years [ASCO abstract]. *J Clin Oncol* 2007, 25(18S):4007.

43. Kuebler JP, Wieand HS, O'Connell MJ, *et al.*: Oxaliplatin combined with weekly bolus fluorouracil and leucovorin as surgical adjuvant chemotherapy for stage II and III colon cancer: results from NSABP C-07. *J Clin Oncol* 2007, 25:2198–2204.

44. Land SR, Kopec JA, Cecchini RS, *et al.*: Neurotoxicity from oxaliplatin combined with weekly bolus fluorouracil and leucovorin as surgical adjuvant chemotherapy for stage II and III colon cancer: NSABP C-07. *J Clin Oncol* 2007, 25:2205–2211.

45. Twelves C, Wong A, Nowacki MP, *et al.*: Capecitabine as adjuvant treatment for stage III colon cancer. *N Engl J Med* 2005, 352:2696–2704.

46. Schmoll HJ, Cartwright T, Tabernero J, *et al.*: Phase III trial of capecitabine plus oxaliplatin as adjuvant therapy for stage III colon cancer: a planned safety analysis in 1,864 patients. *J Clin Oncol* 2007, 25:102–109.

47. Saltz LB, Niedzwiecki D, Hollis D, *et al.*: Irinotecan plus fluorouracil/leucovorin (IFL) versus fluorouracil/leucovorin alone (FL) in stage III colon cancer (Intergroup trial CALGB C89803) [ASCO abstract]. *J Clin Oncol* 2004, 22(14S):3500.

48. Van Cutsem E, Labianca R, Hossfeld D, *et al.*: Randomized phase III trial comparing infused irinotecan/5-fluorouracil (5-FU)/folinic acid (IF) versus 5-FU/FA (F) in stage III colon cancer patients (pts) (PETACC 3) [ASCO abstract]. *J Clin Oncol* 2005, 23(16S):8.

49. Ychou M, Raoul JL, Douillard JY, *et al.*: A phase III randomized trial of LV5FU2+CPT-11 vs. LV5FU2 alone in adjuvant high risk colon cancer (FNCLCC Accord02/FFCD9802) [ASCO abstract]. *J Clin Oncol* 2005, 23(16S):3502.

50. Bartram C, Brown G: Endorectal ultrasound and magnetic resonance imaging in rectal cancer staging. *Gastroenterol Clin North Am* 2002, 31:827–839.

51. Willett CG, Compton CC, Shellito PC, Efird JT: Selection factors for local excision or abdominoperineal resection of early stage rectal cancer. *Cancer* 1994, 73:2716–2720.

52. Sengupta S, Tjandra JJ: Local excision of rectal cancer: what is the evidence? *Dis Colon Rectum* 2001, 44:1345–1361.

53. Capecitabine, Oxaliplatin, and Radiation Therapy in Treating Patients Who Are Undergoing Surgery for Stage I Rectal Cancer. ClinicalTrials.gov. Available at http://www.clinicaltrials.gov/ct/show/NCT00114231?order=1. Accessed April 23, 2008.

54. Cecil TD, Sexton R, Moran BJ, Heald RJ: Total mesorectal excision results in low local recurrence rates in lymph node-positive rectal cancer. *Dis Colon Rectum* 2004, 47:1145–1149; discussion 1149–1150.

55. National Comprehensive Cancer Network, Inc.: Rectal cancer. NCCN Clinical Practice Guidelines in Oncology (Version 2.2007). Available at http://www.nccn.org. Accessed August 2, 2007.

56. Wolmark N, Wieand HS, Hyams DM, *et al.*: Randomized trial of postoperative adjuvant chemotherapy with or without radiotherapy for carcinoma of the rectum: National Surgical Adjuvant Breast and Bowel Project Protocol R-02. *J Natl Cancer Inst* 2000, 92:388–396.

57. O'Connell MJ, Martenson JA, Wieand HS, *et al.*: Improving adjuvant therapy for rectal cancer by combining protracted-infusion fluorouracil with radiation therapy after curative surgery. *N Engl J Med* 1994, 331:502–507.

58. Wagman R, Minsky BD, Cohen AM, *et al.*: Sphincter preservation in rectal cancer with preoperative radiation therapy and coloanal anastomosis: long term follow-up. *Int J Radiat Oncol Biol Phys* 1998, 42:51–57.

59. Bosset JF, Calais G, Daban A, *et al.*: Preoperative chemoradiotherapy versus preoperative radiotherapy in rectal cancer patients: assessment of acute toxicity and treatment compliance. Report of the 22921 randomised trial conducted by the EORTC Radiotherapy Group. *Eur J Cancer* 2004, 40:219–224.

60. Desch CE, Benson AB III, Somerfield MR, *et al.*: Colorectal cancer surveillance: 2005 update of an American Society of Clinical Oncology practice guideline. *J Clin Oncol* 2005, 23:8512–8519.

61. Adam R, Delvart V, Pascal G, *et al.*: Rescue surgery for unresectable colorectal liver metastases downstaged by chemotherapy: a model to predict long-term survival. *Ann Surg* 2004, 240:644–657.

62. Palliative chemotherapy for advanced or metastatic colorectal cancer. Colorectal Meta-analysis Collaboration. *Cochrane Database Syst Rev* 2000, (2):CD001545.

63. Meyerhardt JA, Mayer RJ: Systemic therapy for colorectal cancer. *N Engl J Med* 2005, 352:476–487.

64. Kohne CH, Wils J, Lorenz M, *et al.*: Randomized phase III study of high-dose fluorouracil given as a weekly 24-hour infusion with or without leucovorin versus bolus fluorouracil plus leucovorin in advanced colorectal cancer: European Organization of Research and Treatment of Cancer Gastrointestinal Group Study 40952. *J Clin Oncol* 2003, 21:3721–3728.

65. Efficacy of intravenous continuous infusion of fluorouracil compared with bolus administration in advanced colorectal cancer. Meta-analysis Group In Cancer. *J Clin Oncol* 1998, 16:301–308.

66. Meropol NJ: Turning point for colorectal cancer clinical trials. *J Clin Oncol* 2006, 24:3322–3324.

67. Cassidy J, Clarke S, Diaz-Rubio E, *et al.*: XELOX compared to FOLFOX4: survival and response results from XELOX-1/NO16966, a randomized phase III trial of first-line treatment for patients with metastatic colorectal cancer (MCRC) [ASCO abstract]. *J Clin Oncol* 2007, 25(18S):4030.

68. Saltz L, Clarke S, Diaz-Rubio E, *et al.*: Bevacizumab (Bev) in combination with XELOX or FOLFOX4: updated efficacy results from XELOX-1/NO16966, a randomized phase III trial in first-line metastatic colorectal cancer [ASCO abstract]. *J Clin Oncol* 2007, 25(18S):4028.

69. Kabbinavar F, Hurwitz HI, Fehrenbacher L, *et al.*: Phase II, randomized trial comparing bevacizumab plus fluorouracil (FU)/leucovorin (LV) with FU/LV alone in patients with metastatic colorectal cancer. *J Clin Oncol* 2003, 21:60–65.

70. Pentheroudakis G, Twelves C: The rational development of capecitabine from the laboratory to the clinic. *Anticancer Res* 2002, 22:3589–3596.

71. Van Cutsem E, Twelves C, Cassidy J, *et al.*: Oral capecitabine compared with intravenous fluorouracil plus leucovorin in patients with metastatic colorectal cancer: results of a large phase III study. *J Clin Oncol* 2001, 19:4097–4106.

72. Hoff PM, Ansari R, Batist G, *et al.*: Comparison of oral capecitabine versus intravenous fluorouracil plus leucovorin as first-line treatment in 605 patients with metastatic colorectal cancer: results of a randomized phase III study. *J Clin Oncol* 2001, 19:2282–2292.

73. Van Cutsem E, Hoff PM, Harper P, *et al.*: Oral capecitabine vs intravenous 5-fluorouracil and leucovorin: integrated efficacy data and novel analyses from two large, randomised, phase III trials. *Br J Cancer* 2004, 90:1190–1197.

74. Camidge R, Reigner B, Cassidy J, *et al.*: Significant effect of capecitabine on the pharmacokinetics and pharmacodynamics of warfarin in patients with cancer. *J Clin Oncol* 2005, 23:4719–4725.

75. Raymond E, Faivre S, Chaney S, *et al.*: Cellular and molecular pharmacology of oxaliplatin. *Mol Cancer Ther* 2002, 1:227–235.

76. Giacchetti S, Perpoint B, Zidani R, *et al.*: Phase III multicenter randomized trial of oxaliplatin added to chronomodulated fluorouracil-leucovorin as first-line treatment of metastatic colorectal cancer. *J Clin Oncol* 2000, 18:136–147.

77. de Gramont A, Figer A, Seymour M, *et al.*: Leucovorin and fluorouracil with or without oxaliplatin as first-line treatment in advanced colorectal cancer. *J Clin Oncol* 2000, 18:2938–2947.

78. Rothenberg ML, Oza AM, Bigelow RH, *et al.*: Superiority of oxaliplatin and fluorouracil-leucovorin compared with either therapy alone in patients with progressive colorectal cancer after irinotecan and fluorouracil-leucovorin: interim results of a phase III trial. *J Clin Oncol* 2003, 21:2059–2069.

79. Grothey A: Oxaliplatin-safety profile: neurotoxicity. *Semin Oncol* 2003, 30(Suppl 15):5–13.

80. Tournigand C, Cervantes A, Figer A, *et al.*: OPTIMOX1: a randomized study of FOLFOX4 or FOLFOX7 with oxaliplatin in a stop-and-go fashion in advanced colorectal cancer: a GERCOR study. *J Clin Oncol* 2006, 24:394–400.

81. Pizzolato JF, Saltz LB: The camptothecins. *Lancet* 2003, 361:2235–2242.

82. Saltz LB, Cox JV, Blanke C, *et al.*: Irinotecan plus fluorouracil and leucovorin for metastatic colorectal cancer. Irinotecan Study Group. *N Engl J Med* 2000, 343:905–914.

83. Douillard JY, Cunningham D, Roth AD, *et al.*: Irinotecan combined with fluorouracil compared with fluorouracil alone as first-line treatment for metastatic colorectal cancer: a multicentre randomised trial. *Lancet* 2000, 355:1041–1047.

84. Gupta E, Lestingi TM, Mick R, *et al.*: Metabolic fate of irinotecan in humans: correlation of glucuronidation with diarrhea. *Cancer Res* 1994, 54:3723–3725.

85. Gupta E, Wang X, Ramirez J, Ratain MJ: Modulation of glucuronidation of SN-38, the active metabolite of irinotecan, by valproic acid and phenobarbital. *Cancer Chemother Pharmacol* 1997, 39:440–444.

86. Innocenti F, Undevia SD, Iyer L, *et al.*: Genetic variants in the UDP-glucuronosyltransferase 1A1 gene predict the risk of severe neutropenia of irinotecan. *J Clin Oncol* 2004, 22:1382–1388.

87. Goldberg RM, Sargent DJ, Morton RF, *et al.*: A randomized controlled trial of fluorouracil plus leucovorin, irinotecan, and oxaliplatin combinations in patients with previously untreated metastatic colorectal cancer. *J Clin Oncol* 2004, 22:23–30.

88. Colucci G, Gebbia V, Paoletti G, *et al.*: Phase III randomized trial of FOLFIRI versus FOLFOX4 in the treatment of advanced colorectal cancer: a multicenter study of the Gruppo Oncologico Dell'Italia Meridionale. *J Clin Oncol* 2005, 23:4866–4875.

89. Tournigand C, Andre T, Achille E, *et al.*: FOLFIRI followed by FOLFOX6 or the reverse sequence in advanced colorectal cancer: a randomized GERCOR study. *J Clin Oncol* 2004, 22:229–237.

90. Grothey A, Sargent D, Goldberg RM, Schmoll HJ: Survival of patients with advanced colorectal cancer improves with the availability of fluorouracil-leucovorin, irinotecan, and oxaliplatin in the course of treatment. *J Clin Oncol* 2004, 22:1209–1214.

91. Folkman J: Seminars in medicine of the Beth Israel Hospital, Boston. Clinical applications of research on angiogenesis. *N Engl J Med* 1995, 333:1757–1763.

92. Folkman J: Tumor angiogenesis: therapeutic implications. *N Engl J Med* 1971, 285:1182–1186.

93. Karkkainen MJ, Petrova TV: Vascular endothelial growth factor receptors in the regulation of angiogenesis and lymphangiogenesis. *Oncogene* 2000, 19:5598–5605.

94. Cross MJ, Dixelius J, Matsumoto T, Claesson-Welsh L: VEGF-receptor signal transduction. *Trends Biochem Sci* 2003, 28:488–494.

95. Ferrara N, Hillan KJ, Novotny W: Bevacizumab (Avastin), a humanized anti-VEGF monoclonal antibody for cancer therapy. *Biochem Biophys Res Commun* 2005, 333:328–335.

96. Hurwitz H, Fehrenbacher L, Novotny W, *et al.*: Bevacizumab plus irinotecan, fluorouracil, and leucovorin for metastatic colorectal cancer. *N Engl J Med* 2004, 350:2335–2342.

97. Giantonio BJ, Catalano PJ, Meropol NJ, *et al.*: Bevacizumab in combination with oxaliplatin, fluorouracil, and leucovorin (FOLFOX4) for previously treated metastatic colorectal cancer: results from the Eastern Cooperative Oncology Group Study E3200. *J Clin Oncol* 2007, 25:1539–1544.

98. Giantonio BJ, Catalno PJ, O'Dwyer PJ, *et al.*: Impact of bevacizumab dose reduction on clinical outcomes for patients treated on the Eastern Cooperative Oncology Group's Study E3200 [ASCO abstract]. *J Clin Oncol* 2006, 24(18S):3538.

99. Cunningham D, Humblet Y, Siena S, *et al.*: Cetuximab monotherapy and cetuximab plus irinotecan in irinotecan-refractory metastatic colorectal cancer. *N Engl J Med* 2004, 351:337–345.

100. Saltz LB, Meropol NJ, Loehrer PJ Sr, *et al.*: Phase II trial of cetuximab in patients with refractory colorectal cancer that expresses the epidermal growth factor receptor. *J Clin Oncol* 2004, 22:1201–1208.

101. Saltz L, Rubin MS, Hochster HS: Cetuximab (IMC-C225) plus irinotecan (CPT-11) is active in CPT-11-refractory colorectal cancer (CRC) that expresses epidermal growth factor receptor (EGFR) [abstract]. *Proc Am Soc Clin Oncol* 2001, 20:7.

102. Jennis A, Polikoff J, Mitchell EO, *et al.*: Erbitux (cetuximab) plus FOLFOX for colorectal cancer (EXPLORE): preliminary efficacy analysis of a randomized phase III trial [ASCO abstract]. *J Clin Oncol* 2005, 23(16S):3574.

103. Van Custem E, Nowacki MP, Lang I, *et al.*: Randomized phase III study of irinotecan and 5-FU/FA with or without cetuximab in the first-line treatment of patients with metastatic colorectal cancer (mCRC): the CRYSTAL trial [ASCO abstract]. *J Clin Oncol* 2007, 25(18S):4000.

104. Lenz H, Mayer RJ, Gold PJ: Activity of cetuximab in patients with colorectal cancer refractory to both irinotecan and oxaliplatin [ASCO abstract]. *J Clin Oncol* 2004, 22(14S):3510.

105. Chung KY, Shia J, Kemeny NE, *et al.*: Cetuximab shows activity in colorectal cancer patients with tumors that do not express the epidermal growth factor receptor by immunohistochemistry. *J Clin Oncol* 2005, 23:1803–1810.

106. Perez-Soler R, Saltz L: Cutaneous adverse effects with HER1/EGFR-targeted agents: is there a silver lining? *J Clin Oncol* 2005, 23:5235–5246.

107. Van Cutsem E, Peeters M, Siena S, *et al.*: Open-label phase III trial of panitumumab plus best supportive care compared with best supportive care alone in patients with chemotherapy-refractory metastatic colorectal cancer. *J Clin Oncol* 2007, 25:1658–1664.

108. Giusti RM, Shastri KA, Cohen MH, *et al.*: FDA drug approval summary: panitumumab (Vectibix). *Oncologist* 2007, 12:577–583.

109. Keefe DM, Schubert MM, Elting LS, *et al.*: Updated clinical practice guidelines for the prevention and treatment of mucositis. *Cancer* 2007, 109:820–831.

110. Benson AB III, Ajani JA, Catalano RB, *et al.*: Recommended guidelines for the treatment of cancer treatment-induced diarrhea. *J Clin Oncol* 2004, 22:2918–2926.

111. Hochster HS, Grothey A, Childs BH: Use of calcium and magnesium salts to reduce oxaliplatin-related neurotoxicity. *J Clin Oncol* 2007, 25:4028–4029.

112. Cassidy J, Bjarnason GA, Hickish T, *et al.*: Randomized double blind (DB) placebo (Plcb) controlled phase III study assessing the efficacy of xaliproden (X) in reducing the cumulative peripheral sensory neuropathy (PSN) induced by the oxaliplatin (Ox) and 5-FU/LV combination (FOLFOX4) in first-line treatment of patients (pts) with metastatic colorectal cancer (MCRC) [ASCO abstract]. *J Clin Oncol* 2006, 24(18S):3507.

113. Grothey A: Clinical management of oxaliplatin-associated neurotoxicity. *Clin Colorectal Cancer* 2005, 5(Suppl 1):S38–S46.

114. Hurwitz H, Saini S: Bevacizumab in the treatment of metastatic colorectal cancer: safety profile and management of adverse events. *Semin Oncol* 2006, 33(Suppl 10):S26–S34.

115. Scappaticci FA, Skillings JR, Holden SN, *et al.*: Arterial thromboembolic events in patients with metastatic carcinoma treated with chemotherapy and bevacizumab. *J Natl Cancer Inst* 2007, 99:1232–1239.

116. Skillings JR, Johnson D, Miller K, *et al.*: Arterial thromboembolic events (ATEs) in a pooled analysis of 5 randomized, controlled trials (RCTs) of bevacizumab (BV) with chemotherapy [ASCO abstract]. *J Clin Oncol* 2005, 23(16S):3019.

117. Scappaticci FA, Fehrenbacher L, Cartwright T, *et al.*: Surgical wound healing complications in metastatic colorectal cancer patients treated with bevacizumab. *J Surg Oncol* 2005, 91:173–180.

118. Gordon MS, Cunningham D: Managing patients treated with bevacizumab combination therapy. *Oncology* 2005, 69(Suppl 3):25–33.

119. Segaert S, Van Cutsem E: Clinical signs, pathophysiology and management of skin toxicity during therapy with epidermal growth factor receptor inhibitors. *Ann Oncol* 2005, 16:1425–1433.

120. Ryan DP, Compton CC, Mayer RJ: Carcinoma of the anal canal. *N Engl J Med* 2000, 342:792–800.

121. Cummings BJ: Current management of anal canal cancer. *Semin Oncol* 2005, 32(Suppl 9):S123–S128.

122. Frisch M, Glimelius B, van den Brule AJ, *et al.*: Sexually transmitted infection as a cause of anal cancer. *N Engl J Med* 1997, 337:1350–1358.

123. Arends MJ, Benton EC, McLaren KM: Renal allograft recipients with high susceptibility to cutaneous malignancy have an increased prevalence of human papillomavirus DNA in skin tumours and a greater risk of anogenital malignancy. *Br J Cancer* 1997, 75:722–728.

124. Roka S, Rasoul-Rockenschaub S, Roka J, *et al.*: Prevalence of anal HPV infection in solid-organ transplant patients prior to immunosuppression. *Transpl Int* 2004, 17:366–369.

125. Johnson LG, Madeleine MM, Newcomer LM, *et al.*: Anal cancer incidence and survival: the surveillance, epidemiology, and end results experience, 1973–2000. *Cancer* 2004, 101:281–288.

126. Daling JR, Madeleine MM, Johnson LG, *et al.*: Human papillomavirus, smoking, and sexual practices in the etiology of anal cancer. *Cancer* 2004, 101:270–280.

127. National Comprehensive Cancer Network, Inc.: Anal carcinoma. NCCN Clinical Practice Guidelines in Oncology (Version 1.2007). Available at http://www.nccn.org. Accessed August 2, 2007.

128. Ortholan C, Ramaioli A, Peiffert D, *et al.*: Anal canal carcinoma: early-stage tumors < or =10 mm (T1 or Tis): therapeutic options and original pattern of local failure after radiotherapy. *Int J Radiat Oncol Biol Phys* 2005, 62:479–485.

129. Greenall MJ, Quan SH, Urmacher C, DeCosse JJ: Treatment of epidermoid carcinoma of the anal canal. *Surg Gynecol Obstet* 1985, 161:509–517.

130. Epidermoid anal cancer: results from the UKCCCR randomised trial of radiotherapy alone versus radiotherapy, 5-fluorouracil, and mitomycin. UKCCCR Anal Cancer Trial Working Party. UK Coordinating Committee on Cancer Research. *Lancet* 1996, 348:1049–1054.

131. Bartelink H, Roelofsen F, Eschwege F, *et al.*: Concomitant radiotherapy and chemotherapy is superior to radiotherapy alone in the treatment of locally advanced anal cancer: results of a phase III randomized trial of the European Organization for Research and Treatment of Cancer Radiotherapy and Gastrointestinal Cooperative Groups. *J Clin Oncol* 1997, 15:2040–2049.

132. Flam M, John M, Pajak TF, *et al.*: Role of mitomycin in combination with fluorouracil and radiotherapy, and of salvage chemoradiation in the definitive nonsurgical treatment of epidermoid carcinoma of the anal canal: results of a phase III randomized intergroup study. *J Clin Oncol* 1996, 14:2527–2539.

133. Ajani JA, Winter KA, Gunderson LL, *et al.*: Intergroup RTOG 98-11: a phase III randomized study of 5-fluorouracil (5-FU), mitomycin, and radiotherapy versus 5-fluorouracil, cisplatin and radiotherapy in carcinoma of the anal canal [ASCO abstract]. *J Clin Oncol* 2006, 24(18S):4009.

134. Peddada AV, Smith DE, Rao AR, *et al.*: Chemotherapy and low-dose radiotherapy in the treatment of HIV-infected patients with carcinoma of the anal canal. *Int J Radiat Oncol Biol Phys* 1997, 37:1101–1105.

135. Hoffman R, Welton ML, Klencke B, *et al.*: The significance of pretreatment CD4 count on the outcome and treatment tolerance of HIV-positive patients with anal cancer. *Int J Radiat Oncol Biol Phys* 1999, 44:127–131.

136. Eng C: Anal cancer: current and future methodology. *Cancer Invest* 2006, 24:535–544.

137. Petrelli N, Herrera L, Rustum Y, *et al.*: A prospective randomized trial of 5-fluorouracil versus 5-fluorouracil and high-dose leucovorin versus 5-fluorouracil and methotrexate in previously untreated patients with advanced colorectal carcinoma. *J Clin Oncol* 1987, 5:1559–1565.

138. Poon MA, O'Connell MJ, Wieand HS, *et al.*: Biochemical modulation of fluorouracil with leucovorin: confirmatory evidence of improved therapeutic efficacy in advanced colorectal cancer. *J Clin Oncol* 1991, 9:1967–1972.

139. de Gramont A, Bosset JF, Milan C, *et al.*: Randomized trial comparing monthly low-dose leucovorin and fluorouracil bolus with bimonthly high-dose leucovorin and fluorouracil bolus plus continuous infusion for advanced colorectal cancer: a French Intergroup study. *J Clin Oncol* 1997, 15:808–815.

140. Rougier P, Van Cutsem E, Bajetta E, *et al.*: Randomised trial of irinotecan versus fluorouracil by continuous infusion after fluorouracil failure in patients with metastatic colorectal cancer. *Lancet* 1998, 352:1407–1412.

141. Andre T, Louvet C, Maindrault-Goebel F, *et al.*: CPT-11 (irinotecan) addition to bimonthly, high-dose leucovorin and bolus and continuous-infusion 5-fluorouracil (FOLFIRI) for pretreated metastatic colorectal cancer. GERCOR. *Eur J Cancer* 1999, 35:1343–1347.

142. Giantonio BJ, Catalano PJ, Meropol NJ, *et al.*: High-dose bevacizumab improves survival when combined with FOLFOX4 in previously treated advanced colorectal cancer: results from the Eastern Cooperative Oncology Group (ECOG) study E3200 [ASCO abstract]. *J Clin Oncol* 2005, 23(16S):2.

Head and Neck Cancer

Khaled El-Shami, Arlene A. Forastiere

9

ETIOLOGY AND RISK FACTORS

Cancers of the head and neck, which include cancers of the larynx, paranasal sinuses and nasal cavity, oral cavity, pharynx, salivary glands, and thyroid, comprise approximately 5% of malignancies in the United States, with an estimated incidence of 65,000 cases and about 12,500 deaths annually [1–3]. Excluding thyroid cancer, until recently, African Americans had the highest incidence of head and neck cancer compared with other racial and ethnic groups. Currently, white individuals have the highest incidence of head and neck cancer, although mortality is still highest in African Americans [4]. By virtue of their location and the attendant morbidity of their treatment, these tumors can cause significant functional and cosmetic impairments with substantial impact on quality of life. It is estimated that $3.2 billion is spent in the United States each year on the treatment of head and neck cancer [5]. The incidence of head and neck cancer rises with age—especially after age 50—with the majority of patients being between 50 and 70 years of age at the time of diagnosis. Tobacco and alcohol are the two most significant risk factors. Increasing tobacco consumption is responsible for a rising incidence of head and neck cancer among women. In Asia, tobacco and betel nut chewing is a common risk factor resulting in a high incidence of head and neck cancer. Although alcohol and tobacco are independent risk factors, together they produce a synergistic potentiation of the carcinogenic risk with a clear, quantitative relationship between both the intensity and duration of exposure and cancer risk [1].

Other potential risk factors include nutritional deficiencies, poor dental care, an immunocompromised state, and a genetic predisposition (Table 9-1). Exposure to wood dust, nickel scraps, or textile fibers is associated with adenocarcinoma of the paranasal sinuses. Nasopharyngeal carcinoma is associated with Epstein-Barr virus (EBV) and is endemic in some regions of North Africa and Asia. Human papillomavirus (HPV) is now recognized to play a role in the pathogenesis of a subset of head and neck squamous cell carcinomas (HNSCC), particularly those that arise from the lingual and palatine tonsils of the oropharynx. HPV DNA has been identified in approximately 20% of HNSCC cases. The most commonly detected oncogenic HPV in HNSCC is HPV-16, which has been demonstrated in 90% to 95% of all HPV-positive HNSCC cases, followed by HPV-18, HPV-33, and HPV-35 [6]. Measures of HPV exposure, including sexual behaviors, seropositivity to HPV-16, and oral, high-risk HPV infection, are associated with increased risk for oropharyngeal cancer. HPV infection may be altering the demographics of HNSCC patients, as these patients tend to be younger nonsmokers and nondrinkers. There is sufficient evidence to conclude that a diagnosis of HPV-positive HNSCC has significant prognostic implications; these patients have at least half the risk of death from HNSCC when compared with the HPV-negative patient [7].

Regardless of the inciting environmental factor(s), the mechanism of cancer development appears to be a multistep process involving progressive genetic alterations, mutations, and oncogenic amplifications that alter normal mucosa to dysplastic mucosa to carcinoma in situ and finally to invasive cancer with metastatic potential. These genetic changes include mutational inactivation of p16(ink4A) and p53, hypermethylation of the RASSF1A tumor suppressor gene, amplification of cyclin D1 and epidermal growth factor receptor (EGFR), and deletion of Rb [8]. Intramucosal migration and clonal expansion of transformed cells with formation of abnormal genetic fields appear to be responsible for field cancerization, local recurrences, and development of second primary tumors. Head and neck cancer is typically an environmentally induced disease and avoidance of risk factors is the best prevention. Moreover, the proclivity of head and neck cancer patients to develop second cancers after the index neoplasm is managed successfully is a hallmark of this disease. This feature has important implications in posttherapy surveillance and in the development of strategies for chemoprevention. Therefore, patients at risk should receive a regular physical examination, careful inspection of the oral cavity, discussion about changes in eating habits, and early referral for laryngoscopy if hoarseness or other symptoms persist (Table 9-2).

STAGING AND PROGNOSIS

Head and neck cancer comprises a heterogeneous group of cancers originating from different primary sites. Squamous cell carcinoma, or one of its variants, is by far the most common histologic type in adults. Disease can range from in situ cancers to invasive lesions. Verrucous cancers typically do not invade beyond the basement membrane and are most frequently encountered in the oropharynx and larynx. Ulcerative lesions progress toward infiltration. Infiltrative lesions have a propensity to extend deeply into underlying structures. Exophytic lesions, on the other hand, grow more superficially and metastasize later in the course of the disease than other types. Premalignant lesions fall primarily into two categories. Leukoplakia refers to hyperkeratosis presenting as a white patch of mucosa that occasionally transforms into invasive cancer, whereas erythroplakia is a superficial friable red patch that arises adjacent to normal mucosa and evolves into an invasive cancer in about 40% of cases [9]. Other histologic diagnoses include those of salivary gland origin, adenocarcinoma, adenoid cystic carcinoma, mucoepidermoid carcinoma (low, intermediate, and high grade), and undifferentiated carcinoma of the nasopharynx type. Lymphoma, Hodgkin's disease, sarcoma, esthesioneuroblastoma, neuroendocrine carcinomas, melanoma,

Table 9-1. Risk Factors for Head and Neck Cancer

Tobacco use

Alcohol use

Poor orodental care

Genetic susceptibility

Occupational exposure (*eg*, wood dust, textile fibers, nickel, cadmium, radium)

Smokeless tobacco use (chewing)

Malnutrition

Mechanical irritation

Viruses (*eg*, Epstein-Barr, herpes simplex, human papilloma)

Table 9-2. Prevention and Early Detection

Prevention

Avoid alcohol

Avoid smoking

Avoid combination of alcohol and smoking

Discontinue risk factor exposure after diagnosis to reduce risk of second malignancy

Participate in chemoprevention trials

Early detection

Yearly physical examination with special attention to the upper aerodigestive tract and neck

Digital examination of oral cavity

Refer to ear, nose, and throat specialist for unexplained symptoms lasting > 4 wk

Leukoplakia as possible early sign of transformation; biopsy and frequent follow-up necessary

and cancer of unknown primary site may all arise in the head and neck and must therefore be distinguished [10]. Metastases of lung cancer or gastrointestinal neoplasms may present primarily in the neck. Treatment depends on localization, resectability, and histology. For squamous cell carcinoma, local and regional extension determines the stage and prognosis.

Cancers of the head and neck are staged using the American Joint Committee on Cancer TNM (tumor, node, metastasis) classification [10]. The T-stage classification is specific for the various anatomic sites in the head and neck area. Generally, lesions considered to be T1 and T2 are small primary tumors, whereas T3 and T4 lesions are large, with T4 tumors invading surrounding structures (*eg*, bone, cartilage, skin). Regional lymph nodes are staged uniformly as N1 to N3 for all anatomic sites based on increasing size and number of nodes (Table 9-3). Stages I and II represent T1/N0 and T2/N0 lesions, respectively, whereas stages III and IV represent locally advanced disease (T3, T4) and/or regional involvement (N1–N3). Distant metastases are present in 10% of patients at diagnosis and are included in stage IV. Lung, bone, and liver are the most commonly involved sites [11]. Most patients (60%) have loco-regionally advanced disease (T3 and T4 or N2–N3) at presentation and die of complications of loco-regional disease, indicating the inability of currently available therapy to produce cure consistently. Regional node involvement appears to be the most important prognostic factor (Table 9-4).

Up to 25% of the patients with advanced squamous cell carcinoma relapse with distant metastases, but autopsy series indicate an up to 60% rate of occult metastatic disease. Thirty to 50% of patients with locally advanced disease are cured with surgery and radiation therapy, but cure may be achieved in more patients with multimodality treatment. In early-stage disease, cure rates vary from 60% to 90%. However, a basic principle of head and neck cancer management is that every patient is different and requires an individualized treatment plan based on the anatomic, pathologic, and clinical characteristics of the tumor.

NASOPHARYNGEAL CANCER AND EPSTEIN-BARR VIRUS

Nasopharyngeal cancer with a distinct undifferentiated or poorly differentiated (lymphoepithelial) histology must be considered separately from cancer in the nasopharynx with squamous cell histology. Surgical accessibility is difficult and because of its hidden location, the cancer causes few symptoms. Most patients present with an advanced stage of disease, nodal involvement, and frequently distant metastases. Undifferentiated carcinoma of the nasopharynx is one of the most common tumor types in Southeast Asia. A strong etiologic association has been found for EBV infection [12]. Activation of the viral genome may be caused by frequent consumption of salted fish or nitrosamines. EBV genome and viral protein expression can be detected in most nasopharyngeal tumors.

Nasopharyngeal cancer is exquisitely sensitive to both radiation and chemotherapy, suggesting the usefulness of a combined modality approach. In a randomized trial, three cycles of BEC chemotherapy (bleomycin, epirubicin, cisplatin) followed by radiation were compared with radiotherapy (RT) alone [13]. Despite an excess in toxic deaths in the experimental arm, which correlated with the experience of the treating center, a significantly improved disease-free survival rate but not overall survival was observed for the induction chemotherapy group. In a randomized intergroup trial, concomitant chemoradiotherapy with cisplatin followed by adjuvant chemotherapy with cisplatin and 5-fluorouracil (5-FU) was compared with

standard RT. This trial was closed early after an interim analysis showed a significantly improved outcome for the combined modality treatment (3-year survival 76% for RT vs 46% for radiation and concomitant chemotherapy; $P < 0.001$) [14]. Similarly, a randomized trial from Hong Kong reported improved local control and survival with concomitant cisplatin chemotherapy (40 mg/m^2 weekly) and RT [15]. In the light of these results, all patients should be treated with concurrent cisplatin chemotherapy and radiation. The addition of three cycles of chemotherapy is recommended because of a high risk of distant metastases.

SALIVARY GLAND CANCER

Salivary gland tumors can arise from either the major or minor salivary glands. Salivary gland cancers are different from HNSCC. Histologically, these are commonly adenocarcinoma, adenoid cystic, or mucoepidermoid carcinoma. Low-grade histologies tend to recur loco-regionally with a natural history over many years, whereas high-grade tumors frequently invade adjacent muscle, bone, and nerves. Perineural invasion is particularly common in adenoid cystic carcinoma. Management of these tumors is mainly surgical with adjuvant radiation. Adjuvant RT is typically administered for larger lesions, nodal involvement, positive margins, or other adverse pathologic features.

The role of chemotherapy is largely experimental. Chemotherapy for recurrent or metastatic disease commonly includes an anthracycline-containing regimen (*eg*, CAP [cyclophosphamide, doxorubicin, cisplatin] or FAP [5-FU, doxorubicin, cisplatin]). Mucoepidermoid carcinoma, on the other hand, responds to the same regimens commonly used in treating squamous cell carcinomas (5-FU and cisplatin with or without taxanes). In the most recent review of the literature using multivariate Cox analysis, only the use of platinum-based chemotherapy was identified as an independent predictor of increased survival ($P = 0.01$). This observation was confirmed in a meta-analysis in which median survival was increased by 2.5 months (95% CI, 0.7–4.4) and 4.9 months (95% CI, 0.45–9.4) for patients treated with platinum-based ($P = 0.007$) and anthracycline-based ($P = 0.03$) chemotherapy, respectively [16].

TREATMENT STRATEGY

Stage is the main determinant factor when deciding on a treatment strategy for an individual patient [17]. Patients are best evaluated jointly by a head and neck surgeon, a radiation oncologist, and a medical oncologist. In addition, an experienced radiologist, an oral surgeon, a nutritionist, and a social worker are often valuable resources when determining an overall treatment strategy.

Early-stage cancers can usually be cured equally well with surgery or RT. For locally advanced stages, resectability and the expected morbidity of surgery relative to organ function influences treatment decision making; however, a multimodal approach is necessary for optimal patient care. Local control can be improved by concomitant chemoradiotherapy. Organ preservation with concomitant chemotherapy and RT can be an important goal for compliant patients. Surgery is then reserved for patients failing to

Table 9-3. TNM Staging and Survival*

Stage	Survival rate, %
I	75–90
II	40–70
III	20–50
IV	< 10–30

*TNM (tumor, node, metastasis) stages are defined as follows: early (stage I, II); intermediate (T3/N0, T1–2/N1); loco-regionally advanced (T3, T4, and N2–3); metastatic disease (M1, M2).

Table 9-4. Prognostic Factors

Factor/Tumor location	Comment(s)
Nodal involvement, N stage	Most important prognostic factor; N0 better than N+
Extracapsular spread	Tendency for recurrence in the neck and distant metastases
Tumor size	
Histologic differentiation	Salivary gland cancer only
Hypopharynx	Commonly advanced with poor outcome
Larynx	Overall prognostically better; potential for organ preservation with induction chemotherapy
Nasopharynx	Chemosensitive tumor; tendency for distant metastases; median survival 4–5 y; late relapses frequent

respond or those with recurrent disease. For patients who cannot comply with a lengthy and intensive treatment and regular follow-up, primary surgery remains the treatment of choice. Patients with recurrent or metastatic disease are candidates for palliative chemotherapy [18].

EARLY-STAGE DISEASE

Early-stage cancers (T1 and T2/N0) can be cured with surgery or with RT alone in 60% to 90% of cases. If surgery is performed, it may include elective dissection of the regional lymph nodes based on the pattern of nodal drainage for the specific primary site. This procedure allows more accurate pathologic staging with important prognostic and therapeutic implications. In more than 50% of cases, the pathologic stage will be higher than the clinical stage. A similar outcome in early-stage disease can be achieved with RT. The choice of treatment is based on patient preference and location of the primary cancer. For example, early-stage glottic cancers are generally treated with RT, reserving laryngectomy for salvage treatment of recurrent disease. RT is a lengthy process (> 6 to 7 weeks), with mucositis, xerostomia, and loss of taste as the major secondary effects. This modality should only be chosen for reliable and compliant patients. For early-stage laryngeal cancer, RT is often the first choice; laser resection and partial laryngectomy may be alternative treatments for selected patients.

LOCALLY ADVANCED DISEASE

About 60% of patients present with locally advanced disease (stage III and IV) and, in many, the disease recurs locally or regionally. In locally advanced disease, bimodal therapy with surgery followed by RT has been the historic standard treatment for patients with resectable disease. This approach has resulted in cure rates up to 50%. Depending on the location and size of the primary tumor, surgery may lead to impaired or lost organ function, muscle atrophy, and disfigurement despite advances in reconstruction techniques. New strategies have been developed to improve cure rates and overall survival. Multimodal therapy, with concomitant chemoradiotherapy, improves loco-regional control and survival compared with radiation alone for cancers of the oropharynx, nasopharynx, and unresectable squamous cancers of all sites. Induction chemotherapy allows for organ preservation in patients with hypopharyngeal tumors. Combined modality therapy must now be considered the standard approach for most patients with locally advanced head and neck carcinomas.

INDUCTION CHEMOTHERAPY

RATIONALE

The idea that induction chemotherapy could enhance curability of head and neck cancer and improve organ preservation is based on observations that 5-FU/cisplatin chemotherapy results in objective tumor responses in up to 90% of newly diagnosed HNSCC with pathologic complete responses in up to 50% [19]. Furthermore, induction chemotherapy with 5-FU/cisplatin resulted in a significant proportion of negative margin resections [20]. Induction chemotherapy is generally better tolerated than similar therapy given postoperatively or to irradiated patients. Higher doses can potentially be delivered, thus improving local responses and eradicating micrometastatic disease. Additionally, drug delivery is more effective in untreated, well-vascularized tumors [21].

RANDOMIZED TRIALS

Although induction chemotherapy with cisplatin and 5-FU results in high response rates, it did not translate into a significant loco-regional control and survival advantage in six conclusive randomized trials [22–27]. However, a reduction in distant metastasis was demonstrated, which suggests systemic activity against early micrometastatic disease [22,23,28]. Improved survival was shown for primarily inoperable patients after induction chemotherapy followed by radiation [22]. A survival advantage was also shown by subset analysis for patients with oral cancer and N2 disease after induction and adjuvant chemotherapy [29]. However, a meta-analysis revealed that while the induction trials did not improve survival in patients with head and neck cancer compared with standard therapy, the subset of induction chemotherapy trials that used cisplatin/5-FU chemotherapy resulted in a 5%

improvement in 5-year survival compared with standard therapy [30]. This difference was less substantial than the 8% improvement observed with chemoradiotherapy but was statistically significant ($P = 0.01$).

An improvement over the 5-FU/cisplatin doublet was observed with the addition of docetaxel or paclitaxel. In three completed phase 3 randomized trials [31–33], more than 1000 patients were randomized to receive either 5-FU/cisplatin or the same regimen with the addition of paclitaxel or docetaxel. The addition of a taxane to the doublet resulted in improvement in response rate and overall survival. Thus, paclitaxel or docetaxel combined with cisplatin and 5-FU has emerged as the new standard of care for induction chemotherapy of head and neck cancer. Nonetheless, the role of induction chemotherapy has yet to be defined relative to the standard of care indications for concurrent chemoradiation. Randomized trials evaluating the role of sequential therapy (induction chemotherapy followed by chemoradiation) directly compared with chemoradiation alone are in progress.

ORGAN PRESERVATION

Radiation therapy is the standard organ-preserving treatment modality in head and neck cancer, as these malignancies are generally deemed radiosensitive. More recently, organ function–preserving surgical procedures have been evolving and may be equally effective in achieving local tumor control and preserving primary site function.

Organ preservation has been a primary end point of two randomized trials [23,27]. Patients with stages III and IV larynx cancer [23] and stages II, III, and IV pyriform sinus cancer [27] were treated with three [23] or four [27] cycles of induction chemotherapy with cisplatin and 5-FU. Patients who responded (complete or partial response in the larynx trial; complete response only in the pyriform sinus trial) then received definitive radiation. Surgery was restricted to those with insufficient responsive and as salvage treatment in patients with residual disease after radiation or with recurrent disease. For laryngeal primaries, organ preservation at 3 years was 64%; for hypopharyngeal primaries, the 3-year estimate of survival with a functional larynx was 42% and overall survival was statistically equivalent. The feasibility of organ preservation has also been shown for nonlaryngeal sites [29].

More recently, the Intergroup Radiation Therapy Oncology Group (RTOG) 91-11 trial compared induction chemotherapy followed by radiation in responders versus radiation alone versus concurrent chemoradiation with single-agent cisplatin in patients with resectable stage III and IV laryngeal cancer [34,35]. While no significant difference in larynx preservation and loco-regional control was observed between the induction and RT alone groups, concurrent radiation and single-agent cisplatin was statistically superior for both end points. This study evaluated the contribution of chemotherapy added to RT and the optimal sequencing of these two modalities. The results form the basis of the current standard of care for larynx preservation.

CONCOMITANT CHEMORADIOTHERAPY

CONCEPTS AND RATIONALE

High response rates and a consistently decreased incidence of distant metastases underline the efficacy of chemotherapy in the treatment of HNSCC. Use of chemotherapy as a radiation sensitizer is also well established. The goal of concomitant chemoradiotherapy is to administer both treatment modalities at an optimal dose and schedule simultaneously within a short time. Overall, three different, but similar, concepts have been investigated:

1. Standard and uninterrupted radiation with simultaneous low-dose, single-agent chemotherapy with a pure radiosensitizing objective.
2. Modified radiation therapy schedule with planned treatment breaks and simultaneous, intensified (at systemically active doses) combination chemotherapy.
3. Rapidly alternating sequenced therapy with radiation and combination chemotherapy.

The rationale for concomitant chemotherapy and RT has been reviewed extensively [36,37]. Concomitant chemotherapy may eradicate radiation-resistant tumor cells, presumably by making the tumor cells more susceptible to radiation. Further, chemotherapy may eliminate micrometastatic disease outside the radiation field (spatial cooperation). Although concomitant chemoradiotherapy enhances treatment efficacy, it also adds significant toxicity. Mucositis, neutropenia, and infections can be severe and occasionally cause life-threatening complications [38,39]. Nevertheless, concomitant intensive chemoradiotherapy is the treatment of choice for most patients with advanced head and neck cancer. Because of increased acute toxicities, an experienced and multidisciplinary team should administer these treatments. In addition, most patients require close follow-up and supportive care (*eg*, percutaneous endoscopic gastrostomy).

RANDOMIZED TRIALS

Many well-conducted trials were published in the past few years, all suggesting improved loco-regional control or prolonged survival with concomitant chemoradiotherapy. 5-FU has been widely used with concomitant radiation [40]. In a placebo-controlled trial, 5-FU (1200 mg/m^2 continuous infusion, days 1–3) was added to standard RT on weeks 1 and 3. The 2-year survival with 5-FU was 63% versus 50% ($P = 0.076$) without chemotherapy [41]. There was no impact on the incidence of distant metastases. In an earlier trial, 5-FU bolus (250 mg/m^2) every other day was comparable with hyperfractionated twice-daily RT (1.1 Gy given twice daily) and significantly superior to standard RT alone. Median survival was 85, 84, and 38 months, respectively. Prolonged survival was also shown for cisplatin (50 mg/wk) and standard radiation versus RT alone in the postoperative adjuvant treatment of high-risk patients. The 2-year survival rates were 75% versus 44% ($P < 0.05$) [42]. The combination of cisplatin (12 mg/m^2, days 1–5) and 5-FU (600 mg/m^2, days 1–5) during the first and sixth weeks of hyperfractionated RT was compared with twice-daily hyperfractionated (125 cGy twice daily) RT alone, suggesting an improved 3-year survival (28% vs 15%; $P = 0.06$) and a decreased incidence of distant metastases [43].

In a large, randomized, multicenter trial, concomitant split-course chemoradiotherapy with cisplatin and 5-FU was compared with sequential chemotherapy (induction) followed by radiation. Loco-regional control was improved in the concomitant arm; however, an excess death rate due to complications in the concomitant chemoradiotherapy arm emphasized the increase in toxicity and necessity of center experience [38]. Intergroup 0126 compared standard RT (2 Gy/d, up to 70 Gy) with the same RT and concomitant cisplatin (100 mg/m^2, days 1, 22, and 43) and with split-course RT and three cycles of concomitant cisplatin (75 mg/m^2) and 5-FU (1000 mg/m^2 continuous infusion, days 1–4) chemotherapy [44]. Improved survival was seen with the concomitant administration of chemotherapy and uninterrupted standard RT. However, split-course radiation and a more intensive

combination chemotherapy regimen did not improve survival rates, possibly due to unnecessarily long delays of RT, whereas only 10% of patients underwent the planned surgery. Intensive chemoradiotherapy regimens are required to improve both local control and distant failure rate [45–49].

In a randomized trial, rapidly alternating chemoradiotherapy with cisplatin/bolus 5-FU was compared with standard RT [50]. Of 157 patients with advanced, unresectable head and neck cancer, 41% of the patients treated with combined modalities survived at 3 years but only 23% in the RT alone treatment group survived ($P < 0.05$). Recent and ongoing trials are attempting to improve response and overall outcome by using hyperfractionated RT with chemotherapy or accelerated RT with concomitant combination chemotherapy and amifostine as a cytoprotective agent [51]. The success of adding taxanes to induction chemotherapy led to a randomized phase 2 RTOG study [52] that compared cisplatin/paclitaxel with two other arms consisting of 5-FU/cisplatin and 5-FU/hydroxyurea. The cisplatin/paclitaxel arm showed superior 2-year disease-free survival and overall survival rates of 51% and 67%, respectively, suggesting improvement over existing regimens.

The advent of molecularly targeted therapy has probably been the most important development in combined chemoradiation therapy for head and neck cancer. The landmark study that ushered in this development was a randomized phase 3 study comparing radiation with or without cetuximab for patients with locally advanced HNSCC [53]. The median duration of failure-free survival (defined as loco-regional failure or death) was 24.4 months among patients treated with cetuximab plus RT and 14.9 months among those given RT alone (HR for loco-regional progression or death, 0.68; $P = 0.005$). With a median follow-up of 54.0 months, the median overall survival was 49.0 months among patients treated with combined therapy and 29.3 months among those treated with RT alone (HR for death, 0.74; $P = 0.03$). RT plus cetuximab significantly prolonged progression-free survival (HR for disease progression or death, 0.70; $P = 0.006$). Cetuximab did not significantly add to the acute side effects of RT, offering a real therapeutic advantage to patients who are ineligible to receive standard chemoradiation. As a result of this study, cetuximab was approved by the US Food and Drug Administration/European Medicines Agency in combination with RT to treat HNSCC in February and April 2006. However, this study did not compare cetuximab plus RT with platinum-based RT, which is the current standard of care. Additionally, RT was not uniformly administered among all patients. These shortcomings are currently addressed in the RTOG trial 0522, which has been recently initiated and compares chemoradiation with cisplatin to chemoradiation plus cetuximab.

RECURRENT OR METASTATIC DISEASE

Patients with disease recurrence after primary treatment should be considered for surgical salvage. However, less than 30% of patients who actually present with recurrent disease are candidates for such approach. The ability to obtain tumor-free margin is largely dependent on the tumor location, pattern of recurrence (local vs loco-regional), the anatomy, and the surgical expertise. Therefore, overall survival and disease-free survival rates after salvage surgery are variable [54]. In general, patients with early-stage disease (T1 and T2) who recur have overall survival and disease-free survival of 30% to 60% and 44% to 88%, respectively [54,55]. On the other hand, patients with locally advanced disease (T3 and T4) who recur have limited potential for long-term or disease-free survival [56].

Patients with recurrent disease who are not candidates for surgical salvage or who relapse with metastatic disease are typically offered palliative chemotherapy or enrollment in clinical trials. Combination chemotherapy has demonstrated relatively high response rates in recurrent or metastatic head and neck cancer. Methotrexate, platinum agents, bleomycin, taxanes, and 5-FU are drugs with single-agent activity in the range of 15% to 25%. However, a number of phase 2 and 3 studies comparing combination chemotherapy with single-agent therapy have shown statistically significant improvements in objective responses with combination therapy over single agents [57,58].

Platinum agents are the most widely used agents in the treatment of head and neck cancer (Table 9-5). Cisplatin has been shown to have higher and more rapid response rates when compared with other active agents.

Table 9-5. Current Treatment Regimens for Head and Neck Cancer

Regimen	Response rates, %
Methotrexate 40–60 mg/m^2 IV weekly	10–29
Cisplatin 100 mg/m^2 IV every 3–4 wk	15–27
Cisplatin 100 mg/m^2 + 5-FU 800–1000 mg daily as continuous infusion for 4–5 d; repeat cycle every 3–4 wk	30–80
Carboplatin 300–400 mg/m^2 + 5-FU 800–1000 mg/m^2 daily as continuous infusion for 4–5 d; repeat cycle every 3–4 wk	20–25
Cisplatin 100 mg/m^2 + 5-FU 600–800 mg/m^2 with leucovorin daily as continuous infusion for 4–5 d; repeat cycle every 3–4 wk	15–90
Docetaxel 100 mg/m^2 IV every 3 wk	21–43
Paclitaxel 135–175 mg/m^2 over 3–24 h every 3–4 wk	30–40
Docetaxel 75 mg/m^2 + cisplatin 75 mg/m^2 + 5-FU 750 mg/m^2 daily as continuous infusion for 5 d; repeat cycle every 3 wk	—
Cisplatin, 5-FU, hydroxyurea, and concomitant radiation	70–80

5-FU—5-fluorouracil.

Carboplatin has also been tested in phase 2/3 trials and was found to have acceptable, although lower, response rates.

The cisplatin and 5-FU combination regimen has become the reference regimen because of its relatively good response rate and favorable toxicity profile when compared with other regimens [18,57,58]. This regimen has been tested in multiple trials and has an overall response rate of 30% to 40% in recurrent or metastatic disease and an overall median survival of 6 to 8 months. Taxanes have also been tested in advanced head and neck cancer. No major studies have shown superiority of substituting docetaxel or paclitaxel for cisplatin when combined with 5-FU. One phase 2 study of docetaxel and 5-FU reported an overall response rate of 20% [59]. The combination of taxanes and cisplatin has also been compared with cisplatin/5-FU in a phase 3 randomized trial that enrolled 218 patients [60]. No difference in the overall response rates (26% and 27% in the paclitaxel and 5-FU arms, respectively) or median overall survival (8.1 and 8.7 months in the paclitaxel and 5-FU arms, respectively) was observed.

Attempts to improve response rates and survival achieved with doublets have led to studies testing triple-agent regimens. These studies have yielded higher response rates, both overall and complete, but with increasing toxicity [57,61]. Among the triplet-agent regimens are cisplatin with paclitaxel and 5-FU; docetaxel, cisplatin, and 5-FU; and paclitaxel, ifosfamide, and cisplatin. Overall response and complete response rates for these regimens are comparable (40% to 60% and 12% to 50% respectively), with the highest responses (and toxicities) observed with cisplatin, paclitaxel, and 5-FU. Median survival for patients treated with these regimens ranges between 9 and 14 months [57,61]. As expected, improvements seen in response rates have been associated with increased toxicity, particularly grade 3 to 4 myelosuppression. As such, when considering patients for treatment with triple-agent regimens, the observation of increased toxicity needs to be balanced against potential modest gains in palliation.

The EGFR is overexpressed in 80% to 100% of HNSCC and its overexpression is associated with advanced stage and poor prognosis following conventional therapy [62,63]. Two small molecule inhibitors of tyrosine kinase activity of EGFR, gefitinib and erlotinib, have demonstrated single-agent activity in a small fraction (11% and 5%, respectively) of patients with advanced head and neck cancer [64,65]. Cetuximab is a chimeric murine human monoclonal antibody that targets the extracellular domain of EGFR. Cetuximab was found to have single-agent activity in 15% of patients. In a randomized phase 3 trial of combination cetuximab and cisplatin versus cisplatin alone [66], the response rate in the combined treatment arm was 26% compared with 10% in the cisplatin alone arm ($P = 0.02$). Thus, these data suggest that cetuximab is an active agent in recurrent/metastatic HNSCC.

PREVENTION AND CHEMOPREVENTION

Stopping the use of tobacco and alcohol (the two primary risk factors for HNSCC) is central to any prevention program. Counseling combined with the use of pharmacologic intervention, such as tapering nicotine patch, doubles success rates; however, only a minority of smokers succeed in quitting on their first attempt. Important reasons for smoking cessation that clinicians can discuss with their patients include the fact that the rate of second primary tumors is higher among patients who continue to smoke and that continuing to smoke adversely influences the effectiveness and tolerance of cancer treatment.

The understanding of the stepwise molecular events that define the risk of progression to invasive disease has fueled interest in potential areas for preventive intervention. Testing of retinoids to reverse the processes that ultimately lead to epithelial carcinogenesis began in the mid-1980s. Trials investigating 13-cis-retinoic acid (13cRA) in high and low doses showed that high-dose 13cRA was able to reverse oral intraepithelial neoplasia in approximately two thirds of premalignant lesions and maintain the effect for as long as treatment was continued. However, intolerable side effects precluded chronic long-term dosing [67].

The results of other randomized trials do not show a clear improvement in outcome. No reduction in second primary tumors was found in a study of etretinate (50 mg daily for 1 month followed by 25 mg daily for 24 months) in patients with early-stage disease [68]. In a placebo-controlled intergroup trial of tolerable low-dose isotretinoin in patients with curatively treated stage I or II HNSCC, no effect was observed in the rate of second primary tumors (HR, 1.03; 95% CI, 0.81–1.32) [69]. A large study conducted by the European Organization for Research and Treatment of Cancer found no significant benefit in the rate of second primary tumors, event-free survival, or overall survival when vitamin A and antioxidant therapy (N-acetylcysteine) were used in patients with upper aerodigestive cancers treated with curative intent [70].

In light of these negative randomized trials, no systemic therapy can be recommended, and patients with oral premalignant mucosal changes should be enrolled in clinical trials. Novel approaches in chemoprevention such as bioadjuvant therapy with combination of 13cRA, interferon alfa-2a, and vitamin E as well as approaches targeting the EGFR are currently being explored.

REFERENCES

1. Spitz MR: Epidemiology and risk factors for head and neck cancer. *Semin Oncol* 1994, 21:281–288.

2. Fandi A, Altun M, Azli N, *et al.*: Nasopharyngeal cancer: epidemiology, staging, and treatment. *Semin Oncol* 1994, 21:382–397.

3. American Cancer Society: *Cancer Facts and Figures 2005*. Atlanta: American Cancer Society; 2005.

4. Jemal A, Siegel R, Ward E, *et al.*: Cancer statistics, 2006. *CA Cancer J Clin* 2006, 56:106–130.

5. Brown ML, Riley GF, Schussler N, Etzioni R: Estimating health care costs related to cancer treatment from SEER-Medicare data. *Med Care* 2002, 40(Suppl):IV-104–IV-117.

6. Gillison ML: Human papillomavirus-associated head and neck cancer is a distinct epidemiologic, clinical, and molecular entity. *Semin Oncol* 2004, 31:744–754.

7. Fakhry C, Gillison ML: Clinical implications of human papillomavirus in head and neck cancers. *J Clin Oncol* 2006, 24:2606–2611.

8. Perez-Odonez B, Beauchemin M, Jordan RC: Molecular biology of squamous carcinoma of the head and neck. *J Clin Pathol* 2006, 59:445–453.

9. Neville BW, Day TA: Oral cancer and precancerous lesions. *CA Cancer J Clin* 2002, 52:195–215.

10. Greene FL, Page DL, Fleming ID, *et al.*: *AJCC Cancer Staging Manual*, edn 6. New York: Springer; 2002.

11. Calhoun KH, Fulmer P, Weiss R, Hokanson JA: Distant metastases from head and neck squamous cell carcinomas. *Laryngoscope* 1994, 104:1199–1205.

12. Vokes EE, Liebowitz DN, Weichselbaum RR: Nasopharyngeal carcinoma. *Lancet* 1997, 350:1087–1091.

13. Preliminary results of a randomized trial comparing neoadjuvant chemotherapy (cisplatin, epirubicin, bleomycin) plus radiotherapy vs. radiotherapy alone in stage IV (> N2, M0) undifferentiated nasopharyngeal carcinoma: a positive effect on progression-free survival. *Int J Radiat Oncol Biol Phys* 1996, 35:463–469.

14. Al-Sarraf M, LeBlanc M, Giri PG, *et al.*: Chemoradiotherapy versus radiotherapy in patients with advanced nasopharyngeal cancer: phase III randomized Intergroup study 0099. *J Clin Oncol* 1998, 16:1310–1317.

15. Chan AT, Leung SF, Ngan RK, *et al.*: Overall survival after concurrent cisplatin-radiotherapy compared with radiotherapy alone in locoregionally advanced nasopharyngeal carcinoma. *J Natl Cancer Inst* 2005, 97:536–539.

16. Rizk S, Robert A, Vandenhooft A, *et al.*: Activity of chemotherapy in the palliative treatment of salivary gland tumors: review of the literature. *Eur Arch Otorhinolaryngol* 2007, 264:587–594.

17. Forastiere A, Koch WM, Trotti A, Sidransky D: Medical progress: head and neck cancer. A review. *N Engl J Med* 2001, 345:1890–1900.

18. Browman GP, Cronin L: Standard chemotherapy in squamous cell head and neck cancer: what we have learned from randomized trials. *Semin Oncol* 1994, 21:311–319.

19. Ensley JF, Jacobs JR, Weaver A, *et al.*: Correlation between response to cisplatinum-combination chemotherapy and subsequent radiotherapy in previously untreated patients with advanced squamous cell cancers of the head and neck. *Cancer* 1984, 54:811–814.

20. Haddad R, Tishler R, Wirth L, *et al.*: Rate of pathologic complete responses to docetaxel, cisplatin, and fluorouracil induction chemotherapy in patients with squamous cell carcinoma of the head and neck. *Arch Otolaryngol Head Neck Surg* 2006, 132:678–681.

21. Adelstein DJ: Induction chemotherapy in head and neck cancer. *Hematol Oncol Clin North Am* 1999, 13:689–698, v-vi.

22. Paccagnella A, Orlando A, Marchiori C, *et al.*: Phase III trial of initial chemotherapy in stage III or IV head and neck cancers: a study by the Gruppo di Studio sui Tumori della Testa e del Collo. *J Natl Cancer Inst* 1994, 86:265–272.

23. Induction chemotherapy plus radiation compared with surgery plus radiation in patients with advanced laryngeal cancer. The Department of Veterans Affairs Laryngeal Cancer Study Group. *N Engl J Med* 1991, 324:1685–1690.

24. Laramore GE, Scott CB, al-Sarraf M, *et al.*: Adjuvant chemotherapy for resectable squamous cell carcinomas of the head and neck: report on Intergroup study 0034. *Int J Radiat Oncol Biol Phys* 1992, 23:705–713.

25. Schuller DE, Metch B, Stein DW, *et al.*: Preoperative chemotherapy in advanced resectable head and neck cancer: final report of the Southwest Oncology Group. *Laryngoscope* 1988, 98:1205–1211.

26. Head and Neck Contracts Program: Adjuvant chemotherapy for advanced head and neck squamous carcinoma: final report. *Cancer* 1987, 60:301–311.

27. Lefebvre JL, Chevalier D, Luboinski B, *et al.*: Larynx preservation in pyriform sinus cancer: preliminary results of a European Organization for Research and Treatment of Cancer phase III trial. EORTC Head and Neck Cancer Cooperative Group. *J Natl Cancer Inst* 1996, 88:890–899.

28. Schuller DE, Stein DW, Metch B: Analysis of treatment failure patterns. A Southwest Oncology Group study. *Arch Otolaryngol Head Neck Surg* 1989, 115:834–836.

29. Jacobs C, Makuch R: Efficacy of adjuvant chemotherapy for patients with resectable head and neck cancer: a subset analysis of the Head and Neck Contracts Program. *J Clin Oncol* 1990, 8:838–847.

30. Monnerat C, Faivre S, Temam S, *et al.*: End points for new agents in induction chemotherapy for locally advanced head and neck cancers. *Ann Oncol* 2002, 13:995–1006.

31. Hitt R, Lopez-Pousa A, Martinez-Trufero J, *et al.*: Phase III study comparing cisplatin plus fluorouracil to paclitaxel, cisplatin, and fluorouracil induction chemotherapy followed by chemoradiotherapy in locally advanced head and neck cancer. *J Clin Oncol* 2005, 23:8636–8645.

32. Vermorken JB, Remenar E, van Herpen C, *et al.*: Cisplatin, fluorouracil, and docetaxel in unresectable head and neck cancer. *N Engl J Med* 2007, 357:1695–1704.

33. Posner MR, Hershock DM, Blajman CR, *et al.*: Cisplatin and fluorouracil alone or with docetaxel in head and neck cancer. *N Engl J Med* 2007, 357:1705–1715.

34. Forastiere AA, Goepfert H, Maor M, *et al.*: Concurrent chemotherapy and radiotherapy for organ preservation in advanced laryngeal cancer. *N Engl J Med* 2003, 349:2091–2098.

35. Forastiere AA, Maor M, Weber RS, *et al.*: Long-term results of Intergroup RTOG 91-11: a phase III trial to preserve the larynx. Induction cisplatin/5-FU and radiation therapy versus concurrent cisplatin and radiation therapy versus radiation therapy [ASCO abstract]. *J Clin Oncol* 2006, 24(18S):5517.

36. Stupp R, Weichselbaum RR, Vokes EE: Combined modality therapy of head and neck cancer. *Semin Oncol* 1994, 21:349–358.

37. Vokes EE, Weichselbaum RR: Concomitant chemoradiotherapy: rationale and clinical experience in patients with solid tumors. *J Clin Oncol* 1990, 8:911–934.

38. Denham JW, Abbott RL: Concurrent cisplatin, infusional fluorouracil, and conventionally fractionated radiation therapy in head and neck cancer: dose-limiting mucosal toxicity. *J Clin Oncol* 1991, 9:458–463.

39. Taylor SG, Murthy AK, Vannetzel JM, *et al.*: Randomized comparison of neoadjuvant cisplatin and fluorouracil infusion followed by radiation versus concomitant treatment in advanced head and neck cancer. *J Clin Oncol* 1994, 12:385–395.

40. Stupp R, Vokes EE: 5-fluorouracil plus radiation for head and neck cancer. *J Infus Chemother* 1995, 5:55–60.

41. Browman GP, Cripps C, Hodson DI, *et al.*: Placebo-controlled randomized trial of infusional fluorouracil during standard radiotherapy in locally advanced head and neck cancer. *J Clin Oncol* 1994, 12:2648–2653.

42. Bachaud JM, David JM, Boussin G, Daly N: Combined postoperative radiotherapy and weekly cisplatin infusion for locally advanced squamous cell carcinoma of the head and neck: preliminary report of a randomized trial. *Int J Radiat Oncol Biol Phys* 1991, 20:243–246.

43. Brizel DM, Albers ME, Fisher SR, *et al.*: Hyperfractionated irradiation with or without concurrent chemotherapy for locally advanced head and neck cancer. *N Engl J Med* 1998, 338:1798–1804.

44. Adelstein D, Adams G, Li Y, *et al.*: A phase III comparison of standard radiation therapy (RT) versus RT plus concurrent DDP and 5-fluorouracil (5FU) in patients with unresectable squamous cell head and neck cancer: an Intergroup study [abstract]. *Proc Am Soc Clin Oncol* 2000, 19:411a.

45. Vokes E, Haraf DJ, Mick R, *et al.*: Concomitant chemoradiotherapy for intermediate stage head and neck cancer [abstract]. *Proc Am Soc Clin Oncol* 1994, 13:282.

46. Haraf DJ, Kies M, Rademaker AW, *et al.*: Radiation therapy with concomitant hydroxyurea and fluorouracil in stage II and III head and neck cancer. *J Clin Oncol* 1999, 17:638–644.

47. Kies M, Haraf DJ, Mittal B, *et al.*: Intensive combined therapy with C-DDP, 5-FU, hydroxyurea, and bid radiation (C-FHX) for stage IV squamous cancer (SCC) of the head and neck [abstract]. *Proc Am Soc Clin Oncol* 1996, 15:314.

48. Brockstein B, Haraf DJ, Stenson K, *et al.*: Phase I study of concomitant chemoradiotherapy with paclitaxel, fluorouracil, and hydroxyurea with granulocyte colony-stimulating factor support for patients with poor-prognosis cancer of the head and neck. *J Clin Oncol* 1998, 16:735–744.

49. Brockstein B, Haraf DJ, Stenson K, *et al.*: Distant metastases after concomitant chemoradiotherapy for head and neck cancer: risk is dependent upon pretreatment lymph node stage [abstract]. *Proc Am Soc Clin Oncol* 2000, 19:414a.

50. Merlano M, Vitale V, Rosso R, *et al.*: Treatment of advanced squamous-cell carcinoma of the head and neck with alternating chemotherapy and radiotherapy. *N Engl J Med* 1992, 327:1115–1121.

51. Ozsahin EM, Kutter J, Martinet S, *et al.*: Promising results using weekly concomitant boost accelerated radiotherapy and concomitant full-dose chemotherapy in locally advanced squamous cell carcinoma of the head and neck [abstract]. *Presented at the 5th International Conference on Head and Neck Cancer*. Program and Abstracts Book. 2000:S68.

52. Garden AS, Harris J, Vokes EE, *et al.*: Preliminary results of Radiation Therapy Oncology Group 97-03: a randomized phase II trial of concurrent radiation and chemotherapy for advanced squamous cell carcinomas of the head and neck. *J Clin Oncol* 2004, 22:2856–2864.

53. Bonner JA, Harari PM, Giralt J, *et al.*: Radiotherapy plus cetuximab for squamous-cell carcinoma of the head and neck. *N Engl J Med* 2006, 354:567–578.

54. Wong LY, Wei WI, Lam LK, Yuen AP: Salvage of recurrent head and neck squamous cell carcinoma after primary curative surgery. *Head Neck* 2003, 25:953–959.

55. Ganly I, Patel SG, Matsuo J, *et al.*: Results of surgical salvage after failure of definitive radiation therapy for early-stage squamous cell carcinoma of the glottic larynx. *Arch Otolaryngol Head Neck Surg* 2006, 132:59–66.

56. Gleich LL, Ryzenman J, Gluckman JL, *et al.*: Recurrent advanced (T3 or T4) head and neck squamous cell carcinoma: is salvage possible? *Arch Otolaryngol Head Neck Surg* 2004, 130:35–38.

57. Colevas AD: Chemotherapy options for patients with metastatic or recurrent squamous cell carcinoma of the head and neck. *J Clin Oncol* 2006, 24:2644–2652.

58. Forastiere AA, Metch B, Schuller DE, *et al.*: Randomized comparison of cisplatin plus fluorouracil and carboplatin plus fluorouracil versus methotrexate in advanced squamous-cell carcinoma of the head and neck: a Southwest Oncology Group study. *J Clin Oncol* 1992, 10:1245–1251.

59. Genet D, Cupissol D, Calais G, *et al.*: Docetaxel plus 5-fluorouracil in locally recurrent and/or metastatic squamous cell carcinoma of the head and neck: a phase II multicenter study. *Am J Clin Oncol* 2004, 27:472–476.

60. Gibson MK, Li Y, Murphy B, *et al.*: Randomized phase III evaluation of cisplatin plus fluorouracil versus cisplatin plus paclitaxel in advanced head and neck cancer (E1395): an Intergroup trial of the Eastern Cooperative Oncology Group. *J Clin Oncol* 2005, 23:3562–3567.

61. Glisson BS, Murphy BA, Frenette G, *et al.*: Phase II trial of docetaxel and cisplatin combination chemotherapy in patients with squamous cell carcinoma of the head and neck. *J Clin Oncol* 2002, 20:1593–1599.

62. Mrhalova M, Plzak J, Betka J, Kodet R: Epidermal growth factor receptor: its expression and copy numbers of EGFR gene in patients with head and neck squamous cell carcinomas. *Neoplasma* 2005, 52:338–343.

63. Ongkeko WM, Altuna X, Weisman RA, Wang-Rodriguez J: Expression of protein tyrosine kinases in head and neck squamous cell carcinomas. *Am J Clin Pathol* 2005, 124:71–76.

64. Soulieres D, Senzer NN, Vokes EE, *et al.*: Multicenter phase II study of erlotinib, an oral epidermal growth factor receptor tyrosine kinase inhibitor, in patients with recurrent or metastatic squamous cell cancer of the head and neck. *J Clin Oncol* 2004, 22:77–85.

65. Cohen EE, Rosen F, Stadler WM, *et al.*: Phase II trial of ZD1839 in recurrent or metastatic squamous cell carcinoma of the head and neck. *J Clin Oncol* 2003, 21:1980–1987.

66. Burtness B, Li Y, Flood W, *et al.*: Phase III trial comparing cisplatin (C) + placebo (P) to C + anti-epidermal growth factor antibody (EGFR) C225 in patients with metastatic/recurrent head and neck cancer [abstract]. *Proc Am Soc Clin Oncol* 2002, 21:226a.

67. Hong WK, Lippman SM, Itri LM, *et al.*: Prevention of second primary tumors with isotretinoin in squamous-cell carcinoma of the head and neck. *N Engl J Med* 1990, 323:795–801.

68. Bolla M, Lefur R, Ton Van J, *et al.*: Prevention of second primary tumours with etretinate in squamous cell carcinoma of the oral cavity and oropharynx. Results of a multicentric double-blind randomised study. *Eur J Cancer* 1994, 30A:767–772.

69. Khuri FR, Lee JJ, Lippman SM, *et al.*: Randomized phase III trial of low-dose isotretinoin for prevention of second primary tumors in stage I and II head and neck cancer patients. *J Natl Cancer Inst* 2006, 98:441–450.

70. van Zandwijk N, Dalesio O, Pastorino U, *et al.*: EUROSCAN, a randomized trial of vitamin A and N-acetylcysteine in patients with head and neck cancer or lung cancer. For the European Organization for Research and Treatment of Cancer Head and Neck and Lung Cancer Cooperative Groups. *J Natl Cancer Inst* 2000, 92:977–986.

Lung cancer is the leading cause of cancer-related mortality in both men and women in the United States, accounting for more than 28% of all cancer deaths in 2008. The estimated number of new cases of lung cancer in 2008 is 215,020 with an estimated 161,840 lung cancer deaths [1]. Lung cancer is the third most common cancer type in the United States after prostate and breast cancer but more Americans die from this disease than from breast, prostate, and colorectal cancer combined because of the low 14% cure rate [2]. This low rate can be ascribed almost exclusively to the high propensity for metastatic spread, lack of effective screening measures, and inability of systemic therapy to cure metastatic disease. Most patients present with inoperable stage III disease or with metastasis to distant organs (stage IV) [3]. Patients with stage IV disease are rarely cured with previous chemotherapeutic approaches [3]. A small minority of patients, between 15% and 25%, with advanced regional stage III disease with either small cell lung cancer (SCLC) or non–small cell lung cancer (NSCLC) may be cured with intensive combined-modality approaches. Surgery cures 10% to 80% of operable cases depending on stage [3]. Because most patients develop systemic disease, chemotherapy is indicated for a high percentage of patients. Chemotherapeutic options have improved considerably in recent years, with more effective and less toxic regimens now available. Chemotherapy improves symptoms, quality of life, and survival of lung cancer patients. Other agents such as erlotinib and bevacizumab are uniquely designed to block biologic pathways that are aberrant in lung cancer and are now approved for use in this disease.

ETIOLOGY AND RISK FACTORS

Most lung cancers are caused by carcinogens and tumor promoters derived from cigarette smoking (Table 10-1). Overall, the relative risk of developing lung cancer is increased about 13-fold by active smoking and about 1.5-fold by long-term passive exposure to cigarette smoke [3]. There appears to be a dose-response relationship between the lung cancer death rate and the total amount (often expressed in cigarette pack years) of cigarette smoke, such that the risk increases 60- to 70-fold for a man or woman smoking two packs a day for 20 years compared with findings in a nonsmoker. Conversely, the chance of developing lung cancer decreases with cessation of smoking but never returns to the level of the nonsmoker [4]. For this reason, more than half of all lung cancer diagnoses in the United States are now in former smokers [5].

Cigarette smoking is more common in black than white individuals. In 2006, 23% of American black and 21.9% of white individuals were smokers, although white persons smoked more cigarettes per day. The greatest differences in smoking were seen between educational groups, with a 32.7% incidence in those with less than a high school education compared with 8.5% among college graduates [6,7]. Many countries have launched programs to decrease tobacco use and to educate the public. These programs include legislative activity (*eg*, smoke-free areas, banning of tobacco advertisements), educational activities through mass media and schools, and interventional approaches targeted to groups at highest risk for developing tobacco-related cancer. The greatest impact on decreased smoking habits appears to be the stigma placed on smokers by society. These activities have reduced the percentage of the US population who smoke from a high of about 42% to about 21%. Linkage of cigarette smoking to lung cancer and other diseases has resulted in a decrease in tobacco use among men. As a result, a modest decrease in the death rate due to lung cancer has occurred among US men. The rate of lung cancer among US women finally peaked in 1991 and then plateaued from 1992 through 2004, largely due to trends in women's continued use of cigarettes that lag behind men's by 20 years [8]. Young women continue to take up the habit of cigarette smoking more rapidly than their male counterparts, suggesting that the death rate due to lung cancer will not decrease in US women for many years to come.

A small minority of lung cancer cases may be caused by exposure to other carcinogens [3]. Increases in lung cancer risk accompany exposure to carcinogens such as asbestos, radon, bis(chloromethyl) ether, polycyclic aromatic hydrocarbons, chromium, nickel, and inorganic arsenic compounds. The association with occupational exposure to these agents appears to be independent of cigarette smoking [9]; however, exposure to both increases the risk of lung cancer in an exponential manner.

PATHOLOGY

Four major cell types make up 95% of all primary lung neoplasms [10,11]. These are SCLC, squamous (epidermoid) carcinoma, adenocarcinoma (including bronchoalveolar), and large cell (undifferentiated) carcinoma (Table 10-2). The latter three cell types are often grouped together and referred to as NSCLC. The remaining 5% include carcinoids, bronchial gland tumors, and mesotheliomas. The various cell types have different

Table 10-1. Lung Cancer Etiology

Cause	Percentage
Active tobacco smoking	85
Current smoking	35
Former smoking	50
Passive tobacco exposure	3
Radon	3
Other environmental factors (*eg*, asbestos, arsenic, chloromethyl ester)	0.1–3.0

(*From* Schottenfeld [9] and Blot and Fraumeni [10].)

Table 10-2. Lung Cancer Pathology

Cell type	Frequency, %	Features
Non–small cell lung cancer		
Squamous	35	Central location; more common in men; less metastases; associated with hypercalcemia, clubbing, hypertrophic pulmonary osteoarthropathy
Adenocarcinoma (includes bronchoalveolar)	35	Peripheral in location; equal frequency in both sexes; associated with scars; metastatic potential common; most common type in nonsmokers; hypercoagulable states; associated with filtered cigarettes
Large cell	10	Peripheral in location; equal frequency in both sexes; anaplastic; undifferentiated metastatic potential
Small cell lung cancer	20	Central location; strong relationship with smoking; associated with neuroendocrine features, paraneoplastic syndromes; metastasizes widely; most sensitive to chemotherapy and radiotherapy

(*From* Travis *et al.* [11].)

natural histories and responses to therapy, and thus a correct histologic diagnosis by an experienced pathologist is the first step to correct treatment. Major treatment decisions are made on the basis of the crucial distinction between histologic classification of a tumor as SCLC or NSCLC. Therapy is discussed separately here for SCLC and NSCLC.

At one time, squamous cell carcinoma (SCC) was the most frequent of all lung cancers. SCC arises most frequently in proximal segmental bronchi and is preceded by squamous metaplasia. Because of its central location and ability to exfoliate, squamous cancers can be detected by cytologic examination in an early stage. With further growth, SCC invades the basement membrane and extends into the bronchial lumen, producing obstruction with resultant atelectasis or pneumonia. These tumors tend to be slow growing so that it is estimated that up to 3 or 4 years are required from the development of in situ carcinoma to a clinically apparent tumor. Histologically, the SCC tumor is composed of sheets of epithelial cells, which may be well or poorly differentiated. Most well-differentiated tumors demonstrate keratin pearls.

Adenocarcinoma has become the most frequent lung cancer histology in North America, accounting for about 35% to 40% of all cases of lung cancer. Most such tumors are peripheral in origin, arising from alveolar surface epithelium or bronchial mucosal glands. They also can arise from peripheral scar tumors. Adenocarcinoma appears to have a worse prognosis for operable stages than SCC because of its propensity for early metastases. Histologically, these tumors form glands and produce mucin. Bronchoalveolar carcinoma is a distinct clinicopathologic type of adenocarcinoma. This tumor appears to arise from type II pneumocytes, growing along alveolar septa by lepidic growth, and showing little if any desmoplastic or glandular change. They can present in three different fashions: a solitary peripheral nodule, multifocal disease, or a rapidly progressive pneumonic form that appears to spread from lobe to lobe, ultimately encompassing both lungs.

Large cell carcinoma is the least common of all NSCLC tumor types, accounting for about 15% of all lung cancers. Most are located peripherally and are similar to adenocarcinomas in prognosis.

SCLCs have both biologic and clinical differences from NSCLC tumors. Biologically, SCLCs have neuroendocrine features, which lead to frequent endocrine and neurologic paraneoplastic syndromes. SCLCs also have more rapid growth and a greater propensity for early metastatic spread [12]. More than 90% of patients with SCLC have mediastinal lymph node metastases and more than two thirds of cases have distant organ metastases at the time of diagnosis. SCLC has the most aggressive clinical course of any type of pulmonary tumor, with median survival from diagnosis of only 2 to 4 months without treatment. Because of its propensity for distant metastases, localized forms of treatment (*eg*, radiotherapy or surgical resection) rarely produce long-term survival [12]. SCLCs are more sensitive to chemotherapy than NSCLCs and chemotherapy represents the cornerstone of therapy.

EARLY DETECTION AND SCREENING

No method has been established as effective in early detection or screening for lung cancer [13]. Annual chest radiographs or routine sputum cytology examinations, or a combination of both, were studied in large-scale trials because they were thought to be useful as screening and early detection strategies to reduce lung cancer mortality [14–18]. The Mayo Lung Project (MLP), a randomized controlled trial that was conducted between 1971 and 1983, observed no reduction in lung cancer mortality with an intense regimen of chest radiographs and sputum cytology. Data on an extended median MLP follow-up of 20.5 years continued to demonstrate no decrease in lung cancer mortality rate [19]. Similar results have been obtained in other studies. Thus, these trials did not prove a screening role for either sputum or chest radiographs. Subsequently, the American Cancer Society, the National Cancer Institute, and other organizations resolved that large-scale radiologic and cytologic screening for lung cancer could not be justified [20]. These studies lacked the power to exclude a useful role for chest radiographs and thus, the Prostate, Lung, Colorectal and Ovarian Cancer study is currently examining the role of annual chest radiographs. Although standard sputum cytology may not be sufficiently sensitive for a routine screening examination, it remains an excellent diagnostic test for smokers with symptoms.

The new generation of spiral computed tomography (SCT) scanners has led to faster image acquisition times, with more data being captured and lower radiation exposure [21]. In the Early Lung Cancer Action Project, Henschke *et al.* [22] demonstrated low-dose SCT was superior to chest radiograph in the detection of early or resectable lung cancers. A strong correlation was found between lesion size and likelihood of cancer, with a greater percentage of lung cancers being detected by SCT (2.7%) compared with by chest radiographs (0.7%) [22]. Of those lung cancers detected by SCT, 96% were resectable and 85% were stage I. Although the rate of false-positive findings at baseline screening was high, the annual report screening showed much lower rates [22]. In 2006, the same group published the survival data of patients with stage I lung cancer detected during CT screening. Of the 31,567 patients screened from 1993 until 2005, 484 subjects were diagnosed with lung cancer. Of those patients, 85% had clinical stage I disease. The estimated 10-year survival rate was 88% in this group [23]. However, the study results had inherent biases such as lead time and over-diagnosis [24]. It also did not well define the group of patients who should be routinely screened. Thus, it appears that although SCT scan can detect early lung cancers better than chest radiographs and these patients may live longer, it also detects many nonmalignant nodules that are expensive to evaluate and is not certain to reduce lung cancer–related mortality. The National Lung Cancer Screening Trial is ongoing in an attempt to answer this question. In the trial, subjects are randomized to either SCT or chest x-ray. This type of study is necessary before SCT can be adopted as a routine screening measure.

PREVENTION OF LUNG CANCER

The fact that between 85% and 87% of lung cancers are caused by active tobacco smoking makes primary prevention an essential element of any prevention strategy. Worldwide efforts to limit tobacco usage have been relatively ineffective. In the United States, the percentage of adult smokers declined progressively from the time of the Surgeon General's report on the association between tobacco smoke and lung cancer in 1964 until 1998 when about 24.1% of the population was active smokers [25]. Unfortunately, over the past several years, the percentage of smokers has ceased to decline and may even have increased slightly. Education and public awareness can aid in preventing individuals from starting smoking and thus becoming addicted to nicotine. Other efforts are aimed at helping smokers quit. Smoking cessation efforts including physician and nurse advice and nicotine replacement therapy may increase the rate of successful quitting. Although only a minority of smokers (< 10%) are able to stop smoking successfully for 1 year or more in their first attempt, more than half have been able to stop with the assistance of health professionals [26].

The risk of lung cancer declines within 1 or 2 years after the cessation of smoking and continues to decline through at least 15 years but never reaches that of a nonsmoker [4]. Consequently, about half of the lung cancers now diagnosed in the United States are in former smokers [5]. Thus, secondary preventive measures such as chemoprevention must be considered as well. Epidemiologic evidence has supported a protective association between the consumption of large amounts of carrots and yellow and green leafy vegetables (rich in vitamin A and β-carotene) and the risk of lung cancer [27]. These compounds have relatively little toxicity when given in therapeutic doses and have been the first agents studied for the secondary prevention of lung cancer.

Two large, randomized prevention studies were completed during 1990s, the ATBC (α-Tocopherol, β-Carotene) study in Finland and CARET (β-Carotene and Retinol Efficacy Trial) in the United States. Surprisingly, both studies confirmed an increased risk of lung cancer in the group taking β-carotene [28,29]. To date, studies do not prove that we can prevent lung cancer other than with smoking cessation. However, the potential preventative effects of selenium, nonsteroidal anti-inflammatory drugs (NSAIDs), and diets high in fresh fruits and vegetables are currently under study.

STAGING AND PROGNOSIS

The most important prognostic factors for lung cancer are the stage, the patient's performance status, and the amount of weight loss before diagnosis of lung cancer. The current staging classification for NSCLC is shown in Table 10-3 [30]. The primary tumor is indicated by the T stage, which goes from the smallest lesion (< 3 cm) (T1), to the most extensive lesion with invasion of the mediastinum and great vessels, extensive pleural involvement with pleural effusion, or satellite lesions within the same lobe of the lung (T4). Regional lymph node metastases may be uninvolved (N0), involve hilar or peribronchial nodes (N1) or ipsilateral mediastinal nodes (N2), or may be extensively involved, including high paratracheal, supra-clavicular, or contralateral nodes (N3). Distant spread to other organs indicates metastatic involvement (M1). The T, N, and M designations are then used to divide patients into stages. As shown in Table 10-4, survival rates decline as the stage increases, with a 5-year survival rate of about 67% for pathologic stage IA compared with 1% for stage IV disease.

The stage of disease is based on a combination of clinical (physical examination, radiologic, and laboratory studies) and pathologic (biopsy of lymph nodes, bronchoscopy, mediastinoscopy, or other type of thoracotomy) studies. For asymptomatic patients, a complete history and physical examination, a chest radiograph and CT scan of the chest and upper abdomen to include the liver and adrenals, complete blood count, and blood chemistry are usually all that is required to determine the clinical stage. Additional studies such as magnetic resonance imaging (MRI) scans of the brain or bone scans are only indicated if there is a question of metastatic spread based on patient's symptoms, signs, or laboratory data. Evaluation should include questions regarding weight loss, focal skeletal pain, chest pain, seizures, syncope, extensive weakness, headache, and mental status changes. CT scans of the chest can provide an accurate assessment of the size of lymph nodes in the mediastinum but lymph node size is a poor predictor of cancer involvement. Thus, mediastinoscopy with biopsy of these nodes is indicated in most cases for adequate staging of nodal status. Whole-body positron emission tomography (PET) scanning is an

imaging modality that has been demonstrated to be more accurate than conventional imaging methods in the staging of NSCLC [31]. It is more effective than CT in evaluating the mediastinum, with reported sensitivity of 91% and specificity of 86% with the corresponding values of CT being 75% and 66%, respectively [31]. In a randomized trial, PET scanning was shown to reduce the costs of evaluating and treating early-stage lung cancer patients because it reduces the rate of "futile" thoracotomy.

SCLC is classified as either limited or extensive stage [12]. Limited-stage disease is confined to the hemithorax of origin, the mediastinum, or the supraclavicular lymph nodes, which are encompassable within a "tolerable" radiotherapy port. Radiation therapy cannot be delivered to an entire hemithorax. Therefore, patients with malignant pleural effusions and distant metastases are included in the classification of extensive-stage disease.

Performance status describes the functional ability of patients to carry out their usual daily activity. It is usually scored from 0 to 4 using the Eastern Cooperative Oncology Group (ECOG) scale or from 0% to 100% using the Karnofsky scale. Patients with decreased activity have a poorer prognosis and more toxicity from therapy [32]. Similarly, the degree of weight loss also correlates with a shorter survival [33]. In SCLC, other prognostic factors in addition to stage and performance status include lactate dehydrogenase (LDH) levels and gender. Patients with performance status of 0 or 1, a normal LDH level, and female gender have a better prognosis [12].

THERAPY FOR SMALL CELL LUNG CANCER

Small cell lung cancer accounts for 15% to 25% of the total lung cancer cases in the United States, with the number of cases in 2000 estimated at 34,300. At time of diagnosis, 65% to 70% of patients with SCLC present with extensive disease—metastasis beyond the ipsilateral lung and regional lymph nodes [3,12]. The remaining 30% to 35% of the cases present with limited-stage SCLC—disease confined to one lung, the mediastinum, and

Table 10-3. Staging Classification of Lung Cancer

Classification	Description
Primary tumor (T)	
TX	Primary tumor cannot be assessed or tumor is proven by the presence of malignant cells in sputum or bronchial washings but not visualized by imaging or bronchoscopy
T0	No evidence of primary tumor
Tis	Carcinoma in situ
T1	Tumor ≤ 3.0 cm in greatest diameter and surrounded by lung or visceral pleura, without evidence of invasion more proximal than the lobar bronchus (*ie*, not in the main bronchus)
T2	Tumor with any of the following features of size or extent: > 3.0 cm in greatest dimension; involving the main bronchus, > 2.0 cm or more distal to the carina; invading the visceral pleura; associated with atelactasis or obstructive pneumonitis that extends to the hilar region but does not involve the entire lung
T3	Tumor of any size with direct extension to the chest wall (including superior sulcus tumors), diaphragm, mediastinal pleura, parietal pericardium; tumor in the main bronchus < 2.0 cm distal to the carina but without involvement of the carina; associated atelactasis or obstructive pneumonitis of the entire lung
T4	Tumor of any size that invades any of the following: mediastinum, heart, great vessels, trachea, esophagus, vertebral body, carina; or tumor with a malignant pleura or pericardial effusion or with satellite tumor nodule(s) within the ipsilateral primary tumor lobe of the lung
Nodal involvement (N)	
NX	Regional lymph nodes cannot be assessed
N0	No regional lymph node metastasis
N1	Metastasis in ipsilateral peribronchial and/or ipsilateral hilar lymph nodes, including direct extension
N2	Metastasis in ipsilateral mediastinal and/or subcarinal lymph nodes
N3	Metastasis in contralateral mediastinal, contralateral hilar, ipsilateral or contralateral scalene, or supraclavicular lymph nodes
Distant metastasis (M)	
MX	Presence of distant metastasis cannot be assessed
M0	No distant metastasis
M1	Distant metastasis (beyond the ipsilateral supraclavicular nodes)

ipsilateral or contralateral supraclavicular lymph nodes or both that can be encompassed in a tolerable radiation port. SCLC has distinct histologic, clinical, and biologic features including high response rates to chemotherapy and radiation therapy, high propensity for metastases, neuroendocrine features, and paraneoplastic syndromes [12]. SCLC in general carries a poor prognosis. When untreated, the median survival time after diagnosis is only 2 to 4 months. With first-line multiagent chemotherapy, response rates approximate 80% to 90%, with complete response in 10% to 50% of

patients, depending on disease stage [12]. Survival improves to a median 8 to 12 months for extensive stage and 14 to 20 months for limited stage. Chemotherapy is the cornerstone of therapy for all patients, with concurrent radiation for those with limited stage disease and with surgery for stage I patients.

LIMITED-STAGE SMALL CELL LUNG CANCER

Patients with limited-stage SCLC are currently treated with concurrent chemotherapy and chest irradiation. This bimodal therapy was shown to be superior to either modality alone, resulting in increased complete response rate, decreased local recurrence, and improved survival [34–42]. A meta-analysis of 13 randomized trials showed a modest but significant 14% reduction in the relative mortality rate of patients receiving combined-modality therapy, with 14% of patients alive after 3 years compared with 9% in the chemotherapy-only group [34,35]. Patients receiving chemotherapy and chest irradiation experienced greater toxicity, but the gain in response and survival is thought to outweigh the increased toxicity in most instances.

The most widely used chemotherapy regimen for a combined-modality approach is EP (etoposide and cisplatin; Table 10-5) [36–40]. EP is the standard chemotherapy regimen for SCLC. It replaced the CAV (cyclophosphamide, doxorubicin, vincristine) regimen of the 1970s and the CEA (cyclophosphamide, etoposide, doxorubicin) regimen of the early 1980s largely because it was less toxic and more convenient [41]. New chemotherapy combinations are currently under investigation.

Optimal timing of concurrent radiotherapy remains somewhat undefined. Earlier studies by the National Cancer Institute of Canada (NCIC) supported the early administration of thoracic radiotherapy [42,43]. In one NCIC trial, Murray *et al.* [42] demonstrated that progression-free survival ($P = 0.036$)

Table 10-4. TNM Staging for Lung Cancer 5-Year Survival Rates

Staging	TNM	5-y survival, %
Stage 0	Tis, N0, M0	0
Stage IA	T1, N0, M0	67
Stage IB	T2, N0, M0	57
Stage IIA	T1, N1, M0	34
Stage IIB	T2, N1, M0	24
	T3, N0, M0	22
Stage IIIA	T3, N1, M0	9
	T1–3, N2, M0	13
Stage IIIB	T4, any N, M0	7
	Any T, N3, M0	3

TNM—tumor, node, metastasis.

Table 10-5. Combined Chemotherapy With EP and Thoracic Radiotherapy in Limited-Stage Small Cell Lung Cancer

Study	Chemotherapy dosage schedule	Chest radiotherapy	CR, %	PR, %	MS, *mo*	2-y survival, %	Comments
McCracken *et al.* [36]	Cisplatin 50 mg/m² IV on d 1, 8, 29, 36, 57, and 64; Etoposide 50 mg/m² IV on d 1–5, 29–33, and 57–61; Vincristine 1.4 mg/m² IV on d 15, 22, 43, and 50	45 Gy concurrent as 180 cGy/fr once daily × 25 fr on d 1–25	56	27	17.5	45	Every 4 wk × 3 cycles; PCI 30 Gy; consolidation with vincristine, methotrexate, etoposide alternating with doxorubicin and cyclophosphamide
Turrisi *et al.* [37]	Cisplatin 60 mg/m² IV on d 1; Etoposide 120 mg/m² IV on d 4, 6, and 8	45 Gy concurrent as 150 cGy/fr twice daily × 30 fr on d 1–21	78	18	20	36	Every 3 wk × 2 cycles; PCI 30 Gy; consolidation with EP alternating CAV 6 cycles
Johnson *et al.* [38]	Cisplatin 30 mg/m² IV on d 1–3; Etoposide 120 mg/m² IV on d 1–3	45 Gy alternating, as 150 cGy/fr twice daily × 30 fr on d 8–12, 29–33, and 50–54	59	38	18	44	Every 3 wk × 4 cycles; PCI optional; consolidation with cyclophosphamide/etoposide
Johnson *et al.* [39]	Cisplatin 80 mg/m² IV on d 1; Etoposide 80 mg/m² IV on d 1–3	45 Gy concurrent, as 150 cGy/fr twice daily × 30 fr on d 6–24	74	22	21.3	43	Every 4 wk × 4 cycles; PCI optional; consolidation with CAV × 4 cycles or individualized chemotherapy
Turrisi *et al.* [40]	Cisplatin 60 mg/m² IV on d 1; Etoposide 120 mg/m² IV on d 1–3	45 Gy concurrent, as 180 cGy/fr once daily × 30 fr on d 1–41	46	35.2	19 (8-y follow-up)	41.7 (2 y); 16.5 (5 y)	Every 3 wk × 4 cycles; PCI for patients in CR
	Cisplatin 60 mg/m² IV on d 1; Etoposide 120 mg/m² IV on d 1–3	45 Gy concurrent, as 150 cGy/fr twice daily × 30 fr on d 1–20	52.7	29.1	23 (8-y follow-up)	44.3 (2 y); 26 (5 y)	

CAV—cyclophosphamide, doxorubicin, vincristine; CR—complete response; EP—etoposide, cisplatin; fr—fraction; IV—intravenous; MS—median survival; PCI—prophylactic cranial irradiation; PR—partial response.

and overall survival ($P = 0.008$) were superior by starting radiotherapy concurrent and early in the course of chemotherapy. A subsequent phase 3 randomized trial from the Japan Clinical Oncology Group (JCOG) also favored the early concurrent treatment approach [44]. This group compared an early concurrent (arm C) schedule with conventional consolidative sequential (arm S) radiotherapy after platinum-etoposide therapy. Although the response rates were not significantly different between the two arms (97.4% for arm C vs 90.4% for arm S), the median survival time favored arm C (27.2 vs 19.5 months). The overall survival rates at 2 and 3 years were significantly superior in the C arm (55.3% vs 35.4% and 30.9% vs 20.7%, respectively; $P = 0.057$). Thus, these studies support the evidence that starting radiotherapy concurrent and early in the course of chemotherapy is most beneficial for long-term survival of patients with limited-stage SCLC.

Increasing the frequency of delivery of the radiotherapy by giving it twice daily in fractions that are one half (hyperfractionated) or more than the usual daily dose of accelerated hyperfractionated radiotherapy (AHRT) has also been evaluated. A randomized intergroup trial showed that the AHRT approach produced a significant improvement in local control and a small improvement in survival, but also increased toxicity [40]. The 5-year survival rates increased from 16% to 26% in the AHRT arm. It is not known whether increasing the once-daily therapy to biologically equivalent doses (eg, 65 Gy) would produce the same result. In practice either the twice-daily fractionation or a higher total dose with once-daily therapy should be chosen for good-risk patients. More recent studies adjusted the radiotherapy component by reducing volumes through using ports designed by CT scans and by using postchemotherapy volumes or shrinking fields. These studies suggest volume reductions have reduced toxicity without adversely affecting outcome. Unfortunately, patients with limited-stage SCLC who receive combined-modality therapy still have a high relapse rate at both local and distant sites [45].

Based on these and other related data, it can be concluded that four to six cycles of EP plus a course of radiotherapy (given either once or twice daily beginning with cycle 1 of chemotherapy) is an appropriate therapy for patients with limited-stage SCLC.

For the rare stage IA patient without nodal involvement or distant metastases (T1 N0; T2 N0), surgery followed by chemotherapy with or without radiotherapy appears to be a reasonable treatment option [12,46]. Cure rates exceeding 60% are reported in these instances. For stage IB, II, and III disease, surgery in addition to chemotherapy and radiotherapy failed to improve outcome [47].

EXTENSIVE-STAGE SMALL CELL LUNG CANCER

Several combinations of chemotherapeutic agents have been used over the past 20 to 30 years to manage SCLC [12]. In the 1970s and in the early part of the 1980s, the CAV combination was the most commonly used therapeutic regimen for both limited- and extensive-stage disease. In the latter, CAV demonstrated overall response rates of 55% to 65%, complete response rates of 10% to 15%, and a small number of 5-year survivors (1% to 5%) were also observed [48,49]. However, a relatively high rate of grade 4 myelosuppression, pulmonary toxicity, and neuropathy were noted with the CAV regimen. Furthermore, failure to respond to CAV meant, in general, poor response to second-line chemotherapy, usually less than 10% overall response with a dismal survival of 8 to 12 weeks. It was obvious then that the search for new combination drug regimens active in SCLC was crucial.

EP is a combination regimen demonstrating significant activity in SCLC. It was originally developed in the early 1980s as a salvage treatment for CAV-refractory SCLC [50]. The EP regimen demonstrated a response rate of 50% in patients who relapsed after induction therapy with CAV [50]. A subsequent study showed that the EP regimen used after CAV induction demonstrated significant improvement in survival compared with CAV alone [51]. Another study reported data on the use of EP as a first-line therapy in a small cohort of patients with both extensive- and limited-stage SCLC who were not candidates to receive induction therapy with the CAV regimen due to underlying cardiac history. An overall response rate of 86% (43% complete response, 43% partial response) was reported, with an increased median duration of response and survival time [52].

SCLC is highly sensitive to combination chemotherapy with high initial response rates. However, the number and duration of these responses remain limited because of the emergence of drug-resistant clones of tumor cells. The mathematical model of Goldie and Coldman [53] focuses on development of tumor cell drug resistance. It predicts that the optimal use of chemotherapeutic agents in malignant disease will involve the simultaneous use of all active agents early in the disease process. However, realization of this model is prevented due to the presence of agents with similar toxicities, mainly myelosuppression. To decrease the odds of appearance of multiply resistant tumor clones, the next best option, theoretically, would be alternation of non–cross-resistant combination agents. On this basis, the alternating CAV/EP regimens were developed and tested. In the first NCIC study, significantly higher response rate, progression-free survival, and overall survival were obtained with the alternating chemotherapy regimen. Subsequently, the Southeastern Study Group conducted a phase 3 trial composed of three induction treatment arms: arm 1, EP alone; arm 2, CAV alone; and arm 3, the alternating regimen (CAV/EP) [48]. No significant differences were shown in treatment outcome for any arm of the study in terms of response rate, complete response rate, or median survival. Myelosuppression was the dose-limiting toxicity for all patients, with incident leukopenia/granulocytopenia higher in those treated with CAV or alternating therapy (CAV/EP). The conclusion was that the combination regimens EP and CAV were equally effective induction therapies in extensive SCLC and that alternating therapy provided no therapeutic advantage compared with use of either of the individual regimens alone [48]. In a similar phase 3 Japanese study, Fukuoka et al. [49] reported results that slightly favored the alternating chemotherapy (CAV/EP) over the individual regimens of CAV and EP in a cohort of patients with both limited- and extensive-stage SCLC. In this study, the response rates/complete response rates for the EP, CAV/EP, and CAV were similar: 78%/14%, 76%/16%, and 55%/15%, respectively. Survival was also equivalent except in a subset analysis of limited disease in which the alternating regimen was preferred [49]. The conclusion from these studies is that any of these combinations could be used. Four cycles of EP were most convenient and least toxic.

Activity of carboplatin in SCLC was recognized some time after cisplatin became a standard agent. Carboplatin has the advantage of producing less nephrotoxicity, ototoxicity, neuropathy, nausea, and vomiting, and it is easier to administer. Two randomized trials showed carboplatin to be equivalent in efficacy and less toxic compared with cisplatin [54,55]. Therefore, the etoposide/carboplatin combination regimen is often used by oncologists today.

Irinotecan (CPT-11) is a water-soluble derivative of camptothecin, a potent inhibitor of DNA topoisomerase I that has demonstrated activity in a phase 2 trial conducted by Masuda et al. [56] in refractory or relapsed SCLC. The combination of irinotecan combined with cisplatin is an alternative to EP and is used as standard therapy in Japan. The JCOG demonstrated an improved survival in patients with extensive disease with this regimen [57]. Irinotecan (60 mg/m^2) infused on day 1, 8, and 15 with cisplatin (60 mg/m^2) on day 1 only was compared with EP dosed at 100 mg/m^2 on days 1, 2, and 3 and 80 mg/m^2 on day 1, respectively. Patients receiving the irinotecan combination lived longer (12.8 vs 9.4 months; $P = 0.002$). Myelosuppression was more prominent in the EP arm and diarrhea was reported only in the irinotecan/cisplatin arm. Noda et al. [58] proposed that the irinotecan/cisplatin regimen should be considered a new standard treatment for extensive-stage SCLC because of its superior results ($P > 0.01$). Irinotecan/cisplatin can be considered an acceptable therapy and is added to the standard therapies given later in this chapter. A similar study done in the United States did not demonstrate the survival advantage [59]; however, this study was criticized because the schedule and dose of irinotecan were different than the Japanese study. Reasons for these mixed results are unclear, although the different doses used in the two studies and potential inherent differences between the two populations may explain the lack of survival advantage in the US population. Published results are pending from another US study led by Southwest Oncology Group (SWOG) that is comparing the exact same doses and regimens as the Japanese study.

MAINTENANCE THERAPY

Debate continues about the optimal number of chemotherapy cycles and the role of maintenance therapy. Three large, randomized trials showed that time to progression was longer in the groups receiving maintenance chemotherapy, but no differences in survival rates were found [60–63]. Toxicity was higher in patients receiving the maintenance therapy. At present, both continued exposure to the toxic chemotherapy and the fact that patients whose disease progresses under maintenance chemotherapy tend to do poorly under salvage treatment make the discontinuation of chemotherapy after four to six cycles a preferred approach. Subsequent randomized trials using the biologic agent interferon [64] and topotecan [65] have also failed to show any improvement in survival with maintenance therapy even though in the latter study, topotecan did prolong time to progression.

SECOND-LINE THERAPY

Topotecan is another semisynthetic water-soluble analogue of camptothecin that shares similar activity with the other topoisomerase I inhibitor irinotecan. Both of these drugs stabilize a covalent DNA topoisomerase I complex to yield enzyme-linked DNA single-strand breaks [66]. The recommended starting dose of topotecan as a single agent is 1.5 mg/m^2 [66]. Schiller *et al.* [67] reported an objective response rate, median response duration, and overall median survival of 39% (no complete response), 4.8 months, and 10 months, respectively. This study confirmed the activity of single-agent topotecan in previously untreated SCLC patients.

A phase 2 study involving patients with refractory and sensitive SCLC was conducted by Ardizzoni *et al.* [68]. Refractory patients are those who never responded to first-line therapy or who responded but whose disease progressed within 3 months from the end of treatment. These patients rarely respond to second-line therapy [68]. The sensitive patient population is defined as those who responded to first-line therapy and relapse after a treatment-free interval of 3 or more months. These patients have a reasonable chance of responding to second-line chemotherapy. Ardizzoni *et al.* [68] reported an overall response rate of 6.4% and 37.8% and a median survival of 4.7 months and 6.9 months in the refractory and sensitive groups, respectively. Overall median duration of response was 7.6 months. These data stimulated a subsequent phase 3 trial conducted by von Pawel *et al.* [69] comparing CAV versus topotecan (1.5 mg/m^2) in patients with SCLC who had relapsed at least 60 days after completion of first-line therapy. These authors reported equivalent response rates of 24.3% versus 18.3%, median progression-free survival of 13.3 weeks versus 12.3 weeks, and median survival of 25 weeks versus 24.7 weeks for the topotecan versus CAV regimens, respectively. The differences were not statistically significant. Relief of patients' symptoms was more frequent with topotecan. The authors concluded that topotecan was at least as effective as CAV in the treatment of patients with recurrent SCLC and produced improvement in various symptoms to a greater degree.

THERAPY FOR OLDER PATIENTS AND THOSE IN POOR PHYSICAL CONDITION

Many older patients have several comorbid conditions in addition to SCLC, especially with a long-term history of smoking. Several studies showed that single-agent oral etoposide (VP-16) is well tolerated by this patient population, and that response and survival rates are similar to those reported in younger and healthier patients. However, randomized trials comparing oral etoposide with standard combination regimens showed that the combination regimens produce better quality of life and longer survival without increased toxicity [70,71]. Therefore, standard chemotherapy combinations are the preferred treatment for those with a poorer prognosis.

NEWER AGENTS

Unfortunately, most SCLC patients relapse and die from progressive disease. Extensive-stage SCLC patients who receive chemotherapy have a 5-year survival rate of only 1%. Thus, it has been reasonable to study new agents in untreated extensive-stage SCLC patients. Several chemotherapy agents with novel mechanisms of action have become available over the years. These include the taxanes (paclitaxel, docetaxel), the synthetic vinca alkaloid (vinorelbine), and a novel antimetabolite (gemcitabine). These drugs have demonstrated activity as single agents in SCLC [72].

The two taxanes, paclitaxel (Taxol, Bristol-Myers Squibb, Princeton, NJ) and docetaxel (Taxotere, Sanofi-Aventis, Bridgewater, NJ), are agents with broad-spectrum activity that have shown activity in SCLC. In a phase 2 ECOG study of paclitaxel in patients with extensive-stage SCLC, Ettinger *et al.* [73] reported an overall response rate of 34%. Nonresponders or partial responders subsequently received salvage chemotherapy with EP. In a similar phase 2 study by the North American Cancer Treatment Group, Kirschling *et al.* [74] reported an overall response rate of 53%. However, the response duration was short (median, 3.4 months). These authors concluded that paclitaxel was indeed an active agent in SCLC and thus attractive for use in combination regimens. The European Organization for Research and Treatment of Cancer (EORTC) reported that docetaxel at a dose of 100 mg/m^2 led to an objective response rate of 25% among 28 patients, most of whom had received prior therapy. Of their patients, however, 90% developed grade 4 neutropenia, and a significant minority of the patients developed clinically significant pulmonary effusion, ascites, and edema [75].

In a study from Greece, Mavroudis *et al.* [76] reported data on a randomized trial comparing TEP (paclitaxel, etoposide, cisplatin) with EP in a small cohort of patients with limited- and extensive-stage SCLC. The outcome (survival and response) was not improved in the three-drug combination. The study was closed early due to the increased number of toxic deaths in the TEP treatment arm. Therefore, at the present time, due to the limited number of patients, this and other triple combinations must remain experimental.

PROPHYLACTIC CRANIAL IRRADIATION

Because of the high frequency of brain metastases in SCLC, prophylactic cranial irradiation (PCI) was evaluated and shown to reduce metastases of the central nervous system (CNS). Its effects on survival prolongation were debated until a meta-analysis of all randomized trials was reported in 1999 [77]. In an initial retrospective review of seven studies in which patients had been randomized to PCI versus no PCI while in complete remission after standard induction therapy, neuropsychological impairment was reported in 76% and 15% of these patients, respectively [12]. Other studies have shown no significant difference in long-term neuropsychologic function among those patients randomized to PCI and control arm. These studies suggest that further studies on the optimal dose and schedule of PCI are needed but that it can be offered to patients with a good response to induction therapy. The Prophylactic Cranial Irradiation Overview Collaborative Group reported a 5.4% increase in the rate of survival at 3 years in favor of the treatment group (15.3% in the control group vs 20.7% in the treatment group) [77]. The treatment group was also demonstrated to have a higher rate of disease-free survival and a decrease in the cumulative index of brain metastasis. The meta-analysis also reported a significant trend toward a greater decrease in the risk of brain metastasis with larger doses of radiation. Finally, a significant trend toward a decrease in the risk of brain metastasis was observed with earlier administration of PCI after initiation of induction chemotherapy. This meta-analysis concluded that PCI does indeed improve the overall survival and disease-free survival of patients with SCLC who have achieved a complete remission after standard induction therapy [77].

THERAPY FOR NON–SMALL CELL LUNG CANCER

TREATMENT OF STAGES I AND II NON–SMALL CELL LUNG CANCER

Surgery is the primary therapy for patients with stage I and II NSCLC, with the goal of removing the entire tumor with negative resection margins [3]. Assessment of lung function by simple spirometry remains one of the most important determinants of operability. In general, a forced expiratory volume of 1 second (FEV$_1$) of at least 2.0 L (60% of predicted value), a maximum voluntary ventilatory capacity of more than 50%, or a diffusing capacity of carbon monoxide of more than 60% means that a patient likely has the pulmonary reserve to tolerate a pneumonectomy or lesser resection. For those who do not meet these criteria, smoking cessation, pulmonary rehabilitation, and intensive preoperative respiratory therapies can help. Patients continuing to have poor pulmonary function tests after these measures can still undergo resection if a postoperative predictive FEV_1 of more than 40% or 800 mL is obtained. Most often this requires a lobectomy or a pneumonectomy [3]. The latter is required in only a few cases. When the tumor is centrally located or extends into several lobes, it can only be removed in its entirety by pneumonectomy. Lesser resection, such as wedge resection, segmental resection, or sleeve lobectomy, should be reserved for patients with compromised pulmonary function who could not tolerate a lobectomy. This was shown in a Lung Cancer Study Group (LCSG) study in T1N0 NSCLC comparing limited resection with lobectomy. In this study, a higher local recurrence rate and shorter survival were noted in the limited resection group [78]. Chest wall resection and sleeve resection may be performed for T3 lesions. Sleeve resections are performed for tumors near the carina where a distal bronchus from an uninvolved lobe is sewn into the carina after resection.

Surgical therapy provides excellent results with cure rates exceeding 65% only for stage IA (T1, N0, M0) NSCLC [3,30]. No convincing evidence confirms that any adjuvant therapy including immunotherapy, radiotherapy, or chemotherapy improves survival for these patients. Because most of these patients are cured by surgery, it is probably best to reserve further study of adjuvant chemotherapy until such adjuvant therapy shows value in NSCLC patients at higher risk of relapse. However, stage I lung cancer patients resected for cure have a high risk of developing second primary tumors that exceeds the risk of disease recurrence. Because of this, patients should be encouraged to stop smoking. These patients also serve as excellent subjects for chemoprevention studies.

Most patients with stage IB to IIIA NSCLC have disease recurrence after surgical therapy and most such recurrences are in distant sites [79]. Postoperative radiation therapy in stage IB to IIIA NSCLC has been found to reduce the rate of local recurrence but has no benefit in overall survival [79,80]. A randomized trial by the LCSG investigating the efficacy of postoperative mediastinal irradiation in completely resected SCC of the lung demonstrated a reduction in local recurrence (41% to 3%), but this improvement did not translate into a survival benefit because most of the failures were distant [80]. Meta-analysis of all randomized trials of postoperative radiotherapy showed a worsening of survival, with a 21% increase in the hazard of death and a 7% decrease in the 2-year survival rate [81]. This detrimental effect was more pronounced for patients with stage I/II, N0–N1 disease, whereas for stage IIIA (N2) disease, no clear evidence confirmed any adverse effect [81]. This study has been criticized because many older studies used cobalt radiotherapy and larger ports. Nonetheless, there are no positive randomized trials concluding that radiotherapy should be considered judiciously in select patients; a randomized trial is needed to show some benefit.

The earliest studies of postoperative adjuvant chemotherapy used alkylating agents alone or in combination [82]. These studies showed no benefit for postoperative chemotherapy and in several studies, survival was actually shortened. Meta-analysis of all postoperative adjuvant studies with alkylating agent–based therapy confirmed an increased hazard ratio (HR) for death and a shortened survival [82]. These therapies were also relatively toxic, leading to considerable pessimism for the role of adjuvant chemotherapy.

After cisplatin-based chemotherapy was shown to have activity in advanced NSCLC, it was evaluated as postoperative therapy in resected patients. Many trials used the CAP regimen, comprised of cyclophosphamide, doxorubicin, and low-dose cisplatin (40 mg/m^2). Postoperative compliance was often poor. Some of these studies showed survival advantages for the chemotherapy, whereas others did not [79]. Meta-analysis showed that the cisplatin-based therapy was associated with an absolute increase of 5% in the 5-year survival rate, which was a 13% reduction in the HR of death [82]. Given the small number of patients in these studies, this survival increase was of borderline statistical significance.

The standard of care changed in 2004 with the publication of the International Adjuvant Lung Cancer Trial [83]. This trial randomized more than 1800 patients with stage I to IIIA disease after resection to either observation or cisplatin-based chemotherapy (cisplatin combined with either etoposide, vinorelbine, vinblastine, or vindesine). Patients randomized to

adjuvant therapy had an improved 5-year survival compared with those who were observed (44.5% vs 40.4%; HR for death, 0.86; 95% CI, 0.76–0.98; *P* < 0.03). The 5-year disease-free survival was also improved in those receiving adjuvant chemotherapy (39.4% vs 34.3%). Seven patients died from complications of adjuvant chemotherapy. With these data, cisplatin-based adjuvant chemotherapy is felt to be standard.

Other trials have also proven the benefit of adjuvant cisplatin-based chemotherapy in patients with stage IB to IIIA NSCLC. Two studies supported the use of the combination of cisplatin and vinorelbine as adjuvant chemotherapy: the Intergroup JBR10 trial and the ANITA (Adjuvant Navelbine International Trialist Association) trial. JBR10 randomized 482 patients with stage IB or II NSCLC to either observation or vinorelbine and cisplatin after surgery [84]. The overall survival was significantly prolonged in the adjuvant chemotherapy group (94 vs 73 months; HR for death, 0.69; *P* = 0.04). The 5-year survival was 69% for the chemotherapy group and 54% in the observation group (*P* = 0.03). In the ANITA trial, 840 patients with stage IB to IIIA NSCLC were randomized after surgery to either cisplatin and vinorelbine or observation [85]. The overall 5- and 7-year survival was improved by 8.6% to 8.4% with chemotherapy. The median survival was 65.7 months with chemotherapy and 43.7 months with observation (HR for death, 0.80; 95% CI, 0.66–0.96; *P* = 0.017).

Adjuvant chemotherapy for patients with stage IB NSCLC is somewhat controversial, particularly after the publication of the final results of the Cancer and Leukemia Group B (CALGB) 9633 trial. This trial studied a potentially less toxic combination of paclitaxel and carboplatin and included only stage IB patients [5]. The trial was stopped early after accruing 344 of the 384 patients because the interim analysis documented a significant survival benefit for adjuvant chemotherapy. As published in 2004 with a median follow-up of only 34 months, the 4-year overall survival in the chemotherapy arm was 71% versus 59% in the observation arm. However, reanalysis was performed after 54 months of follow-up. At that point, the HR for survival changed such that chemotherapy for patients with stage IB did not show an improvement in survival. The HR for overall survival changed from 0.62 to 0.8, which was no longer significant. The 5-year survival was 59% for patients receiving chemotherapy and 51% for patients followed by observation. In an unplanned subset analysis, patients with a tumor greater than or equal to 4 cm did benefit from chemotherapy (HR, 0.66; 90% CI, 0.45–0.97; *P* = 0.04). The updated CALGB data did not support adjuvant treatment of all patients with stage IB NSCLC. These data are consistent with subset analyses done in the JBR10 and ANITA trials. In these two trials, subset analysis showed that patients with resected stage IB did not gain a survival advantage if they received adjuvant chemotherapy [84,85].

NEOADJUVANT THERAPY

A phase 2 trial conducted by the Bimodality Lung Oncology Team (BLOT) demonstrated that induction chemotherapy followed by surgery produces high response rates and is safe/feasible in early-stage NSCLC [86]. The BLOT study evaluated two cycles of neoadjuvant paclitaxel and carboplatin with three additional cycles of paclitaxel/carboplatin given to patients undergoing complete resection. The objective response rate to neoadjuvant chemotherapy was 56%, the complete resection rate was 86%, and the pathologic complete response was 6%, with an estimated 1-year survival rate of 85% for all patients. The median survival was not reached, with a projected 4-year survival rate of 65%. In a French randomized phase 3 trial, Depierre *et al.* [87] demonstrated that neoadjuvant chemotherapy offers a survival advantage in resectable NSCLC. Patients with resectable stage I, II, and IIIA NSCLC were randomized to undergo direct surgery or to two cycles of neoadjuvant MIC (mitomycin, ifosfamide, and cisplatin). Two additional cycles of MIC were administered postoperatively for those who obtained objective response. Postoperative thoracic radiotherapy was given to all pT3 or pN2 patients in both arms of the study. The initial pathologic response rate was 64% (11% complete response; 53% partial response). Initial survival data favored the induction chemotherapy arm but the differences did not reach statistical significance. The median survival was 26 months and 36 months for the surgery group and neoadjuvant chemotherapy group, respectively; the 1-, 2-, and 3-year survival rates were 73%, 52%, and 41%

and 77%, 59%, and 49% for each group, respectively. Trials of other third-generation chemotherapy combinations, such as gemcitabine and cisplatin or docetaxel and cisplatin, in the neoadjuvant setting have been performed and demonstrated similar results [88,89]. Although the data are promising, randomized trials comparing neoadjuvant versus adjuvant chemotherapy are required to determine the role of this treatment approach in the routine treatment of early-stage NSCLC.

TREATMENT OF STAGE IIIA–N2 NON–SMALL CELL LUNG CANCER

The 5-year survival rates for patients with clinical stage IIIA to N2 NSCLC treated with surgery alone are poor (10%–15%). Postoperative radiotherapy improves local control but fails to improve survival [81]. The poor survival rate and high rate of distant relapse made studies of preoperative chemotherapy logical. Phase 2 studies of such an approach provided encouraging results. Typical results from some studies are summarized in Table 10-6. The Memorial Sloan-Kettering Cancer Center evaluated two or three cycles of neoadjuvant mitomycin, vinblastine, and cisplatin chemotherapy [90]. The objective response rate to chemotherapy was 77%, the complete resection rate was 78%, the pathologic complete response rate was 14%, and for all the patients, the 5-year survival rate was 17%. Nearly all the 5-year survivors were in the subgroup of patients undergoing complete resection. This subset had a 5-year survival of 26%. A group in Toronto using the same chemotherapy regimen reported a 71% response rate and a 51% complete resection rate [91]. The median survival rate was 21.3 months. The 5-year survival rates were encouraging (< 20%).

A large phase 2 trial by the CALGB evaluated 74 patients with stage IIIA NSCLC treated with two cycles of vinblastine/cisplatin before complete resection, followed by chest irradiation in patients who had incomplete resection or no response to chemotherapy [92] (Table 10-6). The objective response plus stable disease rate was 88%. In the study, 86% of patients were treated with surgery and 36% had complete resection. The 3-year overall survival rate was 23%, with median survivals of 20.9 months in patients undergoing complete resection and 17.8 months in those with incomplete resection compared with 8.5 months in patients whose tumors were not resected. A SWOG phase 2 study was done to assess the feasibility of concurrent chemotherapy and irradiation followed by surgery in locally advanced NSCLC [93]. This study reported 85% resectability for the stage IIIA (N2) group and 80% resectability for the IIIB group (Table 10-6). The 2- and 3-year survival rates were 37% and 27%, respectively. The 6-year outcome from this SWOG trial was later reported by Albain et al. [94]. The long-term survival level was at 20% and was still identical for patients with both bulky IIIA (N2) and IIIB tumors treated with trimodality therapy. Those authors also reported that nearly 50% of patients with T4 N0 to N1 tumors survived 6 years after resection of stable disease. Furthermore, they concurred that clearance of mediastinal nodal involvement remains the strongest favorable outcome predictor for patients with initial N2/N3 disease [94].

Encouraging results of these phase 2 neoadjuvant studies led to two prospective phase 3 randomized trials using neoadjuvant cisplatin-based chemotherapy. In the Spanish trial, Rosell et al. [95,96] compared the MIC chemotherapy regimen for three cycles followed by surgery versus surgery alone. The median survival of 26 versus 8 months and the 3-year survival of 25% vs 0% favored the chemotherapy arm. In the M.D. Anderson Cancer

Center study, Roth et al. [97,98] compared preoperative chemotherapy with cisplatin/cyclophosphamide/etoposide for three cycles followed by surgery versus surgery alone. Postoperative chemotherapy was also administered and postoperative radiotherapy was allowed at the discretion of the physician. Results again favored the chemotherapy arm, with an improved median survival of 64 versus 11 months and 3-year survival of 56% versus 15%. Both these studies had a small number of patients (60 in each study). Further accrual was appropriately halted based on ethical considerations due to the highly statistically significant improvement in survival associated with the chemotherapy arm. Recent data on the 7-year follow-up of patients enrolled in both of these randomized studies revealed that the increase in survival conferred by perioperative chemotherapy was maintained during the period of extended observation [96,98]. Many physicians concluded that these studies showed that single-modality surgical therapy for preoperatively defined N2 disease could no longer be justified.

The optimal combined therapy approach remains undefined. Excellent results have been achieved with chemotherapy plus surgery, with chemotherapy plus radiotherapy, and with all three modalities. The North American Intergroup trial in stage III disease (INT-0139) compared concurrent induction chemotherapy/radiotherapy (61 Gy) with chemotherapy/radiotherapy (45 Gy) followed by surgical resection. This study targeted primarily stage IIIA–N2 patients and required pathologic documentation of N2 involvement [99]. In 2005, Albain et al. [100] presented updated data from this trial. The 5-year progression-free survival was 22.4% for the surgical group and 11.1% for the definitive radiation group (logrank $P = 0.017$). However, the two groups did not differ in their median survival (23.6 vs 22.2 months, respectively; $P = 0.24$). The mortality rate observed on the surgical arm was 7.9% compared with 2.1% on the definitive radiation arm. On the arm of neoadjuvant therapy followed by surgery, patients undergoing pneumonectomy had a 26% postoperative death rate compared with only 1% in patients undergoing a lobectomy.

A major remaining controversy is whether preoperative therapy (chemotherapy or chemotherapy/radiotherapy) should now be considered the standard of care in stage IIIA disease. Experts note that the two major subsets of stage III disease must be considered as separate entities. For unresectable, stage IIIA/bulky N2 or IIIB disease, surgery after chemotherapy/radiotherapy has not been proven to be superior to chemotherapy/radiotherapy alone and thus cannot be considered the standard of care [99]. Conversely, long-term survival data reported in both the Rosell et al. [95] and Roth et al. [97] landmark studies supports consideration of preoperative therapy in selected patients with stage IIIA disease. Patients with minimal stage IIIA disease that is technically resectable appear to be the ideal population to benefit from preoperative therapy, assuming the multimodality team involved is experienced in this approach and works in a collaborative manner to maximize the efficacy and minimize potential toxicities.

TREATMENT OF STAGE IIIB NON–SMALL CELL LUNG CANCER

Radiotherapy was the primary therapy for stage IIIB NSCLC for many years because it alleviated symptoms and because between 5% and 10% of patients survived at 5 years [3]. Survival of patients with locally advanced unresectable NSCLC treated with radiotherapy is poor, with a median survival of only 9 to 10 months. The addition of chemotherapy was tested to evalu-

Table 10-6. Selected Phase 2 Neoadjuvant Results in Stage IIIA Non–Small Cell Lung Cancer

Study	Treatment	Patients, n	Response rate, %	Median survival, mo	Survival*, %
Martini et al. [90]	MVP	136	77	19	17 (5)
Burkes et al. [91]	MVP	55	71	21	20 (5)
Sugarbaker et al. [92]	VP	74	88†	20.9	33 (3)
Albain et al. [93,94]	EP + RT	75	88†	13	20 (6; stage IIA); 22 (6; stage IIIB)

*Percent of patients alive at 1 year indicated in parentheses.
†Includes stable disease and responders.
EP—etoposide, cisplatin; MVP—mitomycin, vinblastine, cisplatin; RT—radiation therapy; VP—vinblastine, cisplatin.

ate its ability to improve local control and eliminate or delay the emergence of metastatic disease. Multiple randomized trials of radiotherapy alone versus radiotherapy plus chemotherapy have been completed, most of which showed survival advantage for the combined approach (Table 10-7).

The CALGB, using sequential chemotherapy–radiotherapy, compared two cycles of cisplatin and vinblastine induction chemotherapy followed by chest irradiation with radiotherapy alone in patients with stage III NSCLC [101]. The median survival rates were 13.8 months and 9.7 months for the combined modality and the radiotherapy group alone, respectively ($P = 0.0066$). Survival rates at 2 and 3 years were 24% and 23% and 14% and 11%, respectively. After more than 7 years of follow-up, long-term survival remained greater for the chemotherapy/radiotherapy group (5-year survival rate of 17% vs 6%) [102]. The superiority of this combined regimen was confirmed by a subsequent Radiation Therapy Oncology Group (RTOG) study that compared standard radiation therapy with induction chemotherapy of cisplatin and vinblastine followed by twice-daily radiation therapy in unresectable NSCLC patients [103]. The combined-modality arm was statistically superior to the other two treatment arms (median and 1-year survival of 13.8 months and 60% compared with 11.4 months and 46% in the standard arm and 12.3 months and 51% in the hyperfractionated arm).

A French group [104] compared the effects of standard radiotherapy alone (arm 1) with those of sequential chemotherapy–radiotherapy (arm 2) in unresectable NSCLC. Patients in arm 2 received three cycles of VCPC (vindesine, cyclophosphamide, cisplatin, and lomustine), with three additional cycles of VCPC administered after radiotherapy to patients with stable disease. The objective response rates were 35% (20% complete response) and 31% (16% complete response) for patients on arms 1 and 2, respectively. The rate of distant metastases at 2 years was 64% in the radiotherapy group compared with 43% in the combined-modality group ($P < 0.001$). The combined-modality therapy was associated with significant improvement in length of survival (median survival, 12 vs 10 months) and reduced incidence of distant disease.

A concurrent combined-modality approach was evaluated in an EORTC phase 3 trial in inoperable, nonmetastatic NSCLC. This study compared split-course radiation therapy alone with split-course radiation therapy combined with cisplatin, given either weekly or daily [105]. Survival significantly improved in the combination group compared with the findings in the radiotherapy-only group ($P = 0.009$). Also noted was improved local control in the daily cisplatin/radiotherapy group ($P = 0.003$), suggesting that this schedule results in maximal radiation enhancement.

A randomized study of hyperfractionated radiation therapy with or without concurrent chemotherapy of carboplatin and etoposide in stage III NSCLC was conducted by Jeremic *et al.* [106]. The median and 3-year survival rates were significantly better for the chemotherapy groups (13 months and 16% in the high-dose carboplatin arm vs 18 months and 23% in the low-dose carboplatin arm vs 8 months and 6.6% in the radiation-only arm). There was a higher incidence of acute and/or late high-grade toxicity in the combined groups; even so, no patients died as a result of treatment-related toxicity. A subsequent study was performed by the same group comparing hyperfractionated radiation therapy with or without concurrent low-dose daily carboplatin (50 mg) and etoposide (50 mg). A significantly longer survival time was found in the group receiving both radiation and chemotherapy (median survival, 22 vs 14 months; 4-year survival rate, 23% vs 9%) [107].

Meta-analysis of 14 randomized trials of combination therapy and radiotherapy alone in locally advanced unresectable NSCLC was subsequently done [108]. Compared with radiotherapy alone, combined chemotherapy/radiotherapy reduced the risk for death by 12% at 1 year, 13% by 2 years, and 17% by 3 years. When considered separately, trials of concurrent and sequential chemotherapy yielded similar treatment effects. The addition of chemotherapy to radiotherapy was associated with a 10% to 20% decrease in the risk for death. When the analysis was restricted only to the trials in which cisplatin was used as part of the chemotherapy regimen, the results were similar. Any absolute benefit should be balanced against the increased toxicity associated with the addition of chemotherapy. A UK study showed an improved quality of life when chemotherapy was added to radiation therapy for patients with localized disease [109]. Meta-analysis showed that the combination of chemotherapy and radiotherapy, either concurrently or sequentially, had a positive effect on survival and quality of life. The optimal approach, however, must be further delineated.

The West Japan Lung Cancer Group data on a randomized trial comparing concurrent versus sequential thoracic radiotherapy in combination with mitomycin, vindesine, and cisplatin in unresectable stage III NSCLC [110] are listed in Table 10-7. This group demonstrated a significantly better response rate and survival with the concurrent chemoradiotherapy regimen compared with sequential therapy. A response rate of 84% versus 66% ($P = 0.0002$) and a median survival of 16.5 months versus 13.3 months ($P = 0.03998$) were reported for the concurrent and sequential arms, respectively. The 2-, 3-, 4-, and 5-year survival rates were also superior for the concurrent group (34.6%, 22.3%, 16.9%, and 15.8%, respectively) compared with findings in the sequential group (27.4%, 14.7%, 10.1%, and 8.9%, respectively). A similar randomized trial by RTOG compared two concurrent cisplatin-based

Table 10-7. Randomized Trials of Sequential or Concurrent Chemotherapy and Radiation Therapy

Study	Patients, *n*	Chemotherapy + RT schedule	Type	Median survival*, *mo*	2-y survival*, %
Dillman *et al.* [101,102]	155	Cisplatin/vinblastine × 2 cycles followed by RT 60 Gy over 6 wk	Sequential	13.8 vs 9.7	24 vs 12 (2 y); 23 vs 11 (3 y); 17 vs 6 (5 y)
Sause *et al.* [103]	452	Cisplatin/vinblastine × 2 cycles followed by RT 60 Gy over 6 wk	Sequential	13.8 vs 11.4	30 vs 19
Le Chevalier *et al.* [104]	353	VCPC × 3 cycles followed by 65 Gy over 5.5 wk then VCPC × 3 cycles	Sequential	12 vs 10	21 vs 14
Schaake-Koning *et al.* [105]	308	Cisplatin + 30 Gy over 2 wk + 25 Gy over 2 wk (split)	Concurrent	13 vs 12	25 vs 13
Takada *et al.* [110]	314	MVP + 28 Gy over 3 wk followed by 28 Gy over 3 wk	Concurrent	16.5	34.6
		MVP followed by 56 Gy	Sequential	13.3	27.4
Curran *et al.* [111]	611	Cisplatin/vinblastine + RT 60 Gy starting d 1	Concurrent	17.0	NR
		Cisplatin/vinblastine followed by RT 60 Gy starting d 50	Sequential	14.6	NR
		Cisplatin/etoposide + RT 69.6 Gy in twice-daily fractions starting d 1	Concurrent (twice-daily RT)	15.6	NR

*Chemotherapy plus RT versus RT alone.
MVP—mitomycin, vinblastine, cisplatin; NR—not reported; RT—radiation therapy; VCPC—vindesine, lomustine, cyclophosphamide, cisplatin.

chemotherapy and thoracic radiotherapy regimens with a standard sequential chemotherapy (cisplatin and vinblastine) combined with radiotherapy approach [111]. With a median follow-up of 40 months, the data revealed a significantly improved median survival time of 17 months for the concurrent therapy arm compared with 14.6 months for the sequential therapy arm. It appears then that, in good performance status patients with unresectable stage III NSCLC, the concurrent approach of chemoradiation therapy yields significantly increased response and enhanced median survival rates when compared with the sequential approach.

Currently in the United States, some of the most common combination chemotherapy and radiotherapy regimens consist of either cisplatin and etoposide or carboplatin and paclitaxel. Concurrent cisplatin and etoposide followed by consolidation chemotherapy has been studied by SWOG in studies S9019 and S9504 [93,112]. The S9019 trial treated patients with stage IIIB disease (T4N0/1, T4, N2 or N3) with combination cisplatin (50 mg/m^2/d on days 1, 8, 29, and 36) and etoposide (50 mg/m^2/d on days 1–5 and 29–33) concurrently with once-daily thoracic radiation (61 Gy), followed by two additional cycles of cisplatin plus etoposide. In the 50 eligible patients, the median survival was 15 months, and the 3- and 5-year survival was 58% and 15%, respectively. The most common toxicity was grade 4 neutropenia (32%), with grade 3/4 esophagitis occurring in 20%. Using the information gained in this study, S9504 was designed to evaluate the use of docetaxel as consolidation chemotherapy instead of cisplatin and etoposide. S9504 used the same concurrent chemoradiation schedule and combination followed by docetaxel (75 mg/m^2 for three cycles). In this study of 83 eligible patients, median survival was 26 months with a 3-year survival rate of 76%.

Concurrent carboplatin and paclitaxel with radiotherapy has also been studied [113]. This trial was a randomized phase 2 study of patients with unresectable IIIA and IIIB disease. Patients were either randomized to sequential induction paclitaxel (200 mg/m^2) and carboplatin (area under the curve [AUC] = 6) for two cycles followed by radiation (63 Gy), induction paclitaxel and carboplatin followed by concurrent paclitaxel (45 mg/m^2) and carboplatin (AUC = 2) once a week with radiation, or the same concurrent chemo-radiation regimen followed by consolidation full-dose paclitaxel and carboplatin. The median overall survival was 13, 12.7, and 16.3 months, respectively, for the three arms; the 3-year survival rates were 17%, 15%, and 17%, respectively. Induction chemotherapy resulted in grade 3/4 neutropenia in 32% to 38% of patients. Grade 3/4 esophagitis occurred in 19% to 28% of the patients treated with concurrent paclitaxel/carboplatin and radiation.

Most physicians feel that survival is improved with combination chemotherapy and radiation. However, several questions remain to be answered: Which chemotherapy regimen is best to combine with radiation and is consolidation chemotherapy needed? The role of consolidation chemotherapy remains to be defined.

THERAPY OF STAGE IV NON–SMALL CELL LUNG CANCER

Until the past several years, considerable pessimism endured about the role of chemotherapy in advanced NSCLC [114,115]. No agent consistently produced objective responses in more than 20% of patients, and no evidence showed that chemotherapy prolonged the survival of these patients. During the 1980s, several randomized trials compared cisplatin-based chemotherapy combinations with best supportive care (BSC). All these studies showed superior survival results with the cisplatin therapy; however, this difference was not always statistically significant. Meta-analysis showed a highly statistically significant survival advantage for patients receiving cisplatin-based therapy. However, the survival advantage was modest [82]. A randomized study by the NCIC showed a median survival of 33 weeks in patients treated with chemotherapy compared with 17 weeks in patients treated with BSC [115]. The 1-year survival rate more than doubled from 10% to more than 20% and symptoms improved in responding patients. In the meta-analysis, cisplatin-based combinations significantly improved median survival by about 2 months with a 10% (from 10%–20%) increase in the percentage of patients alive at 1 year [82]. Combination chemotherapy also improved quality of life and palliated symptoms. A UK study showed that chemotherapy (MIC) significantly improved quality of life in addition to median survival compared with standard treatment in inoperable NSCLC of both stages III and IV [109].

As with SCLC, six novel chemotherapy agents demonstrated significant activity in the treatment of NSCLC. The low response rate and survival benefits from older standard platinum-based regimens (*eg*, EP) made the discovery of these more effective agents imperative. During the 1990s, a series of phase 1/2 clinical trials of these agents alone or in combination with a platinum-containing agent were conducted. The single agent and its combination with a platinum agent demonstrated superior overall response rates and survival gains compared with standard therapy [114,116]. Two randomized trials comparing single-agent paclitaxel and docetaxel to BSC showed significantly improved survival with the taxane and a reduction in the hazard of death of more than 30%, which is superior to the 26% reduction from cisplatin-based therapies [117,118]. Two other randomized trials conducted to compare the combination of vinorelbine or gemcitabine plus cisplatin with single-agent cisplatin both confirmed the superiority of the combination regimen [119,120]. This led to two subsequent randomized studies comparing the standard EP regimen [121] or teniposide/cisplatin [122] with paclitaxel/cisplatin. The reported data favored the paclitaxel/cisplatin arm with superior overall response rate and median survival [121]; there was no significant difference in median survival between arms in the study by Giaccone *et al.* [122]. These optimal results standardized a novel agent plus platinum combination as the primary treatment regimen for patients with advanced-stage NSCLC [114,116].

SWOG subsequently conducted the first randomized trial comparing two novel agents plus cisplatin combinations [123] (Table 10-8). Patients were randomized to vinorelbine/cisplatin or to paclitaxel/carboplatin. The overall response rate (28% vs 25%), median survival time (8 months on both treatment arms), and 1-year survival rates (36% vs 38%) were nearly identical. Both regimens were well tolerated. Either combination regimen was then recommended by SWOG for treatment of advanced-stage NSCLC. A subsequent four-arm randomized phase 3 trial conducted by ECOG compared three two-drug combinations with a cisplatin/paclitaxel control arm [124] (Table 10-8). Patients were randomized to cisplatin/paclitaxel, cispla-

Table 10-8. Randomized Trials of New Drug Combinations

Study	Regimen	Patients, *n*	Response rate, %	Median survival, *mo*	1-y survival, %
Wozniak *et al.* [119]	Cisplatin 100 mg/m^2 every 3 wk + vinorelbine 25 mg/m^2/wk × 3 cycles	214	25	8	33
	Cisplatin 100 mg/m^2 every 4 wk	218	10	6	12
Kelly *et al.* [123]	Paclitaxel 225 mg/m^2 over 3 h + carboplatin (AUC = 6) on d 1	207	27	8	36
	Vinorelbine 25 mg/m^2/wk + cisplatin 100 mg/m^2 every 3 wk	201	27	8	33
Schiller *et al.* [124]	Paclitaxel 135 mg/m^2 over 24 h on d 1 + cisplatin 75 mg/m^2 on d 2 every 3 wk	292	21.3	7.8	31
	Cisplatin 100 mg/m^2 on d 1 + gemcitabine 1000 mg/m^2 on d 1, 8, and 15 every 4 wk	288	21	8.1	36
	Cisplatin 75 mg/m^2 on d 1 + docetaxel 75 mg/m^2 over 1 h on d 1 every 3 wk	293	17.3	7.4	31
	Carboplatin (AUC = 6) on d 1 + paclitaxel 225 mg/m^2 over 3 h on d 1 every 3 wk	290	15.3	8.2	35

AUC—area under the curve.

tin/gemcitabine, cisplatin/docetaxel, and to carboplatin/paclitaxel. Neither the median survival (7.8, 8.1, 7.4, and 8.2 months, respectively), overall response rates (21.3%, 21%, 17.3%, and 15.3%, respectively), nor the 1-year survival rates (31%, 36%, 31%, and 35%, respectively) were significantly different in any of the four arms. Overall toxicity was similar in each treatment arm, except for a higher grade 3/4 thrombocytopenia and anemia rate in the cisplatin/gemcitabine arm compared with the control arm ($P = 0.05$). The carboplatin/paclitaxel combination had significantly less grade 4/5 toxicity. Therefore, all these combination regimens are currently recommended by ECOG for the treatment of advanced-stage NSCLC.

More recently, docetaxel has also been studied in combination with platinum agents. The TAX 326 study group conducted a large, multicenter, phase 3 study randomizing 1218 patients with advanced NSCLC to three arms: docetaxel and cisplatin, docetaxel and carboplatin, and vinorelbine and cisplatin. The docetaxel/cisplatin arm demonstrated a significantly improved median survival time (11.3 vs 10.1 months) and response rate (31.6% vs 24.5%) over the vinorelbine/cisplatin arm. There was no significant difference in survival or response rate between the docetaxel/carboplatin and vinorelbine/cisplatin arms. One- and 2-year survival rates were 46% versus 41%, and 21% versus 14% in the docetaxel/cisplatin and vinorelbine/cisplatin arms, respectively. This study demonstrated that a docetaxel/platinum combination is an effective treatment alternative for first-line use in patients with advanced NSCLC [125].

THREE-DRUG REGIMEN (TRIPLE THERAPY) IN NON–SMALL CELL COMBINATION THERAPY

The SWOG 9805 and ECOG 1594 studies established five acceptable novel agent/platinum combinations for the treatment of advanced NSCLC [123,124]. The next approach is how to use these agents in future trials to improve survival rates in these patients. An established approach has been the addition of a second novel agent to the new double combinations. Although three-drug regimens have not consistently demonstrated superiority over two-drug regimens, introduction of a novel agent has been a reasonable approach. Thus far, only one such agent, bevacizumab, has been approved for use with chemotherapy in patients with metastatic NSCLC. Bevacizumab is a monoclonal antibody that binds vascular endothelial growth factor (VEGF). This antibody is thought to block tumor blood vessel growth and potentially improve chemotherapy delivery to the tumor. In ECOG 4599 [126], bevacizumab (15 mg/kg) was combined with paclitaxel (200 mg/m^2) and carboplatin (AUC = 6) and given together once every 3 weeks for up to six cycles; then bevacizumab was given as maintenance until progression in patients who had stable or responding disease. Patients with nonsquamous histology stage IIIB with effusion or stage IV disease were randomized to chemotherapy alone or chemotherapy plus bevacizumab. The median survival was 12.3 months versus 10.3 months, respectively, for the three-drug combination versus the chemotherapy-alone arm, and the response rate was 35% versus 15%. Despite the increase in toxicities with the bevacizumab arm, particularly hypertension, neutropenia, and bleeding, based on this study, the combination was approved in the United States for patients with metastatic nonsquamous cell NSCLC.

NONPLATINUM DOUBLE THERAPY IN ADVANCED-STAGE NON–SMALL CELL LUNG CANCER

Cisplatin is a highly toxic and inconvenient agent. The development of non-platinum combinations could reduce overall toxicity and increase convenience. Therefore, a series of phase 3 trials of nonplatinum combinations compared with platinum combinations has been conducted. Three studies compared gemcitabine/paclitaxel to platinum combinations [127,128]. The combination of docetaxel/gemcitabine was evaluated by investigators in four phase 3 trials [129–132]. A gemcitabine/vinorelbine combination has also been studied and is a feasible doublet [133–137]. Most trials of the nonplatinum doublet versus a platinum combination revealed similar survival, response, and toxicity rates.

Docetaxel/irinotecan double therapy has also undergone phase 2 evaluation. Takeda *et al.* [138] reported a response rate of 34% with median survival and 1-year survival of 9.8 months and 38%, respectively. A subsequent

randomized phase 3 trial conducted by the West Japan Thoracic Oncology Group [139] compared standard docetaxel/cisplatin double therapy with a docetaxel/irinotecan combination. The reported response rates and median survival were 40.9% and 8.5 months for the docetaxel/cisplatin arm and 35% and 9.8 months for the docetaxel/irinotecan arm, respectively. No statistical interarm difference was found. Thus, docetaxel/cisplatin double therapy has a comparable activity and toxicity profile when compared with docetaxel/irinotecan.

In conclusion, non–platinum-containing doublet therapy appears to have an activity and toxicity profile similar to that of the current standard cisplatin-containing regimens. Therefore, these nonplatinum doublet therapies are standard options for first-line therapy of advanced-stage NSCLC in general oncology practice. Differences in toxicity profiles will help guide each practitioner in choosing which regimen to use in a patient in whom platinum is not an option for first-line therapy.

SECOND-LINE CHEMOTHERAPY FOR REFRACTORY AND RELAPSED NON–SMALL CELL LUNG CANCER

Before the introduction of newer agents into the treatment of advanced NSCLC, no therapy had been proven to improve survival of NSCLC patients in the second-line setting. This situation has now changed because docetaxel, pemetrexed, and erlotinib have been shown to improve survival in this regard. Two randomized studies of second-line docetaxel in patients previously treated with cisplatin-based chemotherapy showed a survival advantage for the taxane arm. In the TAX 320 study [125], patients were randomized to either docetaxel 100 mg/m^2 (D100 arm) or 75 mg/m^2 (D75 arm) versus a control regimen of vinorelbine or ifosfamide. The authors reported significantly different response rates in the docetaxel arms (10.8% with D100 and 6.7% with D75) compared with 0.8% with the control arm. The patients in the docetaxel arms also had a longer time to progression ($P = 0.046$) and longer progression-free survival ($P = 0.005$). The best survival data were obtained in the D75 arm, in which 32% of the patients were alive at 1 year, compared with 21% and 19% in the D100 and control arms, respectively ($P = 0.025$). In a subsequent multicenter, international, randomized phase 3 trial conducted by Shepherd *et al.* [140], patients with similar characteristics were randomized to receive either D100, D75, or BSC. The overall response rate of 7.1% in this trial was similar to that obtained in the TAX 320 trial. The median survival and overall 1-year survival rates were significantly different for the docetaxel patients (7.0 months and 29%) compared with the BSC patients (4.6 months and 19%). Survival data were again significantly better for the D75 patients compared with the BSC patients, with reported median and 1-year survival of 7.5 months and 37% and 4.6 months and 11%, respectively. In conclusion, single-agent docetaxel improves survival of NSCLC patients in the second-line setting. Docetaxel 75 mg/m^2 every 21 days appears to be the optimal dose and has been approved by the US Food and Drug Administration for use in this setting.

Pemetrexed is a novel, multitargeted antifolate agent. This agent is approved for use as second-line treatment based on a phase 3 study comparing it with docetaxel [141]. Patients with previously treated advanced NSCLC were randomized to receive either pemetrexed 500mg/m^2 intravenously (IV) on day 1 or docetaxel 75 mg/m^2 IV on day 1. The overall response rate was 9.1% and 8.8% for pemetrexed and docetaxel, respectively. The median overall survival was 8.3 versus 7.9 months, which was not statistically significant. However, patients treated with pemetrexed had fewer side effects compared with docetaxel. Grade 3/4 neutropenia was experienced in 40.2% of patients treated with docetaxel compared with 5.3% of those treated with pemetrexed. Febrile neutropenia occurred in 12.7% versus 1.9% of patients treated with docetaxel or pemetrexed, respectively. Only 6.4% developed any grade of alopecia if treated with pemetrexed compared with 37.7% treated with docetaxel. Anemia and thrombocytopenia rates were similar. Thus, treatment with pemetrexed had equal efficacy but less toxicity compared with docetaxel in the second-line treatment setting.

Erlotinib is an oral epidermal growth factor receptor (EGFR) tyrosine kinase inhibitor. Erlotinib is approved for use in the second- and third-line setting for NSCLC based on a phase 3 trial comparing erlotinib to placebo in patients with advanced NSCLC whose disease had progressed on at least one prior chemotherapy [142]. The standard erlotinib dosage is 150 mg by mouth once a day. Patients treated with erlotinib had a 9% response rate and an overall survival rate of 6.7 months compared with 4.7 months in patients treated with placebo. The common toxicities of erlotinib include rash and diarrhea. Multiple groups have evaluated ways to predict improved response and survival to erlotinib. Studies from Boston and New York have shown that mutations of the EGFR tyrosine kinase are associated with increased response to EGFR tyrosine kinase inhibitors [143–145]. Tsao *et al.* [146] published data on EGFR staining by immunohistochemistry (IHC), and EGFR gene amplification (fluorescence in situ hybridization [FISH]) using tumor samples from the phase 3 trial of erlotinib versus placebo [146]. Patients with EGFR IHC-positive tumors had a HR for death if treated with erlotinib of 0.68 (95% CI, 0.49–0.95; P = 0.02). Patients with EGFR amplification had a HR of death of 0.44 (95% CI, 0.23–0.82; P = 0.008); however, the patients with EGFR mutations had a HR for death of 0.77 (95% CI, 0.40–1.50; P = 0.45). Thus so far, no one test consistently predicts both improved survival and increased response. Further studies are being performed to refine these techniques and their use in selecting the appropriate patients for EGFR tyrosine kinase inhibitor therapy.

FIRST-LINE THERAPY IN OLDER PATIENTS WITH ADVANCED NON–SMALL CELL LUNG CANCER

Older patients with advanced NSCLC are often unsuitable for cisplatin-based chemotherapy. Therefore, clinical investigators have devoted great efforts to identifying optimal and less toxic chemotherapeutic regimens for such patients with advanced NSCLC. Several subgroup analyses have been performed and reveal that survival is similar between the elderly versus the younger population, although, the elderly population is more prone to toxicities. Few elderly-specific phase 3 trials have been performed to date. Two agents that have been explored in several trials of elderly patients with NSCLC are vinorelbine and gemcitabine.

In a phase 2 study of single-agent vinorelbine, Grldelli *et al.* [147] reported a response rate of 23%, with high rates of symptom regression and improvement in performance status in elderly people with advanced NSCLC. Vinorelbine, as a single agent, was well-tolerated by this patient population. The Elderly Lung Cancer Vinorelbine Italian Study (ELVIS) Group conducted a multicenter randomized study to compare the efficacy of single-agent vinorelbine to supportive care alone in terms of quality of life and survival in older patients with advanced NSCLC [148]. In this trial, vinorelbine prolonged survival and had a positive impact on quality of life compared with supportive care. The median survival increased from 21 to 28 weeks (P = 0.03) in patients receiving vinorelbine, with survival rates at 6 and 12 months of 41% and 14% and 55% and 32% for the control and vinorelbine arms, respectively. The patients treated with vinorelbine also scored better than the control arm on quality-of-life functional scales. They also reported reduced lung cancer–related symptoms.

A subsequent randomized phase 3 trial conducted by the Southern Italy Cooperative Oncology Group compared the impact on survival and quality of life of the gemcitabine/vinorelbine combination with that of single-agent vinorelbine in elderly people with advanced NSCLC [149]. The combination arm was associated with significantly better survival (median survival time, 7.3 months) in comparison with the single-agent vinorelbine arm

(median survival time, 4.5 months). The reported overall response rates were 22% and 15% for the combination and vinorelbine arms, respectively. In addition, the quality-of-life score worsened for 60% of the patients in the vinorelbine arm versus 40% of patients in the gemcitabine/vinorelbine arm. The superior results obtained with this novel combination therapy are rather encouraging, particularly because no significantly different toxicity profile was observed between the two arms.

In conclusion, vinorelbine and gemcitabine have each demonstrated optimal activity and toxicity profiles in older patients with advanced NSCLC. The results of the ELVIS trial are convincing, and in clinical practice single-agent therapy or the doublet therapy should be considered when discussing treatment options with older patients with advanced NSCLC.

CONCLUSIONS

Chemotherapy is a major component of therapy for both SCLC and NSCLC patients. Completely resected stage I NSCLC patients have a high risk of developing second primary tumors and should be encouraged to stop smoking as well as be considered for screening and chemoprevention studies. For resectable NSCLC, stage IB, IIA, and IIB NSCLC patients, randomized trials with preoperative or postoperative chemotherapy have demonstrated an improvement in survival with cisplatin-based combination chemotherapy, although adjuvant therapy for patients with stage IB remains controversial. In this setting, postoperative cisplatin therapy showed a 13% reduction in the hazard rate of death, translating into a 5% absolute increase in 5-year survival. In addition, preoperative cisplatin therapy reduced the hazard rate of death by 23%, which led to a 10% improvement in 5-year survival.

For patients with stage III disease, chemotherapy improves survival in both stage IIIB patients when added to radiotherapy and stage IIIA patients when added to surgery. In stage IIIA N2, single-modality therapy is not sufficient. Randomized trials have shown that combined chemotherapy and radiotherapy is superior to either modality alone in both SCLC and in NSCLC. Chemotherapy plus surgery has also been shown to be superior to surgery alone in stage IIIA NSCLC. It remains unclear which combination is better: chemotherapy plus radiotherapy, chemotherapy plus surgery, or all three in combination. For stage IIIB NSCLC patients, combined chemotherapy and radiotherapy approaches are favored over either modality alone, with median survivals of 14 to 22 months and 5-year survival rates between 15% and 20%.

Meta-analyses of randomized trials showed that chemotherapy prolongs the survival of patients with stage III and stage IV SCLC and NSCLC. In extensive-stage SCLC, chemotherapy improves median survival from 2 months to about 9 to 10 months. In NSCLC, newer agent-based chemotherapy improves survival from 4 months to about 10 months and 1-year survival from 10% to between 40% and 50%. These therapies also improve patients' quality of life and their cost is similar to that of other accepted medical therapies. The addition of bevacizumab to paclitaxel and carboplatin improved the median survival in the nonsquamous cell patient to 12 months. For the second-line therapy of advanced NSCLC, docetaxel, pemetrexed, and erlotinib are all possible therapeutic options. The guidelines of lung cancer therapy of the American Society of Clinical Oncology reflect the contribution of chemotherapy to prolonging the survival of these patients [150]. Thus, it is reasonable to offer chemotherapy to advanced NSCLC patients with good performance status.

ETOPOSIDE AND CISPLATIN IN SMALL CELL LUNG CANCER

Cisplatin, a platinum analogue, is one of the most active antineoplastic agents for lung cancer. It inhibits DNA synthesis by producing intrastrand and interstrand crosslinks, similar to bifunctional alkylating agents. Etoposide exerts its effect on DNA by forming a complex with DNA and the DNA-unwinding enzyme topoisomerase II, which causes strand breakage. The combination of cisplatin and etoposide (EP) is currently considered to be one of the most active drug combinations for SCLC, reaching response rates in up to 90% of patients, with complete remissions in up to 50% [51]. In limited-stage disease, EP combined with chest irradiation has been shown to improve local control and median survival. In fact, a concurrent application of chemotherapy and radiotherapy is preferred by most centers (see Table 10-5) [36–38,40].

CANDIDATES FOR TREATMENT

Limited-stage disease concurrent with, alternated with, or followed by chest irradiation; extensive-stage disease

SPECIAL PRECAUTIONS

Patients with renal dysfunction and impaired hearing function

ALTERNATIVE THERAPIES

Carboplatin and etoposide; irinotecan and cisplatin; taxanes, topotecan, gemcitabine, and irinotecan as single agents or in combination with a platinum compound

TOXICITIES

Myelosuppression, nausea, vomiting, nephrotoxicity with electrolyte wasting, neurotoxicity (peripheral neuropathy), auditory impairment, hypotension, hypersensitivity (including anaphylactic reactions), mucositis, diarrhea, alopecia, asthenia

DRUG INTERACTIONS

Cisplatin: other nephrotoxic and ototoxic drugs (*eg*, aminoglycosides, furosemide); **Etoposide:** not known

NURSING INTERVENTIONS

Hypersensitivity: anaphylactic reactions have been documented with both agents; diphenhydramine and epinephrine should be readily available as well as a crash cart; **Myelosuppression:** monitor blood counts; inquire about symptoms of infection, bleeding, and anemia; **Nausea and vomiting:** give antiemetics before chemotherapy and as needed; assess for delayed nausea and vomiting; **Nephrotoxicity:** monitor renal function indices (serum creatinine, blood urea nitrogen [BUN], CrCl) and electrolytes (especially magnesium and calcium); encourage adequate oral and IV hydration as well as high urine flow during therapy; **Neurotoxicity:** assess for weakness and numbness of legs, feet, arms, and hands; **Hypotension:** usually attributed to fast infusion rate of etoposide (due to vehicle); stop infusion and give supportive care; restart infusion at slower rate or consider change to etoposide phosphate; **Local:** venous spasm and occasionally phlebitis may occur

PATIENT INFORMATION

Drink plenty of fluids and urinate frequently; report immediately symptoms of infection (fever, chills, sore throat), unusual bleeding, bruising, breathing problems, upset stomach, numbness, and tingling; maintain good nutrition and exercise; report any nausea or vomiting

CARBOPLATIN AND ETOPOSIDE IN SMALL CELL LUNG CANCER

Carboplatin, a platinum analogue like cisplatin, inhibits DNA synthesis by causing irreversible intrastrand and interstrand crosslinks. Carboplatin is highly effective in SCLC as a single agent. Etoposide, a topoisomerase II inhibitor, produces irreversible strand breakage. In two randomized studies, the combination of carboplatin and etoposide was shown to be as active but less toxic than the combination of cisplatin and etoposide in patients with limited- and extensive-stage disease [54,55]. Another randomized study comparing carboplatin/etoposide with CAV concluded that carboplatin/etoposide and CAV were equally effective, with the carboplatin/etoposide arms being better tolerated and offering a survival advantage to patients with extensive-stage disease [151]. Nonhematologic forms of toxicity such as neuropathy, renal toxicity, asthenia, nausea, and vomiting compare favorably with those found with the EP regimen. Therefore, carboplatin/etoposide (IV or perioral) is frequently used in older patients with poor performance status and extensive-stage disease, showing a remarkable response rate and survival [152]. Furthermore, when paclitaxel is combined with carboplatin/etoposide, the combination's toxicity profile remains tolerable [153]. Several randomized trials are currently comparing this triple therapy with standard carboplatin/etoposide combination in extensive-stage SCLC.

CANDIDATES FOR TREATMENT

Limited-stage disease with chest irradiation and extensive-stage disease; elderly patients

SPECIAL PRECAUTIONS

Treatment delay and transfusions may be mandatory due to myelosuppression. In case of impaired renal function, consult drug instruction form or consider use of Calvert formula: Total dose (in milligrams) = AUC × (CrCl [mL/min] + 25).

ALTERNATIVE THERAPIES

Carboplatin and etoposide; irinotecan and cisplatin; taxanes, topotecan, gemcitabine, and irinotecan as single agents or in combination with a platinum compound

TOXICITIES

Myelosuppression, nausea, vomiting, alopecia, mucositis, infection, peripheral neuropathy, hypotension, hypersensitivity (including anaphylactic reactions), anorexia, mild renal toxicity.

Continued on the next page

CARBOPLATIN AND ETOPOSIDE IN SMALL CELL LUNG CANCER *(CONTINUED)*

DRUG INTERACTIONS

Other nephrotoxic or ototoxic drugs (*eg*, aminoglycosides, furosemide)

NURSING INTERVENTIONS

Hypersensitivity: anaphylactic reactions have been documented with both agents; diphenhydramine and epinephrine should be readily available as well as crash cart; **Myelosuppression:** monitor blood counts; inquire about symptoms of infection, bleeding, and anemia; **Nausea and vomiting:** give antiemetics before chemotherapy and as needed; **Nephrotoxicity:** monitor renal function indices (serum creatinine, BUN) and magnesium; **Neurotoxicity:** assess for weakness and numbness of legs, feet, arms, and hands; **Hypotension:** usually attributed to fast infusion rate of etoposide (due to vehicle); stop infusion and give supportive care; restart infusion at slower rate or consider change to etoposide phosphate; **Local:** venous spasm and occasionally phlebitis may occur

PATIENT INFORMATION

Report immediately symptoms of infections (fever, chills, sore throat) and unusual bleeding or bruising; report upset stomach, numbness, tingling; maintain good nutrition, fluid intake, and exercise

Experiences and Response Rates: Randomized Carboplatin/Etoposide Trials With Cisplatin-Containing Regimens in Limited- and Extensive-Stage Small Cell Lung Cancer

Study	Patients, *n*	Dosage schedule	Response rates (LD/ED) CR, %	PR, %	Median survival, *mo*	Comments
Wolf *et al.* [54]	129	Doxorubicin/ifosfamide/vincristine alternating with carboplatin 300 mg/m² IV on d 1 + etoposide 120 mg/m² IV on d 1–3	20/17	53/34	12.0 (LD); 9.3 (ED)	Every 4 wk × 4 cycles; chest RT for LD
	133	Doxorubicin/ifosfamide/vincristine alternating with cisplatin 90 mg/m² IV on d 1 + etoposide 150 mg/m² IV on d 1–3	22/14	56/36	14.3 (LD); 9.3 (ED)	
Skarlos *et al.* [55]	72	Carboplatin 300 mg/m² IV on d 1 + etoposide 100 mg/m² IV on d 1	37/19	49/48	11.8 (LD/ED)	Every 3 wk × 6 cycles; chest RT for LD; PCI if complete remission
	71	Cisplatin 50 mg/m² IV on d 1 and 2 + etoposide 100 mg/m² IV on d 1–3	44/10	29/40	12.5 (LD/ED)	
Joos *et al.* [151]	93	Vincristine 1.4 mg/m² on d 1 + doxorubicin 50 mg/m² IV on d 1 + carboplatin 1000 mg/m2 IV on d 1	81/50*		11.7 (LD); 6.4 (ED)	Every 3 wk × 6 cycles
	102	Carboplatin 100 mg/m² IV on d 1 + etoposide 120 mg/m² IV on d 1–3	77/67*		14.0 (LD); 8.4 (ED)	Every 4 wk × 3 cycles

*LD/ED values are for overall response rates.
CR—complete response; ED—extensive-stage disease; IV—intravenous; LD—limited-stage disease; PCI—prophylactic cranial irradiation; PR—partial response; RT—radiation therapy.

Experiences and Response Rates: Nonrandomized Carboplatin/Etoposide Trials in Limited- and Extensive-Stage Small Cell Lung Cancer

Study	Patients, *n*	Dosage schedule	Response rate (LD + ED), %	Median survival, %	Comments
Okamoto *et al.* [152]	36	Carboplatin (AUC = 5) IV on d 1 + etoposide 100 mg/m² IV on d 1–3	75	11.6 (LD); 10.1 (ED)	Every 3 wk × 4 cycles
Hainsworth *et al.* [153]	72	Paclitaxel 200 mg/m² IV on d 1 + carboplatin (AUC = 5) IV on d 1 + etoposide 50 or 100 mg/m² IV every other d on d 1–10	91	NR (LD); 10.0 (ED)	Chest radiation therapy for LD with cycles 3 and 4

AUC—area under the curve; ED—extensive-stage disease; LD—limited-stage disease; NR—not reported.

IRINOTECAN AND CISPLATIN IN SMALL CELL LUNG CANCER

Irinotecan (CPT-11) is a unique, water-soluble, semisynthetic analogue of the alkaloid camptothecin, derived from the *Camptotheca acuminata* tree. It inhibits topoisomerase I, which is an enzyme with swivel-like enzymatic activity that may be required for the elongation phase of DNA replication and RNA transcription. Irinotecan induces protein-linked DNA single-strand breaks that depend on topoisomerase I content in the cell. Inhibition of topoisomerase I activity damages DNA, which leads to cell death. Irinotecan has shown activity as a single agent against SCLC. It has also been demonstrated to have in vitro synergistic activity with cisplatin against SCLC. In a randomized phase 3 trial by the JCOG, combined irinotecan/cisplatin was compared with EP in patients with extensive-stage SCLC [58]. The study demonstrated the irinotecan/cisplatin arm was significantly superior to the EP arm, with response rate and median survival of 83% and 13 months and 68% and 9.6 months, respectively.

CANDIDATES FOR TREATMENT
Patients with extensive-stage SCLC

SPECIAL PRECAUTIONS
Patients with renal dysfunction and impaired hearing function

ALTERNATIVE THERAPIES
EP, carboplatin/etoposide, or paclitaxel, docetaxel, gemcitabine, topotecan, and irinotecan as single agents

TOXICITIES
Myelosuppression, diarrhea, nausea, vomiting, nephrotoxicity with electrolyte wasting, neurotoxicity (peripheral neuropathy), auditory impairment, alopecia

DRUG INTERACTIONS
Cisplatin: other nephrotoxic and ototoxic drugs

NURSING INTERVENTIONS
Hypersensitivity: anaphylactic reactions have been documented with cisplatin; diphenhydramine and epinephrine should be readily available; **Myelosuppression:** associated with both drugs, monitor blood counts, inquire about symptoms of infection, bleeding, and anemia; **Diarrhea:** particularly associated with irinotecan; inquire about diarrhea; give loperamide one or two tablets every 2 hours until diarrhea resolves; check electrolytes, BUN, CrCl levels; **Nausea/vomiting:** give antiemetics before chemotherapy and as needed; **Nephrotoxicity:** monitor renal function indices (serum creatinine, BUN, CrCl), monitor electrolytes, especially magnesium and calcium, encourage oral and IV hydration as well as high levels of urine flow during therapy; **Neurotoxicity:** assess for weakness and numbness of legs, feet, arms, and hands

PATIENT INFORMATION
Drink plenty of fluids; report immediately symptoms of infection (fever, chills, sore throat), unusual bleeding, bruising and breathing problems; report frequency of diarrhea; report nausea/vomiting

PACLITAXEL AND CISPLATIN IN NON–SMALL CELL LUNG CANCER

Paclitaxel is a unique diterpene anticancer agent derived from the bark of the *Taxus brevifola* tree. It exerts its antitumor effect by stabilizing microtubules, rendering them resistant to disassembly. This differs from the other antimicrotubule agents like the vinca alkaloids, which induce microtubule disassembly. Two initial phase 2 studies of paclitaxel as 24-hour infusions showed a response rate of 22% among the 49 patients, with an improved median survival of about 40 weeks. Subsequent studies in combination with cisplatin ensued. The ECOG did a randomized study comparing low- and high-dose paclitaxel with cisplatin to the standard regimen of EP [121]. Both the paclitaxel arms showed a higher response rate (26.5% and 32.1% vs 12.0%) and better 1-y survival rates. The EORTC did a randomized study using a short infusion of paclitaxel and cisplatin compared with teniposide and cisplatin [122]. This study showed a higher response rate (44% vs 30%), reduced toxicity, and improved quality of life in patients receiving paclitaxel. Survival was similar in both treatment groups. SWOG 9805 and ECOG 1594 have both demonstrated the superior activity of this double therapy in the treatment of advanced stage NSCLC [123,124].

CANDIDATES FOR TREATMENT

Patients with stage III and stage IV disease as well as preoperatively in resectable early-stage disease

SPECIAL PRECAUTIONS

Patients with renal dysfunction; a history of cardiac toxicity should caution the caregiver

ALTERNATIVE THERAPIES

Carboplatin/paclitaxel, cisplatin/vinorelbine, cisplatin/gemcitabine, carboplatin/gemcitabine, cisplatin/docetaxel, or vinorelbine, gemcitabine, and paclitaxel as single agents

TOXICITIES

Paclitaxel: myelosuppression (almost exclusively neutropenia; thrombocytopenia is rare), neurotoxicity (peripheral neuropathy, seizures), gastrointestinal (nausea, vomiting, diarrhea, mucositis, neutropenic enterocolitis), cardiac (arrhythmia, ventricular tachycardia, myocardial infarction, bradycardia), anaphylactic and urticarial reactions, and alopecia and radiation pneumonitis (when administered concomitantly with radiation); **Cisplatin:** gastrointestinal (nausea, vomiting, anorexia), renal toxicity (with an elevation of BUN, creatinine, serum uric acid, impairment of endogenous CrCl, and renal tubular damage), ototoxicity (with hearing loss that initially is in the high-frequency range and tinnitus), peripheral neuropathy, and hyperuricemia. Anaphylactic-like reactions (*eg*, facial edema, bronchoconstriction, tachycardia, and hypotension) may occur; myelosuppression often with delayed erythrosuppression is expected; electrolyte disturbances (*eg*, hypomagnesemia and/or hypocalcemia) can occur, resulting in tetany or seizures; subsequent courses should not be given until serum creatinine returns to normal if elevated

DRUG INTERACTIONS

Agents that are nephrotoxic should be given with caution

NURSING INTERVENTIONS

Hypersensitivity: give premedications for prevention of allergic reactions to paclitaxel (dexamethasone, diphenhydramine, and cimetidine); **Myelosuppression:** monitor blood counts; inquire about symptoms of infection, bleeding, and anemia; **Nausea/vomiting:** give antiemetics before chemotherapy and as needed; **Nephrotoxicity:** monitor renal function indices (serum creatinine, BUN), monitor magnesium, give adequate hydration; **Neurotoxicity:** assess for weakness and numbness of legs, feet, arms, and hands

PATIENT INFORMATION

Patient should drink plenty of fluids and urinate frequently; report prolonged upset stomach and symptoms of infection (fever, chills, sore throat) or neurotoxicity (numbness and tingling sensation of hands or toes); report nausea/vomiting

Experiences and Response Rates					
Study	Patients, *n*	Dosage schedule	Response rate, %	Median survival	Comments
Bonomi *et al.* [121]	201	Paclitaxel 135 mg/m^2 IV as continuous infusion over 24 h on d 1 + cisplatin 75 mg/m2 on d 1	25.3	9.5 mo	Phase 3 study every 3 wk
	196	Paclitaxel 250 mg/m^2 IV over 24 h on d 1 +GCSF 5 µg/kg subcutaneously on d 3–10 + cisplatin 75 mg/m2 on d 1	27.7	10 mo	
Giaccone *et al.* [122]	154	Paclitaxel 175 mg/m^2 IV over 3 h on d 1 + cisplatin 80 mg/m2 IV on d 1	44	9.4 mo	Phase 3 study every 3 wk

GCSF—granulocyte colony-stimulating factor; IV—intravenous.

PACLITAXEL AND CARBOPLATIN IN NON–SMALL CELL LUNG CANCER

Due to a higher incidence of peripheral neuropathy associated with the cisplatin/paclitaxel combination, several trials combining carboplatin with paclitaxel (either as a 24-h or 3-h infusion) have been initiated. It appears that short infusion schedules of paclitaxel have similar degrees of efficacy as compared with 24-hour infusion schedules. Shorter infusion schedules result in less myelosuppression, and neuropathy becomes dose limiting. SWOG conducted a study comparing carboplatin and paclitaxel with cisplatin and vinorelbine [123]; and the ECOG conducted a four-arm study comparing docetaxel/cisplatin with paclitaxel/cisplatin to paclitaxel/carboplatin to gemcitabine/cisplatin [124]. All novel agent/platinum combinations studied revealed similar results. Thus, SWOG-9805 and ECOG-1594 have established five acceptable novel-agent/platinum combinations for treatment of advanced NSCLC.

CANDIDATES FOR TREATMENT

Patients with stage III and IV disease who have been untreated or refractory to other regimens

SPECIAL PRECAUTIONS

Patients with renal dysfunction; a history of cardiac toxicity should caution the caregiver

ALTERNATIVE THERAPIES

Cisplatin/paclitaxel, carboplatin/paclitaxel, cisplatin/vinorelbine, cisplatin/gemcitabine, cisplatin/docetaxel, carboplatin/gemcitabine; or single-agent vinorelbine, gemcitabine, and paclitaxel

TOXICITIES

Carboplatin: myelosuppression, nausea, vomiting, and loss of appetite are common; rare toxicities include gross hematuria, hyponatremia, ageusia, allergic reaction, peripheral neuropathy, veno-occlusive disease, liver and kidney damage, hearing loss, dizziness, and blurred vision; **Paclitaxel:** myelosuppression (almost exclusively neutropenia; thrombocytopenia is rare), neurotoxicity (peripheral neuropathy, seizures), gastrointestinal (nausea, vomiting, diarrhea, mucositis, neutropenic enterocolitis), cardiac (arrhythmia, ventricular tachycardia, myocardial infarction, bradycardia), anaphylactic and urticarial reactions, and alopecia and radiation pneumonitis (when administered concomitantly with radiation)

DRUG INTERACTIONS

None known

NURSING INTERVENTIONS

Hypersensitivity: give premedications for prevention of allergic reactions to paclitaxel (dexamethasone, diphenhydramine, and cimetidine); **Myelosuppression:** monitor blood counts; inquire about symptoms of infection, bleeding, and anemia; **Nausea/vomiting:** give antiemetics before chemotherapy and as needed; **Nephrotoxicity:** monitor renal function indices (serum creatinine, BUN) and magnesium; give adequate hydration; **Neurotoxicity:** assess for weakness and numbness of legs, feet, arms, and hands

PATIENT INFORMATION

Patient should drink plenty of fluids and urinate frequently; report prolonged upset stomach and irregularities in heart rhythm, and symptoms of infection (fever, chills, sore throat) or neurotoxicity (tingling or numbness of hands and toes)

Experiences and Response Rates

Study	Patients, *n*	Dosage schedule	Response rate, %	Median survival, *mo*	1-y survival, %
SWOG 9805 [123]	207	Paclitaxel 225 mg/m^2 over 3 h + carboplatin (AUC = 6) on d 1	27	8	36
	201	Vinorelbine 25 mg/m^2/wk + cisplatin 100 mg/m^2 every 3 wk	27	8	33
ECOG 1594 [124]	292	Paclitaxel 135 mg/m^2 over 24 h on d 1 + cisplatin 75 mg/m^2 on d 2 every 3 wk	21.3	7.8	31
	288	Cisplatin 100 mg/m^2 on d 1 + gemcitabine 1000 mg/m^2 on d 1, 8, and 15 every 4 wk	21	8.1	36
	293	Cisplatin 75 mg/m^2 on d 1 + docetaxel 75 mg/m^2 over 1 h on d 1 every 3 wk	17.3	7.4	31
	290	Carboplatin (AUC = 6) on d 1 + paclitaxel 225 mg/m^2 over 3 h on d 1 every 3 wk	15.3	8.2	35

AUC—area under the curve; ECOG—Eastern Cooperative Oncology Group; SWOG—Southwest Oncology Group.

VINORELBINE AND CISPLATIN IN NON–SMALL CELL LUNG CANCER

Vinorelbine is a unique semisynthetic vinca alkaloid. Its mechanism of action is similar to the other vinca alkaloids in that it is an inhibitor of microtubule assembly. It binds to tubulin, resulting in disruption of the mitotic spindle apparatus during metaphase. Vinorelbine has a lesser effect on axonal microtubules, and because neurotoxicity of vinca alkaloids is postulated to derive from damage to axonal microtubules, a more favorable therapeutic index of vinorelbine has been postulated. Preclinical studies with vinorelbine indicate activity against several tumor cell lines representing leukemia, SCLC, NSCLC, breast and colon cancer, and melanoma. Vinorelbine was later demonstrated to have significant activity in previously untreated NSCLC patients. SWOG 9805 established the vinorelbine/cisplatin combination as one of the current standard treatment of advanced NSCLC [123].

CANDIDATES FOR TREATMENT

Preoperative resectable stage II to IIIA as well as stage IIIB and IV disease

SPECIAL PRECAUTIONS

Patients with renal dysfunction; a history of peripheral neuropathy should caution the caregiver

ALTERNATIVE THERAPIES

Carboplatin/paclitaxel, cisplatin/paclitaxel, cisplatin/gemcitabine, carboplatin/gemcitabine, cisplatin/docetaxel; or vinorelbine, paclitaxel, and gemcitabine as single agents

TOXICITIES

Vinorelbine: myelosuppression with neutropenia and leukopenia are the most frequent dose-limiting toxicities (thrombocytopenia is rare; however, thrombocytosis is fairly common); mild to moderate constipation and decreased deep tendon reflexes are the most frequent occurring neurotoxicities; paresthesias occur infrequently; foot drop, peripheral neuropathy, and paralytic ileus have also been observed; mild to moderate nausea and vomiting occur in about 50% of patients; phlebitis characterized by erythema and tenderness extending over the palpable length of the infused vein has been associated with intravenous vinorelbine; mild to moderate alopecia has occurred and is related to duration of treatment; allergic reactions, fatigue, inappropriate antidiuretic hormone syndrome, hemorrhagic cystis, and insomnia have been reported

DRUG INTERACTIONS

None known

NURSING INTERVENTIONS

Myelosuppression: monitor blood counts; ask for symptoms of infection, bleeding, and anemia; **Nausea/vomiting:** give antiemetics before chemotherapy and as needed; **Nephrotoxicity:** monitor renal function indices (serum creatinine, BUN) and magnesium; give adequate hydration; **Neurotoxicity:** assess for weakness and numbness of legs, feet, arms, and hands

Experiences and Response Rates

Study	Patients, *n*	Dosage schedule	Response rate, %	Median survival, *wk*	1-y survival, %	Comments
Wozniak *et al.* [119]	195	Cisplatin 100 mg/m² IV every 3 wk + vinorelbine 25 mg/m²/wk × 3 cycles	26	28	36	Results showed better 1-y survival rate of this combination compared with cisplatin alone
Le Chevalier *et al.* [104]	206	Cisplatin 120 mg/m² IV on d 1 and 28 then every 6 wk + vinorelbine 30 mg/m²/wk × 6 cycles then every 2 wk	30	40	34	Compared with vinorelbine alone and with cisplatin/vindesine, this combination showed higher response and 1-y survival rates with a major difference in survival in stage IV patients

GEMCITABINE AND CISPLATIN IN NON–SMALL CELL LUNG CANCER

Gemcitabine is a deoxycytidine analogue related to cytosine arabinoside (Ara-C) that has been found to have considerable activity in NSCLC. Several phase 2 trials using gemcitabine in advanced, untreated NSCLC patients have shown a favorable overall response rate. The impressive low toxicity profile of gemcitabine adds to its appeal in combining it with other active agents such as cisplatin. Several phase 2 studies in combination with cisplatin have reported an overall response rate of 47% with an average median survival of 57 weeks and 1-year survival rate of 61% (Table 10-8). ECOG 1594 has established the gemcitabine/platinum combination as one of the current standard treatment for advanced-stage NSCLC [124]

CANDIDATES FOR TREATMENT

Patients refractory to standard chemotherapy; patients with stage III and stage IV NSCLC

SPECIAL PRECAUTIONS

Patients with renal dysfunction and impaired liver function

ALTERNATIVE THERAPIES

Etoposide and paclitaxel, etoposide and carboplatin, carboplatin and paclitaxel, cisplatin and vinorelbine, vinorelbine alone, or gemcitabine alone

TOXICITIES

Gemcitabine: myelosuppression is the dose-limiting toxicity; thrombocytopenia occurs occasionally, but thrombocytosis is also reported; abnormalities in liver transaminase enzymes can occur; nausea and vomiting occurs in two thirds of patients; mild proteinuria and hematuria can be present but is not associated with any change in serum creatinine or BUN; a rash is seen in 25% of patients and is associated with pruritus in about 10% of patients; other reported toxicities include a flu-like syndrome, mild to moderate peripheral edema, pulmonary edema, and rarely facial edema

DRUG INTERACTIONS

Cisplatin: other nephrotoxic or ototoxic drugs

NURSING INTERVENTIONS

Myelosuppression: monitor blood counts; inquire about symptoms of infection, bleeding, and anemia; **Nausea/vomiting:** give antiemetics before chemotherapy and as needed; **Nephrotoxicity:** monitor renal function indices (serum creatinine, BUN) and magnesium; give adequate hydration; **Neurotoxicity:** assess for weakness and numbness of legs, feet, arms, and hands

PATIENT INFORMATION

Patients should drink plenty of fluids and urinate frequently; report prolonged upset stomach, symptoms of infection (fever, chills, sore throat), and unusual bleeding or bruising; report nausea/vomiting

DOCETAXEL AND CISPLATIN IN NON–SMALL CELL LUNG CANCER

Docetaxel is synthesized from the extracts of the leaves of *Taxus baccata*. It enhances microtubule assembly and inhibits the depolymerization of tubulin. As with paclitaxel, this can lead to bundles of microtubules in the cell, leading to an inability of the cell to divide. The cell cycle is halted in M-phase. In initial clinical studies, docetaxel produced clinical responses in patients with breast cancer, ovarian cancer, NSCLC, and pancreatic cancer. Single-agent docetaxel has produced favorable response rates in patients with advanced NSCLC. Phase 2 trials of the docetaxel/cisplatin doublet in NSCLC have demonstrated response, median survival, and 1-year survival rates of 35%, 35 weeks, and 58%, respectively (Table 10-8). ECOG 1594 demonstrated docetaxel/cisplatin double therapy to be equivalent in efficacy to cisplatin/paclitaxel, cisplatin/gemcitabine, and carboplatin/paclitaxel [124]

CANDIDATES FOR TREATMENT

Patients with stage IIIB or IV NSCLC

SPECIAL PRECAUTIONS

Patients with renal dysfunction; previous reactions to the taxanes

ALTERNATIVE THERAPIES

Cisplatin/paclitaxel, carboplatin/paclitaxel, cisplatin/vinorelbine, cisplatin/gemcitabine, carboplatin/gemcitabine; or vinorelbine, gemcitabine, and paclitaxel as single agents

TOXICITIES

Docetaxel: dose-limiting neutropenia; thrombocytopenia noted but less frequent; anaphylactic reactions consistent with dyspnea and rash; anxiety noted in a few patients on the first course of treatment. After pretreatment with diphenhydramine and dexamethasone, patients have been able to be treated without difficulty. Other toxicities include phlebitis and alopecia. Pleural effusions and peripheral edema have both been reported. Premedication with dexamethasone as well as the modification of the treatment regimen to lower weekly doses or a maximum dose of 75 mg/m^2 every 3 weeks have decreased the incidence of fluid retention

NURSING INTERVENTIONS

Myelosuppression: monitor blood counts and ask for symptoms of infection, bleeding, and anemia; **Nausea/vomiting:** give antiemetics before chemotherapy and as needed; **Nephrotoxicity:** monitor renal function indices (serum creatinine, BUN), monitor magnesium, give adequate hydration; **Neurotoxicity:** assess for weakness and numbness of legs, feet, arms, and hands; **Fluid retention:** make sure the patient has been premedicated with dexamethasone before docetaxel infusion

The information here is provided as guidance only. Prescribers should always consult the manufacturer's current prescribing information.

BEVACIZUMAB WITH PLATINUM COMBINATION CHEMOTHERAPY IN ADVANCED NON–SMALL CELL LUNG CANCER

Bevacizumab is an antibody to the VEGF. In combination with paclitaxel and carboplatin, bevacizumab increased the response rate and survival in patients with nonsquamous cell advanced NSCLC. The recommended dose in NSCLC is 15 mg/kg IV once every 3 weeks infused on day 1 with chemotherapy [126].

CANDIDATES FOR TREATMENT

Stage IIIB with pleural effusion and stage IV without history of bleeding (including hemoptysis) and no history of brain metastasis

SPECIAL PRECAUTIONS

Treatment delay may be needed for 2+ or greater proteinuria. Hypertension may develop on bevacizumab and may require medical intervention to maintain blood pressure control. If bleeding such as hemoptysis occurs while on therapy, bevacizumab should be stopped immediately. Permanently discontinue bevacizumab in the following conditions: gastrointestinal perforation, fistula formation in the gastrointestinal tract, and/or intra-abdominal abscess; fistula formation involving an internal organ; wound dehiscence requiring medical intervention; serious bleeding; severe arterial thromboembolic event; nephrotic syndrome; hypertensive crisis or hypertensive encephalopathy; and reversible posterior leukoencephalopathy syndrome (RPLS). Do not give bevacizumab at least for 28 days following surgery.

ALTERNATIVE THERAPIES

No other antiangiogenesis agents are approved for use for NSCLC; patients with contraindications for bevacizumab should receive combination chemotherapy alone

TOXICITIES

Bleeding, allergic reaction, hypertension, proteinuria, increased incidence of neutropenia when combined with chemotherapy, increased incidence of neurotoxicity when combined with neurotoxic chemotherapy such as paclitaxel, poor wound healing, gastrointestinal perforation, congestive heart failure, arterial thrombotic events, and RPLS

NURSING INTERVENTIONS

Hypersensitivity: anaphylactic reactions have been documented with bevacizumab so that diphenhydramine and epinephrine should be readily available; **Myelosuppression:** monitor blood counts and ask for symptoms of infection, bleeding, and anemia; **Nephrotoxicity/proteinuria:** monitor urine protein; **Vascular:** monitor blood pressure

PATIENT INFORMATION

Report immediately symptoms of infections (*eg*, fever, chills) and bleeding or unusual bruising; report numbness or tingling; report severe constipation, abdominal pain, or nausea and vomiting; maintain good nutrition and exercise

PEMETREXED

Pemetrexed is a novel multitargeted antifolate agent. This agent is approved for use for second-line treatment based on a phase 3 study comparing it with docetaxel [141]. Pemetrexed is dosed at 500 mg/m^2 IV over 10 minutes once every 21 days.

CANDIDATES FOR TREATMENT

NSCLC: Patients with stage IIIB with pleural effusion and stage IV disease whose tumors have progressed during or after first-line chemotherapy

SPECIAL PRECAUTIONS

In case of impaired renal function, pemetrexed should not be administered to patients with glomerular filtration rate less than 45 mL/min. All patients should be routinely given oral folic acid supplementation (at least 350 mcg orally per day) and a B$_{12}$ injection (1000 mcg intramuscularly once every 9 weeks) starting 5 to 7 days prior to chemotherapy treatment. Dexamethasone premedication is recommended as 4 mg orally twice a day starting the day prior to injection continuing through the day after injection of pemetrexed. Treatment delay and transfusion may be mandatory due to myelosuppression

ALTERNATIVE THERAPIES

Single-agent docetaxel or erlotinib

TOXICITIES

Myelosuppression, fatigue, anorexia, nausea, vomiting, mucositis/stomatitis, infection, hypersensitivity (mainly rash), diarrhea, constipation, rarely alopecia

DRUG INTERACTIONS

NSAIDs impair the renal excretion of pemetrexed. Patients should be advised to discontinue use at least 5 days prior to pemetrexed injection (at least 8 days for long-acting NSAIDs)

NURSING INTERVENTIONS

Hypersensitivity: rash and anaphylactic reactions have been documented so that diphenhydramine and epinephrine should be readily available and confirm that patients have taken their dexamethasone premedication as directed; **Myelosuppression:** monitor blood counts and ask for symptoms of infection, bleeding, and anemia; **Nausea:** give antiemetics as needed

PATIENT INFORMATION

Take folic acid daily as well as dexamethasone premedications as directed; report immediately symptoms of infections, bleeding, rash, or diarrhea; report upset stomach; maintain good nutrition, fluid intake, and exercise

The information here is provided as guidance only. Prescribers should always consult the manufacturer's current prescribing information.

ERLOTINIB

Erlotinib is an oral EGFR tyrosine kinase inhibitor. Erlotinib is approved for use in the second- and third-line setting for NSCLC based on a phase 3 trial comparing erlotinib with placebo in patients with advanced NSCLC whose disease progressed on at least one prior chemotherapy [142]. The dose of erlotinib is 150 mg by mouth once a day.

CANDIDATES FOR TREATMENT

NSCLC: Patients with stage IIIB with pleural effusion and stage IV disease whose tumors have progressed during or aft r first-line chemotherapy or second-line chemotherapy

SPECIAL PRECAUTIONS

Patients with liver dysfunction. Patients should take this drug on an empty stomach; taking erlotinib with food will increase the absorption of erlotinib and increase the toxicities

ALTERNATIVE THERAPIES

Single-agent pemetrexed or docetaxel in the second-line treatment setting

TOXICITIES

Dermatologic: Rash, erythema pruritus, dry skin; **Gastrointestinal:** diarrhea, nausea and vomiting, liver function test abnormalities; **Miscellaneous:** fatigue, conjunctivitis, myocardial infarction; rarely interstitial pneumonitis and alopecia

DRUG INTERACTIONS

With warfarin, erlotinib can increase international normalized ratio (INR) levels. Patients who are on warfarin and start erlotinib should have their INR levels monitored closely. Special attention should be given when administering CYP3A4 inhibitors and inducers (*eg*, St. John's wort or carbamazepine) which can affect the metabolism of erlotinib

NURSING INTERVENTIONS

Rash: if severe, stop erlotinib; if moderate, dose reduction can be attempted; if mild, topical corticosteroids or antibiotic ointments can be used; **Pruritus:** diphenhydramine oral or topical can be used; **Dry skin:** encourage aggressive topical lotion/emollient use up to three times day; **Diarrhea:** inquire about diarrhea, give loperamide one or two tablets every 2 hours until diarrhea resolved, check electrolytes, BUN/CrCl clearance levels; **Nausea:** give antiemetics as needed or encourage patients to take in the evening prior to bedtime

PATIENT INFORMATION

Erlotinib should be taken once daily on an empty stomach (1 hour prior or 2 hours after a meal). Report uncontrolled diarrhea not responding to loperamide immediately. While a rash, dry skin, and itching are to be expected, report severe and/or intolerable rash. Report nausea and vomiting. Report all medication changes as several medications can interact with erlotinib. Patients should be advised to stop smoking since smoking can affect the metabolism of this drug. Patients should also be advised not to eat grapefruit or drink grapefruit juice while taking this drug

REFERENCES

1. Jemal A, Siegel R, Ward E, *et al.*: Cancer statistics. *CA Cancer J Clin* 2008, 58:71–96.

2. Parker SL, Tong T, Bolden S, *et al.*: Cancer statistics, 2000. *CA Cancer J Clin* 2000, 47:5–27.

3. Ginsberg RJ, Vokes EE, Raben A: Non-small cell lung cancer. *Principles and Practice of Oncology*, edn 5. Edited by DeVita VT, Hellman S, Rosenberg SA. Philadelphia, PA: Lippincott-Raven; 1997:858–911.

4. Ockene JK, Kuller LH, Svendsen KH, *et al.*: The relationship of smoking cessation to coronary heart disease and lung cancer in the Multiple Risk Factor Intervention Trial (MRFIT). *Am J Public Health* 1990, 80:954–958.

5. Strauss G, DeCamp M, Dibiccaro E, *et al.*: Lung cancer diagnosis is being made with increasing frequency in former cigarette smokers [abstract]. *Proc Am Soc Clin Oncol* 1995, 14:A1106.

6. American Cancer Society: *Cancer Facts and Figures – 1996*. Atlanta, GA: American Cancer Society; 1996.

7. Centers for Disease Control and Prevention: Smoking and tobacco use: data and statistics. Available at http://www.cdc.gov/tobacco/data_statistics/. Accessed August 12, 2008.

8. American Cancer Society: 2008 Cancer Statistics. Available at http://www.cancer.org/docroot/PRO/content/PRO_1_1_Cancer_Statistics_2008_Presentation.asp. Accessed August 12, 2008.

9. Schottenfeld D: Epidemiology of lung cancer. In *Lung Cancer: Principles and Practice*. Edited by Pass HI, Mitchell JB, Johnson DH, *et al.* Philadelphia: Lippincott-Raven; 1996:305–321.

10. Blot WJ, Fraumeni JF Jr: Lung and pleura. In *Cancer Epidemiology and Prevention*, edn 2. Edited by Schottenfeld D, Fraumeni JF Jr. Philadelphia: WB Saunders; 1982:564–670.

11. Travis WD, James L, Mackey B: Classification, histology, cytology and electron microscopy. In *Lung Cancer; Principles and Practice*. Edited by Pass HI, Mitchell JB, Johnson DH, *et al.* Philadelphia: Lippincott-Raven; 1996:361–395.

12. Cook RM, Miller YE, Bunn PA Jr: Small cell lung cancer: etiology, biology, clinical features, staging, and treatment. *Curr Probl Cancer* 1993, 17:69–141.

13. Berlin NI, Buncher CR, Fontana RS, *et al.*: The National Cancer Institute Cooperative Early Lung Cancer Detection Program. Results of the initial screen (prevalence). Early lung cancer detection: introduction. *Am Rev Respir Dis* 1984, 130:545–549.

14. Shaw GL: Screening for lung cancer. In *Lung Cancer*. Edited by Johnson BE, Johnson DH. New York: Wiley-Liss; 1995:55–72.

15. Early Lung Cancer Cooperative Study Group: Early lung cancer detection: summary and conclusions. *Am Rev Respir Dis* 1984, 130:565–570.

16. Flehinger BJ, Melamed MR, Zaman MB, *et al.*: Early lung cancer detection: results of the initial (prevalence) radiologic and cytologic screening in the Memorial Sloan-Kettering study. *Am Rev Respir Dis* 1984, 130:555–560.

17. Fontana RS, Sanderson DR, Taylor WF, *et al.*: Early lung cancer detection: results of the initial (prevalence) radiologic and cytologic screening in the Mayo Clinic study. *Am Rev Respir Dis* 1984, 130:561–565.

18. Frost JK, Ball WC Jr, Levin ML, *et al.*: Early lung cancer detection: results of the initial (prevalence) radiologic and cytologic screening in the Johns Hopkins study. *Am Rev Respir Dis* 1984, 130:549–554.

19. Marcus PM, Bergstralh EJ, Fagerstrom RM, *et al.*: Lung cancer mortality in the Mayo Lung Project: impact of extended follow-up. *J Natl Cancer Inst* 2000, 92:1308–1316.

20. Eddy DM: Screening for lung cancer. *Ann Intern Med* 1989, 111:232–237.

21. Karp D, Mulshine J, Henschke C, *et al.*: Non-small cell lung cancer: screening, new imaging and prevention. *Am Soc Clin Oncol Educational Book* 2000, 587–601.

22. Henschke CI, McCauley DI, Yankelevitz DF, *et al.*: Early Lung Cancer Action Project: overall design and findings from baseline screening. *Lancet* 1999, 354:99–105.

23. The International Early Lung Cancer Action Program Investigators: Survival of patients with stage I lung cancer detected on CT screening. *N Engl J Med* 2006, 355:1763–1771.

24. Unger M: A pause, progress, and reassessment in lung cancer screening. *N Engl J Med* 2006, 355:1822–1824.

25. US Centers for Disease Control and Prevention: cigarette smoking among adults: United States, 1998. *MMWR Morb Mortal Wkly Rep* 2000, 49:881–884.

26. Hurt RD, Dale LC, Fredrickson PA, *et al.*: Nicotine patch therapy for smoking cessation combined with physician advice and nurse follow-up. One-year outcome and percentage of nicotine replacement. JAMA 1994, 271:595–600.

27. Kvale G, Bjelke E, Gart JJ: Dietary habits and lung cancer risk. *Int J Cancer* 1983, 31:397–405.

28. The effect of vitamin E and beta carotene on the incidence of lung cancer and other cancers in male smokers. The Alpha-Tocopherol, Beta Carotene Cancer Prevention Study Group. *N Engl J Med* 1994, 330:1029–1035.

29. Omenn GS, Goodman GE, Thornquist MD, *et al.*: Risk factors for lung cancer and for intervention effects in CARET, the Beta-Carotene and Retinol Efficacy Trial. *J Natl Cancer Inst* 1996, 88:1550–1559.

30. Mountain CF: Revisions in the International System for Staging Lung Cancer. *Chest* 1997, 111:1710–1717.

31. Pieterman RM, van Putten JW, Meuzelaar JJ, *et al.*: Preoperative staging of non-small-cell lung cancer with positron-emission tomography. *N Engl J Med* 2000, 343:254–261.

32. O'Connell JP, Kris MG, Gralla RJ, *et al.*: Frequency and prognostic importance of pretreatment clinical characteristics in patients with advanced non-small-cell lung cancer treated with combination chemotherapy. *J Clin Oncol* 1986, 4:1604–1614.

33. Dewys WD, Begg C, Lavin PT, *et al.*: Prognostic effect of weight loss prior to chemotherapy in cancer patients. Eastern Cooperative Oncology Group. *Am J Med* 1980, 69:491–497.

34. Warde P, Payne D: Does thoracic irradiation improve survival and local control in limited-stage small-cell carcinoma of the lung? A meta-analysis. *J Clin Oncol* 1992, 10:890–895.

35. Pignon JP, Arriagada R, Ihde DC, *et al.*: A meta-analysis of thoracic radiotherapy for small-cell lung cancer. *N Engl J Med* 1992, 327:1618–1624.

36. McCracken JD, Janaki LM, Crowley JJ, *et al.*: Concurrent chemotherapy/radiotherapy for limited small-cell lung carcinoma: a Southwest Oncology Group Study. *J Clin Oncol* 1990, 8:892–898.

37. Turrisi AT, Wagner H, Glover B, *et al.*: Limited small cell lung cancer (LSCLC): concurrent BID thoracic radiotherapy (TRT) with platinum-etoposide (PE): an ECOG study [abstract]. *Proc Am Soc Clin Oncol* 1990, 9:A887.

38. Johnson DH, Turrisi AT, Chang AY, *et al.*: Alternating chemotherapy and twice-daily thoracic radiotherapy in limited-stage small-cell lung cancer: a pilot study of the Eastern Cooperative Oncology Group. *J Clin Oncol* 1993, 11:879–884.

39. Johnson BE, Bridges JD, Sobczeck M, *et al.*: Patients with limited-stage small-cell lung cancer treated with concurrent twice-daily chest radiotherapy and etoposide/cisplatin followed by cyclophosphamide, doxorubicin, and vincristine. *J Clin Oncol* 1996, 14:806–813.

40. Turrisi AT III, Kim K, Blum R, *et al.*: Twice-daily compared with once-daily thoracic radiotherapy in limited small-cell lung cancer treated concurrently with cisplatin and etoposide. *N Engl J Med* 1999, 340:265–271.

41. Albain KS, Crowley JJ, LeBlanc M, *et al.*: Determinants of improved outcome in small-cell lung cancer: an analysis of the 2,580-patient Southwest Oncology Group data base. *J Clin Oncol* 1990, 8:1563–1574.

42. Murray N, Coy P, Pater JL, *et al.*: Importance of timing for thoracic irradiation in the combined modality treatment of limited-stage small-cell lung cancer. The National Cancer Institute of Canada Clinical Trials Group. *J Clin Oncol* 1993, 11:336–344.

43. Murray N, Coldman C: The relationship between thoracic irradiation timing and long term survival in combined modality therapy of limited stage small cell lung cancer [abstract]. *Proc Am Soc Clin Oncol* 1995, 14:A1099.

44. Goto K, Nishiwaki Y, Takada M, *et al.*: Final results of a phase III study of concurrent versus sequential thoracic radiotherapy (TRT) in combination with cisplatin (P) and etoposide (E) for limited stage small cell lung cancer (LSSCLC): the Japan Clinical Oncology Group (JCOG) Study [abstract]. *Proc Am Soc Clin Oncol* 1999, 18:468a.

45. Janaki LM, Rector D, Turrisi AT, *et al.*: Patterns of failure and second malignancies from SWOG 8269: Concurrent cisplatin, etoposide vincristine and once daily radiotherapy for the treatment of limited small cell lung cancer [abstract]. *Proc Am Soc Clin Oncol* 1994, 13, 331:abstract 29.

46. Shepherd FA, Ginsberg RJ, Feld R, *et al.*: Surgical treatment for limited small-cell lung cancer. The University of Toronto Lung Oncology Group experience. *J Thorac Cardiovasc Surg* 1991, 101:385–393.

47. Lad T, Piantadosi S, Thomas P, *et al.*: A prospective randomized trial to determine the benefit of surgical resection of residual disease following response of small cell lung cancer to combination chemotherapy. *Chest* 1994, 106:320S–323S.

48. Roth BJ, Johnson DH, Einhorn LH, *et al.*: Randomized study of cyclophosphamide, doxorubicin, and vincristine versus etoposide and cisplatin versus alternation of these two regimens in extensive small-cell lung cancer: a phase III trial of the Southeastern Cancer Study Group. *J Clin Oncol* 1992, 10:282–291.

49. Fukuoka M, Furuse K, Saijo N, *et al.*: Randomized trial of cyclophosphamide, doxorubicin, and vincristine versus cisplatin and etoposide versus alternation of these regimens in small-cell lung cancer. *J Natl Cancer Inst* 1991, 83:855–861.

50. Evans WK, Osoba D, Feld R, *et al.*: Etoposide (VP-16) and cisplatin: an effective treatment for relapse in small-cell lung cancer. *J Clin Oncol* 1985, 3:65–71.

51. Einhorn LH, Crawford J, Birch R, *et al.*: Cisplatin plus etoposide consolidation following cyclophosphamide, doxorubicin, and vincristine in limited small-cell lung cancer. *J Clin Oncol* 1988, 6:451–456.

52. Evans WK, Shepherd FA, Feld R, *et al.*: VP-16 and cisplatin as first-line therapy for small-cell lung cancer. *J Clin Oncol* 1985, 3:1471–1477.

53. Goldie JH, Coldman AJ: A mathematic model for relating the drug sensitivity of tumors to their spontaneous mutation rate. *Cancer Treat Rep* 1979, 63:1727–1733.

54. Wolf M, Drings P, Hans K, *et al.*: Alternating chemotherapy with adriamycin/ifosfamide/vincristine (AIO) and either cisplatin/etoposide (PE) or carboplatin/etoposide (CE) in small cell lung cancer (SCLC) [abstract]. *Lung Cancer* 1991, 7(Suppl):A527.

55. Skarlos DV, Samantas E, Kosmidis P, *et al.*: Randomized comparison of etoposide-cisplatin vs. etoposide-carboplatin and irradiation in small-cell lung cancer. A Hellenic Co-operative Oncology Group study. *Ann Oncol* 1994, 5:601–607.

56. Masuda N, Fukuoka M, Kusunoki Y, *et al.*: CPT-11: a new derivative of camptothecin for the treatment of refractory or relapsed small-cell lung cancer. *J Clin Oncol* 1992, 10:1225–1229.

57. Noda K, Nishiwaki Y, Kawahara M, *et al.*: Irinotecan plus cisplatin compared with etoposide plus cisplatin for extensive small-cell lung cancer. *N Engl J Med* 2002, 346:85–91.

58. Noda K, Nishiwaki Y, Kawahara M, *et al.*: Randomized phase III study of irinotecan (CPT-11) and cisplatin versus etoposide and cisplatin in extensive-disease small cell lung cancer: Japan Clinical Oncology Group study (JCOG-9511) [abstract]. *Proc Am Soc Clin Oncol* 2000, 19:483a.

59. Hanna N, Bunn PA Jr, Langer C, *et al.*: Randomized phase III trial comparing irinotecan/cisplatin with etoposide/cisplatin in patients with previously untreated extensive-stage disease small-cell lung cancer. *J Clin Oncol* 2006, 24:2038–2043.

60. Bunn PA, Cullen MR, Fukuola M, *et al.*: Chemotherapy in small cell lung cancer. A consensus report of the International Association for the Study of Lung Cancer Workshop. *Lung Cancer* 1989, 5:127–134.

61. Giaccone G, Dalesio O, McVie GJ, *et al.*: Maintenance chemotherapy in small-cell lung cancer: long-term results of a randomized trial. European Organization for Research and Treatment of Cancer Lung Cancer Cooperative Group. *J Clin Oncol* 1993, 11:1230–1240.

62. Spiro SG, Souhami RL, Geddes DM, *et al.*: Duration of chemotherapy in small cell lung cancer: a Cancer Research Campaign trial. *Br J Cancer* 1989, 59:578–583.

63. Bleehen NM, Fayers PM, Girling DJ, *et al.*: Controlled trials of twelve versus six courses of chemotherapy in small cell lung cancer. *Br J Cancer* 1989, 59:584–590.

64. Kelly K, Crowley JJ, Bunn PA Jr, *et al.*: Role of recombinant interferon alfa-2a maintenance in patients with limited-stage small-cell lung cancer responding to concurrent chemoradiation: a Southwest Oncology Group study. *J Clin Oncol* 1995, 13:2924–2930.

65. Johnson DH, Adak S, Schiller JH, *et al.*: Topotecan (T) vs observation (OB) following cisplatin (P) plus etoposide (E) in extensive stage small cell lung cancer (ES SCLC) (E7593): a phase III trial of the Eastern Cooperative Oncology Group (ECOG) [abstract]. *Proc Am Soc Clin Oncol* 2000, 19:482a.

66. Rowinsky EK, Grochow LB, Hendricks CB, *et al.*: Phase I and pharmacologic study of topotecan: a novel topoisomerase I inhibitor. *J Clin Oncol* 1992, 10:647–656.

67. Schiller JH, Kim K, Hutson P, *et al.*: Phase II study of topotecan in patients with extensive-stage small-cell carcinoma of the lung: an Eastern Cooperative Oncology Group Trial. *J Clin Oncol* 1996, 14:2345–2352.

68. Ardizzoni A, Hansen H, Dombernowsky P, *et al.*: Topotecan, a new active drug in the second-line treatment of small-cell lung cancer: a phase II study in patients with refractory and sensitive disease. The European Organization for Research and Treatment of Cancer Early Clinical Studies Group and New Drug Development Office, and the Lung Cancer Cooperative Group. *J Clin Oncol* 1997, 15:2090–2096.

69. von Pawel J, Schiller JH, Shepherd FA, *et al.*: Topotecan versus cyclophosphamide, doxorubicin, and vincristine for the treatment of recurrent small-cell lung cancer. *J Clin Oncol* 1999, 17:658–667.

70. Harper PG, Underhill C, Ruiz de Elvira MC, *et al.*: A randomized study of oral etoposide versus combination chemotherapy in poor prognosis small cell lung cancer. *J Clin Oncol* 1996, 14:1750.

71. Clark PI, Thatcher N, Lallenand G, *et al.*: Updated results of a randomized trial confirm that oral etoposide alone is inadequate palliative chemotherapy for small cell lung cancer (SCLC). *Lancet Oncol* 1996, 348:563–566.

72. Kelly K: New chemotherapy agents for small cell lung cancer. *Chest* 2000, 117:156S–162S.

73. Ettinger D, Finkelstein D, Sarma R, *et al.*: Phase II study of paclitaxel in patients with extensive disease small-cell lung cancer: an Eastern Cooperative Oncology Group study. *J Clin Oncol* 1995, 13:1430–1435.

74. Kirschling RJ, Grill JP, Marks RS, *et al.*: Paclitaxel and G-CSF in previously untreated patients with extensive stage small-cell lung cancer: a phase II study of the North Central Cancer Treatment Group. *Am J Clin Oncol* 1999, 22:517–522.

75. Bunn PA Jr: Future directions in therapeutic approaches for small cell lung cancer. *Semin Oncol* 1996, 23:136–138.

76. Mavroudis D, Papadakis E, Veslemes M, *et al.*: A multi-center randomized phase III study compared paclitaxel-cisplatin-etoposide versus cisplatin-etoposide as front line treatment in patients with small cell lung cancer [abstract 1894]. *Proc Am Soc Clin Oncol* 2000, 19:484a.

77. Auperin A, Arriagada R, Pignon JP, *et al.*: Prophylactic cranial irradiation for patients with small-cell lung cancer in complete remission. Prophylactic Cranial Irradiation Overview Collaborative Group. *N Engl J Med* 1999, 341:476–484.

78. Ginsberg RJ, Rubinstein L: The comparison of limited resection to lobectomy for T1N0 non-small cell lung cancer. LCSG 821. *Chest* 1994, 106:318S–319S.

79. Bunn PA Jr: The treatment of non-small cell lung cancer: current perspectives and controversies, future directions. *Semin Oncol* 1994, 21:49–59.

80. Effects of postoperative mediastinal radiation on completely resected stage II and stage III epidermoid cancer of the lung. The Lung Cancer Study Group. *N Engl J Med* 1986, 315:1377–1381.

81. Postoperative radiotherapy for non-small cell lung cancer. PORT Meta-Analysis Trialists Group. *Cochrane Database Syst Rev* 2000, 2:CD002142.

82. Non-Small Cell Lung Cancer Collaborative Group: Chemotherapy in non-small cell lung cancer: a meta-analysis using updated data on individual patients from 52 randomized clinical trials. *Br Med J* 1995, 311:899–909.

83. Arriagada R, Bergman B, Dunant A, *et al.*; International Adjuvant Lung Cancer Trial Collaborative Group: Cisplatin-based adjuvant chemotherapy in patients with completely resected non-small cell lung cancer. *N Engl J Med* 2004, 350:351–360.

84. Winton T, Livingston R, Johnson D, *et al.*: Vinorelbine plus cisplatin vs. observation in resected non-small-cell lung cancer. *N Engl J Med* 2005, 352:2589–2597.

85. Douillard JY, Rosell R, De Lena M, *et al.*: Adjuvant vinorelbine plus cisplatin versus observation in patients with completely resected stage IB-IIIA non-small-cell lung cancer (Adjuvant Navelbine International Trialist Association [ANITA]): a randomised controlled trial. *Lancet Oncol* 2006, 7:719–727.

86. Pisters K, Ginsberg R, Bunn PA, *et al.*: Induction chemotherapy before surgery for early-stage lung cancer: a novel approach. *J Thorac Cardiovasc Surg* 2000, 119:429–439.

87. Depierre A, Milleron B, Moro D, *et al.*: Phase III trial of neoadjuvant chemotherapy in resectable stage I (except T1N0), II, IIIA NSCLC: the French experience [abstract]. *Proc Am Soc Clin Oncol* 1999, 18:465a.

88. Betticher DC, Hsu Schmitz SF, Totsch M, *et al.*: Mediastinal lymph node clearance after docetaxel-cisplatin neoadjuvant chemotherapy is prognostic of survival in patients with stage IIIA pN2 non-small-cell lung cancer: a multicenter phase II trial. *J Clin Oncol* 2003, 21:1752–1759.

89. Van Zandwijk N, Smit EF, Kramer GW, *et al.*: Gemcitabine and cisplatin as induction regimen for patients with biopsy-proven stage IIIA N2 non-small-cell lung cancer: a phase II study of the European Organization for Research and Treatment of Cancer Lung Cancer Cooperative Group (EORTC 08955). *J Clin Oncol* 2000, 18:2658–2664.

90. Martini N, Kris MG, Flehinger BJ, *et al.*: Preoperative chemotherapy for stage IIIa (N2) lung cancer: the Sloan-Kettering experience with 136 patients. *Ann Thorac Surg* 1993, 55:1365–1373; discussion 1373–1374.

91. Burkes RL, Ginsberg RJ, Shepherd FA, *et al.*: Induction chemotherapy with mitomycin, vindesine, and cisplatin for stage III unresectable non-small-cell lung cancer: results of the Toronto phase II trial. *J Clin Oncol* 1992, 10:580–586.

92. Sugarbaker DJ, Herndon J, Kohman LJ, *et al.*: Results of Cancer and Leukemia Group B protocol 8935. A multi-institutional phase II trimodality trial for stage IIIA (N2) non-small-cell lung cancer. Cancer and Leukemia Group B Thoracic Surgery Group. *J Thorac Cardiovasc Surg* 1995, 109:473–483; discussion 483–485.

93. Albain KS, Rusch VW, Crowley JJ, *et al.*: Concurrent cisplatin/etoposide plus chest radiotherapy followed by surgery for stages IIIA (N2) and IIIB non-small-cell lung cancer: mature results of Southwest Oncology Group phase II study 8805. *J Clin Oncol* 1995, 13:1880–1892.

94. Albain KS, Rusch VW, Crowley J, *et al.*: Long term survival after concurrent cisplatin/etoposide (PE) plus chest radiotherapy (RT) followed by surgery in bulky stage IIIA (N2) and IIIB non-small cell lung cancer: 6-year outcome from Southwest Oncology Group Study 8805 [abstract]. *Proc Am Soc Clin Oncol* 1999, 18:467a.

95. Rosell R, Gomez-Codina J, Camps C, *et al.*: A randomized trial comparing preoperative chemotherapy plus surgery with surgery alone in patients with non-small-cell lung cancer. *N Engl J Med* 1994, 330:153–158.

96. Rosell R, Gomez-Codina J, Camps C, *et al.*: Preresectional chemotherapy in stage IIIA non-small-cell lung cancer: a 7-year assessment of a randomized controlled trial. *Lung Cancer* 1999, 26:7–14.

97. Roth JA, Fossella F, Komaki R, *et al.*: A randomized trial comparing perioperative chemotherapy and surgery with surgery alone in resectable stage IIIA non-small-cell lung cancer. *J Natl Cancer Inst* 1994, 86:673–680.

98. Roth JA, Atkinson EN, Fossella F, *et al.*: Long-term follow-up of patients enrolled in a randomized trial comparing perioperative chemotherapy and surgery with surgery alone in resectable stage IIIA non-small-cell lung cancer. *Lung Cancer* 1998, 21:1–6.

99. Gandara DR, Leigh B, Vallieres E, *et al.*: Preoperative chemotherapy in stage III non-small cell lung cancer: long-term outcome. *Lung Cancer* 1999, 26:3–6.

100. Albain KS, Swann RS, Rusch VR, *et al.*: Phase III study of concurrent chemotherapy and radiotherapy (CT/RT) vs CT/RT followed by surgical resection for stage IIIA (pN2) non-small cell lung cancer (NSCLC). Outcomes update of North American Intergroup 0139 (RTOG 9309) [abstract]. *Proc Am Soc Clin Oncol* 2005, 23:624s.

101. Dillman RO, Seagren SL, Propert KJ, *et al.*: A randomized trial of induction chemotherapy plus high-dose radiation versus radiation alone in stage III non-small-cell lung cancer. *N Engl J Med* 1990, 323:940–945.

102. Dillman RO, Herndon J, Seagren SL, *et al.*: Improved survival in stage III non-small-cell lung cancer: seven-year follow-up of Cancer and Leukemia Group B (CALGB) 8433 trial. *J Natl Cancer Inst* 1996, 88:1210–1215.

103. Sause WT, Scott C, Taylor S, *et al.*: Radiation Therapy Oncology Group (RTOG) 88-08 and Eastern Cooperative Oncology Group (ECOG) 4588: preliminary results of a phase III trial in regionally advanced, unresectable non-small-cell lung cancer. *J Natl Cancer Inst* 1995, 87:198–205.

104. Le Chevalier T, Brisgand D, Soria JC, *et al.*: Long-term analysis of survival in the European randomized trial comparing vinorelbine/cisplatin to vindesine/cisplatin and vinorelbine alone in advanced non-small cell lung cancer. *Oncologist* 2001, 6(suppl 1):8–11.

105. Schaake-Koning C, van den Bogaert W, Dalesio O, *et al.*: Effects of concomitant cisplatin and radiotherapy on inoperable non-small-cell lung cancer. *N Engl J Med* 1992, 326:524–530.

106. Jeremic B, Shibamoto Y, Acimovic L, *et al.*: Randomized trial of hyperfractionated radiation therapy with or without concurrent chemotherapy for stage III non-small-cell lung cancer. *J Clin Oncol* 1995, 13:452–458.

107. Jeremic B, Shibamoto Y, Acimovic L, *et al.*: Hyperfractionated radiation therapy with or without concurrent low-dose daily carboplatin/etoposide for stage III non-small-cell lung cancer: a randomized study. *J Clin Oncol* 1996, 14:1065–1070.

108. Pritchard RS, Anthony SP: Chemotherapy plus radiotherapy compared with radiotherapy alone in the treatment of locally advanced, unresectable, non-small-cell lung cancer. A meta-analysis. *Ann Intern Med* 1996, 125:723–729.

109. Cullen MH, Billingham LJ, Woodroffe CM, *et al.*: Mitomycin, ifosfamide, and cisplatin in unresectable non-small-cell lung cancer: effects on survival and quality of life. *J Clin Oncol* 1999, 17:3188–3194.

110. Takada Y, Furuse K, Fukuoka YH, *et al.*: A randomized phase III study of concurrent versus sequential thoracic radiotherapy (TRT) in combination with mitomycin, vindesine and cisplatin in unresectable stage III non-small cell lung cancer (NSCLC) [abstract]. *Lung Cancer* 1997, 18(Suppl 1):A294.

111. Curran WJ, Scott C, Langer C, *et al.*: Phase III comparison of sequential vs concurrent chemotherapy for PTS with unresectable stage III non-small cell lung cancer (NSCLC): initial report of Radiation Therapy Oncology Group (RTOG) 9410 [abstract 1891]. *Proc Am Soc Clin Oncol* 2000, 19:484a.

112. Gandara DR, Chansky K, Albain KS, *et al.*: Consolidation docetaxel after concurrent chemoradiotherapy in stage IIIB non-small-cell lung cancer: phase II Southwest Oncology Group Study S9504. *J Clin Oncol* 2003, 21:2004–2010.

113. Belani CP, Choy H, Bonomi P, *et al.*: Combined chemoradiotherapy regimens of paclitaxel and carboplatin for locally advanced non-small-cell lung cancer: a randomized phase II locally advanced multi-modality protocol. *J Clin Oncol* 2005, 23:5883–5891.

114. Bunn PA Jr, Kelly K: New chemotherapeutic agents prolong survival and improve quality of life in non-small cell lung cancer: a review of the literature and future directions. *Clin Cancer Res* 1998, 4:1087–1100.

115. Rapp E, Pater JL, Willan A, *et al.*: Chemotherapy can prolong survival in patients with advanced non-small-cell lung cancer: report of a Canadian multicenter randomized trial. *J Clin Oncol* 1988, 6:633–641.

116. Kelly K: Future directions for new cytotoxic agents in the treatment of advanced stage non-small cell lung cancer. *Am Soc Clin Oncol Educational Book* 2000, 357–367.

117. Thatcher N, Ranson M, Anderson H, *et al.*: Phase III study of paclitaxel versus supportive care in inoperative NSCLC [abstract]. *Ann Oncol* 1998, 9(Suppl):1.

118. Roszkowski K: Taxotere versus best supportive care in chemonaive patients with unresectable NSCLC: final results of the phase III study [abstract]. *Eur J Cancer* 1999, 35:246.

119. Wozniak AJ, Crowley JJ, Balcerzak SP, *et al.*: Randomized trial comparing cisplatin with cisplatin plus vinorelbine in the treatment of advanced non-small-cell lung cancer: a Southwest Oncology Group study. *J Clin Oncol* 1998, 16:2459–2465.

120. Sandler AB, Nemunaitis J, Denham C, *et al.*: Phase III trial of gemcitabine plus cisplatin versus cisplatin alone in patients with locally advanced or metastatic non-small-cell lung cancer. *J Clin Oncol* 2000, 18:122–130.

121. Bonomi P, Kim K, Fairclough D, *et al.*: Comparison of survival and quality of life in advanced non-small-cell lung cancer patients treated with two dose levels of paclitaxel combined with cisplatin versus etoposide with cisplatin: results of an Eastern Cooperative Oncology Group trial. *J Clin Oncol* 2000, 18:623–631.

122. Giaccone G, Postmus P, Debruyne C, *et al.*: Final results of an EORTC phase III study of paclitaxel vs. teniposide, in combination with cisplatin in advanced NSCLC [abstract]. *Proc Am Soc Clin Oncol* 1997, 16:460a.

123. Kelly K, Crowley JJ, Bunn PA, *et al.*: A randomized phase III trial of paclitaxel plus carboplatin (PC) versus vinorelbine plus cisplatin (VC) in untreated advanced non-small cell lung cancer (NSCLC): Southwest Oncology Group (SWOG) Trial [abstract]. *Proc Am Soc Clin Oncol* 1999, 18:461a.

124. Schiller JH, Harrington D, Sandler A, *et al.*: A randomized phase III trial of four chemotherapy regimens in advanced non-small cell lung cancer (NSCLC). ECOG 1594 [abstract]. *Proc Am Soc Clin Oncol* 2000, 19:1a.

125. Fossella FV, DeVore R, Kerr RN, *et al.*: Randomized phase III trial of docetaxel versus vinorelbine or ifosfamide in patients with advanced non-small-cell lung cancer previously treated with platinum-containing chemotherapy regimens. The TAX 320 Non-Small Cell Lung Cancer Study Group. *J Clin Oncol* 2000, 18:2354–2362.

126. Sandler A, Gray R, Perry MC, *et al.*: Paclitaxel-carboplatin alone or with bevacizumab for non-small-cell lung cancer. *N Engl J Med* 2006, 355:2542–2550.

127. Kosmidis P, Mylonakis N, Nicolaides C, *et al.*: Paclitaxel plus carboplatin versus gemcitabine plus paclitaxel in advanced non-small-cell lung cancer: a phase III randomized trial. *J Clin Oncol* 2002, 20:3578–3585.

128. Smit EF, van Meerbeeck JP, Lianes P, *et al.*: Three-arm randomized study of two cisplatin-based regimens and paclitaxel plus gemcitabine in advanced non-small-cell lung cancer: a phase III trial of the European Organization for Research and Treatment of Cancer Lung Cancer Group: EORTC 08975. *J Clin Oncol* 2003, 21:3909–3917.

129. Georgoulias V, Papadakis E, Alexopoulos A, *et al.*: Platinum-based and non-platinum-based chemotherapy in advanced non-small-cell lung cancer: a randomised multicentre trial. *Lancet* 2001, 357:1478–1484.

130. Kakolyris S, Tsiafaki X, Agelidou A, *et al.*: Preliminary results of a multi-center randomized phase III trial of docetaxel plus gemcitabine (DG) versus vinorelbine plus cisplatin (VC) in patients with advanced non-small cell lung cancer [abstract]. *Proc Am Soc Clin Oncol* 2002, 21:296a.

131. Rigas J, Carey M, Cole B, *et al.*: Multicenter web-based phase III study to test the survival equivalence of non-platinum based (NPB) vs platinum-based (PB) therapy for advanced non-small cell lung cancer (NSCLC): The Dartmouth NPB Chemotherapy Trial (D0112) [abstract]. *Proc Am Soc Clin Oncol* 2004, 22:634s.

132. Pujol JL, Breton JL, Gervais R, *et al.*: Gemcitabine-docetaxel versus cisplatin-vinorelbine in advanced or metastatic non-small-cell lung cancer: a phase III study addressing the case for cisplatin. *Ann Oncol* 2005, 16:602–610.

133. Gridelli C, Gallo C, Shepherd FA, *et al.*: Gemcitabine plus vinorelbine compared with cisplatin plus vinorelbine or cisplatin plus gemcitabine for advanced non-small-cell lung cancer: a phase III trial of the Italian GEMVIN Investigators and the National Cancer Institute of Canada Clinical Trials Group. *J Clin Oncol* 2003, 21:3025–3034.

134. Tan EH, Szczesna A, Krzakowski M, *et al.*: Randomized study of vinorelbine/gemcitabine versus vinorelbine/carboplatin in patients with advanced non-small cell lung cancer. *Lung Cancer* 2005, 49:233–240.

135. Greco FA, Spigel DR, Kuzur ME, *et al.*: Paclitaxel/carboplatin/gemcitabine versus gemcitabine/vinorelbine in advanced non-small-cell lung cancer: a phase II/III study of the Minnie Pearl Cancer Research Network. *Clin Lung Cancer* 2007, 8:483–487.

136. Laack E, Dickgreber N, Muller T, *et al.*: Randomized phase III study of gemcitabine and vinorelbine versus gemcitabine, vinorelbine, and cisplatin in the treatment of advanced non-small-cell lung cancer: from the German and Swiss Lung Cancer Study Group. *J Clin Oncol* 2004, 22:2348–2356.

137. Alberola V, Camps C, Provencio M, *et al.*: Cisplatin plus gemcitabine versus a cisplatin-based triplet versus nonplatinum sequential doublets in advanced non-small-cell lung cancer: a Spanish Lung Cancer Group phase III randomized trial. *J Clin Oncol* 2003, 21:3207–3213.

138. Takeda K, Negoro S, Masuda N, *et al.*: Phase I study of docetaxel (Doc) and irinotecan (CPT-11) for previously untreated advanced non-small cell lung cancer (NSCLC) [abstract]. *Proc Am Soc Clin Oncol* 1999, 18:524a.

139. Takeda K, Yamamoto N, Negoro S, *et al.*: Randomized phase III study of docetaxel (DOC) plus cisplatin (CDDP) versus DOC plus irinotecan in advanced non-small-cell lung cancer (NSCLC): a West Japan Thoracic Oncology Group (WJTOG) study [abstract]. *Proc Am Soc Clin Oncol* 2000, 19:497a.

140. Shepherd FA, Dancey J, Ramlau R, *et al.*: Prospective randomized trial of docetaxel versus best supportive care in patients with non-small-cell lung cancer previously treated with platinum-based chemotherapy. *J Clin Oncol* 2000, 18:2095–2103.

141. Hanna N, Shepherd FA, Fossella FV, *et al.*: Randomized phase III trial of pemetrexed versus docetaxel in patients with non-small-cell lung cancer previously treated with chemotherapy. *J Clin Oncol* 2004, 22:1589–1597.

142. Shepherd FA, Rodrigues Pereira J, Ciuleanu T, *et al.*: Erlotinib in previously treated non-small-cell lung cancer. *N Engl J Med* 2005, 353:123–132.

143. Paez JG, Janne PA, Lee JC, *et al.*: EGFR mutations in lung cancer: correlation with clinical response to gefitinib therapy. *Science* 2004, 304:1497–1500.

144. Lynch TJ, Bell DW, Sordella R, *et al.*: Activating mutations in the epidermal growth factor receptor underlying responsiveness of non-small-cell lung cancer to gefitinib. *N Engl J Med* 2004, 350:2129–2139.

145. Pao W, Miller V, Zakowski M, *et al.*: EGF receptor gene mutations are common in lung cancers from "never smokers" and are associated with sensitivity of tumors to gefitinib and erlotinib. *Proc Natl Acad Sci U S A* 2004, 101:13306–13311.

146. Tsao MS, Sakurada A, Cutz JC, *et al.*: Erlotinib in lung cancer: molecular and clinical predictors of outcome. *N Engl J Med* 2005, 353:133–144.

147. Gridelli C, Perrone F, Gallo C, *et al.*: Vinorelbine is well tolerated and active in the treatment of elderly patients with advanced non-small cell lung cancer. A two-stage phase II study. *Eur J Cancer* 1997, 33:392–397.

148. Gridelli C, Perron F, Gallo C, *et al.*: Effects of vinorelbine on quality of life and survival of elderly patients with advanced NSCLC: the Elderly Lung Cancer Vinorelbine Italian Study (ELVIS) Group. *J Natl Cancer Inst* 1999, 91:66–72.

149. Frasci G, Lorusso V, Panza N, *et al.*: Gemcitabine + vinorelbine (GV) yields better survival than vinorelbine alone in elderly NSCLC patients: final analysis of a Southern Italy Cooperative Oncology Group (SICOG) phase III trial [abstract]. *Proc Am Soc Clin Oncol* 2000, 19:485a.

150. Pfister DG, Johnson DH, Azzoli CG, *et al.*: American Society of Clinical Oncology treatment of unresectable non-small-cell lung cancer guideline: update 2003. *J Clin Oncol* 2004, 22:330–353.

151. Joos G, Pinson P, Van Renterghem D, *et al.*: A randomized study comparing vincristine, Adriamycin, cyclophosphamide (VAC) to carboplatin, etoposide (CE) in previously untreated small cell lung cancer (SCLC) [abstract]. *Proc Am Soc Clin Oncol* 1999, 18:470a.

152. Okamoto H, Watanabe K, Nishiwaki Y, *et al.*: Phase II study of area under the plasma-concentration-versus-time curve-based carboplatin plus standard-dose intravenous etoposide in elderly patients with small-cell lung cancer. *J Clin Oncol* 1999, 17:3540–3545.

153. Hainsworth JD, Gray JR, Stroup SL, *et al.*: Paclitaxel, carboplatin, and extended-schedule etoposide in the treatment of small-cell lung cancer: comparison of sequential phase II trials using different dose-intensities. *J Clin Oncol* 1997, 15:346–370.

Neoplasms of the skin account for the greatest percentage of human malignancies. Nonmelanoma neoplasms chiefly are comprised of squamous cell carcinomas (SCC) and basal cell carcinomas (BCC), which evolve slowly, demonstrate predominantly local growth with rare metastasis, and are typically cured with local treatments. Melanoma is a less common, but more aggressive, cutaneous neoplasm that often manifests regional and distant spread. Rarely, melanoma arises from noncutaneous sites, including the mucosa, the acral and subungual regions of the hands and feet, the uveal tract of the eye, and the leptomeninges. Clinically, the natural course and response to treatment of these varied melanomas are distinct. Recently, the possibility of distinguishing melanomas of cutaneous and various noncutaneous origins by molecular and genetic features, such as activating mutations of BRAF kinase, has been proposed [1–3]. The incidence of melanoma has risen annually for the past 30 years, and now ranks as the sixth leading cancer diagnosis. An estimated 60,000 people were diagnosed with melanoma in 2007, with an approximate 8000 deaths. The estimated lifetime risk of melanoma among white Americans is 1 in 49 men and 1 in 73 women [4]. The following chapter addresses the epidemiology, pathology, staging, and management of cutaneous melanoma as well as of BCC and SCC, the predominant skin cancers that confront the clinician.

MELANOMA

Over the past several decades, the incidence of melanoma has increased at a rate of approximately 3% per year. A rise has been demonstrated not only in adults, but in adolescents and children as well [5,6]. This broad range in patient age is one of many unique characteristics of melanoma. Other distinctive characteristics include well-defined genetic and environmental risk factors, a clear epidemiologic association with ultraviolet (UV) exposure, and a host immune response that can be enhanced to treat the disease in some patients. In this discussion, we will divide the risk factors for melanoma into host (*ie*, genetics) and nonhost (*ie*, UV exposure) (Table 11-1).

The mainstay of treatment for a primary melanoma, after the diagnosis has been establihsed with a biopsy, is wide local excision of the primay site. In patients who have primary tumors with a Breslow thickness 1 mm or greater or those less than 1 mm thick but with a Clark level IV or greater, ulceration, or other worrisome features, lymphatic mapping and sentinel lymph node (SLN) biopsy at the time of wide local excision are considered standard of care. In stage I and II patients, SLN status is the most important predictor of disease-specific survival [7]. With advances in our understanding of distinct molecular and genetic abnormalities in melanoma, our knowledge of this heterogeneous disease is improving and will likely impact therapeutic decisions in the future.

ETIOLOGY AND RISK FACTORS

Host

The majority of melanomas, approximately 90%, are sporadic [8]. While familial melanoma syndromes are rare, families also share heritable risk factors. Extensive research supports that darkly pigmented individuals are at less risk for melanoma than lightly pigmented individuals [9,10]. The "at-risk" phenotype includes not only fair skin color, but light hair and eye color, the presence of freckling and nevi, and sun sensitivity (penchant for burning rather than tanning). It is clear that the presence of nevi, or moles, is one of the strongest risk factors for melanoma. Multiple moles, as well as atypical mole features, further increase an individual's risk. Additionally, the presence of one or more dysplastic nevi is considered an independent risk factor for melanoma [9,11]. Dysplastic nevi were first described in familial melanoma kindreds. Patients with these findings should have a thorough assessment of family history and be followed closely by a dermatologist.

A family history of melanoma is a strong independent risk factor, especially in association with dysplastic nevi. The primary germline genetic abnormality associated with familial melanoma is of the *CDKN2A* gene (also known as *p16INK4a*), localized to chromosome 9p21 [12]. The 9p21 locus encodes two distinct tumor suppressor proteins, p16INK4a and p14ARF (produced via alternative splicing), which regulate cell cycle progression via the retinoblastoma and p53 pathways, respectively. Mutations in *p16INK4a* have been documented in 20% to 40% of familial melanoma, and appear to enhance the risk for pancreatic cancer [13,14]. Another high-risk, although less common, mutation associated with familial melanoma is of the *CDK4* gene, which is also involved in cell cycle regulation [15]. Due to variable penetrance, the lifetime risk of melanoma in these kindreds can vary [12]. At this time, performing genetic testing on individuals with known risk factors for melanoma will not impact their clinical management or that of their family members if they are under appropriate dermatologic surveillance.

Table 11-1. Risk Factors of Melanoma and Nonmelanoma Skin Cancers

Risk factor	Cancer type
Nevi (moles) (multiple, atypical, dysplastic)	Melanoma
Family history of melanoma	Melanoma
Familial melanoma syndromes	Melanoma
9p21 mutations (CDKN2A or p16INK4a)	
12q14 mutation (CDK4)	
Skin type (tanning ability)	Melanoma/SCC/BCC
Degree of pigmentation (light skin/hair/eye color)	Melanoma/SCC/BCC
Prior melanoma	Melanoma/SCC/BCC
Immunosuppression	Melanoma/SCC/BCC
HIV/AIDS	
Prior organ transplantation	
Immunosuppressive medication	
Xeroderma pigmentosum	Melanoma/SCC/BCC
Sun/ultraviolet (UV) exposure	Melanoma/SCC/BCC
Arsenic	Melanoma/SCC/BCC
Methoxsalen (psoralen) and UVA treatment	Melanoma/SCC/BCC
Tanning bed use	Melanoma/SCC
Ionizing radiation exposure	SCC/BCC
Polycyclic aromatic hydrocarbons	SCC/BCC
Human papillomavirus infection	SCC/BCC
Cigarette smoking	SCC/BCC
Albinism	SCC/BCC
Chronic wounds	SCC
Chronic inflammatory conditions (epidermodysplasia verruciformis)	SCC
Precancerous lesions (SCC in situ, actinic keratosis, Bowen's disease, other precursor lesions)	SCC
Nevoid BCC (Gorlin's) syndrome	BCC
Rombo syndrome	BCC
Bazex-Dupre-Christol syndrome	BCC

BCC—basal cell carcinoma; SCC—squamous cell carcinoma.
(*Data from* Tucker and Goldstein [9], Pho *et al.* [12], Zuo *et al.* [15], Gallagher *et al.* [42], Alam and Ratner [142], Rubin *et al.* [143], and IARC Working Group [148].)

Molecular and genetic profiling of various cancers is being vigorously pursued in an effort to improve classification, therapeutics, and ultimately outcomes. The mitogen-activated protein kinase (MAPK) signal transduction pathway has received much attention given its involvement in cell proliferation, survival, and invasion [16,17]. This pathway is comprised of RAS, RAF, MEK, and ERK tyrosine kinases. Mutations in RAS and RAF have been described in a variety of malignancies. A recent groundbreaking finding was the documentation of activating mutations in the BRAF kinase in 66% of primary melanomas [18]. This same BRAF mutation was found later to be present in up to 82% of benign nevi [19]. While it appears to be insufficient for in vivo malignant transformation in isolation, the exact role of BRAF in melanoma remains to be clarified. Mutant BRAF does appear to correlate with UV exposure, albeit indirectly. The most common mutation of BRAF (V600E) is not characteristic of UV-induced DNA damage [18]. BRAF mutations are found much more frequently in cutaneous melanomas that occur on intermittently sun-exposed skin as compared with those melanomas on chronically sun-exposed skin or non–sun-exposed sites [1,20]. Further, BRAF mutations are not seen in congenital nevi [21], are not associated with familial melanoma [22], and are rare in other noncutaneous melanomas [23,24]. Patterns of mutations in other pathways, including PI3K and c-KIT, also have been reported [1,2]. Various therapeutic agents targeted at molecular pathways are being developed and tested in mela-noma, including sorafenib (BAY 43-9006, Nexavar; Bayer, West Haven CT and Onyx, Richmond, CA).

The evidence for host immune reactivity against melanoma includes spontaneous partial and complete regression of primary and metastatic lesions [25], development of vitiligo-like hypopigmentation in various stages of melanoma [26], documentation of endogenous antibodies against mela-noma antigens [27], and development of autoimmune diseases in response to successful immunotherapies [28–30]. Indeed, a small number of stage IV patients appear to be cured with high-dose interleukin-2 (IL-2) therapy [31,32]. Histologically, the presence of tumor-infiltrating lymphocytes in primary lesions correlates with improved survival [33]. Additionally, aside from an individual's genetic and constitutional risk factors, many conditions associated with impaired cell-mediated immunity correlate with an increased risk of cutaneous melanoma and nonmelanoma skin cancers as well as more aggressive disease courses. These conditions include some hematologic malignancies [34,35], organ transplantation [36], and HIV/AIDS [37].

NONHOST

Sun and UV radiation exposure clearly play a role in development of mela-noma and nonmelanoma skin cancers [38]. While a direct effect has not been established, epidemiologic studies have provided strong indirect evidence to support the role of these exposures in melanomagenesis [39,40]. However, the relationship is not straightforward. It appears that intense, intermittent sun exposure, as opposed to chronic or cumulative exposure, carries the greatest risk of melanoma [41]. As previously discussed, molecular and genetic studies also support the concept of distinct subtypes of melanoma that may, in part, be related to type of sun exposure [1,2]. As expected, it is difficult to quantify sun and UV radiation exposure in an individual or across studies. These same issues have plagued studies attempting to evaluate tanning bed use and melanoma risk. A recent meta-analysis concluded that tanning bed use does increase the risk of melanoma but that the amount of use needed to produce this effect is unclear [42].

CLINICAL AND PATHOLOGIC APPEARANCE

The clinical characteristics of skin lesions considered of concern for melanoma have been well described and include the "ABCDE" criteria of asymmetry, border, color, diameter greater than 6 mm, and evolution or change noted by the patient or another individual [43]. Bleeding and/or development of an overlying blister or scab can correlate with histologic ulceration of the primary lesion, conveying a poorer prognosis. Evolution of a skin lesion, including the sensation of itching, should prompt investigation and possible biopsy. As previously mentioned, melanomas may arise from prior nevi or de novo. A variety of morphologic subtypes of cutaneous melanoma can be distinguished, including superficial spreading, nodular, lentigo maligna, acral lentiginous (including subungual), and desmoplastic. While these subtypes may have distinct clinical behavior (*eg*, lentigo maligna melanomas often present as thinner lesions), they do not have independent prognostic value [44].

STAGING, DIAGNOSIS, AND PROGNOSIS

In the past few decades, melanoma classification has evolved from the general groupings of local resectable disease, regionally advanced and resectable disease, and disseminated disease to the current American Joint Commission on Cancer (AJCC) staging system (Table 11-2 and Table 11-3), which was revised in 2002 [45]. The most significant changes with this revision included the addition of ulceration to T (tumor) classification, changing the thresholds of Breslow thickness to whole number increments, the characterization of nodal involvement according to tumor burden (clinically occult/microscopic or clinically evident/macroscopic) as well as number of involved nodes, and the classification of metastatic disease into distinct subsets according to organ site involvement and serum lactate dehydrogenase (LDH) level [46]. In general terms, stage I and II encompass localized disease of low and intermediate recurrence risk, stage III encompasses disease with lymph node involvement at high recurrence risk, and stage IV includes distant metastatic disease. In stage III disease, the most important variables affecting local and distant recurrence risk are the extent (microscopic vs macroscopic) of lymph node

Table 11-2. AJCC TNM Classification for Melanoma

T Classification	Tumor thickness, *mm*	Ulceration status
Tis	In situ	—
T1	< 1.0	a: Without ulceration and Clark's level II/III
		b: With ulceration or Clark's level IV/V
T2	1.01–2.0	a: Without ulceration
		b: With ulceration
T3	2.01–4.0	a: Without ulceration
		b: With ulceration
T4	> 4.0	a: Without ulceration
		b: With ulceration
N Classification	**Metastatic nodes, *n***	**Nodal metastatic mass**
N1	1 node	a: Micrometastases
		b: Macrometastases
N2	2–3 nodes	a: Micrometastases
		b: Macrometastases
		c: Satellite(s)/in-transit metastases without metastatic node(s)
N3	≥ 4 nodes, or matted nodes, or satellite(s)/in-transit metastases with metastatic nodes	—
M Classification	**Site**	**Serum lactate dehydrogenase**
M1a	Distant skin, subcutaneous, or node	Normal
M1b	Lung	Normal
M1c	All other visceral sites	Normal
	Any distant metastases	Elevated

AJCC—American Joint Committee on Cancer; TNM—tumor, node, metastasis. (*Adapted from* Balch [45].)

involvement, the number of involved nodes, and the presence or absence of gross extracapsular extension [47].

A work-up for primary melanoma includes a history and physical examination with attention to skin pigmentation, including the presence of hypopigmentation, other skin lesions, and lymph nodes. Hypopigmentation may reflect a regressing or regressed primary site or a paraneoplastic vitiligo-like destruction of the normal melanocytes in the skin. The detection of a primary melanoma or a cutaneous recurrence or metastasis hinges upon an awareness of an individual's known skin lesions, recognition of any change in a lesion, or development of new lesions. Photographic evaluation is useful in providing a frame of reference for follow-up of patients with numerous or varied lesions [48]. The proper initial evaluation of a lesion suspected to be a melanoma should include an excisional biopsy, if feasible, in order to establish as accurate diagnosis and assessment of tumor thickness. If not, a partial biopsy, such as an incisional, punch, or deep shave (saucerization) biopsy, may be used [49]. Shallow shave biopsies are discouraged as these may transect the primary melanoma, and nonsurgical treatment, such as electrocautery, is contraindicated. If a diagnosis of melanoma is made, the next step is to proceed to wide local excision with or without a SLN biopsy, where the features of the primary tumor (thickness, level of invasion, ulceration) will determine the margins of excision and need for SLN biopsy (Table 11-4). Re-biopsy is recommended if a specimen is insufficient to establish a diagnosis of melanoma or to assess the features of a primary melanoma, such as tumor thickness. Repeat wide local excision, if feasible, is recommended if inadequate margins are obtained.

If a patient presents with nodal or metastatic disease in the absence of an obvious primary tumor, less obvious cutaneous sites should be examined, including the scalp, perineal area, the palms and soles, and subungual surfaces. A work-up of potential noncutaneous primary sites of melanoma, including mucosal surfaces and the uveal tract of the eye, should be guided by the history and physical examination. A rectal examination, including a gynecologic examination in women, should be performed, as anorectal and

vaginal primaries are frequent sites of primary mucosal melanoma [50]. More invasive procedures, such as upper and lower endoscopies, should be pursued in the setting of concerning signs or symptoms, such as gastrointestinal bleeding or iron deficiency anemia. An ophthalmologic examination can evaluate for a primary uveal melanoma.

A chest radiograph and liver function tests, including LDH, may be performed on initial evaluation for stage IB to III melanoma to screen for clinically occult metastatic disease in these two organs, although neither test is highly sensitive [51]. These evaluations are not recommended in earlier-stage melanomas because the risk of dissemination is minimal. In regionally advanced and metastatic settings, full body evaluation with either computed tomography (CT) of the chest/abdomen/pelvis or whole body positron emission tomography fused with CT (PET/CT) is indicated, as is magnetic resonance imaging of the brain [52].

In the past, elective complete lymphadenectomy (ELND) was performed for the drainage basin at greatest risk according to the anatomic location of the primary. However, ELND has shown no survival benefit in any of several large, randomized controlled trials [53]. Lymphoscintigraphy and SLN biopsy was developed to ascertain the drainage of primary melanomas and other tumors and to detect early lymphatic spread in patients without clinical evidence of lymphatic involvement [54]. SLN biopsy offers accurate evaluation with lower morbidity for staging of regional lymph node basins than lymphadenectomy [55]. SLN status has been shown to be the most important predictor of disease-free survival and risk of relapse in stage I/II melanoma [7]. SLN biopsy is considered a diagnostic procedure, but not definitively therapeutic. However, recently published results of the third planned interim analysis (of a planned five) of the Multicenter Selective Lymphadenectomy Trial I (MSLT-1) lend support to it being therapeutic as well [56]. This was a randomized phase 3 study of patients with intermediate-thickness melanoma (1.2–3.5 mm) who received either wide local excision with SLN biopsy and immediate completion lymph node dissection (CLND) if the SLN was positive versus wide local excision and observation, with a CLND performed at the time of nodal relapse. As of this latest analysis, the overall survival and melanoma-specific survival for the two arms were not significantly different. However, the 5 year disease-free survival of the SLN/CLND arm was greater than that of the observation arm (78% vs 73%; hazard ratio [HR] for death, 0.74; *P* = 0.009). On subgroup analysis, the patients with nodal metastases who underwent SLN and immediate CLND had an improved 5-year survival compared with the observation group (72% vs 52%; hazard ratio for death, 0.51; *P* = 0.004). The current standard of care for patients with lymph node metastases, either microscopic or macroscopic, is an immediate CLND. Whether or not immediate CLND is beneficial in the setting of microscopically positive SLN metastasis [57] is the question being addressed by the MSLT-II. This ongoing, randomized phase 3 study is evaluating melanoma-specific survival in SLN-positive patients who undergo immediate CLND versus observation with serial ultrasound with CLND only if they develop clinically evident lymph node metastasis. There is no role for lymphoscintigraphy or SLN biopsy in patients with clinically evident lymphadenopathy concerning for metastases. These patients should have a fine-needle aspiration or core biopsy performed to evaluate for metastatic melanoma. Again, if regional lymph node involvement is confirmed in the absence of distant metastases, CLND

Table 11-3. AJCC Stage Groupings for Cutaneous Melanoma

Clinical staging				Pathologic staging			
0	Tis	N0	M0	0	Tis	N0	M0
IA	T1a	N0	M0	IA	T1a	N0	M0
IB	T1b	N0	M0	IB	T1b	N0	M0
	T2a	N0	M0		T2a	N0	M0
IIA	T2b	N0	M0	IIA	T2b	N0	M0
	T3a	N0	M0		T3a	N0	M0
IIB	T3b	N0	M0	IIB	T3b	N0	M0
	T4a	N0	M0		T4a	N0	M0
IIC	T4b	N0	M0	IIC	T4b	N0	M0
III	Any T	Any N	M0	IIIA	T1–4a	N1a	M0
					T1–4a	N2a	M0
				IIIB	T1–4b	N1a	M0
					T1–4b	N2a	M0
					T1–4a	N1b	M0
					T1–4a	N2b	M0
					T1–4a/b	N2c	M0
				IIIC	T1–4b	N1b	M0
					T1–4b	N2b	M0
					T1–4b	N2c	M0
					Any T	N3	M0
IV	Any T	Any N	Any M	IV	Any T	Any N	Any M

AJCC—American Joint Committee on Cancer.
(*Adapted from* Balch [45].)

Table 11-4. Recommended Margins for Wide Local Excision*

Tumor thickness, *mm*	Recommended clinical margins, *cm*
In situ	0.5
≤ 1.0	1.0
1.01–2	1–2
2.01–4	2.0
> 4	2.0

*Margins may be modified to accommodate individual anatomic or cosmetic considerations. For in situ melanomas, pathologic confirmation of a negative peripheral margin is important.
(Reproduced with permission from the National Comprehensive Cancer Network [52].)

is recommended. Likewise, if distant metastases are suspected, pathologic confirmation of metastatic melanoma via biopsy is recommended to determine correct staging and treatment.

Follow-up for melanoma varies by stage and should include surgical and/or medical oncologic evaluations as well as dermatologic assessments. Table 11-5 outlines the recommended surveillance schedules for all stages of melanoma. These recommendations are adapted from the National Comprehensive Cancer Network (NCCN) guidelines [52], and should be adjusted for each individual patient according to his or her disease, risk factors, signs and symptoms, and other factors. These follow-ups, which do not account for treatment visits, should also include patient education regarding self skin-examination. Of note, there are no recommendations for routine CT or PET/CT imaging in these patients, although it is often done in practice. Additionally, there are no established guidelines for follow-up of patients with stage IV who have no evidence of disease (NED); the authors' recommendations are included in Table 11-5. All patients with a history of melanoma stage 0 to IV, if NED, require at least an annual dermatologic examination for life because of the risk of late recurrence and/or another primary melanoma [52].

Prognostic factors predictive of survival include microstage of disease as defined by tumor thickness (Breslow depth), presence or absence of ulceration, and in stage I patients, skin layer penetration (Clark level). Mitotic rate, presence of satellite lesions, and other features are prognostically important histologic factors [58]. Younger patients, females, and patients with primaries on an extremity have a better prognosis compared with older patients, males, or those with primaries on the trunk or head

and neck. It now appears that younger patients may have a higher likelihood of a positive sentinel node [59].

TREATMENT

SURGERY

The surgical treatment of primary melanoma is well established. Consensus from the published studies indicates that a wide local excision should be performed for all primary lesions, including in situ melanomas. The recommended margins of excision are dependent upon tumor thickness, hence the importance of the initial biopsy (Table 11-4). In patients with primary tumors 1 mm or more in thickness or those less than 1 mm in thickness but with a Clark level IV or greater or with ulceration, lymphoscintigraphy and SLN biopsy at the time of wide local excision should be performed. As aforementioned, therapeutic CLND is the current standard of care for regional lymph node metastases, identified on SLN biopsy or clinically, in the absence of distant disease. Limited resection of distant metastases, including cutaneous, nodal, or other organ metastases, has a role in palliation of symptomatic lesions. Patients with solitary brain metastases, and patients with solitary or oligometastatic disease involving lung, liver, adrenal gland, or cutaneous tissue, may obtain significant benefit from surgical resection, with prolonged disease-free intervals beyond 2 years [60–62].

RADIATION

Radiation therapy is used in a few particular circumstances in the management of melanoma. In stage III disease following appropriate surgical management, local control of an involved lymph node basin can be improved by

Table 11-5. Recommendations for Follow-Up

Stage	Follow-up*	Blood work		Imaging	
		Work-up[†]	In follow-up	Work-up	In follow-up
0	H&P (emphasis on nodes and skin); at least annual skin exam for life; consider educating patient in monthly self skin exam	None	None	None	None
IA	H&P (emphasis on nodes and skin) every 3–12 mo to follow-up for specific signs and symptoms; at least annual skin exam for life; consider educating patient in monthly self skin and lymph node exam	None	None	Further imaging to evaluate specific signs and symptoms (CT scan, PET, MRI)	None
IB–II	H&P (emphasis on nodes and skin) every 3–6 mo for 3 y, then every 4–12 mo for 2 y, then annually as clinically indicated; at least annual skin exam for life; consider educating patient in monthly self skin and lymph node exam	None specified	LDH, CBC, LFT every 3–12 mo (optional)	Chest x-ray (optional); CT scan, PET, MRI to evaluate specific signs and symptoms for stage IIB, IIC patients	Chest x-ray every 3–12 mo (optional); CT scan to follow-up for specific signs and symptoms
III	H&P (emphasis on nodes and skin) every 3–6 mo for 3 y, then every 4–12 mo for 2 y, then annually as clinically indicated; at least annual skin exam for life; consider educating patient in monthly self skin and lymph node exam	LDH (optional)	LDH, CBC, LFT every 3–12 mo (optional)	Chest x-ray (optional); pelvic CT if inguinofemoral nodes positive (clinically positive nodes); further imaging (CT ± PET, MRI) to evaluate specific signs and symptoms	Chest x-ray every 3–12 mo (optional); CT scan to follow-up for specific signs and symptoms
IV	As indicated according to systemic disease and response to treatment	LDH	As indicated for therapy	Chest x-ray and/or chest CT; consider abdominal/pelvic CT or head MRI and/or PET; further imaging to evaluate specific signs and symptoms	As indicated for therapy
IV (NED)[‡]	H&P (emphasis on nodes and skin) every 3–6 mo for 3 y, then every 4–12 mo for 2 y, then annually as clinically indicated; at least annual skin exam for life; consider educating patient in monthly self skin and lymph node exam	LDH	LDH, CBC, LFT every 3–12 mo (optional)	Chest x-ray and/or chest CT; consider abdominal/pelvic CT or head MRI and/or PET; further imaging to evaluate specific signs and symptoms	Chest x-ray every 3–12 mo (optional); CT scan to follow-up for specific signs and symptoms

*Schedule influenced by risk of recurrence, prior primary melanoma, and family history of melanoma and includes other factors, such as dysplastic nevus syndrome and patient anxiety.
[†]Other blood work may be done at the discretion of the physician.
[‡]For patients with stage IV melanoma who are rendered disease free by any modality, a follow-up schedule similar to stage III disease was felt to be appropriate.
CBC—complete blood count; CT—computed tomography; H&P—history and physical exam; LDH—lactate dehydrogenase; LFT—liver function tests; MRI—magnetic resonance imaging; NED—no evidence of disease; PET—positron emission tomography.
(Reproduced with permission from the National Comprehensive Cancer Network [52].)

irradiation of the dissected basin when four or more lymph nodes contain metastatic melanoma, if the lymph nodes are matted or demonstrate gross extracapsular extension, of if the nodal recurrence occurred in a previously dissected nodal basin [63]. In stage IV disease, radiation is a palliative modality for metastatic sites, particularly for the brain or painful bone metastases. In the setting of metastatic brain involvement, steroid treatment is usually necessary to alleviate cerebral edema and the associated symptoms of increased intracranial pressure. Patients with brain metastasis may benefit from whole brain irradiation (WBI), intensive focal radiation (gamma knife or stereotactic radiosurgery [SRS]), or a combination of both. Patients with a solitary brain metastasis accompanied by no or low-volume extracranial metastases should be considered for neurosurgery [64–66]. Data on the best utilization of SRS continues to evolve. SRS does improve survival over WBI alone, when feasible [67]. These techniques are useful treatments for brain metastases that are unresectable, isolated, or of a limited number (≤ 4) and size (< 3 cm) [68]. WBI has been used palliatively when surgery or SRS is not indicated. A recent prospective study to evaluate WBI in conjunction with SRS versus SRS alone in patients with up to four brain metastases from varied malignancies demonstrated no survival benefit, but did show reduced risk of central nervous system (CNS) relapse [69]. For patients who have undergone surgical resection of a brain metastasis, at a minimum, radiation to the resection bed is recommended [70].

SYSTEMIC THERAPY

ADJUVANT SETTING

The risk of relapse in patients with stage I melanoma is quite low; greater than 90% will be surgically cured [46]. Patients with stage IIA melanoma are at intermediate risk of relapse or death, roughly 10% to 30%. At this time, there is no role for adjuvant therapy in these patient groups. Patients at high risk of relapse, generally at or exceeding 50% in the first 5 years of follow-up, include those with stage IIB through stage IIIC melanoma. It is this group of high-risk patients that have been the focus for adjuvant therapy clinical trials including chemotherapy and immunotherapy. Except for high-dose interferon alfa-2b, no agent has proven to be of benefit in the adjuvant setting. High-dose interferon alfa-2b is the only agent with US Food and Drug Association (FDA) approval for the adjuvant treatment of stage IIB, IIC, and III melanoma. This approval was based on the results of Eastern Cooperative Oncology Group (ECOG) protocol 1684 comparing 1 year of high-dose interferon alfa-2b with observation in patients with surgically treated stage IIB, IIC, or III disease. The study showed a relapse-free survival (RFS) benefit (median, 1.72 vs 0.98 years) and an overall survival benefit (median, 3.82 vs 2.78 years) for the high-dose interferon alfa-2b arm at a median follow-up of 6.9 years [71]. The high-dose interferon alfa-2b regimen consisted of 20 million units (MU)/m^2/d given intravenously Monday through Friday for 4 weeks followed by 10 MU/m^2/d given subcutaneously three times per week for 11 months. Disappointingly, at a median follow-up of 12.6 years, the overall survival benefit was lost, although there was still a statistically significant RFS benefit [72].

The ECOG performed two larger follow-up studies of high-dose interferon alfa-2b. In ECOG protocol 1690, 642 patients were randomized to high-dose interferon alfa-2b, low-dose interferon, or observation. At a median follow up of 6.6 years, there was a statistically significant RFS advantage for high-dose interferon alfa-2b but no overall survival benefit [72,73]. In ECOG 1694, 800 high-risk patients were randomized between high-dose interferon alfa-2b and a GM2-ganglioside vaccine. The study did show overall survival benefit for high-dose interferon alfa-2b, but the results are difficult to interpret because of a lack of a control arm and a short follow-up that has not been updated [74].

Associated toxicities at this interferon dose and schedule are significant and will necessitate dose reductions in approximately 75% of patients [75]. Side effects include fatigue, anorexia, flu-like symptoms, depression, liver abnormalities, and cytopenias. Numerous trials have evaluated less toxic schedules of low-, intermediate-, or protracted-dose interferon. None of these schedules have shown an overall survival benefit. Eggermont *et al.* [76] recently showed that 5 years of pegylated interferon-α improved RFS but not overall survival in stage III patients. A meta-analysis of adjuvant interferon randomized trials again supported a significant RFS improvement in patients treated with high-dose interferon alfa-2b (four studies) compared with controls (HR, 0.83; 95% CI, 0.77–0.90) [77]. Any overall survival benefit to high-dose interferon alfa-2b remains in question as the confidence interval in this meta-analysis crossed 1.0 (HR, 0.93; 95% CI, 0.85–1.02). On subgroup analysis, the degree of RFS benefit appeared to correlate directly with the dose of interferon alfa-2b, supporting the concept that only the high-dose, year-long course provides measurable benefit.

A number of cancer vaccines have been studied in melanoma in both the adjuvant and metastatic settings. The goal of cancer vaccines is to initiate a specific cell-mediated, antitumor response, with or without a humoral antitumor response. While immunologic responses to cancer vaccines are often induced, it has been difficult to demonstrate measurable clinical benefit [78]. Many different vaccine formulations, schedules, and delivery methods have been attempted. An improved understanding of the complexities of the human immune system has led to the development of more sophisticated vaccines currently in phase 1, 2, and 3 trials. These include gene-transfected whole cell vaccines, peptide vaccines, various formulations of dendritic cells (the most potent antigen-presenting cells), naked DNA, and heat shock proteins [79]. An in-depth discussion of vaccines is beyond the scope of this chapter; the reader is referred to other extensive reviews [79]. Here we will highlight some of the vaccines that have been evaluated in large randomized trials.

All large, randomized phase 3 studies of melanoma vaccines in the adjuvant setting have had negative results thus far. These include trials of the Newcastle disease virus melanoma oncolysate [80] and a cell lysate vaccine combined with detoxified lipid A (Melacine, Corixa Corporation, Seattle, WA) [81]. In a retrospective analysis, patients who were human leukocyte antigen (HLA)-A2 or -C3 positive appeared to benefit from Melacine, but no follow-up studies have been done or are planned [82]. In ECOG protocol 1694, a GM2 ganglioside vaccine was inferior to high-dose interferon alfa-2b [74]. More recently, Canvaxin (CancerVax, Carlsbad, CA), an allogeneic whole cell vaccine composed of three highly antigenic, irradiated melanoma cell lines given with Bacillus Calmette-Guérin (BCG) was no more effective than BCG alone in stage III and stage IV NED patients [83].

Some of the initial work in whole cell vaccines centered on the use of autologous tumor cells. This technique ensures a relevant mix of antigens but has many inherent difficulties, including the need for adequate tumor tissue. M-VAX (AVAX Technologies, Philadelphia, PA) is an autologous, irradiated, whole-cell melanoma vaccine modified by the hapten dinitrophenol. A phase 3 study in metastatic melanoma is currently ongoing based on the results of a phase 2 study that showed improved disease-free and overall survival correlating with the development of a delayed-type hypersensitivity response in stage III melanoma patients, where historical controls served as the reference [84,85].

Since the discovery that melanomas express HLA-restricted peptide antigens that can elicit a cytotoxic T-cell response, a great deal of work has gone into developing allogeneic peptide vaccines [86]. Many of these short (9-10) amino acid peptides have now been identified and classified into three large groups: 1) differentiation or lineage-specific antigens (mainly associated with melanin formation); 2) cancer testis antigens, which refer to a series of melanoma antigens (MAGE 1,2,3; NY-ESO-1; HO-MEL-40) specified by X-linked genes and expressed only in certain cancers and in normal testis and ovarian tissue; and 3) mutated tumor antigens [87]. Allogeneic peptide vaccines are easier to manufacture and more generalizable that autologous vaccines, but require that patients be HLA matched. Thus far, clinical trials have utilized 1-4 epitope peptide vaccines with little success [79]. More recent research is using HLA class I restricted multi-epitope vaccines alone or in combination with class II restricted epitope vaccines [79]. By using greater numbers of epitopes, it is speculated that the vaccines will target all tumor cells in a particular melanoma and induce a more robust T-cell response. Research has shown that there are multiple natural inhibitory mechanisms (*eg*, cytotoxic T-lymphocyte antigen-4 [CTLA-4], T-regulatory cells) in the human immune system that prevent autoimmunity, but also inhibit responses to immunotherapy [88]. These mechanisms are being taken into consideration in the design of future melanoma vaccines.

In summary, management discussions with patients regarding adjuvant treatment decisions following resection of stage IIB to III melanoma are challenging and time consuming. Overall, the treatment options in the adjuvant setting are threefold: participation in a clinical trial, high-dose interferon alfa-2b, or observation. Given the current limited treatment options, discussing and referring patients for clinical trial participation is imperative. While controversy still exists regarding high-dose interferon alfa-2b in high-risk melanoma patients, it is an option that should be discussed, as it has shown a consistent RFS benefit in multiple studies. Of course, the adjuvant therapy decision must be individualized to each patient and will depend upon several factors, including comorbid conditions, availability of trials, and patient preference. Stage IV patients who have been surgically rendered NED should be observed or referred for clinical trials since they have no standard therapy options.

METASTATIC SETTING

Exciting clinical research in melanoma over the past several years has centered around two very different classes of therapeutics: agents targeted at molecular pathways, such as sorafenib, and agents targeted at inhibitory immunologic pathways, namely antibodies against CTLA-4. The data are interesting and may likely affect standard clinical practice in the near future. Dacarbazine and high-dose IL-2 are the only FDA-approved therapies for treatment of metastatic melanoma in the United States. Unfortunately, to date, no survival benefit has been demonstrated for any therapeutic agent, either alone or in combination with other agents [89]. In this section, the discussion will be divided into two sections: 1) chemotherapeutics and molecularly targeted agents and 2) immunotherapeutics. Before presenting newer data, we will review the current standard agents.

CHEMOTHERAPY

Dacarbazine (DTIC), an alkylating agent that requires hepatic conversion to its active intermediate, has consistently shown complete and partial responses as a single agent in 5% to 20% of patients [90,91].The list of single agents evaluated in the setting of metastatic melanoma is long, and includes interferon-α [92], cisplatin [93], carboplatin [94], carmustine (BCNU) [95], vindesine [96], paclitaxel [97], docetaxel [98], and vinorelbine [99]. None of these single agents has shown superiority over single-agent dacarbazine. Various two- and three-drug combinations have not yet yielded superior results to single-agent dacarbazine either [89]. Two multidrug chemotherapy regimens initially achieved higher response rates than single agents but have not conveyed improved survival and are associated with greater toxicities. Early studies of both the Dartmouth regimen (dacarbazine, carmustine, cisplatin, and tamoxifen) and the BOLD regimen (bleomycin, vincristine, lomustine, and dacarbazine) showed response rates greater than 40% [100,101]. Upon further evaluation in larger, multicenter, randomized trials, the response rates were not as dramatic and no incremental improvement in survival for combination therapy was seen [91,102,103]. Therefore, single-agent dacarbazine remains the standard option. Another chemotherapeutic option is single-agent temozolomide, an orally bioavailable prodrug that is spontaneously converted to the same active intermediate as dacarbazine. Temozolomide was compared with dacarbazine in a randomized phase 3 study and showed equivalent survival [104]. It was not FDA approved as it did not show superiority; therefore, temozolomide may not be reimbursed fully by insurance. Temozolomide may be dosed on two different schedules: 150 to 200 mg/m^2 orally on days 1 to 5 in a 28-day cycle or 75 mg/m^2 orally every day for 6 weeks followed by a 2-week break. As it penetrates the blood-brain barrier, temozolomide is the preferred treatment for patients with CNS involvement. If concurrent external-beam radiation to the CNS or elsewhere is planned, the extended dosing regimen should also be considered as temozolomide is radiosensitizing [105]. In the clinical management of patients taking temozolomide, prophylaxis against *Pneumocystis jiroveci* (formerly *Pneumocystis carinii*) pneumonia should be considered because selective CD4+ lymphopenia can occur [106]. This is more common with the extended regimen, and concomitant steroids and/or radiation increase the risk.

MOLECULARLY TARGETED AGENTS

Molecularly targeted agents have created a new class of cancer therapeutics. These agents interfere with molecular pathways involved in cellular functions, such as cell growth and division. It is these same pathways that are aberrant, for a variety of reasons, in malignancies. The actual drugs may be small molecules (such as sorafenib), antibodies (such as bevacizumab [Avastin, Genentech, South San Francisco, CA]), or even antisense oligonucleotides (such as oblimersen sodium [Genasense, Genta International Inc, Berkeley Heights, NJ]) that inhibit the translation of proteins from RNA. Because these agents do not target cells in the same manner as chemotherapy, the side effect profile is quite different. Ultimately, we may elucidate agents that, either alone or in combination with other molecular agents/chemotherapy/immunotherapy, specifically inhibit the initiation, maintenance, or progression of cancer. Within the field of melanoma, sorafenib has garnered the most attention due to the potentially pivotal role of BRAF in this tumor. Sorafenib, a multitargeted tyrosine kinase inhibitor, inhibits mutant and wild-type BRAF as well as vascular endothelial growth factor receptor-2 and -3, platelet-derived growth factor receptor, c-KIT, and others [107]. Despite high expectations, sorafenib proved ineffective as a single agent in advanced melanoma [108]. In a randomized phase 2 study in melanoma of dacarbazine alone versus dacarbazine and sorafenib, a significant difference in response rate (12% vs 24%) and 6-month progression-free survival (18% vs 41%) was seen [109]. In a phase 1/2 study in cutaneous melanoma of sorafenib in combination with carboplatin and paclitaxel, a response rate of 27% was reported, including one complete response [110]. An astounding 73% of patients at 6 months had a complete response, partial response, or stable disease. A phase 3 randomized trial sponsored by ECOG was rapidly initiated and recently completed accrual. This trial was designed to compare sorafenib to placebo in combination with carboplatin and paclitaxel in chemotherapy-naive patients, with overall survival as the primary end point. Given the design, the trial was continued despite the announcement that the corporate drug company–sponsored, international, randomized phase 3 trial in melanoma comparing the same arms—but aimed at chemotherapy-refractory patients—failed to demonstrate improved progression-free survival, their primary end point [111]. Additionally, drugs that target BRAF more specifically, other members of the MAPK pathway, as well as multiple other pathways, are currently in clinical trials [3].

The Bcl-2 antisense oligonucleotide oblimersen sodium is designed to block prosurvival mechanisms, thereby increasing the effects of chemotherapy. Overexpression of Bcl-2 previously has been shown in melanoma [112]. Oblimersen was combined with dacarbazine in a large, randomized phase 3 study in advanced melanoma. This combination showed a small improvement in response rate (13.5% vs 7.5%; *P* = 0.007), complete response (2.8% vs 0.8%), and progression-free survival (median, 2.6 vs 1.6 months; *P* < 0.001) compared with dacarbazine alone [113]. Based on these data, oblimersen did not receive approval in this setting from the FDA. Due to evidence of a survival benefit in patients with normal serum LDH on subset analysis, the AGENDA (A Phase 3 Randmonized, Double-Blind, Placebo-Controlled Trial of Genasense Plus Dacarbazine vs Dacarbazine Alone in Advanced Melanoma) randomized phase 3 study of oblimersen with dacarbazine versus dacarbazine alone in patients with unresectable advanced melanoma and normal serum LDH was initiated and is accuring. Also of note, clinical studies exploring the efficacy of imatinib (Gleevec, Novartis, Basel, Switzerland) in advanced melanoma are of renewed interest despite two negative phase 2 trials [114,115]. This interest is due to a recent report demonstrating the detection of genetic abnormalities in c-kit (targeted by imatinib) in distinct clinical subtypes of melanoma, specifically acral melanoma, mucosal melanoma, and melanomas arising from chronically sun-exposed skin [2]. These changes were not seen in melanomas that arose from skin without chronic sun damage. This highlights the importance of continued research into the unique molecular and genetic features of melanomas and individual tumors so that the proper patient, or subset of patients, may be selected for the appropriate treatments [3]. As we continue to develop and test these targeted agents, we will better understand how to measure response, limit toxicity, and best utilize them.

IMMUNOTHERAPY

Interleukin-2, or T-cell derived growth factor, has been employed since 1984 in the treatment of patients with melanoma [116]. The high-dose bolus regimen, one cycle consisting of 600,000 to 720,000 units/kg given intravenously every 8 hours to a maximum of 14 doses, has achieved response rates of up to 20%, with a subset of patient (5%–6%) experiencing a durable complete response [31,32]. IL-2 is thought to enhance cell-mediated immunity through elaboration of tumor-specific cytotoxic T-lymphocytes; however, there may be additional mechanisms of action that remain to be elucidated. Treatment with IL-2 requires a motivated patient, experienced clinicians and ancillary staff, as well as intensive monitoring due to the significant side effects during and after drug administration requiring supportive care. The most prominent adverse effects include vascular leak syndrome, hypotension, cardiac arrhythmias, renal and hepatic dysfunction, and electrolyte disturbance [117]. Contraindications to high-dose IL-2 treatment include brain metastases, coronary artery disease, cardiac arrhythmias, renal insufficiency, advanced age, poor functional status, pleural or pericardial effusions, and active infections [117]. Lower, less toxic doses of IL-2 have not been proven to be effective [118]. Adoptive transfer of lymphokine-activated killer cells or tumor-infiltrating lymphocytes with high-dose IL-2 is not more effective than high-dose IL-2 alone [119]. Yet, Dudley *et al.* [120] recently reported a 51% objective response rate among 35 refractory metastatic melanoma patients receiving nonmyeloablative, lymphodepleting chemotherapy followed by high-dose IL-2 and selected T-cell infusion.

Inappropriate tolerance to tumor cells is believed to be a means of tumor escape, progression, and resistance to treatment. Newer immunologic strategies seek to interfere with regulatory host immune signals that create tolerance. CD28, a costimulatory receptor present on T cells, provides the necessary positive stimulus to initiate a T-cell immune response when bound by CD80 or CD86, ligands present on antigen-presenting cells or tumor cells. CTLA-4, a homologue of CD28, is a negative regulator of T-cell function expressed on the surface of activated T cells. Possessing a much higher affinity for CD80/CD86 than CD28, CTLA-4 inhibits T-cell activation when bound. CTLA-4 promotes peripheral tolerance and prevents autoimmunity and can also inhibit an effective antitumor immunologic response [88]. Antagonist antibodies to CTLA-4 have shown antitumor activity in phase 1 and 2 clinical trials, despite the incidence of severe autoimmune toxicities [121,122]. Interestingly, the development of autoimmunity correlates with clinical response [30]. Response rates range from 10% to 15%, including some complete and durable responses. Some responses may be delayed and occur after initial tumor enlargement [123].

BIOCHEMOTHERAPY

The combination of IL-2–based immunotherapy and cisplatin-based chemotherapy are the basic building blocks of various biochemotherapy regimens that have been studied in the metastatic, neoadjuvant, and now adjuvant settings. Many early studies reported very high response rates, including complete responses, in metastatic melanoma [124,125]. Surprisingly, a much lower response rate with no survival advantage was seen in a large phase 3 trial [126]. In the adjuvant setting, the Southwest Oncology Group protocol S0008 is evaluating three cycles of biochemotherapy against 1 year of high-dose interferon alfa-2b. The neoadjuvant setting may prove to be the most advantageous time for biochemotherapy given the potentially high response rate, but this requires further investigation [127,128].

ISOLATED LIMB PERFUSION

Isolated limb perfusion (ILP) with melphalan has been applied for many years and has gone through a resurgence of interest with the advent of isolated limb infusion (ILI), a less invasive procedure pioneered at the Sydney Melanoma Unit [129]. ILP/ILI are reasonable options in patients with locally advanced melanoma that is confined to one limb. ILP yields objective response rates of 47% to 82%, with a median duration of 9 months for complete responders [130]. There have been no direct comparisons between the two procedures, but similar response rates have been reported with lower toxicities for ILI [131,132]. Neither the addition of tumor necrosis factor-α nor interferon-γ to melphalan administered by ILP appears to improve outcomes [133,134].

Risk factors predictive of survival in metastatic disease include initial site of metastases (cutaneous and nodal sites fare better than lung involvement; other visceral sites portend the worst survival), disease-free interval prior to distant metastases, stage of disease preceding distant metastases,

and serum levels of LDH, alkaline phosphatase, and platelets [135]. In long-term survivors, prior immunotherapy, younger age, and female gender tended to correlate with improved survival. Also significant was that long-term surviving patients had resectable metastatic disease or manifested a complete or partial response with initial chemotherapy or immunotherapy.

UVEAL MELANOMA

Arising from the pigmented epithelium of the eye, a diagnosis of uveal (or ocular) melanoma typically is prompted by new visual disturbances. Uveal melanoma is rare (accounting for 5% of all melanomas), with an annual incidence of six cases per million population [136,137]. Caucasian individuals in the fifth to seventh decade of life are most commonly affected. Clinically evident metastatic disease at the time of initial diagnosis is uncommon. Primary uveal melanomas are classified as small, medium, or large based on established height and width criteria [45]. Initial work-up involves an ophthalmologic examination, including visual acuity, ocular ultrasound, and blood work. Biopsies are not required to establish a diagnosis given the straightforward clinical features, limited differential diagnoses, and difficulties inherent in such a procedure. Treatment decisions are based on tumor size and configuration and location in the uvea (choriod, ciliary body, iris). The two treatment options for primary choroidal melanoma include enucleation or radioactive plaque therapy. The Collaborators of the Ocular Melanoma Study (COMS), supported by the National Eye Institute and the National Cancer Institute, was a large, multicenter study that established the current guidelines for evaluation, treatment, and management of uveal melanoma. In medium-sized melanomas localized to the choroid, the COMS study demonstrated that there was equal efficacy of enucleation and plaque therapy [138]. Unfortunately, even with successful therapy of the primary, the risk of subsequent relapse with distant metastases is approximately 50% [137]. Large tumors, or those involving the ciliary body have a greater risk of metastasis and enucleation is recommended. Additionally, poor prognostic chromosomal and molecular/genetic features have been identified and include monosomy 3, amplification of 8q, expression of c-myc, or expression of p53, cyclin D1, and MDM2 [137,139]. Recurrence is characterized by distant organ involvement, often in the liver. Metastatic spread is predominantly hematogenous due to minimal, if any, lymphatic drainage of the eye. Metastases from ocular melanoma are more resistant to systemic chemotherapy or immunotherapy than those from cutaneous melanoma [140]. Alternative strategies for managing metastatic sites include liver-directed approaches, including chemo-embolization, radiofrequency ablation, and clinical trials of liver infusion or perfusion with chemotherapy [140,141].

NONMELANOMA SKIN CANCERS

The most frequent neoplasms in the Caucasian population are nonmelanoma skin cancers. While difficult to measure, more than 1 million new cases of BCC and SCC were estimated for 2007, where BCC accounts for the majority (80%) [4]. There is a clear, dominant relationship between UV exposure and incidence of these tumors [142,143]. As in melanoma, phenotypic features including degree of pigmentation and skin type also impact the risk of nonmelanoma skin cancers. Most tumors occur at sun-exposed skin; the head and neck is the most common site for both SCC and BCC. Other risk factors, including immunosuppression, are listed in Table 11-1. Current recommendations state that immunosuppressed individuals should undergo regular screening for skin cancers [144]. Overall, nonmelanoma tumors are easily cured and controlled with local therapies, as these are predominantly locally aggressive tumors. Of the two, SCC is more likely to metastasize than BCC. When metastatic, the most common sites are regional lymph nodes [142]. Rarely, liver, lung, bone, or brain metastases are found. Deaths due to these tumors are extremely infrequent.

The primary treatment for nonmelanoma skin tumors is local ablative therapy. This may consist of electrodesiccation and curettage, cryosurgery, simple excision, excision with skin grafting or flap rotation, Mohs' surgery, or radiation therapy. Many issues will influence the choice of treatment, including, but not limited to, tumor site, tumor size, risk for recurrence or metastasis, cosmesis, comorbid illnesses, and patient preference. Local recurrence is the major risk; therefore, surgical excision with adequate margins offers the best chance for cure. Of note, the margin of excision needed to control BCC and SCC is less than that needed for melanoma [144,145]. Moh's surgery is a specialized surgical technique designed to surgically excise a tumor while preserving as much normal skin as possible. This procedure is quite useful in the management of BCC and SCC, although it requires special training and is time-consuming and costly. Moh's surgery has no role in the treatment melanoma, where frozen sections are notoriously unreliable in assessing the presence of disease and wide margins are required.

Since the 1970s, topical 5-fluorouracil has been used to treat superficial BCC, SCC in situ, and actinic keratoses [146]. Other topical treatments for these conditions include photodynamic therapy and imiquimod (Aldara, 3M Pharmaceuticals, St. Paul, MN). Imiquimod, an immune response modifier that binds and stimulates Toll-like receptor 7, is FDA approved for treatment of superficial BCC and actinic keratoses [147]. Imiquimod is thought to exert its antitumor effects by stimulating cell-mediated immunity via the elaboration of cytokines from stimulated macrophages, monocytes, and dendritic cells [147]. Radiation therapy is perhaps best used in patients with areas involved by too numerous to resect lesions, such as in immunocompromised patients. It may be used in older patients as a second choice if the patient is deemed not a surgical candidate. Topical treatments are a good option in patients with multiple BCCs or actinic keratoses, in which surgical removal is difficult or not feasible. The NCCN recently issued thorough guidelines for the care and management of nonmelanoma skin cancers [144].

INTERFERON ALFA-2B

High-dose interferon alfa-2b has shown consistent RFS benefit as a single agent in the adjuvant setting in patients with high-risk melanoma. An overall survival benefit has been inconsistently demonstrated in clinical trials. Those patients with the smallest degree of nodal involvement may derive the most benefit.

DOSAGE AND SCHEDULE

Induction: 20 MU/m^2 daily IV for 5 d × 4 wk
Maintenance: 10 MU/m^2/d 3 × per week subcutaneously × 48 wk

DOSAGE MODIFICATION

Interferon should be held for a granulocyte count below 500/μL, aspartate transaminase (AST) or alanine transaminase (ALT) rise above five times the upper limit of normal (ULN), or platelet count below 50,000/μL. Interferon can be resumed at a 33% to 50% dose reduction once the abnormal laboratory values normalize [75].

ELIGIBLE PATIENTS

Resected stage II: primary melanoma > 4 mm, and no nodal involvement
Resected stage III: any nodal involvement

No established role in resected stage IIIC disease with in-transit lesions or satellitosis

MONITORING

Complete blood count, basic metabolic panel, and hepatic panel weekly × 4 wk, and then monthly for 11 mo

TOXICITIES

Systemic: fevers, chills, myalgias and arthralgias, fatigue, headache; **Hematologic:** neutropenia, anemia, thrombocytopenia (not dose limiting unless severe); **Hepatic:** hyperbilirubinemia, elevated transaminases, hepatic necrosis (rare); **Renal:** proteinuria, elevated creatinine or blood urea nitrogen (BUN); **Psychiatric:** depression, inattention, anxiety; **Autoimmune manifestations:** vitiligo-like dermatosis, hypothyroidism [75]

ALTERNATIVE THERAPIES

Adjuvant therapy clinical trials (vaccines, chemotherapeutics, biologic or molecular agents) or close observation according to guidelines

CONTRAINDICATIONS

Psychiatric disorder, hepatic or renal insufficiency, patient preference

HIGH-DOSE BOLUS INTERLEUKIN-2

High-dose bolus IL-2 can induce durable complete remissions in a small percentage of patients with metastatic melanoma [31,32]. Must be administered in specialized medical centers by trained oncologists and ancillary staff with intensive monitoring.

DOSAGE AND SCHEDULE

600,000 to 720,000 units/kg every 8 hours IV × 14 doses. The next cycle begins 9 to 14 d after hospital discharge from prior cycle. Response is evaluated every 2 cycles.

DOSAGE MODIFICATION

Doses may be held during the treatment course according to specific parameters for heart rate, blood pressure, pressor requirements; cardiac, renal, and hepatic dysfunction; cytopenias; altered mental status; electrolyte abnormalities. Significant toxicities, such as lethal cardiac arrhythmias, require complete cessation.

ELIGIBLE PATIENTS

Unresectable stage III or IV melanoma with no brain metastases, no pleural or pericardial effusions, no renal insufficiency, no history of cardiac disease. Patients older than 50 must have normal findings on stress thallium testing and good pulmonary function; age 65 years or younger; ECOG performance status 0–1

TOXICITIES

Systemic: Fevers, chills, myalgias and arthralgias, fatigue, headache, anasarca; **Hematologic:** neutropenia, anemia, thrombocytopenia; **Hepatic:** elevated transaminases, hyperbilirubinemia; **Renal:** elevated creatinine and/or BUN, electrolyte abnormalities; **Cardiovascular:** vascular leak syndrome, cardiac arrhythmias, cardiac ischemia, myocardial necrosis (rare); **Neurologic:** altered mental status; **Autoimmune:** vitiligo-like dermatosis, hypothyroidism, hyperthyroidism (rare and typically self-limited) [117]

ALTERNATIVE THERAPIES

Chemotherapy, biochemotherapy, clinical trials

ISOLATED LIMB PERFUSION WITH MELPHALAN

Locoregional spread of melanoma within an extremity, without distant dissemination, occurs in ~ 10% of patients. Despite the localized nature, these patients may develop significant local complications that are difficult to manage related to in-transit and/or satellite lesions. Regional delivery of chemotherapy via ILP can provide complete response rates of 40% to 55%, with a 9-month median duration of response [130]. Must be performed in a specialized medical center with surgeons and ancillary staff trained in the procedure and after-procedure management. The procedure is done under anesthesia and a hospital stay of ~ 1 wk is required.

ELIGIBLE PATIENTS

Patients with advanced locoregional melanoma of an extremity, accompanied by in-transit or satellite lesions (stage IIIC)

TOXICITIES

Wound healing, lymphatic fistulas, fever, pain and erythema of the extremity, compartment syndrome possibly requiring amputation

ALTERNATIVE THERAPIES

Systemic chemotherapy or immunotherapy, clinical trials

The information here is provided as guidance only. Prescribers should always consult the manufacturer's current prescribing information.

REFERENCES

1. Curtin JA, Fridlyand J, Kageshita T, *et al.*: Distinct sets of genetic alterations in melanoma. *N Engl J Med* 2005, 353:2135–2147.

2. Curtin JA, Busam K, Pinkel D, *et al.*: Somatic activation of KIT in distinct subtypes of melanoma. *J Clin Oncol* 2006, 24:4340–4346.

3. Fecher LA, Cumming SD, Keefe MJ, *et al.*: Toward a molecular classification of melanoma. *J Clin Oncol* 2007, 25:1606–1620.

4. Jemal A, Siegel R, Ward E, *et al.*: Cancer statistics, 2007. *CA Cancer J Clin* 2007, 57:43–66.

5. Strouse JJ, Fears TR, Tucker MA, *et al.*: Pediatric melanoma: risk factor and survival analysis of the Surveillance, Epidemiology, and End Results database. *J Clin Oncol* 2005, 23:4735–4741.

6. de Vries E, Steliarova-Foucher E, Spatz A, *et al.*: Skin cancer incidence and survival in European children and adolescents (1978–1997). Report from the Automated Childhood Cancer Information System Project. *Eur J Cancer* 2006, 42:2170–2182.

7. Gershenwald JE, Thompson W, Mansfield PF, *et al.*: Multi-institutional melanoma lymphatic mapping experience: the prognostic value to sentinel lymph node status in 612 stage I or II melanoma patients. *J Clin Oncol* 1999,17:976–983.

8. Hayward NK: Genetics of melanoma predisposition. *Oncogene* 2003, 22:3053–3062.

9. Tucker MA, Goldstein AM: Melanoma etiology: where are we? *Oncogene* 2003, 22:3042–3052.

10. Berwick M, Wiggins C: The current epidemiology of cutaneous malignant melanoma. *Front Biosci* 2006, 11:1244–1254.

11. Elwood M, Aitken J, English D: Prevention and screening. In *Cutaneous Melanoma*, edn 4. Edited by Balch CM, Houghton A, Sober A, Soong SJ. St. Louis: Quality Medical Publishing, Inc; 2003:93–120.

12. Pho L, Grossman D, Leachman S: Melanoma genetics: a review of genetic factors and clinical phenotypes in familial melanoma. *Curr Opin Oncol* 2006, 18:173–179.

13. Whelan AJ, Bartsch D, Goodfellow PJ: A familial syndrome of pancreatic cancer and melanoma with a mutation in the CDKN2a tumor-suppressor gene. *N Engl J Med* 1995, 333:970–974.

14. Goldstein AM, Cham M, Harland M, *et al.*: High-risk melanoma susceptibility genes and pancreatic cancer, neural system tumors, and uveal melanoma across GenoMEL. *Cancer Res* 2006, 66:9818–9828.

15. Zuo L, Weger J, Yang Q, *et al.*: Germline mutations in the p16INK4a binding domain of CDK4 in familial melanoma. *Nat Genet* 1996, 12:97–99.

16. Giehl K: Oncogenic Ras in tumour progression and metastasis. *Biol Chem* 2005, 386:193–205.

17. Beeram M, Patnaik A, Rowinsky EK: Raf: a strategic target for therapeutic development against cancer. *J Clin Oncol* 2005, 23:6771–6790.

18. Davies H, Bignell GR, Cox C, *et al.*: Mutations of the BRAF gene in human cancer. *Nature* 2002, 417:949–954.

19. Pollock PM, Harper UL, Hansen KS, *et al.*: High frequency of BRAF mutations in nevi. *Nat Genet* 2003, 33:19–20.

20. Maldonado JL, Fridlyand J, Patel H, *et al.*: Determinants of BRAF mutations in primary melanomas. *J Natl Cancer Inst* 2003, 95:1878–1890.

21. Bauer J, Curtin JA, Pinkel D, *et al.*: Congenital melanocytic nevi frequently harbor NRAS mutations but no BRAF mutations. *J Invest Dermatol* 2007, 127:179–182.

22. Meyer P, Klaes R, Schmitt C, *et al.*: Exclusion of BRAFV599E as a melanoma susceptibility mutation. *Int J Cancer* 2003, 106:78–80.

23. Cohen Y, Rosenbaum E, Begum S, *et al.*: Exon 15 BRAF mutations are uncommon in melanomas arising in nonsun-exposed sites. *Clin Cancer Res* 2004, 10:3444–3447.

24. Wong CW, Fan YS, Chan TL, *et al.*: BRAF and NRAS mutation are uncommon in melanomas arising in diverse internal organs. *J Clin Pathol* 2005, 58:640–644.

25. High WA, Stewart D, Wilbers CR, *et al.*: Completely regressed primary cutaneous malignant melanoma with nodal and/or visceral metastases: a report of 5 cases and assessment of the literature and diagnostic criteria. *J Am Acad Dermatol* 2005, 53:89–100.

26. Nordlund JJ, Kirkwood JM, Forget BM, *et al.*: Vitiligo in patients with metastatic melanoma: a good prognostic sign. *J Am Acad Dermatol* 1983, 9:689–896.

27. Kitamura K, Livingston PO, Fortunato SR, *et al.*: Serological response patterns of melanoma patients immunized with a GM2 ganglioside conjugate vaccine. *Proc Natl Acad Sci* 1995, 92:2805–2809.

28. Gogas H, Ioannovich J, Dafni U, *et al.*: Prognostic significance of autoimmunity during treatment of melanoma with interferon. *N Engl J Med* 2006, 354:709–718.

29. Phan GQ, Attia P, Steinberg SM, *et al.*: Factors associated with response to high-dose interleukin-2 in patients with metastatic melanoma. *J Clin Oncol* 2001, 19:3477–3482.

30. Attia P, Phan GQ, Maker AV, *et al.*: Autoimmunity correlates with tumor regression in patients with metastatic melanoma treated with anti-cytotoxic T-lymphocyte antigen-4. *J Clin Oncol* 2005, 23:6043–6053.

31. Rosenberg SA, Yang JC, White DE, *et al.*: Durability of complete responses in patients with metastatic cancer treated with high-dose interleukin-2: identification of the antigens mediating response. *Ann Surg* 1998, 228:307–319.

32. Atkins MB, Lotze MT, Dutcher JP, *et al.*: High-dose recombinant interleukin-2 therapy for patients with metastatic melanoma: analysis of 270 patients treated from 1985–1993. *J Clin Oncol* 1999, 17:2105.

33. Clemente CG, Mihm MC Jr, Bufalino R, *et al.*: Prognostic value of tumor infiltrating lymphocytes in the vertical growth phase of primary cutaneous melanoma. *Cancer* 1996, 77:1303–1310.

34. Licata AG, Wilson LD, Braverman IM, *et al.*: Malignant melanoma and other second cutaneous malignancies in cutaneous T-cell lymphoma. The influence of additional therapy after total skin electron beam radiation. *Arch Dermatol* 1995, 131:432–435.

35. Otley CC: Non-Hodgkin lymphoma and skin cancer: a dangerous combination. *Australas J Dermatol* 2006, 47:231–236.

36. Berg D, Otley C: Skin cancer in organ transplant recipients: epidemiology, pathogenesis, and management. *J Am Acad Dermatol* 2002, 47:1–17.

37. Wilkins K, Turner R, Doley JC, *et al.*: Cutaneous malignancy and human immunodeficiency virus disease. *J Am Acad Dermatol* 2006, 54:189–206.

38. Armstrong BK, Kricker A: The epidemiology of UV induced skin cancer. *J Photochem Photobiol B* 2001, 63:8–18.

39. Jhappan C, Noonan FP, Merlino G: Ultraviolet radiation and cutaneous malignant melanoma. *Oncogene* 2003, 22:3099–3112.

40. Ivry GB, Ogle CA, Shim EK: Role of sun exposure in melanoma. *Dermatol Surg* 2006, 32:481–492.

41. Elwood JM, Jopson J: Melanoma and sun exposure: an overview of published studies. *Int J Cancer* 1997, 73:198–203.

42. Gallagher RP, Spinelli JJ, Lee TK: Tanning beds, sunlamps, and risk of cutaneous malignant melanoma. *Cancer Epidemiol Biomarkers Prev* 2005, 14:562–566.

43. Abbasi NR, Shaw HM, Rigel DS, *et al.*: Early diagnosis of cutaneous melanoma: revisiting the ABCD criteria. *JAMA* 2004, 292:2771–2776.

44. Balch CM: Cutaneous melanoma: prognosis and treatment results worldwide. *Semin Surg Oncol* 1992, 8:400–414.

45. Balch CM: *AJCC Cancer Staging Manual*, edn 6. Edited by Greene FL, Page DL, Fleming ID, *et al.* New York: Springer-Verlag: 2002.

46. Balch CM, Buzaid AC, Soong SJ, *et al.*: Final version of the American Joint Committee on Cancer staging system for cutaneous melanoma. *J Clin Oncol* 2001, 19:3635–3648.

47. Balch CM, Soong SJ, Gershenwald JE, *et al.*: Prognostic factors analysis of 17,600 melanoma patients: validation of the American Joint Committee on Cancer melanoma staging system. *J Clin Oncol* 2001, 19:3622–3634.

48. Halpern AC: Total body skin imaging as an aid to melanoma detection. *Semin Cutan Med Surg* 2003, 22:2–8.

49. Balch CM, Miller SJ: Biopsy. In *Cutaneous Melanoma*, edn 4. Edited by Balch CM, Houghton A, Sober A, Soong SJ. St. Louis: Quality Medical Publishing, Inc: 2003:163–170.

50. Tomicic J, Wanebo HJ: Mucosal melanoma. *Surg Clin North Am* 2003, 83:237–252.

51. Wang TS, Johnson TM, Cascade PN, *et al.*: Evaluation of staging chest radiographs and serum lactate dehydrogenase for localized melanoma. *J Am Acad Dermatol* 2004, 51:399–405.

52. The NCCN (V.2.2007) Melanoma Clinical Practice Guidelines in Oncology. National Comprehensive Cancer Network, 2007. Available at http://www.nccn.org. Accessed September 18, 2007. To view the most recent and complete version of the guideline, go online to www.nccn.org.

53. Balch CM, Cascinelli N, Sim FH: Elective lymph node dissection: results of prospective randomized surgical trials. In *Cutaneous Melanoma*, edn 4. Edited by Balch CM, Houghton A, Sober A, Soong SJ. St. Louis: Quality Medical Publishing, Inc.; 2003:379–395.

54. Morton DL, Wen DR, Wong JH, *et al.*: Technical details of intraoperative lymphatic mapping for early stage melanoma. *Arch Surg* 1992, 127:393–399.

55. Morton DL, Cochran AJ, Thompson, JF, *et al.*: Sentinel node biopsy for early melanoma: accuracy and morbidity in MSLT-I, an international multi-center trial. *Ann Surg* 2005, 242:302–313.

56. Morton DL, Thompson JF, Cochran AJ, *et al.*: Sentinel-node biopsy or nodal observation in melanoma. *N Engl J Med* 2006, 355:1307–1317.

57. Wong SL, Morton DL, Thompson JF, *et al.*: Melanoma patients with positive sentinel nodes who did not undergo completion lymphadenectomy: a multi-institutional study. *Ann Surg Oncol* 2006, 13:809–816.

58. Crowson AN, Magro CM, Mihm MC: Prognosticators of melanoma, the melanoma report, and the sentinel lymph node. *Mod Pathol* 2006, 19:S71–S87.

59. Paek SC, Griffith KA, Johnson TM, *et al.*: The impact of factors beyond Breslow depth on predicting sentinel lymph node positivity in melanoma. *Cancer* 2007, 109:100–108.

60. Wornom IL III, Smith JW, Soong SJ, *et al.*: Surgery as palliative treatment for distant metastases of melanoma. *Ann Surg* 1986, 204:181–185.

61. Wong JH, Skinner KA, Kim KA, *et al.*: The role of surgery in the treatment of nonregionally recurrent melanoma. *Surgery* 1993, 113:389–394.

62. Karakousis CP, Velez A, Driscoll DL, *et al.*: Metastasectomy in malignant melanoma. *Surgery* 1994, 115:295–302.

63. Strom EA, Ross MI: Adjuvant radiation therapy after axillary lymphadenectomy for metastatic melanoma: toxicity and local control. *Ann Surg Oncol* 1995, 2:445–449.

64. Sampson JH, Carter JH, Friedman AH, *et al.*: Demographics, prognosis, and therapy in 702 patients with brain metastases from malignant melanoma. *J Neurosurg* 1998, 88:11–20.

65. Lagerwaard FJ, Levendag PC, Nowak PJ, *et al.*: Identification of prognostic factors in patients with brain metastases: a review of 1292 patients. *Int J Radiat Oncol Biol Phys* 1999, 43:795–803.

66. Fife KM, Colman MH, Stevens GN, *et al.*: Determinants of outcome in melanoma patients with cerebral metastases. *J Clin Oncol* 2004, 22:1293–1300.

67. Kondziolka D, Patel A, Lunsford LD, *et al.*: Stereotactic radiosurgery plus whole brain radiotherapy versus radiotherapy alone for patients with multiple brain metastases. *Int J Radiat Oncol Biol Phys* 1999, 45:427–434.

68. Gaudy-Marqueste C, Regis JM, Muracciole X, *et al.*: Gamma-knife radiosurgery in the management of melanoma patients with brain metastases: a series of 106 patients without whole-brain radiotherapy. *Int J Radiat Oncol Biol Phys* 2006, 65:809–816.

69. Aoyama H, Shirato H, Tago M, *et al.*: Stereotactic radiosurgery plus whole-brain radiation therapy vs stereotactic radiosurgery alone for treatment of brain metastases: a randomized controlled trial. *JAMA* 2006, 295:2483–2491.

70. Patchell RA, Tibbs PA, Regine WF: Postoperative radiotherapy in the treatment of single metastases to the brain: a randomized trial. *JAMA* 1998, 280:1485–1489.

71. Kirkwood JM, Strawderman MH, Ernstoff MS, *et al.*: Interferon alfa-2b adjuvant therapy of high-risk resected cutaneous melanoma: the Eastern Cooperative Oncology Group Trial EST1684. *J Clin Oncol* 1996, 14:7–17.

72. Kirkwood JM, Manola J, Ibrahim J, *et al.*: A pooled analysis of Eastern Cooperative Oncology Group and intergroup trials of adjuvant high-dose interferon for melanoma. *Clin Cancer Res* 2004, 10:1670–1677.

73. Kirkwood JM, Ibrahim JG, Sondak VK, *et al.*: High- and low-dose interferon alfa-2b in high-risk melanoma: first analysis of Intergroup trial E1690/S9111/C9190. *J Clin Oncol* 2000, 18:2444–2458.

74. Kirkwood JM, Ibrahim JG, Sosman JA, *et al.*: High-dose interferon alfa-2b significantly prolongs relapse-free and overall survival compared with GM2-KLH/QS-21 vaccine in patients with resected stage IIB-III melanoma: results of Intergroup trial E1694/S9512/C509801. *J Clin Oncol* 2001, 19:2370–2380.

75. Kirkwood JM, Bender C, Agarwala S, *et al.*: Mechanisms and management of toxicities associated with high-dose interferon alfa-2b therapy. *J Clin Oncol* 2002, 20:3703–3718.

76. Eggermont AM, Suciu S, Santinami M, *et al.*: EORTC 18991: long-term adjuvant pegylated interferon-alpha2b (PEG-IFN) compared to observation in resected stage III melanoma, final results of a randomized phase III trial [ASCO abstract]. *J Clin Oncol* 2007, 25(18S):8504.

77. Wheatley K, Ives N, Hancock B, *et al.*: Does adjuvant interferon-alfa for high-risk melanoma provide a worthwhile benefit? A meta-analysis of the randomized trials. *Cancer Treat Rev* 2003, 29:241–252.

78. Rosenberg SA, Yang JC, Restifo NP: Cancer Immunotherapy: moving beyond current vaccines. *Nat Med* 2004, 10:909–915.

79. Terando AM, Faries MB, Morton DL: Vaccine therapy for melanoma: current status and future directions. *Vaccine* 2007, 25(Suppl):B14–B16.

80. Wallack MK, Sivanandham M, Balch CM, *et al.*: A phase III randomized, double-blind, multi-institutional trial of vaccine melanoma oncolysate-active specific immunotherapy for patients with stage II melanoma. *Cancer* 1995, 75:34–42.

81. Sondak VK, Liu PY, Tuthill RJ, *et al.*: Adjuvant immunotherapy of resected, intermediate-thickness, node-negative melanoma with an allogeneic tumor vaccine: overall results of a randomized trial of the Southwest Oncology Group. *J Clin Oncol* 2002, 20:2058–2066.

82. Sosman JA, Unger JM, Liu PY, *et al.*: Adjuvant immunotherapy of resected, intermediate-thickness, node-negative melanoma with an allogeneic tumor vaccine: impact of HLA class I antigen expression on outcome. *J Clin Oncol* 2002, 20:2067–2075.

83. Morton DL, Mozzillo N, Thompson JF, *et al.*: An international, randomized, phase III trial of bacillus Calmette-Guerin (BCG) plus allogeneic melanoma vaccine (MCV) or placebo after complete resection of melanoma metastatic to regional or distant sites [ASCO abstract]. *J Clin Oncol* 2007, 25(18S):8508.

84. Berd D, Maguire HC Jr, Schuchter LM, *et al.*: Autologous hapten-modified melanoma vaccine as postsurgical adjuvant treatment after resection of nodal metastases. *J Clin Oncol* 1997, 15:2359–2370.

85. Berd D, Sato T, Maguire HC Jr, *et al.*: Immunopharmacologic analysis of an autologous, hapten-modified human melanoma vaccine. *J Clin Oncol* 2004, 22:403–415.

86. van der Bruggen P, Traversari C, Chomez P, *et al.*: A gene encoding an antigen recognized by cytolytic T lymphocytes on a human melanoma. *Science* 1991, 254:1643–1647.

87. Novellino L, Castelli C, Parmiani G: A listing of human tumor antigens recognized by T cells: March 2004 update. *Cancer Immunol Immunother* 2005, 54:187–207.

88. Waldmann TA: Effective cancer therapy through immunomodulation. *Annu Rev Med* 2006, 57:65–81.

89. Gogas H, Kirkwood J, Sondak VK: Chemotherapy for metastatic melanoma: time for a change? *Cancer* 2007, 109:455–464.

90. Hill GJ II , Krementz ET, Hill HZ: Dimethyl triazeno imidazole carboxamide and combination therapy for melanoma. IV. Late results after complete response to chemotherapy (Central Oncology Group protocols 7130, 7131, and 7131A). *Cancer* 1984, 53:1299–1305.

91. Chapman PB, Einhorn LH, Meyers ML, *et al.*: Phase III multicenter randomized trial of the Dartmouth regimen versus dacarbazine in patients with metastatic melanoma. *J Clin Oncol* 1999, 17:2745–2751.

92. Creagan ET, Ahmann DL, Green SJ, *et al.*: Phase II study of recombinant leukocyte A interferon (rIFN-alpha A) in disseminated malignant melanoma. *Cancer* 1984, 54:2844–2849.

93. Song SY, Chary KK, Higby DJ, *et al.*: Cisdiamminedichloride (II) in the treatment of metastatic malignant melanoma. *Clin Res* 1977, 25:411.

94. Evans LM, Casper ES, Rosenbluth R: Phase II trial of carboplatin in advanced malignant melanoma. *Cancer Treat Rep* 1987, 71:171–172.

95. Ramirez G, Wilson W, Grage T, *et al.*: Phase II evaluation of 1,3-bis(2-chloroethyl)-1-nitrosourea (BCNU; NSC-409962) in patients with solid tumors. *Cancer Chemother Rep* 1972, 56:787–790.

96. Retsas S, Newton KA, Westbury G: Vindesine as a single agent in the treatment of advanced malignant melanoma. Cancer *Chemother Pharmacol* 1979, 2:257–260.

97. Legha SS, Ring S, Papadopoulos N, *et al.*: A phase II trial of Taxol in metastatic melanoma. *Cancer* 1990, 65:2478–2481.

98. Einzig AI, Schuchter LM, Recio A, *et al.*: Phase II trial of docetaxel (Taxotere) in patients with metastatic melanoma previously untreated with cytotoxic chemotherapy. *Med Oncol* 1996, 13:111–117.

99. Feun LG, Savaraj N, Hurley J, *et al.*: A clinical trial of intravenous vinorelbine tartrate plus tamoxifen in the treatment of patients with advanced malignant melanoma. *Cancer* 2000, 88:584–588.

100. Seigler HF, Lucas VS, Pickett NJ, *et al.*: DTIC, CCNU, bleomycin and vincristine (BOLD) in metastatic melanoma. *Cancer* 1980, 46:2346–2348.

101. Del Prete SA, Maurer LH, O'Donnell J, *et al.*: Combination chemotherapy with cisplatin, carmustine, dacarbazine and tamoxifen in malignant melanoma. *Cancer Treat Rep* 1984, 68:1403–1405.

102. The Prudente Foundation Melanoma Study Group: Chemotherapy of disseminated melanoma with bleomycin, vincristine, CCNU, and DTIC (BOLD regimen). *Cancer* 1989, 63:1676–1680.

103. Rustoven JJ, Quirt IC, Iscoe NA, *et al.*: Randomized, double-blind, placebo-controlled trial comparing the response rates of carmustine, dacarbazine, and cisplatin with and without tamoxifen in patients with metastatic melanoma. *J Clin Oncol* 1996, 14:2083–2090.

104. Middleton MR, Grob JJ, Aaronson N, *et al.*: Randomized phase III study of temozolomide versus dacarbazine in the treatment of patients with advanced metastatic malignant melanoma. *J Clin Oncol* 2000, 18:158–166.

105. Margolin K, Atkins B, Thompson A, *et al.*: Temozolomide and whole brain irradiation in melanoma metastatic to the brain: a phase II trial of the Cytokine Working Group. *J Cancer Res Clin Oncol* 2002, 128:214–218.

106. Su YB, Sohn S, Krown SE, *et al.*: Selective CD4+ lymphopenia in melanoma patients treated with temozolomide: a toxicity with therapeutic implications. *J Clin Oncol* 2004, 22:610–616.

107. Wilhelm SM, Carter C, Tang L, *et al.*: BAY 43-9006 exhibits broad spectrum oral antitumor activity and targets the RAF/MEK/ERK pathway and receptor tyrosine kinases involved in tumor progression and angiogenesis. *Cancer Res* 2004, 64:7099–7109.

108. Eisen T, Ahmad T, Flaherty KT, *et al.*: Sorafenib in advanced melanoma: a phase II randomised discontinuation trial analysis. *Br J Cancer* 2006, 95:581–586.

109. McDermott D, Sosman J, Hodi F, *et al.*: Randomized phase II study of dacarbazine with and without sorafenib in patients with advanced melanoma [ASCO abstract]. *J Clin Oncol* 2007, 25(18S):8511.

110. Flaherty KT, Brose M, Schuchter L, *et al.*: Phase I/II trial of BAY 43-9006, carboplatin (C) and paclitaxel (P) demonstrates preliminary antitumor activity in the expansion cohort of patients with metastatic melanoma [ASCO abstract]. *J Clin Oncol* 2004, 22(14S):7507.

111. Bayer Pharmaceuticals Corporation & Onyx Pharmaceuticals: Phase III trial of Nexavar in patients with advanced melanoma does not meet primary endpoint [press release]. Onyx Pharmaceuticals; December 4, 2006. http://www.onyx-pharm.com/wt/page/pr_1165242111.

112. Soengas M, Lowe S: Apoptosis and melanoma chemoresistance. *Oncogene* 2003, 22:3138–3151.

113. Bedikian AY, Millward M, Pehamberger H, *et al.*: Bcl-2 antisense (oblimersen sodium) plus dacarbazine in patients with advanced melanoma: the Oblimersen Melanoma Study Group. *J Clin Oncol* 2006, 24:4738–4745.

114. Ugurel S, Hildenbrand R, Zimpfer A, *et al.*: Lack of clinical efficacy of imatinib in metastatic melanoma. *Br J Cancer* 2005, 92:1398–1405.

115. Wyman K, Atkins MB, Prieto V, *et al.*: Multicenter phase II trial of high-dose imatinib mesylate in metastatic melanoma: significant toxicity with no clinical efficacy. *Cancer* 2006, 106:2005–2011.

116. Rosenberg SA, Lotze MT, Muul LM, *et al.*: Observations on the systemic administration of autologous lymphokine-activated killer cells and recombinant interleukin-2 to patients with metastatic cancer. *N Engl J Med* 1985, 313:1485–1492.

117. Schwartzentruber DJ: Guidelines for the safe administration of high-dose interleukin-2. *J Immunother* 2001, 24:287–293.

118. Marincola F, White D, Wise A, *et al.*: Combination therapy with interferon alfa-2a and interleukin-2 for the treatment of metastatic cancer. *J Clin Oncol* 1995, 13:1110–1122.

119. Rosenberg SA, Lotze MT, Yang JC, *et al.*: Prospective randomized trial of high-dose interleukin-2 alone or in conjunction with lymphokine-activated killer cells for the treatment of patients with advanced cancer. *J Natl Cancer Inst* 1993, 85:622–632.

120. Dudley ME, Wunderlich JR, Yang JC, *et al.*: Adoptive cell transfer therapy following non-myeloablative but lymphodepleting chemotherapy for the treatment of patients with refractory metastatic melanoma. *J Clin Oncol* 2005, 23:2346–2357.

121. Phan GQ, Yang JC, Sherry RM, *et al.*: Cancer regression and autoimmunity induced by cytotoxic T lymphocyte-associated antigen-4 blockade in patients with metastatic melanoma. *Proc Natl Acad Sci U S A* 2003, 100:8372–8377.

122. Ribas A, Camacho LH, Lopez-Berestein G, *et al.*: Antitumor activity in melanoma and anti-self responses in a phase I trial with the anti-cytotoxic T lymphocyte-associated antigen 4 monoclonal antibody CP-675,206. *J Clin Oncol* 2005, 23:8968–8977.

123. Hamid O, Urba WJ, Yellin M, *et al.*: Kinetics of response to ipilimumab [ASCO abstract]. *J Clin Oncol* 2007, 25(18S):abstract 8525.

124. Richards JM, Mehta N, Ramming K, *et al.*: Sequential chemoimmunotherapy in the treatment of metastatic melanoma. *J Clin Oncol* 1992, 10:1338–1343.

125. Legha SS, Ring S, Eton O, *et al.*: Development of a biochemotherapy regimen with concurrent administration of cisplatin, vinblastine, dacarbazine, interferon alfa, and interleukin-2 for patients with metastatic melanoma. *J Clin Oncol* 1998, 16:1752–1759.

126. Atkins MB, Lee S, Flaherty LE, *et al.*: A prospective randomized phase III trial of concurrent biochemotherapy (BCT) with cisplatin, vinblastine, dacarbazine (CVD), IL-2 and interferon alpha-2b (INF) versus CVD alone in patients with metastatic melanoma (E3695): an ECOG coordinated intergroup trial [abstract]. *Proc Am Soc Clin Oncol* 2003, 22:abstract 2847.

127. Buzaid AC, Colome M, Bedikian A, *et al.*: Phase II study of neoadjuvant concurrent biochemotherapy in melanoma patients with local-regional metastases. *Melanoma Res* 1998, 8:549–556.

128. Lewis KD, Robinson WA, McCarter M, *et al.*: Phase II multicenter study of neoadjuvant biochemotherapy for patients with stage III malignant melanoma. *J Clin Oncol* 2006, 24:3157–3163.

129. Thompson JF, Kam PC, Waugh RC: Isolated limb infusion with cytotoxic agents: a simple alternative to isolated limb perfusion. *Semin Surg Oncol* 1998, 14:238–247.

130. Cumberlin R, De Moss E, Lassus M, *et al.*: Isolated limb perfusion for malignant melanoma of the extremity: a review. *J Clin Oncol* 1985, 3:1022–1031.

131. Lindner P, Doubrovsky A, Kam PC, *et al.*: Prognostic factors after isolated limb infusion with cytotoxic agents for melanoma. *Ann Surg Oncol* 2002, 9:127–136.

132. Brady MS, Brown K, Patel A, *et al.*: A phase II trial of isolated limb infusion with melphalan and dactinomycin for regional melanoma and soft tissue sarcoma of the extremity. *Ann Surg Oncol* 2006, 13:1123–1129.

133. Cornett WR, McCall LM, Petersen RP, *et al.*: Randomized multicenter trial of hyperthermic isolated limb perfusion with melphalan alone compared with melphalan plus tumor necrosis factor: American College of Surgeons Oncology Trial Z0020. *J Clin Oncol* 2006, 24:4196–4201.

134. Lienard D, Eggermont AM, Koops HS, *et al.*: Isolated limb perfusion with tumor necrosis factor-alpha and melphalan with or without interferon-gamma for the treatment of in-transit melanoma metastases: a multicenter randomized phase II study. *Melanoma Res* 1999, 9:491–502.

135. Manola J, Atkins M, Ibrahim J, Kirkwood J: Prognostic factors in metastatic melanoma: a pooled analysis of Eastern Cooperative Oncology Group trials. *J Clin Oncol* 2000, 18:3782–3793.

136. McLaughlin CC, Wu XC, Jemal A, *et al.*: Incidence of noncutaneous melanomas in the U.S. *Cancer* 2005, 103:1000–1007.

137. Singh A, Bergman L, Seregard S: Uveal melanoma: epidemiologic aspects. *Ophthalmol Clin N Am* 2005, 18:75–84.

138. Collaborative Ocular Melanoma Study Group: The COMS randomized trial of iodine 125 brachytherapy for choroidal melanoma. V. Twelve-year mortality rates and prognostic factors: COMS report no. 28. *Arch Ophthalmol* 2006, 124:1684–1693.

139. Damato B, Duke C, Coupland SE, *et al.*: Cytogenetics of uveal melanoma: a 7-year clinical experience. *Ophthalmology* 2007, 114:1925–1931.

140. Bedikian AY: Metastatic uveal melanoma therapy: current options. *Int Ophthalmol Clin* 2006, 46:151–166.

141. Pingpank JF, Libutti SK, Chang R, *et al.*: Phase I study of hepatic arterial melphalan infusion and hepatic venous hemofiltration using percutaneously placed catheters in patients with unresectable hepatic metastases. *J Clin Oncol* 2005, 23:3465–3474.

142. Alam M, Ratner D: Cutaneous squamous cell carcinoma. *N Engl J Med* 2001, 344:975–983.

143. Rubin AI, Chen EH, Ratner D: Basal-cell carcinoma. *N Engl J Med* 2005, 353:2262–2269.

144. Miller SJ, Alam M, Andersen A, *et al.*: Basal cell and squamous cell skin cancers. National Comprehensive Cancer Network (NCCN) Practice Guidelines in Oncology v.1.2007.

145. Brodland DG, Zitelli JA: Surgical margins for excision of primary cutaneous squamous cell carcinoma. *J Am Acad Dermatol* 1992, 27:241–248.

146. Ashton H, Beveridge GW, Stevenson CJ: Topical treatment of skin tumors with 5-flourouracil. *Br J Dermatol* 1970, 82:207–209.

147. Gupta AK, Cherman AM, Tyring SK: Viral and nonviral uses of imiquimod: a review. *J Cutan Med Surg* 2004, 8:338–352.

148. International Agency for Reseach on Cancer Working Group on artificial ultraviolet (UV) light and skin cancer: The association of use of sunbeds with cutaneous malignant melanoma and other skin cancers: a systematic review. Int J Cancer 2007, 120:2526.

Sarcomas are a heterogeneous group of connective tissue tumors that are relatively rare, representing only 1% of all adult tumors and 15% of pediatric neoplasms. Approximately 9500 new cases of soft tissue sarcoma (STS) and 2500 cases of bone sarcoma are diagnosed in the United States each year [1], making the incidence of sarcoma similar to testicular cancer and Hodgkin's lymphoma. More than half of sarcoma patients will die of their disease by 5 years, highlighting the need for more effective therapeutics.

ADULT SOFT TISSUE SARCOMAS

ETIOLOGY AND GENETICS

Most sarcomas have an unclear etiology. Mutations in genes such as *RB1* and *p53* have been implicated in the development of sarcomas [2,3], and patients with syndromes such as familial adenomatous polyposis and neurofibromatosis are at increased risk. Soft tissue and bone sarcomas can arise in fields of prior radiation exposure. Lymphedema is associated with develop of lymphangiosarcoma, most commonly in postmastectomy post-irradiated breast cancer, a phenomenon originally described by Stewart and Treves [4]. Recurrent cytogenetic abnormalities exist that occur in some STS, usually high-grade tumors [5,6] (Table 12-1).

PATHOLOGIC CLASSIFICATION, GRADE, AND STAGING

Sarcomas are classified according to the differentiated tissue they most resemble histologically. The latest World Health Organization (WHO) classification of STS was introduced in late 2002 and has gained widespread acceptance [7]. More than 50 different subtypes of STS have been identified. Although each subtype has distinct histologic features, tumor grade is the best predictor of the biologic aggressiveness for adult STS [8]. The American Joint Commission on Cancer (AJCC) revised its grading system in 2002 and relies on tumor size (T), the presence or absence of nodal (N)

or distant metastases (M), as well as histologic grade (G) [9,10] (Table 12-2 and Table 12-3). Low-grade lesions carry a low risk for developing distant metastases (< 15%) and have an excellent survival rate, whereas high-grade lesions are associated with greater than 50% risk for developing distant metastases. The Memorial Sloan-Kettering Cancer Center (MSKCC) developed a postoperative nomogram to help predict 12-year sarcoma-specific death [11,12]. The nomogram uses a point system and formulates probability of death from disease at 12 years based on size, site, histology, and age. Because of the strong influence of tumor grade on prognosis, staging, and therapy of sarcoma patients, all sarcoma specimens should be reviewed by an experienced sarcoma pathologist.

DIAGNOSIS AND WORK-UP

Sixty percent of all STS arise in the extremities, with retroperitoneal and intraperitoneal (20%) and truncal (10%) lesions accounting for the majority of other sites [5]. Patients typically present with a painless enlarging mass. Magnetic resonance imaging (MRI) provides the best anatomic imaging and is preferred for primary extremity lesions and for distinguishing between benign and malignant lesions [13]. Computed tomography (CT) scans of the chest, abdomen, and pelvis should be obtained to assess for metastatic disease [14]. Recently, attention has focused on whether the Response Evaluation Criteria in Solid Tumors (RECIST) criteria are adequate in evaluating the response of STS to therapy, especially with regard to gastrointestinal stromal tumors (GIST). Benjamin *et al.* [15] proposed that Choi criteria might be more appropriate for evaluating the responsiveness of GIST (and potentially other STS) than RECIST.

A [^{18}F]-fluoro-2-deoxy-D-glucose positron emission tomography (FDG-PET) scan can be useful for prognostication and for grading and assessing response to chemotherapy [16]. Recent studies have demonstrated the val-

Table 12-1. Chromosomal and Molecular Alterations in Soft Tissue Sarcoma

Tumor type	Cytogenetic abnormality	Molecular alteration
Synovial sarcoma	t(X;18)(p11;q11)	SSX1 or SSX2, SYT fusion
Myxoid or round cell liposarcoma	t(12;16)(p13;q11)	FUS-DDIT3 fusion
	t(12;16)(p13;q12)	EWS-DDIT3 fusion
Ewing's sarcoma or PNET	t(11;22)(q24;q12)	EWS-FLI1 fusion
	t(21;22)(q22;q12)	EWS-ERG fusion
	t(2;22)(q33;q12)	EWS-FEV fusion
	t(7;22)(p22;q12)	EWS-ETV1 fusion
	t(17;22)(q12;q12)	EWS-E1AF fusion
Desmoplastic small round cell tumor	t(11;22)(p13;q12)	EWS-WT1 fusion
Alveolar rhabdomyosarcoma	t(2;13)(q35;q14)	PAX3-FOXO1A fusion
	t(1;13)(p36;q14)	PAX7-FOXO1A fusion
Extraskeletal myxoid chondrosarcoma	t(9;22)(q22;q12)	EWS-NOR1 fusion
Clear cell sarcoma	t(9;17)(q22;q11)	TAFZN-NOR1 fusion
	t(12;22)(q13;q12)	EWS-ATF1 fusion
Alveolar soft part sarcoma	t(X;17)(p11;q25)	TFE-ASPL fusion
Dermatofibrosarcoma or giant cell fibroblastoma	t(17;22)(q22;q13)	COL1A1-PDGFB fusion
Infantile fibrosarcoma	t(12;15)(p13;q25)	ETV6-NTRK3 fusion
Well-differentiated liposarcoma	Ring form of chromosome 12	Amplification of mdm2
Gastrointestinal stromal tumor	Monosomies 14 and 22	KIT mutation
	Deletion of 1p	

ue of FDG-PET scan in evaluating response to neoadjuvant chemotherapy in patients with high-grade extremity STS and prediction of outcome in liposarcoma [17].

Biopsy and pathologic examination of the tumor tissue are imperative for devising a treatment plan. In most cases, core-needle biopsy is the procedure of choice, whereas fine-needle aspiration can be used in hard to access areas like the lung parenchyma. Surgical biopsies may become necessary if the other, less invasive biopsies do not provide adequate data. It is recommended that biopsies be obtained by a trained orthopedic surgical oncologist or radiologist and preferably at a multidisciplinary sarcoma treatment center. The biopsy site should be chosen so that the track will lay in the field of future en bloc resection [5]. The accuracy of core-needle biopsy in the diagnosis of soft tissue masses has been addressed by several investigators [18–20]. If a retroperitoneal tumor is resectable and a diagnosis of sarcoma is suspected, a biopsy should not be obtained. The risk of transperitoneal spread and track implantation are too high [21]; however, if neoadjuvant therapy is entertained, CT-guided core biopsy is preferred.

TREATMENT MODALITIES

SURGERY

Surgery is the most effective modality in the treatment of localized STS. The goal of surgical excision should be complete removal of the tumor with a margin of normal tissue. Both pathologists and surgeons should note the margins when evaluating a case. Margins less than 1 cm should be reevaluated carefully for consideration of reexcision or other adjuvant therapy. If

adequate margins cannot be obtained, patients should be considered for neoadjuvant radiation or chemotherapy. In cases in which the tumor abuts major neurovascular structures, every attempt at conservation should be made, but not at the expense of adequate resection. Amputation, once the standard for surgical control of extremity STS, should only be applied in select cases of advanced or recurrent local regional disease [22]. Local control rates with limited wide local excision (limb-sparing surgery [LSS]) and adjuvant radiotherapy now approach those obtained historically with amputation [23], and more than 95% of all patients with extremity STS are managed with LSS. Amputations should be considered under the following situations: patient preference, extensive soft tissue mass and skin involvement, major arterial or nerve involvement, extensive bony involvement that requires whole bone resection, failure of preoperative therapies, and recurrence after prior resections and radiation [24]. Surgery is also the primary therapy for retroperitoneal tumors. En bloc resection of adjacent viscera is frequently required, and complete resection (with negative margins) is often impossible. Most tumors will recur, emphasizing the urgent need for better adjuvant therapies [25–27].

CHEMOTHERAPY

The role of adjuvant chemotherapy for the treatment of STS is controversial. An interim analysis of a randomized phase 3 trial presented by the European Organisation for Research and Treatment of Cancer (EORTC) at the American Society of Clinical Oncology (ASCO) 2007 meeting failed to show a survival advantage for adjuvant chemotherapy in STS. Currently, there are only two agents that reproducibly demonstrate a greater than 20% response rate in metastatic sarcoma: doxorubicin and ifosfamide. Doxorubicin is the single most effective agent against STS, with response rates reported from 9% to 70% [28–30]. Sarcoma response to doxorubicin may be dependent on the dose intensity. Unfortunately, increasing the doxorubicin dose is limited by severe myelosuppression, mucositis, and cardiotoxicity. Ifosfamide also has activity as a single agent in the treatment of STS [31,32] and is active in patients who have failed doxorubicin-based therapy [33]. The severe hemorrhagic cystitis associated with the use of ifosfamide has been greatly reduced by the uroprotective agent mesna [34]. Dacarbazine (DTIC) is another agent frequently used in combination regimens for the treatment of STS.

To improve response rates seen with single-agent therapies, several important randomized trials of combination chemotherapy have been conducted by the large cooperative groups [29,30,35–39]. The Eastern Cooperative Oncology Group (ECOG) conducted a series of randomized trials comparing single-agent doxorubicin with combination regimens. Higher response rates were observed for regimens combining doxorubicin with ifosfamide and doxorubicin with dacarbazine. However, the combination therapies offered no survival advantage and were associated with significantly higher toxicity [30,37]. The EORTC performed a phase 3 randomized trial comparing doxorubicin (50 mg/m^2) and ifosfamide (5 g/m^2) with doxorubicin (75 mg/m^2), a 50% increase in the doxorubicin dose, and ifosfamide (5 g/m^2) with granulocyte-macrophage colony-stimulating factor (GM-CSF) (250 µg/m^2) support. There was no apparent difference in response rate or survival [40]. At this time, due to lack of substantial evidence supporting the use of adjuvant chemotherapy in the treatment of resected STS, only treatment in the clinical trial setting is recommended.

Newer agents with proven efficacy against other solid tumors have been evaluated in STS. Paclitaxel and docetaxel have been evaluated and are minimally active as single agents [41–45]. Based on phase 2 data [46,47],

Table 12-2. AJCC Classification for Soft Tissue Sarcoma

Stage	Definition
Primary tumor (T)	
TX	Primary tumor cannot be assessed
T0	No evidence of primary tumor
T1	Tumor < 5 cm
T1a	Superficial tumor*
T1b	Deep tumor*
T2	Tumor > 5 cm
T2a	Superficial tumor*
T2b	Deep tumor*
Regional lymph nodes (N)	
NX	Regional lymph nodes cannot be assessed
N0	No regional lymph node metastasis
N1	Regional lymph node metastasis (presence of N1 is considered stage IV)
Distant metastasis (M)	
MX	Distant metastasis cannot be assessed
M0	No distant metastasis
M1	Distant metastasis
Histologic grade (G)	
GX	Grade cannot be assessed
G1	Well differentiated
G2	Moderately differentiated
G3	Poorly differentiated
G4	Poorly differentiated or undifferentiated (4-tiered systems only)

*Superficial tumor is located exclusively above the superficial fascia without invasion of the fascia; deep tumor is located beneath the superficial fascia, superficial to the fascia but invasive of the fascia, or superficial yet beneath the fascia. Retroperitoneal, mediastinal, and pelvic sarcomas are all classified as deep.
AJCC—American Joint Committee on Cancer.

Table 12-3. AJCC Stage Groupings for Soft Tissue Sarcoma

Stage I	T1a, T1b, T2a, T2b	N0	M0	G1–2	G1	Low
Stage II	T1a, T1b, T2a	N0	M0	G3–4	G2–3	High
Stage III	T2b	N0	M0	G3–4	G2–3	High
Stage IV	Any T	N1	M0	Any G	Any G	High or low
	Any T	N0	M1	Any G	Any G	High or low

AJCC—American Joint Committee on Cancer.

gemcitabine is also minimally effective as a single agent. Maki *et al.* [48] recently published results from a phase 2 trial using gemcitabine and docetaxel as a combination therapy compared with gemcitabine alone. The combination therapy had a RECIST response rate of 16%, compared with 8% in the single-agent arm. Neither of these response rates is as good as those seen with doxorubicin or ifosfamide.

RADIATION THERAPY
Definitive radiotherapy doses that do not exceed normal tissue tolerance rarely achieve local STS control. Even with doses equaling or exceeding 6400 cGy, local control is only 44%, although the smallest tumors (< 5 cm) had a local control of 88% [49]. Therefore, radiotherapy is likely to be most effective in combination with surgery. One randomized trial compared LSS plus postoperative radiotherapy to amputation and found that local failure was 0% for amputation compared with 15% for LSS with radiotherapy (*P* = 0.06), with no difference in overall survival [50]. A subsequent trial of low- and high-grade extremity STS patients compared LSS plus postoperative radiotherapy versus LSS alone. Patients with high-grade STS also received chemotherapy, which was given concurrently in those randomized to the radiotherapy arm. Local control was excellent on the radiotherapy arm (4% local failure for low-grade lesions and 0% for high-grade lesions at 10 years) but significantly worse on the surgery-alone arm (37% local failure for low-grade lesions and 22% for high-grade tumors). No differences in overall survival were observed [51].

A randomized trial conducted by the National Cancer Institute of Canada (NCIC) tested preoperative radiotherapy of 5000 cGy in 25 fractions against postoperative radiotherapy of 6600 cGy in 33 fractions. In the preoperative radiotherapy arm, the minority with positive margins received a postoperative boost of an additional 1600 cGy. The trial showed equal rates of local control, but toxicities were different between the two arms. Wound healing complications were more common in the preoperative arm (35% vs 17%) and were especially high among patients with lower extremity tumors [52]. However, whereas limb function was better initially in postoperative radiotherapy patients, differences between the two arms of the study disappeared after 6 weeks [53], and late effects (fibrosis, joint stiffness, and edema) were less pronounced at 2 years among patients in the preoperative radiotherapy arm [54]. Whether factors such as tumor size, surgical margin width, location, or grade can be used to select patients for LSS without radiotherapy has been the subject of multiple retrospective reports [55–57] without firm conclusions. LSS plus radiotherapy remains the standard local therapy for extremity STS.

The preoperative and postoperative doses used in the NCIC trial are typical of those used in standard practice. The treatment volume typically encompasses the preoperative tumor or postoperative tumor bed with 5-cm longitudinal margins and 2-cm radial margins to a dose of 5000 cGy. The longitudinal margins are reduced when boost doses are given (*ie*, in preoperative radiotherapy cases with positive resection margins and in postoperative cases routinely).

STAGE-SPECIFIC TREATMENT RECOMMENDATIONS

STAGE I SOFT TISSUE SARCOMA (LOW GRADE)
Low-grade (T1a–1b, N0, M0) STS have low metastatic potential. Surgical resection with negative tissue margins of at least 2 cm or more in all directions is the desired treatment. Small tumors generally have a favorable outcome with surgery alone [22]. Local recurrence is the greatest risk; therefore, if the surgical margins are less than 1 cm, reexcision or postoperative radiation therapy should be considered [51]. Adjuvant chemotherapy is generally not indicated.

STAGE II, III SOFT TISSUE SARCOMA (HIGH GRADE)
The surgical management of high-grade localized STS is usually LSS that involves wide local excision combined with preoperative or postoperative radiation therapy. Adjuvant chemotherapy for patients with high-grade STS remains controversial, and the two largest trials do not support the use of adjuvant chemotherapy because neither showed a statistically significant improvement in overall survival [58,59]. Neoadjuvant chemotherapy may offer advantages such as early treatment of microscopic metastatic disease, ability to monitor the primary tumor in vivo to gauge responsiveness

to particular agents, and shrinkage of advanced local tumors that may allow limb salvage. An M.D. Anderson Cancer Center retrospective analysis of 46 patients who received doxorubicin-based neoadjuvant chemotherapy found significantly improved disease-free and overall survival in patients whose primary tumors responded [60]. However, a prospective trial at MSKCC of 29 patients with large (> 10 cm) high-grade extremity sarcomas failed to demonstrate improved survival compared with historical controls [61]. A recently completed multi-institutional study of neoadjuvant therapy supports the single-institution data [62].

STAGE IV SOFT TISSUE SARCOMA
The most frequent site of metastases for STS is the lung. If possible, patients with limited pulmonary metastases should be considered for curative-intent surgery by resection of the primary and pulmonary metastectomy [63–65]. In a retrospective study of more than 3000 patients, the important prognostic variables that were associated with a better outcome with metastectomy were metastasis size, metastasis number, and primary tumor histologic grade [66]. Chemotherapy should be considered for those patients with metastatic disease. Alternatively, for asymptomatic stage IV patients, "watchful waiting" may be reasonable. For symptomatic patients, proceeding to palliative therapeutic options is appropriate. Chemotherapy, radiation therapy, palliative surgery, or interventional techniques like radiofrequency ablation or cryotherapy are all reasonable approaches.

RECURRENT DISEASE
Patients with locally recurrent disease should be treated similarly to patients with primary local disease, with attempts at re-resection to achieve negative margins and consideration given to additional adjuvant radiotherapy [63,67]. Despite adequate treatment of their primary tumors, many patients with high-grade extremity sarcomas will recur locally. The link between local recurrence and the development of distant metastases is unclear. Retrospective data correlate local recurrence with increased risk of developing distant metastases and decreased overall survival [63,64]. Yet in two prospective, randomized trials, better local control rates did not translate into improved survival [51,68]. It appears that survival is dictated by the biologic aggressiveness of the tumor and the presence of microscopic metastatic disease at the time of diagnosis. In cases of multifocal recurrence or previous maximum radiotherapy, amputation may be necessary.

RHABDOMYOSARCOMA

PATHOLOGIC CLASSIFICATION, GRADE, AND STAGING
Rhabdomyosarcoma is the most common STS of childhood, accounting for 5% to 8% of childhood cancers [69]. There are two major identified histologic variants: embryonal and alveolar. Embryonal rhabdomyosarcoma is subdivided into solid and botryoid variants, accounts for 57% of rhabdomyosarcoma cases, typically arises in the head and neck region or in the genitourinary tract, and usually affects children between 3 and 12 years of age. Alveolar rhabdomyosarcoma accounts for 19% of cases, is more frequent in the trunk and extremities, and usually affects patients between 6 and 21 years of age [69]. Embryonal rhabdomyosarcoma carries a more favorable prognosis than alveolar.

Recurrent translocations have been identified in alveolar rhabdomyosarcoma. In 55% of cases, a translocation between chromosomes 2 and 13, t(2;13)(q35;q14), is seen, and in 22% of cases a similar translocation involving chromosome 1, t(1;13)(p36;q14), is identified [70]. These translocations involve related transcription factor genes, *PAX3* and *PAX7*, respectively. In each case, the DNA binding domain of the *PAX* gene is fused to the transactivation domain of the *FKHR* gene. Disruption of *PAX* genes leads to abnormal muscle development [71], suggesting a direct etiologic relationship between the translocation and development of malignancy. Patients with the PAX3-FKHR translocation appear to have a poorer prognosis than patients with PAX7-FKHR [72]. No similar molecular changes have yet been identified in embryonal rhabdomyosarcoma.

Rhabdomyosarcoma is staged using a tumor-specific TNM staging system that incorporates the site of the primary tumor, reflecting prognostic differences between favorable and unfavorable anatomic locations (Table 12-4) [73]. Patients are also assigned a so-called "clinical group," which accounts for extent of locoregional spread and sufficiency of surgery (Table 12-5).

Patients are classified as high-, intermediate-, or low-risk based on clinical group and stage, and treatment is based on this assessment of risk.

PRESENTATION AND DIAGNOSIS

Signs and symptoms present at diagnosis depend on the primary tumor site. Typically, patients present with an asymptomatic mass, although involvement of cortical bone may cause pain, and genitourinary disease may present with hematuria or urinary retention. Head and neck sites, including orbit and parameningeal primaries, account for 40% of cases, trunk and extremity sites account for 25% to 30% of cases, and genitourinary sites account for 20% [70]. The most common sites of metastasis are the lungs, lymph nodes, cortical bone, and bone marrow.

TREATMENT

The choice of local therapy in rhabdomyosarcoma is influenced by whether an oncologic resection is feasible and whether it is able to preserve form and function. The location of the primary site, a major determinant of outcome [74], correlates with clinical factors such as size, invasiveness, and regional spread and therefore influences the choice of local therapy. Guidelines for the use of local radiotherapy depend on the clinical group. A retrospective analysis of clinical group I patients treated in the Intergroup Rhabdomyosarcoma Study (IRS)-I, -II, and -III showed a significant failure-free and overall survival benefit with the use of radiotherapy in patients with alveolar and undifferentiated histology tumors [75]. Radiotherapy for clinical group II patients has been routinely employed in the IRS studies, with local and regional failure rates of 8% and 4% at 5 years [76]. These observations support the IRS policy for definitive radiotherapy in clinical group III patients. Good local control has been reported historically with radiotherapy for these patients: in the more recent IRS trials, local failure was 19% at 5 years on IRS-III [77] and 13% at 5 years on IRS-IV [78]. Certain cooperative groups have attempted to minimize the impact of local therapy by withholding radiotherapy in clinical group III patients with favorable response to chemotherapy or patients whose disease is resected following induction chemotherapy, but this approach is associated with unfavorable local control [79] and possibly decreased survival in many primary site groups [80].

The specifics of systemic chemotherapy vary depending on risk stratification. For low-risk patients, current standard therapy consists of four cycles of VAC (vincristine, actinomycin, cyclophosphamide), followed by four cycles of VA (vincristine, actinomycin) for the lowest-risk patients and 12 cycles of VA for patients with slightly higher-risk tumors. For intermediate-risk patients, standard treatment consists of 14 cycles of VAC. Currently, the Children's Oncology Group (COG) is conducting a clinical trial comparing this with 14 cycles of alternating VAC and VI (vincristine and irinotecan). A recently completed COG study with a VI window prior to standard therapy for high-risk patients showed an excellent 70% response rate to the window treatment. For high-risk patients, the current COG protocol treats patients with two cycles of VI, followed by six cycles of alternating VDC (vincristine, doxorubicin, cyclophosphamide) and I/E (ifosfamide, eto-

poside), then six cycles of intermixed VI, I/E, and VDC, finally followed with six cycles of alternating VAC and VI.

Because of the dismal prognosis for patients presenting with metastatic rhabdomyosarcoma, autologous peripheral blood stem cell transplant (PBSCT) has been used; however, its role is not established. PBSCT for high-risk rhabdomyosarcoma patients should be reserved for clinical trials.

NONEXTREMITY AND ATYPICAL SOFT TISSUE SARCOMAS

VISCERAL AND RETROPERITONEAL SARCOMAS

The relatively rare retroperitoneal sarcomas present additional treatment challenges. These patients will often present with large, bulky tumors. The differential diagnosis of retroperitoneal masses should include lymphoma, sarcoma, and, in the male patient, metastatic testicular cancer. Complete surgical resection is often difficult because of the anatomic location, compromising the ability to achieve desired surgical margins. Unlike extremity tumors, survival from retroperitoneal sarcomas is most dependent on locoregional control. Every attempt should be made to completely resect the tumor with negative margins at initial exploration because this is the only potentially curative therapy. Whenever necessary, adjacent viscera involved with the tumor should be removed en bloc with the specimen. Conversely, uninvolved organs should not be removed. Resectability of retroperitoneal sarcomas has been reported to be between 50% and 80% and despite complete resection, local recurrence will develop in 40% to 50% of patients [81–83].

Given the high recurrence rates in retroperitoneal sarcomas, combined modality approaches are standard, but lack evidence-based data to prove an overall survival advantage [81]. Local recurrences are managed by successive surgical resections. Unfortunately, efforts to improve local control with adjuvant radiotherapy are limited by the radiosensitivity of overlying viscera. Attempts to minimize the dose of radiotherapy to normal tissue by means of intraoperative delivery of radiotherapy have been successful in decreasing local failure rates but do not appear to improve survival [84,85].

BONE SARCOMAS

PATHOLOGIC CLASSIFICATION, GRADE, AND STAGING

Three common types of sarcoma arise from bone: osteosarcoma, chondrosarcoma, and Ewing's sarcoma. Ewing's sarcoma and osteosarcoma are more common in adolescents, and chondrosarcoma is more common in older adults.

Ewing's sarcoma is a small round blue cell tumor, and the tumor cells characteristically express the cell surface antigen CD99. Ewing's sarcoma is also characterized by the presence of a reciprocal translocation—t(11;22)(q24;q12)—that fuses a gene known as *EWS* with the ets family transcription factor FLI-1 and is found in 85% of such tumors [86]. In contrast, osteosarcoma is characterized by spindle cells and osteoid deposition. There are several histologic subtypes of osteosarcoma, including osteoblastic, fibroblastic, chondroblastic, and telangiectatic. There does not appear to be prognostic significance to these distinctions. Unlike Ewing's sarcoma, recurrent chromosomal translocations have not been identified in osteosarcoma. Chondrosarcomas tend to be lobulated tumors

Table 12-4. TNM Staging of Rhabdomyosarcoma					
Stage	Sites	T	Size	N	M
1	Orbit; head and neck; GU (not prostate or bladder); biliary tract	Any	a or b	Any	M0
2	Bladder; prostate; extremity; cranial; parameningeal; trunk; retroperitoneum	Any	a	N0 or NX	M0
3	Bladder; prostate; extremity; cranial; parameningeal; trunk; retroperitoneum	Any	a	N1	M0
			b	Any	M0
4	All	Any	a or b	N0 or N1	M1

GU—genitourinary; TNM—tumor, node, metastasis.

Table 12-5. Clinical Group Classification of Rhabdomyosarcoma	
Group	Definition
I	Localized disease completely resected
IIa	Gross total resection with microscopic residual disease
IIb	Regionally involved lymph nodes, completely resected with the primary
IIc	Regional disease with involved nodes, totally resected with either microscopic residual disease or histologic evidence of involvement of the most distant lymph node in the dissection
III	Incomplete resection
IV	Distant metastases

with varying degrees of cellularity and differentiation. Histologic grading of chondrosarcomas has prognostic significance. Well-differentiated (grade I) chondrosarcomas have chondrocytes that appear differentiated and mitoses are absent. Grade II tumors have more cellularity and less matrix than well-differentiated tumors, and mitoses are present, although rarely. High-grade tumors have even more cellularity and the matrix is often myxoid. A mesenchymal subtype also exists; this variant is particularly aggressive. Bone sarcomas are staged simply as localized or metastatic.

PRESENTATION AND DIAGNOSIS

Pain and swelling are the most common presenting symptoms of Ewing's sarcoma, occurring in 84% and 63% of patients, respectively [87]. These symptoms are often longstanding, with a delay between onset of symptoms and diagnosis in excess of 6 months in more than half of patients [88]. Ewing's sarcoma shows a predilection for the lower extremity (46%) and pelvis (20%) [89]. Approximately 25% of patients present with metastases. Of these, half have metastases to the lungs, one quarter to other bones, and one fifth to bone marrow [87].

The most common presenting complaint of a patient with osteosarcoma is pain [69]. On plain radiograph, a mixed osteolytic/sclerotic lesion with disorganized soft tissue calcification is seen. At diagnosis, the disease is localized in 80% of cases. Osteosarcoma arises most frequently in the limbs (80% of cases), with the femur being the most commonly affected bone [90]. It occurs predominantly in the metaphysis of long bones, arising from the medullary cavity and invading into the epiphysis, even in the presence of a growth plate.

Chondrosarcomas tend to present as a painless mass with symptoms based on location. Because of their slow growth, there is a prolonged duration of symptoms, with one study reporting a mean duration of symptoms of 27 months for skull base lesions [91].

Definitive diagnosis of a bone sarcoma requires a biopsy, and this procedure should be performed with consideration for the definitive surgical procedure to follow. Poorly placed biopsies will limit future limb-sparing options. In general, core-needle biopsy is the preferred technique and will yield an adequate specimen for diagnosis in most cases [92].

TREATMENT

The treatment for high-grade bone sarcomas is multidisciplinary and includes surgery, chemotherapy, and often radiotherapy. Low-grade chondrosarcoma is treated primarily surgically, although radiation and chemotherapy are sometimes also required.

Ewing's sarcoma and osteosarcoma are both treated with neoadjuvant chemotherapy followed by local control and adjuvant chemotherapy. The current standard chemotherapy regimen includes cycles of vincristine, doxorubicin, and cyclophosphamide alternating with cycles of ifosfamide and etoposide [93]. Four neoadjuvant cycles are administered followed by 10 adjuvant cycles. The most recent cooperative group trial randomized patients with localized disease to receive cycles of chemotherapy every 2 or 3 weeks. Unpublished results from this study show a significant survival advantage for patients treated every 2 weeks, making this the current recommended treatment interval.

Surgery is used as local control for primary tumors of expendable bones (*eg*, fibula, small bones of the hands/feet, ribs, and clavicle) or when good reconstructive options exist [94]. Patients treated with surgery alone fare better than patients treated with radiotherapy. This likely reflects selection bias, as patients with smaller tumors or tumors in accessible locations are more commonly treated with surgery, as seen in the contemporary Intergroup 0091 trial [93] and multiple European cooperative group trials [95]. A local control analysis of Intergroup 0091 restricted to patients with pelvic Ewing's sarcoma and adjusted for tumor size showed no difference regardless of whether local therapy consisted of radiotherapy alone, surgery alone, or surgery and radiotherapy [96]. Intergroup 0091 results also suggest that local control is improved with optimized chemotherapy: patients were randomized to standard chemotherapy with vincristine, doxorubicin, cyclophosphamide, and actinomycin versus the same chemotherapy alternating with ifosfamide and etoposide, and a significant benefit in event-free

and overall survival (54% vs 69% and 61% vs 72%) seen in nonmetastatic patients was primarily due to improved local control (85% vs 95%) [93].

The total radiotherapy dose for Ewing's sarcoma is 5580 cGy [97] given following 3 to 4 months of induction chemotherapy. The initial treatment volume encompasses the initial tumor volume with a 3-cm margin to 4500 cGy, followed by a boost for an additional 1080 cGy to the postchemotherapy, preradiotherapy volume [93]. Historically, the entire bone was irradiated, but a randomized trial (Pediatric Oncology Group [POG] 8346) comparing whole-bone versus involved-field radiotherapy demonstrated no differences in local control or event-free survival [98]. Adjuvant radiotherapy is applied in lesions resected to a positive margin. A dose of 4500 cGy is typically given for microscopic disease, and 5580 cGy for gross residual disease. In the Cooperative Ewing Sarcoma Study (CESS)-81 [99], a 5-year local failure of 17% was observed with a postoperative radiotherapy dose of 36 Gy compared with approximately 5% in CESS-86 [100], suggesting a dose-response relationship [94]. When delineating involved-field treatment volumes, the radiation oncologist should be mindful of the cortical and medullary as well as extraosseous components of the tumor, and bone scintigraphy, CT, and MRI should be jointly employed.

Treatment for patients with metastatic disease is the same as that for patients with localized disease. For patients with metastatic disease, autologous PBSCT has been investigated to improve outcomes. One of the earliest and largest reports of high-dose therapy investigated the use of total body irradiation with autologous PBSCT as consolidation therapy for high-risk Ewing's sarcoma patients. Promising results have been reported from a review of European Bone Marrow Transplant Registry data. While disease-free survival rates for patients with Ewing's sarcoma metastatic to bone or bone marrow who underwent PBSCT between 1982 and 1992 was only 21% [101], 5-year overall survival was 44% for the patients treated with a busulfan-containing regimen, compared with 23% for patients treated without this drug [102]. Although there are no randomized trials, retrospective data appear to support a survival advantage for patients treated with regimens incorporating high doses of alkylating agents, especially busulfan.

Whole lung radiotherapy (WLRT) is important for the management of patients with lung metastases at presentation. A retrospective joint analysis of CESS-81, CESS-86, and European Intergroup CESS (EICESS)-92 demonstrated significantly better event-free survival for 75 patients who received WLRT (15–18 Gy depending on age) versus 25 patients who did not (38% vs 27% at 5 years) [103]. A dose-response has also been suggested [104]. WLRT is also currently used as part of salvage therapy for patients with pulmonary relapse. A retrospective analysis of patients treated at St. Jude Children's Research Hospital for isolated pulmonary recurrence demonstrated significantly higher postrecurrence survival in patients who received WLRT versus those who did not (30% vs 17% at 5 years) [105].

Therapy for osteosarcoma follows the same paradigm as Ewing's sarcoma. Standard neoadjuvant chemotherapy consists of high-dose methotrexate, doxorubicin, and cisplatin. With modern surgical techniques, the vast majority of patients are able to undergo local control with a limb-salvage approach. Performing definitive surgery after administration of chemotherapy allows the tumor's chemosensitivity to be evaluated. This has led to the recognition that tumor necrosis is a strong prognostic indicator. Patients with a good histologic response (> 90% tumor necrosis) had 68% overall survival at 5 years, compared with 52% survival in poor responders [106]. Based on this finding, there have been several attempts to improve survival by augmenting chemotherapy for the poor responders. No such attempt has shown a statistically significant benefit [107]. Thus, standard adjuvant therapy remains methotrexate, doxorubicin, and cisplatin, and is the same for patients with localized or metastatic disease, despite the vast difference in prognosis between these groups.

Osteosarcoma is considered a radioresistant malignancy [108]. Radiotherapy as the definitive local modality should not replace surgery when wide surgical margins can be achieved. Sites in which an appropriate resection is difficult to achieve, such as the pelvis, spine, and head and neck, are therefore unfavorable [109] and may require radiotherapeutic management. A retrospective report from Massachusetts General Hospital described the outcome of 41 such patients whose local treatment included radiotherapy. Local control at 5 years was 78% among 27 patients who underwent postoperative radiotherapy after gross total resection to close or positive margins and 78% among nine patients who underwent postoperative radiotherapy after subtotal resection. Local control was only 40% among five patients who underwent definitive radiotherapy [109]. Similar results with definitive radiotherapy were observed retrospectively in a report from Russia regarding 31 patients who underwent induction chemotherapy and refused surgery. With a median dose of 60 Gy, 5-year local progression-free survival was 56%. Response to induction chemotherapy was a major determinant of local control with radiotherapy [110].

GASTROINTESTINAL STROMAL TUMORS

GIST is the most common mesenchymal neoplasm of the gastrointestinal tract. Most, but not all, GISTs are CD-117 (c-kit) positive. They can arise anywhere along the gastrointestinal tract, but are most common in the stomach (50%) and small bowel (24%) [111]. GISTs most commonly metastasize to the liver or disseminate throughout the abdominal cavity. Work-up is similar to other abdominal sarcomas. Because biopsies can cause tumor hemorrhage and increased risk for dissemination of disease, if the tumor is easily resectable it may be preferential to resect rather than biopsy. However, if preoperative therapy is being considered, biopsy is necessary to confirm the diagnosis.

At least 50% of patients will develop recurrence or metastasis following complete resection; the 5-year survival is about 50% [112,113]. As a result, alternative treatment approaches are being explored. Imatinib mesylate, a selective inhibitor of the c-kit protein tyrosine kinase, has produced clinical benefit and objective responses in more than 50% of patients [114–116]. The suggested starting dose of imatinib is 400 mg/d; however, in patients treated with 800 mg/d, improved progression-free survival has been observed [117]. PET scans allow for rapid assessment of tumor response to imatinib. Baseline CT with or without MRI followed by subsequent PET-CT about 2 to 4 weeks after initiating therapy can be performed to assess therapeutic effect [118].

There are several ongoing clinical trials to assess the efficacy of adjuvant imatinib. At the 2007 ASCO conference, DeMatteo *et al.* [119] presented their phase 3 adjuvant trial evaluating imatinib mesylate in patients with completely resected localized primary GIST (North American Intergroup phase 3 trial ACOSOG Z9001). Of 644 evaluable patients, the recurrence-free survival at 1 year was 97% in the treatment arm versus 83% in the control arm.

HEAD AND NECK SARCOMAS

Sarcomas arising in the head and neck region are uncommon, representing less than 5% of all sarcomas. Although any sarcoma can arise within the head and neck tissues, angiosarcoma has a head and neck preference. Treatment of these lesions is similar to sarcomas in other locations and surgery remains the mainstay of therapy [120]. Local failure is a significant problem for head and neck sarcomas, given the difficulty of obtaining wide surgical margins in this region. Successful treatment is predicted by the grade and size of the primary tumor, status of the surgical margins,

and presence or absence of bony invasion [121]. As with other sarcomas, lymph node metastases are rare, and routine lymphadenectomy is not recommended. Five-year survival has been reported to vary from 20% to 68%. Angiosarcomas have a poorer prognosis than other sarcomas in the head and neck region. They also have a higher lymph node metastasis incidence than other sarcomas, with a rate of 10% to 15% [122].

DESMOID TUMOR

Desmoid tumors, also known as aggressive fibromatoses, usually present as well-circumscribed collections of proliferating fibroblastic cells. More often then not, they are locally invasive, despite being termed "benign" [123]. The most common sites are the abdominal wall, mesentery, and extremities. Desmoid tumors may be a component of familial adenomatous polyposis, and in patients who have had prophylactic colectomy, desmoids can sometimes become the main cause of future morbidity. Desmoids rarely metastasize, and the primary treatment should be wide local excision. If adequate margins are obtained, treatment can stop with resection. If close or positive margins are obtained, re-resection can be considered or adjuvant radiation therapy can be given. There have been recent data to support the use of cytostatic agents like tamoxifen and imatinib [124,125], or nonsteroidal anti-inflammatory agents, like sulindac [126], because these agents can halt progression. Cytotoxic regimens including doxorubicin or vinblastine plus methotrexate have been used with some success [127–130].

BREAST SARCOMA

Primary STS of the breast is rare, accounting for approximately 1% of all breast malignancies. They usually present as a painless mass without any associated findings on mammography. As with other STS, the treatment approach should be surgery with an attempt at wide excision and generous margins. One study reported 25 patients treated with surgery with or without radiation therapy. The overall 5-year survival rate was 61%. The five patients in the study who received adjuvant radiation therapy had no local recurrence [131].

KAPOSI'S SARCOMA

Kaposi's sarcoma is an unusual vascular tumor associated with human herpes virus-8 (HHV-8). There are four different classifications: classic, which occurs in the skin of elderly men of Mediterranean or Jewish origin; African variant, which occurs in all parts of equatorial Africa and is not associated with an immunocompromised state; organ transplant–associated Kaposi's; and HIV/AIDS-related Kaposi's sarcoma [132]. Treatment strategies vary depending on the clinical scenario in which the tumor arises. If the patient is immunocompromised secondary to HIV, the first treatment strategy should be starting or optimizing the patient's highly active antiretroviral therapy medications [133]. If the patient is symptomatic from disease and a more immediate intervention is needed, systemic chemotherapy can be used; excellent responses have been noted with single-agent vincristine, doxorubicin, vinblastine, and the taxanes. There are currently ongoing trials using more targeted agents, like imatinib.

MAI (MESNA, DOXORUBICIN, IFOSFAMIDE) FOR ADVANCED SOFT TISSUE SARCOMA

Doxorubicin is the most effective single agent in the treatment of STS in the adult. Ifosfamide has been shown to also have good activity as a single agent. The combination regimen of doxorubicin and ifosfamide with or without dacarbazine (DTIC) has been shown to have higher response rates than treatment with single agents. Unfortunately, overall survival has not been shown to be improved by combination regimens. Moreover, toxicity is significantly greater. Efforts to limit myelosuppressive toxicity and increase the dose of doxorubicin in these regimens have been investigated but do not change overall survival.

INDICATIONS

Doxorubicin is the only drug with a labeled indication for the treatment of STS. Combination regimens incorporating ifosfamide with mesna and/or dacarbazine have been shown in randomized trials to improve response rates in STS. Currently little data exist to support the use of these drugs in the adjuvant setting outside of clinical trials; for patients with advanced disease, single-agent doxorubicin may provide palliative benefit. The greater response rates with combination regimens should be balanced against the increased toxicity.

CANDIDATES FOR TREATMENT

Patients with advanced STS who have normal renal and cardiac function

TOXICITIES

Combination regimen: enhanced myelosuppression; administration of hematopoietic growth factors may blunt severe neutropenia; severe nausea and emesis is common; alopecia is to be expected; **Doxorubicin:** cardiac toxicity is the single most important concern with the incidence increasing the higher the dose; may also tinge urine red-orange color; hyperpigmentation and creasing of nail beds may occur; should be administered through central venous line because local extravasation will result in severe cellulitis, vesication, and tissue necrosis; **Ifosfamide:** severe hemorrhagic cystitis; should only be administered with vigorous hydration in combination with uroprotective agent mesna; neurologic manifestations (eg, somnolence, confusion, hallucinations, to frank coma)

DRUG INTERACTIONS

Administration of live vaccines should be avoided in all patients receiving myelosuppressive chemotherapy; **Doxorubicin:** cyclosporine may induce coma and/or seizures; phenobarbital increases elimination of doxorubicin; phenytoin levels may be decreased by coadministration of doxorubicin; **Ifosfamide:** no specific interactions cited in literature; physician should be alert to possible combined drug interactions

NURSING INTERVENTIONS

Strict sterile technique when accessing central venous devices should be practiced; general supportive measures, including prophylactic antiemetics and mouth care to minimize symptoms from stomatitis; vigorous hydration with administration of ifosfamide; immediately report any symptoms of infection, bleeding, chemotherapy extravasation, or shortness of breath

PATIENT INFORMATION

Common side effects from administration of these agents include nausea, vomiting, and stomatitis; in addition, doxorubicin may have direct cardiac toxicity manifested by acute left ventricular failure; immunosuppression is expected and occurs at a maximum of 10–14 d after therapy; patients should notify their physician immediately if they develop a fever, abnormal bleeding, or shortness of breath.

AVAILABILITY

Doxorubicin: Supplied as generic by multiple manufacturers as 10-mg, 50-mg, and 100-mg vials. Reconstitute with sterile sodium chloride (0.9%) to final concentration of 2 mg/mL. Reconstituted solution is stable up to 24 h at room temperature and 48 h under refrigeration (2°C–8°C)

Ifosfamide: (Ifex, Bristol-Myers Squibb, Princeton, NJ) supplied as 1-g or 3-g single- or multiple-dose vials in combination packages with mesna (Mesnex). Should be reconstituted in sterile water to final concentration of 50 mg/mL. Should be refrigerated and used within 24 h of reconstitution.

EXPERIENCES AND RESPONSE RATES

Study	Regimen	Doxorubicin dose	Patients, *n*	RR, %	CR, %
Antman and Elias [33]	MAID	60 mg/m²/course	108	47	10
Hicks *et al.* [134]	MAID + GM-CSF	75 mg/m²/course	13	—	—
Le Cesne *et al.* [40]	Doxorubicin + ifosfamide + GM-CSF	60 mg/m²/course	145	45	10

CR—complete response; GM-CSF—granulocyte-macrophage colony-stimulating factor; MAID—mesna, doxorubicin, ifosfamide, dacarbazine; RR—response rate.

REFERENCES

1. Jemal A, Siegel R, Ward E, *et al.*: Cancer statistics, 2007. *CA Cancer J Clin* 2007, 57:43–66.
2. Strong LC, Williams WR, Tainsky MA: The Li-Fraumeni syndrome: from clinical epidemiology to molecular genetics. *Am J Epidemiol* 1992, 135:190–199.
3. Wong FL, Boice JD Jr, Abramson DH, *et al.*: Cancer incidence after retinoblastoma. Radiation dose and sarcoma risk. *JAMA* 1997, 278:1262–1267.
4. Jessner M, Zak FG, Rein CR: Angiosarcoma in postmastectomy lymphedema (Stewart-Treves syndrome). *AMA Arch Derm Syphilol* 1952, 65:123–129.
5. Clark MA, Fisher C, Judson I, *et al.*: Soft-tissue sarcomas in adults. *N Engl J Med* 2005, 353:701–711.
6. Rubin BP, Goldblum JR: Pathology of soft tissue sarcoma. *J Natl Compr Canc Netw* 2007, 5:411–418.
7. Fletcher CD: The evolving classification of soft tissue tumours: an update based on the new WHO classification. *Histopathology* 2006, 48:3–12.
8. Gaynor JJ, Tan CC, Casper ES, *et al.*: Refinement of clinicopathologic staging for localized soft tissue sarcoma of the extremity: a study of 423 adults. *J Clin Oncol* 1992, 10:1317–1329.
9. Kotilingam D, Lev DC, Lazar AJ, *et al.*: Staging soft tissue sarcoma: evolution and change. *CA Cancer J Clin* 2006, 56:282–291; quiz 314–315.
10. Wittekind C, Compton CC, Greene FL, *et al.*: TNM residual tumor classification revisited. *Cancer* 2002, 94:2511–2516.

11. Kattan MW, Leung DH, Brennan MF: Postoperative nomogram for 12-year sarcoma-specific death. *J Clin Oncol* 2002, 20:791–796.

12. Eilber FC, Brennan MF, Eilber FR, *et al.*: Validation of the postoperative nomogram for 12-year sarcoma-specific mortality. *Cancer* 2004, 101:2270–2275.

13. Sanders TG, Parsons TW III: Radiographic imaging of musculoskeletal neoplasia. *Cancer Control* 2001, 8:221–231.

14. Demas BE, Heelan RT, Lane J, *et al.*: Soft-tissue sarcomas of the extremities: comparison of MR and CT in determining the extent of disease. *AJR Am J Roentgenol* 1988, 150:615–620.

15. Benjamin RS, Choi H, Macapinlac HA, *et al.*: We should desist using RECIST, at least in GIST. *J Clin Oncol* 2007, 25:1760–1764.

16. Eary JF, Conrad EU: PET imaging: update on sarcomas. *Oncology (Williston Park)* 2007, 21:249–252.

17. Brenner W, Eary JF, Hwang W, *et al.*: Risk assessment in liposarcoma patients based on FDG PET imaging. *Eur J Nucl Med Mol Imaging* 2006, 33:1290–1295.

18. Barth RJ Jr, Merino MJ, Solomon D, *et al.*: A prospective study of the value of core needle biopsy and fine needle aspiration in the diagnosis of soft tissue masses. *Surgery* 1992, 112:536–543.

19. Ball AB, Fisher C, Pittam M, *et al.*: Diagnosis of soft tissue tumours by Tru-Cut biopsy. *Br J Surg* 1990, 77:756–758.

20. Heslin MJ, Lewis JJ, Woodruff JM, *et al.*: Core needle biopsy for diagnosis of extremity soft tissue sarcoma. *Ann Surg Oncol* 1997, 4:425–431.

21. Clark MA, Thomas JM: Portsite recurrence after laparoscopy for staging of retroperitoneal sarcoma. *Surg Laparosc Endosc Percutan Tech* 2003, 13:290–291.

22. Geer RJ, Woodruff J, Casper ES, *et al.*: Management of small soft-tissue sarcoma of the extremity in adults. *Arch Surg* 1992, 127:1285–1289.

23. Spiro IJ, Rosenberg AE, Springfield D, *et al.*: Combined surgery and radiation therapy for limb preservation in soft tissue sarcoma of the extremity: the Massachusetts General Hospital experience. *Cancer Invest* 1995, 13:86–95.

24. Clark MA, Thomas JM: Amputation for soft-tissue sarcoma. *Lancet Oncol* 2003, 4:335–342.

25. Alektiar KM, Velasco J, Zelefsky MJ, *et al.*: Adjuvant radiotherapy for margin-positive high-grade soft tissue sarcoma of the extremity. *Int J Radiat Oncol Biol Phys* 2000, 48:1051–1058.

26. Rossi CR, Deraco M, De Simone M, *et al.*: Hyperthermic intraperitoneal intraoperative chemotherapy after cytoreductive surgery for the treatment of abdominal sarcomatosis: clinical outcome and prognostic factors in 60 consecutive patients. *Cancer* 2004, 100:1943–1950.

27. Sindelar WF, Kinsella TJ, Chen PW, *et al.*: Intraoperative radiotherapy in retroperitoneal sarcomas. Final results of a prospective, randomized, clinical trial. *Arch Surg* 1993, 128:402–410.

28. Verweij J, van Oosterom AT, Somers R, *et al.*: Chemotherapy in the multidisciplinary approach to soft tissue sarcomas. EORTC Soft Tissue and Bone Sarcoma Group studies in perspective. *Ann Oncol* 1992, 3(Suppl 2):S75–S80.

29. Borden EC, Amato DA, Edmonson JH, *et al.*: Randomized comparison of doxorubicin and vindesine to doxorubicin for patients with metastatic soft-tissue sarcomas. *Cancer* 1990, 66:862–867.

30. Edmonson JH, Ryan LM, Blum RH, *et al.*: Randomized comparison of doxorubicin alone versus ifosfamide plus doxorubicin or mitomycin, doxorubicin, and cisplatin against advanced soft tissue sarcomas. *J Clin Oncol* 1993, 11:1269–275.

31. Stuart-Harris R, Harper PG, Kaye SB, et al.: High-dose ifosfamide by infusion with mesna in advanced soft tissue sarcoma. *Cancer Treat Rev* 1983, 10(Suppl A):163–164.

32. Stuart-Harris RC, Harper PG, Parsons CA, *et al.*: High-dose alkylation therapy using ifosfamide infusion with mesna in the treatment of adult advanced soft-tissue sarcoma. *Cancer Chemother Pharmacol* 1983, 11:69–72.

33. Antman KH, Elias A: Dana-Farber Cancer Institute studies in advanced sarcoma. *Semin Oncol* 1990, 17:7–15.

34. Elias AD, Eder JP, Shea T, *et al.*: High-dose ifosfamide with mesna uroprotection: a phase I study. *J Clin Oncol* 1990, 8:170–178.

35. Antman K, Crowley J, Balcerzak SP, *et al.*: An intergroup phase III randomized study of doxorubicin and dacarbazine with or without ifosfamide and mesna in advanced soft tissue and bone sarcomas. *J Clin Oncol* 1993, 11:1276–1285.

36. Schoenfeld DA, Rosenbaum C, Horton J, *et al.*: A comparison of Adriamycin versus vincristine and Adriamycin, and cyclophosphamide versus vincristine, actinomycin-D, and cyclophosphamide for advanced sarcoma. *Cancer* 1982, 50:2757–2762.

37. Borden EC, Amato DA, Rosenbaum C, *et al.*: Randomized comparison of three Adriamycin regimens for metastatic soft tissue sarcomas. *J Clin Oncol* 1987, 5:840–850.

38. Baker LH, Frank J, Fine G, *et al.*: Combination chemotherapy using Adriamycin, DTIC, cyclophosphamide, and actinomycin D for advanced soft tissue sarcomas: a randomized comparative trial. A phase III, Southwest Oncology Group Study (7613). *J Clin Oncol* 1987, 5:851–861.

39. Santoro A, Tursz T, Mouridsen H, *et al.*: Doxorubicin versus CYVADIC versus doxorubicin plus ifosfamide in first-line treatment of advanced soft tissue sarcomas: a randomized study of the European Organization for Research and Treatment of Cancer Soft Tissue and Bone Sarcoma Group. *J Clin Oncol* 1995, 13:1537–1545.

40. Le Cesne A, Judson I, Crowther D, *et al.*: Randomized phase III study comparing conventional-dose doxorubicin plus ifosfamide versus high-dose doxorubicin plus ifosfamide plus recombinant human granulocyte-macrophage colony-stimulating factor in advanced soft tissue sarcomas: a trial of the European Organization for Research and Treatment of Cancer/Soft Tissue and Bone Sarcoma Group. *J Clin Oncol* 2000, 18:2676–2684.

41. Verweij J, Lee SM, Ruka W, *et al.*: Randomized phase II study of docetaxel versus doxorubicin in first- and second-line chemotherapy for locally advanced or metastatic soft tissue sarcomas in adults: a study of the European Organization for Research and Treatment of Cancer Soft Tissue and Bone Sarcoma Group. *J Clin Oncol* 2000, 18:2081–2086.

42. Amodio A, Carpano S, Paoletti G, *et al.*: Phase II study of docetaxel in patients with advanced stage soft tissue sarcoma [in Italian]. *Clin Ter* 1998, 149:121–125.

43. Edmonson JH, Ebbert LP, Nascimento AG, *et al.*: Phase II study of docetaxel in advanced soft tissue sarcomas. *Am J Clin Oncol* 1996, 19:574–576.

44. Balcerzak SP, Benedetti J, Weiss GR, *et al.*: A phase II trial of paclitaxel in patients with advanced soft tissue sarcomas. A Southwest Oncology Group study. *Cancer* 1995, 76:2248–2252.

45. Casper ES, Waltzman RJ, Schwartz GK, *et al.*: Phase II trial of paclitaxel in patients with soft-tissue sarcoma. *Cancer Invest* 1998, 16:442–446.

46. Merimsky O, Meller I, Flusser G, *et al.*: Gemcitabine in soft tissue or bone sarcoma resistant to standard chemotherapy: a phase II study. *Cancer Chemother Pharmacol* 2000, 45:177–181.

47. Amodio A, Carpano S, Manfredi C, *et al.*: Gemcitabine in advanced stage soft tissue sarcoma: a phase II study [in Italian]. *Clin Ter* 1999, 150:17–20.

48. Maki RG, Wathen JK, Patel SR, *et al.*: Randomized phase II study of gemcitabine and docetaxel compared with gemcitabine alone in patients with metastatic soft tissue sarcomas. *J Clin Oncol* 2007, 25:2755–2763.

49. Tepper JE, Suit HD: Radiation therapy alone for sarcoma of soft tissue. *Cancer* 1985, 56:475–479.

50. Rosenberg SA, Tepper J, Glatstein E, *et al.*: The treatment of soft-tissue sarcomas of the extremities: prospective randomized evaluations of (1) limb-sparing surgery plus radiation therapy compared with amputation and (2) the role of adjuvant chemotherapy. *Ann Surg* 1982, 196:305–315.

51. Yang JC, Chang AE, Baker AR, *et al.*: Randomized prospective study of the benefit of adjuvant radiation therapy in the treatment of soft tissue sarcomas of the extremity. *J Clin Oncol* 1998, 16:197–203.

52. O'Sullivan B, Davis AM, Turcotte R, *et al.*: Preoperative versus postoperative radiotherapy in soft-tissue sarcoma of the limbs: a randomised trial. *Lancet* 2002, 359:2235–2241.

53. Davis AM, O'Sullivan B, Bell RS, *et al.*: Function and health status outcomes in a randomized trial comparing preoperative and postoperative radiotherapy in extremity soft tissue sarcoma. *J Clin Oncol* 2002, 20:4472–4477.

54. Davis AM, O'Sullivan B, Turcotte R, *et al.*: Late radiation morbidity following randomization to preoperative versus postoperative radiotherapy in extremity soft tissue sarcoma. *Radiother Oncol* 2005, 75:48–53.

55. Fabrizio PL, Stafford SL, Pritchard DJ: Extremity soft-tissue sarcomas selectively treated with surgery alone. *Int J Radiat Oncol Biol Phys* 2000, 48:227–232.

56. Khanfir K, Alzieu L, Terrier P, *et al.*: Does adjuvant radiation therapy increase loco-regional control after optimal resection of soft-tissue sarcoma of the extremities? *Eur J Cancer* 2003, 39:1872–1880.

57. Fleming JB, Berman RS, Cheng SC, *et al.*: Long-term outcome of patients with American Joint Committee on Cancer stage IIB extremity soft tissue sarcomas. *J Clin Oncol* 1999, 17:2772–2780.

58. Alvegard TA, Sigurdsson H, Mouridsen H, *et al.*: Adjuvant chemotherapy with doxorubicin in high-grade soft tissue sarcoma: a randomized trial of the Scandinavian Sarcoma Group. *J Clin Oncol* 1989, 7:1504–1513.

59. Bramwell V, Rouesse J, Steward W, *et al.*: Adjuvant CYVADIC chemotherapy for adult soft tissue sarcoma: reduced local recurrence but no improvement in survival: a study of the European Organization for Research and Treatment of Cancer Soft Tissue and Bone Sarcoma Group. *J Clin Oncol* 1994, 12:1137–1149.

60. Pezzi CM, Pollock RE, Evans HL, *et al.*: Preoperative chemotherapy for soft-tissue sarcomas of the extremities. *Ann Surg* 1990, 211:476–481.

61. Casper ES, Gaynor JJ, Harrison LB, *et al.*: Preoperative and postoperative adjuvant combination chemotherapy for adults with high grade soft tissue sarcoma. *Cancer* 1994, 73:1644–1651.

62. Kraybill WG, Harris J, Spiro IJ, *et al.*: Phase II study of neoadjuvant chemotherapy and radiation therapy in the management of high-risk, high-grade, soft tissue sarcomas of the extremities and body wall: Radiation Therapy Oncology Group Trial 9514. *J Clin Oncol* 2006, 24:619–625.

63. van Geel AN, Pastorino U, Jauch KW, *et al.*: Surgical treatment of lung metastases: the European Organization for Research and Treatment of Cancer-Soft Tissue and Bone Sarcoma Group study of 255 patients. *Cancer* 1996, 77:675–682.

64. Casson AG, Putnam JB, Natarajan G, *et al.*: Five-year survival after pulmonary metastasectomy for adult soft tissue sarcoma. *Cancer* 1992, 69:662–668.

65. Putnam JB Jr, Roth JA: Surgical treatment for pulmonary metastases from sarcoma. *Hematol Oncol Clin North Am* 1995, 9:869–887.

66. Weiser MR, Downey RJ, Leung DH, *et al.*: Repeat resection of pulmonary metastases in patients with soft-tissue sarcoma. *J Am Coll Surg* 2000, 191:184–190; discussion 190–191.

67. Singer S, Antman K, Corson JM, *et al.*: Long-term salvageability for patients with locally recurrent soft-tissue sarcomas. *Arch Surg* 1992, 127:548–553; discussion 553–554.

68. Pisters PW, Harrison LB, Leung DH, *et al.*: Long-term results of a prospective randomized trial of adjuvant brachytherapy in soft tissue sarcoma. *J Clin Oncol* 1996, 14:859–868.

69. Pizzo PA, Poplack DG: *Principles and Practice of Pediatric Oncology*, edn 4. Philadelphia: Lippincott Williams & Wilkins: 2002.

70. McDowell HP: Update on childhood rhabdomyosarcoma. *Arch Dis Child* 2003, 88:354–357.

71. Seale P, Sabourin LA, Girgis-Gabardo A, *et al.*: Pax7 is required for the specification of myogenic satellite cells. *Cell* 2000, 102:777–786.

72. Lam PY, Sublett JE, Hollenbach AD, *et al.*: The oncogenic potential of the Pax3-FKHR fusion protein requires the Pax3 homeodomain recognition helix but not the Pax3 paired-box DNA binding domain. *Mol Cell Biol* 1999, 19:594–601.

73. Meza JL, Anderson J, Pappo AS, *et al.*: Analysis of prognostic factors in patients with nonmetastatic rhabdomyosarcoma treated on intergroup rhabdomyosarcoma studies III and IV: the Children's Oncology Group. *J Clin Oncol* 2006, 24:3844–3851.

74. Crist WM, Anderson JR, Meza JL, *et al.*: Intergroup rhabdomyosarcoma study-IV: results for patients with nonmetastatic disease. *J Clin Oncol* 2001, 19:3091–3102.

75. Wolden SL, Anderson JR, Crist WM, *et al.*: Indications for radiotherapy and chemotherapy after complete resection in rhabdomyosarcoma: a report from the Intergroup Rhabdomyosarcoma Studies I to III. *J Clin Oncol* 1999, 17:3468–3475.

76. Smith LM, Anderson JR, Qualman SJ, *et al.*: Which patients with microscopic disease and rhabdomyosarcoma experience relapse after therapy? A report from the Soft Tissue Sarcoma Committee of the Children's Oncology Group. *J Clin Oncol* 2001, 19:4058–4064.

77. Wharam MD, Meza J, Anderson J, *et al.*: Failure pattern and factors predictive of local failure in rhabdomyosarcoma: a report of group III patients on the third Intergroup Rhabdomyosarcoma Study. *J Clin Oncol* 2004, 22:1902–1908.

78. Donaldson SS, Meza J, Breneman JC, *et al.*: Results from the IRS-IV randomized trial of hyperfractionated radiotherapy in children with rhabdomyosarcoma: a report from the IRSG. *Int J Radiat Oncol Biol Phys* 2001, 51:718–728.

79. Stevens MC, Rey A, Bouvet N, *et al.*: Treatment of nonmetastatic rhabdomyosarcoma in childhood and adolescence: third study of the International Society of Paediatric Oncology–SIOP Malignant Mesenchymal Tumor 89. *J Clin Oncol* 2005, 23:2618–2628.

80. Donaldson SS, Anderson JR: Rhabdomyosarcoma: many similarities, a few philosophical differences. *J Clin Oncol* 2005, 23:2586–2587.

81. Heslin MJ, Lewis JJ, Nadler E, *et al.*: Prognostic factors associated with long-term survival for retroperitoneal sarcoma: implications for management. *J Clin Oncol* 1997, 15:2832–2839.

82. Dalton RR, Donohue JH, Mucha P Jr, *et al.*: Management of retroperitoneal sarcomas. *Surgery* 1989, 106:725–732; discussion 732–733.

83. Aques DP, Coit DG, Hajdu SI, *et al.*: Management of primary and recurrent soft-tissue sarcoma of the retroperitoneum. *Ann Surg* 1990, 212:51–59.

84. Kinsella TJ, Sindelar WF, Lack E, *et al.*: Preliminary results of a randomized study of adjuvant radiation therapy in resectable adult retroperitoneal soft tissue sarcomas. *J Clin Oncol* 1988, 6:18–25.

85. Ballo MT, Zagars GK, Pollock RE, *et al.*: Retroperitoneal soft tissue sarcoma: an analysis of radiation and surgical treatment. *Int J Radiat Oncol Biol Phys* 2007, 67:158–163.

86. Delattre O, Zucman J, Melot T, *et al.*: The Ewing family of tumors: a subgroup of small-round-cell tumors defined by specific chimeric transcripts. *N Engl J Med* 1994, 331:294–299.

87. Grier HE: The Ewing family of tumors. Ewing's sarcoma and primitive neuroectodermal tumors. *Pediatr Clin North Am* 1997, 44:991–1004.

88. Pritchard DJ, Dahlin DC, Dauphine RT, *et al.*: Ewing's sarcoma. A clinicopathological and statistical analysis of patients surviving five years or longer. *J Bone Joint Surg Am* 1975, 57:10–16.

89. Kissane JM, Askin FB, Foulkes M, *et al.*: Ewing's sarcoma of bone: clinicopathologic aspects of 303 cases from the Intergroup Ewing's Sarcoma Study. *Hum Pathol* 1983, 14:773–779.

90. Dahlin DC: Osteosarcoma of bone and a consideration of prognostic variables. *Cancer Treat Rep* 1978, 62:189–192.

91. Korten AG, ter Berg HJ, Spincemaille GH, *et al.*: Intracranial chondrosarcoma: review of the literature and report of 15 cases. *J Neurol Neurosurg Psychiatry* 1998, 65:88–92.

92. Mankin HJ, Lange TA, Spanier SS: The hazards of biopsy in patients with malignant primary bone and soft-tissue tumors. *J Bone Joint Surg Am* 1982, 64:1121–1127.

93. Grier HE, Krailo MD, Tarbell NJ, *et al.*: Addition of ifosfamide and etoposide to standard chemotherapy for Ewing's sarcoma and primitive neuroectodermal tumor of bone. *N Engl J Med* 2003, 348:694–701.

94. Hristov B, Shokek O, Frassica DA: The role of radiation treatment in the contemporary management of bone tumors. *J Natl Compr Canc Netw* 2007, 5:456–466.

95. Schuck A, Ahrens S, Paulussen M, *et al.*: Local therapy in localized Ewing tumors: results of 1058 patients treated in the CESS 81, CESS 86, and EICESS 92 trials. *Int J Radiat Oncol Biol Phys* 2003, 55:168–177.

96. Yock TI, Krailo M, Fryer CJ, *et al.*: Local control in pelvic Ewing sarcoma: analysis from INT-0091: a report from the Children's Oncology Group. *J Clin Oncol* 2006, 24:3838–3843.

97. Paulino AC, Nguyen TX, Mai WY, *et al.*: Dose response and local control using radiotherapy in non-metastatic Ewing sarcoma. *Pediatr Blood Cancer* 2007, 49:145–148.

98. Donaldson SS, Torrey M, Link MP, *et al.*: A multidisciplinary study investigating radiotherapy in Ewing's sarcoma: end results of POG #8346. Pediatric Oncology Group. *Int J Radiat Oncol Biol Phys* 1998, 42:125–135.

99. Jurgens H, Bier V, Dunst J, *et al.*: The German Society of Pediatric Oncology Cooperative Ewing Sarcoma Studies CESS 81/86: report after 6 1/2 years [in German]. *Klin Padiatr* 1988, 200:243–252.

100. Dunst J, Jurgens H, Sauer R, *et al.*: Radiation therapy in Ewing's sarcoma: an update of the CESS 86 trial. *Int J Radiat Oncol Biol Phys* 1995, 32:919–930.

101. Ladenstein R, Lasset C, Pinkerton R, *et al.*: Impact of megatherapy in children with high-risk Ewing's tumours in complete remission: a report from the EBMT Solid Tumour Registry. *Bone Marrow Transplant* 1995, 15:697–705.

102. Ladenstein R, Hartmann O, Pinkerton R, *et al.*: A multivariate and matched pair analysis on high-risk Ewing tumor (ET) patients treated by megatherapy (MGT) and stem cell reinfusion (sCR) in Europe [abstract]. *Proc Annu Meet Am Soc Clin Oncol* 1999, 18:555.

103. Paulussen M, Ahrens S, Craft AW, *et al.*: Ewing's tumors with primary lung metastases: survival analysis of 114 (European Intergroup) Cooperative Ewing's Sarcoma Studies patients. *J Clin Oncol* 1998, 16:3044–3052.

104. Dunst J, Paulussen M, Jurgens H: Lung irradiation for Ewing's sarcoma with pulmonary metastases at diagnosis: results of the CESS-studies. *Strahlenther Onkol* 1993, 169:621–623.

105. Rodriguez-Galindo C, Billups CA, Kun LE, *et al.*: Survival after recurrence of Ewing tumors: the St. Jude Children's Research Hospital experience, 1979–1999. *Cancer* 2002, 94:561–569.

106. Bacci G, Bertoni F, Longhi A, *et al.*: Neoadjuvant chemotherapy for high-grade central osteosarcoma of the extremity. Histologic response to preoperative chemotherapy correlates with histologic subtype of the tumor. *Cancer* 2003, 97:3068–3075.

107. Bacci G, Ferrari S, Bertoni F, *et al.*: Long-term outcome for patients with nonmetastatic osteosarcoma of the extremity treated at the Istituto Ortopedico Rizzoli according to the Istituto Ortopedico Rizzoli/Osteosarcoma-2 protocol: an updated report. *J Clin Oncol* 2000, 18:4016–4027.

108. Gaitan-Yanguas M: A study of the response of osteogenic sarcoma and adjacent normal tissues to radiation. *Int J Radiat Oncol Biol Phys* 1981, 7:593–595.

109. DeLaney TF, Park L, Goldberg SI, *et al.*: Radiotherapy for local control of osteosarcoma. *Int J Radiat Oncol Biol Phys* 2005, 61:492–498.

110. Machak GN, Tkachev SI, Solovyev YN, *et al.*: Neoadjuvant chemotherapy and local radiotherapy for high-grade osteosarcoma of the extremities. *Mayo Clin Proc* 2003, 78:147–155.

111. Miettinen M, Monihan JM, Sarlomo-Rikala M, *et al.*: Gastrointestinal stromal tumors/smooth muscle tumors (GISTs) primary in the omentum and mesentery: clinicopathologic and immunohistochemical study of 26 cases. *Am J Surg Pathol* 1999, 23:1109–1118.

112. DeMatteo RP, Lewis JJ, Leung D, *et al.*: Two hundred gastrointestinal stromal tumors: recurrence patterns and prognostic factors for survival. *Ann Surg* 2000, 231:51–58.

113. Eisenberg BL, Judson I: Surgery and imatinib in the management of GIST: emerging approaches to adjuvant and neoadjuvant therapy. *Ann Surg Oncol* 2004, 11:465–475.

114. Verweij J, Casali PG, Zalcberg J, *et al.*: Progression-free survival in gastrointestinal stromal tumours with high-dose imatinib: randomised trial. *Lancet* 2004, 364:1127–1134.

115. Verweij J, van Oosterom A, Blay JY, *et al.*: Imatinib mesylate (STI-571 Glivec, Gleevec) is an active agent for gastrointestinal stromal tumours, but does not yield responses in other soft-tissue sarcomas that are unselected for a molecular target. Results from an EORTC Soft Tissue and Bone Sarcoma Group phase II study. *Eur J Cancer* 2003, 39:2006–2011.

116. Demetri GD, von Mehren M, Blanke CD, *et al.*: Efficacy and safety of imatinib mesylate in advanced gastrointestinal stromal tumors. *N Engl J Med* 2002, 347:472–480.

117. Zalcberg JR, Verweij J, Casali PG, *et al.*: Outcome of patients with advanced gastro-intestinal stromal tumours crossing over to a daily imatinib dose of 800 mg after progression on 400 mg. *Eur J Cancer* 2005, 41:1751–1757.

118. Van den Abbeele AD, Badawi RD: Use of positron emission tomography in oncology and its potential role to assess response to imatinib mesylate therapy in gastrointestinal stromal tumors (GISTs). *Eur J Cancer* 2002, 38(Suppl 5):S60–S65.

119. DeMatteo R, Owzar K, Maki R, *et al.*: Adjuvant imatinib mesylate increases recurrence of free survival (RFS) in patients with completely resected localized primary gastrointestinal stromal tumor (GIST): North American Intergroup Phase III trial ACOSOG 29001 [abstract]. Presented at the 43rd Annual Metting of the American Society of Clinical Oncology; June 1–5, 2007; Chicago, IL. Abstract 10079.

120. McIntosh BC, Narayan D: Head and neck angiosarcomas. *J Craniofac Surg* 2005, 16:699–703.

121. Farhood AI, Hajdu SI, Shiu MH, *et al.*: Soft tissue sarcomas of the head and neck in adults. *Am J Surg* 1990, 160:365–369.

122. Tran LM, Mark R, Meier R, *et al.*: Sarcomas of the head and neck. Prognostic factors and treatment strategies. *Cancer* 1992, 70:169–177.

123. Tolan S, Shanks JH, Loh MY, *et al.*: Fibromatosis: benign by name but not necessarily by nature. *Clin Oncol (R Coll Radiol)* 2007, 19:319–326.

124. Mace J, Sybil Biermann J, Sondak V, *et al.*: Response of extraabdominal desmoid tumors to therapy with imatinib mesylate. *Cancer* 2002, 95:2373–2379.

125. Chao AS, Lai CH, Hsueh S, *et al.*: Successful treatment of recurrent pelvic desmoid tumour with tamoxifen: case report. *Hum Reprod* 2000, 15:311–313.

126. Hansmann A, Adolph C, Vogel T, *et al.*: High-dose tamoxifen and sulindac as first-line treatment for desmoid tumors. *Cancer* 2004, 100:612–620.

127. Seiter K, Kemeny N: Successful treatment of a desmoid tumor with doxorubicin. *Cancer* 1993, 71:2242–2244.

128. Patel SR, Evans HL, Benjamin RS: Combination chemotherapy in adult desmoid tumors. *Cancer* 1993, 72:3244–3247.

129. Lynch HT, Fitzgibbons R Jr, Chong S, *et al.*: Use of doxorubicin and dacarbazine for the management of unresectable intra-abdominal desmoid tumors in Gardner's syndrome. *Dis Colon Rectum* 1994, 37:260–267.

130. Gega M, Yanagi H, Yoshikawa R, *et al.*: Successful chemotherapeutic modality of doxorubicin plus dacarbazine for the treatment of desmoid tumors in association with familial adenomatous polyposis. *J Clin Oncol* 2006, 24:102–105.

131. North JH Jr, McPhee M, Arredondo M, *et al.*: Sarcoma of the breast: implications of the extent of local therapy. *Am Surg* 1998, 64:1059–1061.

132. Schwartz RA: Kaposi's sarcoma: an update. *J Surg Oncol* 2004, 87:146–151.

133. Holkova B, Takeshita K, Cheng DM, *et al.*: Effect of highly active antiretroviral therapy on survival in patients with AIDS-associated pulmonary Kaposi's sarcoma treated with chemotherapy. *J Clin Oncol* 2001, 19:3848–3851.

134. Hicks LG, Balcerzak SP, Zalupski M: GM-CSF did not allow doxorubicin dose escalation in the MAID regimen: a phase I trial. A Southwest Oncology Group study. *Cancer Invest* 1996, 14:507–512.

Genitourinary Cancer

Roberto Pili, Janet R. Walczak, Michael A. Carducci, Samuel R. Denmeade

In the past 10 to 15 years, significant advances have been made in the treatment of genitourinary malignancies. New findings in cell and molecular biology, biochemistry, pharmacology, immunology, and radiobiology continue to broaden and deepen our understanding of the pathobiology that has led to a number of new treatment paradigms. This chapter summarizes the present medical and surgical therapies used for testicular, prostate, urinary bladder, and renal cancers. In particular, salient basic and clinical observations that have formed the foundation of the current therapeutic strategies in genitourinary cancers are highlighted.

TESTICULAR CANCER

ETIOLOGY AND RISK FACTORS

Germ cell cancers arise from pleuripotent cells capable of differentiating along five different embryonic lines. These tumors commonly arise in the testes but can also occasionally occur in extragonadal primary sites, where they are managed the same as those arising in the testes. Although germ cell tumors are uncommon—with approximately 8000 new cases per year in the United States—they are the most common solid tumor in men between 15 and 34 years of age [1]. These tumors are classified as seminomatous and nonseminomatous. Seminomas arise from the spermatocyte, the earliest cell with the greatest ability to differentiate into embryonic or placental tissue. Nonseminomas are often mixed and can contain elements of embryonal cells, yolk sac, choriocarcinoma, and teratoma. Teratomas are considered either mature or immature depending on whether adult or fetal cell types are found. Nonseminoma is the more clinically aggressive tumor. When both seminoma and elements of nonseminoma are present, the management follows that for a nonseminoma.

For unknown reasons, worldwide incidence of germ cell tumors has more than doubled in the past 40 years. Identified risk factors include a prior history of a germ cell tumor, a positive family history, testicular dysgenesis, and Klinefelter's syndrome. Cryptorchidism is the most important predisposing factor, with a relative risk of 7 or more in some series [2]. Screening for early-stage testicular malignancies has not proved to be beneficial [3].

STAGING AND PROGNOSIS

Diagnostic and therapeutic approaches to germ cell tumors of the testis must take into consideration the stage, histologic type, anatomy of lymphatic drainage, and levels of serum markers. While a solid, painless testicular mass is pathognomonic for testicular cancer, patients frequently present with testicular pain or swelling. These patients receive a trial of antibiotics to treat suspected epididymitis or orchitis. Persistent swelling or palpable mass requires further evaluation using testicular ultrasound to help with the diagnosis and define the lesion.

When testicular malignancy is suspected, a routine battery of laboratory and radiologic evaluations should be performed. Laboratory tests include β-human chorionic gonadotropin (β-hCG), α-fetoprotein (AFP), and lactate dehydrogenase (LDH). These markers are critical in making the diagnosis, determining prognosis, and assessing response to therapy. Some patients with seminoma and nonseminoma can present with negative markers at any stage. AFP is produced by nonseminomatous embryonal carcinoma and yolk sac tumor cells and, therefore, only nonseminomas can make AFP, which has a half-life of 5 to 7 days. In contrast, serum concentrations of hCG, which has a half-life of 1 to 3 days, can be elevated in patients with either seminoma or nonseminoma. Although LDH is a nonspecific marker, elevated levels suggest the presence of bulky lymph node involvement.

Computed tomography (CT) scans of chest, abdomen, and pelvis should be subsequently performed if a testicular tumor is found at orchiectomy. Brain magnetic resonance imaging (MRI) or bone scan should be considered if clinically indicated. While not recommended for screening, positron emission tomography (PET) scans should be considered in the evaluation of residual masses following appropriate therapy.

Several staging systems are used to classify patients with metastatic disease into prognostic groups [4–6]. These include the TNM (tumor, node, metastasis) system (Table 13-1), the Memorial Sloan-Kettering classification, the Indiana classification, and the International Germ Cell Consensus

Table 13-1. Staging of Testicular Cancer

Stage/Marker	Description
Primary tumor (pT)	
pTis	Intratubular germ cell neoplasia (carcinoma in situ)
pT1	Tumor limited to the testis and epididymis without vascular/lymphatic invasion; tumor may invade into the tunica albuginea but not the tunica vaginalis
pT2	Tumor limited to the testis and epididymis with vascular/lymphatic invasion, or tumor extending through the tunica albuginea with involvement of the tunica vaginalis
pT3	Tumor invades the spermatic cord with or without vascular/lymphatic invasion
pT4	Tumor invades the scrotum with or without vascular/lymphatic invasion
Regional lymph nodes (N)	
NX	Regional lymph nodes cannot be assessed
N0	No regional lymph nodes
N1	Lymph node mass ≤ 2 cm in greatest dimension, or multiple lymph nodes all < 2 cm in greatest dimension
N2	Lymph node mass(es) > 2 cm and ≤ 5 cm
N3	Lymph node mass > 5 cm in greatest dimension
Distant metastasis (M)	
M0	No distant metastasis
M1	Distant metastasis
M1a	Nonregional nodes or pulmonary metastasis
M1b	Metastasis to other sites
Serum tumor markers (S)	
SX	Markers not available or performed
S0	Markers within normal limits
S1	LDH < 1.5 × ULN and β-hCG < 5000 mIU/mL and AFP < 1000 ng/mL
S2	LDH 1.5–10 × ULN and β-hCG 5000–50,000 mIU/mL and AFP 1000–10,000 ng/mL
S3	LDH 1.5–10 × ULN and β-hCG > 50,000 mIU/mL and AFP > 10,000 ng/mL

Stage Groupings

Stage 0	pTis	N0	M0	S0
Stage IA	pT1	N0	M0	S0
Stage IB	pT2–T4	N0	M0	S0
Stage IS	Any pT	N0	M0	S1–3
Stage IIA	Any pT	N1	M0	S0 or S1
Stage IIB	Any pT	N2	M0	S0 or S1
Stage IIC	Any pT	N3	M0	S0 or S1
Stage III	Any pT	Any N	M1	S0–S3

AFP—α-fetoprotein; hCG—human chorionic gonadotropin; LDH—lactate dehydrogenase; ULN—upper limit of normal.

classification. In general, patients can be classified as good risk, intermediate risk, or poor risk on the basis of primary tumor location, location of metastases, and marker levels (Table 13-2). Overall, more than 90% of patients diagnosed with germ cell tumors are cured, including 70% to 80% of patients with advanced or metastatic tumors who are treated with chemotherapy. Standard therapeutic regimens have been established for all stages of disease management and these regimens must be closely/strictly followed to preserve the high potential for cure.

PRIMARY THERAPY

Inguinal orchiectomy is considered primary treatment for most patients presenting with a suspicious testicular mass. Transscrotal biopsy should not be performed because it may lead to loco-regional recurrences in as many as one fourth of patients and may also disrupt the normal lymphatic drainage pattern of the testes. An open inguinal biopsy of the contralateral testes should be considered in patients with a cryptorchid or markedly atrophied testes or if a suspicious lesion is observed on ultrasound. Sperm banking should be discussed with all patients prior to orchiectomy and should be considered before undergoing any intervention that may compromise fertility, including retroperitoneal lymph node dissection (RPLND), radiation, or chemotherapy.

ADJUVANT THERAPY FOR SEMINOMATOUS TUMORS

Patients with stage I seminoma are typically treated with 20 to 30 Gy of infradiaphragmatic radiation therapy to include the para-aortic with or without ipsilateral iliac nodes [7–10]. Surveillance or single-agent carboplatin can be considered in patients with a horseshoe or pelvic kidney, prior radiation, or inflammatory bowel disease. Patients who are stage IIA or IIB are also treated with radiation at higher dose of 35 to 40 Gy with inclusion of the ipsilateral iliac nodes [10]. Select patients with IIB disease (multiple large nodes) should be considered for chemotherapy with four cycles of EP (etoposide and cisplatin) [10]. Patients with good-risk stage IIC or III disease receive either four cycles of EP or three cycles of BEP (bleomycin, etoposide, and cisplatin). Patients with intermediate-risk disease receive BEP for four cycles [11–14]. No patients with seminoma are considered poor risk.

ADJUVANT THERAPY FOR NONSEMINOMATOUS TUMORS

The algorithms for the treatment of nonseminomas are somewhat more complicated than those for seminoma [15]. For stage I patients, therapy may involve surveillance, nerve-sparing RPLND, or chemotherapy. Surveillance studies suggest disease progression occurs in 30% of patients and frequently presents with bulkier disease. Embryonal and choriocarcinomatous histologic elements are highly prone to metastatic spread. Patients with venous or lymphatic invasion or tumors outside the tunica albuginea may be poor candidates for surveillance.

Patients with stage I disease are frequently treated with RPLND. The major morbidity associated with this procedure is retrograde ejaculation, which results in infertility. Nerve dissection techniques (ie, nerve-sparing) preserve antegrade ejaculation in 90% of patients [16]. Open nerve-sparing RPLND is the standard approach. While laparoscopic RPLND may be less morbid to the patient, concerns about the inadequacy of lymph node sampling have limited its use.

STAGE I DISEASE

Patients with stage IA disease can be offered surveillance (in compliant patients) or RPLND. The cure rate for either approach is 95%. This high cure rate in the patients receiving surveillance depends on close follow-up and chemotherapy for the approximately 25% of patients who experience relapse. Surveillance recommendations are outlined in Table 13-3. RPLND is usually performed within 4 weeks of CT scan and with 7 days of repeat serum marker testing. If the lymph nodes are not involved, no adjuvant chemotherapy is given. If nodes are involved, the decision to treat with chemotherapy depends on the extent of nodal involvement and is preferred in patients with pN2 or pN3 disease. Recommended chemotherapy is two cycles of EP for patients with pN1 to N2 disease and either four cycles of EP or three cycles of BEP for patients with pN3 disease. Patients with stage IB disease are offered similar treatment options with the exception of upfront treatment with two cycles of BEP followed by RPLND or surveillance. Surveillance is not recommended for patients with T2 disease and vascular invasion due to a 50% chance of relapse. Patients with stage IS disease have persistent marker elevation after orchiectomy but no other radiographic evidence of disease. These patients almost always have disseminated disease and therefore receive chemotherapy with either EP for four cycles or BEP for three cycles instead of RPLND [17,18].

STAGE IIA AND IIB DISEASE

Treatment for patients with stage IIA and IIB disease depends on tumor marker levels and radiographic findings. Patients with stage IIA disease with persistent marker elevation are treated with chemotherapy followed by RPLND or surveillance. When tumor markers are negative, the patient can either undergo upfront chemotherapy with two cycles of EP or BEP or have RPLND followed by chemotherapy or surveillance based on number of positive lymph nodes [19]. Chemotherapy is preferred for patients with pN2 to pN3 disease and results in a nearly 100% relapse-free survival rate [20]. Patients with stage IIB (pN2) with negative markers and CT findings showing nodes within the normal lymphatic drainage of the testes can be offered either RPLND followed by chemotherapy based on findings or receive primary chemotherapy with four cycles of EP or three cycles of BEP. If CT findings show more distal nodal disease, primary chemotherapy is recommended.

STAGE IIC AND III DISEASE

Treatment of patients with stages IIC and III disease consists of primary chemotherapy. The extent and type of chemotherapy depends on the risk category (good, intermediate, poor) as defined by the International Germ Cell Consensus classification [21]. Standard treatment for good-risk diseases is either four cycles of EP or three cycles of BEP [22–24]. Patients receiving BEP should have prescreening baseline pulmonary function tests that can be repeated during the treatment course if decreased function is suspected. Either regimen cures approximately 90% of patients in this good-risk category [24,25]. Intermediate-risk patients are treated with four cycles of BEP, which produces a cure rate of about 70%. For poor-risk patients, less than half achieve complete response to this regimen; these patients should be considered for clinical trials [26].

Postchemotherapy patients should undergo CT scans and have tumor markers measured. Patients with complete radiographic response and negative markers can be followed closely or undergo RPLND. Patients with residual disease and normal markers should have resection of residual disease. If only debris or teratoma is found, no further treatment except observation is indicated. If residual cancer is found, patients can be treated with two additional cycles of chemotherapy that includes EP, TIP (paclitaxel, ifosfamide, cisplatin), or VeIP (vinblastine, ifosfamide, cisplatin).

Table 13-2. International Germ Cell Consensus Classification

Risk class	Nonseminoma	Seminoma
Good risk	Primary tumor in testes or retroperitoneum and only pulmonary metastases and good marker status (S1)	Any primary site and only pulmonary metastases
Intermediate risk	Good risk tumor status (primary tumor in testes or retroperitoneum and only pulmonary metastases) and intermediate marker status (S2)	Any primary site and nonpulmonary visceral metastases
Poor risk	Primary tumor in mediastinum or nonpulmonary visceral metastases or poor marker status (S3)	No patients classified as poor risk

SALVAGE THERAPY

Patients who do not achieve complete response to first-line therapy are treated with salvage therapy (Table 13-4). Patients with favorable prognostic factors (testicular primary, prior complete response, low serum markers and disease volume [27]) are treated with four cycles of ifosfamide and cisplatin combined with either vinblastine or paclitaxel [28–30]. Patients who do not achieve complete response with salvage chemotherapy should be considered for high-dose chemotherapy with autologous stem cell support [31,32]. This treatment should also be considered for patients with unfavorable prognostic factors or those requiring a third-line salvage. Clinical trials should also be considered. Third-line therapy with two cycles of high-dose carboplatin and etoposide with or without cyclophosphamide or ifosfamide results in durable complete response in 15% to 20% of patients [31]. Patients who do not respond to high-dose chemotherapy have incurable disease and should receive palliative therapy and supportive care.

PROSTATE CANCER

ETIOLOGY AND RISK FACTORS

Prostate cancer is the leading cause of cancer in men in the United States—approximately 215,000 men were diagnosed in 2007 (33% of cancers in men)—and the second leading cause of cancer deaths in men, with an estimated 27,050 deaths (9% of cancer deaths) [1]. In autopsy studies, 30% of men between 50 and 70 years of age with no overt evidence of prostate cancer before death had evidence of prostate carcinoma [33]. Age is the major risk factor for prostate cancer. Other risk factors include ethnic background, with African Americans having the highest rate of prostate cancer in the world, and early prostate cancer diagnosed before age 65 in a first-degree relative [34,35]. Eating a Western diet high in fat and red meat may also be a possible risk factor. The Health Professionals Follow-Up Study evaluated prostate cancer risk factors in 51,529 US male health professionals. This study documented findings in other studies regarding positive family history and African-American race [35]. In addition, low intake of tomato sauce and high intake of α-linolenic acid were also risk factors; cigarette smoking and increased body mass index were not associated with increased risk.

Chronic inflammation has been shown to contribute to the development of several human cancers and medical conditions. Recently, scientists have begun to consider inflammation in the etiology of prostate cancer, in part due to the frequent observation of inflammatory infiltrates near putative prostate cancer precursor lesions [36–38]. Proposed sources of intraprostatic inflammation include infections, such as sexually transmitted infections and other urogenital infections, and chemical or physical intraluminal irritants [38]. Emerging evidence from epidemiologic studies suggests that use of aspirin and other nonsteroidal anti-inflammatory drugs may reduce the risk of developing prostate cancer [38].

SCREENING

Men in the United States have an approximate one in six chance of being diagnosed with prostate cancer and a one in 30 chance of eventually dying as a result [39]. The advent of prostate-specific antigen (PSA) testing has led to significant controversy over early detection recommendations. This is due to the fact that not all men with prostate cancer will die of the disease and treatment is not necessary in some patients. In addition, the PSA test itself has limitations in regard to specificity and sensitivity for detecting prostate cancer in the general population. The American Cancer Society and the American Urological Association were the first groups to advise men to obtain an annual digital rectal examination (DRE) and serum PSA test beginning at age 50 in the absence of risk factors and earlier for those in high-risk groups. In contrast, given that no prospective, randomized trial has shown an unequivocal benefit with a decrease in disease-specific mortality, other groups such as the US Preventive Services Task Force and the American College of Physicians do not recommend routine PSA screening for prostate cancer, instead preferring to recommend physicians to first discuss the implications of the PSA test with patients beginning at age 50. In the face of this controversy, it is clear that the introduction of early detection screening via DRE and PSA has resulted in a downward migration of prostate cancer staging over the past decade. This migration has required the creation of a new stage, T1c, to indicate men with prostate cancer diagnosed only on the basis of elevated PSA (Table 13-5). Over the period of 1992 to 2002, there has been a 75% decrease in the rate of metastatic disease at presentation and 70% to 80% of prostate cancers are now pathologically organ confined at diagnosis [39].

One of the main diagnostic dilemmas remains the discrimination of prostate cancer from benign prostatic hyperplasia (BPH) based on PSA level and urinary symptoms without the need for prostatic biopsy. Numerous studies have shown that a PSA level above 4 ng/mL increases the chance of detection of prostate cancer at biopsy to 30% to 35%, whereas PSA levels greater than 10 ng/mL increase the chances to more than 67% [40,41]. Recent studies have assessed the predictive value of evaluating men with PSA in the 2 to 4.0 ng/mL range [42]. Carter *et al.* [43] first demonstrated that the PSA velocity (the rate of change in PSA over time) can increase the specificity of PSA for cancer detection. Recent analysis of data from the Baltimore Longitudinal Study on Aging has suggested that PSA velocity may be able to identify men at risk of prostate cancer 10 to 15 years before diagnosis is made [44]. Other methods for improving the predictive value of PSA include the use of age- and race-specific PSA ranges and the evaluation of different isoforms of PSA in the serum. The latter is based on studies demonstrating that the ratio of free, inactive PSA in the blood to PSA complexed to protease inhibitors could improve the predictive value [45,46]. Other isoforms of PSA under evaluation include B-PSA, a form of PSA produced by BPH tissue, and proPSA species, which may be produced at higher levels by prostate cancer cells [47].

Table 13-3. Primary Chemotherapy Regimens for Metastatic Germ Cell Tumor in Previously Untreated Patients

Risk classification	Treatment regimen
Good risk	EP:
	Etoposide 100 mg/m² IV daily × 5 d
	Cisplatin 20 mg/m² IV daily × 5 d
	Four cycles administered at 21-d intervals
	or
	BEP:
	Etoposide 100 mg/m² IV daily × 5 d
	Cisplatin 20 mg/m² IV daily × 5 d
	Bleomycin 30 units IV weekly on d 1, 8, and 15
	Three cycles administered at 21-d intervals
Intermediate or poor risk	BEP for four cycles administered at 21-d intervals

---

Table 13-4. Salvage Chemotherapy Regimens for Metastatic Germ Cell Tumor in Previously Treated Patients

VeIP:

Vinblastine 0.11 mg/kg IV × 2 d

Ifosfamide 1200 mg/m² IV daily × 5 d

Mesna 400 mg/m² IV every 8 h × 5 d

Cisplatin 20 mg/m² IV daily × 5 d

Cycle administered at 21-d intervals

or

TIP:

Paclitaxel 250 mg/m² IV on d 1

Ifosfamide 1500 mg/m² IV on d 2–5

Mesna 500 mg/m² IV before and 4 h and 8 h after each ifosfamide dose

Cisplatin 25 mg/m² IV on d 2–5

Cycle administered at 21-d intervals

STAGING AND PROGNOSIS

As mentioned above, the introduction of early detection screening via DRE and PSA has resulted in a downward migration of prostate cancer staging over the past decade. Clinical stage (Table 13-5), PSA level, and Gleason score have been incorporated into validated nomograms (*eg*, Partin tables) to make predictions regarding the likelihood of organ-confined disease, extracapsular extension, seminal vesicle invasion, and lymph node metastases [48,49]. Imaging studies such as ultrasound and MRI have yet to be accepted as adjuncts to staging. Bone scans have limited value in men with PSA levels less than 10 ng/mL but can be appropriate for men with PSA levels greater than 20 ng/mL or with Gleason scores 8 or above.

In addition to PSA level, several factors have been identified to determine risk for distant disease after prostatectomy, such as pathologic tumor category (T1c or T2a), positive nodal and margin status, and Gleason score of 8 to 10. Positive lymph nodes/seminal vesicles and a Gleason score of 8 to 10 have been associated with distant disease at the time of prostatectomy and therefore are less likely to benefit from local salvage therapy [50]. In addition, PSA kinetics have been correlated with clinical outcomes [51]. Multivariate analyses have demonstrated several predictors of survival or benefit from local salvage therapy. Initially, Pound *et al.* [52] and more recently Freedland *et*

al. [53] demonstrated increased rates of distant metastases and death for men with brief intervals to PSA relapse (< 3 years), rapid PSA doubling time (< 10 months), and a Gleason score of 8 to 10. Following radiation therapy, patients who had a PSA doubling time less than 8 months and a rising PSA within the first year after radiation therapy had the highest rates of distant spread [54].

TREATMENT OF EARLY-STAGE PROSTATE CANCER

Initial treatment recommendations depend on clinical staging, radiographic findings, level of serum PSA, and pathology on biopsy characterized by the Gleason scoring system. Men with Gleason score of 5 or less are increasingly managed with "watchful waiting." Treatment modalities for men with higher Gleason scores or clinical stage include surgery via radical prostatectomy, external-beam radiation therapy, and brachytherapy using implantable, radioactive seeds. Radical prostatectomy and external-beam radiation appear to produce equivalent results in matched patients; however, randomized trials comparing these two modalities have never been performed. Additional modalities that are used to treat localized prostate cancer include robotic prostatectomy, cryoablation of the prostate, and other methods of radiation therapy that include high-dose rate radiation. Clinical experience with these modalities is more limited and, therefore, their effectiveness compared with more standard approaches is not known.

BIOCHEMICAL RELAPSE

When PSA becomes detectable after radical prostatectomy or rises above the nadir on three occurrences after radiation therapy, recurrence of prostate cancer is suspected (Table 13-6). What constitutes biochemical failure has varying definitions. After prostatectomy, failure may be defined as any rising PSA or a PSA level greater than 0.2 or 0.4 ng/mL [55]. Also, after radiation, there is an additional requirement of three consecutive rises at least 2 weeks apart [56,57]. Unfortunately, the PSA is not specific enough used alone to determine whether the recurrence is of clinical significance.

A small fraction of these men may have a local recurrence only. Local recurrence may be suspected in men with the following: 1) only a rising PSA and pretreatment factors of PSA less than 10 ng/mL, clinical stage of T1c or T2a, and PSA velocity in the year prior to diagnosis of less than 2 ng/mL; 2) pathologic factors of Gleason below 7, positive surgical margins, and negative lymph nodes and seminal vesicles; or 3) more than 3 years to PSA relapse, PSA doubling time greater than 12 months, and PSA level of less than 1 ng/mL before beginning salvage local therapy [54]. Postsurgery patients can be offered external-beam radiation. Patients who have undergone radiation have limited options given concerns regarding treatment modalities such as salvage prostatectomy, further external radiation therapy, and cryotherapy. For patients who have received radiation therapy alone, there is always the question as to whether the disease is local or not. Unfortunately, imaging studies including [^{18}F]fluoro-2-deoxy-D-glucose (FDG)-PET and capromab pendetide (ProstaScint, Cytogen Corp., Princeton, NJ) are not necessarily sensitive enough for diagnosing a local recurrence or persistence of disease and have not been very helpful in definitively aiding in treatment decisions [58,59]. If distant disease is present, local salvage therapy is likely to have little if any impact on survival.

ANDROGEN ABLATION THERAPY

Standard therapy for men presenting with metastatic disease is androgen ablation therapy through medical castration using luteinizing hormone–releasing hormone (LHRH) agonists (leuprolide, goserelin, or triptorelin)

Table 13-5. Staging of Prostate Cancer

Stage/Marker	Description
Primary tumor (T)	
T1	Nonpalpable, nonimageable tumor
T1a	Tumor incidental in ≤ 5% tissue
T1b	Tumor incidental in > 5% tissue
T1c	Elevated PSA and positive needle biopsy
T2	Tumor confined within the prostate
T2a	Tumor involves ≤ 50% of one lobe
T2b	Tumor involves > 50% of one lobe
T2c	Tumor involves both lobes
T3	Tumor extends through the prostatic capsule
T3a	Extracapsular extension
T3b	Seminal vesicle invasion
T4	Tumor fixed or invades adjacent structures
Regional lymph nodes (N)	
N0	No regional lymph nodes
N1	Regional lymph nodes
Distant metastasis (M)	
M0	No distant metastasis
M1	Distant metastasis
Grade (G)	
G1	Well differentiated (Gleason 2–4)
G2	Moderately differentiated (Gleason 5–6)
G3	Poorly differentiated (Gleason 7–10)

Stage Groupings

Stage I	T1a	N0	M0	G1
Stage II	T1a	N0	M0	G2
	T1b–T2	N0	M0	Any G
Stage III	T3	N0	M0	Any G
Stage IV	T4	N0	M0	Any G
	Any T	N1	M1	Any G

PSA—prostate-specific antigen.

Table 13-6. Criteria for Biochemical Relapse

Occurrence	Criteria
After prostatectomy	PSA level > 0.2 ng/mL or 4 ng/mL
	Minimum of 3 consecutive rising PSA levels
After radiation therapy	Minimum of 3 consecutive rising PSA levels over PSA nadir level at least 2 weeks apart

PSA—prostate-specific antigen.
(*Data from* Amling *et al.* [55], ASTRO panel [56], and Horwitz *et al.* [57].)

or surgical castration. While each approach achieves the same end point of inhibiting testicular production, medical castration with a LHRH agonist causes an initial immediate increase in testosterone. Thus, when initiating therapy for men with known metastatic disease, the addition of an antiandrogen (bicalutamide, flutamide, or nilutamide) for 2 to 4 weeks will block the surge in testosterone levels associated with the initial dose of the LHRH agonist. An antiandrogen is recommended to prevent the potential flare reaction, particularly in men with bony disease or obstructive symptoms. Numerous side effects are associated with androgen ablation and include those associated with decreased testosterone. Loss of libido, erectile dysfunction, and hot flashes (55%–80%) are the most frequently reported side effects. Less commonly recognized side effects include gynecomastia, loss of muscle mass/strength, osteoporosis, weight gain (increase in body fat), anemia, fatigue, microgenitalia, and neurocognitive changes [60,61]. Recently, metabolic effects of androgen deprivation have been reported, resulting in an increased risk for hyperglycemia and insulin resistance that can lead to cardiovascular disease and mortality [62].

When clinical or traditional radiographic evidence of disease (bone scan or CT scan) is present, the benefits of initiating therapy outweigh the risks. Blocking testosterone production will induce decreased tumor burden with an associated decrease in the PSA and treat areas of metastatic disease. Unfortunately, the beneficial effects do not persist indefinitely; most patients experience progression within 2 to 3 years. Over time, resistance emerges with proliferation of androgen-independent cells. Clinically, androgen independence is demonstrated by the rise in PSA despite the continued androgen deprivation and castrate testosterone levels.

For men who have a rising PSA without symptoms or clinical or radiographic evidence of metastatic disease after local therapy, the choice is not so clear. Whether or not to begin androgen ablation therapy or pursue active surveillance is a difficult choice without a well-defined standard. Given that all men with recurrence have a preexisting androgen-independent component to their disease, androgen ablation remains strictly palliative and not curative. Therefore, the decision to initiate androgen ablation for a potential palliative benefit must be weighed with the certain risk of the side effects for more years. The duration of response varies but is similar to that experienced by men with metastatic disease. Because prostate cancer is a slow-growing disease that may be present for decades before diagnosis, it remains unproven that "early" initiation of androgen ablative therapy versus deferred therapy has any effect on survival except in select situations, such as those in which androgen deprivation is used in the neoadjuvant setting prior to radiation or in postradical prostatectomy where positive lymph nodes are present. In these select situations, survival benefits of early therapy have been identified [63,64]. Early hormonal therapy will decrease the PSA and delay the time to progression to clinically or radiographically evident metastatic disease, but there are little reported data demonstrating any impact on survival. However, the added exposure to the long-term effects of the therapy is present.

Ultimately, the decision to start androgen ablation therapy in the setting of biochemical failure is based on one of several trigger points used in the clinical setting (*eg*, a predetermined PSA level that will trigger the initiation of therapy, such as an arbitrary PSA level of about 10, or a PSA doubling time less than a year). The PSA doubling time enables an assessment of the likelihood of progression. This can be useful to discuss with patients in deciding when to initiate hormone therapy. There is an increased rate of metastatic disease when the interval between primary treatment and PSA failure is short (< 2 years) with a rapid PSA doubling time (< 10 months) [20]. Unfortunately, there are no real data to aid in this decision-making process. Often it is simpler to begin therapy; however, caution regarding impact on quality of life and clinical benefit must be considered. Patients who opt for active surveillance will require ongoing discussions regarding the risks and benefits of deferred therapy. Clinical trials would be optimal to help address this dilemma.

Although it remains investigational, intermittent androgen ablation therapy is being used more frequently because it is potentially a mechanism for maintaining improved control of the disease and quality of life. In our practice, we reserve this approach for men choosing hormone therapy with no radiographic evidence of disease. Initial treatment consists of a LHRH agonist 6 to 9 months until the PSA nadirs, then treatment is stopped until the patient's PSA reaches a predetermined level, such as 10 ng/mL. Recovery of testicular function is variable and can often be delayed for many months, particularly in elderly men. However, this approach enables men to have periods in which testosterone production resumes and side effects, particularly hot flashes and impotence, abate. There are currently three ongoing clinical trials to address this issue: the European multicenter EC507 trial, comparing intermittent hormone therapy with continuous hormone therapy for PSA relapse postprostatectomy; the Southwest Oncology Group (SWOG) JPR7 trial sponsored by the National Cancer Institute of Canada (NCIC), comparing overall survival for intermittent versus continuous therapy for PSA failure after radiation therapy; and the SWOG 9436 trial for men with new bone metastases (D2 disease) [65].

ANDROGEN-INDEPENDENT DISEASE

Androgen-independent disease is defined as when PSA begins to rise while on androgen suppression with castrate testosterone levels. Patients may still be responsive to manipulation of second-line hormone therapy, but these are often short-lived effects (Table 13-7). The goal of second-line hormonal therapy is to treat any remaining androgen-sensitive cancer cells by decreasing the level or effect of circulating androgens produced by the adrenal gland. This has been the most widely used approach in men with only a rising PSA or with asymptomatic progression of metastatic disease, but these therapies tend to have PSA responses that are short lived and survival benefit has never been documented. Adding antiandrogens (bicalutamide, nilutamide, flutamide) to block any circulating testosterone at the receptor site can produce a PSA response in approximately 20% to 30% of patients. Inhibition of steroid synthesis of cortisol and androgens by the adrenal gland using high-dose ketoconazole has resulted in higher reported response rates in up to 70% of patients in phase 2 trials but is less well tolerated and requires hydrocortisone at replacement levels [66]. When the PSA begins to rise on the combined androgen blockade, withdrawal of the antiandrogen may cause the PSA to decrease in up to 10% to 35% of patients, particularly those on flutamide. In up to 50% of patients on combined androgen blockade, the antiandrogens may alter the activity and expression of the androgen receptor, causing the PSA to no longer respond to the combined blockade [67,68].

CHEMOTHERAPY

Chemotherapy has become the new standard for men with androgen-independent disease who have metastatic or progressing disease. Previously, only mitoxantrone and prednisone were approved for treating advanced symptomatic prostate cancer and resulted in palliation of pain symptoms rather than a survival benefit [69,70] (Table 13-8). In the 1990s, phase 2 studies were undertaken to evaluate the taxanes, which had demonstrated

Table 13-7. Treatment Options for Men With Androgen-Independent Disease

Consider clinical trials at each stage

Second-line hormone therapy

   Antiandrogen therapy (bicalutamide, nilutamide, flutamide)

   Ketoconazole + hydrocortisone

   Estrogens (oral vs parenteral)

   Glucocorticoids

Antiandrogen withdrawal

Chemotherapy

   Docetaxel shown to have modest survival benefit

   Mitoxantrone/prednisone: palliative, no survival benefit

Radiation therapy

   External beam to painful sites

   Systemic radioisotopes for palliation of pain

activity in vitro and in vivo. The taxane/taxoids potently inhibit microtubule disassembly by promoting polymerization of the tubules. The ultimate result is that cells arrest in G2/M phase and apoptosis occurs. Docetaxel (Taxotere, Sanofi Aventis, Bridgewater, NJ) rapidly moved from phase 2 studies into phase 3 studies: TAX327 and SWOG 9916, both of which compared docetaxel with mitoxantrone. SWOG 9916 compared docetaxel/estramustine with mitoxantrone/prednisone and TAX327 compared docetaxel/prednisone with mitoxantrone/prednisone but also had two different treatment schedules of the docetaxel component (weekly versus every 3 weeks) (Table 13-8). Both trials demonstrated a relatively small but significant survival benefit with docetaxel (SWOG 9916: 17.5 months for docetaxel vs 15.6 months for mitoxantrone; $P = 0.01$; TAX327: 18.9 months for every-3-weeks docetaxel vs 16.4 months for mitoxantrone; $P = 0.009$ [the weekly docetaxel was not statistically significant in prolonging survival]) [71,72]. With these trials completed and showing a survival benefit with acceptable toxicity, docetaxel alone has become the standard regimen for first-line chemotherapy for patients with metastatic disease (symptomatic or asymptomatic). Estramustine has been virtually eliminated due to added toxicity (nausea, vomiting, thrombosis) without added benefit. Docetaxel is now being investigated in combination with investigational novel drugs with different mechanisms of action and varying toxicities in an effort to improve the single-agent response and survival. Some of the agents being tested with docetaxel are bevacizumab (Cancer and Leukemia Group B [CALGB] 90401 trial), calcitriol (AIPC Study of Calcitriol Enhancing Taxotere [ASCENT] II trial), and atrasentan (SWOG 0421 trial). Additionally, docetaxel is being investigated in earlier-stage disease, such as in adjuvant therapy for men with high risk of relapse or those with only biochemical relapse (TAX3501 trial) and in men with a rising PSA in combination with androgen ablation (ChemoHormonal Therapy vs Androgen Ablation Randomized Trial for Extensive Disease [CHAARTED] Eastern Cooperative Oncology Group [ECOG] 5805 trial).

BISPHOSPHONATES

Skeletal events are common in men with androgen-independent prostate cancer. These events include osteoporosis and the resulting fractures from prolonged androgen deprivation as well as bone metastases that are primarily osteosclerotic, with osteoblastic bone growth preceding osteoclastic stimulation that ultimately results in bone pain [73]. Bisphosphonates bind to bone surfaces to block osteoclast resorption and inhibit cancer cells from adhering to bone. Zoledronic acid is a potent bisphosphonate and has demonstrated significant reduction in the risk for skeletal events ($P = 0.02$), such as pathologic fracture, spinal cord compression, surgery or radiation to the bone, or change in antitumor therapy to treat new bone pain. Such results were demonstrated in a randomized, double-blind, placebo-controlled study of men with metastatic androgen-independent prostate cancer. This trial concluded that zoledronic acid is well tolerated, with a toxicity profile consistent with other bisphosphonates except for serum creatinine elevations. This renal effect could be reduced with a prolonged infusion time of 15 minutes [74]. Osteonecrosis of the jaw associated with prolonged bisphosphonate use has recently been reported as a rare side effect of therapy [75,76]. Ongoing assessment of dental health as well as kidney function is indicated for safety. Zoledronic acid is approved for treatment of bone metastases in men who have progressive disease despite hormone therapy. The optimal frequency and duration of therapy is still being defined as is the utility of bisphosphonates in preventing skeletal events earlier in the disease process [77]. Zoledronic acid is indicated if there is a decrease in bone density or as approved for bone metastases in hormone-refractory disease. However, many extrapolate the data in more advanced disease (hormone-refractory metastatic) and use zoledronic acid earlier, when hormone therapy is initiated.

RADIATION THERAPY

The use of radiation therapy for palliation of symptoms from metastatic disease is an established treatment for advanced prostate cancer. Radiation therapy can be delivered via two modalities: using external-beam radiation to treat a single painful site of bone metastasis or an obstructing mass or lymph nodes or using systemic radioisotopes to treat multiple painful sites. Strontium-89 and samarium-153 are the radioisotopes most commonly used. Both are β-emitters that may kill prostate cancer cells and relieve bone pain. Strontium-89 has demonstrated significant improvement in pain and quality of life when compared with placebo when given with local radiation, but without change in survival [78]. However, with a half-life of almost 2 months in the bone, bone marrow toxicity can be a problem, especially when given to patients who are candidates for chemotherapy. Samarium, on the other hand, has a shorter half-life, causing less marrow toxicity with similar efficacy results [79]. While the effectiveness of both isotopes has been demonstrated, many believe that samarium's shorter half-life with minimal bone marrow toxicity makes it the preferred radioisotope for the treatment of bony metastatic disease, particularly in men who are also candidates for chemotherapy [78–80]. It is currently being investigated in combination with docetaxel in hormone-refractory, symptomatic bone metastases. Because of the marrow toxicity when used late in the disease process, it may be of more benefit when used earlier.

BLADDER CANCER

ETIOLOGY AND RISK FACTORS

Bladder cancer is a common disease, with an estimated 60,000 new cases diagnosed annually in the United States [1]. Three major histologic types of cancers arise from the urothelium. Transitional cell carcinoma is the most common type and the focus of this review. Squamous cell carcinomas and adenocarcinomas of the bladder present a different clinical and therapeutic problem and are not discussed here. The major risk factor for transitional cell carcinoma remains tobacco use, particularly in association with a slow acetylator phenotype [81,82]. Although dietary factors have been implicated in bladder cancer formation, there is no definitive evidence to date [81,83]. Animal studies have suggested that saccharin consumption is associated with the development of bladder tumors in the rat, but recent meta-analyses do not implicate this substance in bladder tumor formation in humans [81].

Transitional cell cancer may develop anywhere transitional epithelium is present. More than 90% originate in the bladder, whereas 8% originate in the renal pelvis and 2% begin in the ureter and urethra. The majority

---

Table 13-8. Results of Randomized Chemotherapy Trials in Men With Hormone-Refractory Metastatic Prostate Cancer

Trial/Study	Patients, *n*	Regimen(s)	PSA response, %	Pain response, %	Median survival, *mo*
CALGB 9182 [69]	242	Mitoxantrone + hydrocortisone	37.5	NR	12.3
		Hydrocortisone	21	NR	12.6
Tannock *et al.* [70]	161	Mitoxantrone + prednisone	33	29	No difference in survival
		Prednisone	12	12	
TAX327 [71]	1006	Docetaxel + prednisone every 3 wk	45	35	18.9 ($P = 0.009$)
		Docetaxel + prednisone 1 wk	48	31	17.4 (no difference)
		Mitoxantrone + prednisone	32	22	16.5
SWOG 9916 [72]	770	Docetaxel/estramustine + prednisone every 3 wk	50	NR	17.5 ($P = 0.01$)
		Mitoxantrone + prednisone	27	NR	15.6

CALGB—Cancer and Leukemia Group B; NR—not reported; PSA—prostate-specific antigen; SWOG—Southwest Oncology Group.

(65%–80%) of bladder cancers are stage Ta/T1/Tis at presentation, and the natural history of non–muscle-invasive bladder cancer (NMIBC) is unique in its propensity for local recurrence during the course of a patient's life. Following transurethral resection, anywhere from 50% to 90% of NMIBCs will eventually recur. The significance of these recurrences can be variable; however, 10% to 30% of cases progress to a more advanced stage and 10% to 50% progress to a more advanced stage and/or grade [84]. The rationale for early detection of disease, primary or recurrent, is illustrated by 5-year survival rates for noninvasive, locally invasive, and metastatic disease of roughly 94%, 50%, and 6%, respectively [85].

A combination of methods has become the established means of detecting bladder cancer, as no single procedure is 100% sensitive. Exophytic lesions are readily identified with cystoscopy, but flat lesions, in particular carcinoma in situ, can be more difficult to detect. In addition, upper tract urothelial cancers in the ureter or renal pelvis elude detection by cystoscopic examination alone. Since its introduction in 1945 by Papanicolau and Marshall, the microscopic examination of urinary cytology has been used as an adjunct to cystoscopy. Urinary cytology is highly specific for bladder cancer, with overall specificities of more than 90% in contemporary reviews [86,87]. The sensitivity of cytology is somewhat more problematic, in particular for low-grade lesions. The overall sensitivity of cytology has been reported to be in the range of 40% to 60% versus detection rates of 80% to 95% for high-grade lesions [86,87]. In addition, cytology suffers from limitations because of interobserver variability and the need for specialized laboratory personnel. The ability of cytology to detect high-grade disease has clear clinical relevance, but its overall poorer performance has supported interest in the development of novel urinary markers for bladder cancer detection [85].

EARLY DETECTION

Bladder cancer presents a unique opportunity for early detection due to the ability to easily sample patients' urine. The field of urine-based biomarker discovery and development for bladder cancer is a very active area of investigation, with dozens of candidate markers in various stages of development and several tests approved for use in clinical practice (Table 13-9). Some markers are being developed as enhancements to the current standard of care (cytology and cystoscopy), whereas others are being developed for the potential of actually modifying the standard of care [85]. Differences between the goals and limitations of screening and primary detection versus surveillance for recurrent disease affect the evaluation and development of urinary markers for bladder cancer detection. Urinary markers for bladder cancer are not, at this point in time, sufficiently specific for use in population screening [85]. Given the relatively low prevalence of bladder cancer, screening the general population with existing approved urine-based markers would probably yield unacceptable numbers of false-positive tests, prompting unnecessary anxiety and costly and invasive evaluations. Nonetheless, some authors have studied the performance of

screening tests in selected cohorts, for instance individuals with high-risk industrial or environmental exposures, with encouraging results [88]. Several US Food and Drug Administration (FDA)-approved markers are in use in the clinical setting for surveillance of recurrent bladder cancer, whereas other promising markers are in earlier phases of clinical development (Table 13-9) [89–92].

STAGING AND PROGNOSIS

Transitional cell carcinoma of the bladder may be distinguished according to whether the tumor is superficial or invasive (Table 13-10). Superficial tumors of the bladder represent local disease with little or no capability for metastasis and thus can be treated with local therapies. Histologic grading, tumor type (papillary or carcinoma in situ), muscle invasion, and differentiation are important clinicopathologic features that should be evaluated.

Recurrence of superficial tumors (stage 0 or 1) and the need for intravesical therapy are determined by grade, tumor size, and whether multiple tumors are present [93]. True squamous differentiation in the tumor usually predicts for poor response to systemic chemotherapy. Indices of proliferation and genetic markers are being studied as indicators for progression of superficial tumors (ECFr, p53, pRB, c-erg-2, nuclear matrix, metalloproteinases, and E-cadherin) [94,95]. Nuclear accumulation of p53 has been associated with tumor recurrences and tumor progression in transitional cell carcinoma of the bladder. A multivariable analysis of grade, pathologic

Table 13-9. Urinary Markers in the Detection of Bladder Cancer

FDA-approved markers

Nuclear matrix protein 22

ImmunoCyt (DiagnoCure, Inc., Quebec, Canada)

Fluorescent in situ hybridization

Markers under development

Telomerase

Bladder cancer antigen 4

Cytokeratin 20

Soluble Fas

Epidermal growth factor receptor

Fibroblast growth factor receptor

FDA—US Food and Drug Administration.

Table 13-10. Staging of Bladder Cancer

Stage	Description		
Primary tumor (T)			
Ta	Noninvasive papillary tumor		
Tis	Carcinoma in situ		
T1	Tumor invades subepithelial connective tissue		
T2	Tumor invades muscle		
T2a	Invades superficial muscle		
T2b	Invades deep muscle		
T3	Tumor invades perivesical tissue		
T3a	Evident microscopically		
T3b	Extravesical mass		
T4	Tumor invades adjacent tissues		
T4a	Invades into prostate, uterus, vagina		
T4b	Invades pelvic wall, abdominal wall		
Regional lymph nodes (N)			
N0	No regional lymph nodes		
N1	Metastasis in single node ≤ 2 cm		
N2	Metastasis in node(s) > 2 cm and ≤ 5 cm		
N3	Metastasis in node(s) > 5 cm		
Distant metastasis (M)			
M0	No distant metastasis		
M1	Distant metastasis		
Stage Groupings			
Stage 0	Ta	N0	M0
Stage 0a	Tis	N0	M0
Stage I	T1	N0	M0
Stage II	T2a or T2b	N0	M0
Stage III	T3a, T3b, or T4a	N0	M0
Stage IV	T4b	N0	M0
	Any T	N1–3	M1

stage, lymph node status, and nuclear p53 status has confirmed p53 over-expression as an independent predictor [94].

PRIMARY DISEASE THERAPY

Most uroepithelial tumors present with either gross or microscopic hematuria. Urinary cytology is an important part of the evaluation. Full assessment of the uroepithelium is indicated and is accomplished with cystoscopy and intravenous (IV) or retrograde pyelography. Transurethral resection of the bladder tumor (TURB) is the initial treatment. Intravesical therapy is usually considered for high-grade tumors, carcinoma in situ, or recurrent low-grade tumors.

Treatment for superficial bladder cancers is directed not only at tumor regression but also at reduction of the subsequent recurrence rate and prevention of tumor invasion. TURB alone, for low-grade papillary transitional cell carcinoma, or in combination with intravesical chemotherapy and immunotherapy, can control local superficial tumor and prevent recurrences and invasion. Many therapeutic agents have been used in the treatment of superficial disease [96]. Bacillus Calmette-Guérin (BCG) is considered the best of these agents, although its use is not without associated morbidity.

Herr *et al.* [97] performed a 10-year follow-up of a prospective, randomized controlled trial comparing TURB alone versus TURB and intravesical BCG. The median time to progression had not been reached in the BCG-treated group, and 10-year progression-free survival (PFS) was 61.9% versus 38% in the TURB-alone group. It should be noted that all patients who received BCG experienced cystitis. A published 15-year update of this study found no significant differences with regard to overall progression rates and disease-specific survival [98]. In addition, there was a 31% incidence of upper tract tumors after a median or 7.3 years of follow-up. Although small (86 patients), this study demonstrates the necessity of close follow-up for extended periods, despite the initial advantage shown in the BCG-treated group.

Thiotepa, mitomycin C, and doxorubicin have been evaluated as intravesicular chemotherapy and have been shown to be effective and safe agents. The low molecular weight of thiotepa allows absorption across the bladder epithelium and can result in suppression, whereas the use of doxorubicin is associated with bladder contractures [99,100]. Mitomycin C has minimal systemic absorption and a low incidence of myelosuppression. Mitomycin C appears to give the same clinical results as thiotepa, with less risk of leukoneutropenia but with increased risk for bladder irritation. On this basis, mitomycin C is recommended as first-line intravesicular therapy in BCG-refractory patients with early-stage disease. In a randomized, prospective trial of 337 patients with high-risk superficial bladder tumors, Krege *et al.* [101] compared TURB alone versus resection with BCG or resection with mitomycin C. All patients underwent complete resection before starting intravesical therapy. Both groups treated with intravesical therapy had a lower relative risk of recurrence. Although there was no significant difference in the rates of progression between the two treatment groups, mitomycin C demonstrated an initial modest advantage in patients with recurrent tumors. Side effects were more common with BCG. Thus, it seems reasonable to consider mitomycin C for intravesical therapy, especially in the context of recurrence [101].

Other forms of intravesical immunotherapy, specifically interferon-α (IFN-α), also appear to have benefits in superficial bladder cancer [102]. Use of high-dose intravesical IFN-α has also been explored in superficial bladder cancer. Little toxicity has been observed and although it is inferior to BCG or mitomycin C as first-line therapy, its role as a single agent or in combination with other agents is still being explored [102]. Other agents and methods for intravesical therapies that are being explored include use of targeting antibodies, genetically modified BCG, and newer chemotherapy drugs [102].

ADJUVANT THERAPY FOR REGIONAL DISEASE

The current standard therapy for locally invasive transitional cell carcinoma of the bladder remains cystectomy. The patient's risk of relapse depends on the depth of invasion into the wall of the bladder. Overall, there is a 40% to 60% chance of failure from cystectomy alone, raising the question of the need and effectiveness of adjuvant therapies. New pathologic techniques

are becoming available to help distinguish metastatic potential of invasive bladder cancers, which include measurements of p53, NM23 RNA levels, DNA ploidy, and expression of the antigen T138 on the cell surface. Much recent work has been published regarding the use of concomitant chemotherapy with radiation and TURB as a means of providing effective local and systemic therapy while preserving an intact bladder. Primary radiation therapy has a 5-year survival of 10% to 20% and results in poor local control [103]. Based on in vitro data, the NCIC tested cisplatin plus radiation versus radiation alone in a randomized clinical trial [104]. Patients randomized to the chemotherapy group received three cycles of concomitant cisplatin at 100 mg/m² every 21 days with their radiation. There were no significant differences between the groups with regard to response, overall survival, or PFS, but there was significantly better local control with concomitant cisplatin and a trend toward better bladder preservation.

The role of radiotherapy combined with multiagent chemotherapy has been explored by Kaufman *et al.* [105]. A pilot study of 53 patients demonstrated a 77% survival rate at 54 months [106]. Pilot data from a protocol of complete transurethral resection and outpatient multidrug chemotherapy followed by a short course of high-dose split-fraction radiotherapy has shown similar excellent results, with a 70% complete response rate [107]. The Radiation Therapy Oncology Group (RTOG) reported a phase 2 trial evaluating bladder preservation for invasive disease, using two cycles of MCV (methotrexate, cisplatin, and vinblastine) after incomplete resection followed by concomitant radiation and cisplatin in 91 patients [108]. Patients not entering a complete remission went to immediate cystectomy. If complete remission was achieved, the patient received a third cycle of cisplatin with consolidating radiation. The complete remission rate was 80% in this study, with an actuarial 4-year survival of 62% and an actuarial survival at 4 years of 44% with the bladder intact. Cystectomy ultimately was required in 40% (37 of 91 patients). However, toxicity was high, with a 12% rate of leukopenia and 16 cases of severe delayed toxicity.

Although large, multicenter phase 3 trials have not definitively answered questions regarding the ultimate utility of these combined-modality bladder-preserving approaches, it seems reasonable to offer such an approach to patients unable or unwilling to undergo cystectomy. Common features of success from the trials performed include resection of as much visible tumor as possible, completion of chemotherapy as possible (given the toxicity), early stage (*ie*, T2), and lack of hydronephrosis and carcinoma in situ. If the patient does not experience a complete remission, reconsideration of cystectomy is mandated. Although theoretical concerns regarding surgery after chemoradiation rationally exist, no current studies demonstrate an increased complication rate, and none were reported in the above trials [108,109].

ADJUVANT THERAPY

The role of adjuvant or neoadjuvant chemotherapy has not been definitively proven because no randomized comparisons of adequate sample size have shown a definite survival benefit. Preliminary reports of randomized trials suggest that cisplatin-based multiagent chemotherapy may have a significant impact on the treatment of high-risk invasive bladder cancer. Stockle *et al.* [110] reported a study of 49 patients with pathologically staged T3b and T4a bladder cancer with or without lymph node involvement randomized to receive methotrexate, vinblastine (or epirubicin), doxorubicin, and cisplatin following cystectomy or cystectomy alone. Although time of follow-up was limited, only three of 18 patients treated with adjuvant chemotherapy had relapse compared with 18 of 23 patients in the control arm. Freiha *et al.* [111] conducted a randomized controlled trial comparing radical cystectomy alone to radical cystectomy followed by four cycles of MCV-like chemotherapy in patients with pT3b or pT4 disease with or without nodal involvement. Twenty-five patients from each group were evaluable at 5 years. Of note, patients in the observation group received MCV therapy at first sign of recurrence. The recurrence rate in the adjuvant group was 48% (12 of 25 patients) versus 76% in the observation group. Although there was significant freedom from progression in the chemotherapy group, no difference was found in rates of overall survival. The authors contributed the latter finding to the crossover allowed in the design, indicating the benefit from chemotherapy may have also been seen with delayed treatment. Trials involving neoadjuvant multiagent, cisplatin-based chemotherapy have been completed [112–114]. In a moderately sized randomized clinical trial, the RTOG evaluated the role of two cycles of neoadjuvant MCV in muscle-invading bladder cancer treated with bladder-preserving radiation. Patients received either MCV before radiation/cisplatin therapy or radiation/cisplatin therapy alone. Survival rates for the two arms were identical (5-year actuarial survival rates were 48% and 49%, respectively). A major criticism of the study is that, overall, only 74% of the patients completed the course of therapy: 67% in the neoadjuvant arm and 81% in the radiation/cisplatin alone arm [114]. In a study of 976 patients with stage T2, G3, T3, T4a N0 to NX, or N0 disease who received either cystectomy or radiation for primary treatment with or without three cycles of MCV neoadjuvant therapy, no improvement in 3-year survival rate was seen. Median follow-up in this study was 4 years [113].

These data suggest that the adjuvant or neoadjuvant therapy for invasive bladder cancer requires four or more cycles of multiagent chemotherapy with currently available agents. Newer agents, particularly gemcitabine and the taxanes, have encouraging activity in metastatic disease and should be tested in the adjuvant setting. Patients with pathologic stage T2 or less with no nodal involvement are low risk and do not necessarily require adjuvant therapy. No data are available to support the use of adjuvant therapy in patients with nontransitional cell carcinomas.

CHEMOTHERAPY FOR ADVANCED DISEASE

Patients with unresectable or metastatic bladder cancer are generally treated with multiagent systemic chemotherapy [115,116]. Until recently, the most commonly used combinations were MVAC (methotrexate, vinblastine, doxorubicin, cisplatin) and MCV. MVAC was found to be superior to cisplatin alone (objective response rates of 39% vs 12%, respectively) in a randomized ECOG trial evaluating the treatment of metastatic bladder cancer [117]. Other randomized chemotherapy trials for metastatic bladder cancer are also outlined in Table 13-11 [117–121].

More recent studies have documented the activity of three drug types in the treatment of advanced bladder cancer: cisplatin, gemcitabine, and the taxanes (paclitaxel and docetaxel) [115,116]. Combinations of two or three of these drugs have shown clinical benefit. The combination of gemcitabine and cisplatin has emerged as a first-line choice for patients with advanced disease. In a randomized trial in 405 patients, gemcitabine/cisplatin was found to be equivalent to MVAC therapy with regard to overall response, survival, and time to treatment failure, but gemcitabine/cisplatin had a more favorable toxicity profile [121] (Table 13-11). Other newer combinations with activity include cisplatin/paclitaxel, gemcitabine/paclitaxel, gemcitabine/docetaxel, carboplatin/paclitaxel, cisplatin/gemcitabine/paclitaxel, and cisplatin/gemcitabine/docetaxel [115,116]. These combinations have not been compared with reference regimens such as MVAC. While response rates of 50% to 60% have been reported for these combinations, complete responses are not common and the duration of response is often short. At present, there is an international phase 3 trial coordinated by the European

Organisation for Research and Treatment of Cancer comparing paclitaxel, gemcitabine, and cisplatin with gemcitabine and cisplatin. The aim of the study is to enroll 305 patients in each group and assess overall survival as an end point. Differences in PFS, response rates, duration of response, and toxic effects will also be assessed [115].

RENAL CELL CARCINOMA
ETIOLOGY AND RISK FACTORS

In 2007 an estimated 51,000 Americans were diagnosed with kidney cancer and approximately 13,000 died of the disease [1]. For unknown reasons, the rate of renal cell carcinoma (RCC) has increased 2% per year for the past 65 years. Approximately 90% of renal tumors are RCC, the majority being of clear cell pathology [122]. Other less common cell types include papillary, chromophobe, and collecting duct tumors. Medullary renal carcinoma is a variant of collecting duct and was initially described as occurring in patients who are sickle-trait positive. The etiology of this association is not known.

Smoking and obesity are the major risk factors for development of RCC. Other risk factors include end-stage renal failure, acquired cystic disease, analgesic abuse, and asbestos exposure [123–127]. Molecular genetic evaluation has documented that the most common chromosomal abnormality is loss of heterozygosity of 3p13-26, which is found in 66% to 98% of clear cell RCC tumors but is not observed in papillary tumors [124]. Several hereditary types of RCC exist. The most common predisposing hereditary disorder is Von Hippel-Lindau disease (VHL), caused by a mutation in the *VHL* gene [128,129]. Loss of heterozygosity of the *VHL* locus is observed in 80% to 98% of sporadic RCC, with *VHL* gene mutations detectable in approximately 50% to 60% of the cases analyzed [128]. Silencing of the *VHL* gene by hypermethylation of the promoter region is also observed in a significant proportion of RCC [130].

STAGING AND PROGNOSIS

Staging for renal cancer is presented in Table 13-12. Recent changes to the staging system include T1 size increased to include tumors 7 cm or less and the modification of the definition of T3b tumors in recognition of the prognostic importance of tumor extension into the renal vein or its segmental (muscle-containing) branches. Patients with the sarcomatoid variant of RCC have a worse prognosis, with survival less than 1 year. Poor performance status, short disease-free interval between initial nephrectomy and development of metastases, hypercalcemia, and the presence of nonpulmonary metastases are common poor prognostic factors [128]. The estimated 5-year survival rates for patients with RCC are 96% for stage I, 82% for stage II, 64% for stage III, and 23% for stage IV [128].

PRIMARY DISEASE THERAPY

Surgical resection remains the only potentially curative therapy for clinically localized RCC. Radical nephrectomy, with removal of the kidney, perirenal

Table 13-11. Randomized Chemotherapy Trials for Metastatic Bladder Cancer

Study	Regimen	Patients, *n*	Response rate, %	Median survival, *mo*	Superior arm?
Loehrer *et al.* [117]	MVAC	126	39	12.5	MVAC
	Cisplatin	120	12	8.2	
Logothetis *et al.* [118]	MVAC	65	65	12.6	MVAC
	CISCA	55	46	10.0	
Bamias *et al.* [119]	MVAC	109	54	14.2	MVAC
	Docetaxel/cisplatin	111	37	9.3	
Sternberg *et al.* [120]	MVAC	129	50	14.1	MVAC ~ high-dose MVAC
	High-dose MVAC	134	62	14.5	
von der Maase *et al.* [121]	MVAC	202	46	14.8	MVAC ~ gemcitabine/cisplatin
	Gemcitabine/cisplatin	203	49	13.8	

CISCA—cisplatin, cyclophosphamide, doxorubicin; MVAC—methotrexate, vinblastine, doxorubicin, cisplatin.

fat, regional lymph nodes, and the ipsilateral adrenal gland, is the preferred treatment, particularly if the tumor extends into the vena cava [131]. The lymph node dissection in this case is not therapeutic but does provide prognostic information [132]. Almost all patients with nodal involvement subsequently relapse with distant metastases and may be candidates for clinical trials assessing the role of adjuvant therapy. Nephron-sparing therapy (ie, partial nephrectomy) was originally only considered in patients who would be made functionally anephric by the surgery, necessitating dialysis. However, the nephron-sparing approach has been used increasingly in patients with T1 tumors and a contralateral kidney [131]. Outcomes in these patients have been equivalent to radical nephrectomy [131]. Nephron sparing is used for patients with tumors that are in the upper or lower pole, or in patients with a hereditary form of RCC such as VHL. Stereotactic radiation or gamma knife has been increasingly used for central nervous system (CNS) metastases and as primary therapy for elderly or infirm patients with small tumors. Otherwise, radiation therapy for RCC is used to palliate metastatic sites.

After surgical excision, 20% to 30% of patients with localized (ie, stage I–III) tumors relapse, with lung metastases being the most common site of distal recurrence. Adjuvant therapy after nephrectomy has no established role in patients who have undergone complete tumor resection. Adjuvant radiation therapy after nephrectomy is not beneficial even in patients with nodal involvement or incomplete resection [128]. Adjuvant systemic therapy with biologic agents interleukin (IL)-2 (low or high dose) and IFN-α have not resulted in improved time to relapse or survival [133,134]. The new class of tyrosine kinase inhibitors is currently under evaluation in the adjuvant setting in phase 3 clinical trials.

Table 13-12. Staging of Renal Cancer

Stage	Description
Primary tumor (T)	
T1	Tumor ≤ 7 cm limited to kidney
T1a	Tumor ≤ 4 cm limited to kidney
T1b	Tumor > 4 cm but ≤ 7 cm limited to kidney
T2	Tumor > 7 cm limited to kidney
T3	Tumor extends into major veins, adrenal gland not beyond Gerota's fascia
T3a	Invades adrenal or perirenal and/or renal sinus fat
T3b	Grossly extends into renal vein or segmental (muscle-containing) branches or vena cava below diaphragm
T3c	Grossly extends into vena cava above diaphragm
T4	Tumor invades beyond Gerota's fascia
Regional lymph nodes (N)	
N0	No regional lymph nodes
N1	Metastasis in single regional node
N2	Metastasis in > 1 regional node
Distant metastasis (M)	
M0	No distant metastasis
M1	Distant metastasis

Stage Groupings

Stage I	T1	N0	M0
Stage II	T2	N0	M0
Stage III	T1 or T2	N1	M0
Stage IV	T3	N0 or N1	M0
	T4	N0 or N1	M0
	Any T	N2	M0
	Any T	Any N	M1

ADVANCED DISEASE THERAPY

Select patients with metastatic RCC are also candidates for surgery. A small subset of patients with surgically respectable primary RCC and a solitary respectable metastasis to lung, bone, or brain may be candidates for nephrectomy and surgical metastectomy [135]. Most patients who undergo resection of a solitary metastasis have recurrence at the primary or another metastatic site, but long-term survival has been reported in some patients.

Randomized trials performed by SWOG (SWOG 8949) and the EORTC demonstrated a benefit for cytoreductive nephrectomy followed by interferon therapy in patients with metastatic RCC [136,137]. A combined analysis of these trials demonstrated a median survival of 13.6 months for patients treated with surgery plus interferon compared with 7.8 months for those treated with interferon alone [138]. Patients who are most likely to benefit from this approach are those with good performance status, lung-only metastasis, and good prognostic features [136–138].

Until recently, limited systemic treatment options were available for patients with metastatic RCC. Cytokine therapy had been the mainstay of treatment based on multiple randomized studies evaluating interferon and IL-2 in various combinations and dosing schedules [139–143]. Low-dose schedules of interferon and IL-2 suggest a response rate from 10% to 20%. Higher-dose IL-2 results in higher response rates compared with low-dose IL-2 and has been approved by the FDA for the treatment of metastatic RCC [140]. The toxicity of high-dose IL-2 is significant and consideration should be given to administering this therapy only in centers with experience and ability to aggressively manage patients with noninvasive and invasive monitoring, fluid replacement, low-dose pressors, antiemetics, antihistamines, and antibiotics.

The recognition that higher levels of vascular endothelial growth factor (VEGF)—the best-characterized proangiogenic factor—are correlated with more aggressive disease in kidney cancer, and that regulation of the VHL/hypoxia-inducible factor-1 (HIF-1) oxygen-sensing pathway is disrupted in RCC has intensified interest in drug development for approaches aimed at the angiogenesis axis in the treatment of RCC [144]. Recently, the clinical efficacy of antiangiogenic therapy in RCC has led to the FDA approval of three antiangiogenesis drugs, sunitinib malate, sorafenib tosylate, and temsirolimus, for the treatment of advanced kidney cancer. A fourth agent, bevacizumab, has shown benefit in a pivotal phase 3 trial (Table 13-13).

Sunitinib (SU11248) is a multitargeted receptor tyrosine kinase inhibitor that inhibits a number of kinases including VEGF (ie, VEGFR1–3) and platelet-derived growth factor (PDGF; α, β) receptors [145]. In a multicenter phase 2 trial, patients with metastatic RCC and progression on first-line cytokine therapy received sunitinib monotherapy in repeated 6-week cycles of daily oral therapy for 4 weeks, followed by a 2-week recovery period [146]. Overall response rate was the primary end point, and time to progression and safety were secondary end points. In this study, 25 of 63 (40%) patients treated with sunitinib achieved partial responses; 17 additional patients (27%) demonstrated stable disease lasting at least 3 months. The median time to progression in the 63 patients was 8.7 months. Dosing was generally tolerated with manageable toxicities. Based on this study and an additional phase 2 study demonstrating antitumor activity as second-line therapy in metastatic RCC, the FDA approved sunitinib for the treatment of advanced kidney cancer in early 2006.

Because sunitinib demonstrated activity in two uncontrolled phase 2 studies in patients with metastatic RCC, a comparison of the drug with IFN-α in a multicenter, randomized phase 3 trial was performed in 750 patients with previously untreated, metastatic RCC. Patients received either repeated 6-week cycles of sunitinib (at a dose of 50 mg given orally once daily for 4 weeks, followed by 2 weeks without treatment) or IFN-α at a dose of 9 MU given subcutaneously three times weekly [147]. The primary end point was PFS. Secondary end points included the objective response rate, overall survival, patient-reported outcomes, and safety. The median PFS was significantly longer in the sunitinib group (11 months) than in the IFN-α group (5 months). Sunitinib was also associated with a higher objective response rate than was IFN-α. The proportion of patients with grade 3 or 4 treatment-related fatigue was significantly higher in the group treated with IFN-α, whereas diarrhea was more frequent in the sunitinib group.

Patients in the sunitinib group reported a significantly better quality of life than did patients in the IFN-α group. On the basis of the statistically significant improvement in PFS and its tolerability, sunitinib was given a category 1 recommendation for first-line treatment of patients with relapsed or medically unresectable stage IV clear cell RCC by the National Comprehensive Cancer Center Network Practice guidelines.

Sorafenib (BAY 43-9006) is an oral kinase inhibitor targeting both tumor cells and the tumor vasculature. It was originally developed as an inhibitor of Raf-1, a member of the Raf/MEK/ERK signaling pathway [148,149]. Sorafenib was subsequently found to have activity against B-Raf, VEGFR-2, PDGF receptor, Fms-like tyrosine kinase-3 (Flt-3), and stem cell growth factor (c-KIT) [150]. A multicenter, placebo-controlled, randomized discontinuation trial was performed to determine whether sorafenib inhibits tumor growth in patients with metastatic RCC who maintain stable disease after a 12-week run-in period [151]. After 12 weeks, patients with changes in bidimensional tumor measurements that were less than 25% from baseline were randomized to sorafenib or placebo for an additional 12 weeks. Patients with 25% or greater tumor shrinkage continued open-label sorafenib, whereas patients with 25% or greater tumor growth discontinued treatment. Of 202 patients treated during the run-in period, 73 patients had tumor shrinkage of 25% or greater. Sixty-five patients with stable disease at 12 weeks were randomly assigned to sorafenib ($n = 32$) or placebo ($n = 33$). At 24 weeks, 50% of the sorafenib-treated patients were progression free versus 18% of the placebo-treated patients. Median PFS from randomization was significantly longer with sorafenib (24 weeks) than placebo (6 weeks).

The positive results from the phase 2 study led to a phase 3 randomized, double-blind, placebo-controlled trial of sorafenib known as TARGET (Treatment Approaches in RCC Global Evaluation Trial) in patients with advanced clear cell RCC [152]. Nine hundred three patients with RCC that was resistant to cytokine therapy were randomly assigned to receive continuous treatment with oral sorafenib (400 mg twice daily) or placebo. The primary end point was overall survival. After planned analysis demonstrated a PFS benefit, crossover was permitted from placebo to sorafenib. In the placebo arm assessed at the time of crossover, the median survival was 14.3 months compared with 19.3 months for sorafenib.

Because these two trials were conducted in patients after progression on prior cytokine therapy, an additional trial was performed to assess the efficacy of sorafenib versus interferon in previously untreated patients with metastatic clear cell RCC. In this trial, the median PFS was similar between the two groups (5.7 vs 5.6 months); the incidence of adverse events was also similar. The most common side effects associated with sorafenib were diarrhea, rash, fatigue, and hand–foot skin reactions. Hypertension and cardiac ischemia were rare serious adverse events that were more common in patients receiving sorafenib than in those receiving placebo. As compared with placebo, treatment with sorafenib prolonged PFS in patients with advanced clear cell RCC in whom previous therapy had failed. Based on these data, the FDA approved sorafenib in December 2005 for the treatment of advanced kidney cancer.

Temsirolimus (CCI-779) is a novel mammalian target of rapamycin (mTOR) kinase inhibitor. It has been shown to bind with high affinity to the immunophilin FKBP, and this complex inhibits mTOR kinase activity [153,154]. In addition, the mTOR pathway appears to be involved in the development of a hereditary form of RCC seen in patients with tuberous sclerosis. mTOR activation increases *HIF-1* gene expression at both the levels of mRNA translation and protein stabilization [155]. Thus, inhibition of mTOR by temsirolimus could also prevent the enhanced angiogenesis associated with sporadic RCC and loss of *VHL* function.

In a phase 2 study, patients ($n = 111$) were randomly assigned to receive temsirolimus 25, 75, or 250 mg weekly as a 30-minute IV infusion [156]. Patients were evaluated for tumor response, time to tumor progression, survival, and adverse events. Temsirolimus produced an objective response rate of 7% (one complete response and seven partial responses) and minor responses in 26% of these advanced RCC patients. Median time to tumor progression was 5.8 months and median survival was 15.0 months. The most frequently occurring adverse events of all grades were maculopapular rash (76%), mucositis (70%), asthenia (50%), and nausea (43%). The most frequently occurring grade 3 or 4 adverse events were hyperglycemia (17%), hypophosphatemia (13%), anemia (9%), and hypertriglyceridemia (6%). Neither toxicity nor efficacy was significantly influenced by the temsirolimus dose level.

The promising data led to a multicenter, phase 3 trial in which 626 patients with previously untreated, poor-prognosis metastatic RCC were randomly assigned to receive 25 mg of IV temsirolimus weekly, 3 million U of IFN-α (with an increase to 18 million U) subcutaneously three times weekly, or combination therapy with 15 mg of temsirolimus weekly plus 6 million U of IFN-α three times weekly [157]. The primary end point was overall survival in comparisons of the temsirolimus group and the combination therapy group with the IFN-α group. Patients who received temsirolimus alone had longer overall survival (HR for death, 0.73) and PFS than did patients who received IFN-α alone. Overall survival in the combination therapy group did not differ significantly from that in the IFN-α group (HR, 0.96). Median overall survival times in the IFN-α group, the temsirolimus group, and the combination therapy group were 7.3, 10.9, and 8.4 months, respectively. Rash, peripheral edema, hyperglycemia, and hyperlipidemia were more common in the temsirolimus group, whereas asthenia was more common in the IFN-α group. There were fewer patients with serious adverse events in the temsirolimus group than in the IFN-α group. As compared with IFN-α, temsirolimus improved overall survival among patients with metastatic RCC and a poor prognosis. The addition of temsirolimus to IFN-α did not improve survival. These recent data led the FDA to approved temsirolimus for the treatment of advanced kidney cancer in May 2007.

Bevacizumab is an anti–VEGF-A recombinant monoclonal antibody that binds and neutralizes circulating VEGF-A. In a phase 2 randomized, placebo-controlled, double-blind study, patients with measurable metastatic clear cell RCC were treated with low (3 mg/kg) or high (10 mg/kg) doses of bevacizumab or placebo [158,159]. Beginning 1 week after a loading dose of 150% of the assigned dose, treatment was given by IV infusion every 2 weeks. The primary end points were time to tumor progression (by World Health Organization criteria) and response rate. Survival was a secondary

Table 13-13. New Therapies in the Treatment of Metastatic Renal Cancer

Agent	Dosing	Toxicities
Sunitinib	50 mg orally once daily × 4 wk followed by 2 wk off	Neutropenia, thrombocytopenia, hyperamylasemia, hand-foot syndrome, mucositis, diarrhea, hypertension, nausea, vomiting, fatigue, anemia, neutropenia, left ventricular dysfunction
Sorafenib	400 mg orally twice daily	Rash, hand-foot skin reaction, alopecia, nausea, diarrhea, abdominal pain, fatigue, hypertension, increased amylase and lipase, headache, cardiac ischemia (rare)
Temsirolimus	25 mg IV over 30–60 min once weekly; premedicate with diphenhydramine IV 30 min prior to each dose	Edema, rash, hyperglycemia, hyperlipidemia, hypertriglyceridemia, hypophosphatemia, decreased hemoglobin, decreased lymphocyte count, asthenia, loss of appetite, nausea, hypersensitivity
Bevacizumab	10 mg/kg IV every 2 wk	Hypertension, hematuria, epistaxis, alopecia, headache, asymptomatic proteinuria, asthenia, abdominal pain; discontinue if gastrointestinal perforation, wound dehiscence requiring intervention, serious bleeding, severe arterial thromboembolic event, nephrotic syndrome, hypertensive crisis, or reversible posterior leukoencephalopathy syndrome occur

end point, because crossover from placebo to 3 mg/kg of bevacizumab was allowed for patients progressing with placebo. Minimal toxic effects were seen, with hypertension and asymptomatic proteinuria predominating. The trial was stopped after the interim analysis met the criteria for early stopping. With 116 patients randomly assigned to treatment groups (40 to placebo, 37 to low-dose antibody, and 39 to high-dose antibody), there was a significant prolongation of the time to progression of disease in the high-dose–antibody group as compared with the placebo group (HR, 2.55). There was a small difference, of borderline significance, between the time to progression of disease in the low-dose–antibody group and that in the placebo group (HR, 1.26). The probability of being progression-free for patients given high-dose antibody, low-dose–antibody, and placebo was 64%, 39%, and 20%, respectively, at 4 months and 30%, 14%, and 5% at 8 months. In this trial, there were four partial responses (10% response rate) and a highly substantial prolongation of time to tumor progression in patients receiving the higher dose of bevacizumab. There were no significant differences in overall survival between groups.

In view of the positive results from the phase 2 study, a phase 3 trial (Avastin for Renal Cell Cancer [AVOREN]) was conducted to evaluate the efficacy and safety of IFN-α with or without bevacizumab as first-line treatment in metastatic [160]. Nephrectomized patients with clear cell RCC, Karnofsky's performance status of 70%, no CNS metastases, and adequate organ function received IFN-α (9 MIU three times per week for up to 1 year) plus bevacizumab (10 mg/kg every 2 weeks) or placebo until disease progression. Tumor assessments were performed every 8 weeks until week 32 and every 12 weeks thereafter. Between June 2004 and October 2006, 649 patients were randomized (641 treated) at 101 centers in 18 countries. The addition of bevacizumab to IFN-α significantly increased PFS (10.2 vs 5.4 months; HR, 0.63) and objective tumor response rate (30.6% vs 12.4%). A trend toward improved overall survival was observed with the addition of bevacizumab to IFN-α. These data suggest that bevacizumab improves PFS when combined with IFN-α in RCC. No unexpected safety events were observed. These results were presented at the American Society of Clinical Oncology plenary session in 2008; FDA approval of bevacizumab is expected soon.

Although sorafenib, sunitinib, temsirolimus, and bevacizumab have added greatly to the therapeutic armamentarium for patients with advanced renal cancer, as single agents, these drugs produce partial and not complete responses in a minority of patients, require long-term administration for continued disease control, and have side effects. Treatment resistance typically develops within 6 to 12 months, and tumors often progress quickly once treatment is stopped. Reasons for these results can be multifold: 1) optimal dosing has not been achieved; 2) the signaling pathway is not sufficiently understood; and 3) tumor heterogeneity is responsible for different dependences from the targeted pathway among patients. Combination therapy has been proposed as a way of potentially producing more durable benefit. Although critically important, testing of combination regimens must proceed cautiously due to the potential for synergistic toxicity and/or countervailing activity inherent with these multitargeted agents [154]. Approaches to combination therapy currently being investigated include "vertical" combinations, in which the HIF/VEGF pathway is blocked at several steps, and "horizontal" combinations, in which multiple separate signaling pathways are blocked simultaneously [161].

REFERENCES

1. Jemal A, Siegel R, Ward E, *et al.*: Cancer statistics, 2007. *CA Cancer J Clin* 2007, 57:43–66.

2. Pinczowski D, McLaughlin JK, Lackgren G, *et al.*: Occurrence of testicular cancer in patients operated on for cryptorchidism and inguinal hernia. *J Urol* 1991, 146:1291–1294.

3. Sladden M, Dickinson J: Testicular cancer: how effective is screening? *Aust Fam Physician* 1993, 22:1350–1356.

4. Birch R, Williams S, Cone A, *et al.*: Southeastern Cancer Group: prognostic factors for favorable outcome in disseminated germ cell tumors. *J Clin Oncol* 1986, 4:400–407.

5. Aass N, Klepp O, Cavallin-Stahl E, *et al.*: Prognostic factors in unselected patients with nonseminomatous metastatic testicular cancer: a multicenter experience. *J Clin Oncol* 1991, 9:818–826.

6. Sesterhenn IA, Weiss BB, Mostofi FK, *et al.*: Prognosis and other clinical correlates of pathologic review in stage I and II testicular carcinoma: a report from the Testicular Cancer Intergroup Study. *J Clin Oncol* 1992, 10:69–78.

7. Jones WG, Fossa SD, Mead GM, *et al.*: Randomized trial of 30 versus 20 Gy in the adjuvant treatment of stage I testicular seminoma: a report on Medical Research Council Trial TE18, European Organisation for the Research and Treatment of Cancer trial 30942 (ISRCTN18525328). *J Clin Oncol* 2005, 23:1200–1208.

8. Warde P, Gospodarowicz MK, Panzarella T, *et al.*: Stage I testicular seminoma: results of adjuvant irradiation and surveillance. *J Clin Oncol* 1995, 13:2255–2262.

9. Alomary I, Samant R, Gallant V: Treatment of stage I seminoma: a 15 year review. *Urol Oncol* 2006, 24:180–183.

10. Gospodarowicz M, Sturgeon JF, Jewitt MA: Early stage and advanced seminoma: role of radiation therapy, surgery, and chemotherapy. *Semin Oncol* 1998, 25:160–173.

11. de Wit R, Roberts JT, Wilkinson PM, *et al.*: Equivalence of three or four cycles of bleomycin, etoposide, and cisplatin chemotherapy and of a 3- or 5-day schedule in good-prognosis germ cell cancer: a randomized study of the European Organization for Research and Treatment of Cancer Genitourinary Tract Cancer Cooperative Group and the Medical Research Council. *J Clin Oncol* 2001, 19:1629–1640.

12. Loehrer PJ Sr, Johnson D, Elson P, *et al.*: Importance of bleomycin in favorable-prognosis disseminated germ cell tumors: an Eastern Cooperative Oncology Group trial. *J Clin Oncol* 1995,13:470–476.

13. Bajorin DF, Sarosdy MF, Pfister DG, *et al.*: Randomized trial of etoposide and cisplatin versus etoposide and carboplatin in patients with good-risk germ cell tumors: a multi-institutional study. *J Clin Oncol* 1993, 11:598–606.

14. Kondagunta GV, Bacik J, Bajorin D, *et al.*: Etoposide and cisplatin chemotherapy for metastatic good-risk germ cell tumors. *J Clin Oncol* 2005, 23:9290–9294.

15. National Comprehensive Cancer Network: NCCN guidelines for treatment of testicular, prostate, bladder and renal carcinoma. NCCN website. http://www.nccn.org. Accessed July 8, 2008.

16. Carver BS, Sheinfeld J: The current status of laparoscopic retroperitoneal lymph node dissection for non-seminomatous germ-cell tumors. *Nat Clin Pract Urol* 2005, 2:330–35.

17. Davis BE, Herr HW, Fair WR, *et al.*: The management of patients with nonseminomatous germ-cell tumors of the testis with serologic disease only after orchiectomy. *J Urol* 1994, 152:111–114.

18. Culine S, Theodore C, Terrier-Lacombe MJ, Droz JP: Primary chemotherapy in patients with nonseminomatous germ cell tumors of the testis and biological disease only after orchiectomy. *J Urol* 1996, 155:1296–1298.

19. Foster R, Bihrle R: Current status of retroperitoneal lymph node dissection and testicular cancer: when to operate. *Cancer Control* 2002, 9:277–283.

20. Motzer RJ, Sheinfeld J, Mazumdar M, *et al.*: Etoposide and cisplatin adjuvant therapy for patients with pathologic stage II germ-cell tumors. *Classic Papers and Current Comments* 1998b, 2:455–459.

21. International Germ Cell Cancer Collaborative Group: International germ-cell consensus classification: a prognostic factor-based staging system for metastatic germ-cell cancers. *J Clin Oncol* 1997, 15:594–603.

22. Loehrer PJ Sr, Johnson D, Elson P, *et al.*: Importance of bleomycin in favorable-prognosis disseminated germ cell tumors: an ECOG trial. *J Clin Oncol* 1995, 13:470–476.

23. Xiao H, Mazumdar M, Bajorin DF, *et al.*: Long-term follow-up of patients with good-risk germ cell tumors treated with etoposide and cisplatin. *J Clin Oncol* 1997, 15:2553–2558.

24. Saxman SB, Finch D, Gonin R, Einhorn LH: Long-term follow-up of a phase III study of three versus four cycles of bleomycin, etoposide, and cisplatin in favorable-prognosis germ-cell tumors: the Indiana University Experience. *J Clin Oncol* 1998, 16:702–706.

25. Jones RH, Vasey PA: Part II: testicular cancer—management of advanced disease. *Lancet Oncol* 2003;4:738–747.

26. Toner GC, Motzer RJ: Poor prognosis germ-cell tumors: current status and future directions. *Semin Oncol* 1998, 25:194–202.

27. Motzer RJ, Geller NL, Tan CC, *et al.*: Salvage chemotherapy for patients with germ-cell tumors. The Memorial Sloan-Kettering Cancer Center experience (1979–1989). *Cancer* 1991, 67:1305–1310.

28. McCaffrey JA, Mazumdar M, Bajorin DF, *et al.*: Ifosfamide + cisplatin regimens as first-line salvage therapy in germ-cell tumors: response and survival [abstract]. *Proc Am Soc Clin Oncol* 1996, 14:250.

29. Loehrer PJ, Gonin R, Nichols CR, *et al.*: Vinblastine plus ifosfamide plus cisplatin as initial salvage therapy in recurrent germ-cell tumor. *J Clin Oncol* 1998, 16:2500–2504.

30. Kondagunta GV, Bacik J, Donadio A, *et al.*: Combination of paclitaxel, ifosfamide, and cisplatin is an effective second-line therapy for patients with relapsed testicular germ cell tumors. *J Clin Oncol* 2005, 23:6549–6555.

31. Motzer RJ, Bosl GJ: High-dose chemotherapy for resistant germ cell tumors: recent advances and future directions. *J Natl Cancer Inst* 1992, 84:1703–1709.

32. Beyer J, Kramer A, Mandanas R, *et al.*: High-dose chemotherapy as salvage treatment in germ-cell tumors: a multivariate analysis of prognostic factors. *J Clin Oncol* 1996, 14:2638–2645.

33. Byar DP, Mostofi FK: Cancer of the prostate in men less than 50 years old: an analysis of 51 cases. *J Urol* 1969, 102:726–733.

34. Platz EA, Rimm EB, Willett WC, *et al.*: Racial variation in prostate cancer incidence and in hormonal system markers among male health professionals. *J Natl Cancer Inst* 2000, 92:2009–2017.

35. Giovannucci E, Liu Y, Platz EA, *et al.*: Risk factors for prostate cancer incidence and progression in the health professionals follow-up study. *Int J Cancer* 2007, 121:1571–1578.

36. De Marzo AM, Platz EA, Sutcliffe S, *et al.*: Inflammation in prostate carcinogenesis. *Nat Rev Cancer* 2007, 7:256–269.

37. De Marzo AM, DeWeese TL, Platz EA, *et al.*: Pathological and molecular mechanisms of prostate carcinogenesis: implications for diagnosis, detection, prevention, and treatment. *J Cell Biochem* 2004, 91:459–477.

38. Sutcliffe S, Platz EA: Inflammation in the etiology of prostate cancer: an epidemiologic perspective. *Urol Oncol* 2007, 25:242–249.

39. Ries LA, Melbert D, Krapcho M, *et al.*: SEER Cancer Statistics Review, 1975-2004, National Cancer Institute: Bethesda, MD. http://seer.cancer.gov/csr/1975_2004/, based on November 2006 SEER data submission. Posted to the SEER website, 2007.

40. Gann PH, Hennekens CH, Stampfer MJ: A prospective evaluation of plasma prostate-specific antigen for detection of prostatic cancer. *JAMA* 1995, 273:289–294.

41. Catalona WJ, Smith DS, Ratliff TL, *et al.*: Detection of organ-confined prostate cancer is increased through prostate-specific antigen-based screening. *JAMA* 1993, 270:984–954.

42. Horninger W. Cheli C, Babaian RJ, *et al.*: Complexed prostate specific antigen for early detection of prostate cancer in men with serum prostate-specific antigen levels of 2-4 nanograms per milliliter. *Urology* 2002, 60(Suppl 4A):31–35.

43. Carter HB, Pearson JD, Metter EJ, *et al.*: Longitudinal evaluation of prostate-specific antigen levels in men with and without prostate disease. *JAMA* 1992, 267:2215–2220.

44. Carter HB, Ferrucci L, Kettermann A, *et al.*: Detection of life-threatening prostate cancer with prostate-specific antigen velocity during a window of curability. *J Natl Cancer Inst* 2006, 98:1521–1527.

45. Partin AW, Brawer MK, Subong EN, *et al.*: Prospective evaluation of percent free-PSA and complexed-PSA for early detection of prostate cancer. *Prostate Cancer Prostatic Dis* 1998, 1:197–203.

46. Partin AW, Brawer MK, Bartsch G, *et al.*: Complexed prostate specific antigen improves specificity for prostate cancer detection: results of a prospective multicenter clinical trial. *J Urol* 2003, 170:1787–1791.

47. Denmeade SR, Isaacs JT: The role of prostate-specific antigen in the clinical evaluation of prostatic disease. *BJU Int* 2004, 93(Suppl 1):10–15.

48. Makarov DV, Trock BJ, Humphreys EB, *et al.*: Updated nomogram to predict pathologic stage of prostate cancer given prostate-specific antigen level, clinical stage, and biopsy Gleason score (Partin tables) based on cases from 2000 to 2005. *Urology* 2007, 69:1095–1101.

49. Partin AW, Yoo J, Carter HB, *et al.*: The use of prostate specific antigen, clinical stage and Gleason score to predict pathological stage in men with localized prostate cancer. *J Urol* 1993, 150:110–114.

50. Roberts WW, Bergstralh EJ, Blute ML, *et al.*: Contemporary identification of patients at high risk of early prostate cancer recurrence after radical retropubic prostatectomy. *Urology* 2001, 57:1033–1037.

51. D'Amico AV, Chen MH, Roehl KA, Catalona WJ: Preoperative PSA velocity and the risk of death from prostate cancer after radical prostatectomy. *N Engl J Med* 2004, 351:125–135.

52. Pound CR, Partin AW, Eisenberger MA, *et al.*: Natural History of progression after PSA elevation following radical prostatectomy. *JAMA* 1999, 281:1591–1597.

53. Freedland SJ, Humphreys EB, Mangold LA, *et al.*: Risk of prostate cancer-specific mortality following biochemical recurrence after radical prostatectomy. *JAMA* 2005, 294:433–439.

54. Lee AK, D'Amico AV: Utility of prostate-specific antigen kinetics in addition to clinical factors in the selection of patients for salvage local therapy. *J Clin Oncol* 2005, 23:8193–8197.

55. Amling CL, Bergstralh EJ, Blute ML, *et al.*: Defining prostate specific antigen progression after radical prostatectomy: what is the most appropriate cut point? *J Urol* 2001, 165:1146–1151.

56. Consensus statement: guidelines for PSA following radiation therapy: American Society for Therapeutic Radiology and Oncology Consensus Panel. *Int J Radiol Oncol Biol Phys* 1997, 37:1035–1041.

57. Horwitz EM, Vicini FA, Ziaja EL, *et al.*: The correlation between the ASTRO Consensus Panel definition of biochemical failure and clinical outcome for patients with prostate cancer treated with external beam radiation: American Society of Therapeutic Radiology and Oncology. *Int J Radiat Oncol Biol Phys* 1998, 41:267–272.

58. Hofer C, Laubenbacher C, Block T, *et al.*: Fluorine-18-fluorodeoxyglucose positron emission tomography is useless for the detection of local recurrence after radical prostatectomy. *Eur Urol* 1999, 36:31–35.

59. Seltzer MA, Barbaric Z, Belldegrun A, *et al.*: Comparison of helical computerized tomography, positron emission tomography and monoclonal antibody scans for evaluation of lymph node metastases in patients with prostate specific antigen relapse after treatment for localized prostate cancer. *J Urol* 1999, 162:1322–1328.

60. Thompson CA, Shanafelt TD, Loprinzi CL: Andropause: symptom management for prostate cancer patients treated with hormonal ablation. *Oncologist* 2003, 8:474–487.

61. Higano CS: Side effects of androgen deprivation therapy: Monitoring and minimizing toxicity. *Urology* 2003, 61(Suppl 2A):32–38.

62. Basaria S, Muller DC, Carducci MA, *et al.*: Hyperglycemia and insulin resistance in men with prostate carcinoma who receive androgen-deprivation therapy. *Cancer* 2006, 106:581–588.

63. D'Amico AV, Manola J, Loffredo M, *et al.*: 6-month androgen suppression plus radiation therapy vs radiation therapy alone for patients with clinically localized prostated cancer: a randomized controlled trial. *JAMA* 2004, 292:821–827.

64. Messing EM, Sarosdy M, Wilding G, *et al.*: Immediate hormone therapy compared with observation after radical prostatectomy and pelvic lymphadenectomy in men with node positive prostate cancer: results at 10 years of ECOG3886 [abstract]. *Proc Amer Urol Assoc* 2003:abstract 1480.

65. Bhandari MS, Crook J, Hussain M: Should intermittent androgen deprivation be used in routine clinical practice. *J Clin Oncol* 2005, 23:8212–8218.

66. Small EJ, Baron AD, Fippin L, Apodaca D: Ketoconazole retains activity in advanced prostate cancer patients with progression despite flutamide withdrawal. *J Urol* 1997, 157:1204–1207.

67. Culag Z, Hoffmann, Erdel M, *et al.*: Switch from antagonist to agonist of the androgen receptor bicalutamide is associated with prostate tumour progression in a new model. *Br J Cancer* 1999, 81:242–251.

68. Scher HI, Kelly WK: The flutamide withdrawal syndrome: its impact on clinical trials in hormone-refractory prostate cancer. *J Clin Oncol* 1993, 11:1566–1572.

69. Kantoff PW, Halabis S, Conaway M, *et al.*: Hydrocortisone with or without mitoxantrone in men with hormone-refractory prostate cancer: results of the cancer and leukemia group B 9182 study. *J Clin Oncol* 1993, 17:2506–2513.

70. Tannock IF, Osoba D, Stockler MR, *et al.*: Chemotherapy with mitoxantrone plus prednisone or prednisone alone for symptomatic hormone-resistant prostate cancer: a Canadian randomized trial with palliative end points. *J Clin Oncol* 1996, 14:1756–1764.

71. Tannock IF, de Wit R, Berry WR, *et al.*: Docetaxel plus prednisone or mitoxantrone plus prednisone for advanced prostate cancer. *N Engl J Med* 2004, 351:1502–1512.

72. Petrylak DP, Tangen CM, Hussain MH, *et al.*: Docetaxel and estramustine compared with mitoxantrone and prednisone for advanced refractory prostate cancer. *N Engl J Med* 2004, 351:1513–1520.

73. Walczak JR, Carducci MA: Pharmacological treatments for prostate cancer. *Expert Opin Investig Drugs* 2002, 11:1737–1748.

74. Saad F, Gleason DM, Murray R, *et al.*: A randomized, placebo-controlled trial of zoledronic acid in patients with hormone-refractory metastatic prostate carcinoma. *J Natl Cancer Inst* 2002, 94:1458–1468.

75. Ruggiero SL, Mehrotra B, Rosenberg TJ, Engroff SL: Osteonecrosis of the jaws associated with the use of bisphosphonates: a review of 63 cases. *J Oral Maxillofac Surg* 2004, 62:527–534.

76. Greenberg MS: Intravenous bisphosphonates and osteonecrosis. *Oral Surg Oral Med Oral Pathol Radiol Endod* 2004, 62:259–260.

77. Michaelson MD, Smith MR: Bisphosphonates for treatment and prevention of bone metastases. *J Clin Oncol* 2005, 23:8219–8224.

78. Porter AT, McEwan AJ, Powe JE, *et al.*: Results of a randomized phase-III trial to evaluate the efficacy of strontium-89 adjuvant to local field external beam irradiation in the management of endocrine resistant metastatic prostate cancer. *Int J Radiat Oncol Biol Phys* 1993, 25:805–813.

79. Sartor O, Reid RH, Hoskin PJ, *et al.*: Quadramet 424SM10/11 Study Group: Samarium-153-Lexidronam complex for treatment of painful bone metastases in hormone-refractory prostate cancer. *Urology* 2004, 63:940–945.

80. Loberg RD, Logothetis CJ, Evan TK, Pienta KJ: Pathogenesis and treatment of prostate cancer bone metastases: targeting the lethal phenotype. *J Clin Oncol* 2005, 23:8232–8241.

81. Pelucchi C, Bosetti C, Negri E, *et al.*: Mechanisms of disease: the epidemiology of bladder cancer. *Nat Clin Pract Urol* 2006, 3:327–340.

82. Sanderson S, Salanti G, Higgins J: Joint effects of the N-acetyltransferase 1 and 2 (NAT1 and NAT2) genes and smoking on bladder carcinogenesis: a literature-based systematic HuGE review and evidence synthesis. *Am J Epidemiol* 2007, 166:741–751.

83. Vena IE, Graham S, Freudenheim J, *et al.*: Diet in the epidemiology of bladder cancer in western New York. *Nutr Cancer* 1992, 18:255–264.

84. Holmang S, Hedelin H, Anderstrom C, *et al.*: The relationship among multiple recurrences, progression and prognosis of patients with stages Ta and T1 transitional cell cancer of the bladder followed for at least 20 years. *J Urol* 1995, 153:1823–1826.

85. Nielsen ME, Schaeffer EM, Veltri RW, *et al.*: Urinary markers in the detection of bladder cancer: what's new? *Curr Opin Urol* 2006, 16:350–355.

86. van Rhijn BW, van der Poel HG, van der Kwast TH: Urine markers for bladder cancer surveillance: a systematic review. *Eur Urol* 2005, 47:736–748.

87. Glas AS, Roos D, Deutekom M, *et al.*: Tumor markers in the diagnosis of primary bladder cancer. A systematic review. *J Urol* 2003; 169:1975–1982.

88. Hemstreet GP III, Yin S, Ma Z, *et al.*: Biomarker risk assessment and bladder cancer detection in a cohort exposed to benzidine. *J Natl Cancer Inst* 2001, 93:427–436.

89. Grossman HB, Messing E, Soloway M, *et al.*: Detection of bladder cancer using a point-of-care proteomic assay. *JAMA* 2005, 293:810–816.

90. Messing EM, Teot L, Korman H, *et al.*: Performance of urine test in patients monitored for recurrence of bladder cancer: a multicenter study in the United States. *J Urol* 2005, 174:1238–1241.

91. Degtyar P, Neulander E, Zirkin H, *et al.*: Fluorescence in situ hybridization performed on exfoliated urothelial cells in patients with transitional cell carcinoma of the bladder. *Urology* 2004, 63:398–401.

92. Skacel M, Fahmy M, Brainard JA, *et al.*: Multitarget fluorescence in situ hybridization assay detects transitional cell carcinoma in the majority of patients with bladder cancer and atypical or negative urine cytology. *J Urol* 2003, 169:2101–2105.

93. Tachibana M, Deguchi N, Baba S, *et al.*: Prognostic significance of bromodeoxyuridine high labeled bladder cancer measured by flow cytometry: does flow cytometric determination predict the prognosis of patients with transitional cell carcinoma of the bladder? *J Urol* 1993, 149:739–743.

94. Esrig D, Elmajian D, Groshen S, *et al.*: Accumulation of nuclear p53 and tumor progression in bladder cancer. *N Engl J Med* 1994, 331:1259–1264.

95. Lacombe L, Dalbagni G, Zhang Z, *et al.*: Overexpression of p53 in a high-risk population of patients with superficial bladder cancer before and after Bacillus Calmette-Guerin therapy: correlation to clinical outcome. *J Clin Oncol* 1996, 14:2646–2652.

96. Dalbagni G: The management of superficial bladder cancer. *Nat Clin Pract Urol* 2007, 4:254–260.

97. Herr HW, Schwalb BM, Zhang Z, *et al.*: Intravesical Bacillus Calmette-Guerin therapy prevents tumor progression and death from superficial bladder cancer: ten-year follow-up of a prospective randomized trial. *J Clin Oncol* 1995, 13:1404–1408.

98. Cookson MS, Herr HW, Zhang Z, *et al.*: The treated natural history of high-risk superficial bladder cancer: 15-year outcome. *J Urol* 1997, 158:62–67.

99. Burnand KG, Boyd PJ, Mayo ME, *et al.*: Single dose intravesical thiotepa as adjuvant to cystodiathermy in the treatment of transitional cell bladder carcinoma. *Br J Urol* 1976, 48:55–59.

100. Lamm OL, Crissman J, Blumenstein B, *et al.*: Adriamycin versus BCG in superficial bladder cancer: a Southwest Oncology Group study. *Prog Clin Biol Res* 1989, 310:263–270.

101. Krege S, Giani G, Meyer R, *et al.*: A randomized multicenter trial of adjuvant therapy in superficial bladder cancer: transurethral resection only versus transurethral resection plus mitomycin-C versus transurethral resection plus Bacillus Calmette-Guerin. *J Urol* 1996, 156:962–966.

102. Witjes JA: Management of BCG failures in superficial bladder cancer: a review. *Eur Urol* 2006, 49:790–797.

103. Einstein AB Jr, Wolf M, Halliday KR, *et al.*: Combination transurethral resection, systemic chemotherapy and pelvic radiotherapy for invasive (T2-T4) bladder cancer unsuitable for cystectomy: a phase I/II SWOG study. *Urology* 1996, 47:652–657.

104. Coppin CM, Gospodarowica MK, James K, *et al.*: Improved local control of invasive bladder cancer by concurrent cisplatin and preoperative or definitive radiation: the NCI Canada Trials Group. *J Clin Oncol* 1996, 14:2901–2907.

105. Kaufman OS, Shipley WU, Griffin PP, *et al.*: Selective bladder preservation by combination treatment of invasive bladder cancer [see comments]. *N Engl J Med* 1993, 329:1377–1382.

106. Shipley WU, Kaufman DS, Heney NM, *et al.*: The integration of chemotherapy, radiotherapy and transurethral surgery in bladder-sparing approaches for patients with invasive tumors. *Prog Clin Biol Res* 1990, 353:85–94.

107. Zietman AL, Shipley WU, Kaufman DS: The combination of cisplatin based chemotherapy and radiation in the treatment of muscle invading transitional cell cancer of the bladder. *Int J Radiat Oncol Biol Phys* 1993. 27:161–170.

108. Tester W, Caplan R, Heany NM, *et al.*: Neoadjuvant combined modality program with selective organ preservation for invasive bladder cancer: results of RTOG phase II trial 8802. *J Clin Oncol* 1996, 14:119–126.

109. Kachnic LA, Kaufman DS, Heney NM, *et al.*: Bladder preservation by combined modality therapy for invasive bladder cancer. *J Clin Oncol* 1997, 15:1022–1029.

110. Stockle M, Meyenburg W, Wellek S, *et al.*: Advanced bladder cancer (stages pT3b, pT4a, pN1, pN2): improved survival after radical cystectomy and 3 adjuvant cycles of chemotherapy. Results of a controlled prospective study. *J Urol* 1992, 148:302–306.

111. Freiha F, Reese I, Torti FM: A randomized trial of radical cystectomy versus radical cystectomy plus cisplatin, vinblastine, and methotrexate chemotherapy for muscle invasive bladder cancer. *J Urol* 1996, 155:495–499.

112. Mead GM, Russel M, Clark P, *et al.*: A randomized trial comparing methotrexate and vinblastine (MV) with cisplatin, methotrexate and vinblastine (CMV) in advanced transitional cell carcinoma: results and a report on prognostic factors, in a Medical Research Council study. MRC Advanced Bladder Cancer Working Party. *Br J Cancer* 1998, 78:1067–1075.

113. Neoadjuvant cisplatin, methotrexate, and vinblastine chemotherapy for muscle-invasive bladder cancer: a randomized controlled trial [international collaboration of trialists]. *Lancet* 1999, 354:526–527.

114. Shipley WU, Winter KA, Kaufman DS, *et al.*: Phase III trial of neoadjuvant chemotherapy in patients with invasive bladder cancer treated with selective bladder preservation by combined radiation therapy and chemotherapy: initial results of Radiation Therapy Oncology Group 8903. *J Clin Oncol* 1999, 17:1327–1328.

115. Hussain SA, James ND: The systemic treatment of advanced and metastatic bladder cancer. *Lancet Oncol* 2003, 4:489–497.

116. Rosenberg JE, Carroll PR, Small EJ: Update on chemotherapy for advanced bladder cancer. *J Urol* 2005, 174:14–20.

117. Loehrer PJ Sr, Einhorn LH, Elson PJ, *et al.*: A randomized comparison of cisplatin alone or in combination with methotrexate, vinblastine, and doxorubicin in patients with metastatic urothelial carcinoma: a cooperative group study. *J Clin Oncol* 1992, 10:1066–1073.

118. Logothetis CJ, Dexeus F, Finn L, *et al.*: A prospective randomized trial comparing CISCA to MVAC chemotherapy in advanced metastatic urothelial tumors. *J Clin Oncol* 1990, 8:1050–1055.

119. Bamias A, Aravantinos G, Deliveliotis C: Docetaxel and cisplatin with granulocyte colony-stimulating factor (G-CSF) versus M-VAC with G-CSF in advanced urothelial carcinoma: a multicenter, randomized, phase III study from the Hellenic Cooperative Oncology Group. *J Clin Oncol* 2004, 22:220–228.

120. Sternberg CN, de Mulder PH, Schornagel JH, *et al.*; the European Organization for Research and Treatment of Cancer Genitourinary Tract Cancer Cooperative Group: Randomized phase III trial of high-dose-intensity methotrexate, vinblastine, doxorubicin, and cisplatin (MVAC) chemotherapy and recombinant human granulocyte colony-stimulating factor versus classic MVAC in advanced urothelial tract tumors: European Organization for Research and Treatment of Cancer Protocol no. 30924. *J Clin Oncol* 2001, 19:2638–2646.

121. von der Maase H, Hansen SW, Roberts JT, *et al.*: Gemcitabine and cisplatin versus methotrexate, vinblastine, doxorubicin and cisplatin in advanced or metastatic bladder cancer: results of a large, randomized, multinational, multicenter phase III study. *J Clin Oncol* 2000, 17:3068–3077.

122. Karumanchi SA, Merchan J, Sukhatme VP: Renal cancer: molecular mechanisms and newer therapeutic options. *Curr Opin Nephrol Hypertens* 2002, 11:37–42.

123. McCredie M, Stewart JH: Risk factors for kidney cancer in New South Wales: IV. Occupation. *J Indust Med* 1993, 50:349–354.

124. van der Hout AH, van den Berg E, van der Vlies P, *et al.*: Loss of heterozygosity at the short arm of chromosome 3 in renal-cell cancer correlates with the cytological tumor type. *Int J Cancer* 1993, 53:353–357.

125. McCredie M, Stewart JH, Day NE: Different roles for phenacetin and paracetamol in cancer of the kidney and renal pelvis. *Int J Cancer* 1993, 53:245–249.

126. McCredie M, Stewart JH: Risk factors for kidney cancer in New South Wales: I. Cigarette smoking. *Eur J Cancer* 1992, 28A:2050–2054.

127. La Vecchia C, Negri E, D'Avanzo B, Franceschi S: Smoking and renal cell carcinoma. *Cancer Res* 1990, 50:5231–5233.

128. DeVita VT Jr, Hellman S, Rosenberg SA, *et al.*: *Cancer Principles and Practice of Oncology*, 7th ed. Philadelphia, PA: Lippincott Williams & Wilkins: 2004.

129. Choyke PL: Hereditary renal cancers. *Radiology* 2003, 226:33–46.

130. Herman JG, Latif F, Weng Y, *et al.*: Silencing of the VHL tumor-suppressor gene by DNA methylation in renal carcinoma. *Proc Natl Acad Sci U S A* 1994, 91:9700–9404.

131. Thiel DD, Winfield HN: State-of-the-art surgical management of renal cell carcinoma. *Expert Rev Anticancer Ther* 2007, 7:1285–1294.

132. Zisman A, Pantuck AJ, Wieder J, *et al.*: Risk assessment and clinical outcome algorithm to predict the natural history of patients with surgically resected renal cell carcinoma. *J Clin Oncol* 2002, 20:4559–4566.

133. Messing EM, Manola J, Wilding G, *et al.*; Eastern Cooperative Oncology Group/Intergroup: Phase III study of interferon alfa-NL as adjuvant treatment for resectable renal cell carcinoma: an Eastern Cooperative Oncology Group/Intergroup trial. *J Clin Oncol* 2003, 21:1214–1222.

134. Clark JI, Atkins MB, Urba WJ, *et al.*: Adjuvant high-dose bolus interleukin-2 for patients with high-risk renal cell carcinoma: a Cytokine Working Group randomized trial. *J Clin Oncol* 2003, 21:3133–3140.

135. Kavolius JP, Mastorakos DP, Pavlovich C, *et al.*: Resection of metastatic renal cell carcinoma. *J Clin Oncol* 1998, 16:2261–2266.

136. Flanigan RC, Salmon SE, Blumenstein BA, *et al.*: Nephrectomy followed by interferon-alfa-2b compared with interferon alfa-2b alone for metastatic renal-cell cancer. *N Engl J Med* 2001, 345:1655–1659.

137. Mickisch GH, Garin A, van Poppel H, *et al.*: Radical nephrectomy plus interferon-alfa-based immunotherapy compared with interferon alfa alone in metastatic renal-cell carcinoma: a randomised trial. *Lancet* 2001, 358:966–970.

138. Flanigan RC, Mickisch GH, Sylvester R, *et al.*: Cytoreductive nephrectomy in patients with metastatic renal cancer: a combined analysis. *J Urol* 2004, 171:1071–1076.

139. Negrier S, Escudier B, Lasset C, *et al.*: Recombinant human interleukin-2, recombinant human interferon alfa-2a, or both in patients with metastatic renal-cell carcinoma. *N Engl J Med* 1998, 338:1273–1278.

140. Yang JC, Topalian SL, Parkinson D, *et al.*: Randomized comparison of high-dose and low-dose intravenous interleukin-2 for the therapy of metastatic renal cell carcinoma: an interim report. *J Clin Oncol* 1994, 12:1572–1576.

141. Quesada JR, Swanson DA, Gutterman JU: Phase II study of interferon alpha in metastatic renal cell carcinoma: a progress report. *J Clin Oncol* 1985, 3:1086–1092.

142. Kirkwood JM, Harris JE, Vera R, *et al.*: A randomized study of low and high doses of leukocyte alpha-interferon in metastatic renal cell carcinoma: the American Cancer Society Collaborative Trial. *Cancer Res* 1985, 45:863–871.

143. Atkins MB, Sparano J, Fisher RI, *et al.*: Randomized phase II trial of high-dose interleukin-2 either alone or in combination with interferon alfa-2b in advanced renal cell carcinoma. *J Clin Oncol* 1993, 11:661–670.

144. Ebbinghaus SW, Gordon MS: Renal cell carcinoma: rationale and development of therapeutic inhibitors of angiogenesis. *Hematol Oncol Clin North Am* 2004, 18:1143–1159.

145. Faivre S, Demetri G, Sargent W, Raymond E: Molecular basis for sunitinib efficacy and future clinical development. *Nat Rev Drug Discov* 2007, 6:734–745.

146. Motzer RJ, Michaelson MD, Redman BG, *et al.*: Activity of SU11248, a multitargeted inhibitor of vascular endothelial growth factor receptor and platelet-derived growth factor receptor, in patients with metastatic renal cell carcinoma. *J Clin Oncol* 2006, 24:16–24.

147. Motzer RJ, Hutson TE, Tomczak P, *et al.*: Sunitinib versus interferon alfa in metastatic renal-cell carcinoma. *N Engl J Med* 2007, 356:115–124.

148. Wilhelm S, Chien DS: BAY 43-9006: preclinical data. *Curr Pharm Des* 2002, 8:2255–2257.

149. Hilger RA, Scheulen ME, Strumberg D: The Ras-Raf-MEK-ERK pathway in the treatment of cancer. *Onkologie* 2002, 25:511–518.

150. Wilhelm SM, Carter C, Tang L, *et al.*: BAY 43-9006 exhibits broad spectrum oral anti-tumor activity and targets the Raf/MEK/ERK pathway and receptor tyrosine kinases involved in tumor progression and angiogenesis. *Cancer Res* 2004, 64:7099–7109.

151. Ratain MJ, Eisen E, Stadler WM, *et al.*: Phase II placebo-controlled randomized discontinuation Trial of sorafenib in patients with metastatic renal cell carcinoma. *J Clin Oncol* 2006, 24:2505–2512.

152. Escudier B, Eisen T, Stadler WM, *et al.*; TARGET Study Group: Sorafenib in advanced clear-cell renal-cell carcinoma. *N Engl J Med* 2007, 356:125–134.

153. Dudkin L, Dilling MB, Cheshire PJ, *et al.*: Biochemical correlates of mTOR inhibition by the rapamycin ester CCI-779 and tumor growth inhibition. *Clin Cancer Res* 2001, 7:1758–1764.

154. Neshat MS, Mellinghoff IK, Tran C, *et al.*: Enhanced sensitivity of PTEN-deficient tumors to inhibition of FRAP/mTOR. *Proc Natl Acad Sci U S A* 2001, 98:10314–10319.

155. Hudson CC, Liu M, Chiang GG, *et al.*: Regulation of hypoxia-inducible factor 1alpha expression and function by the mammalian target of rapamycin. *Mol Cell Biol* 2002, 22:7004–7014.

156. Atkins MB, Hidalgo M, Stadler WM, *et al.*: Randomized phase II study of multiple dose levels of CCI-779, a novel mammalian target of rapamycin kinase inhibitor, in patients with advanced refractory renal cell carcinoma. *J Clin Oncol* 2004, 22:909–918.

157. Hudes G, Carducci M, Tomczak P, *et al.*; Global ARCC Trial: Temsirolimus, interferon alfa, or both for advanced renal-cell carcinoma. *N Engl J Med* 2007, 356:2271–2281.

158. Yang JC, Haworth L, Sherry RM, *et al.*: A randomized trial of bevacizumab, an anti-vascular endothelial growth factor antibody, for metastatic renal cancer. *N Engl J Med* 2003, 349:427–434.

159. Yang YC: Bevacizumab for patients with metastatic renal cancer: an update. *Clin Cancer Res* 2004, 10:6367S–6370S.

160. Escudier B, Koralewski P, Pluzanska A, *et al.*; AVOREN investigators: A randomized, controlled, double-blind phase III study (AVOREN) of bevacizumab/interferon-alpha2a vs placebo/interferon-alpha2a as first-line therapy in metastatic renal cell carcinoma [abstract]. *J Clin Oncol* 2007, 25(18S):3.

161. Kaelin WG: The von Hippel-Lindau tumor suppressor protein and kidney cancer. *Clin Cancer Res* 2004, 10:6290S–6295S.

Tumors of the female reproductive tract vary greatly in epidemiology, histology, natural history, clinical behavior, and methods of diagnosis and treatment. Optimal treatment outcome requires close communication between the gynecologist, gynecologic oncologist, medical and radiation oncologists, and imaging specialists. Tumor types discussed in this section include epithelial ovarian cancer, cervical cancer, and uterine cancer (Table 14-1).

EPITHELIAL OVARIAN CANCER

ETIOLOGY, RISK FACTORS, AND SCREENING

The lifetime incidence for ovarian malignancies is approximately 1 in 70 (1%–2% lifetime risk) for women in the United States [1]. Cancers of the fallopian tube and primary peritoneal carcinomas have a similar etiology, natural history, and response to treatment as ovarian cancer; thus, the information provided here is applicable to all three malignancies. Epithelial tumors comprise approximately 95% of all ovarian malignancies, occurring most commonly in the sixth and seventh decades of life. While a clear etiologic factor responsible for the development of ovarian cancer has not been identified, the risk of the disease is inversely proportional to the number of lifetime ovulations. Thus factors associated with suppression of ovulation, such as increasing number of full-term pregnancies, longer duration of lactation, and oral contraceptive use, are associated with a decrease in ovarian cancer. Factors associated with increased lifetime ovulation such as nulliparity or prolonged exposure to ovarian hormones with menopausal hormone replacement therapy increase risk [2]. Inflammatory conditions also appear to affect ovarian cancer risk; endometriosis increases risk whereas tubal ligation and hysterectomy without oophorectomy (procedures that alter ovarian environmental exposure) reduce risk. While these hormonal, reproductive, and environmental factors mildly alter ovarian cancer risk, genetic factors have the most potent impact on ovarian cancer risk.

ROLE OF GENETIC MUTATIONS

Approximately 10% of epithelial ovarian cancers are associated with inheritance of an autosomal dominant genetic aberration, which confers cancer predisposition with a high penetrance. Perhaps the most important new dimension in understanding the etiology of some cancers of the ovary was the discovery of the role of mutations in the BRCA genes. The BRCA1 gene, located on chromosome 17q, and the BRCA2 gene located on chromosome 13q are tumor suppressor genes. Inheritance of a deleterious mutation in one of these BRCA genes is associated with a 45% to 85% lifetime risk of breast cancer and a 27% to 44% lifetime risk of ovarian cancer compared with 1.6% in the general population. The age of onset of ovarian cancer is significantly earlier in women with a BRCA1 mutation compared with a BRCA2 mutation, whereas overall ovarian cancer risk is slightly lower in women with a BRCA2 mutation [3]. It is estimated that between 1/300 and 1/800 non-Ashkenazi white women harbor a BRCA mutation. However the BRCA mutation carrier rate is higher in certain populations, most notably, in the Ashkenazi Jewish population, in whom the carrier rate is 2.1% [4].

In addition to mutations in the BRCA genes, a higher incidence of ovarian cancer is observed in women who are members of families characterized by the Lynch II syndrome (hereditary nonpolyposis colorectal cancer [HNPCC]). These families are characterized by a higher incidence and earlier onset of carcinomas of the colon, gastrointestinal tract, ovary, and uterus. The HNPCC syndrome is characterized by mutations in any of four mismatch repair genes (hMSH2, hMLH1, hPMS1, and hPMS2) [3]. Risk factors for ovarian cancer are shown in Table 14-2.

SCREENING FOR OVARIAN CANCER

Screening the general population is neither cost-effective nor practical; however, certain subpopulations of patients—primarily those defined by the genetic risk factors described above—may be candidates for ovarian cancer screening. Three screening tests are currently employed: bimanual pelvic examination, cancer antigen (CA)-125, and transvaginal ultrasound. The pelvic examination is cost-effective and reliable when done by experienced hands, but it lacks adequate sensitivity and specificity as a screening test. It is estimated that physical examination detects only 1 in 10,000 ovarian carcinomas in asymptomatic women. The radioimmunoassay for CA-125, a tumor-specific antigen, is elevated in 80% of ovarian carcinomas, but only in 50% of women with cancer limited to the ovary. It may also be elevated in women with benign ovarian disease and in otherwise healthy women, which limits its specificity.

Ultrasound techniques are not only expensive but also limited in their specificity and sensitivity. In one published study, 4526 high-risk women underwent ultrasound every 6 months. There were 49 invasive surgical procedures, 37 for benign tumors and 12 for gynecologic malignancies. The detected malignancies were ovarian, peritoneal, or fallopian tube carcinoma in 10 women, all stage III, and stage IA endometrial adenocarcinoma in two women [5]. The authors concluded that ultrasound was of limited value for detection of early-stage epithelial ovarian cancer in asymptomatic high-risk women. Thus, although no data demonstrate that screening reduces the mortality of the disease even in the higher-risk groups, women who are at the highest risk should at least have an annual bimanual pelvic examination, assay for CA-125, and transvaginal ultrasound. Prophylactic oophorectomy is the most definitive risk reduction for ovarian cancer and

Table 14-1. Common Tumors of the Female Genital Tract

Ovary

Epithelial

Stromal

Germ cell

Metastatic

Cervix

Squamous cell carcinoma

Adenocarcinoma

Adenosquamous carcinoma

Uterus

Adenocarcinoma

Sarcoma

  Leiomyosarcoma

  Mixed mesodermal tumors/Carcinosarcoma

  Endometrial stromal sarcoma

Table 14-2. Risk Factors for Development of Ovarian Cancer

Increased risk	Decreased risk
Increasing age	Multiparity
Nulliparity	Lactation
Infertility	Hysterectomy
Menopausal HRT	Oral contraceptive use
Endometriosis	Tubal ligation
BRCA mutation	
Hereditary nonpolyposis colorectal cancer	

HRT—hormone replacement therapy.

should be considered in women with a known deleterious *BRCA* mutation who have completed childbearing.

DIAGNOSIS AND MANAGEMENT OF OVARIAN CANCER

MANAGEMENT OF THE ADNEXAL MASS

Detection of an adnexal mass either by physical or radiographic examination requires a management strategy. Although most are benign, between 13% and 21% of women undergoing surgery for a suspicious mass will have an ovarian malignancy. Recommendation for surgery depends on the degree of suspicion that this mass may be malignant; factors that should be considered include age, menopausal status, family history, size and complexity of the mass, associated symptoms, CA-125, unilaterality versus bilaterality, and characteristics on ultrasound. Management may include observation with repeat examination, further radiographic imaging, and laparoscopy or laparotomy depending on the clinical circumstances.

SURGERY FOR EPITHELIAL OVARIAN CANCER

While ovarian cancer can spread hematogenously or via the lymphatic system, the bulk of the tumor will be found on peritoneal surfaces. This peritoneal disease results from shedding of ovarian tumor cells into the peritoneal cavity, circulation of these cells throughout the abdomen and pelvis, and eventual implantation onto peritoneal surfaces. Viability and growth of these cells and successful tumor growth is further dependent upon the development of sufficient neovasculature to support cell survival and tumor growth.

This unique pattern of spread within the relatively accessible peritoneal cavity has led to attempts at surgical cytoreduction before administration of systemic chemotherapy. Dating back more than 30 years, nearly every study has demonstrated an inverse correlation between volume of tumor remaining at the completion of initial surgery and overall survival for patients with ovarian cancer [6]. While these data are almost exclusively retrospective, the consistency of the observation of improved outcome with surgical debulking has led to the goal of "optimal" tumor cytoreduction to no macroscopic visible disease with initial diagnostic surgery. Patients who have had only a biopsy, paracentesis, or incomplete debulking may be referred to an experienced gynecologic oncologist for consideration for reoperation given the effect of initial surgery on clinical outcome. It should be recognized that it is unique among solid tumors to attempt maximal surgical cytoreduction in the presence of widespread disease outside of the organ of origin.

The goals of initial surgery in ovarian cancer are thus to diagnose and stage disease and to provide therapeutic benefit with cytoreduction. Precise histologic diagnosis and accurate staging are required before treatment.

Table 14-3. Staging and Prognosis of Ovarian Carcinoma

Stage	Characteristics	3-y survival, %
I	Disease confined to the ovaries	92.4
IA	One ovary, capsule intact, no ascites	
IB	Both ovaries, capsule intact, no ascites	
IC	IA or IB plus ascites or washings, capule ruptures, tumor on ovarian surface	
II	Disease confined to the pelvis	71.4
III	Disease confined to the abdominal cavity, including surface of the liver, pelvic, inguinal, or para-aortic lymph node, omentum, or bowel	29.8
IIIA	Negative nodes, plus microscopic seeding of peritoneal surfaces	
IIIB	Negative nodes, peritoneal implants ≤ 2 cm	
IIIC	Positive nodes and/or abdominal implants > 2 cm	
IV	Spread to liver parenchyma, lung, pleura, or other extra-abdominal site	10.4

(*Adapted from* International Federation of Gynecology and Obstetrics [7], and http://seer.cancer.gov/csr/1975_2004/results_merged/sect_21_ovary.pdf.)

The International Federation of Gynecology and Obstetrics (FIGO) staging system of 1989 [7] is outlined in Table 14-3. Staging laparotomy requires thorough inspection of the entire peritoneal cavity including the gutters, pelvis, and domes of the diaphragm, total abdominal hysterectomy and bilateral salpingo-oophorectomy, liver palpation and biopsy, lymph node sampling, omentectomy, and peritoneal washings. If surgical debulking is incomplete, the surgeon must estimate the size and extent of residual tumor.

TREATMENT OF EARLY-STAGE (STAGES I AND II) OVARIAN CARCINOMA

Specific ovarian carcinoma treatment recommendations are dependent on the stage of the disease and extent of surgical debulking. Approximately 25% of women with ovarian cancer have disease confined to one or both ovaries (FIGO stage I) or to the pelvis (FIGO stage II). Even among this good-prognosis group, the failure rate is high enough to warrant adjuvant chemotherapy in many patients. The Gynecologic Oncology Group (GOG) has attempted to precisely define the subgroups that would benefit from adjuvant therapy and determine the optimal form of therapy for these patients. Studies over the past three decades have shown that patients with stage Ia or Ib disease (growth limited to one or both ovaries with no ascites and negative peritoneal washings) and with well- or moderately differentiated histology have a 5-year disease-free survival rate of 91% and overall survival rate of 94% with surgery alone; thus this subset of patients does well and should not receive adjuvant therapy. In contrast, chemotherapy improves progression-free survival for patients with stage Ia or Ib poorly differentiated disease, stage IC disease, or stage II disease, and these patients should receive adjuvant chemotherapy [8].

The rarity of early-stage ovarian cancer has made it difficult to perform studies in this group of patients. The most recently reported phase 3 study in this population compared three versus six cycles of paclitaxel and carboplatin [9]. The 5-year probability of recurrence was 20.1% for six cycles versus 25.4% for three cycles, a 24% reduction in recurrence risk. However, the overall survival was similar for both regimens and the decrease in recurrence risk did not reach statistical significance. Based on this study, most recommend a minimum of three cycles of paclitaxel and carboplatin for early-stage patients who are treated with adjuvant chemotherapy.

TREATMENT OF ADVANCED-STAGE (STAGES III AND IV) OVARIAN CARCINOMA

Approximately 75% of women with ovarian carcinoma present with stage III or IV disease [10]. As noted above, prognosis correlates with extent of residual disease following primary debulking surgery. While this is best documented in patients with stage III disease, even patients with stage IV disease have an improved prognosis with optimal debulking. The contemporary definition for optimal disease is no residual implant greater than 1 cm. It is clear that this is a continuum with those with the least tumor burden following surgery having the best prognosis and with prognosis worsening as the diameter of the smallest residual lesion increases [6].

TREATMENT OF OPTIMALLY DEBULKED DISEASE

The long-term overall survival rate for women with optimally debulked stage III disease is approximately 25%; thus, an appreciable cure rate is found in women treated with aggressive initial surgery followed by platinum-based chemotherapy. Following surgery, all women should receive at least six cycles of platinum-based therapy with either cisplatin or carboplatin in combination with a taxane, usually paclitaxel. If cisplatin is used, patients require careful monitoring of renal function, electrolytes, and neurologic status. Because nephrotoxicity and neurotoxicity are cumulative, cisplatin dosing should be modified early if there is any indication of renal dysfunction or for progressive sensory neuropathy. Based on the results of GOG protocol 158, systemic treatment with carboplatin and 3-hour paclitaxel is equivalent to cisplatin and 24-hour paclitaxel, with an improved toxicity profile [11].

For women with optimally debulked ovarian cancer, the major controversy concerns the route, intravenous (IV) or intraperitoneal (IP), by which the drug is to be optimally administered. Three randomized trials comparing IV with IP chemotherapy have shown a clinical benefit for use of the IP approach. The first trial, led by the Southwest Oncology Group, used IV cyclophosphamide in combination with cisplatin administered either IP or IV. This study showed a survival advantage for the group receiving IP cisplatin (49 vs 41 months; $P = 0.02$; relative risk [RR] 0.76), and there was a significant reduction in sensory neuropathy with IP therapy [12]. The second study compared a standard IV paclitaxel and cisplatin regimen with two cycles of high-dose carboplatin IV at an area under the curve (AUC) of 9 followed by six cycles of IV paclitaxel and IP cisplatin. This study showed an improvement in progression-free survival (28 vs 22 months; P = 0.01; RR 0.78) and overall survival (63 vs 52 months; P = 0.05; RR 0.81) for the IP regimen [13]. The third study compared the same standard IV paclitaxel and cisplatin to an intensive regimen of IV paclitaxel with IP cisplatin and IP paclitaxel. This study also showed an improvement in progression-free survival (24 vs 18 months; P = 0.80; RR 0.80) and overall survival (66 vs 50 months; P = 0.03; RR 0.75) for the IP regimen [14]. The latter two studies showed increased toxicity for the IP regimen compared with the IV regimen and fewer patients able to complete assigned IP therapy compared with those assigned to IV therapy. However, the consistency of improvement across these studies led to a clinical alert from the National Cancer Institute about the use of IP therapy in optimally debulked disease [15]. Current efforts are focusing on ways to improve tolerability of IP using contemporary supportive care measures, modification of the regimens, and use of carboplatin in place of cisplatin for IP administration. It should be noted that the use of IP therapy for suboptimally debulked disease has not been widely accepted. Most such patients will still receive systemic therapy, which is considered next.

TREATMENT OF SUBOPTIMAL STAGE III AND STAGE IV DISEASE

Women who have residual disease larger than 1 cm after initial debulking surgery have a substantially worse prognosis than those with optimally debulked disease. Nevertheless, a small proportion of these women will have long-term disease-free survival. In contrast, women with disease outside the abdominal cavity or in the liver parenchyma, making them stage IV, have a worse prognosis and rarely have long-term disease-free survival. In addition to residual tumor volume, other factors associated with a poor prognosis include advanced age, mucinous or clear cell histology, large-volume ascites, grade 3 histology, aneuploidy, and increased S-phase.

Evidence clearly demonstrates that chemotherapy prolongs survival in women with stage III disease, whether optimally or suboptimally debulked, and possibly in stage IV disease. Thus, women in these disease categories should be encouraged to receive chemotherapy as a treatment option following surgery. Although there are many active agents for treatment of ovarian cancer, the standard of care is combination therapy that includes a taxane and a platinum compound.

Fifteen years ago, combination chemotherapy with paclitaxel plus cisplatin as administered in GOG 111 became the standard of care for patients with advanced ovarian cancer [16]. The superiority of this regimen over the older cyclophosphamide and cisplatin regimen was confirmed in a European Organization for Research and Treatment of Cancer (EORTC) study [17]. The latter trial used 3-hour paclitaxel with cisplatin and demonstrated an increased incidence of high-grade neurotoxicity. Based on the notable differences in neurotoxicity between these two trials, the standard of care is to use a prolonged 24-hour paclitaxel infusion when combined with cisplatin to decrease neurotoxicity.

A subsequent study, GOG 132, compared treatment with high-dose cisplatin 100 mg/m² as a single agent with high-dose paclitaxel 200 mg/m² as a single agent, versus paclitaxel 135 mg/m² plus cisplatin 75 mg/m² administered concurrently. All regimens were given every 3 weeks for six cycles to women with suboptimally debulked disease [18]. Results of this trial failed to demonstrate the same median survival for women treated with the combination as in GOG 111. Furthermore, women who received cisplatin as a single agent or in combination with paclitaxel had equivalent survival rates, whereas women receiving paclitaxel alone had an inferior result. This is the only study in the current era using a non–platinum-containing treatment for newly diagnosed patients and it demonstrates the superiority of platinum-based therapies. Given that the combination of cisplatin and paclitaxel was less toxic than cisplatin alone, and that more patients were able to complete therapy, the combination was considered the treatment of choice.

Docetaxel was examined as a replacement for paclitaxel in the Scottish Randomised Trial in Ovarian Cancer (SCOTROC) study. This study compared carboplatin AUC 5 with either paclitaxel 175 mg/m² every 3 hours

or docetaxel 75 mg/m²/h. There were no differences in progression-free survival (14.8 vs 15 months) or in 2-year survival (68.9% vs 64.2%) for paclitaxel/carboplatin compared with docetaxel/carboplatin, respectively [19]. There were more myelosuppression and hypersensitivity reactions on the docetaxel arm and more neurotoxicity and arthralgia/myalgia on the paclitaxel arm. The conclusion from the study was that docetaxel/carboplatin was an alternative first-line chemotherapy regimen for ovarian cancer.

More recently, the GOG and the Gynecologic Cancer Intergroup evaluated the addition of a third drug to the paclitaxel/carboplatin backbone for initial therapy of ovarian cancer. More than 4000 women with newly diagnosed stage III or IV ovarian cancer were randomized to receive carboplatin/paclitaxel or one of four experimental regimens containing a third drug: a triplet of carboplatin/paclitaxel and gemcitabine; a triplet of carboplatin/paclitaxel and liposomal doxorubicin; a sequential doublet of carboplatin/topotecan followed by carboplatin/paclitaxel; or a sequential doublet of gemcitabine/carboplatin followed by carboplatin/paclitaxel. There was no difference in median progression-free survival (15.3–16.4 months) or median overall survival (39.1–42.8 months) for any of the experimental regimens compared with carboplatin/paclitaxel [20].

Some controversy exists regarding the appropriate doses of carboplatin and paclitaxel to use in this setting. The above trials have used carboplatin at an AUC ranging from 4 to 7.5 and paclitaxel at 150 to 175 mg/m² over 3 hours or 135 mg/m² over 24 hours. While some have argued that there is a dose-response effect for carboplatin, the overall comparable results from these trials argue against this point. Most now use an AUC of 6 for initial chemotherapy. A summary of results from randomized trials of taxane and platinum therapy are shown in Table 14-4 [9,11,13,14,16,19–22].

DURATION OF THERAPY AND EVALUATION OF THE PATIENT ON THERAPY

Other considerations in the treatment of these patients must include the following findings. Before treatment, levels of the ovarian tumor marker CA-125 should be measured and, if elevated, should be used as adjunctive evidence of response to therapy. Levels should be measured routinely during the course of treatment. A consistent rise in CA-125 can be used as a measure of failure of treatment in the absence of radiographic and clinical changes. Likewise, a linear fall in serum levels of CA-125 can be used as a measure of treatment success in the absence of radiographic and clinical changes. Incorporation of CA-125 is a critical element in treatment. Levels of carcinoembryonic antigen (CEA) and CA-19 may be elevated in women with mucinous carcinomas and may be potentially useful in following the course of the disease.

Treatment should consist of six to eight cycles of therapy administered every 3 weeks or monthly. Residual disease should be measured before beginning therapy by visual inspection at the time of surgery, by CT scan if bulk disease remains, or by physical examination or chest radiograph when appropriate. Levels of CA-125 are followed as already described. If these levels rise or fail to decrease, resistance to treatment should be suspected. The role of positron emission tomography (PET) scanning is currently being investigated and may add to the therapeutic investigation of these patients.

EVALUATION OF THE PATIENT AFTER INITIAL THERAPY

Following six to eight cycles of initial chemotherapy, patients who are clinically responding should be reevaluated regularly with physical examination and CA-125 levels. CT scanning is sometimes used as an adjunct for follow-up, particularly in patients in whom CA-125 is not a reliable marker. Patients whose disease has clinically progressed through initial therapy have a very poor prognosis [23]. Options for these patients include further treatment with a non–platinum-containing regimen as for platinum-resistant disease, or investigational therapy.

TREATMENT OF RECURRENT OVARIAN CANCER

Once recurrent ovarian cancer is diagnosed, the goals of therapy should be carefully reviewed. In the recurrent setting, excessively aggressive therapy can limit future treatment options, impair quality of life, and lead to a compromise in drug dose and schedule. Patients may be under the impression that aggressive treatment can still result in cure. Unfortunately, the cumulative experience with recurrent ovarian cancer is that, while it is highly treatable, it is generally not curable. Patients with an early, platinum-resistant relapse rarely achieve a complete response from any therapy and will likely be on some type of treatment for the majority of their remaining life. Even patients who relapse late and respond completely to second-line therapy will have a second remission that is shorter than the first in more than 95% of cases [24]. The goals of treatment of recurrent ovarian cancer are thus to prolong survival, to delay time to progression, to control disease-related symptoms, to minimize treatment-related symptoms, and to maintain or improve quality of life.

Patients with recurrent disease are commonly characterized as platinum sensitive or platinum resistant. While this definition is useful for clinical trial purposes and to determine the optimal approach to treatment, it does have limitations. The definition of platinum-resistant disease includes patients who progress while receiving initial chemotherapy (sometimes called platinum refractory), or within 6 months of completing initial platinum-based chemotherapy. This definition has been used to determine eligibility for clinical trials, most of which require disease that is measurable using traditional imaging modalities such as CT. Thus, most of the data regarding efficacy of treatment in this group of patients are limited to those meeting this criteria. Patients who are determined to recur based solely on more sensitive criteria such as CA-125 or PET imaging generally have lower volume disease and may respond better than those with larger-volume, traditionally measurable disease.

TREATMENT OF PLATINUM-SENSITIVE RECURRENT OVARIAN CANCER

Platinum-sensitive patients are defined by relapse six or more months after completion of initial chemotherapy. Platinum-sensitive disease is a spectrum ranging from relatively less platinum-sensitive patients who relapse shortly after the 6-month benchmark, to those recurring more than 12 to 18 months after completing initial treatment. A common observation is that the response to platinum retreatment increases with a longer interval from prior platinum. Because there are compelling data that cytoreductive surgery improves survival for patients with newly diagnosed ovarian cancer, the issue of surgery is appropriate to address in a highly platinum-sensitive recurrent patient with potentially resectable disease.

Recent randomized trials have compared single-agent platinum with platinum-based combinations in this group of patients. The first study was from the International Collaborative Ovarian Neoplasm (ICON) Group and Arbeitsgemeinschaft Gynakologische Onkologie Studiengruppe Ovarialkarzinom (AGO-OVAR) comparing single-agent platinum with paclitaxel plus platinum chemotherapy [25]. Compared with the carboplatin arm, the paclitaxel/platinum arm had an improvement in response rate (54% vs 66%), time to progres-

sion (9 vs 12 months), 1-year progression-free survival rate (40% vs 50%), median survival (24 vs 29 months), and 2-year survival (50% vs 57%).

A second study, AGO-OVAR 2.5, randomized platinum-sensitive patients to carboplatin (AUC 4 on day 1) with gemcitabine (1000 mg/m^2 on days 1 and 8) or carboplatin alone (AUC 5) [26]. Compared with single-agent carboplatin, the combination arm had an improved response rate (31% vs 47%) and an improved progression-free survival (5.8 vs 8.6 months). However, there were no significant differences in overall survival for the two arms (17.3 vs 18 months). The improved outcome for the gemcitabine/carboplatin arm provides an alternative to taxane/carboplatin therapy with less neurotoxicity and alopecia, which are toxicities that can negatively impact quality of life for many patients.

A third randomized study in recurrent platinum-sensitive ovarian cancer has completed accrual but has not yet been reported for therapeutic efficacy. The CALYPSO GCIG (Gynecologic Cancer Intergroup) study compared paclitaxel (175 mg/m^2) and carboplatin (AUC = 5) every 21 days with the combination of pegylated liposomal doxorubicin (30 mg/m^2) and carboplatin (AUC = 5) every 28 days. Toxicity has been reported for the first 500 patients in the study [27]. This showed more myelosuppression, mucositis, and hand-foot syndrome for patients treated with pegylated liposomal doxorubicin and carboplatin, and more alopecia, neuropathy, and hypersensitivity/allergic reactions in patients treated with paclitaxel and carboplatin. Overall, there were fewer drug-related adverse events and less early termination of therapy in the carboplatin/pegylated liposomal doxorubicin arm. Progression-free survival was the primary end point for this trial and results of this analysis are awaited. The recommendations for treatment of recurrent, platinum-sensitive ovarian cancer are summarized in Table 14-5.

TREATMENT OF RECURRENT PLATINUM-RESISTANT OVARIAN CANCER

Most recurrent ovarian cancer patients will eventually develop platinum-resistant disease. In general, platinum-resistant patients will be treated with sequential single agents rather than combination therapy. Table 14-6 lists common chemotherapy agents used in the treatment of recurrent platinum-resistant ovarian cancer. Topotecan was first used as a "daily × 5" regimen using the drug for five consecutive days on a 3-week schedule [28]. This regimen results in a high degree of myelosuppression and is poorly tolerated past second- or third-line therapy. More recently, weekly topotecan has been documented to be active in platinum-resistant disease [29]. The weekly topotecan regimen has much less myelosuppression and alopecia than the "daily × 5" regimen, and is better tolerated as treatment in more

Table 14-4. Randomized Trials of Taxane and Platinum Therapy in Ovarian Cancer

Study	Population	Treatment	PFS*	OS*
Bell *et al.* [9] (GOG 157)	Stage I and II	IV paclitaxel + IV carboplatin for 6 cycles	80% (5 y)	83% (5 y)
		IV paclitaxel + IV carboplatin for 3 cycles	75% (5 y)	82% (5 y)
Armstrong *et al.* [14] (GOG 172)	Optimal stage III	IV paclitaxel + IP cisplatin + IP paclitaxel	24 mo	66 mo
		IV paclitaxel + IV cisplatin	18 mo	50 mo
Markman *et al.* [13] (GOG 114)	Optimal stage III	IV carboplatin + IV paclitaxel + IP cisplatin	28 mo	63 mo
		IV pacitaxel + IV cisplatin	22 mo	52 mo
Ozols *et al.* [11] (GOG 158)	Optimal stage III	IV paclitaxel + IV carboplatin	22 mo	57 mo
		IV paclitaxel + IV cisplatin	19 mo	49 mo
McGuire *et al.* [16] (GOG 111)	Suboptimal stage III and IV	IV paclitaxel + IV cisplatin	18 mo	38 mo
Rose *et al.* [22] (GOG 152)	Suboptimal stage III and IV	IV paclitaxel + IV cisplatin	11 mo	34 mo
Spriggs *et al.* [21] (GOG 162)	Suboptimal stage III and IV	IV paclitaxel + IV cisplatin	12 mo	30 mo
Vasey *et al.* [19] (SCOTROC)	Stage IC–IV	IV docetaxel + IV carboplatin	15 mo	23 mo
		IV paclitaxel + IV carboplatin	15 mo	23 mo
Bookman *et al.* [20] (GOG 182)	All stage III and IV	IV paclitaxel + IV carboplatin for 8 cycles	16 mo	40 mo

*Months indicate median values.
GOG—Gynecologic Oncology Group; IP—intraperitoneal; IV—intravenous; OS—overall survival; PFS—progression-free survival; SCOTROC—Scottish Randomised Trial in Ovarian Cancer.

heavily pretreated patients. The weekly topotecan regimen has not been directly compared with the "daily × 5" regimen to formally compare efficacy; however, the improved tolerance of the weekly regimen has led to the more common use of this schedule.

Pegylated liposomal doxorubicin also has documented efficacy in recurrent platinum-resistant ovarian cancer [28]. It has unique toxicities of hand-foot syndrome and mucositis, although these toxicities are not common and do not usually limit therapy. The convenience of the once-every-28-days treatment and the relative lack of myelosuppression make this a favored regimen in treatment of recurrent disease. Pegylated liposomal doxorubicin and topotecan have been compared in a randomized phase 3 trial [28]. Results showed similar response rates in patients with platinum-resistant disease with no significant differences in response, progression-free survival, or overall survival.

Gemcitabine has been compared with pegylated liposomal doxorubicin in a randomized phase 3 trial in patients who recurred within 12 months of completion of initial chemotherapy [30]. In this trial, 56% of patients were platinum refractory, having relapsed within 6 months of completing initial chemotherapy. Compared with the pegylated liposomal doxorubicin, the gemcitabine arm had an improved response rate (29% vs 16%); however, this did not reach statistical significance ($P = 0.06$). The median progression-free survival was 20 weeks for gemcitabine and 16 weeks for pegylated liposomal doxorubicin ($P = 0.4$). In spite of the higher response rate and progression-free survival for the gemcitabine arm, the pegylated liposomal doxorubicin arm had an improved median overall survival compared with the gemcitabine arm (55 vs 50 weeks), which reached statistical significance ($P = 0.048$).

Oral etoposide has significant activity in platinum-refractory ovarian cancer [31] but is not commonly used, possibly because of secondary hematologic malignancies associated with its use [32]. Alternative taxanes have been shown to be active in platinum- and paclitaxel-resistant ovarian cancer. Weekly paclitaxel and doctaxel are both active [33,34]. This would seem to indicate that resistance to standard, every-3-week paclitaxel does not necessarily confer resistance to an alternate paclitaxel schedule using weekly administration or to an alternative taxane, docetaxel. Based on these studies, retreatment with an alternative taxane is reasonable to consider in platinum- and paclitaxel-resistant ovarian cancer.

The major focus of current clinical trials for treatment of recurrent ovarian cancer is the use of targeted biologic agents. While several families of agents have been tried, the greatest success to date has been in the use of agents that target the vascular endothelial growth factor (VEGF) family. Bevacizumab is the most extensively tested agent and, in contrast to most other solid tumors, it has significant single-agent activity in ovarian cancer [35]. Based on this activity, current clinical trials are testing bevacizumab or other VEGF-targeted agents in combination with chemotherapy for both newly diagnosed and recurrent ovarian cancer.

CARCINOMA OF THE UTERINE CERVIX

GENERAL PRINCIPLES

Cervical cancer has a biphasic age distribution with peaks in the fourth and fifth decades and in the eighth and ninth decades of life. It affects approximately 12,000 women annually in the United States. Cervical cancer is more commonly found in poor women, women who have first intercourse early, have had multiple sexual partners, and have had multiple pregnancies. It is found less often in women who are nulliparous and those who are sexually inactive. A close association exists between infection with specific subtypes of human papillomavirus (HPV), specifically types 16 and 18, and the development of cervical cancer and carcinoma in situ. The development of vaccines against HPV should impact the incidence of premalignant cervical lesions and invasive cervical cancer. If females in the developing world have access to these vaccines, the impact would be even greater because cervical cancer ranks higher in incidence and in cancer-related mortality in developing countries. The association with HIV infection is appreciable but has not been fully defined. Risk factors for cervical cancer are listed in Table 14-7.

SCREENING, EARLY DETECTION, AND DIAGNOSIS

The Papanicolaou (Pap) smear, or cytologic evaluation of cells obtained from the cervix, is one of the most sensitive, specific, and cost-effective screening tests for human cancers. International studies have demonstrated a significant reduction in the death rate from cervical cancer with introduction of this test. False-negative results are usually related to poor preparation of the smears or inadequate sampling. Combined with the relatively slow rate of development of invasive cervical cancer from the dysplastic lesions of the cervix, regular Pap smear has a good probability of preventing the development of invasive cancer.

Management of patients with dysplastic lesions of the cervix is complex and beyond the scope of this chapter. Low-grade lesions require careful follow-up, although most regress spontaneously. Management of high-grade lesions is more controversial. Carcinoma in situ has an unacceptable rate of progression to invasive disease and requires either close follow-up or immediate surgical management. Entry of these patients into chemoprevention studies with novel agents may also be appropriate.

Diagnosis of invasive cervical cancer requires examination of tissue obtained from a cervical biopsy specimen. In the case of an abnormal Pap smear result, either a colposcopic biopsy or cone biopsy should be done. For lesions that can be appreciated visually on speculum examination, a punch biopsy is adequate for diagnosis.

APPROACH TO THE PATIENT WITH EARLY-STAGE DISEASE

Goals of treatment in early-stage disease are cure, and in late-stage disease to prevent pain, preserve renal function, and prevent disease progression that can result in fistula formation, malodorous discharge, and thromboembolic events. Unlike carcinoma of the ovary, diagnosis is usually straightforward, because the cervix can be visually inspected and subjected to

---

Table 14-5. Treatment Recommendations for Platinum-Sensitive Ovarian Cancer

Consider surgery for appropriate patients

Platinum retreatment is the standard of care for chemotherapy

Platinum-based combination therapy improves response rate, progression-free survival, and possibly overall survival

Prior and persistent toxicities should be considered when choosing therapy

---

Table 14-6. Common Chemotherapy Regimens in Recurrent Platinum-Resistant Ovarian Cancer

Topotecan daily × 5 days; 21-day cycle

Weekly topotecan on days 1, 8, and 15; 28-day cycle

Pegylated liposomal doxorubicin on day 1; 28-day cycle

Gemcitabine on days 1 and 8; 21-day cycle

Oral etoposide 14/21 days or 14–21/28 days

Weekly paclitaxel on days 1, 8, and 15; 28-day cycle

Docetaxel on day 1; 21-day cycle

Table 14-7. Risk Factors for Cervical Cancer

Lower socioeconomic status

Underdeveloped countries

First coitus at early age

Multiple sexual partners

Human papillomavirus types 16, 18, 31, 33, and 35

Cigarette smoking

AIDS-related malignancy

Cervical carcinoma in situ

easy biopsy. Thus, 75% of cervical cancers are diagnosed at early stages, whereas only 25% of ovarian carcinomas are diagnosed before they have spread to the abdomen. Unlike ovarian cancer, staging for cervical cancer is based on clinical findings. Examination is optimally conducted with the patient under anesthesia. Other tests may be employed including cervical biopsy, cystoscopy, proctosigmoidoscopy, chest radiography, IV pyelography, CT scan, or PET scan. Precise staging is required as this correlates well with prognosis. Furthermore, accurate staging is the foundation for further approaches to therapy. Table 14-8 shows the staging of cervical cancer and the prognosis based on stage.

For patients receiving radiation therapy to the pelvis, combination treatment with chemotherapy and radiation therapy is recommended and—based on evidence from five randomized controlled trials—was the subject of an alert from the National Cancer Institute in February 1999. The benefits of chemoradiation over radiation alone were demonstrated when used as primary therapy, as neoadjuvant therapy, and adjuvant therapy. The common denominator in the chemotherapy regimens used in the five trials was cisplatin; thus, a weekly dose of 40 mg/m^2 is most commonly used. Radiation consists of external-beam therapy at doses of 5000 to 6000 cGy, sometimes followed by brachytherapy to deliver 6500 to 7200 cGy to point A (*ie*, the bulkiest portion of the tumor).

For stages I to IIA (minimal local disease), either surgery or chemoradiation can be used and treatment is individualized based on clinical and pathologic parameters. For stages IIB to IVA (extensive local disease) chemoradiation is preferred whereas chemotherapy alone is used in metastatic stage IVB disease. There are several classes of hysterectomy that can be used as surgical treatment, but radical hysterectomy usually includes, in addition to total hysterectomy, en bloc resection of the parametrial connective tissues and the upper vagina, ureteral dissection, and total pelvic lymphadenectomy.

For patients with positive findings in the para-aortic lymph nodes, therapy remains controversial. Treatment of microscopic disease in para-aortic nodes with extended-field radiation therapy did prolong survival in one study [36]. However, this does not necessarily imply a clinical benefit for patients with macroscopic involvement. When involvement of para-aortic nodes is confirmed intraoperatively, the planned hysterectomy is usually abandoned. Whether PET or other sensitive imaging techniques can accurately aid in preoperative determination of surgical feasibility is a topic of ongoing debate.

TREATMENT OF METASTATIC OR RECURRENT DISEASE

Patients in whom local radiation therapy fails and who have no evidence of pelvic sidewall involvement or distant disease may be candidates for pelvic exenteration. This procedure is associated with high rates of morbidity but is curative in approximately 25% of carefully selected patients. Pelvic exenteration should only be attempted by a gynecologic oncologist with relevant expertise. Partial exenterative procedures (anterior or posterior) may be associated with lower rates of morbidity. Reconstructive procedures include construction of continent conduits, creation of a neovagina, and low rectal anastomosis.

CHEMOTHERAPY FOR METASTATIC OR RECURRENT DISEASE

Patients in whom local therapy fails or who present de novo with disease at distant sites, such as liver, bone, or lung, are candidates for systemic therapy. Usefulness of single-agent therapy is limited; a selected list of active agents is shown in Table 14-9 [37]. Combination chemotherapy in cervical cancer is frequently used for initial therapy. Cisplatin-based combination therapy with topotecan [38] or paclitaxel [39] can be used but it is now clear that response to these combinations is decreased when patients have a short disease-free interval from primary therapy or have received prior cisplatin as a radiosensitizer. A recent four-arm randomized trial comparing cisplatin with either paclitaxel, vinorelbine, topotecan, or gemcitabine was stopped early because a futility analysis indicated that there would be no significant differences in the study arms. Although the combination of paclitaxel and carboplatin has not been subject to the rigors of a randomized phase 3 trial in cervical cancer, retrospective [40] and phase 2 studies have documented activity of the regimen and, particularly in patients who have a poor performance status or compromised renal function, it may be a preferred regimen. After initial therapy, it is most appropriate to use single-agent therapy. Recently, bevacizumab was shown to have activity in cervical cancer [41]. Given the critical role for HPV in cervical cancer pathogenesis, ongoing trials are attempting to use HPV as a target in therapeutic vaccines in cervical cancer.

ENDOMETRIAL CARCINOMA

GENERAL PRINCIPLES

Cancer of the endometrium is the most common tumor type of the female genital tract, accounting for approximately 35,000 cases of cancer annually in the United States. Because endometrial carcinoma is usually detected in early stages, this disease accounts for fewer deaths than carcinoma of the ovary. This disease is usually easily diagnosed; thus at time of diagnosis, 80% of cases will be stage I disease, confined to the uterine corpus.

SCREENING, EARLY DETECTION, AND DIAGNOSIS

Risk factors for endometrial cancer are described in Table 14-10. Routine screening of asymptomatic, postmenopausal women is not warranted; however, women with postmenopausal bleeding, morbid obesity, Lynch II syndrome (HNPCC), or a history of endometrial hyperplasia require evaluation and screening because of their increased risk. Provocative data on risk for endometrial carcinoma come from the National Surgical Adjuvant Breast and Bowel Project (NSABP) trials in women receiving long-term tamoxifen both for breast cancer therapy and as breast cancer chemoprevention [42]. The incidence of endometrial cancer increased among those women receiving tamoxifen, likely as a result of tamoxifen's estrogenic action on uterine tissue. However, the risk increase is almost exclusively in women older than 50 years of age. With the advent of aromatase inhibitors for treatment of postmenopausal breast cancer, tamoxifen use has decreased in this demographic group.

There is also a familial risk factor for endometrial carcinoma. Endometrial carcinoma is part of the HNPCC or Lynch II familial cancer syndrome (see earlier description of this syndrome in this chapter in the section on ovarian carcinoma). Endometrial cancer may be more common than colorectal

Table 14-8. Staging and Prognosis of Cervical Cancer

Stage	Characteristics	5-y survival, %
I	Microscopic or macroscopic disease confined to the cervix	75–95
II	Disease confined to the pelvis but not involving the pelvic sidewall or the lower one third of the vagina	65–80
III	Disease that has spread to the pelvic sidewall or the lower one third of the vagina or presents with hydronephrosis	35–45
IV	Disease that has involved the mucosa of the bladder or rectum or has spread outside the pelvis	10–20

Table 14-9. Advanced Cervical Cancer Single-Agent Response Rates

Drug	Response rate, %
Cisplatin	17–38
Carboplatinum	15–28
Paclitaxel	17–31
Docetaxel	0–34
Doxorubicin	17–20
Ifosfamide	11–50
Topotecan	13–19
Vinorelbine	17–18

(*Adapted from* Long HJ III [37].)

cancer in women with this syndrome and prophylactic hysterectomy once childbearing is complete is increasingly recommended.

The peak age group for the development of endometrial carcinoma is in patients between 60 and 70 years of age. The disease is associated with obesity and diabetes, which makes these patients somewhat older and less healthy than other patients with gynecologic malignancies. The typical presentation of endometrial carcinoma is postmenopausal bleeding, which occurs in 80% of patients. Other symptoms include vaginal discharge and leukorrhea. Evaluation of postmenopausal bleeding includes fractional dilatation and curettage, with separation of cervical and endometrial specimens.

SURGERY FOR UTERINE CANCER

Patients should undergo a biopsy before hysterectomy. For patients with disease confined to the uterine corpus, the treatment is total abdominal hysterectomy and bilateral salpingo-oophorectomy. The ovaries are removed because of occasional implants on ovaries or fallopian tubes. Peritoneal washings should be obtained. Lymph node evaluation should be done in women with deep myometrial invasion or high-grade tumors. Unfortunately, depth of invasion is difficult to predict intraoperatively and final pathology may differ from preoperative biopsy. Any suspicious nodes noted at surgery should be excised. If there is any indication of pelvic node involvement, a para-aortic lymph node dissection is indicated.

Table 14-10. Risk Factors for Endometrial Carcinoma

Risk factor	Relative risk
Endometrial hyperplasia	29
Familial cancer syndrome (Lynch II)	20–30
Obesity	3–10
Unopposed estrogen use	9.5
Diabetes	2.8
Late menopause	2.4
Long-term tamoxifen use	2.5
Infertility	2–3
Nulliparity	2
Early menarche	1.5–2
Hypertension	1.5

Table 14-11. 1988 FIGO Surgical Staging for Endometrial Cancer

Stage	Description
Stage I	
IA	Tumor limited to endometrium
IB	Invasion < 50% myometrium
IC	Invasion > 50% myometrium
Stage II	
IIA	Endocervical gland involvement
IIB	Endocervical stromal invasion
Stage III	
IIIA	Serosa, adenexae, cytology
IIIB	Vaginal involvement
IIIC	Pelvic/aortic lymph node metastases
Stage IV	
IVA	Bladder/bowel mucosal invasion
IVB	Distant metastasis, inguinal lymph node metastases

FIGO—International Fenderation of Gynecology and Obstetrics.

STAGING AND PROGNOSIS

Staging of endometrial carcinoma is described in Table 14-11. Factors that adversely affect survival include clear cell, papillary, or adenosquamous histologies; increased grade; increased uterine size; myometrial invasion; positive peritoneal cytology; positive pelvic or para-aortic lymph nodes; or adnexal spread. A high percentage of patients present with favorable factors; therefore, survival rates in endometrial carcinoma are higher than those of ovarian carcinoma.

POOR-RISK SUBTYPES OF ENDOMETRIAL ADENOCARCINOMA

Uterine papillary serous carcinoma (UPSC) is well recognized as a more aggressive variant that clinically behaves more like an aggressive ovarian carcinoma than the generally more indolent endometrial adenocarcinomas. Specifically, UPSC tends to metastasize earlier with involvement of the peritoneal cavity. Clear cell, poorly differentiated adenocarcinomas, undifferentiated tumors, and squamous cell carcinoma of the endometrium also have more aggressive clinical courses with a poorer outcome.

ADJUVANT THERAPY FOR ENDOMETRIAL CANCER

Adjuvant radiation therapy is recommended in selected circumstances for endometrial cancer. Vaginal brachytherapy can be used alone for low-risk disease and whole pelvic radiation therapy, with or without brachytherapy, can be used for higher-risk disease. For low- and intermediate-risk patients, radiation improves local control and disease-free survival but has minimal impact on survival. Recently, there has been a gradual shift in the use of chemotherapy with or without radiation therapy for intermediate- and high-risk patients. This is based largely on the results of GOG protocol 122 that showed that chemotherapy with doxorubicin and cisplatin was superior to whole abdominal radiation therapy in women with resected stage III and IV disease, significantly improving 5-year disease-free and overall survival [43]. A major difficulty in comparing trials has been a lack of consensus in the definition of risk and heterogeneous patient populations, frequently lacking nodal staging.

THERAPY FOR ADVANCED UTERINE CARCINOMA

Endometrial cancer is highly curable when it is confined to the uterus, but the prognosis for metastatic or recurrent endometrial cancer is poor. The median survival for recurrent or metastatic endometrial cancer is only approximately 12 months. Hormonal therapy may benefit a small subgroup of women with endometrial cancer; it is most successful in patients with a long disease-free interval before recurrence (*ie*, 2 years or more), in well-differentiated tumors, and progesterone receptor–positive tumors. The most commonly employed agent is the progestational agent megestrol acetate (Megace; Bristol-Myers Squibb, Princeton, NJ), which is usually given at 160 mg/d. Toxicities with progestational agents are modest, with the most common side effects of fluid retention and weight gain. Response rates range from 11% to 16% but can be durable over months or years. The antiestrogenic agent tamoxifen has been tested in combination with progestational agents with response rates of 27% to 33% [44]. Table 14-12 summarized the data from four GOG trials of hormonal therapy for endometrial cancer [45–48].

Given the limited response to hormonal therapy, chemotherapy is most commonly used as initial treatment for women with metastatic or recurrent disease, particularly those with high-grade tumors or significant visceral disease. Table 14-13 lists the single agents and combination regimens commonly used for treatment of endometrial cancer. The combination of paclitaxel, doxorubicin, and cisplatin (TAP) was compared with doxorubicin

Table 14-12. Hormonal Therapy of Endometrial Cancer

Study	Agent	Response rate, %
GOG 168 [45]	Anastrozole	9
GOG 159 [46]	Goserelin acetate	12
GOG 153 [47]	Megestrol acetate/tamoxifen	27
GOG 119 [48]	Tamoxifen/medroxyprogesterone	33

GOG—Gynecologic Oncology Group.

and cisplatin (AC) in a randomized phase 3 trial [49,50]. The TAP regimen significantly improved response rate and progression-free and overall survival but was associated with increased neuropathy and required the use of white cell growth factor. More recently, TAP has been compared with the combination of paclitaxel and carboplatin in advanced measurable disease but results of that study are not yet available. It should be noted that greater use of chemotherapy in the adjuvant setting may have a significant impact on options for treatment of recurrent disease.

TREATMENT OF UTERINE SARCOMAS

Sarcomas of the uterus include leiomyosarcoma, carcinosarcoma (malignant mixed Mullerian tumor [MMMT]), and endometrial stromal sarcoma.

Table 14-13. Chemotherapy for Endometrial Cancer

Treatment	Response rate, %
Single-agent chemotherapy	
Cisplatin	20–25
Carboplatin	13–33
Doxorubicin	26
Paclitaxel	36
Topotecan	
First line	20
Second line	9
Liposomal doxorubicin	11
Combination chemotherapy*	
Doxorubicin and cisplatin	33–81
Doxorubicin and paclitaxel	43
Cyclophosphamide, doxorubicin, and platinum	31–56
Doxorubicin and cyclophosphamide	31–46
Paclitaxel, doxorubicin, and cisplatin	57
Paclitaxel and carboplatin	50–78

*Combination chemotherapy data are primarily from patients with no prior chemotherapy. (*Adapted from* Carey *et al.* [50].)

These are uncommon tumors, accounting for fewer than 5% of all uterine malignancies. These have a variable natural history but can be aggressive tumors. Interpretation of the pathologic specimen is sometimes problematic in tumors with mixed histologies. Standard treatment for uterine sarcomas is total abdominal hysterectomy with bilateral salpingo-oophorectomy with or without lymph node dissection. External-beam radiation therapy can be used for stage I or II leiomyosarcoma or carcinosarcoma. Most studies show that radiation will decrease the local (pelvic) relapse rate but it has not been shown to consistently impact survival. Adjuvant chemotherapy has not been shown to impact survival in any of these diseases.

For patients with advanced recurrent or metastatic disease, systemic therapy is used. Endometrial stromal sarcomas are most commonly treated with hormonal agents such as megestrol acetate, medroxyprogesterone, tamoxifen, or gonadotropin-releasing hormone analogues. Table 14-14 shows the response of leiomyosarcoma and carcinosarcoma to different chemotherapy drugs and regimens from recent and historical studies [51]. The MAID (mesna, doxorubicin, ifosfamide, dacarbazine) regimen is sometimes used in leiomyosarcoma, but with the identification of gemcitabine and docetaxel as an active combination that can be given in the outpatient setting, it is less frequently used.

Table 14-14. Chemotherapy for Uterine Sarcomas

Disease	Drug/regimen	Response rate, %
Leiomyosarcoma	Liposomal doxorubicin	16
	Gemcitabine	20
	Gemcitabine + docetaxel	36–53
	Temozolomide	8–13
	MAID	9–47
Carcinosarcoma	Paclitaxel	18
	Paclitaxel + carboplatin	80
	Ifosfamide + paclitaxel	45
	Ifosfamide + cisplatin	54
	Topotecan	10

MAID—mesna, doxorubicin, ifosfamide, dacarbazine. (*Adapted from* Gadducci *et al.* [51].)

DEDICATION

This edition of the chapter on gynecologic malignancies is dedicated to the memory of Dr. Scott Wadler, author of the previous edition of this chapter, who devoted his professional life to improving the care of cancer patients.

REFERENCES

1. SEER (Surveillance, Epidemiology, and End Results): SEER stat fact sheet: cancer of the ovary. Available at http://seer.cancer.gov/statfacts/html/ovary.html. Accessed April 22, 2007.

2. Salehi F, Dunfield L, Phillips KP, *et al.*: Risk factors for ovarian cancer: an overview with emphasis on hormonal factors. *J Toxicol Environ Health B Crit Rev* 2008, 11:301–321.

3. Russo A, Calò V, Bruno L, *et al.*: Hereditary ovarian cancer. *Crit Rev Oncol Hematol* 2008, [Epub ahead of print].

4. Satagopan JM, Boyd J, Kauff ND, *et al.*: Ovarian cancer risk in Ashkenazi Jewish carriers of BRCA1 and BRCA2 mutations. *Clin Cancer Res* 2002, 8:776–781.

5. Fishman DA, Cohen L, Blank SV, *et al.*: The role of ultrasound evaluation in the detection of early-stage epithelial ovarian cancer. *Am J Obstet Gynecol* 2005, 192:1214–1221; discussion 1221–1222.

6. Bristow RE, Tomacruz RS, Armstrong DK, *et al.*: Survival effect of maximal cytoreductive surgery for advanced ovarian carcinoma during the platinum era: a meta-analysis. *J Clin Oncol* 2002, 20:1248–1259.

7. International Federation of Gynecology and Obstetrics: Annual report on the results of treatment in gynecologic cancer. *Int J Gynecol Obstet* 1989, 28:189–190.

8. Young RC, Walton LA, Ellenberg SS, *et al.*: Adjuvant therapy in stage I and stage II epithelial ovarian cancer: results of two prospective randomized trials. *N Engl J Med* 1990, 322:1021–1027.

9. Bell J, Brady MF, Young RC, *et al.*: Randomized phase III trial of three versus six cycles of adjuvant carboplatin and paclitaxel in early stage epithelial ovarian carcinoma: a Gynecologic Oncology Group study. *Gynecol Oncol* 2006, 102:432–439.

10. Chan JK, Zhang M, Hu JM, *et al.*: Racial disparities in surgical treatment and survival of epithelial ovarian cancer in United States. *J Surg Oncol* 2008, 97:103–107.

11. Ozols RF, Bundy BN, Greer BE, *et al.*: Phase III trial of carboplatin and paclitaxel compared with cisplatin and and paclitaxel in patients with optimally resected stage III ovarian cancer: a Gynecologic Oncology Group study. *J Clin Oncol* 2003, 21:3194–3200.

12. Alberts DS, Liu PY, Hannigan EV, *et al.*: Intraperitoneal cisplatin plus intravenous cyclophosphamide versus intravenous cisplatin plus intravenous cyclophosphamide for stage III ovarian cancer. *N Engl J Med* 1996, 335:1950–1955.

13. Markman M, Bundy BN, Alberts DS, *et al.*: Phase III trial of standard-dose intravenous cisplatin plus paclitaxel versus moderately high-dose carboplatin followed by intravenous paclitaxel and intraperitoneal cisplatin in small-volume stage III ovarian carcinoma: an intergroup study of the Gynecologic Oncology Group, Southwestern Oncology Group, and Eastern Cooperative Oncology Group. *J Clin Oncol* 2001, 19:1001–1007.

14. Armstrong DK, Bundy BN, Wenzel L, *et al.*: Intraperitoneal cisplatin and paclitaxel in ovarian cancer. *N Engl J Med* 2006, 354:34–43.

15. US National National Library of Medicine, National Institutes of Health: Clinical advisory: NCI issues clinical announcement for preferred method of treatment for advanced ovarian cancer. Available at http://www.nlm.nih.gov/databases/alerts/ovarian_ip_chemo.html. Accessed September 1, 2008.

16. McGuire WP, Hoskins WJ, Brady MF, *et al.*: Cyclophosphamide and cisplatin compared with paclitaxel and cisplatin in patients with stage III and stage IV ovarian cancer. *N Engl J Med* 1996, 334:1–6.

17. Piccart MJ, Bertelsen K, James K, *et al.*: Randomized intergroup trial of cisplatin-paclitaxel versus cisplatin-cyclophosphamide in women with advanced epithelial ovarian cancer: three-year results. *J Natl Cancer Inst* 2000, 92:699–708.

18. Muggia FM, Braly PS, Brady MF, *et al.*: Phase III randomized study of cisplatin versus paclitaxel versus cisplatin and paclitaxel in patients with suboptimal stage III or IV ovarian cancer: a Gynecologic Oncology Group study. *J Clin Oncol* 2000, 18:106–115.

19. Vasey PA, Jayson GC, Gordon A, *et al.*: Phase III randomized trial of docetaxel-carboplatin versus paclitaxel-carboplatin as first-line chemotherapy for ovarian carcinoma. *J Natl Cancer Inst* 2004, 96:1682–1691.

20. Bookman MA: GOG0182-ICON5: 5-arm phase III randomized trial of paclitaxel (P) and carboplatin (C) vs combinations with gemcitabine (G), PEG-liposomal doxorubicin (D), or topotecan (T) in patients (pts) with advanced-stage epithelial ovarian (EOC) or primary peritoneal (PPC) carcinoma [abstract]. *J Clin Oncol* 2006, 24(18S):abstract 5002.

21. Spriggs D, Brady M, Vacarello L, *et al.*: A phase III randomized trial of IV cisplatin plus a 24-or 96-hour infusion of paclitaxel in epithelial ovarian cancer: a Gynecologic Oncology Group study. *J Clin Oncol* 2007, 25:4466–4471.

22. Rose PG, Nerenstone S, Brady M, *et al.*: Secondary surgical cytoreduction in advanced ovarian carcinoma: a Gynecologic Oncology Group study. *N Engl J Med* 2004, 351:2489–2497.

23. Eisenhauer EA, Vermorken JB, van Glabbeke M: Predictors of response to subsequent chemotherapy in platinum pretreated ovarian cancer: a multivariate analysis of 704 patients. *Ann Oncol* 1997, 8:963–968.

24. Markman M, Markman J, Webster K, *et al.*: Duration of response to second-line, platinum-based chemotherapy for ovarian cancer: implications for patient management and clinical trial design, *J Clin Oncol* 2004, 22:3120–3125.

25. Parmar MK, Ledermann JA, Colombo N, *et al.*: Paclitaxel plus platinum-based chemotherapy versus conventional platinum-based chemotherapy in women with relaped ovarian cancer: the ICON4/AGO-OVAR-2.2 trial. *Lancet* 2003, 361:2099–2106.

26. Pfisterer J, Plante M, Vergote I, *et al.*: Gemcitabine plus carboplatin compared with carboplatin in patients with platinum-sensitive recurrent ovarian cancer: an intergroup trial of the AGO-OVAR, the NCIC CTG, and the EORTC GCG. *J Clin Oncol* 2006, 24:4699–4707.

27. Âvall-Lundqvist E, Wimberger P, Gladieff L, *et al.*: Pegylated liposomal doxorubicin (PLD)-carboplatin (C) (C-D) vs paclitaxel-carboplatin (C-P) in relapsing sensitive ovarian cancer (OC): a 500-patient interim safety analysis of the CALYPSO GCIG intergroup phase III study [abstract]. *J Clin Oncol* 2008, 26(Suppl):abstract 5565.

28. Gordon AN, Fleagle JT, Guthrie D, *et al.*: Recurrent epithelial ovarian carcinoma: a randomized phase III study of pegylated liposomal doxorubicin versus topotecan. *J Clin Oncol* 2001, 19:3312–3322.

29. Abushahin F, Singh DK, Lurain JR, *et al.*: Weekly topotecan for recurrent platinum resistant ovarian cancer. *Gynecol Oncol* 2008, 108:53–57.

30. Ferrandina G, Ludovisi M, Lorusso D, *et al.*: Phase III trial of gemcitabine compared with pegylated liposomal doxorubicin in progressive or recurrent ovarian cancer. *J Clin Oncol* 2008, 26:890–896.

31. Rose PG, Blessing JA, Mayer AR, *et al.*: Prolonged oral etoposide as second-line therapy for platinum-resistant and platinum-sensitive ovarian carcinoma: a Gynecologic Oncology Group study. *J Clin Oncol* 1998, 16:405–410.

32. Yagita M, Ieki Y, Onishi R, *et al.*: Therapy-related leukemia and myelodysplasia following oral administration of etoposide for recurrent breast cancer. *Int J Oncol* 1998, 13:91–96.

33. Markman M, Blessing J, Rubin SC, *et al.*: Phase II trial of weekly paclitaxel (80 mg/m2) in platinum and paclitaxel-resistant ovarian and primary peritoneal cancers: a Gynecologic Oncology Group study. *Gynecol Oncol* 2006, 101:436–440.

34. Rose P, Blessing JA, Ball HG, *et al.*: A phase II study of docetaxel in paclitaxel-resistant ovarian and peritoneal cancer: a Gynecologic Oncology Group study. *Gynecol Oncol* 2003, 88:130–135.

35. Burger RA, Sill MW, Monk BJ, *et al.*: Phase II trial of bevacizumab in persistent or recurrent epithelial ovarian cancer or primary peritoneal cancer: a Gynecologic Oncology Group study. *J Clin Oncol* 2007, 25:5165–5171.

36. Rotman M, Pajak TF, Choi K, *et al.*: Prophylactic extended-field irradiation of para-aortic lymph nodes in stages IIB and bulky IB and IIA cervical carcinomas. Ten-year treatment results of RTOG 79-20. *JAMA* 1995, 274:387–393.

37. Long HJ III: Management of metastatic cervical cancer: review of the literature. *J Clin Oncol* 2007, 25:2966–2974.

38. Long HJ III, Bundy BN, Grendys EC Jr, *et al.*; Gynecologic Oncology Group study: randomized phase III trial of cisplatin with or without topotecan in carcinoma of the uterine cervix: a Gynecologic Oncology Group study. *J Clin Oncol* 2005, 23:4626–4633.

39. Moore DH, Blessing JA, McQuellon RP, *et al.*: Phase III study of cisplatin with or without paclitaxel in stage IVB, recurrent, or persistent squamous cell carcinoma of the cervix: a Gynecologic Oncology Group study. *J Clin Oncol* 2004, 22:3113–3119.

40. Moore KN, Herzog TJ, Lewin S, *et al.*: A comparison of cisplatin/paclitaxel and carboplatin/paclitaxel in stage IVB, recurrent or persistent cervical cancer. *Gynecol Oncol* 2007, 105:299–303.

41. Monk BJ, Sill MW, Burger RA, *et al.*: Phase II trial of bevacizumab in the treatment of recurrent squamous cell carcinoma of the cervix: a Gynecologic Oncology Group study [abstract]. *Gynecol Oncol* 2008, 108(Suppl):abstract 45.

42. Goldstein SR: The effect of SERMs on the endometrium. *Ann N Y Acad Sci* 2001, 949:237–242.

43. Randall ME, Filiaci VL, Muss H, *et al.*; Gynecologic Oncology Group Study: Randomized phase III trial of whole-abdominal irradiation versus doxorubicin and cisplatin chemotherapy in advanced endometrial carcinoma: a Gynecologic Oncology Group Study. *J Clin Oncol* 2006, 24:36–44.

44. Herzog TJ: What is the clinical value of adding tamoxifen to progestins in the treatment of advanced or recurrent endometrial cancer? *Gynecol Oncol* 2004, 92:1–3.

45. Rose PG, Brunetto VL, VanLe L, *et al.*: A phase II trial of anastrozole in advanced recurrent or persistent endometrial cancer: a Gynecologic Oncology Group study. *Gynecol Oncol* 2000, 78:212–216.

46. Asbury RF, Brunetto VL, Lee RB, *et al.*: Gosereline acetate as treatment for recurrent endometrial carcinoma: a Gynecologic Oncology Group study. *Am J Clin Oncol* 2002, 25:557–560.

47. Fiorica JV, Brunetto VL, Hanjani P, *et al.*: Phase II trial of alternating courses of megestrol acetate and tamoxifen in advanced endometrial carcinoma: a Gynecologic Oncology Group study. *Gynecol Oncol* 2004, 92:10–14.

48. Whitney CW, Brunetto VL, Zaino R, *et al*.: Phase II study of medroxypro-gesterone acetate plus tamoxifen in advanced endometrial carcinoma: a GOG study. *Gynecol Oncol* 2004, 92:4–9.

49. Fleming GF, Brunetto VL, Cella D, *et al*.: Phase III trial of doxorubicin plus cisplatin with or without paclitaxel plus filgrastim in advanced endome-trial carcinoma: a Gynecologic Oncology Group study. *J Clin Oncol* 2004, 22:2159–2166.

50. Carey MS, Gawlik C, Fung-Kee-Fung M, *et al*., and Cancer Care Ontario Practice Guidelines Initiative Gynecology Cancer Disease Site Group: Sys-tematic review of systemic therapy for advanced or recurrent endometrial cancer. *Gynecol Oncol* 2006, 101:158–167.

51. Gadducci A, Cosio S, Romanini A, Genazzani AR: The management of patients with uterine sarcoma: a debated clinical challenge. *Crit Rev Oncol Hematol* 2008, 65:129–142.

Erin M. Dunbar, John Laterra

Primary central nervous system (CNS) tumors represent a diverse set of difficult-to-treat neoplasms. Affecting both children and adults, these tumors may either be indolent and slow-growing lesions or rapidly proliferative lesions that cause death within less than a year. Well-demarcated, noninvasive tumors are potentially curable with surgery alone, in contrast to the poorly demarcated invasive lesions, which represent the most common primary brain tumors in adults, namely infiltrative gliomas. This chapter reviews the diagnosis and treatment of the latter, focusing on gliomas and, specifically, the astrocytoma and oligodendroglioma subtypes.

EPIDEMIOLOGY

In 2007, primary malignant CNS (brain and other nervous system) tumors in the United States were diagnosed in an estimated 20,500 men and women (11,170 men and 9330 women); of those, 12,740 were expected to die per the American Cancer Society's "Cancer Facts and Figures" report [1]. Per the Surveillance, Epidemiology, and End Results (SEER) database for 1975–2004, primary malignant CNS tumors in the United States currently have an estimated combined incidence of 6.6 per 100,000 persons per year, with an estimated mortality of 4.6 per 100,000 persons per year. The SEER database also reports that primary malignant CNS tumors remain the leading causes of cancer death for children younger than age 15 and for men up to age 34. They are also the fourth cause of cancer death in women between the ages of 15 and 34. The average age of onset for all primary CNS tumors is 54 years, and is slightly higher in the more malignant phenotypes, such as glioblastoma multiforme (GBM) [2].Gliomas, the focus of this chapter, usually constitute approximately 49% of primary CNS tumors. The incidence of gliomas has remained relatively stable over the past few decades [2], likely accounted for by the balancing of an aging population with improved diagnostics and treatments.

Identification of risk factors has been difficult because of tumor heterogeneity, retrospective exposure analyses, and uncertain latency periods. Ionizing radiation is a clear, noninherited risk factor for primary brain tumors [3,4]. Radiotherapy, used historically to treat tinea capitis, skin hemangiomas, and pituitary adenomas, has been associated with an increased risk of meningioma and glioma. An elevated risk of subsequent primary brain tumors has been observed after radiotherapy for childhood tumors (other than leukemia). In contrast, atomic bomb survivors in Japan have not shown an increased risk of CNS tumors [4]. Similarly, recent meta-analyses have not shown a statistically significant increase of brain tumors in response to electromagnetic field exposure [5–7]. Several recent international studies also have not demonstrated any elevated risk from cell phone use [8,9]. Several studies conducted to evaluate the risk of certain occupations and industries have come to inconsistent conclusions, at least partly due to a lack of an identified causal agent(s), relatively low exposures, and a slow incidence of diagnosis. These industries include pesticide and fertilizer manufacturing, synthetic rubber processing, vinyl chloride industries, and petrochemical and oil refineries [3,4]. Chemicals of continued investigative interest include N-nitroso compounds, organochlorides, nitrates and nitrites, formaldehyde, and vinyl chloride. Acquired immunosuppressive conditions, including severe combined immunodeficiency disorder, organ transplantation, and HIV/AIDS, can result in both a higher incidence and early onset of CNS tumors, primarily lymphomas and gliomas.

DIAGNOSTIC IMAGING

Magnetic resonance imaging (MRI) is more sensitive than computed tomography (CT) for detecting initial tumor, defining extent of tumor, and monitoring therapeutic response. CT is particularly less sensitive for evaluating lesions in the posterior fossa and skull base due the "beam-hardening" artifacts generated by adjacent bony structures. MRI has the additional advantage of imaging in multiple planes, thereby improving the differentiation of intra-axial and extra-axial lesions (*eg*, meningioma). Hydrogen protons in water generate low signal intensity on T1-weighted magnetic resonance sequences and high intensity on T2-weighted sequences. Tissue contrast from pathologic processes is usually most apparent on T2-weighted images compared with the intermediate signal intensity of normal brain parenchyma. T2 fluid attenuation inversion recovery (FLAIR) magnetic resonance sequences provide valuable information about peritumor inflammation, edema, and treatment changes. However, since a wide variety of pathologic processes such as tumor, infection, inflammation, and infarct all produce increased extracellular water, MRI cannot always definitively distinguish tumor from these other processes. Diffusion-weighted MRI, if performed within 7 to 10 days of the presenting clinical event, is helpful for distinguishing acute infarction from tumor. If diffusion imaging is unavailable, follow-up imaging with routine MRI in 10 days and then by 3 months can be extremely helpful, as infarctions demonstrate a unique temporal pattern of initial rapid new contrast enhancement and mass effect followed by later resolution. Another unique temporal pattern can be seen occasionally in the acute plaques of "tumefactive" demyelination, where plaques initially demonstrate mass effect, contrast enhancement, and vasogenic edema. Follow-up MRI imaging of these plaques in 6 to 8 weeks usually demonstrates a distinct spontaneous improvement. Lastly, the radiographic pattern of nontumor pathologic processes can be unique. For instance, cerebral abscesses typically have a much thinner and more uniform rim of contrast enhancement (see below) when compared with the pattern of enhancement typically surrounding zones of necrosis within a malignant glioma.

Since their introduction in 1988, MRI contrast agents have had a tremendous impact on CNS tumor evaluation. Gadolinium, a rare earth metal with seven unpaired electrons, is the most commonly used MRI contrast agent. The unpaired electrons enable nearby protons to realign more quickly with the main magnetic field, thus shortening T1 relaxation time to generate higher signal intensity compared with the precontrast T1 sequences. Normal brain capillaries with an intact blood-brain barrier are impermeable to gadolinium complexes. Postgadolinium contrast enhancement results from the abnormal vascular permeability typical of malignant brain tumors. A notable exception to this is the low-grade pilocytic astrocytoma, which classically demonstrates intense contrast enhancement, a reflection of a prominent permeable vasculature. Also notable, the pituitary gland, pineal gland, choroid plexus, and dura lack a blood-brain barrier and will normally enhance after gadolinium infusion.

Low-grade (World Health Organization [WHO] grade II) and high-grade (WHO grade III–IV) gliomas are diffusely infiltrating neoplasms that impart mass effect and compress adjacent structures. These features are reflected in imaging characteristics. Currently, it is not possible to predict glioma subtype or histologic grade based on MRI appearance [10], as exemplified by the above-mentioned pilocytic astrocytoma. Oligodendroglioma is supratentorial 90% of the time, most commonly involves peripheral cortex, and typically extends into the adjacent white matter. The peripheral cortex involvement explains why oligodendroglioma presents with epileptic seizures more often than any other glioma. Oligodendroglioma is the most common brain tumor to have calcification, which is better visualized by CT than MRI. Given their usual slow growth, oligodendroglioma can often present with mass effect out of proportion to neurologic deficit and occasionally with adjacent calvarial erosion. Contrast enhancement is variable, particularly for intermediate grade (III) lesions. Nearly all GBM (WHO grade IV) and most grade III glioma contain regions of intense contrast enhancement. Most low-grade (WHO grade II) gliomas do not enhance. Approximately 20% of nonenhancing gliomas are found to be high grade at pathologic diagnosis. It is not unusual for low-grade oligodendroglioma to demonstrate subtle often punctate regions of contrast enhancement that can fluctuate in the absence of therapy. Hemorrhage is more commonly seen in the higher-grade lesions. A characteristic pattern of GBM is radiographic spread across the white matter tracts of the corpus callosum, a reflection of infiltration involving the contralateral cerebral hemisphere (*ie*, the "butterfly" appearance).

Over the past decade, major efforts have been undertaken to evaluate newer imaging technologies with the goal of improved noninvasive differentiation of tumor histology, grade, and therapeutic response. One of these is magnetic resonance spectroscopy (MRS). Regions of interest are evaluated for intracellular metabolites, most commonly choline-containing compounds, creatine, and N-acetyl aspartate. Neoplasms typically contain elevated choline and diminished N-acetyl aspartate. Radiation injury is characterized by low levels of all three metabolites [11,12]. Limiting its utility, current MRS technology is unable to reliably distinguish neoplasms from acute demyelinating lesions that also reveal elevated choline/creatine ratios. Imaging technologies of positron emission tomography (PET), which uses [18F]fluoro-2-deoxy-D-glucose (FDG) to detect regions of hypermetabolism, as well as coregistration MRI and MRS, can improve the diagnostic accuracy of gliomas. One frequent application of these imaging technologies includes identifying tumor regions for biopsy that are most likely to yield definitive diagnostic information [13,14].

HISTOPATHOLOGY

Infiltrative gliomas are categorized by the WHO into grades II through IV, with each grade manifesting increasing pleiomorphism, proliferation (mitosis), endothelial proliferation, and necrosis. The WHO grade I noninfiltrating gliomas represent distinct entities most commonly seen in children and will not be discussed here. For either astrocytic or oligodendroglial tumors, grade II represents "low-grade gliomas" and grade III (anaplastic) and IV (GBM) are categorized as "high-grade gliomas" or "malignant gliomas." Importantly, these grades predict prognosis and guide treatment strategies. The cell(s) of origin for the gliomas remains unknown. Current theory and experimental evidence suggest a pleuripotent neural stem cell origin [15].

Molecular and genetic discoveries are advancing the understanding of how these malignancies develop and are increasingly influencing clinical practice. Malignant gliomas can arise from more than one molecular and genetic pathway. Some cases of GBM, called "secondary GBM," progress from lower-grade astrocytoma. Secondary GBM often contain mutations in the p53 gene, overexpression of platelet-derived growth factor receptors, and loss of heterozygosity (LOH) at 17p, 19q, and 10q. In contrast, "primary GBM" originate de novo and often contain loss of all or a portion of chromosome 10 and amplification/overexpression of epidermal growth factor receptor (EGFR) and PTEN mutations [16]. Less is known regarding how oligodendroglioma arise; however, they share a natural history for a tendency to malignantly transform. The presence of 1p/19q co-deletion (1p/19q-LOH) in oligodendroglioma is an independent prognostic feature of improved survival and predicts increased responsiveness to cytotoxic therapeutics [17,18]. Silencing of the promoter for O6-methylguanine–DNA methyltransferase (MGMT) by epigenetic methylation has been shown to confer increased sensitivity to alkylating agents (temozolomide, carmustine [BCNU]) and to confer improved median and overall survival in patients with malignant astrocytoma [19,20]. It is not yet known if MGMT silencing has similar implications in WHO grade II glioma. The coexpression of wild-type PTEN and the constitutively active EGFR variant vIII (EGFRvIII) deletion mutation has been found in a small series to predict sensitivity of WHO grade III and IV astrocytoma to EGFR kinase inhibitors [21]. While many questions remain regarding the application of these and other molecular/genetic markers for clinical decision making, the field is moving rapidly in this direction.

TREATMENT

Tumor histology, anatomic location, comorbidities, and, in some cases, molecular/genetic profile greatly impact prognosis and treatment strategies. In general, the goals of surgery are to obtain as much tissue as possible for accurate diagnosis and to maximally reduce tumor burden. The goal of postoperative external-beam radiation is to minimize residual tumor burden and/or delay the time of tumor recurrence. Up until recently, chemotherapy was predominantly used as "salvage" treatment at recurrence. However, chemotherapy is now proven to prolong survival when used with radiation therapy in patients with newly diagnosed GBM. Chemotherapy is increasingly being considered for low-grade gliomas, although definitive efficacy in this setting remains controversial.

Numerous retrospective studies support the view that the most aggressive safe tumor resection impacts favorably on performance status, by reducing mass effect and prolonging patient survival [22–27]. It remains unresolved whether this simply reflects the fact that more favorable tumors are more amenable to gross total resection. However, whenever possible, maximal safe surgical resection is preferred over stereotactic or excisional biopsy. Numerous new technical modalities exist to aid safe maximal resection. Intraoperative suites with "real-time" imaging can guide the evolving resection. Awake craniotomies with frameless computer-guided stereotaxis and intraoperative cortical/subcortical electrophysiologic mapping allow the surgical team to avoid injuring eloquent areas. The precise extent of surgical resection that clearly confers a survival benefit has not been delineated beyond what is termed *subtotal resection*. However, the surgical literature often refers to more than 90% resection as the surgical goal [22,24,27].

Phase 3 studies support the survival benefit of external-beam radiotherapy over "best palliative care" in malignant glioma [28–35]. The use of three-dimensional conformal technique administered in single daily fractions, 5 days per week, to a maximum dose of 54 to 60 Gy, is considered the standard of care in the United States. The modern target-volume of external-beam radiation includes the region of T2 elevation (tumor and edema) and an additional 2-cm margin because about 80% of malignant gliomas recur within approximately 2 cm of the original tumor margins [36]. The use of whole-brain irradiation technique, with the goal of killing microscopic tumor cells known to infiltrate well beyond the identifiable tumor margin, has an increased risk of delayed neurocognitive toxicity, yet without an improved survival beyond the more conformal techniques [36].

Attempts to increase the radiation dose beyond the modern standard of care dose range of 54 to 60 Gy have not proven to be superior to 60 Gy; rather they have proven to increase toxicity. Similarly, numerous attempts to increase the physiologic radiation intensity at a given radiation dose have been largely unsuccessful. These include the use of radiation sensitizers and various dose-fractionation techniques such as hypofractionation. Despite several radiation dose-intensity trials yielding mixed results, they continue to be investigated [37]. A recent phase 3 trial (Radiation Therapy Oncology Group [RTOG] 9305) showed no benefit of upfront stereotactic radiosurgery in newly diagnosed GBM [38]. Although still controversial, the use of stereotactic radiosurgery boosts at the time of recurrence may offer some benefit [39–44]. Gliasite (Cytyc Surgical Products, Marlborough, MA), an inflatable balloon catheter inserted at the time of surgical resection and designed to receive a liquid I-125 radioisotope, was approved by the US Food and Drug Administration (FDA) in 2003 as a device for treating recurrent malignant glioma [45]. Efficacy is yet to be established. Similarly, numerous trials with radiosensitizers have been performed, including the notable phase 3 trial evaluating the treatment of recurrent anaplastic astrocytoma tumors using radiation plus PCV chemotherapy (procarbazine, lomustine, and vincristine) with or without the putative radiosensitizer bromodeoxyuridine. Responses were not superior compared with standard radiation strategies alone [46].

The goals and use of chemotherapy are evolving. Adjuvant chemotherapy has been shown to improve survival in an increasing portion of patients [47]. Three chemotherapies have been FDA approved over the past 30 years for the treatment of malignant brain tumors: systemic BCNU, approved in 1977; implantable polymeric BCNU (Gliadel, MGI Pharma, Inc., Bloomington, MN), approved in 1995; and oral temozolomide (Temodar, Schering-Plough Corp., Kenilworth, NJ), approved in 2005. Historically, the chemotherapy most often used was single-agent intravenous BCNU, which was frequently not used in older patients secondary to poor tolerability. Overall, the median survival remains relatively unchanged for individuals with high-grade glioma with or without adjuvant BCNU, but younger patients with otherwise favorable prognostic factors and individuals with anaplastic tumors do appear to have a slight 2-year survival advantage with adjuvant chemotherapy [48]. The surgically placed polymeric BCNU, approved for recurrent malignant gliomas in 1995 [48] and for newly diagnosed high-grade gliomas in 2003 [49], has similar efficacy to systemic BCNU and has less systemic toxicities.

Temozolomide, an oral alkylating agent, has recently become the standard adjuvant chemotherapy for newly diagnosed GBM. This adjuvant chemotherapy, used as part of an "up-front" (postoperative) regimen, consists of daily low-dose temozolomide (75 mg/m^2/d) for 6 weeks during radiation therapy, followed by six sequential 28-day cycles of temozolomide (200 mg/m²/d) on cycle days 1 through 5. This regimen was proven more effective than radiation followed by best standard of care in a landmark prospective, controlled trial of 573 patients at 85 international centers conducted by the European Organisation for Research and Treatment of Cancer (EORTC)/National Cancer Institute of Canada [50]. Patients in the combination radiation plus temozolomide group experienced a median survival of 14.6 months versus 12.1 months with radiotherapy alone (*P* < 0.001). The 2-year overall survival rate was 26.5% with radiotherapy plus temozolomide versus 10.4% with radiotherapy alone (*P* < 0.001). The most common side effects were hematologic toxicity (myelosuppression) and associated immunosuppression, with a 7% frequency of grade 3 or 4 National Cancer Institute Common Toxicity Criteria (NCI-CTC) toxicities. Patients with epigenetic silencing of the DNA repair enzyme MGMT had preferentially improved median survival (21.7 vs 15.3 months for those receiving radiotherapy alone) [18]. This treatment regimen is now frequently offered to patients with grade III glioma without objective evidence of improved efficacy in these somewhat less-aggressive malignancies. To date, no chemotherapy combination has proven more efficacious than single-agent therapy in the adjuvant setting, including the PCV regimen. In numerous phase 3 trials, PCV was no better than radiotherapy alone or BCNU [51] in the adjuvant setting. Combinations using temozolomide are currently being investigated.

In contrast to the WHO grade IV GBM, the use of adjuvant chemotherapy has not consistently been shown to improve outcomes for patients with WHO grade III anaplastic astrocytomas and anaplastic oligodendrogliomas. In general, these malignant gliomas have a slightly longer median survival of approximately 4 to 5 years [28,32,51–53] and have similar prognostic factors to the WHO grade IV GBMs. Although there has recently been an increased effort to separate WHO grade III anaplastic gliomas from grade IV GBMs as distinct prognostic entities in clinical trials, they frequently receive the same standard treatment. Outside of a clinical trial, postoperative radiotherapy (54–60 Gy, usually divided into 1.8–2.0 Gy fractions) remains the standard therapy for most patients. However, in recent years, several prospective phase 2 trials of exclusively anaplastic tumors have supported numerous retrospective reviews of anaplastic subsets within larger trials, in the conclusion that adjuvant chemotherapy may yield a slight survival advantage [51,54]. A large, retrospective pooled analysis of four RTOG protocols of 432 patients with anaplastic astrocytomas and anaplastic oligodendrogliomas showed no benefit from adjuvant PCV regimen over BCNU chemotherapy [55]. There have only been a few prospective, randomized trials of adjuvant chemotherapy for WHO grade III gliomas. To date, none of these have demonstrated an unequivocal survival benefit, although one prospective trial suggested some additional benefit with BCNU [56]. The historical limitations related to the absence of an adequately sized, prospective phase 3 trial of exclusively anaplastic tumors are being addressed by renewed interest in clinical trials modeling the encouraging trials of combination temozolomide plus radiation in GBM.

For anaplastic oligodendrogliomas, there is also a lack of definitive evidence that adjuvant chemotherapy improves survival over postoperative radiotherapy alone. This is best exemplified by results of the intergroup RTOG 9402 trial, in which 289 patients with anaplastic oligodendroglioma and anaplastic oligoastrocytoma were randomly assigned to (neoadjuvant) PCV chemotherapy followed by radiotherapy versus postoperative radiotherapy alone. Of those who progressed after radiotherapy alone, 80% subsequently received chemotherapy. At 3-year follow-up, there was no statistical difference in median survival (4.9 years for PCV followed by radiotherapy vs 4.7 years for radiotherapy alone; *P* = 0.26). There was a slight increase in progression-free survival (2.6 years for PCV followed by radiotherapy vs 1.7 years for radiotherapy alone; *P* = 0.004). This small benefit was at the expense of grade 3 or 4 toxicity in 65% of patients and one death. Although the efficacy of PCV was not impressive, this was one of the first studies to demonstrate the correlation of 1p/19q-LOH with improved outcomes, regardless of treatment (> 7-year median survival if co-deleted vs 2.8 years without; *P* = 0.001) [57]. Just as with the anaplastic astrocytomas, the improved outcomes seen in GBMs with temozolomide have inspired clinical trials using temozolomide in the adjuvant setting of anaplastic oligodendrogliomas. Results are eagerly anticipated. However,

until these results are available, the standard treatment for anaplastic oligodendrogliomas remains maximal safe resection followed by postoperative radiation and reservation of chemotherapy until recurrence.

TREATMENT AT RELAPSE

Despite the varied survival benefit afforded by adjuvant therapies for WHO grade III and IV gliomas, most patients will experience recurrence. Frequently complicating matters, the adjuvant treatments described above can result in the development of radiation necrosis ("pseudo-recurrence"), which can radiographically and clinically mimic true tumor recurrence. This is a critical distinction and has important implications for the patient's treatment options and prognosis. Once true tumor recurrence has been determined, and assuming the individual has an adequate performance status, treatment strategies for WHO III to IV gliomas include the sequential use of surgery, chemotherapy, reirradiation, and investigational agents. Patients are generally believed to be good candidates for surgery if they are candidates for a substantial resection, have an adequate performance status, have symptoms able to be ameliorated by surgery, and have additional therapeutic options available to them, either at the time of surgery (*eg*, interstitial polymer-based drug delivery) or following surgery [24,58–61]. Systemic chemotherapy can either be used in combination with surgery or radiotherapy, as in a multimodality strategy, or alone, as in a single-modality strategy [62,63]. Agents include one of the "front-line" chemotherapies not yet utilized, such as temozolomide, systemic BCNU, implantable polymeric BCNU (Gliadel), or Gliasite radiotherapy. International brain cancer centers offer numerous investigational agents for these patients. Considerable attention is currently focused on angiogenesis inhibitors (*eg*, bevacizumab) and small molecule tyrosine kinase inhibitors that target oncogenic signaling pathways, either as single agents or with concurrent chemotherapy. Survival after tumor recurrence is extremely variable, and remains on average about 6 months.

LOW-GRADE GLIOMA

Although the focus of this chapter is malignant glioma, referring to the WHO grade III and IV "high-grade" glioma, the WHO grade II "low-grade" glioma deserves mention in this chapter. Like the high-grade glioma, the grade II glioma is highly infiltrative and not routinely curable with surgery. The natural history of low-grade glioma is to recur with a high propensity for progression to a higher-grade lesion. The low-grade glioma encompasses a wide variety of histologies, including fibrillary and protoplasmic astrocytoma, oligodendroglioma, mixed oligoastrocytoma, and others. With such a diverse spectrum of histologic subtypes, variations in clinical presentation and treatment approaches exist. In general, these tumors present in younger adults, often in the setting of new-onset seizures or a variety of neurologic symptoms resulting from slowly increasing mass effect.

As discussed for high-grade glioma, maximum safe surgical resection is preferable to optimize pathologic diagnosis and reduce tumor burden. Extent of surgical resection has been correlated with improved survival in retrospective studies [25,64]. Biases within patient selection and retrospective analysis have made it impossible to confirm these retrospective conclusions in lieu of a prospective, randomized trial. However, given the significant associated benefits of relieving symptoms and obtaining sufficient tissue to confirm the diagnosis, maximum safe surgical resection should be attempted whenever possible. Distinct from high-grade glioma, a subset of grade II low-grade gliomas can be observed after initial diagnosis without adjuvant therapy. Once a decision to treat is made, options are remarkably similar to those discussed for high-grade glioma: radiation, chemotherapy, the combination of radiation plus chemotherapy (in some cases), and investigational therapies [65,66]. Prognostic factors used to select between treatment options include both tumor-specific and patient-specific factors. The former include histology, grade, MRI contrast enhancement, location, and molecular/genetic markers; the latter include performance status, age, and symptoms (especially seizures) [67]. On average, low-grade gliomas occurring in patients older than 50 years of age are more likely to be biologically aggressive and more likely to undergo malignant transformation to higher-grade glioma. Therefore, these patients should be considered for immediate postoperative treatment, particularly in the setting of bulky residual disease [65]. Survival following the diagnosis of low-grade glioma is very variable and survival curves typically have a long tail. Median life expectancy is approximately 7 years for low-grade astrocytoma and more than 10 years for oligodendroglioma [2]. The eventual natural history of low-grade glioma includes a series of relapses, with shorter periods of progression-free survival at each relapse. Most patients eventually die of tumor progression and often after malignant progression to higher-grade lesions including GBM.

The diversity in presentation of low-grade glioma is reflective of the diversity of literature regarding treatment options. Although there is general consensus that surgical resection is more beneficial than radiation as the first therapeutic option whenever possible, there remains controversy regarding both the optimal timing of the first therapeutic option (*ie*, whether at diagnosis or at time of clinical and/or radiographic progression) and the preferred first postsurgical treatment (*ie*, radiation vs chemotherapy). Some initially symptomatic gliomas may require upfront treatment [63,68]. For the latter, some studies strongly suggest that early intervention with radiotherapy improves outcome, whereas others suggest that intervention later in the course of the disease will yield an equivalent outcome [69–74]. Low-grade glioma can often be discovered incidentally or following a first seizure. Findings from a recent EORTC trial demonstrated that radiation therapy can be safely delayed for patients with no evidence of ongoing tumor growth [74]. In this study, 157 patients were randomly assigned to either postoperative radiotherapy (54 Gy) versus radiotherapy deferred until the time of clinical and/or radiographic progression. Although the median progression-free survival was 5.3 years in the postoperative radiotherapy group and 3.4 years in the deferred radiotherapy group (*P* < 0.0001), the median overall survival was similar between groups (7.4 years in the postoperative radiotherapy group and 7.2 years in the deferred radiotherapy group; *P* = 0.872). This study found improved seizure control within the postoperative radiotherapy group at 1 year. The latter finding is consistent with other small prospective series demonstrating improved seizure control in medically uncontrollable seizures in glioma patients receiving radiotherapy [75]. Low-grade glioma patients with no evidence of ongoing tumor growth can be successfully observed with serial imaging, often for numerous years, before they require treatment for clinical and/or radiographic progression. Delaying the potential neurocognitive toxicity of radiation is an important goal, particularly in young patients who will likely experience long-term survival. Current studies are now investigating how the timing of therapy affects both quality of life and other clinical symptoms. Whenever radiation is utilized, radiotherapy is given to the tumor area and a margin surrounding it, often incorporating the entire T2/FLAIR abnormality. It is not entirely clear what the optimal dose should be for treatment; however, in most cases, a dose of 54 Gy is used. Lower doses in some recent prospective studies appear to be similar in efficacy as 54 Gy, whereas other retrospective series suggest that higher doses are superior [69,70,73,76].

The use of chemotherapy for low-grade glioma is evolving. The efficacy of temozolomide in high-grade glioma has stimulated interest in the potential benefits of chemotherapy in low-grade glioma, including the neoadjuvant setting (before the "definitive" surgery or radiation), the adjuvant setting (with or without radiation), or in lieu of surgery and/or radiation. A growing number of retrospective and small phase 2 trials of adjuvant chemotherapy have demonstrated modest activity, as defined by a partial response or disease stability, especially for subsets expressing co-deletion of 1p/19q [18,77,78]. However, there is currently no evidence that the routine use of adjuvant chemotherapy significantly prolongs survival in patients with low-grade glioma [74]. Long-term follow-up studies, performed in the 1990s, of oligodendroglioma patients who initially reported response to PCV chemotherapy have subsequently been shown to largely reflect the subset of these oligodendroglioma tumors expressing co-deletion of 1p/19q. To date, chemotherapy is generally deferred until clinical and/or radiographic progression. When chemotherapy is used, the standard chemotherapy for progressive or recurrent low-grade glioma is temozolomide [18,79]. Ongoing obstacles to achieving definitive results from low-grade glioma chemotherapy trials remain the characteristics inherent to low-grade gliomas, including heterogeneous histologies, hetero-

geneous approaches to the timing of chemotherapy in the course of disease, and heterogeneous response criteria across trials. Overall, low-grade glioma outcomes are gradually improving as clinicians are better learning how to combine sequential treatments (radiation, surgery, chemotherapy) and more agents are becoming available for clinical trial. Our hope is that the results of two ongoing phase 3 trials in patients with newly diagnosed low-grade glioma will lead to further improvements in the use of chemotherapy. In the EORTC trial, patients are randomized to receive either temozolomide chemotherapy or radiation at diagnosis, whereas in the RTOG trial, patients deemed "unfavorable" are randomized to receive either radiation plus PCV chemotherapy versus radiation alone.

EMERGING TREATMENTS

A comprehensive discussion of emerging agents, technologies, and delivery systems is beyond the scope of this chapter; however, a few promising treatments will be briefly addressed. The goals of agents that target the increased angiogenic capacity of the high-grade glioma include reversing the glioma's ability to create new tumor vasculature, reversing impaired drug delivery, and reversing tumor-related vascular dysfunction. One such antiangiogenic agent, bevacizumab (Avastin, Genentech Inc., San Francisco, CA), a neutralizing anti–vascular endothelial growth factor monoclonal antibody, is currently undergoing phase 2 testing as a single agent or in combination with irinotecan in highly pretreated malignant glioma patients. Initial results are promising, with approximately 70% radiographic response rates and approximately 30% prolonged response rates. Subsets of end-stage patients appear to clearly benefit for at least a few months from bevacizumab-based regimens, predominantly from decreased cerebral edema, mass effect, and contrast-enhancement abnormalities. Effects on survival remain undetermined. The goals of agents that target epidermal growth factor receptor (EGFR) amplification and constitutively active EGFRvIII deletion mutation that occur frequently in high-grade glioma are to reverse the resultant increased cell proliferation, decreased cell death, and tumor invasion [80]. Small series suggest that small molecule EGFR inhibitors (*eg*, erlotinib [Tarceva, Genentech, Inc.]) can be active in appropriately selected patient subsets [21]. Numerous other agents against oncogenic targets that are amplified, overexpressed, or constitutively activated in glioma subsets are under investigation [81]. The goals of agents that target the blood-brain barrier and blood-tumor barrier that occur in gliomas are to reverse the historical limitations of drug delivery, drug safety, and drug efficacy. Attempts to circumvent these barriers include intra-arterial and direct intratumoral drug infusion, blood-brain barrier disruption via hyperosmolar solutions or biomolecules, and implantation of drugs embedded in controlled-release delivery systems. The goal of agents that target the dysfunctional immune system with anticancer vaccines is to stimulate the patient's immune system to selectively recognize and destroy the "foreign" tumor cells. Three of many current vaccines strategies being investigated include the use of autologous (individual patient) tumor-derived heat shock protein, autologous glioma lysate-derived dendritic cell vaccine, and autologous natural killer cell–based vaccines [82–85].

CONCLUSIONS

Malignant glioma poses unique dilemmas to both researchers and patients. The biology of these tumors is being intensely investigated worldwide, both within the laboratory and in the clinic. The information gathered thus far supports a highly complicated, genetically heterogeneous tumor biology that currently exceeds optimal translation of these investigations into successful treatments. However, the pace and volume of basic and translational research is challenging clinical researchers to design more efficient and provocative clinical trials with which to encourage individuals to enroll. The empiricism of the past is now fortunately replaced by molecularly and genetically driven models that we hope will result in improved treatment responses, longer survival, and improved quality of life. Overcoming the compromised immune system, enhancing drug delivery, and optimizing the design and interpretation of both clinical and radiographic response criteria are active areas of research. Clearly, patients with malignant glioma have many more options for participation in clinical trials than ever before. Referral to specialized centers to discuss these options is highly recommended.

REFERENCES

1. Ries LG, Melbert D, Krapcho M, *et al*.: Brain and other nervous system section. In *SEER Cancer Statistics Review, 1975–2004*. Bethesda: National Cancer Institute. http://seer.cancer.gov/csr/1975_2004/. Based on November 2006 SEER data submission, posted to the SEER web site, 2007.

2. American Cancer Society: *Cancer Facts and Figures 2007*. Atlanta: American Cancer Society; 2007. http://www.cancer.org/downloads/STT/CAFF-2007PWSecured.pdf.

3. Wrensch M, Bondy ML, Wiencke J, *et al*.: Environmental risk factors for primary malignant brain tumors: a review. *J Neurooncol* 1993, 17:47–64.

4. Preston-Martin S: Epidemiology of primary CNS neoplasms. *Neurol Clin* 1996, 14:273–290.

5. Kaletsch U, Kaatsch P, Meinert R, *et al*.: Childhood cancer and residential radon exposure: results of a population-based case-control study in Lower Saxony (Germany). *Radiat Environ Biophys* 1999, 38:211– 215.

6. Meinert R, Michaelis J: Meta-analyses of studies on the association between electromagnetic fields and childhood cancer. *Radiat Environ Biophys* 1996, 35:11–18.

7. Kheifets LI, Afifi AA, Buffler PA, *et al*.: Occupational electric and magnetic field exposure and brain cancer: a meta-analysis [see comments]. *J Occup Environ Med* 1995, 37:1327–1341.

8. Lönn S, Ahlbom A, Hall P, *et al*.: Long-term mobile phone use and brain tumor risk. *Am J Epidemiol* 2005, 161:526–535.

9. Lahkola A, Auvinen A, Raitanen J, *et al*.: Mobile phone use and risk of glioma in 5 North European countries. *Int J Cancer* 2007, 120:1769–1775.

10. Kondziolka D, Lunsford LD, Martinez AJ: Unreliability of contemporary neurodiagnostic imaging in evaluating suspected adult supratentorial (low-grade) astrocytoma. *J Neurosurg* 1993, 79:533–536.

11. Wald LL, Nelson SJ, Day MR, *et al*.: Serial proton magnetic resonance spectroscopy imaging of glioblastoma multiforme after brachytherapy. *J Neurosurg* 1997, 87:525–534.

12. Nelson SJ, Huhn S, Vigneron DB, *et al*.: Volume MRI and MRSI techniques for the quantitation of treatment response in brain tumors: presentation of a detailed case study. *J Magn Reson Imaging* 1997, 7:1146–1152.

13. Pirotte B, Goldman S, Massager N, *et al*.: Comparison of 18F-FDG and 11C-methionine for PET-guided stereotactic brain biopsy of gliomas. *J Nucl Med* 2004, 45:1293-1298.

14. Herminghaus S, Dierks T, Pilatus U, *et al*.: Determination of histopathological tumor grade in neuroepithelial brain tumors by using spectral pattern analysis of in vivo spectroscopic data. *J Neurosurg* 2003, 98:74–81.

15. Nader S, Alvarez-Buylla A, Berger M: Neural stem cells and the origin of gliomas. *N Engl J Med* 2005, 353:811–822.

16. Kleihues P, Ohgaki H: Primary and secondary glioblastomas: from concept to clinical diagnosis [review]. *Neuro-oncol* 1999, 1:44–51.

17. McDonald JM, See SJ, Tremont IW, *et al*.: The prognostic impact of histology and 1p/19q status in anaplastic oligodendroglial tumors. *Cancer* 2005, 104:1468–1477.

18. Kaloshi G, Benouaich-Amiel A, Diakite F, *et al*.: Temozolomide for low-grade gliomas: predictive impact of 1p/19q loss on response and outcome. *Neurology* 2007, 68:1831–1836.

19. Esteller M, Garcia-Foncillas J, Andion E, *et al*.: Inactivation of the DNA-repair gene MGMT and the clinical response of gliomas to alkylating agents. *N Engl J Med* 2000, 343:1350–1354.

20. Hegi ME, Diserens A, Gorlia T, *et al*.: MGMT gene silencing and benefit from temozolomide in Glioblastoma. *N Engl J Med* 2005, 352:997–1003.

21. Mellinghoff IK, Wang MY, Vivanco V, *et al*.: Molecular determinants of the response of glioblastomas to EGFR kinase inhibitors. *N Engl J Med* 2005, 353:2012–2024.

22. Curran WJ Jr, Scott CB, Horton J, *et al*.: Recursive partitioning analysis of prognostic factors in three Radiation Therapy Oncology Group malignant glioma trials. *J Natl Cancer Inst* 1993, 85:704–710.

23. Ammirati M, Vick N, Liao YL, *et al*.: Effect of the extent of surgical resection on survival and quality of life in patients with supratentorial glioblastomas and anaplastic astrocytomas. *Neurosurgery* 1987, 21:201–206.

24. Barker FG II, Chang SM, Gutin PH, *et al*.: Survival and functional status after resection of recurrent glioblastoma multiforme. *Neurosurgery* 1998, 42:709–720.

25. Berger MS, Deliganis AV, Dobbins J, *et al*.: The effect of extent of resection on recurrence in patients with low-grade cerebral hemisphere gliomas. *Cancer* 1994, 74:1784–1791.

26. Keles, GE, Lamborn, KR, Berger, MS: Low-grade hemispheric gliomas in adults: a critical review of extent of resection as a factor influencing outcome. *J Neurosurg* 2001, 95:735–745.

27. Keles GE, Chang EF, Lamborn KR, *et al*.: Volumetric extent of resection and residual contrast enhancement on initial surgery as predictors of outcome in adult patients with hemispheric anaplastic astrocytoma. *J Neurosurg* 2006, 105:34–40.

28. Fine HA: The basis for current treatment recommendations for malignant gliomas. *J Neurooncol* 1994, 20:111–120.

29. Gaspar LE, Fisher BJ, Macdonald DR, *et al*.: Supratentorial malignant glioma: patterns of recurrence and implications for external beam local treatment. *Int J Radiat Oncol Biol Phys* 1992, 24:55–57.

30. Leibel SA, Scott CB, Loeffler JS: Contemporary approaches to the treatment of malignant gliomas with radiation therapy. *Semin Oncol* 1994, 21:198–219.

31. Papsdorf K, Wolf U, Hildebrandt G, *et al*.: Outcome and side effects in radiotherapy of glioblastoma: conventional fractionation versus accelerated hyperfractionation. *Front Radiat Ther Oncol* 1999, 33:158–165.

32. Prados MD, Larson DA, Lamborn K, *et al*.: Radiation therapy and hydroxyurea followed by the combination of 6-thioguanine and BCNU for the treatment of primary malignant brain tumors. *Int J Radiat Oncol Biol Phys* 1998, 40:57–63.

33. Prados MD, Berger MS, Wilson CB: Primary central nervous system tumors: advances in knowledge and treatment. *CA Cancer J Clin* 1998, 48:331–360.

34. Scott CB, Scarantino C, Urtasun R, *et al*.: Validation and predictive power of Radiation Therapy Oncology Group (RTOG) recursive partitioning analysis classes for malignant glioma patients: a report using RTOG 90-06. *Int J Radiat Oncol Biol Phys* 1998, 40:51–55.

35. Surawicz TS, Davis F, Freels S, *et al*.: Brain tumor survival: results from the National Cancer Data Base. *J Neurooncol* 1998, 40:151–160.

36. Hochberg FH, Pruitt A: Assumptions in the radiotherapy of glioblastoma. *Neurology* 1980, 9:907–911.

37. Radiation Therapy Oncology Group: RTOG 0513: a phase I/II trial of temozolomide, motexafin gadolinium, and 60 Gy fractionated radiation for newly diagnosed supratentorial glioblastoma multiforme. http://www.rtog.org. Published online December 9, 2005; updated February 24, 2006.

38. Souhami L, Seiferheld W, Brachman D, *et al*.: Randomized comparison of stereotactic radiosurgery followed by conventional radiotherapy with carmustine to conventional radiotherapy with carmustine for patients with glioblastoma multiforme: report of Radiation Therapy Oncology Group 93–05 protocol. *Int J Radiat Oncol Biol Phys* 2004, 60:853–860.

39. Larson DA, Gutin PH, McDermott M, *et al*.: Gamma knife for glioma: selection factors and survival. *Int J Radiat Oncol Biol Phys* 1996, 36:1045–1053.

40. Prados MD, Gutin PH, Phillips TL, *et al*.: Interstitial brachytherapy for newly diagnosed patients with malignant gliomas: the UCSF experience. *Int J Radiat Oncol Biol Phys* 1992, 24:593–597.

41. Sneed PK, Gutin PH, Prados MD, *et al*.: Brachytherapy of brain tumors. *Stereotact Funct Neurosurg* 1992, 59:157–165.

42. Sneed PK, McDermott MW, Gutin PH: Interstitial brachytherapy procedures for brain tumors. *Semin Surg Oncol* 1997, 13:157–166.

43. Gutin PH, Prados MD, Phillips TL, *et al*.: External irradiation followed by an interstitial high activity iodine-125 implant "boost" in the initial treatment of malignant gliomas: NCOG study 6G-82-2. *Int J Radiat Oncol Biol Phys* 1991, 21:601–606.

44. Ulm AJ III, Friedman WA, Bradshaw P: Radiosurgery in the treatment of malignant gliomas: the University of Florida experience. *Neurosurgery* 2005, 57:512–517.

45. Tatter SB, Shaw EG, Rosenblum ML, *et al.*: An inflatable balloon catheter and liquid 125-I radiation source (GliaSite Radiation Therapy System) for treatment of recurrent malignant glioma: multicenter safety and feasibility trial. *J Neurosurg* 2003, 99:297–303.

46. Prados MD, Seiferheld W, Sandler HM, *et al.*: Phase 3 randomized study of radiotherapy plus procarbazine, lomustine, and vincristine with or without BUdR for treatment of anaplastic astrocytoma: final report of RTOG 9404. *Int J Radiat Oncol Biol Phys* 2004, 58:1147–1152.

47. Stewart LA: Chemotherapy in adult high-grade glioma: a systematic review and meta-analysis of individual patient data from 12 randomized trials. *Lancet* 2002, 359:1011–1018.

48. Brem H, Piantadosi S, Burger PC, *et al.*: Placebo-controlled trial of safety and efficacy of intraoperative controlled delivery by biodegradable polymers of chemotherapy for recurrent gliomas. The Polymer-brain Tumor Treatment Group. *Lancet* 1995, 345:1008–1012.

49. Westphal M, Hilt DC, Bortey E, *et al.*: A phase 3 trial of local chemotherapy with biodegradable carmustine (BCNU) wafers (Gliadel wafers) in patients with primary malignant glioma. *Neuro-oncol* 2003, 2:79–88.

50. Stupp R, Mason WP, van den Bent MJ, *et al.*: Radiotherapy plus concomitant and adjuvant temozolomide for glioblastoma. *N Engl J Med* 2005, 352:987–996.

51. Levin VA, Silver P, Hannigan J, *et al.*: Superiority of post-radiotherapy adjuvant chemotherapy with CCNU, procarbazine, and vincristine (PCV) over BCNU for anaplastic gliomas: NCOG 6G61 final report. *Int J Radiat Oncol Biol Phys* 1990, 18:321–324.

52. Prados MD, Scott C, Sandler H, *et al.*: A phase 3 randomized study of radiotherapy plus procarbazine, CCNU, and vincristine (PCV) with or without BUdR for the treatment of anaplastic astrocytoma: a preliminary report of RTOG 9404. *Int J Radiat Oncol Biol Phys* 1999, 53:1109–1115.

53. Levin VA, Prados MR, Wara WM, *et al.*: Radiation therapy and bromodeoxyuridine chemotherapy followed by procarbazine, lomustine, and vincristine for the treatment of anaplastic gliomas. *Int J Radiat Oncol Biol Phys* 1995, 32:75–83.

54. Brandes AA, Nicolardi L, Tosoni A, *et al.*: Survival following adjuvant PCV or temozolomide for anaplastic astrocytoma. *Neuro-oncol* 2006, 3:253–260.

55. Prados MD, Scott C, Curran WJ Jr, *et al.*: Procarbazine, lomustine, and vincristine (PCV) chemotherapy for anaplastic astrocytoma: a retrospective review of Radiation Therapy Oncology Group protocols comparing survival with carmustine or PCV adjuvant chemotherapy. *J Clin Oncol* 1999, 17:3389–3395.

56. Walker MD, Green SB, Byar DP, *et al.*: Randomized comparisons of radiotherapy and nitrosoureas for the treatment of malignant glioma after surgery. *N Engl J Med* 1980, 303:1323–1329.

57. Cairncross GJ, Berkey B, Shaw E, *et al.*: Phase III trial of chemotherapy plus radiotherapy compared with radiotherapy alone for pure and mixed anaplastic oligodendroglioma: Intergroup Radiation Therapy Oncology Group Trial 9402. *J Clin Oncol* 2006, 24:2707–2714.

58. Brem H, Tamargo R, Olivi A, *et al.*: Biodegradable polymers for controlled delivery of chemotherapy with and without radiotherapy in the monkey brain. *J Neurosurg* 1994, 80:283–290.

59. Brem H, Ewend M, Piantadosi S, *et al.*: The safety of interstitial chemotherapy with BCNU-loaded polymer followed by radiotherapy in the treatment of newly diagnosed malignant gliomas. *J Neurooncol* 1995, 26:111–123.

60. Scharfen CO, Sneed PK, Wara WM, *et al.*: High activity iodine-125 interstitial implant for gliomas. *Int J Radiat Oncol Biol Phys* 1992, 24:583–591.

61. Sneed PK, Stauffer PR, Gutin PH, *et al.*: Interstitial irradiation and hyperthermia for the treatment of recurrent malignant brain tumors. *Neurosurgery* 1991, 28:206–215.

62. Burton E, Prados M: New chemotherapy options for the treatment of malignant gliomas. *Curr Opin Oncol* 1999, 11:157–161.

63. Chang SM, Prados MD: Chemotherapy for gliomas. *Curr Opin Oncol* 1995, 7:207–213.

64. Lote K, Egeland T, Hager B, *et al.*: Survival, prognostic factors, and therapeutic efficacy in low-grade glioma: a retrospective study in 379 patients. *J Clin Oncol* 1997, 15:3129–3140.

65. Bauman G, Lote K, Larson D, *et al.*: Pretreatment factors predict overall survival for patients with low-grade glioma: a recursive partitioning analysis. *Int J Radiat Oncol Biol Phys* 1999, 45:923–929.

66. Cairncross JG, Laperriere NJ: Low-grade glioma. To treat or not to treat? *Arch Neurol* 1989, 46:1238–1239.

67. Stupp R, Janzer RC, Hegi ME, *et al.*: Prognostic factors for low-grade gliomas. *Semin Oncol* 2003, 30(Suppl 19):23–28.

68. Prados MD, Edwards MS, Rabbitt J, *et al.*: Treatment of pediatric low-grade gliomas with a nitrosourea-based multiagent chemotherapy regimen. *J Neurooncol* 1997, 32:235–241.

69. Karim AB, Maat B, Hatlevoll R, *et al.*: A randomized trial on dose response in radiation therapy of low-grade cerebral glioma: European Organization for Research and Treatment of Cancer (EORTC) study 22844. *Int J Radiat Oncol Biol Phys* 1996, 36:549–556.

70. Karim AB, Bleehen N, Afra D, *et al.*: Immediate postoperative radiotherapy in low-grade glioma improves progression-free survival but not overall survival: preliminary results of an EORTC/MRC randomized trial [abstract]. *Proc ASCO* 1998, 17:400.

71. Shaw EG: The low-grade glioma debate: evidence defending the position of early radiation therapy. *Clin Neurosurg* 1995, 42:488–494.

72. Shaw E, Arusell R, Scheithauer B, *et al.*: A prospective randomized trial of low-versus high-dose radiation therapy in adults with supratentorial low-grade glioma: initial report of a NCCTG/RTOG/ECOG study [ASCO abstract]. *J Clin Oncol* 2002, 20:2267–2276.

73. Shaw EG, Berkey B, Coons SW, *et al.*: Radiation therapy oncology group (RTOG) protocol 9802: radiation therapy (RT) alone versus RT + PCV chemotherapy in adult low-grade glioma (LGG). *Neuro-oncol* 2006, 8:489.

74. van den Bent MJ, Afra D, de Witte O, *et al.*: Long-term efficacy of early versus delayed radiotherapy for low-grade astrocytoma and oligodendroglioma in adults: the EORTC 22845 randomised trial. *Lancet* 2005, 366:985–990.

75. Rogers LR, Morris HH, Lupica K: Effect of cranial irradiation on seizure frequency in adults with low-grade astrocytoma and medically intractable epilepsy. *Neurology* 1993, 43:1599–1601.

76. Shaw EG, Scheithauer BW, Gilbertson DT, *et al.*: Postoperative radiotherapy of supratentorial low-grade gliomas. *Int J Radiat Oncol Biol Phys* 1989, 16:663–668.

77. Wen PY, DeAngelis LM: Chemotherapy for low-grade gliomas: emerging consensus on its benefits. *Neurology* 2007, 68:1762–1763.

78. Brada M, Viviers L, Abson C, *et al.*: Phase II study of primary temozolomide chemotherapy in patients with WHO grade II gliomas. *Ann Oncol* 2003, 14:1715–1721.

79. Hoang-Xuan K, Capelle L, Kujas M, *et al.*: Temozolomide as initial treatment for adults with low-grade oligodendrogliomas or oligoastrocytomas and correlation with chromosome 1p deletions. *J Clin Oncol* 2004, 22:3133–3138.

80. Lal A, Glazer CA, Martinson HM, *et al.*: Mutant epidermal growth factor receptor up-regulates molecular effectors of tumor invasion. *Cancer Res* 2002, 62:3335–3339.

81. Sathornsumetee S, Reardon DA, Desjardins A, *et al.*: Molecularly targeted therapy for malignant glioma. *Cancer* 2007, 110:13–24.

82. Yamanaka R: Novel immunotherapeutic approaches to glioma, *Curr Opin Mol Ther* 2006, 8:46–51.

83. Yamanaka R, Itoh K: Peptide-based immunotherapeutic approaches to glioma: a review. *Exp Opin Biol Ther* 2007, 7:645–649.

84. Parajuli P, Mathupala S, Mittal S, *et al.*: Dendritic cell-based active specific immunotherapy for malignant glioma. *Exp Opin Biol Ther* 2007, 7:439–448.

85. Ishikawa E, Tsuboi K, Saijo K, *et al.*: Autologous natural killer cell therapy for human recurrent malignant glioma. *Anticancer Res* 2004, 24:1861–1871.

This chapter reviews the current diagnosis and therapy of some of the diverse group of cancers affecting the endocrine glands. The first sections focus on thyroid cancer, the predominant endocrine cancer. Subsequent sections discuss adrenal cancers (adrenal cortical carcinoma and malignant pheochromocytoma/paraganglioma) and gastroenteropancreatic endocrine tumors. Because a number of these endocrine cancers occur in hereditary syndromes as well as sporadic forms, diagnosis, genetic testing issues, and special management considerations for these familial forms are also discussed.

THYROID CANCER

EPIDEMIOLOGY

In 2008, approximately 37,340 new cases of thyroid cancer will be diagnosed in the United States, with a female:male ratio of 3.2:1 [1]. Thyroid cancer is now the sixth most common incident cancer in American women. New cases of thyroid cancer increased from 3.6 per 100,000 persons in 1973 to 8.7 per 100,000 in 2002—a 2.4-fold increase [2]. Explanations for the remarkable increase in thyroid cancer are diverse, but the dramatic increase in neck imaging, especially ultrasound, computed tomography (CT), and positron emission tomography (PET), is responsible for incidental detection of many clinically occult thyroid cancers. Most thyroid cancers are papillary (PTC; 80%); follicular (FTC; 15%), medullary (MTC; 4%), and anaplastic (ATC; 1%) thyroid cancers account for the remainder (Table 16-1) [3]. PTC and FTC (including its common variant, Hurthle cell cancer) are conventionally classed as differentiated thyroid cancer (DTC). Remarkably, thyroid cancer accounts for 94% of new endocrine cancer diagnoses in the United States and 65% of endocrine cancer deaths. The ratio of new cases to deaths (23.5) is greater than other noncutaneous epithelial cancers, including testicular cancer (21.2) [1]. One of the most important challenges in thyroid cancer management is identification of the small subset of patients who require more intensive surgical and adjuvant therapy.

Radiation exposure in childhood is one recognized risk factor for thyroid cancer. Sources of radiation exposure include nuclear accidents such as Chernobyl, in which the youngest children were most sensitive. The minimal latent period for thyroid cancer development after exposure was about 4 years. The most common genetic abnormality associated with childhood iodine-131 (^{131}I) exposure appears to be the RET-PTC3 rearrangement. Table 16-2 lists other molecular abnormalities in thyroid cancer [4]. Therapeutic external radiation in childhood is also a major risk factor for thyroid cancer. For example, standardized incidence ratios of thyroid cancer following treatment of childhood Hodgkin's lymphoma and non-Hodgkin's lymphoma were 52.5 and 40.4, respectively [5]. Childhood radiation treatments formerly used for benign conditions, including acne and tonsillar enlargement, are also associated with increased rates of thyroid cancer, often with prolonged latency. Graves disease, with associated thyroid-stimulating antibodies, is associated with a higher incidence of occult and clinically aggressive thyroid cancers [6]. In addition, thyroid cancer incidence increases with age, with outcomes distinctly worse for patients presenting after age 50.

Several genetic syndromes are also associated with thyroid cancer. Approximately 5% of DTC cases are familial. Gardner syndrome, hereditary polyposis coli, and Cowden disease are all recognized as having DTC as a minor component. Individuals in whom DTC and thyroid nodules are the predominant components are referred to as having familial nonmedullary thyroid cancer. No DNA-based tests are currently available for this syndrome. In comparison with DTC, 25% of MTC cases are familial, inherited as one of the three syndromes comprising MEN2. MEN2 stems from characteristic germline-activating mutations in the Ret proto-oncogene, which can be identified in presymptomatic testing. The three MEN2 syndromes include familial isolated MTC, MEN2A (MTC plus ~ 50% prevalence of pheochromocytoma and 15% hyperparathyroidism), and MEN2B (aggressive early-onset MTC with pheochromocytoma and mucosal ganglioneuromatosis). Each of these syndromes has characteristic *Ret* gene mutations and varying MTC penetrance. An international consensus statement has summarized recommendations for MEN2 testing and treatment [7]. Other than MEN2, no other familial or environmental factors are known for MTC.

ATC is the rarest and most aggressive form of thyroid cancer, with a median survival of less than 6 months. Approximately 25% of anaplastic cases have a preceding history of PTC, but most occur de novo as rapidly expanding anterior neck masses in older patients.

DIAGNOSTIC METHODS

Thyroid cancer may present with a palpable thyroid nodule or cervical adenopathy or rarely with distant metastases. Nearly 50% of thyroid cancers are now detected incidentally in the imaging work-up for other disorders—a mode of presentation common in oncology practices. Carotid ultrasound, neck and chest CT, and [^{18}F]fluoro-2-deoxy-D-glucose (FDG)-PET scanning are the most common modalities. In the case of FDG-PET, approximately 27% to 45% of patients with focal uptake within the thyroid gland have been found to harbor thyroid cancer on further evaluation [8]. Overall though, thyroid nodules discovered by examination or by imaging carry a similar risk of malignancy, about 5% in the overall population. Patients with multiple thyroid nodules do not appear to have a significantly lower risk of thyroid cancer than patients with solitary nodules. Thyroid cancer risk should be assessed on a "nodule by nodule" basis.

Thyroid ultrasound evaluation is recommended in all patients with palpable or incidentally discovered thyroid nodules. Ultrasound is useful because on examination many patients with solitary nodules will prove to have multiple nodules on sonography. Sonographically suspicious features such as microcalcification and irregular margins can also be identified. Serum thyroid-stimulating hormone (TSH) is useful to screen patients for the possibility of a hyperfunctioning nodule, in which case thyroid cancer risk is low. The role of routine serum calcitonin assay is currently controversial. The presence of a significant calcitonin elevation (> 100 pg/mL) provides strong evidence for MTC; lower level elevations may be difficult

Table 16-1. Types of Thyroid Cancer	
Cancer	**Incidence, %**
Papillary	80
Follicular (including Hurthle)	15
Medullary	3
Anaplastic	2
Thyroid lymphoma	< 1

Table 16-2. Molecular Abnormalities in Thyroid Cancer	
Mutations	**Thyroid cancer type**
Activating mutations	
BRAF (V600E)	Papillary, anaplastic
Ret rearrangement	Papillary
Ras	Follicular
Ret point mutation	Sporadic medullary (somatic)
	MEN2 (germline) syndrome
Inactivating mutations	
p53	Anaplastic
p18	Medullary

to interpret. Fine-needle aspiration (FNA) is the most accurate and cost-effective method for evaluating thyroid nodules. Suspicious or diagnostic biopsies warrant surgery; benign biopsies warrant conservative follow-up. Cytologically indeterminate nodules should generally be considered for limited surgery (lobectomy) [9]. For an inadequate sample, nondiagnostic biopsies should be repeated. Although large nodules may be biopsied by direct palpation, ultrasound-guided FNA offers distinct advantages for smaller or partially cystic lesions and generally is the technique of choice.

Patients with a cytologically proven diagnosis of DTC are recommended to have preoperative neck ultrasound with FNA of suspicious cervical nodes. In the case of cytologically proven MTC, a more extensive biochemical and staging work-up is recommended for most patients. In addition to a detailed family history, Ret proto-oncogene DNA analysis is recommended to exclude hereditary MTC. If Ret testing is positive or unavailable, patients should be screened preoperatively for pheochromocytoma (*eg*, plasma and/or 24-hour urine metanephrines) and hyperparathyroidism (calcium and parathyroid hormone [PTH]). All MTC patients should have preoperative calcitonin and carcinoembryonic antigen (CEA) levels measured. Additional imaging work-up to consider includes neck ultrasound, neck and chest CT, abdominal magnetic resonance imaging (MRI) or arterial-venous phase CT, and bone imaging.

TREATMENT

SURGERY

Thyroidectomy is recommended as initial treatment for DTC and MTC patients, but not in most cases of ATC [9]. The extent of surgery chosen in most cases of DTC is total or near-total thyroidectomy. However, a lobectomy/isthmusectomy is frequently elected in patients with unilateral indeterminate cytologic findings such as follicular neoplasm, often followed by completion thyroidectomy if the surgical pathology proves to contain thyroid cancer. In DTC, the presence of significant lymph node metastasis on preoperative neck ultrasound confirmed with FNA would prompt a compartment-oriented cervical node dissection, frequently comprising levels 2, 3, 4, and 6 (less commonly including level 5). In typical sporadic cases of MTC, surgery includes total thyroidectomy and central (level 6) and ipsilateral modified radical neck dissection (levels 2–5). (The high frequency of cervical node involvement in MTC tumors greater than 1 cm usually warrants ipsilateral neck dissection, even in the absence of neck imaging findings.) Bilateral modified neck dissections may be considered in some cases. For ATC, surgery is focused on securing the airway, plus obtaining enteral access and adequate tissue for diagnosis. Primary resections of ATC have often proved ineffective in sustaining local control. Some centers continue to recommend thyroidectomy in ATC when feasible, either upfront or following initial response to chemoradiation (see below).

ADJUVANT TREATMENT OF DTC

Standard adjuvant therapy options in DTC include radioactive iodine ablation of the thyroid gland remnant and TSH suppression by L-thyroxine. The goals for radioactive iodine therapy are to destroy residual thyroid tissue to facilitate long-term surveillance with stimulated thyroglobulin measurements and sometimes radioiodine whole body scans. A secondary goal is to identify and potentially treat loco-regional residual disease, lung metastases, or other sites such as bone, liver, or brain. Several retrospective studies indicate a significant reduction in the rates of disease recurrence and thyroid cancer–related death in subsets of DTC patients following radioiodine [9]. Patients with small, unifocal tumors (< 1.5 cm) limited to the thyroid have no significant improvements in survival or recurrence and may be followed without adjuvant radioiodine. In the most recent American Thyroid Association guidelines, adjuvant radioiodine is recommended for patients with stages III and IV disease (according to the American Joint Committee on Cancer staging system), all patients with stage II disease younger than 45 years of age, and most patients with stage II disease 45 years of age or older. Radioiodine is especially warranted in patients with multifocal disease, nodal metastases, extrathyroidal or vascular invasion, and/or more aggressive histologies [9]. Doses of ^{131}I between 30 and 100 mCi generally achieve comparable levels of remnant ablation. Patients may be prepared for radioiodine with an iodine-restricted diet and either

thyroid hormone withdrawal (allowing the TSH to rise spontaneously) or with recombinant human TSH (Thyrogen, Genzyme Corp., Cambridge, MA) injections. Known side effects of radioiodine therapy include xerostomia, sialadenitis, and taste alterations, all of which are usually transient. After remnant ablation, a posttreatment scan is obtained and patients are treated with L-thyroxine. The L-thyroxine dose is selected to produce mild or moderate reductions in TSH, depending on the severity of thyroid cancer. High-risk patients are usually suppressed to a TSH level below 0.1 mU/L, whereas low-risk patients' TSH levels are maintained at or slightly below the lower limit of normal (0.1–0.5 mU/L). The risks of thyroid hormone overtreatment, especially in the elderly, are well known, and include atrial fibrillation and accelerated bone loss.

Postoperative surveillance in DTC includes periodic TSH and thyroglobulin testing, plus cervical ultrasound, and further imaging in some patients. The sensitivity of thyroglobulin as a measure of persistent thyroid remnant or thyroid cancer is enhanced by recombinant TSH treatment. One widely used scheme for surveillance includes a cervical ultrasound and thyroxine-suppressed thyroglobulin at 6 months, and recombinant TSH-stimulated thyroglobulin at 12 months. After the initial posttreatment diagnostic whole body scan is negative outside of the thyroid bed area, patients typically do not require routine diagnostic whole body scanning during follow-up [9]. Long-term surveillance includes periodic TSH and thyroglobulin testing and cervical ultrasound; the most appropriate time intervals have not been established. Because late recurrences may occur, including very rare progression to ATC, patients in remission are generally followed indefinitely.

PERSISTENT AND RECURRENT DTC

Patients discovered to have macroscopic cervical lymph node involvement during follow-up are frequently treated with additional surgery, even if radioiodine uptake exists. Patients with significant persistent thyroglobulin elevations but negative anatomic imaging, as well as patients with inoperable metastases, are investigated to determine whether there is radioiodine uptake or not. For the thyroglobulin-positive/scan-negative patient, we typically employ an empiric radioiodine treatment to determine whether there is significant uptake on the higher-activity posttreatment scan.

For radioiodine treatment of inoperable metastases, one can use empiric fixed doses, doses determined by the upper bound limit of blood and body dosimetry, or doses identified by quantitative tumor dosimetry. No clear overall preference exists [9]. In the case of pulmonary metastases, high remission rates are reported in younger patients and patients with micrometastases. Rates are much lower for macroscopic lesions or in patients older than 50 years of age. Indicators of response include reductions in thyroglobulin and lesion size. Changes in radioiodine uptake in serial studies must be correlated carefully with anatomic studies such as CT. After partial response, radioiodine treatment may be repeated at a 6- to 12-month interval. Little consensus exists regarding dose, interval, or cumulative tolerable dose. There is a low, dose-related risk of secondary malignancies (including bone and soft tissue, colorectal, and salivary gland cancers and leukemia) in long-term thyroid cancer survivors treated with higher lifetime doses of radioactive iodine [10]. Radioiodine-refractory DTC is operationally defined as tumors that persist after high cumulative doses of radioactive iodine (> 600–800 mCi), or tumors defined by anatomic imaging that have scant or absent uptake on an appropriate posttreatment whole body scan. High FDG uptake on PET scanning at follow-up is a predictor of both radioiodine-refractory DTC and greater risk of death [11].

Neck external-beam radiation therapy may be considered in older patients with grossly visible extrathyroidal extension at the time of surgery and a high likelihood of microscopic residual disease, and for those patients with gross residual tumor in whom further surgery or radioactive iodine would likely be ineffective [9]. An additional role for external-beam radiotherapy is in patients with painful bone lesions, especially if these lesions do not take up radioiodine. Surgery may also be considered for these painful or potentially unstable bone lesions. Brain metastases are also seen in older patients with widespread DTC. If possible, resection followed by external-beam radiotherapy is the treatment of choice.

No data currently support the use of cytotoxic chemotherapy in DTC [9]. Doxorubicin and other agents have been used as radiosensitizers in

ATC patients undergoing concurrent radiotherapy [12]. Higher-risk radio-iodine-refractory DTC patients with progression should be considered for a systemic therapy trial. A variety of targeted agents are currently being studied in phase 2 and 3 clinical trials in DTC (Table 16-3). The most common therapeutic target is vascular endothelial growth factor receptor (VEGFR). A number of multifunction tyrosine kinase inhibitors are currently under study. The investigational VEGFR kinase inhibitor axitinib exhibited significant single-agent activity in thyroid cancer, with best responses in FTC (33% partial response, 87% partial response or stable disease) [13]. Among the US Food and Drug Administration (FDA)-approved tyrosine kinase inhibitors, sunitinib and sorafenib are both currently in clinical trials for use in thyroid cancer. As of 2008, with no approved or proven thyroid cancer indications, the use of targeted therapies in thyroid cancer patients should generally be within the context of a clinical trial whenever possible. Recent progress in DTC clinical trials has been reviewed [14,15].

PERSISTENT AND RECURRENT MTC

For MTC, postoperative surveillance includes periodic calcitonin and CEA measurement, plus imaging in selected patients, generally those with significant calcitonin elevations greater than approximately 300 pg/mL (nL < 8). Only about 30% of sporadic MTC patients are biochemically cured by surgery. Most have residual cancer with fairly indolent progression. Imaging options include neck ultrasound, neck and chest CT, liver MRI (or arterial-venous phase CT), and bone imaging [16]. There is no role for radioiodine treatment in MTC, and only a limited role for external-beam radiation—painful bone metastases, or possibly in resected patients at high risk for cervical recurrence based on positive tumor margins or extranodal extension [17].

The natural history of MTC predicts approximately 75% 10-year survival with stage III (nodal disease) and 25% in stage IV, with some patients having long indolent courses despite distant metastases. The calcitonin and CEA doubling times have proven to be powerful prognostic indicators, even independent of clinical stage, with doubling times under 6 months predicting accelerated mortality [18]. Similar to DTC, cytotoxic chemotherapy has little benefit in MTC, with response rates below 25% and no proven impact on overall survival. Combinations based on dacarbazine or doxorubicin have been tested most frequently. Patients with inoperable, progressive MTC should be considered for enrollment in clinical trials. In addition to VEGFR, a second outstanding target in MTC is the Ret tyrosine kinase, which is activated by mutation in MEN2 and, in up to 50% of sporadic cases, as an acquired somatic mutation [19]. A number of phase 2 and 3 trials are examining the efficacy of combined VEGFR2 and Ret inhibition (Table 16-3). Recent progress in MTC trials has been summarized in several reviews [19,20].

ATC PROGNOSIS AND THERAPY

ATC is among the most aggressive solid tumor types, with growth observed over days to weeks. In Surveillance Epidemiology and End Results data, mortality was 68% at 6 months and 81% at 1 year [21]. Direct extrathyroidal invasion into structures including the larynx, trachea, esophagus, and soft tissues of the neck can be seen in more than 90% of patients at presentation. The current approach to ATC focuses on airway management, frequently with tracheostomy. Once the cytologic diagnosis has been made and the airway secured, combined chemoradiation is usually employed with doxorubicin and hyperfractionated radiotherapy. Sometimes local debulking surgery appears to be effective after initial improvements with chemoradiation. Using this approach, Tennvall et al. [12] reported improved local control in a majority of patients and rare 2-year survivors (9%). Paclitaxel is also reported to have activity in ATC, although with little impact on survival [22]. Several clinical trials are currently under way in ATC, including those using a vascular-disrupting agent (combretastatin) or a peroxisome proliferator–activated receptor (PPAR)-γ agonist in combination with chemotherapy (Table 16-3).

Although DTC frequently can be eradicated by a combination of surgery, radioiodine, and L-thyroxine, the subset of thyroid cancer patients referred to oncologists often has radioiodine-refractory DTC with progressive metastatic disease, or progressive MTC, or ATC. In the absence of standard effective systemic therapies (or even effective loco-regional control therapies in the case of ATC), many patients with advanced thyroid cancer should be considered for clinical trials. The off-label use of cytotoxic chemotherapy or oral tyrosine kinase inhibitors, while a conceivable option, is less attractive compared with clinical trials. Given the indolent course and good performance status of many patients with DTC and MTC, judicious watchful waiting may also be a valid approach for individual patients.

ADRENAL CORTICAL CARCINOMA AND MALIGNANT PHEOCHROMOCYTOMA

EPIDEMIOLOGY AND DIAGNOSTIC METHODS

Malignant tumors of the adrenal glands are uncommon, with an incidence of approximately 1 case per 1 million per year for adrenal cortical carcinoma (ACC) and an even lower rate for malignant pheochromocytoma. ACC has two age ranges of peak incidence: children younger than 10 years of age and adults in their 40s and 50s. There are no known environmental risk factors for ACC. A small minority of ACC patients have inherited cancer predisposition syndromes including Li-Fraumeni (p53 mutation) or Beckwith-Wiedemann syndrome. The most common age of presentation is the fourth and fifth decade of life. Most patients with ACC are discovered to have a large asymptomatic adrenal mass via imaging, sometimes with metastatic involvement of the liver, abdominal lymph nodes, and lung. ACC tumors may be hormonally silent (55%) or have detectable increases in glucocorticoids, androgens, or rarely, aldosterone. Androgen excess is detectable only in women. Men rarely may experience feminizing symptoms such as gynecomastia, testicular atrophy, and low sperm count. Clinical outcomes appear to be worse in hormonally active ACC [23]. ACC tumors have imaging characteristics that usually allow them to be distinguished from benign adrenocortical adenomas, pheochromocytomas, or metastatic tumors from an extra-adrenal source. CT characteristics include large size (> 4 cm), irregular shape, central necrosis and hemorrhage, high un-enhanced Hounsfield unit density, and delay in contrast medium washout. Although CT-guided FNA may be obtained after ruling out pheochromocytoma with biochemical testing, cytology cannot distinguish between benign adrenocortical adenoma and ACC. In some instances, FNA is useful to exclude metastatic tumors of extra-adrenal origin. Hormonal evaluation in ACC patients includes a 24-hour urinary free cortisol to exclude significant hypercortisolism, and androgens including DHEAS (adrenal-specific), testosterone, and androstenedione (gonadal plus adrenal origin).

Table 16-3. Investigational Therapies in Thyroid Cancer

Characteristic/class	Agent(s)	Thyroid cancer type
Mixed-function TKI	Vandetanib	Differentiated
	XL184	Medullary
	Sorafenib	Differentiated
	Sunitinib	Differentiated
	Pazopanib	Differentiated
	PTK787	Differentiated
	Motesanib	Differentiated and medullary
VEGFR-specific TKI	Axitinib	Differentiated
Vascular disrupting	Combretastatin/ paclitaxel carboplatin	Anaplastic
	Lenalidomide	Differentiated
MEK inhibitor	AZD6244	Differentiated
PPAR-γ agonist	CS7017/paclitaxel	Anaplastic
Radioimmunotherapy	Anti-CEA	Medullary
Cytotoxic	Irinotecan	Medullary
	Bortezomib	Differentiated

CEA—carcinoembryonic antigen; PPAR—peroxisome proliferator–activated receptor; TKI—tyrosine kinase inhibitor; VEGFR—vascular endothelial growth factor receptor.

Pheochromocytomas account for about 0.2% of all hypertensive patients. Although it was believed for many years that 10% of pheochromocytomas are malignant, more recent studies indicate a 13% to 15% malignancy rate at presentation and 6% to 23% recurrence rate with prolonged follow-up, for an overall rate of 20% to 30% [24]. In addition to malignant pheochromocytoma, paragangliomas (derived from sympathetic and parasympathetic ganglia rather than the adrenal medulla) have a higher rate of malignancy, especially in the defined hereditary paraganglioma syndromes of succinate dehydrogenase subunit B and D (SDHB and SDHD, respectively), stemming from inactivating mutations in SDH isoenzyme genes (Table 16-4). In contrast, virtually all pheochromocytomas associated with MEN2, and 90% or more associated with Von Hippel-Lindau (VHL) disease and type 1 neurofibromatosis (NF-1), are benign [25]. Diagnosis of pheochromocytoma is based on the presence of characteristic adrenergic signs and symptoms (hypertension, diaphoresis, tachycardia, pallor, orthostatic blood pressure changes), the presence of elevated plasma and urine catecholamines and metabolites, and characteristic imaging findings. Among the possible biochemical tests for pheochromocytoma, plasma metanephrines and urine metanephrines have proven to be most sensitive and specific, although small elevations (< 2.5-fold) must be interpreted with caution. Malignant pheochromocytoma differs from benign pheochromocytoma in several key aspects. Malignant tumors have a median diameter of 9.4 cm versus 5.9 cm for benign tumors, a nearly 25% frequency of extra-adrenal primary site (*eg*, paraganglioma) compared with 7.7% for benign tumors, and a significantly lower frequency of classic adrenergic symptoms and hypertension [26]. Imaging for pheochromocytoma typically begins with CT or MRI. Meta-iodobenzylguanine (MIBG) scintigraphy may be helpful, especially for documenting metastases or paragangliomas. Recently FDG-PET has been shown to have superior imaging properties for paragangliomas associated with the *SDHB* mutation. The most common metastatic sites for malignant pheochromocytoma and paragangliomas are abdominal and pelvic lymph nodes, bone liver, and lung [27]. FNA is contraindicated in pheochromocytoma, but typical contrast administration is permitted.

TREATMENT

Treatment of ACC is initially aimed at surgical resection or nearly complete debulking if metastases are present at the time of operation. Recurrence is likely even after complete resection. Within 2 years after diagnosis, approximately 27% of patients with stage I, 46% of those with stage II, and 63% of those with stage III ACC develop metastasis [23]. Based on the high rates of recurrence, there has been long-standing interest in adjuvant therapy for ACC. The adrenolytic DDT derivative mitotane has been studied as adjuvant therapy for ACC, with some studies showing benefit and others not. A recent retrospective study of 177 ACC patients who underwent surgery in Germany and Italy showed that adjuvant mitotane (1–5 g/d) was associated with a significantly longer recurrence-free survival compared with control groups (median recurrence-free survival of 42 months vs 10 and 25 months in Italian and German control patients, respectively). Overall survival was also superior for the mitotane group versus the control groups (110 vs 52 and 67 months) [28]. The unbalanced nature of the two control groups and lack of a prospective design limit the broad applicability of this trial; howev-

er, adjuvant low-dose mitotane (1–3 g) may be considered in ACC following surgery. The optimal duration remains unclear. Side effects include gastrointestinal and neurologic effects, and are strongly dose related. Serum mitotane levels are important predictors of response and side effects. A target therapeutic range of 14 to 20 mcg/mL can be reached after several months. Patients treated with mitotane develop adrenocortical insufficiency and require initial glucocorticoid replacement (typically prednisone 5–7.5 mg/d) and within 1 to 2 months, mineralocorticoid replacement (typically fludrocortisone 0.1 mg/d). Coordination with an endocrinologist may be helpful in managing symptoms of adrenal insufficiency and excess.

Adjuvant radiation is also controversial in ACC. The available small studies do not support a role for this modality. Although local recurrence may be impacted, overall survival and disease-free survival do not appear to improve with radiation [29]. There is a need for larger prospective studies combining adjuvant radiation with mitotane.

Treatment of patients with persistent or recurrent locally advanced ACC is difficult. Based on limited data, surgical debulking of loco-regional disease in the adrenal bed, abdominal lymph nodes, or liver may help significantly in controlling hypercortisolism, or otherwise remove a majority of the remaining tumor. Single-agent mitotane in this setting has been relatively disappointing. Improved response rates have been reported with patients tolerating mitotane levels above 14 mg/L [30].

For patients with stage IV disease or refractory loco-regional ACC, chemotherapy combinations with mitotane have been frequently used. Monthly etoposide, doxorubicin, and cisplatin plus oral mitotane (4 g daily) was associated with an overall response rate of 49% (7% complete response, 42% partial response) [31]. Median time to progression in responding patients was 24 months. Smaller studies have reported overall response rates of 33% for cisplatin, etoposide, and mitotane [32]; 36% for streptozocin and mitotane [33]; and 14% for etoposide, doxorubicin, vincristine, and mitotane [34]. Combinations lacking mitotane generally have been ineffective for this disorder. A large, multicenter European trial, FIRM-ACT (First International Randomized Trial in Locally Advanced and Metastatic Adrenocortical Carcinoma Treatment), is currently under way to evaluate etoposide, doxorubicin, and cisplatin plus mitotane versus streptozocin and mitotane. FIRM-ACT protocols are available online (http://www.firm-act.org/).

For malignant pheochromocytoma and paraganglioma, initial treatment is surgery after appropriate α- and β-blockade. Surgical manipulations, anesthesia induction, or embolization procedures (sometimes used preoperatively in paraspinal paragangliomas) all carry a risk of excessive catecholamine release. α-Blockade (for example with phenoxybenzamine) should precede β-blocker treatment to avoid paradoxical worsening of hypertension caused by β-2 adrenergic inhibition. For patients with massive tumors or in whom complete resection is impossible, additional preparation with the catecholamine synthesis inhibitor α-methyl paratyrosine (metyrosine) is an option. Principal treatment choices for stage IV and locally advanced malignant pheochromocytoma are ^{131}I-MIBG and combination chemotherapy, usually CVD (cyclophosphamide, vincristine, dacarbazine) (see Scholz *et al.* [25] for review).

Patients are selected for ^{131}I-MIBG therapy on the basis of tumoral uptake of this catecholamine precursor-like agent, compared with uptake of

Table 16-4. Pheochromocytoma/Paraganglioma: Familial Syndromes

Syndrome	Phenotype	Associated lesions	Gene
Von Hippel-Lindau	Pheo-Pgl (> 90% benign)	Retinal hemangioma, pancreatic NET, renal calcium, CNS hemangioblastoma	*VHL* *
MEN2	Pheo (> 99% benign)	Medullary thyroid cancer, hyperparathyroidism, gastrointestinal ganglioneuromas	*Ret* *
Type 1 neurofibromatosis	Pheo-Pgl (90% benign)	Café au lait lesions, neurofibromas	*NF1*
SDHB	Pgl-Pheo (60% malignant)	None	*SDHB* *
SDHD	Pgl, especially carotid Pheo (20%–30% malignant)	None	*SDHD* *

*DNA testing commercially available.
CNS—central nervous system; NET—neuroendocrine tumor; Pgl—paraganglioma; Pheo—pheochromocytoma; SDHB—succinate dehydrogenase subunit B; SDHD—succinate dehydrogenase subunit D.

FDG-PET or anatomic studies such as CT and MRI. Patients with all or most of their lesions MIBG-avid on a diagnostic study (either ^{123}I or ^{131}I-MIBG) are candidates for high-dose therapy. Several studies have now reported efficacy in this patient subset, with 25% complete responses (durations 24 to > 101 months) and 58% partial responses (6–47 months) in the most promising results to date [35]. These subjects were treated intensively with a median dose of 800 mCi, inpatient admission, thyroidal protection with iodide, bladder irrigation, and marrow support for pancytopenia. Re-treatment may be indicated for partial responders. This therapy is being studied in a limited number of US centers.

Chemotherapy for malignant pheochromocytoma is the first choice in patients whose tumors lack significant MIBG uptake. CVD is effective in a significant proportion of patients, although responses longer than 2 years are uncommon. Averbuch *et al.* [36] reported an overall response rate of 57% in a small study of 14 patients using this regimen. Because of the potential for excessive catecholamine release during a tumor lysis syndrome, patients should be appropriately treated with adrenergic-blocking agents and/or metyrosine. CVD may be considered as front-line therapy in patients with rapidly progressive malignant pheochromocytoma [25]. Experience with other chemotherapeutic agents is very limited [25].

GASTROENTEROPANCREATIC ENDOCRINE TUMORS

EPIDEMIOLOGY AND DIAGNOSIS

The group of endocrine tumors affecting the pancreas, stomach, and intestines is very diverse (Table 16-5). Gastroenteropancreatic endocrine tumors may occur sporadically or as part of inherited MEN 1 (combined with hyperparathyroidism and sometimes pituitary tumors) or VHL (pancreatic neuroendocrine tumors combined with retinal angiomas, pheochromocytoma/paraganglioma, occasionally central nervous system lesions, and renal cell carcinoma). While germline testing is possible for both disorders, testing for MEN1 is only approximately 70% sensitive, with no strong genotype-phenotype predictions, whereas VHL testing can be highly informative. It is difficult to estimate the combined prevalence of gastroenteropancreatic endocrine tumors. Carcinoid tumors are the most common, with an overall incidence of 2 to 4 per 100,000 per year in the United States. Metastatic carcinoid tumors are most likely with small intestinal and colonic sites; gastric and rectal primary sites are more likely to be localized [37]. Carcinoid tumors may present with bowel obstruction, abdominal pain, or weight loss. Only 5% to 7% of patients with small intestinal carcinoid tumors present with a classic carcinoid syndrome (including flushing, secretory diarrhea, carcinoid heart disease, and niacin deficiency). Classic carcinoid syndrome is rarely seen at other primary sites in the gastrointestinal tract. The presence of the carcinoid syndrome or of significant elevations of serotonin (or its urinary metabolite 5'HIAA) frequently indicates that a small intestinal carcinoid tumor has metastasized, commonly to the liver. Intestinal carcinoid tumors may be identified on high-resolution CT based on the characteristic desmoplastic changes in the surrounding mesentery. Liver metastases can be seen with combined arterial-venous contrast CT or gadolinium-enhanced MRI. Octreotide scanning is also useful.

Other gastroenteropancreatic endocrine tumors may be identified on the basis of a characteristic endocrine syndrome: fasting hypoglycemia in insulinoma; glucose intolerance and necrolytic migratory erythema in glucagonoma; peptic ulcer disease and secretory diarrhea in gastrinoma; watery diarrhea, hypokalemia, and hypochlorhydria in vasoactive intestinal peptide tumors; and diabetes, steatorrhea, and cholelithiasis in somatostatinoma. The recent World Health Organization classification system deemphasizes the hormone-secretory properties and classifies gastroenteropancreatic tumors in the following classes: 1a) well-differentiated neuroendocrine tumor; 1b) well-differentiated neuroendocrine cancer, a low-grade malignancy; and 2) poorly differentiated neuroendocrine cancer. Overall, 50% to 75% of duodenal neuroendocrine neoplasms are class 1a, 25% to 50% are well-differentiated carcinomas, and 0% to 3% are poorly differentiated neuroendocrine cancers. Serotonin- and gastrin-producing tumors can be classified as 1a or 1b. Supporting this revised classification is the frequent production of more than one hormone by an individual tumor. Duodenal neuroendocrine tumors have recently been extensively reviewed [38]. Malignant insulinoma accounts for 5% to 10% of all insulinomas. These tumors tend to be larger (mean diameter, 6 cm) and recur after initial surgery at a median interval of 2.8 years. Ten-year survival of 29% is reported in malignant insulinoma [39].

TREATMENT

For islet cell tumors, which may include insulin, glucagon, gastrin, somatostatin, and nonsecretory tumors, primary pancreatic surgery is indicated, usually even in the presence of liver metastases. Patients with extrapancreatic disease confined to the liver may be candidates for liver surgery, radiofrequency ablation (tumors < 3 cm), or hepatic artery chemoembolization. Unresectable patients, including patients with significant extrahepatic disease, may be considered for clinical trials or for combination chemotherapy, which has achieved limited success. Active agents include streptozocin, 5-fluorouracil, capecitabine, temozolomide, and α-interferon. Octreotide (150 mcg subcutaneous 3 times daily) has significant palliative action in limiting hormone secretion for glucagon and gastrin; however, efficacy in insulinoma is mixed [39]. If subcutaneous octreotide is well tolerated and patients have a symptomatic response, octreotide long-acting depot 20 mg given monthly as an intramuscular injection can be used. Gastrin hypersecretion is managed symptomatically with proton pump inhibitors. In the setting of MEN1, multifocal gastrin-secreting tumors in the small intestine and stomach make surgical cure difficult; therefore, proton pump inhibitor therapy is often the primary treatment choice.

For gastrointestinal carcinoid tumors with unresectable or residual/metastatic disease, patients are evaluated for presence of the carcinoid syndrome. Useful tumor markers include plasma serotonin, 24-hour urine 5'HIAA, and chromogranin A. Patients with carcinoid syndrome or elevated markers should be evaluated with echocardiography to exclude right-sided heart disease. To date, control of serotonin excess has not resulted in slower progression of carcinoid heart disease [40]. Hepatic regional options include wedge resection/partial hepatectomy, radiofrequency ablation, and hepatic chemoembolization. Symptomatic management incorporates octreotide and octreotide long-acting depot. Patients with progressive disease should be considered for clinical trials.

Table 16-5. Gastroenteropancreatic Endocrine Tumors

Carcinoid (multiple sites)

Insulinoma

Glucagonoma

Gastrinoma

Vasoactive intestinal peptide–producing

Somatostatin-producing

Pancreatic neuroendocrine tumor, not otherwise specified

REFERENCES

1. Jemal A, Siegel R, Ward E, *et al.*: Cancer statistics, 2008. *CA Cancer J Clin* 2008, 58:71–96.

2. Davies L, Welch HG: Increasing incidence of thyroid cancer in the United States, 1973–2002. *JAMA* 2006, 295:2164–2167.

3. Kondo T, Ezzat S, Asa SL: Pathogenetic mechanisms in thyroid follicular-cell neoplasia. *Nat Rev Cancer* 2006, 6:292–306.

4. Adeniran AJ, Zhu Z, Gandhi M, *et al.*: Correlation between genetic alterations and microscopic features, clinical manifestations, and prognostic characteristics of thyroid papillary carcinomas. *Am J Surg Pathol* 2006, 30:216–222.

5. Maule M, Scelo G, Pastore G, *et al.*: Risk of second malignant neoplasms after childhood leukemia and lymphoma: an international study. *J Natl Cancer Inst* 2007, 99:790–800.

6. Pellegriti G, Belfiore A, Giuffrida D, *et al.*: Outcome of differentiated thyroid cancer in Graves' patients. *J Clin Endocrinol Metab* 1998, 83:2805–2809.

7. Brandi ML, Gagel RF, Angeli A, *et al.*: Guidelines for diagnosis and therapy of MEN type 1 and type 2. *J Clin Endocrinol Metab* 2001, 86:5658–5671.

8. Kang KW, Kim SK, Kang HS, *et al.*: Prevalence and risk of cancer of focal thyroid incidentaloma identified by 18F-fluorodeoxyglucose positron emission tomography for metastasis evaluation and cancer screening in healthy subjects. *J Clin Endocrinol Metab* 2003, 88:4100–4104.

9. Cooper DS, Doherty GM, Haugen BR, *et al.*: Management guidelines for patients with thyroid nodules and differentiated thyroid cancer. *Thyroid* 2006, 16:109–142.

10. Rubino C, de Vathaire F, Dottorini ME, *et al.*: Second primary malignancies in thyroid cancer patients. *Br J Cancer* 2003, 89:1638–1644.

11. Wang W, Larson SM, Fazzari M, *et al.*: Prognostic value of [18F]fluorodeoxyglucose positron emission tomographic scanning in patients with thyroid cancer. *J Clin Endocrinol Metab* 2000, 85:1107–1113.

12. Tennvall J, Lundell G, Wahlberg P, *et al.*: Anaplastic thyroid carcinoma: three protocols combining doxorubicin, hyperfractionated radiotherapy and surgery. *Br J Cancer* 2002, 86:1848–1853.

13. Kim S, Rosen LS, Cohen EE, *et al.*: A phase II study of axitinib (AG-013736), a potent inhibitor of VEGFRs, in patients with advanced thyroid cancer [abstract]. *J Clin Oncol* 2006, 24(18S):5529.

14. Baudin E, Schlumberger M: New therapeutic approaches for metastatic thyroid carcinoma. *Lancet Oncol* 2007, 8:148–156.

15. Deshpande HA, Gettinger SN, Sosa JA: Novel chemotherapy options for advanced thyroid tumors: small molecules offer great hope. *Curr Opin Oncol* 2008, 20:19–24.

16. Ball DW: Medullary thyroid cancer: monitoring and therapy. *Endocrinol Metab Clin North Am* 2007, 36:823–837.

17. Brierley J, Tsang R, Simpson WJ, *et al.*: Medullary thyroid cancer: analyses of survival and prognostic factors and the role of radiation therapy in local control. *Thyroid* 1996, 6:305–310.

18. Barbet J, Campion L, Kraeber-Bodere F, *et al.*: Prognostic impact of serum calcitonin and carcinoembryonic antigen doubling-times in patients with medullary thyroid carcinoma. *J Clin Endocrinol Metab* 2005, 90:6077–6084.

19. Ball DW: Medullary thyroid cancer: therapeutic targets and molecular markers. *Curr Opin Oncol* 2007, 19:18–23.

20. Schlumberger M, Carlomagno F, Baudin E, *et al.*: New therapeutic approaches to treat medullary thyroid carcinoma. *Nat Clin Pract Endocrinol Metab* 2008, 4:22–32.

21. Kebebew E, Greenspan FS, Clark OH, *et al.*: Anaplastic thyroid carcinoma. Treatment outcome and prognostic factors. *Cancer* 2005, 103:1330–1335.

22. Ain KB, Egorin MJ, DeSimone PA: Treatment of anaplastic thyroid carcinoma with paclitaxel: phase 2 trial using ninety-six-hour infusion. Collaborative Anaplastic Thyroid Cancer Health Intervention Trials (CATCHIT) Group. *Thyroid* 2000, 10:587–594.

23. Abiven G, Coste J, Groussin L, *et al.*: Clinical and biological features in the prognosis of adrenocortical cancer: poor outcome of cortisol-secreting tumors in a series of 202 consecutive patients. *J Clin Endocrinol Metab* 2006, 91:2650–2655.

24. Goldstein RE, O'Neill JA Jr, Holcomb GW III, *et al.*: Clinical experience over 48 years with pheochromocytoma. *Ann Surg* 1999, 229:755–764; discussion 764–756.

25. Scholz T, Eisenhofer G, Pacak K, *et al.*: Clinical review: current treatment of malignant pheochromocytoma. *J Clin Endocrinol Metab* 2007, 92:1217–1225.

26. Glodny B, Winde G, Herwig R, *et al.*: Clinical differences between benign and malignant pheochromocytomas. *Endocr J* 2001, 48:151–159.

27. Zelinka T, Timmers HJ, Kozupa A, *et al.*: Role of positron emission tomography and bone scintigraphy in the evaluation of bone involvement in metastatic pheochromocytoma and paraganglioma: specific implications for succinate dehydrogenase enzyme subunit B gene mutations. *Endocr Relat Cancer* 2008, 15:311–323.

28. Terzolo M, Angeli A, Fassnacht M, *et al.*: Adjuvant mitotane treatment for adrenocortical carcinoma. *N Engl J Med* 2007, 356:2372–2380.

29. Fassnacht M, Hahner S, Polat B, *et al.*: Efficacy of adjuvant radiotherapy of the tumor bed on local recurrence of adrenocortical carcinoma. *J Clin Endocrinol Metab* 2006, 91:4501–4504.

30. Baudin E, Pellegriti G, Bonnay M, *et al.*: Impact of monitoring plasma 1,1-dichlorodiphenildichloroethane (o,p'DDD) levels on the treatment of patients with adrenocortical carcinoma. *Cancer* 2001, 92:1385–1392.

31. Berruti A, Terzolo M, Sperone P, *et al.*: Etoposide, doxorubicin and cisplatin plus mitotane in the treatment of advanced adrenocortical carcinoma: a large prospective phase II trial. *Endocr Relat Cancer* 2005, 12:657–666.

32. Bonacci R, Gigliotti A, Baudin E, *et al.*: Cytotoxic therapy with etoposide and cisplatin in advanced adrenocortical carcinoma. Reseau Comete INSERM. *Br J Cancer* 1998, 78:546–549.

33. Khan TS, Imam H, Juhlin C, *et al.*: Streptozocin and o,p'DDD in the treatment of adrenocortical cancer patients: long-term survival in its adjuvant use. *Ann Oncol* 2000, 11:1281–1287.

34. Abraham J, Bakke S, Rutt A, *et al.*: A phase II trial of combination chemotherapy and surgical resection for the treatment of metastatic adrenocortical carcinoma: continuous infusion doxorubicin, vincristine, and etoposide with daily mitotane as a P-glycoprotein antagonist. *Cancer* 2002, 94:2333–2343.

35. Rose B, Matthay KK, Price D, *et al.*: High-dose 131I-metaiodobenzylguanidine therapy for 12 patients with malignant pheochromocytoma. *Cancer* 2003, 98:239–248.

36. Averbuch SD, Steakley CS, Young RC, *et al.*: Malignant pheochromocytoma: effective treatment with a combination of cyclophosphamide, vincristine, and dacarbazine. *Ann Intern Med* 1988, 109:267–273.

37. Modlin IM, Lye KD, Kidd M: A 5-decade analysis of 13,715 carcinoid tumors. *Cancer* 2003, 97:934–959.

38. Hoffmann KM, Furukawa M, Jensen RT: Duodenal neuroendocrine tumors: classification, functional syndromes, diagnosis and medical treatment. *Best Pract Res Clin Gastroenterol* 2005, 19:675–697.

39. Grant CS: Insulinoma. *Best Pract Res Clin Gastroenterol* 2005, 19:783–798.

40. Moller JE, Connolly HM, Rubin J, *et al.*: Factors associated with progression of carcinoid heart disease. *N Engl J Med* 2003, 348:1005–1015.

Leukemia

Erica D. Warlick, B. Douglas Smith

ACUTE MYELOID LEUKEMIA

Acute myeloid leukemia (AML) describes a group of heterogeneous disorders characterized by malignant transformation, involving maturation and apoptotic defects, of hematopoietic stem cells that leads to an overabundance of immature myeloid cells and suppression of normal hematopoiesis. Although AML affects people of all ages, the median age at diagnosis is between 62 and 65 years, with a prevalence of five in every 100,000 patients older than 60 years of age. AML is more common in white individuals (1.5–3 per 100,000) and men [1].

CLASSIFICATION AND PROGNOSIS

Biologically, AML is a heterogeneous array of disorders comprising the French-American-British (FAB) classification system of M0–M7. It can arise de novo or secondarily as a consequence of exposure to environmental toxins such as benzene, ionizing radiation, or previous chemotherapy (topoisomerase II inhibitors or alkylating agents). Although the complexities of genetic abnormalities resulting in AML are yet to be fully characterized, it is well established that abnormal expression of oncogenes and tumor suppressor control within a pluripotent stem cell leads to abnormal myeloid maturation and resistance to apoptosis [2].

Prognosis depends upon a number of factors, including age at diagnosis, specific cytogenetic abnormalities, white blood cell (WBC) count at time of presentation, previous chemotherapy or exposure to toxins, and previous hematologic problems. Cytogenetic abnormalities such as inversion of chromosome 16, t(8;21), and t(15;17) are associated with a good prognosis, whereas abnormalities involving loss of chromosome 5 or 7, partial deletions of 5 or 7, and complex cytogenetics are associated with a poor prognosis. Characteristic cytogenetic abnormalities are seen in treatment-related AML, such as unbalanced translocations or deletions of chromosomes 5 and 7 with alkylating agent exposure and balanced translocations involving the 11q23 mixed-lineage leukemia (MLL) gene with topoisomerase II inhibitor exposure. In addition, AML associated with multilineage dysplasia is associated with a poor prognosis [3].

Efforts to expand the prognostic data beyond traditional cytogenetics have focused on the role of molecular mutations and the information that they may provide. Presently, the best-studied mutation with important prognostic information is the internal tandem duplication (ITD) of the receptor tyrosine kinase FLT3. This receptor tyrosine kinase is structurally similar to the platelet-derived growth factor receptor subfamily of tyrosine kinases and is mainly expressed on hematopoietic and neural tissues [4]. FLT3 signaling is associated with cell growth and apoptosis inhibition, and the ITD mutation results in a constitutively activated kinase. Interestingly, the clinical presentation of patients with FLT3-ITD–mutated AML mirrors this biology; patients often have markedly elevated WBC counts and packed marrow spaces. There are now multiple series confirming the presence of FLT3-ITD as a universally poor prognostic marker in AML [5–8]. More recently, mutations of the nucleophosmin gene (ie, NPM) have been identified in more than 50% of AML cases with normal cytogenetics [9–11]. Normally, nucleophosmin is a phosphoprotein expressed in most tissues [12] that shuttles continuously between the nucleus and the cytoplasm [13,14]. Nucleophosmin plays important roles in the biogenesis and nuclear export of ribosomes [15] and in maintaining genomic stability [16,17]; it also interacts with p53 and p19ARF to impact cell proliferation and apoptosis [18]. NPM mutations result in aberrant cytoplasmic expression and irregular trafficking of the mutated NPM proteins. Mutations of the NPM gene have been associated with a favorable prognosis in patients with normal-karyotype AML [11,19,20], although the individual processes involved in this remain under study. Both molecular findings have the ability to contribute to treatment planning for many patients with AML; however, there remains a significant challenge in developing and making available reliable testing for most centers treating AML patients.

TREATMENT

Treatment of AML is divided into three stages: induction, postremission or consolidation therapy, and therapy at the time of relapse (Table 17-1). The goal of induction therapy is to achieve a complete remission (CR) and then to proceed with postremission therapy in an attempt to achieve maximal disease-free survival (DFS) and cure. Of note, induction therapy for M3 AML, acute promyelocytic leukemia, should be considered distinct and is discussed below. Standard induction therapy for all other types of AML includes the combination of cytarabine (cytosine arabinoside, Ara-C) with an anthracycline. Typically, patients receive cytarabine as a continuous infusion of 100 to 200 mg/m²/d for 7 days [21]. This infusion is combined with an anthracycline (eg, daunorubicin, idarubicin) or mitoxantrone for 3 days [21,22]. An overview of randomized trials published by the AML Collaborative Group comparing idarubicin and daunorubicin suggest improved induction remission rates and overall survival with idarubicin, with slightly higher nonrelapse mortality in the idarubicin arms, thus creating a similar DFS between the two agents [23]. As a class, anthracyclines are associated with accumulative cardiotoxicity; those patients exceeding well-recognized dosing thresholds are at particularly high risk. This often limits the treatment options in patient with multiple-relapsed leukemias or those with treatment-related AML and prior exposures. Combination chemotherapy is associated with an induction CR rate of approximately 60% to 70% in patients younger than 60 years of age and 40% in patients older than 60 years of age [24,25].

Alternative induction regimens include high-dose cytarabine [26], high-dose cyclophosphamide plus etoposide [27], or standard-dose cytarabine plus etoposide [28]. In a single-institution trial, the addition of high-dose cytarabine following a standard "7 + 3" regimen (cytarabine plus daunorubicin) improved the remission rate in patients with AML to 86% in patients younger than 63 years of age [29]. This regimen has not been directly compared with the standard "7 + 3" regimen in a randomized study. Additionally, timed-sequential therapy strategies have been investigated, and although no overall difference has been shown in event-free and overall survival, a subset analysis in specific trials has shown improved relapse-free intervals in patients younger than age 50 [30]. Debate exists about whether older patients (> 70 years of age) and patients with secondary AML benefit from intensive induction approaches because in these populations the CR rates

Table 17-1. Chemotherapy Treatment Regimens for Acute Myeloid Leukemia

Study	Regimen type	Chemotherapy
Mitus et al. [29]	Induction	"7 + 3":
		Daunorubicin 50 mg/m² IV on d 1, 3, and 5 or idarubicin 12 mg/m²
		Cytarabine 100–200 mg/m²/d as continuous infusion for 7 d
Mayer et al. [36]	Consolidation	HIDAC:
		Cytarabine 3 g/m² twice daily on d 1, 3, and 5
Yavuz et al. [37]	Salvage	FLAG-IDA:
		Fludarabine 25–30 mg/m² on d 1–5
		Cytarabine 2000 mg/m² on d 1–5
		Idarubicin 10–12 mg/m² on d 2–4
		Granulocyte colony-stimulating factor starting on d 6

remain low and the treatment-related toxicity is significant [31]. Low-dose cytarabine (10–20 mg/m²/d) has been advocated by some in the treatment of older patients in an attempt to avoid the acute side effects associated with standard induction [32]. Although responses can be seen with low-dose cytarabine, many weeks of therapy may be required, and complications related to prolonged pancytopenia can be noted just as when following standard induction chemotherapy. New agents are being tested for initial treatment of elderly AML patients. Tipifarnib, a farnesyltransferase inhibitor, is one of the newer agents showing tolerability and activity [33]. Although the common belief is that older patients are not able to tolerate aggressive induction therapy, a large Southwest Oncology Group (SWOG) trial actually showed a CR rate in elderly patients (median age, 68 years) with favorable or normal cytogenetics comparable with younger patients, suggesting that the elderly may also benefit from more aggressive induction regimens [34]. In addition, a focus on clinical trials for alternative regimens treating elderly AML patients should be stressed.

It is estimated that residual leukemia cells on the order of 109 remain even when patients are in CR. Consequently, postremission or consolidation chemotherapy is required to remove this microscopic disease [35] and may include reiterations of standard-dose cytarabine and anthracycline for two more courses or the use of high-dose cytarabine. In a prospective trial, the Cancer and Leukemia Group B (CALGB) compared three different doses of cytarabine as postremission therapy. Patients received cytarabine 100 mg/m² for 5 days, 400 mg/m² for 5 days, or 3 g/m² every 12 hours for a total of six doses, each given four times over 4 to 6 months. This was followed by four more cycles of subcutaneous cytarabine at 100 mg/m² twice daily for 10 doses and daunorubicin 45 mg/m². Patients younger than 60 years of age receiving the high-dose cytarabine arm had a superior DFS compared with the other groups, whereas there was no difference between arms in patients older than 60 years of age [36].

Despite remission after induction and consolidation chemotherapy, the risk of recurrence is approximately 50% to 60% [1]. Patients with a remission interval of more than 1 year may respond to the same induction regimen at the time of relapse, whereas patients with a shorter duration of remission should be considered for alternative regimens. Patients who are considered poorer risk in terms of cytogenetic abnormalities or age may be offered other treatment modalities. Numerous salvage chemotherapy options for relapsed patients are available. Examples include the FLAG-IDA regimen (fludarabine, cytarabine, granulocyte colony-stimulating factor, idarubicin) [37]; high-dose cytarabine; mitoxantrone plus etoposide [38]; high-dose cyclophosphamide plus etoposide [27]; or gemtuzumab ozogamicin (Mylotarg, Wyeth, Philadelphia, PA), the monoclonal antibody against CD33 conjugated to calicheamicin. However, much of the current excitement extends to more biologically targeted agents, such as FLT3 inhibitors, farnesyltransferase inhibitors, histone deacetylase inhibitors, DNA methyltransferase inhibitors, and Raf kinase inhibitors [35].

ALLOGENEIC BONE MARROW TRANSPLANTATION

Allogeneic bone marrow transplantation (BMT) is a treatment modality considered to be a possible curative option for patients with AML. It is typically reserved for patients with higher-risk AML, including those with high-risk cytogenetics, with relapsed or refractory disease, or whose age and performance status permit the increased intensity of the treatment. According to the Center for International Blood and Marrow Transplant Research data, outcomes for a human leukocyte antigen (HLA)–matched sibling transplant for patients older than 20 years of age in first CR showed 50% to 60% survival at 5 years, and a 40% to 45% survival rate at 5 years in second CR. For a matched–unrelated donor transplant, survival outcomes were slightly lower at 30% at 5 years for both first and second CR. Limitations of allogeneic BMT as a treatment modality include requirements for matched donor, age limitations, treatment-related complications (*eg*, graft-versus-host disease), and infectious complications. Because of these limitations, transplantation is not an option for everyone and alternative treatment strategies need to be investigated.

AUTOLOGOUS BONE MARROW TRANSPLANTATION

Autologous BMT is an option for patients without an HLA-matched sibling and for older patients. The treatment-related mortality associated with

autologous transplantation is lower than allogeneic BMT, approaching 2% to 5%; however, subsequent relapse remains the most significant complication of this approach. Both regimens containing chemotherapy only and those including total-body irradiation appear to be equally effective. Purging of the bone marrow to remove minimal residual disease can be performed by the use of either monoclonal antibodies, which are directed to antigens expressed on the surface of leukemia cells, or by incubation of the marrow in cytotoxic drugs such as 4-hydroperoxycyclophosphamide [39,40]. To date, no clear benefit has been demonstrated by the purging of bone marrow by either technique. Long-term disease-free remission can be obtained in 30% to 50% of patients who receive autologous BMT in second or subsequent relapse.

ACUTE PROMYELOCYTIC LEUKEMIA

Acute promyelocytic leukemia (APL) represents a distinct subgroup of AML characterized by promyelocytic blasts containing the 15;17 chromosomal translocation. This leads to the generation of the fusion transcript comprised of the retinoic acid receptor (a-RAR) and a sequence called PML. Prior to the recognition of this molecular abnormality, retinoic acid had been clinically observed to induce differentiation of blasts in patients with APL, and investigators in France and China used retinoic acid to treat these patients [41]. All-trans-retinoic acid was found to be superior to cis-retinoic acid both in vitro and in vivo in APL and was capable of inducing CR in patients with APL [42]. The current standard of care for APL treatment is the combination of all-trans-retinoic acid and chemotherapy, which generates CR rates in more than 85% of patients [43]. Additionally, the use of all-trans-retinoic acid reduces the complications of disseminated intravascular coagulation associated with induction chemotherapy in APL patients. Approximately 20% of patients treated with all-trans-retinoic acid may develop the "retinoic acid syndrome" or "differentiation syndrome" characterized by fever, pulmonary infiltrates, and hypoxemia with and without leukocytosis [44]. Therefore, it is important to distinguish APL from other subtypes of AML because all-trans-retinoic acid should be used as part of the treatment regimen. Postremission therapy for patients with APL has not been standardized; however, recent efforts have focused on the use of anthracyclines as the main cytotoxic agent for consolidation cycles based on the recognized drug sensitivity patterns in APL. Studies suggest that prolonged maintenance therapy with all-trans-retinoic acid and low-dose chemotherapy improves durable remission rates [45]. In patients who relapse or the rare patient found to be refractory to all-trans-retinoic acid, arsenic trioxide is the standard second-line therapy, with CR rates of 80% to 90% [46]. For patients in second CR with no molecular evidence of disease, there are now studies supporting the use of both autologous and allogeneic BMT in the hope of extending survival. Gemtuzumab has also shown efficacy in refractory and relapsed disease [46].

ACUTE LYMPHOBLASTIC LEUKEMIA

ETIOLOGY AND RISK FACTORS

Acute lymphoblastic leukemia (ALL) is common in children but rare in the adult population. Several factors, such as higher socioeconomic status; genetic factors, as evident by increased risk in monozygotic twins [47], Down syndrome [48], and inherited diseases with increased chromosomal fragility such as Fanconi anemia [49]; radiation exposure [50]; and exposure to industrial chemicals [51], have been associated with ALL. However, the etiology is unknown in the majority of cases. Additionally, Epstein-Barr virus infection has been associated with Burkitt lymphoma and mature B-cell ALL. Lastly, ALL development after chemotherapy exposure with topoisomerase II inhibitors has been noted with the cytogenetic abnormality of t(4;11)(9q21;q23) [52].

CLASSIFICATION AND PROGNOSIS

ALL is a heterogeneous disease with distinct clinical features displayed by various subtypes. As with AML, the FAB classification was the original system used to classify ALL, with three subtypes, L1–L3, described. Expanding knowledge of immunophenotyping and cytogenetic analysis has allowed correlation with clinical outcome and behavior, often trumping the ability of FAB subtype to predict outcome. As a result, the World Health Organization recommendations have abandoned the L1–3 classification [3].

Immunophenotyping allows lineage determination for the vast majority of ALL blasts and divides them into the following categories: pre-B ALL, mature B-cell ALL, and T-lineage ALL. Terminal deoxynucleotidyl transferase testing distinguishes pre-B ALL and T-cell ALL (positive) from mature B-cell ALL (negative). Additionally, pre-B ALL is marked by cytoplasmic immunoglobulin, whereas mature B-cell ALL is marked by surface immunoglobulin and T-cell ALL is marked with cytoplasmic Cd3+ [53]. Approximately 25% of adult ALLs are of T-cell lineage. Although earlier studies have suggested a worse prognosis associated with the T-cell phenotype, recent studies have not confirmed this finding.

Recurring cytogenetic abnormalities have also been demonstrated in ALL. The most common cytogenetic abnormality is the Philadelphia chromosome (Ph) 9;22 translocation, which occurs in about 15% to 30% of adult ALL [54,55]. Approximately one half of patients produce a fusion protein p190, whereas the remaining patients demonstrate a p210 phenotype similar to patients with chronic myeloid leukemia. Although remission rates are similar between Ph-positive and Ph-negative patients, Ph-positive patients have substantially worse prognosis, with almost complete relapse and few long-term survivors. Thus, these patients typically attempt allogeneic BMT in first remission if a donor is available [55]. Abnormalities of chromosome 9p21 are also found in approximately 15% of patients and effect/inactivate a number of the cyclin-dependent kinase inhibitors (*eg*, p16INK4a, p15INK4b). Deletions involving 9p range in prognostic effects; 9p deletion is considered a poor risk factor in B-cell ALL but only in T-cell ALL if the deletion is homozygous [56]. However, these prognostic associations are more consistent in childhood ALL [53,54]. Rearrangements of 11q23 are also prevalent in ALL involving the *MLL* gene, with more than 20 different reciprocal translocations. Interestingly, coexpression of myeloid markers is common and prognosis with 11q23 abnormalities is poor [57]. Another cytogenetic abnormality is 19p13, in which prognosis is dependent on the type of ALL and therapy used, with those patients with pro-B ALL and those receiving aggressive therapy doing better than those with pre-B ALL or standard therapy [53]. A cryptic translocation not routinely found on conventional cytogenetics is translocation 12;21, which is present in upwards of 30% of pediatric ALL cases [58] but uncommon and thus prognostically undefined in adults [59]. In addition to cytogenetic abnormalities, several clinical variables have also been associated with prognosis, including age, sex, time to remission, and WBC count at presentation [60].

TREATMENT

The hallmark of chemotherapy regimens for the treatment of ALL is multi-agent chemotherapy (Table 17-2) with both dose and time intensity. Multi-agent chemotherapy has numerous goals: 1) to work toward eradication of leukemia while preventing the development of resistance subclones, 2) to supply adequate prophylaxis to sanctuary sites such as the central nervous system (CNS) and testicles, 3) to eliminate minimal residual disease, and ultimately 4) to restore normal hematopoiesis [61–64]. ALL chemotherapy is multistaged and composed of induction, intensified consolidation, and maintenance therapy. With multidrug chemotherapy, the majority of adults with ALL achieve a CR [62], with long-term DFS in approximately 30% to 40% of patients [53,63]. The basis for ALL induction regimens has histori-

cally been a combination of steroids, vincristine, and anthracyclines, with high CR rates and a DFS rate of approximately 18 months [65]. Subsequent trials have added cyclophosphamide [66] and dose-intense asparaginase, based on its importance in pediatric regimens; however, its role in adults is not as well defined [61,67]. CNS prophylaxis is another standard component of ALL therapy given that CNS disease occurs in a large percentage of patients without CNS treatment. Prophylaxis can consist of intrathecal chemotherapy, high-dose systemic chemotherapy (*eg*, high-dose methotrexate), or cranial irradiation. Intensified consolidation is the third component of therapy used in ALL and can be comprised of a modified induction schedule, various rotational chemotherapy regimens, or stem cell transplantation. Prolonged maintenance therapy with weekly methotrexate, daily 6-mercaptopurine, and pulses of vincristine and prednisone given every 1 to 3 months is the final component of ALL therapy. This has been shown to prevent relapse in children but has yet to be proven effective in adults. Treatment for mature B-cell ALL differs in that response to short-duration cycles of high intensity with no maintenance therapy appears effective, with few relapses beyond remission of 1 year [63]. Additionally, for Ph-positive ALL, the ideal maintenance therapy is imatinib.

Despite aggressive induction, the majority of adults who have ALL relapse. A second remission may be obtained with chemotherapy in 10% to 70% of patients depending on the regimen used. If relapse occurs after a prolonged remission, reinduction with similar agents used at the time of presentation may be used. Alternative salvage regimens include Hyper-CVAD (fractionated cyclophosphamide, vincristine, doxorubicin, dexamethasone), if not used as initial therapy. Additionally, newer studies indicate activity of the purine analogues clofarabine in ALL and nelarabine in T-cell ALL [68]. However, the durability of second and subsequent remissions is poor, and these patients should be considered candidates for BMT.

ALLOGENEIC BONE MARROW TRANSPLANTATION

Allogeneic BMT for adults with ALL in first CR yields 5-year DFS rates of approximately 40% to 70%, with the majority of benefit seen in patients with high-risk disease. Unfortunately, although relapses are decreased in ALL patients undergoing allogeneic BMT during first CR, treatment-related mortality is substantial [69]. As a result, allogeneic BMT has traditionally been reserved for high-risk patients (*eg*, adverse cytogenetics, Ph-positive, high WBC at diagnosis, or delayed time to first CR) who are in first CR [70,71]. However, the role of allogeneic BMT for all patients in first remission still remains unclear. In historic reports comparing allogeneic BMT in patients with ALL in first remission to the results of chemotherapy alone, no clear benefit of early BMT was demonstrated. The overall 5-year leukemia-free survival was 44% for patients undergoing BMT in first CR versus 38% for patients receiving chemotherapy only. Additionally, the treatment-related mortality in the patients undergoing BMT was higher [72]. However, results from a newer study by the Medical Research Council/Eastern Cooperative Oncology Group (E2993 study), challenge the prior belief that only high-risk ALL patients benefit from allogeneic BMT. In this study, all patients with an HLA-matched sibling donor who achieved a CR after induction were chosen to undergo allogeneic BMT while those without a donor were randomized to either consolidation/maintenance therapy or autologous BMT. In this trial, 5-year event-free survival rates for the allogeneic BMT group versus the randomized groups were 54% and 34%, respectively. Additionally, in the standard-risk group, the 5-year event-free survival in the allogeneic BMT group was 66% compared with 45% in the randomized

Table 17-2. Studies of Multi-Agent Regimens for Acute Lymphoblastic Leukemia

Study	Chemotherapy regimen	Complete remission, %	Median duration response, *mo*
Kantarjian *et al.* [137]	VAD (vincristine, doxorubicin, dexamethasone)	75–90	18
Rowe *et al.* [138]	MRC/ECOG E2993 (2-phase induction therapy*)		
Kantarjian *et al.* [64]	Hyper-CVAD (fractionated cyclophosphamide, vincristine, doxorubicin, dexamethasone)		

*Phase 1 of induction therapy included daunorubicin, vincristine, L-asparaginase, prednisone, and methotrexate. Phase 2 included cyclophosphamide, cytarabine, 6-mercaptopurine, and methotrexate.
ECOG—Eastern Cooperative Oncology Group; MRC—Medical Research Council.

group [73]. Although this study indicates that all groups can benefit from allogeneic BMT in first CR, the standard approach remains to reserve first CR allogeneic BMT for high-risk patients and as salvage therapy for relapsing patients obtaining second CR. Alternative donor sources for patients with no HLA-matched sibling include matched–unrelated donors, umbilical cord blood transplants, and mini-haploidentical transplants.

AUTOLOGOUS BONE MARROW TRANSPLANTATION

Autologous BMT provides an alternative source of stem cells for patients for whom no donor can be identified. Recent studies have shown that the residual leukemia cells infused at the time of marrow infusion can contribute to relapse [74]. A variety of approaches have been attempted to reduce the risk of marrow contamination by tumor cells, including immunologic purging using monoclonal antibodies, long-term culture strategies, and chemical purging in vitro. To date, no purging strategy has proved superior to the others, and some have been associated with prolonged time to engraftment [75].

Uncontrolled trials of autologous BMT in first and second remission have produced results superior to the DFS often seen with chemotherapy alone. Prospective, multicenter trials have not demonstrated a clear benefit in favor of autologous BMT in the treatment of adult patients in first remission. In one study, 96 patients were randomly assigned to autologous BMT and 96 patients received chemotherapy alone. There was no significant difference in the incidence of treatment-related mortality, relapse, CR duration, or survival, with a DFS of approximately 35% at 3 years [76]. When autologous BMT is compared with allogeneic BMT, the treatment-related mortality associated with autologous BMT is much lower; however, the risk of relapse is significantly higher.

CHRONIC MYELOID LEUKEMIA

ETIOLOGY AND RISK FACTORS

Chronic myeloid leukemia (CML) is a malignant clonal hematopoietic stem cell disorder with defined t(9;22) chromosomal rearrangement of the BCR/ABL (breakpoint-cluster region/Abelson leukemia virus) that causes a constitutively activated tyrosine kinase. This chromosomal abnormality is termed the *Philadelphia chromosome* (Ph-positive). The median age of patients at the time of diagnosis is 55, but CML can be seen in both children and young adults. The causative factor in the majority of CML cases is not known, but ionizing radiation is associated with the development of CML.

CLASSIFICATION AND PROGNOSIS

Patients with CML have an elevated WBC count and are often asymptomatic at the time of presentation. The peripheral blood smear demonstrates mature leukocytes and left-shifted myeloid precursors (particularly basophils), whereas the bone marrow is hypercellular with a myeloid predominance with normal or increased megakaryocytes, many of which may be hypolobated. Chronic-phase CML is characterized by a WBC count that is stable or easily controlled with chemotherapy and bone marrow without a significant number of blasts. The median survival for patients in stable phase is approximately 4 years. Patients eventually progress to an accelerated phase characterized by an increasingly difficult-to-control WBC count, organomegaly, the possible development of further cytogenetic abnormalities, and the potential development of myelofibrosis. Blast crisis is the final phase. Similar to acute leukemia, it is associated with bone pain, weight loss, increasing blast percentage with marrow failure, and likely clonal evaluation. The majority of patients in blast crisis have a myeloid phenotype; however, approximately 20% to 30% of cases are lymphoid in derivation. In both scenarios, blasts are poorly differentiated and the median survival after developing blast crises is only 3 months. Chemotherapy agents appro-

priate to the derivation of the leukemia (myeloid or lymphoid) are used to treat blast crisis. If remission is obtained, it is often of short duration.

TREATMENT

Historically, treatment for chronic-phase CML was aimed at cytoreduction. While the first agents used, busulfan and hydroxyurea, were effective at inducing hematologic responses, cytogenetic responses were rare and molecular responses nonexistent [77]. In the 1980s, interferon-α, often in conjunction with cytarabine, became more widely used. Several randomized studies revealed an improved 5-year survival ranging from 50% to 59% compared with busulfan and hydroxyurea, with the majority of patients achieving a hematologic response and cytogenetic responses approaching 19% [78]. Moreover, about half of the patients who achieve a complete cytogenetic response appear to remain in cytogenetic CR after stopping interferon and may in fact be cured [79,80]. It is also important to appreciate that the time to maximal cytogenetic response can be prolonged. Although interferon provides improved cytogenetic responses, side effects including leukopenia, thrombocytopenia, anemia, and flu-like symptoms (*eg*, fever, chills, myalgias, malaise, nausea, vomiting, and diarrhea) [81] prevent a significant proportion of patients from completing therapy and obtaining this clinical benefit.

Imatinib mesylate, a rationally designed selective and potent inhibitor of the protein tyrosine kinase of the BCR-ABL fusion protein, is the current standard of care for the treatment of CML patients in chronic phase. Initial standard dosing is 400 mg/d. Clinical outcomes are vastly superior to any of the historical treatments above, with hematologic responses nearing 95% and complete cytogenetic responses approaching 76% [82] (Table 17-3). Although the complete cytogenetic response rate is substantial, few patients achieve a complete molecular response, indicating that imatinib therapy is not likely curative, and resistance to imatinib therapy has emerged through mechanisms such as gene amplification of the BCR-ABL transcript, point mutations, and increased expression of *MDR1* [83]. For patients developing resistance, the dose of imatinib can be increased; however, if not successful, second-generation tyrosine kinase inhibitors, such as the newly US Food and Drug Administration–approved dasatinib, are being developed.

Although allogeneic BMT remains the only known curative treatment for CML, the pattern of its use has changed since the emergence of imatinib treatment successes. Historically, allogeneic BMT was recommended as first-line therapy in younger patients, with interferon recommended for older patients at higher risk for transplant-related complications. Since the widespread use of imatinib as first-line therapy, transplant use in chronic phase 1 has decreased dramatically beginning in 2001, although its frequency has increased in chronic phase 2/accelerated phase and remained the same in blast [84]. Based on studies reporting inferior overall survival in patients not achieving a complete cytogenetic response at the completion of 12 months of maximal imatinib therapy [85], consensus recommendations for patients in chronic phase are to consider allogeneic BMT at that time [86]. Prospective studies comparing matched-sibling donor transplants with unrelated-donor transplants have shown a 5-year DFS (depending on patient's age) ranging from 57% to 68% (matched-sibling donor) and 46% to 61% (unrelated-donor) in chronic-phase CML patients transplanted within a year from diagnosis [87]. Unrelated-donor transplants more than 1 year from diagnosis or in a CML phase other than chronic were associated with increased graft-versus-host disease and risk of graft failure in patients [87]. The graft-versus-leukemia effect is significant in CML, and T-cell–depleted transplants are associated with a higher incidence of relapse after transplant [88]. When relapse occurs after allogeneic BMT, the use of donor lymphocyte

Table 17-3. Chemotherapy Treatment Regimens for Chronic Myeloid Leukemia

Study	Chemotherapy regimen	CHR, %	CCR, %
O'Brien *et al.* [82]	Interferon-α (target dose 5 MU/m² every d) + cytarabine 20 mg/m² × 10 d every mo	55 (at median 19-mo follow-up)	14.5 (at median 19-mo follow-up)
Druker *et al.* [139]	Imatinib 400 mg orally every d (starting dose)	96 (at 12 mo)	69 (at 12 mo)

CCR—complete cytogenetic response; CHR—complete hematologic response.

infusion is a powerful treatment. Response rates depend on the CML phase at time of administration (hematologic, cytogenetic, or molecular relapse or chronic, accelerated, blast), cell dose, and degree of histocompatibility between donor and recipient [89]. When it is administered at the time of cytogenetic or molecular relapse, donor lymphocyte infusion leads to complete cytogenetic response in more than 70% of patients [89–91].

When transplant is used in patients with CML, the timing is important and—with the introduction of imatinib as first-line therapy—the decision is challenging. Historically, patients treated in early chronic phase (< 1 y after diagnosis) appeared to have an improved DFS compared with those treated in late chronic phase [84], and DFS rates were lower when patients underwent transplantation in the second chronic phase (accelerated or blastic phase) compared with the early chronic phase. Since the widespread, first-line use of imatinib, the use of allogeneic BMT in first chronic phase has declined, while its use in second chronic phase has increased and its use in the accelerated phase has remained the same [84]. Current consensus guidelines are based on data showing inferior long-term survival in patients who have not achieved a complete cytogenetic response within 1 year of imatinib therapy [85]. For patients presenting in chronic phase who have not achieved a complete cytogenetic response at 1 year with maximal imatinib therapy, allogeneic transplant should be considered. For patients presenting with more advanced disease, initiation of imatinib is recommended with planned allogeneic BMT as available [86].

CHRONIC LYMPHOCYTIC LEUKEMIA

ETIOLOGY AND RISK FACTORS

Chronic lymphocytic leukemia (CLL) is a clonal B-cell disorder characterized by CD5+, CD19+, CD23+, and FMC7- circulating lymphocytes [92]. It is the most common leukemia in the United States, occurring most frequently in patients older than 60 years of age. Presenting symptoms can include asymptomatic lymphocytosis, lymphadenopathy, splenomegaly, cytopenias, and constitutional symptoms [93–95]. No etiology of CLL is known; thus, CLL represents the only known leukemia not associated with radiation, drug, or chemical exposure, although familial clustering has been reported [95].

CLASSIFICATION AND PROGNOSIS

Two historical systems have been used to classify and offer prognostic information in CLL. The initial classification system was developed by Rai *et al.* [96] (stages 0, I, II, III, and IV) and the second was proposed by Binet *et al.* [97] (stages A, B, and C). Both systems stage patients in terms of the presence of lymphadenopathy, splenomegaly, hepatomegaly, anemia, or thrombocytopenia in conjunction with the lymphocytosis. Stage increases and prognosis worsens as number of abnormalities increase. Patients with lymphocytosis only (Rai stage 0 or Binet stage A) have a median survival of more than 10 years from diagnosis. Patients presenting in more advanced stages have shorter survival expectancies (median survival: Rai stage I or II, 7 years; Rai stage III or IV, 4 years) [98]. Newer potential prognostic tools are emerging in CLL and include cytogenetic alterations (poor 17p deletion [99] or 11q deletion; favorable 13q deletion if in isolation [100]), mutational status of immunoglobulin variable heavy chain (for which both CD38 [101] and ZAP-70 [102] have been cited as potential surrogates), and serologic factors such as β_2 microglobulin level [103]. Continued research will be required to determine if these prognostic markers should direct earlier treatment intervention.

TREATMENT

The potential indications to initiate treatment for CLL include progressive systemic symptoms, worsening marrow failure, autoimmune cytopenias unresponsive to steroids, progressive splenomegaly or lymphadenopathy, worsening lymphocytosis (defined as a doubling time < 6 months or > 50% increase over 2 months), or Richter's transformation. There is no benefit derived from treating patients solely to control the WBC count because leukostasis is infrequent even with very high counts [98,98,104]. Historically, alkylator therapy with chlorambucil with or without prednisone delivered responses, predominantly partial, from 40% to 80% [105–108]. Additional comparisons of chlorambucil alone versus combination therapy (CHOP [cyclophosphamide, doxorubicin, vincristine, prednisone], CVP [cyclophosphamide, vincristine, prednisone], CAP [cyclophosphamide, doxorubicin, cisplatin]) yielded similar results [109,110]. Due to improved overall response (OR), complete response rates, and longer response duration, purine analogues, primarily fludarabine, have more recently replaced chlorambucil as first-line therapy for CLL [111] (Table 17-4). Single-agent fludarabine has shown OR rates from 60% to 80% and CR rates of 20% to 40%, and despite its similar efficacy to combination chemotherapy (CAP, CHOP) has shown improved CR rates and time to next treatment [112,113]. Additionally, combinations of fludarabine and cyclophosphamide have yielded improved response rates (OR 70%–94%; CR 22%–24%; progression-free survival 41–48 months) compared with fludarabine alone (OR 50%–83%; CR 6%–7% [lower than previously reported trials]; progression-free survival 18–20 months) [114,115]. Innate to fludarabine are some unique toxicities, such as profound marrow suppression with significant depression of cellular immunity, particularly CD4+ cells. Thus, *Pneumocystis jiroveci* (previously known as *Pneumocystis carinii*) prophylaxis should be continued until recovery of the CD4+ count, which can sometimes be prolonged to more than a year from therapy, and an extended interval of viral prophylaxis should be considered [116]. In addition, autoimmune hemolytic anemia is associated with CLL itself, but can also be worsened or precipitated after fludarabine therapy. Lastly, for patients who develop

Table 17-4. Studies of Chemotherapy Regimens for Chronic Lymphocytic Leukemia

Chemotherapy	Study	Regimen(s)	OR, %	CR, %
Chlorambucil	Montserrat *et al.* [105]	0.4 mg/kg on d 6 + prednisone 60 mg/m² on d 1–5	40–80	Few
	Keller *et al.* [106]	30 mg/m² + prednisone 80 mg/d × 5 cycles		
	Rai *et al.* [107], Sawitsky *et al.* [108]	Various other schedules		
Fludarabine	Rai *et al.* [107], Leporrier *et al.* [112], Jonhson *et al.* [113], Eichhorst *et al.* [114]	25 mg/m² every d on d 1–5 for 28 d	60–80	Varying reports (6–40)
Fludarabine + cyclophosphamide	Eichhorst *et al.* [114]	Fludarabine 30 mg/m² every d on d 1–3 + cyclophosphamide 250 mg/m² every d on d 1–3 for 28 d	70–94	22–24
Fludarabine + cyclophosphamide + rituximab	Keating *et al.* [125], Wierda *et al.* [126]	Fludarabine 25 mg/m² on d 2–4 (cycle 1) then on d 1–3 (cycle 2–6) + cyclophosphamide 250 mg/m² on d 2–4 (cycle 1) then on d 1–3 (cycle 2–6) + rituximab 375 mg/m² on d 1 (cycle 1) then 500 mg/m² on d 1 (cycle 2–6)	Nearing 100	70
Rituximab	Byrd *et al.* [117]	375 mg/m² three times a week	45	3
	Hainsworth *et al.* [118,119]	375 mg/m² weekly × 4 cycles then maintenance	46–73	9–37

CR—complete remission; OR—overall response.

recurrent bacterial infections due to hypogammaglobulinemia, the use of intravenous immunoglobulin is suggested.

Monoclonal anti-CD20 and anti-CD52 antibody therapy has also been extensively studied and successful in treating CLL. Specifically, the anti-CD20 antibody rituximab (Rituxan, Biogen Idec, Inc. and Genentech, Inc., San Francisco, CA) has shown significant activity and is used in many clinical scenarios either as monotherapy, in combination with chemotherapy, or in an induction and maintenance schedule. Significant infusional reactions seen in initial studies prompted dosing alterations; a thrice-weekly schedule is the most commonly used and produces OR rates of 45% (CR 3%; partial remission 42%) [117]. Using rituximab induction weekly for four cycles with maintenance of varying time periods has led to OR rates of 46% to 73%, with CR rates varying from 9% to 37% [118,119]. Combining fludarabine with various iterations of rituximab schedules has yielded OR rates from 77% to 93% [120–123]. Further studies evaluating the combination of fludarabine, cyclophosphamide, and rituximab have shown OR rates approaching 100% and CR rates approximating 70% in treatment-naive patients, with continued response in patients with relapsed disease (OR 73%–95%; CR 14%–25%) [124–126]. Despite the improving OR and complete response rate with fludarabine combination treatments, no regimen has shown improved overall survival and thus decision making regarding when and who to treat is challenging. Alemtuzumab, an anti-CD52 monoclonal antibody, has also shown activity in treatment-naive and relapsed/refractory CLL. It has shown the most pronounced effects in the peripheral blood and bone marrow; however, it is generally not used as first-line therapy. Due to its profound immunosuppressive effects, antibacterial, antiviral, and possibly antifungal prophylaxis should be used [127].

Lastly, due to the preponderance of new prognostic marker information under investigation, decision making regarding transplantation and its timing is in transition. Younger patients with poor risk factors as well as patients with fludarabine-refractory CLL have particularly poor outcomes and should be considered for allogeneic BMT or clinical trials of novel approaches.

HAIRY CELL LEUKEMIA

Hairy cell leukemia (HCL) is a chronic lymphoproliferative disorder most commonly presenting in middle-aged men with pancytopenia [128], splenomegaly [129], and a dry marrow aspiration. Although described as a "leukemia" due to blood and marrow involvement, its biology behaves in a manner more consistent with a low-grade lymphoma. HCL can also occur in the context of other clonal hematopoietic and autoimmune disorders. Diagnosis is based on morphologic evidence of hairy cells, with fine or hair-like cytoplasmic projections on peripheral smear that are typically tartrate-resistant acid phosphatase (Trap stain) positive and express CD25 and CD103, all in the clinical context of cytopenias and splenomegaly [130]. Classic HCL is very responsive to therapy and typically involves younger patients with splenomegaly and monocytopenia, whereas variant HCL occurs most often in older patients without splenomegaly or monocytopenia and responds poorly to conventional therapy.

TREATMENT

Treatment is indicated for worsening cytopenias and complications thereof, worsening visceral involvement, significant bulky adenopathy, and significant autoimmune disorders. Historically, options for patients with HCL have included splenectomy, chlorambucil, androgens, and interferons. Current standard of care for initial treatment of HCL includes the purine analogues cladribine (2-CdA) and pentostatin [130,131] (Table 17-5). While it is not clear that nucleoside analogues cure classic HCL, they do provide significant improvements in long-term survival. A number of cladribine treatment schedules exist, including the most standard 0.1 mg/kg/d as a single continuous infusion over 7 days versus 0.14 mg/kg/d over 2 hours daily on 5 consecutive days. The most frequent toxicities from cladribine include myelosuppression and infectious complications [132]. Chadha et al. [133] recently published their long-term follow-up from a study using the 7-day continuous infusion and showed an OR rate of 100% and an overall survival of 87% at 12 years. For the 36% of patients who had relapsed at a median of 9.7 years, the study also demonstrated that an additional cycle of cladribine could induce a CR in 52% of those retreated. Pentostatin, 2'-DCF, is an alternative purine analogue used to treat HCL, dosed at 4 mg/m² and given every 2 weeks until maximum response. Bone marrow suppression and dermatologic changes are the most common toxicities; however, hepatic, renal, neurologic, and gastrointestinal side effects can also occur. Comparative analysis of outcomes from cladribine versus pentostatin have shown a similar CR rate of 82% and 81%, an OR rate of 100% and 96%, and median DFS of 11+ and 15 years, respectively. Neither purine analogue cures patients; relapse rates at 10 years are 48% and 42%, respectively [134]. Options for relapsed or refractory disease depend on the timing of relapse posttransplant, but include retreatment with the initial purine analogue (if long remission), an alternative purine analogue, or rituximab, which has been shown to induce a CR in 13% to 53% of standard cases and has also shown efficacy in case reports of variant HCL [135,136].

ACKNOWLEDGMENTS

The authors would like to thank Dr. Edward D. Ball, author of this textbook's original chapter on leukemia, for his thoughtful review and guidance on the current chapter.

Table 17-5. Chemotherapy Treatment Regimens for Hairy Cell Leukemia

Study	Chemotherapy regimen	OR, %	CR, %
Cheson *et al.* [132]	Cladribine 0.1 mg/kg/d as continuous infusion × 7 d	87–100	50–79
Chadha *et al.* [133]	Cladribine 0.14 mg/kg over 2 h every d × 5 d		
Else *et al.* [134]	Pentostatin 4 mg/m² every 2 wk until maximum response	96	81
Thomas *et al.* [135], Quach *et al.* [136]	Rituximab 375 mg/m² every wk × 8 cycles	—	13–53

CR—complete remission; OR—overall response.

REFERENCES

1. Schumacher HR, Alvares CJ, Blough RI, Mazzella F: Acute leukemia. *Clin Lab Med* 2002, 22:153–192, vii.

2. Godwin JE, Smith SE: Acute myeloid leukemia in the older patient. *Crit Rev Oncol Hematol* 2003, 48:S17–S26.

3. Harris NL, Jaffe ES, Diebold J, *et al.*: World Health Organization classification of neoplastic diseases of the hematopoietic and lymphoid tissues: report of the Clinical Advisory Committee meeting—Airlie House, Virginia, November 1997. *J Clin Oncol* 1999, 17:3835–3849.

4. Lyman SD, Jacobsen SE: c-kit ligand and Flt3 ligand: stem/progenitor cell factors with overlapping yet distinct activities. *Blood* 1998, 91:1101–1134.

5. Kiyoi H, Naoe T, Nakano Y, *et al.*: Prognostic implication of FLT3 and N-RAS gene mutations in acute myeloid leukemia. *Blood* 1999, 93:3074–3080.

6. Iwai T, Yokota S, Nakao M, *et al.*: Internal tandem duplication of the FLT3 gene and clinical evaluation in childhood acute myeloid leukemia. The Children's Cancer and Leukemia Study Group, Japan. *Leukemia* 1999, 13:38–43.

7. Abu-Duhier FM, Goodeve AC, Wilson GA, *et al.*: FLT3 internal tandem duplication mutations in adult acute myeloid leukaemia define a high-risk group. *Br J Haematol* 2000, 111:190–195.

8. Sheikhha MH, Awan A, Tobal K, *et al.*: Prognostic significance of FLT3 ITD and D835 mutations in AML patients. *Hematol J* 2003, 4:41–46.

9. Boissel N, Renneville A, Biggio V, *et al.*: Prevalence, clinical profile, and prognosis of NPM mutations in AML with normal karyotype. *Blood* 2005, 106:3618–3620.

10. Suzuki T, Kiyoi H, Ozeki K, *et al.*: Clinical characteristics and prognostic implications of NPM1 mutations in acute myeloid leukemia. *Blood* 2005, 106:2854–2861.

11. Schnittger S, Schoch C, Kern W, *et al.*: Nucleophosmin gene mutations are predictors of favorable prognosis in acute myelogenous leukemia with a normal karyotype. *Blood* 2005, 106:3733–3739.

12. Cordell JL, Pulford KA, Bigerna B, *et al.*: Detection of normal and chimeric nucleophosmin in human cells. *Blood* 1999, 93:632–642.

13. Borer RA, Lehner CF, Eppenberger HM, Nigg EA: Major nucleolar proteins shuttle between nucleus and cytoplasm. *Cell* 1989, 56:379–390.

14. Yun JP, Chew EC, Liew CT, *et al.*: Nucleophosmin/B23 is a proliferate shuttle protein associated with nuclear matrix. *J Cell Biochem* 2003, 90:1140–1148.

15. Yu Y, Maggi LB Jr, Brady SN, *et al.*: Nucleophosmin is essential for ribosomal protein L5 nuclear export. *Mol Cell Biol* 2006, 26:3798–3809.

16. Grisendi S, Bernardi R, Rossi M, *et al.*: Role of nucleophosmin in embryonic development and tumorigenesis. *Nature* 2005, 437:147–153.

17. Colombo E, Bonetti P, Lazzerini DE, *et al.*: Nucleophosmin is required for DNA integrity and p19Arf protein stability. *Mol Cell Biol* 2005, 25:8874–8886.

18. Ye K: Nucleophosmin/B23, a multifunctional protein that can regulate apoptosis. *Cancer Biol Ther* 2005, 4:918–923.

19. Dohner K, Schlenk RF, Habdank M, *et al.*: Mutant nucleophosmin (NPM1) predicts favorable prognosis in younger adults with acute myeloid leukemia and normal cytogenetics: interaction with other gene mutations. *Blood* 2005, 106:3740–3746.

20. Thiede C, Koch S, Creutzig E, *et al.*: Prevalence and prognostic impact of NPM1 mutations in 1485 adult patients with acute myeloid leukemia (AML). *Blood* 2006,107:4011–4020.

21. Burnett AK: Treatment of acute myeloid leukaemia in younger patients. *Best Pract Res Clin Haematol* 2001, 14:95–118.

22. Goldstone AH, Burnett AK, Wheatley K, *et al.*: Attempts to improve treatment outcomes in acute myeloid leukemia (AML) in older patients: the results of the United Kingdom Medical Research Council AML11 trial. *Blood* 2001, 98:1302–1311.

23. A systematic collaborative overview of randomized trials comparing idarubicin with daunorubicin (or other anthracyclines) as induction therapy for acute myeloid leukaemia. AML Collaborative Group. *Br J Haematol* 1998, 103:100–109.

24. Smith M, Barnett M, Bassan R, *et al.*: Adult acute myeloid leukaemia. *Crit Rev Oncol Hematol* 2004, 50:197–222.

25. Visani G, Olivieri A, Malagola M, *et al.*: Consolidation therapy for adult acute myeloid leukemia: a systematic analysis according to evidence based medicine. *Leuk Lymphoma* 2006, 47:1091–1102.

26. Phillips GL, Reece DE, Shepherd JD, *et al.*: High-dose cytarabine and daunorubicin induction and postremission chemotherapy for the treatment of acute myelogenous leukemia in adults. *Blood* 1991, 77:1429–1435.

27. Brown RA, Herzig RH, Wolff SN, *et al.*: High-dose etoposide and cyclophosphamide without bone marrow transplantation for resistant hematologic malignancy. *Blood* 1990, 76:473–479.

28. Bishop JF, Lowenthal RM, Joshua D, *et al.*: Etoposide in acute nonlymphocytic leukemia. Australian Leukemia Study Group. *Blood* 1990, 75:27–32.

29. Mitus AJ, Miller KB, Schenkein DP, *et al.*: Improved survival for patients with acute myelogenous leukemia. *J Clin Oncol* 1995, 13:560–569.

30. Castaigne S, Chevret S, Archimbaud E, *et al.*: Randomized comparison of double induction and timed-sequential induction to a "3 + 7" induction in adults with AML: long-term analysis of the Acute Leukemia French Association (ALFA) 9000 study. *Blood* 2004, 104:2467–2474.

31. Estey EH: How I treat older patients with AML. *Blood* 2000, 96:1670–1673.

32. Tilly H, Bastard C, Bizet M, *et al.*: Low-dose cytarabine: persistence of a clonal abnormality during complete remission of acute nonlymphocytic leukemia. *N Engl J Med* 1986, 314:246–247.

33. Lancet JE, Gojo I, Gotlib J, *et al.*: A phase 2 study of the farnesyltransferase inhibitor tipifarnib in poor-risk and elderly patients with previously untreated acute myelogenous leukemia. *Blood* 2007, 109:1387–1394.

34. Estey E, Thall P, Beran M, *et al.*: Effect of diagnosis (refractory anemia with excess blasts, refractory anemia with excess blasts in transformation, or acute myeloid leukemia [AML]) on outcome of AML-type chemotherapy. *Blood* 1997, 90:2969–2977.

35. Hiddemann W, Spiekermann K, Buske C, *et al.*: Towards a pathogenesis-oriented therapy of acute myeloid leukemia. *Crit Rev Oncol Hematol* 2005, 56:235–245.

36. Mayer RJ, Davis RB, Schiffer CA, *et al.*: Intensive postremission chemotherapy in adults with acute myeloid leukemia. Cancer and Leukemia Group B. *N Engl J Med* 1994, 331:896–903.

37. Yavuz S, Paydas S, Disel U, Sahin B: IDA-FLAG regimen for the therapy of primary refractory and relapse acute leukemia: a single-center experience. *Am J Ther* 2006, 13:389–393.

38. Lazzarino M, Morra E, Alessandrino EP, *et al.*: Mitoxantrone and etoposide: an effective regimen for refractory or relapsed acute myelogenous leukemia. *Eur J Haematol* 1989, 43:411–416.

39. Robertson MJ, Soiffer RJ, Freedman AS, *et al.*: Human bone marrow depleted of CD33-positive cells mediates delayed but durable reconstitution of hematopoiesis: clinical trial of MY9 monoclonal antibody-purged autografts for the treatment of acute myeloid leukemia. *Blood* 1992, 79:2229–2236.

40. Selvaggi KJ, Wilson JW, Mills LE, *et al.*: Improved outcome for high-risk acute myeloid leukemia patients using autologous bone marrow transplantation and monoclonal antibody-purged bone marrow. *Blood* 1994, 83:1698–1705.

41. Degos L: All-trans-retinoic acid in the treatment of acute promyelocytic leukemia [in French]. *Presse Med* 1990, 19:1483–1484.

42. Warrell RP Jr, Frankel SR, Miller WH Jr, *et al.*: Differentiation therapy of acute promyelocytic leukemia with tretinoin (all-trans-retinoic acid). *N Engl J Med* 1991, 324:1385–1393.

43. Tallman MS, Andersen JW, Schiffer CA, *et al.*: All-trans-retinoic acid in acute promyelocytic leukemia. *N Engl J Med* 1997, 337:1021–1028.

44. Fenaux P, Wang ZZ, Degos L: Treatment of acute promyelocytic leukemia by retinoids. *Curr Top Microbiol Immunol* 2007, 313:101–128.

45. Fenaux P, Chastang C, Chevret S, *et al.*: A randomized comparison of all transretinoic acid (ATRA) followed by chemotherapy and ATRA plus chemotherapy and the role of maintenance therapy in newly diagnosed acute promyelocytic leukemia. The European APL Group. *Blood* 1999, 94:1192–1200.

46. Tallman MS: Treatment of relapsed or refractory acute promyelocytic leukemia. *Best Pract Res Clin Haematol* 2007, 20:57–65.

47. Pombo de Oliveira MS, Awad el Seed FE, Foroni L, *et al.*: Lymphoblastic leukaemia in Siamese twins: evidence for identity. *Lancet* 1986, 2:969–970.

48. Taub JW: Relationship of chromosome 21 and acute leukemia in children with Down syndrome. *J Pediatr Hematol Oncol* 2001, 23:175–178.

49. Janik-Moszant A, Bubala H, Stojewska M, Sonta-Jakimczyk D: Acute lymphoblastic leukemia in children with Fanconi anemia [in Polish]. *Wiad Lek* 1998, 51(Suppl 4):285–288.

50. Preston DL, Kusumi S, Tomonaga M, *et al.*: Cancer incidence in atomic bomb survivors. Part III. Leukemia, lymphoma and multiple myeloma, 1950–1987. *Radiat Res* 1994, 137:S68–S97.

51. Shore DL, Sandler DP, Davey FR, *et al.*: Acute leukemia and residential proximity to potential sources of environmental pollutants. *Arch Environ Health* 1993, 48:414–420.

52. Pedersen-Bjergaard J: Acute lymphoid leukemia with t(4;11) (q21;q23) following chemotherapy with cytostatic agents targeting at DNA-topoisomerase II. *Leuk Res* 1992, 16:733–735.

53. Faderl S, Jeha S, Kantarjian HM: The biology and therapy of adult acute lymphoblastic leukemia. *Cancer* 2003, 98:1337–1354.

54. Faderl S, Kantarjian HM, Talpaz M, Estrov Z: Clinical significance of cytogenetic abnormalities in adult acute lymphoblastic leukemia. *Blood* 1998, 91:3995–4019.

55. Faderl S, Garcia-Manero G, Thomas DA, Kantarjian HM: Philadelphia chromosome-positive acute lymphoblastic leukemia: current concepts and future perspectives. *Rev Clin Exp Hematol* 2002, 6:142–160.

56. Heerema NA, Sather HN, Sensel MG, et al.: Association of chromosome arm 9p abnormalities with adverse risk in childhood acute lymphoblastic leukemia: a report from the Children's Cancer Group. *Blood* 1999, 94:1537–1544.

57. Mancini M, Scappaticci D, Cimino G, et al.: A comprehensive genetic classification of adult acute lymphoblastic leukemia (ALL): analysis of the GIMEMA 0496 protocol. *Blood* 2005, 105:3434–3441.

58. Crist WM, Carroll AJ, Shuster JJ, et al.: Poor prognosis of children with pre-B acute lymphoblastic leukemia is associated with the t(1;19)(q23;p13): a Pediatric Oncology Group study. *Blood* 1990, 76:117–122.

59. Raynaud S, Mauvieux L, Cayuela JM, et al.: TEL/AML1 fusion gene is a rare event in adult acute lymphoblastic leukemia. *Leukemia* 1996, 10:1529–1530.

60. Vitale A, Guarini A, Chiaretti S, Foa R: The changing scene of adult acute lymphoblastic leukemia. *Curr Opin Oncol* 2006, 18:652–659.

61. Larson RA, Dodge RK, Burns CP, et al.: A five-drug remission induction regimen with intensive consolidation for adults with acute lymphoblastic leukemia: Cancer and Leukemia Group B study 8811. *Blood* 1995, 85:2025–2037.

62. Larson RA: Recent clinical trials in acute lymphocytic leukemia by the Cancer and Leukemia Group B. *Hematol Oncol Clin North Am* 2000, 14:1367–1379.

63. Jabbour EJ, Faderl S, Kantarjian HM: Adult acute lymphoblastic leukemia. *Mayo Clin Proc* 2005, 80:1517–1527.

64. Kantarjian HM, O'Brien S, Smith TL, et al.: Results of treatment with hyper-CVAD, a dose-intensive regimen, in adult acute lymphocytic leukemia. *J Clin Oncol* 2000, 18:547–561.

65. Kantarjian HM, O'Brien S, Smith T, et al.: Acute lymphocytic leukaemia in the elderly: characteristics and outcome with the vincristine-Adriamycin-dexamethasone (VAD) regimen. *Br J Haematol* 1994, 88:94–100.

66. Annino L, Vegna ML, Camera A, et al.: Treatment of adult acute lymphoblastic leukemia (ALL): long-term follow-up of the GIMEMA ALL 0288 randomized study. *Blood* 2002, 99:863–871.

67. Nagura E, Kimura K, Yamada K, et al.: Nation-wide randomized comparative study of doxorubicin, vincristine and prednisolone combination therapy with and without L-asparaginase for adult acute lymphoblastic leukemia. *Cancer Chemother Pharmacol* 1994, 33:359–365.

68. Gandhi V, Plunkett W: Clofarabine and nelarabine: two new purine nucleoside analogs. *Curr Opin Oncol* 2006, 18:584–590.

69. Martin TG, Gajewski JL: Allogeneic stem cell transplantation for acute lymphocytic leukemia in adults. *Hematol Oncol Clin North Am* 2001, 15:97–120.

70. Thomas X, Boiron JM, Huguet F, et al.: Outcome of treatment in adults with acute lymphoblastic leukemia: analysis of the LALA-94 trial. *J Clin Oncol* 2004, 22:4075–4086.

71. Sebban C, Lepage E, Vernant JP, et al.: Allogeneic bone marrow transplantation in adult acute lymphoblastic leukemia in first complete remission: a comparative study. French Group of Therapy of Adult Acute Lymphoblastic Leukemia. *J Clin Oncol* 1994, 12:2580–2587.

72. Horowitz MM, Messerer D, Hoelzer D, et al.: Chemotherapy compared with bone marrow transplantation for adults with acute lymphoblastic leukemia in first remission. *Ann Intern Med* 1991, 115:13–18.

73. Rowe JM, Richards SM, Burnett AK, et al.: Favorable results of allogeneic bone marrow transplantation (BMT) for adults with Philadelphia (Ph)-chromosome-negative acute lymphoblastic leukemia (ALL) in first complete remission (CR): results from the International ALL Trial (MRC UKALL XII/ECOG E2993) [abstract]. *Blood* 2001, 98:2009a.

74. Brenner MK, Rill DR, Moen RC, et al.: Gene-marking to trace origin of relapse after autologous bone-marrow transplantation. *Lancet* 1993, 341:85–86.

75. Gilmore MJ, Hamon MD, Prentice HG, et al.: Failure of purged autologous bone marrow transplantation in high risk acute lymphoblastic leukaemia in first complete remission. *Bone Marrow Transplant* 1991, 8:19–26.

76. Fiere D, Lepage E, Sebban C, et al.: Adult acute lymphoblastic leukemia: a multicentric randomized trial testing bone marrow transplantation as postremission therapy. The French Group on Therapy for Adult Acute Lymphoblastic Leukemia. *J Clin Oncol* 1993, 11:1990–2001.

77. Hehlmann R, Heimpel H, Hasford J, et al.: Randomized comparison of interferon-alpha with busulfan and hydroxyurea in chronic myelogenous leukemia. The German CML Study Group. *Blood* 1994, 84:4064–4077.

78. Silver RT, Woolf SH, Hehlmann R, et al.: An evidence-based analysis of the effect of busulfan, hydroxyurea, interferon, and allogeneic bone marrow transplantation in treating the chronic phase of chronic myeloid leukemia: developed for the American Society of Hematology. *Blood* 1999, 94:1517–1536.

79. Bonifazi F, de Vivo A, Rosti G, et al.: Chronic myeloid leukemia and interferon-alpha: a study of complete cytogenetic responders. *Blood* 2001, 98:3074–3081.

80. Mahon FX, Delbrel X, Cony-Makhoul P, et al.: Follow-up of complete cytogenetic remission in patients with chronic myeloid leukemia after cessation of interferon alfa. *J Clin Oncol* 2002, 20:214–220.

81. Ozer H, George SL, Schiffer CA, et al.: Prolonged subcutaneous administration of recombinant alpha 2b interferon in patients with previously untreated Philadelphia chromosome-positive chronic-phase chronic myelogenous leukemia: effect on remission duration and survival: Cancer and Leukemia Group B study 8583. *Blood* 1993, 82:2975–2984.

82. O'Brien SG, Guilhot F, Larson RA, et al.: Imatinib compared with interferon and low-dose cytarabine for newly diagnosed chronic-phase chronic myeloid leukemia. *N Engl J Med* 2003, 348:994–1004.

83. Deininger M, Buchdunger E, Druker BJ: The development of imatinib as a therapeutic agent for chronic myeloid leukemia. *Blood* 2005, 105:2640–2653.

84. Giralt SA, Arora M, Goldman JM, et al.: Impact of imatinib therapy on the use of allogeneic haematopoietic progenitor cell transplantation for the treatment of chronic myeloid leukaemia. *Br J Haematol* 2007, 137:461–467.

85. Roy L, Guilhot J, Krahnke T, et al.: Survival advantage from imatinib compared with the combination interferon-alpha plus cytarabine in chronic-phase chronic myelogenous leukemia: historical comparison between two phase 3 trials. *Blood* 2006, 108:1478–1484.

86. Baccarani M, Saglio G, Goldman J, et al.: Evolving concepts in the management of chronic myeloid leukemia: recommendations from an expert panel on behalf of the European LeukemiaNet. *Blood* 2006, 108:1809–1820.

87. Weisdorf DJ, Anasetti C, Antin JH, et al.: Allogeneic bone marrow transplantation for chronic myelogenous leukemia: comparative analysis of unrelated versus matched sibling donor transplantation. *Blood* 2002, 99:1971–1977.

88. Sehn LH, Alyea EP, Weller E, et al.: Comparative outcomes of T-cell-depleted and non-T-cell-depleted allogeneic bone marrow transplantation for chronic myelogenous leukemia: impact of donor lymphocyte infusion. *J Clin Oncol* 1999, 17:561–568.

89. Simula MP, Marktel S, Fozza C, et al.: Response to donor lymphocyte infusions for chronic myeloid leukemia is dose-dependent: the importance of escalating the cell dose to maximize therapeutic efficacy. *Leukemia* 2007, 21:943–948.

90. Kolb HJ, Schattenberg A, Goldman JM, et al.: Graft-versus-leukemia effect of donor lymphocyte transfusions in marrow grafted patients. European Group for Blood and Marrow Transplantation Working Party Chronic Leukemia. *Blood* 1995, 86:2041–2050.

91. Huff CA, Fuchs EJ, Smith BD, et al.: Graft-versus-host reactions and the effectiveness of donor lymphocyte infusions. *Biol Blood Marrow Transplant* 2006, 12:414–421.

92. Oscier D, Fegan C, Hillmen P, et al.: Guidelines on the diagnosis and management of chronic lymphocytic leukaemia. *Br J Haematol* 2004, 125:294–317.

93. Pangalis GA, Vassilakopoulos TP, Dimopoulou MN, et al.: B-chronic lymphocytic leukemia: practical aspects. *Hematol Oncol* 2002, 20:103–146.

94. Molica S, Levato D, Dattilo A: Natural history of early chronic lymphocytic leukemia. A single institution study with emphasis on the impact of disease-progression on overall survival. *Haematologica* 1999, 84:1094–1099.

95. Yee KW, O'Brien SM: Chronic lymphocytic leukemia: diagnosis and treatment. *Mayo Clin Proc* 2006, 81:1105–1129.

96. Rai KR, Sawitsky A, Cronkite EP, *et al.*: Clinical staging of chronic lymphocytic leukemia. *Blood* 1975, 46:219–234.

97. Binet JL, Auquier A, Dighiero G, *et al.*: A new prognostic classification of chronic lymphocytic leukemia derived from a multivariate survival analysis. *Cancer* 1981, 48:198–206.

98. Cheson BD, Bennett JM, Grever M, *et al.*: National Cancer Institute-sponsored Working Group guidelines for chronic lymphocytic leukemia: revised guidelines for diagnosis and treatment. *Blood* 1996, 87:4990–4997.

99. Dohner H, Fischer K, Bentz M, *et al.*: p53 gene deletion predicts for poor survival and non-response to therapy with purine analogs in chronic B-cell leukemias. *Blood* 1995, 85:1580–1589.

100. Dohner H, Stilgenbauer S, Benner A, *et al.*: Genomic aberrations and survival in chronic lymphocytic leukemia. *N Engl J Med* 2000, 343:1910–1916.

101. Krober A, Seiler T, Benner A, *et al.*: V(H) mutation status, CD38 expression level, genomic aberrations, and survival in chronic lymphocytic leukemia. *Blood* 2002, 100:1410–1416.

102. Chen L, Widhopf G, Huynh L, *et al.*: Expression of ZAP-70 is associated with increased B-cell receptor signaling in chronic lymphocytic leukemia. *Blood* 2002, 100:4609–4614.

103. Montillo M, Hamblin T, Hallek M, *et al.*: Chronic lymphocytic leukemia: novel prognostic factors and their relevance for risk-adapted therapeutic strategies. *Haematologica* 2005, 90:391–399.

104. Kasamon YL, Flinn IW: Management of symptomatic, untreated chronic lymphocytic leukemia. *Blood Rev* 2007, 21:143–156.

105. Montserrat E, Alcala A, Parody R, *et al.*: Treatment of chronic lymphocytic leukemia in advanced stages. A randomized trial comparing chlorambucil plus prednisone versus cyclophosphamide, vincristine, and prednisone. *Cancer* 1985, 56:2369–2375.

106. Keller JW, Knospe WH, Raney M, *et al.*: Treatment of chronic lymphocytic leukemia using chlorambucil and prednisone with or without cycle-active consolidation chemotherapy. A Southeastern Cancer Study Group Trial. *Cancer* 1986, 58:1185–1192.

107. Rai K, Peterson B, Elias L, *et al.*: A randomized comparison of fludarabine and CLB for patients with previously untreated chronic lymphocytic leukemia: a CALGB, SWOG,CTG/NCI-C and ECOG intergroup study [abstract]. *Blood* 1996, 88:141a.

108. Sawitsky A, Rai KR, Glidewell O, Silver RT: Comparison of daily versus intermittent chlorambucil and prednisone therapy in the treatment of patients with chronic lymphocytic leukemia. *Blood* 1977, 50:1049–1059.

109. The French Cooperative Group on Chronic Lymphocytic Leukemia: A randomized clinical trial of chlorambucil versus COP in stage B chronic lymphocytic leukemia. The French Cooperative Group on Chronic Lymphocytic Leukemia. *Blood* 1990, 75:1422–1425.

110. Raphael B, Andersen JW, Silber R, *et al.*: Comparison of chlorambucil and prednisone versus cyclophosphamide, vincristine, and prednisone as initial treatment for chronic lymphocytic leukemia: long-term follow-up of an Eastern Cooperative Oncology Group randomized clinical trial. *J Clin Oncol* 1991, 9:770–776.

111. Rai KR, Peterson BL, Appelbaum FR, *et al.*: Fludarabine compared with chlorambucil as primary therapy for chronic lymphocytic leukemia. *N Engl J Med* 2000, 343:1750–1757.

112. Leporrier M, Chevret S, Cazin B, *et al.*: Randomized comparison of fludarabine, CAP, and ChOP in 938 previously untreated stage B and C chronic lymphocytic leukemia patients. *Blood* 2001, 98:2319–2325.

113. Johnson S, Smith AG, Loffler H, *et al.*: Multicentre prospective randomised trial of fludarabine versus cyclophosphamide, doxorubicin, and prednisone (CAP) for treatment of advanced-stage chronic lymphocytic leukaemia. The French Cooperative Group on CLL. *Lancet* 1996, 347:1432–1438.

114. Eichhorst BF, Busch R, Hopfinger G, *et al.*: Fludarabine plus cyclophosphamide versus fludarabine alone in first-line therapy of younger patients with chronic lymphocytic leukemia. *Blood* 2006, 107:885–891.

115. Flinn IW, Kumm E, Grever MR, *et al.*: Fludarabine and cyclophosphamide produces a higher complete response rate and more durable remissions than fludarabine in patients with previously untreated CLL: Intergroup Trial E2997 [abstract]. *Blood* 2004, 104:139a.

116. Keating MJ, O'Brien S, Lerner S, *et al.*: Long-term follow-up of patients with chronic lymphocytic leukemia (CLL) receiving fludarabine regimens as initial therapy. *Blood* 1998, 92:1165–1171.

117. Byrd JC, Murphy T, Howard RS, *et al.*: Rituximab using a thrice weekly dosing schedule in B-cell chronic lymphocytic leukemia and small lymphocytic lymphoma demonstrates clinical activity and acceptable toxicity. *J Clin Oncol* 2001, 19:2153–2164.

118. Hainsworth JD, Litchy S, Barton JH, *et al.*: Single-agent rituximab as first-line and maintenance treatment for patients with chronic lymphocytic leukemia or small lymphocytic lymphoma: a phase II trial of the Minnie Pearl Cancer Research Network. *J Clin Oncol* 2003, 21:1746–1751.

119. Hainsworth JD, Litchy S, Burris HA III, *et al.*: Rituximab as first-line and maintenance therapy for patients with indolent non-Hodgkin's lymphoma. *J Clin Oncol* 2002, 20:4261–4267.

120. Schulz H, Klein SK, Rehwald U, *et al.*: Phase 2 study of a combined immunochemotherapy using rituximab and fludarabine in patients with chronic lymphocytic leukemia. *Blood* 2002, 100:3115–3120.

121. Byrd JC, Peterson BL, Morrison VA, *et al.*: Randomized phase 2 study of fludarabine with concurrent versus sequential treatment with rituximab in symptomatic, untreated patients with B-cell chronic lymphocytic leukemia: results from Cancer and Leukemia Group B 9712 (CALGB 9712). *Blood* 2003, 101:6–14.

122. Byrd JC, Rai K, Peterson BL, *et al.*: Addition of rituximab to fludarabine may prolong progression-free survival and overall survival in patients with previously untreated chronic lymphocytic leukemia: an updated retrospective comparative analysis of CALGB 9712 and CALGB 9011. *Blood* 2005, 105:49–53.

123. Del Poeta G, Del Principe MI, Consalvo MA, *et al.*: The addition of rituximab to fludarabine improves clinical outcome in untreated patients with ZAP-70-negative chronic lymphocytic leukemia. *Cancer* 2005, 104:2743–2752.

124. Tam CS, Wolf M, Prince HM, *et al.*: Fludarabine, cyclophosphamide, and rituximab for the treatment of patients with chronic lymphocytic leukemia or indolent non-Hodgkin lymphoma. *Cancer* 2006, 106:2412–2420.

125. Keating MJ, O'Brien S, Albitar M, *et al.*: Early results of a chemoimmunotherapy regimen of fludarabine, cyclophosphamide, and rituximab as initial therapy for chronic lymphocytic leukemia. *J Clin Oncol* 2005, 23:4079–4088.

126. Wierda W, O'Brien S, Wen S, *et al.*: Chemoimmunotherapy with fludarabine, cyclophosphamide, and rituximab for relapsed and refractory chronic lymphocytic leukemia. *J Clin Oncol* 2005, 23:4070–4078.

127. Liu NS, O'Brien S: Monoclonal antibodies in the treatment of chronic lymphocytic leukemia. *Med Oncol* 2004, 21:297–304.

128. Zuzel M, Cawley JC: The biology of hairy cells. *Best Pract Res Clin Haematol* 2003, 16:1–13.

129. Flandrin G, Sigaux F, Castaigne S, *et al.*: Hairy cell leukemia: study of the development of 211 cases [in French]. *Presse Med* 1984, 3:2795–2799.

130. Wanko SO, de Castro C: Hairy cell leukemia: an elusive but treatable disease. *Oncologist* 2006, 11:780–789.

131. Gidron A, Tallman MS: Hairy cell leukemia: towards a curative strategy. *Hematol Oncol Clin North Am* 2006, 20:1153–1162.

132. Cheson BD, Sorensen JM, Vena DA, *et al.*: Treatment of hairy cell leukemia with 2-chlorodeoxyadenosine via the Group C protocol mechanism of the National Cancer Institute: a report of 979 patients. *J Clin Oncol* 1998, 16:3007–3015.

133. Chadha P, Rademaker AW, Mendiratta P, *et al.*: Treatment of hairy cell leukemia with 2-chlorodeoxyadenosine (2-CdA): long-term follow-up of the Northwestern University experience. *Blood* 2005, 106:241–246.

134. Else M, Ruchlemer R, Osuji N, *et al.*: Long remissions in hairy cell leukemia with purine analogs: a report of 219 patients with a median follow-up of 12.5 years. *Cancer* 2005, 104:2442–2448.

135. Thomas DA, O'Brien S, Bueso-Ramos C, *et al.*: Rituximab in relapsed or refractory hairy cell leukemia. *Blood* 2003, 102:3906–3911.

136. Quach H, Januszewicz H, Westerman D: Complete remission of hairy cell leukemia variant (HCL-v) complicated by red cell aplasia post treatment with rituximab. *Haematologica* 2005, 90(Suppl):ECR26.

137. Kantarjian HM, Waters RS, Keating MJ, *et al.*: Results of the vincristine, doxorubicin, and dexamethasone regimen in adults with standard- and high-risk acute lymphocytic leukemia. *J Clin Oncol* 1990, 8:994–1004.

138. Rowe JM, Buck G, Burnett AK, *et al.*: Induction therapy for adults with acute lymphoblastic leukemia: results of more than 1500 patients from the international ALL trial: MRC UKALL XII/ECOG E2993. *Blood* 2005, 106:3760–3767.

139. Druker BJ, Guilhot F, O'Brien SG, *et al.*: Five-year follow-up of patients receiving imatinib for chronic myeloid leukemia. *N Engl J Med* 2006, 355:2408–2417.

Hodgkin's lymphoma is a B-cell malignancy that comprises approximately 30% of all lymphomas in Western countries [1,2]. This chapter focuses on current management strategies for Hodgkin's lymphoma in adults.

PATHOLOGY

The World Health Organization defines two general categories of Hodgkin's lymphoma: classical Hodgkin's lymphoma, which represents about 95% of cases and is further divided into nodular sclerosis, mixed cellularity, lymphocyte-rich, and lymphocyte-depleted subtypes; and nodular lymphocyte-predominant (LP) Hodgkin's lymphoma [2]. The distinction between classical and LP Hodgkin's lymphoma is important because their natural histories and management strategies differ.

Hodgkin's lymphoma is histologically characterized by the presence of large, abnormal, binucleate or multinucleate cells with prominent nucleoli (Reed-Sternberg cells) or their mononuclear variants (Hodgkin cells) [2]. Hodgkin cells in LP Hodgkin's lymphoma may have less conspicuous nucleoli. However, except in the rare lymphocyte-depleted type, nearly the entire tumor in Hodgkin's lymphoma is composed of a heterogeneous, benign inflammatory infiltrate, with a minority of interspersed malignant cells [2]. The B-cell origin of Hodgkin's lymphoma has only recently been widely appreciated [3,4]. Although a direct causal relationship has not been established, Epstein-Barr virus (EBV) is detectable in tumor tissue in approximately 25% to 50% of Hodgkin's lymphoma cases [5,6] and has potential prognostic significance [7].

PRESENTATION

Hodgkin's lymphoma is usually a disease affecting younger individuals but has a bimodal age distribution, with one peak in the 20s and a second peak after age 60 or 70 [1]. Classical Hodgkin's lymphoma typically presents with painless cervical lymphadenopathy, with or without constitutional symptoms such as fevers, night sweats, weight loss, and generalized pruritus. Hodgkin's lymphoma most frequently involves cervical, supraclavicular, and/or mediastinal lymph nodes; axillary, hilar, para-aortic, and splenic involvement is also common [8]. Massive mediastinal disease may be symptomatic or incidentally discovered. The lymphoma usually first spreads contiguously to involve adjacent nodal sites, but about 10% to 15% of new patients have dissemination to extranodal sites such as bone marrow, lung, liver, and bone [8].

LP Hodgkin's lymphoma usually presents with asymptomatic, low-volume, early-stage disease in peripheral lymph nodes. In a multicenter, retrospective study, the median age was 35 years, most patients were male, approximately

80% had stage I to II disease, and 10% had B symptoms [9]. The behavior of LP Hodgkin's lymphoma can parallel that of an indolent non-Hodgkin's lymphoma (NHL): the disease tends to be slowly progressive, relapses tend to be late, and multiple relapses can occur over the course of years despite the high likelihood of remission with primary therapy [9–11]. Approximately 3% of cases transform to an aggressive, large B-cell NHL [9,12].

EVALUATION

An incisional or excisional lymph node biopsy specimen is almost always necessary to establish the initial diagnosis with certainty. Treatment on the basis of fine-needle aspirate is discouraged because it often provides insufficient material or architectural information to render a definitive diagnosis. Hodgkin's lymphoma must be differentiated from NHL, including diffuse large B-cell lymphoma and anaplastic large cell lymphoma (which may have a similar histologic appearance or clinical presentation), and from thymoma or other cancers in the case of a mediastinal presentation.

Immunohistochemical stains for cell surface markers assist in establishing the diagnosis. The Reed-Sternberg cells in classical Hodgkin's lymphoma are characteristically positive for CD30 and usually positive for CD15. Unlike most B-cell NHLs, they lack surface immunoglobulin expression and usually lack CD20. In contrast, the Reed-Sternberg cells in LP Hodgkin's lymphoma mark as B cells with expression of CD20 and lack CD15 and CD30. However, in most cases, these tumors can still be readily distinguished from B-cell NHL by the histologic pattern and, in particular, the relative scarcity of neoplastic cells.

The distinction between limited- and advanced-stage disease is essential for planning treatment. Staging is based upon the Cotswolds revision of the Ann Arbor staging system (Table 18-1) [13]. Laparotomy and lower-extremity lymphangiogram, once popular for Hodgkin's lymphoma staging, have largely been abandoned for this purpose. On history and physical examination, particular attention is given to palpable masses, organomegaly, cardiac and respiratory status, and the presence of B symptoms. Baseline laboratory evaluations include a complete blood count with differential; comprehensive chemistries, including lactic acid dehydrogenase; erythrocyte sedimentation rate (an adverse prognostic factor if elevated); and HIV antibody (given the increased risk of developing Hodgkin's lymphoma in HIV-infected individuals) [14]. Chest x-ray and computed tomography of the chest, abdomen, and pelvis are increasingly complemented by [18F]fluoro-2-deoxy-D-glucose positron emission tomography (FDG-PET). Bone marrow biopsy is justifiable regardless of presentation, but is more likely to be positive in older individuals or those with B symptoms, cytopenias, or pelvic or clinical stage III to

Table 18-1. Staging of Hodgkin's Lymphoma (Cotswolds Modification)

Stage/Designation	Description
Stage I	Single lymph node region or lymphoid structure, or single extralymphatic site (IE)
Stage II	≥ 2 lymph node regions or lymphoid structures on same side of diaphragm, or extralymphatic involvement on one side of diaphragm by limited direct extension from an adjacent nodal site (IIE)
Stage III	Lymph node regions or lymphoid structures on both sides of diaphragm, which may be accompanied by limited contiguous involvement of one extralymphatic site (IIIE)
Stage III$_1$	Subdiaphragmatic disease limited to spleen, splenic hilar, celiac, or portal nodes
Stage III$_2$	Subdiaphragmatic disease including para-aortic, iliac, or mesenteric nodes
Stage IV	Extranodal disease beyond that designated "E"
A	No constitutional symptoms
B	Unexplained fevers > 38°C, drenching night sweats, or unexplained > 10% weight loss in preceding 6 months
X	Bulky disease

(*Adapted from* Lister *et al.* [13].)

IV disease [15]. Before chemotherapy, pulmonary function testing, including diffusion capacity, is indicated (prior to bleomycin). Assessment of ejection fraction (prior to anthracycline) is also indicated in selected patients.

PROGNOSTIC FACTORS

The International Prognostic Score (IPS) [16] consists of seven factors that independently predict outcome in advanced Hodgkin's lymphoma: albumin less than 4 g/dL, hemoglobin less than 10.5 g/dL, male sex, age 45 years or older, stage IV disease, white blood cell count 15,000/mm^3 or greater, and lymphocytopenia (lymphocyte count < 600/mm^3 or < 8% of the white blood cell count). The 5-year estimated freedom from progression ranges from 84% among patients with no risk factors to 42% among those with at least five factors. The IPS may aid in study design and analysis as well as in managing individual patients.

For early-stage disease, cooperative groups have employed other criteria for risk stratification and treatment selection [17–19] (Table 18-2). Stage IIB bulky disease (a mass > 10 cm or a mediastinal mass ≥ one third the maximum intrathoracic diameter) may be regarded as advanced disease.

Residual masses are frequent after Hodgkin's lymphoma therapy, but their size correlates poorly with survival outcomes [20]. FDG-PET enhances the ability to distinguish between fibrosis and viable tumor in residual masses, and when performed midtreatment is also highly informative about the quality of the treatment response. Achievement of a negative FDG-PET after only two or three cycles of first-line chemotherapy predicts durable remission, whereas a persistently abnormal FDG-PET is associated with a high risk of treatment failure [21,22]. FDG-PET complements and is potentially superior to the IPS [22]. How to tailor treatment on the basis of this information is the subject of current trials.

TREATMENT OF CLASSICAL HODGKIN'S LYMPHOMA

EARLY-STAGE DISEASE: COMBINED MODALITY THERAPY

Most patients with early-stage Hodgkin's lymphoma are cured with combined modality therapy. Hodgkin's lymphoma is usually a radiosensitive tumor, and radiation was the first modality demonstrated to have curative potential. However, it is the rare patient with classical Hodgkin's lymphoma

in whom radiation alone is now considered appropriate. It might, for example, be considered in elderly patients with early-stage disease who are not candidates for chemotherapy [23], or in patients with low-risk, stage IA disease confined to a single lymph node in the high neck region [19]. However, in most cases, early-stage classical Hodgkin's lymphoma is treated with abbreviated-course chemotherapy (typically four cycles) followed by involved-field radiation therapy (IFRT) [17]. While radiation was historically delivered to more extensive fields, recognition of its late and cumulative toxicities led to a reduction in both field and dose, such that IFRT is now standard in combined modality approaches. Adding chemotherapy to radiation permits less radiation to be delivered without compromise in cure rates [17,24–26], and has produced superior outcomes in early-stage disease compared with radiation alone [17,27,28].

The lowest acceptable radiation dose that minimizes long-term toxicity while preserving cure rates is being defined. On interim analysis, no significant difference in failure-free survival (FFS) was seen with six cycles of EBVP (epirubicin, bleomycin, vinblastine, prednisone) followed by 36- versus 20-Gy IFRT in a European Organisation for Research and Treatment of Cancer (EORTC) trial for early favorable disease [29]. Similarly, on interim analysis of the German Hodgkin Study Group (GHSG) HD10 trial for early favorable Hodgkin's lymphoma, no significant differences were seen between two and four cycles of ABVD (doxorubicin, bleomycin, vinblastine, dacarbazine), or between 20- and 30-Gy IFRT [30]. In the GHSG HD11 trial for early unfavorable Hodgkin's lymphoma, no significant differences were seen on interim analysis of four cycles of ABVD versus baseline BEACOPP (bleomycin, etoposide, doxorubicin, cyclophosphamide, vincristine, procarbazine, prednisone) followed by 20- versus 30-Gy IFRT [31]. More mature results are pending.

EARLY-STAGE, NONBULKY DISEASE: CHEMOTHERAPY ALONE

Extended-course chemotherapy alone has recently emerged as a viable option for those with nonbulky stage I or II disease (Table 18-3). Its appropriateness is a matter of debate [32,33]. The move to chemotherapy alone stems from concerns about the late toxicities of radiation. To date, no study has conclusively demonstrated a statistically significant overall survival difference with the omission of radiation. A randomized study that suggested an overall sur-

Table 18-2. Risk Groups in Early Hodgkin's Lymphoma

Risk group	EORTC-GELA criteria [17]	GHSG criteria [18]	NCIC-ECOG criteria [19]
Very favorable or low risk	All of the following: A. Supradiaphragmatic stage IA B. No large mediastinal mass (ratio < 0.35) C. Female, age < 40 y D. Lymphocyte predominant or nodular sclerosis histology E. ESR < 50 mm/h	—	All of the following: A. Stage IA B. Single lymph node confined to high neck or epitrochlear region C. Bulk < 3 cm D. Lymphocyte predominant or nodular sclerosis histology E. ESR < 50 mm/h
Early favorable	Supradiaphragmatic stage I–II, without the following risk factors: A. Large mediastinal mass (ratio ≥ 0.35 the greatest thoracic cross-sectional diameter) B. Age ≥ 50 y C. ESR ≥ 50 mm/h without, or ≥ 30 mm/h with B symptoms D. ≥ 4 involved regions	Stage I–II, without the following risk factors: A. Large mediastinal mass (> 10 cm or ratio ≥ one third) B. Extranodal disease C. ESR ≥ 50 mm/h without, or ≥ 30 mm/h with B symptoms D. ≥ 3 involved regions	Nonbulky stage I–IIA, without the following risk factors: A. Mixed cellularity or lymphocyte-depleted histology B. Age ≥ 40 y C. ESR ≥ 50 mm/h D. ≥ 4 involved regions
Early unfavorable	Supradiaphragmatic stage I–II, with risk factor(s)	Stage I or IIA with risk factor(s), or stage IIB with C/D but not A/B*	Stage I–IIA with risk factor(s); bulky disease excluded

*Stage IIB with A/B is categorized as advanced disease, along with stage III–IV.
EORTC-GELA—European Organisation for Research and Treatment of Cancer – Groupe d'Études des Lymphomes de l'Adulte; ESR—erythrocyte sedimentation rate; GHSG—German Hodgkin Study Group; NCIC-ECOG—National Cancer Institute of Canada – Eastern Cooperative Oncology Group.

vival advantage to radiation after complete response to six cycles of ABVD was inconclusive due to the heterogeneity of cases [34]. In the National Cancer Institute of Canada/Eastern Cooperative Oncology Group (NCIC-ECOG) HD6 trial of nonbulky stage I to IIA Hodgkin's lymphoma, there was a statistically significant 6% absolute decrease in progression-free survival associated with the omission of radiation on median 4+ years of follow-up, but no difference in overall survival [19]. In a Memorial Sloan-Kettering trial, on median 5+ years of follow-up, no statistically significant difference in event-free or overall survival was detected with ABVD plus radiation versus full-course ABVD alone. However, the study was underpowered to detect a less than 20% difference [35]. In the EORTC-Groupe d'Études des Lymphomes de l'Adulte (GELA) H9-F trial [29], the no-radiation arm was closed due to an excess of treatment failures; however, this may reflect the inadequacy of the chemotherapy regimen, as marked by the 4-year FFS rate of only 69% in early favorable patients who had achieved a complete response.

In summary, although chemoradiation remains the gold standard, full-course chemotherapy alone is an option in patients with localized, nonbulky disease. It should especially be considered in patients who are younger or in whom mediastinum, lung, or breast tissue (in the case of young females) would be included in the radiation field. Although radiation is now given at lower doses than were given historically, the impact of this change on long-term toxicities is not yet defined. On the other hand, the risks of radiation must be weighed against the risks of more chemotherapy cycles and the potentially greater risk of relapse. Postchemotherapy PET scans may very well guide the decision, although there are not yet published clinical trials in this regard.

Bulky disease is associated with an increased risk of local failure. The contribution of consolidative radiotherapy has not been adequately tested in limited-stage bulky disease. Combined modality therapy remains the standard for such cases, which have been excluded from randomized studies involving chemotherapy alone.

ADVANCED DISEASE

All modern Hodgkin's lymphoma regimens contain an anthracycline. ABVD is the present standard against which newer regimens are to be compared. Advanced disease is treated with six to eight cycles. In representative phase 3 studies of advanced or intermediate-advanced Hodgkin's lymphoma, ABVD produced 5-year FFS rates of 63% to 78% and 5-year overall survival rates of 75% to 90% [36,37].

Until the development of MOPP (mechlorethamine, vincristine, procarbazine, prednisone) in the 1960s, advanced Hodgkin's lymphoma had been largely fatal. In a representative study of stage III to IV disease, MOPP produced a 67% complete response and a 50% FFS rate at 5 years [37]. The activity of ABVD, introduced in the 1970s, was demonstrated in MOPP-resistant Hodgkin's lymphoma and then in newly diagnosed patients [38].

In randomized trials, ABVD or ABVD-MOPP combinations yielded superior outcomes compared with MOPP alone [37,39]. The MOPP-ABV (doxorubicin, bleomycin, vinblastine) hybrid is more effective than sequential MOPP followed by ABVD [40] and as effective as ABVD alone [36]. However, ABVD is less toxic, including fewer acute toxicities, fewer cases of myelodysplasia and leukemia, and less sterility [36].

Stanford V is a newer regimen consisting of abbreviated chemotherapy over a 12-week course (doxorubicin, vinblastine, vincristine, bleomycin, nitrogen mustard or cyclophosphamide, etoposide, prednisone) followed by modified IFRT to sites of initial disease 5 cm or greater and to initial macroscopic splenic disease [41]. Myelotoxic and nonmyelotoxic agents alternate, with maintenance of dose intensity and less cumulative exposure to anthracycline and bleomycin. Mature phase 2 data were promising, with no treatment-related deaths and a 5-year freedom from progression rate of 89% overall and 75% for those with an IPS of 3 or higher [41]. Yet in an Italian multicenter trial, a modified Stanford V regimen was inferior to ABVD (5-year freedom from progression of 73% vs 85%, and 5-year FFS of 54% vs 78%) and to a MOPP-containing combination [42]. However, this modified regimen was less aggressive with radiation therapy. The data suggest that Stanford V should be viewed as a combined modality regimen, perhaps with radiation delivered according to the original criteria. Results of a US Intergroup trial of ABVD versus Stanford V are pending.

Introduced in the 1990s by the GHSG, escalated (increased-dose) BEACOPP is an intensive and effective first-line regimen for patients 15 to 65 years of age with advanced Hodgkin's lymphoma. In the GHSG HD9 trial of approximately 1200 patients with stage IIB to IV Hodgkin's lymphoma, escalated BEACOPP yielded superior 5-year FFS and overall survival rates compared with baseline (standard-dose) BEACOPP and with COPP-ABVD (cyclophosphamide, vincristine, procarbazine, prednisone plus ABVD) [43]. Each regimen was followed by radiation to sites of initially bulky ($\geq$ 5 cm) or residual disease. The benefit of escalated BEACOPP was statistically significant across IPS risk groups, but appeared most pronounced in those with four or more risk factors (5-year FFS 82% and 59% and 5-year overall survival 82% and 67% for escalated BEACOPP vs COPP-ABVD in the high-risk group, respectively). Subset analysis suggested benefit in all age groups with the possible exception of patients 60 to 65 years of age. However, escalated BEACOPP is more toxic, including more acute hematologic toxicities, infertility [44], and potentially more secondary myelodysplasia/leukemia. This was evidenced by nine cases in 466 patients (1.9%) after escalated BEACOPP versus one case in 260 patients (0.4%) after COPP-ABVD. Nevertheless, on subsequent follow-up, a statistically significant overall survival advantage at 10 years was retained with escalated BEACOPP [45]. Risk- and response-adapted strategies involving BEACOPP are being investigated to define the optimal types of patients for

Table 18-3. Chemotherapy Versus Chemoradiation for Early Hodgkin's Lymphoma

Study	Cohort	Evaluable patients, n	Chemotherapy	Radiation	FFP, %	FFS, %	OS, %
NCIC-ECOG HD6 [19]	Nonbulky stage IA–IIA	203	None (if very low risk) or ABVD × 2 cycles	Subtotal nodal irradiation	93 (5 y)*	88 (5 y)†	94 (5 y)
		196	ABVD × 4–6 cycles	None	87 (5 y)	86 (5 y)	96 (5 y)
EORTC-GELA H9-F [29]	Early favorable stage I–II with complete response only	239	EBVP × 6 cycles	36-Gy IFRT	—	88 (4 y)*	98 (4 y)
		209	EBVP × 6 cycles	20-Gy IFRT	—	85 (4 y)*	100 (4 y)
		130	EBVP × 6 cycles	None	—	69 (4 y)	98 (4 y)
Straus et al. [35]	Nonbulky stage I–II or nonbulky stage IIIA (13%)	76	ABVD × 6 cycles	IFRT or modified EFRT	86 (5 y)‡	—	97 (5 y)§
		76	ABVD × 6 cycles	None	81 (5 y)	—	90 (5 y)

*Statistically significant compared with no-radiation arm.
†$P = 0.06$.
‡$P = 0.61$; powered to detect a 20% difference.
§$P = 0.08$.
ABVD—doxorubicin, bleomycin, vinblastine, dacarbazine; EBVP—epirubicin, bleomycin, vinblastine, prednisone; EFRT—extended-field radiation therapy; EORTC-GELA—European Organisation for Research and Treatment of Cancer–Groupe d'Études des Lymphomes de l'Adulte; FFP—freedom from progression; FFS—failure-free survival; IFRT—involved-field radiation therapy; NCIC-ECOG—National Cancer Institute of Canada–Eastern Cooperative Oncology Group; OS—overall survival.

this regimen. The relative efficacy of escalated BEACOPP compared with ABVD has not yet been established.

Following chemotherapy for advanced disease, the overall data concerning consolidative radiation therapy to sites of tumor bulk are variable. For example, in a randomized trial of stage III to IV Hodgkin's lymphoma patients with complete response after chemotherapy, there were no significant differences in 5-year event-free or overall survival with the addition of radiation, and there was a trend toward inferior survival in the radiation arm [46]. Similarly, in a meta-analysis of chemotherapy versus chemoradiation for advanced Hodgkin's lymphoma, overall survival was statistically significantly inferior with the addition of radiation [47]. In another study of stage III to IV Hodgkin's lymphoma patients with complete response after chemotherapy, no differences in remission duration or overall survival were noted with radiation, although on subset analysis a statistically significant improvement in disease control was found in patients with nodular sclerosis or bulky lymphoma [48]. On interim analysis of the four-arm GHSG HD12 trial for advanced Hodgkin's lymphoma (escalated BEACOPP for eight cycles with and without radiation vs four escalated and four baseline cycles of BEACOPP with and without radiation), no significant differences between the radiation and no-radiation groups were seen on median 2.5-year follow-up [49]. Thus, there is no one standard and practices vary. The approach to radiation based on radiographic response criteria is limited in that the size of a residual mass does not reliably indicate the presence or absence of viable tumor. New response criteria that incorporate metabolic response have recently been proposed [50], and consolidative radiation that is restricted to residually PET-positive tumor foci is under investigation.

SALVAGE THERAPY

Hodgkin's lymphoma that relapses after radiation alone can be effectively treated with standard front-line chemotherapy such as ABVD. In contrast, high-dose (myeloablative) therapy with blood or bone marrow transplantation (BMT) is the standard approach for most patients whose classical Hodgkin's lymphoma progresses or relapses despite primary chemotherapy or chemoradiation. One potential exception is the patient who has a long disease-free interval after primary therapy. Another potential exception is the patient with early-stage disease who relapses after primary chemotherapy. Whether it is better to pursue radiation or BMT in this situation is unclear, as chemotherapy alone has only recently been considered for early-stage Hodgkin's lymphoma. Age and performances status, extent of disease, and length of initial remission are factored into the decision. BMT is not considered for early intensification of primary therapy in responding patients [51].

Autologous BMT yields an approximately 50% to 60% event-free survival rate at 3 years, although relapses continue to occur beyond this point [52–55]. In a multicenter study [53], 161 patients with relapsed Hodgkin's lymphoma were randomized to receive Dexa-BEAM (dexamethasone, carmustine, etoposide, cytarabine, melphalan) for four cycles, or Dexa-BEAM for two cycles followed by high-dose BEAM with autologous BMT, provided that the disease was chemosensitive. On median 3+ years of follow-up, 3-year freedom from treatment failure was superior in the high-dose therapy arm (55% vs 34%), although there was no statistically significant overall survival advantage. On longer follow-up [30], a significantly better 7-year freedom from treatment failure rate was maintained with BMT (49% vs 32%). Subgroup analysis indicated an advantage to BMT in patients with either early or late first relapse but not in multiple-relapsed patients.

Autologous BMT has been more widely applied for relapsed Hodgkin's lymphoma than allogeneic BMT. However, allogeneic BMT is a viable alternative for younger, healthy patients and has the potential for better disease control, particularly in poor-risk disease such as refractory relapse. Allogeneic BMT is more toxic and has a higher treatment-related mortality, but may confer a lower relapse risk due to a potential graft-versus-lymphoma effect [52].

We usually recommend two to three cycles of standard-dose salvage chemotherapy as a bridge toward high-dose therapy with autologous or allogeneic BMT. Some examples of common salvage regimens include ICE (ifosfamide, carboplatin, etoposide), ESHAP (etoposide, methylprednisolone, high-dose cytarabine, cisplatin), and gemcitabine-based regimens. GVD

(gemcitabine, vinorelbine, pegylated liposomal doxorubicin) is a newer salvage regimen that had promising activity and a favorable toxicity profile in a phase 1/2 Cancer and Leukemia Group B (CALGB) trial [56]. The salvage chemotherapy serves to 1) reduce disease burden and stabilize or improve the patient's overall condition prior to intensive therapy; and 2) establish whether the disease is chemosensitive or chemorefractory, which is centrally important in shaping prognosis and guiding choice of BMT (autologous or allogeneic). For example, we would prioritize a related-donor allogeneic transplant over an autologous transplant for chemorefractory relapse. If radiation is to be delivered (*eg*, localized relapse in a patient with a history of early-stage disease and no prior radiation), it is advisable to postpone that radiation until after BMT to minimize transplant toxicities. For those who are ineligible for or relapse despite of myeloablative transplantation, nonmyeloablative (reduced intensity) allogeneic transplantation has been increasingly pursued, with promising outcomes in a subset of patients [57–59].

For palliative therapy of relapsed or refractory classical Hodgkin's lymphoma, steroids can be beneficial. Rituximab had modest single-agent activity in a pilot study [60]. Therefore, it has been studied with gemcitabine for relapsed disease [61] and with ABVD in newly diagnosed patients [62], with promising early results. Other monoclonal antibodies, mostly directed against CD30, have had minimal or no clinical activity in early-phase trials of relapsed or refractory Hodgkin's lymphoma [63–65] and continue to be investigated. Bortezomib has had minimal or no clinical activity in this setting [66]. Adoptive immunotherapy of EBV-positive Hodgkin's lymphoma has generated interesting results in early-phase trials [67,68], as it has in posttransplant lymphoproliferative disease [69]. Participation in clinical trials is encouraged.

TREATMENT OF LYMPHOCYTE-PREDOMINANT HODGKIN'S LYMPHOMA

There are no randomized clinical trials to guide the therapy of LP Hodgkin's lymphoma. However, the treatment paradigm differs from that of classical Hodgkin's lymphoma. Reported 10-year overall survival rates have ranged from 70% to 93%, with second cancers, cardiovascular disease, and lymphoma being the leading causes of mortality [70]. Given its indolent natural history, a watch-and-wait strategy has been proposed but has not been widely adopted. Although chemotherapy or combined modality therapy can be considered for stage I to II LP Hodgkin's lymphoma, radiation alone is a standard and effective approach [10,71]. Advanced disease is generally treated with ABVD.

Rituximab has clinical activity in LP Hodgkin's lymphoma. In small phase 2 trials of newly diagnosed or relapsed LP Hodgkin's lymphoma, rituximab (375 mg/m^2 weekly for 4 cycles) produced response rates of 94% to 100%, complete response rates of 46% to 53%, and an estimated median time to progression of 10 to 33 months [72,73]. Rituximab is being investigated as primary therapy. Concerns have been raised as to whether rituximab increases the risk of large cell transformation [73]. Large cell transformations are generally treated along an aggressive NHL paradigm.

TREATMENT TOXICITIES

The monitoring for acute treatment-related complications must include vigilance for signs of bleomycin pulmonary toxicity. This is a well-recognized complication that may present acutely or subacutely, either during treatment or up to 6 months afterward [74]. In a representative analysis of 141 patients with newly diagnosed Hodgkin's lymphoma, bleomycin pulmonary toxicity was found in 18%, with a mortality rate of 4% overall and 24% in those with respiratory symptoms and interstitial infiltrates [75]. Notably, in addition to age above 40 years, the use of granulocyte colony-stimulating factor was associated with a significantly increased risk of bleomycin toxicity [75]; this was also evident in preclinical studies [76]. Bleomycin must be withheld if pulmonary toxicity develops and high-dose corticosteroids must be considered [74]. Generally, the same other drugs are continued but with permanent omission of bleomycin, which does not appear to compromise disease control based on small numbers of patients [75,77]. ABVD and AVD (doxorubicin, vinblastine, dacarbazine) are being compared as part of a GHSG trial for early-stage Hodgkin's lymphoma. Other acute toxicities to be monitored include hematologic, infectious, gastrointestinal, neurologic, and cardiac sequelae.

Late side effects of treatment are a major cause of morbidity and mortality in survivors of Hodgkin's lymphoma. On long-term follow-up of Hodgkin's lymphoma patients treated between the 1960s and 1980s, all-cause mortality from diseases other than lymphoma was approximately five to seven times greater than that of the general population [78]. Secondary solid tumors (particularly breast and lung cancer) [79,80], leukemias [81,82], and premature cardiovascular disease [83,84] are among the leading concerns. The risk of secondary cancers continues after 15 to 20 years—without evidence of a plateau—and is most pronounced after combined modality therapy and more extensive radiation [80]. Hypothyroidism and thyroid cancer are also increased after radiation [85]. Leukemia and infertility are related to the type and cumulative amount of chemotherapy; both occur less frequently after ABVD than after MOPP. It is expected that newer risk-adapted treatment approaches and less aggressive radiation strategies [86] will reduce some of these late complications.

ABVD (DOXORUBICIN, BLEOMYCIN, VINBLASTINE, DACARBAZINE)

ABVD is the most standard chemotherapy regimen for early- and advanced-stage Hodgkin's lymphoma and is given alone or followed by radiation depending on the presentation.

DOSAGE MODIFICATIONS

Dosage modifications may be required for hyperbilirubinemia, elevated creatinine, and hematologic or nonhematologic toxicities. Bleomycin is discontinued if pulmonary toxicity develops

CANDIDATES FOR TREATMENT

Classical or LP Hodgkin's lymphoma, as first-line systemic therapy

SPECIAL PRECAUTIONS

Patients with abnormal left ventricular function or history of coronary artery disease (doxorubicin); significantly impaired respiratory function (bleomycin); impaired renal function (bleomycin, dacarbazine); hepatic dysfunction (doxorubicin, vinblastine, dacarbazine); neuropathy (vinblastine)

ALTERNATIVE THERAPIES

Stanford V, BEACOPP (baseline or escalated)

DOSAGE AND SCHEDULING

Doxorubicin 25 mg/m^2 IV on d 1 and 15

Vinblastine 6 mg/m^2 IV on d 1 and 15

Bleomycin 10 units/m^2 IV on d 1 and 15

Dacarbazine 375 mg/m^2 IV on d 1 and 15

• 28-d cycle

• Advanced disease: maximum 8 cycles

EXPERIENCES AND RESPONSE RATES: ADVANCED DISEASE*

Study	Stage	Evaluable patients, n	Regimen	CR, %	FFS, %	OS, %	Comments
Canellos et al. [37]	III$_2$A, IIIB, or IV	123	MOPP	67[†]	50 (5 y)[†]	66 (5 y)	Includes relapses after primary RT; no further RT permitted
		115	ABVD	82	61 (5 y)	73 (5 y)	
		123	MOPP-ABVD	83	65 (5 y)	75 (5 y)	
Duggan et al. [36]	III$_2$A, IIIB, or IV	433	ABVD	76	63 (5 y)	82 (5 y)	Includes relapses after primary RT; no further RT permitted. More treatment-related deaths and leukemia with MOPP-ABV
		419	MOPP-ABV	80	66 (5 y)	81 (5 y)	
Johnson et al. [87]	I/II bulky or B, III, or IV	394	ABVD	92	75 (3 y)	90 (3 y)	Includes relapses after primary RT; RT given to initially bulky or residual disease
		394	Two multidrug regimens	92	75 (3 y)	88 (3 y)	

*See also Gobbi *et al.* [42].
[†]Statistically significant compared with ABVD and MOPP-ABVD.
ABV—doxorubicin, bleomycin, vinblastine; ABVD—doxorubicin, bleomycin, vinblastine, dacarbazine; CR—complete response; FFS—failure-free survival; MOPP—mechlorethamine, vincristine, procarbazine, prednisone; OS—overall survival; RT—radiation therapy.

STANFORD V

Stanford V is an abbreviated regimen of weekly chemotherapy over 12 weeks, alternating between myelotoxic and nonmyelotoxic drugs, followed by radiation depending on disease bulk and location.

DOSAGE MODIFICATIONS

Dosage modifications may be required for hyperbilirubinemia, elevated creatinine, and hematologic or nonhematologic toxicities. Bleomycin is discontinued if pulmonary toxicity develops

CANDIDATES FOR TREATMENT

Classical Hodgkin's lymphoma, as first-line systemic therapy

SPECIAL PRECAUTIONS

Patients with abnormal left ventricular function or history of coronary artery disease (doxorubicin); significantly impaired respiratory function (bleomycin); impaired renal function (bleomycin, etoposide); hepatic dysfunction (doxorubicin, vinblastine, vincristine, etoposide); neuropathy (vinblastine, vincristine)

ALTERNATIVE THERAPIES

ABVD, BEACOPP (baseline or escalated)

DOSAGE AND SCHEDULING

Doxorubicin 25 mg/m^2 IV on d 1 of wk 1, 3, 5, 7, 9, and 11

Vinblastine 6 mg/m^2 IV* on d 1 of wk 1, 3, 5, 7, 9, and 11

Vincristine 1.4 mg/m^2 IV† (maximum 2 mg) on d 1 of wk 2, 4, 6, 8, 10, and 12

Bleomycin 5 units/m^2 IV on d 1 of wk 2, 4, 6, 8, 10, and 12

Nitrogen mustard 6 mg/m^2 IV (or cyclophosphamide 650 mg/m^2 IV if nitrogen mustard is unavailable) on d 1 of wk 1, 5, and 9

Etoposide 60 mg/m^2 IV on d 1–2 of wk 3, 7, and 11

Prednisone 40 mg/m^2 orally every other d of wk 1–9, then tapered

- Chemotherapy is followed by involved-field radiation therapy to initial disease ≥ 5 cm or initial macroscopic nodular splenic disease

*If age > 50 y, reduce vinblastine to 4 mg/m^2 for wk 9 and 11.
†If age > 50 y, reduce vincristine to 1 mg for wk 10 and 12.
Regimen from the E2496 Intergroup trial.

EXPERIENCES AND RESPONSE RATES

Study	Stage	Evaluable patients, *n*	Regimen	CR, %	5-y FFP, %	5-y FFS, %	5-y OS, %
Horning *et al.* [41]	Locally extensive I–II, or III–IV	142	Stanford V	—	89	—	96
Gobbi *et al.* [42]	Bulky II, III–IV	107*	Modified Stanford V	76	73	54	82
		122	ABVD	89†	85†	78†	90
		106	MOPP-EBV-CAD	94†	94†	81†	89

*Total of 354 patients in all arms were included in intent-to-treat analysis.
†*P* < 0.01 for Stanford V versus other regimens.
ABVD—doxorubicin, bleomycin, vinblastine, dacarbazine; CR—complete response; FFP—freedom from progression; FFS—failure-free survival; MOPP-EBV-CAD—mechlorethamine, vincristine, procarbazine, prednisone, epirubicin, bleomycin, vinblastine, lomustine, doxorubicin, vindesine; OS—overall survival.

BEACOPP (BLEOMYCIN, ETOPOSIDE, DOXORUBICIN, CYCLOPHOSPHAMIDE, VINCRISTINE, PROCARBAZINE, PREDNISONE)

BEACOPP is a multidrug regimen that, in its dose-escalated version, has yielded quite promising outcomes in advanced Hodgkin's lymphoma. Its efficacy must be balanced against its greater toxicity. The optimal regimen for advanced Hodgkin's lymphoma—ABVD versus escalated BEACOPP—is a matter of debate. Dose-dense BEACOPP (BEACOPP-14) is also under clinical investigation. BEACOPP may be followed by radiation where appropriate.

DOSAGE MODIFICATIONS

Dosage modifications may be required for hyperbilirubinemia, elevated creatinine, and hematologic or nonhematologic toxicities. Bleomycin is discontinued if pulmonary toxicity develops

CANDIDATES FOR TREATMENT

Classical Hodgkin's lymphoma, as first-line therapy; escalated BEACOPP considered particularly with poor-risk, advanced disease in patients younger than 60 years of age

SPECIAL PRECAUTIONS

Patients with abnormal left ventricular function or history of coronary artery disease (doxorubicin); significantly impaired respiratory function (bleomycin); impaired renal function (bleomycin, etoposide, procarbazine); hepatic dysfunction (etoposide, doxorubicin, vincristine); neuropathy (vincristine); glucose-6-phosphate dehydrogenase deficiency (procarbazine). Procarbazine has a number of drug-drug and drug-food interactions

ALTERNATIVE THERAPIES

ABVD, Stanford V

DOSAGE AND SCHEDULING

Baseline BEACOPP:

Bleomycin 10 mg/m^2 IV on d 8

Etoposide 100 mg/m^2 IV on d 1–3

Doxorubicin 25 mg/m^2 IV on d 1

Cyclophosphamide 650 mg/m^2 IV on d 1

Vincristine 1.4 mg/m^2 IV (maximum 2 mg) on d 8

Procarbazine 100 mg/m^2 orally on d 1–7

Prednisone 40 mg/m^2 orally on d 1–14

• 21-d cycle

• Maximum 8 cycles

Escalated BEACOPP:

Bleomycin 10 mg/m^2 IV on d 8

Etoposide 200 mg/m^2 IV on d 1–3

Doxorubicin 35 mg/m^2 IV on d 1

Cyclophosphamide 1250 mg/m^2 IV on d 1

Vincristine 1.4 mg/m^2 IV (maximum 2 mg) on d 8

Procarbazine 100 mg/m^2 orally on d 1–7

Prednisone 40 mg/m^2 orally on d 1–14

Granulocyte colony-stimulating factor starting on d 8

• 21-d cycle

• Maximum 8 cycles

EXPERIENCES AND RESPONSE RATES

Study	Stage	Evaluable patients, *n*	Regimen*	CR, %	5-y FFS, %	5-y OS, %
GHSG HD9 [43]	IIB bulky, selected III, or IV	260	COPP-ABVD	85	69	83
		469	Baseline BEACOPP	88	76[†]	88
		466	Escalated BEACOPP	96	87[‡]	91[§]

*Each regimen was followed by radiation to initial disease > 5 cm and to residual disease.
[†]*P* = 0.04 compared with COPP-ABVD.
[‡]*P* < 0.001 compared with either other regimen.
[§]*P* = 0.002 compared with COPP-ABVD and *P* = 0.06 compared with baseline BEACOPP.
ABVD—doxorubicin, bleomycin, vinblastine, dacarbazine; BEACOPP—bleomycin, etoposide, doxorubicin, cyclophosphamide, vincristine, procarbazine, prednisone; COPP—cyclophosphamide, vincristine, procarbazine, prednisone; CR—complete response; FFS—failure-free survival; GHSG—German Hodgkin Study Group; OS—overall survival.

REFERENCES

1. Nakatsuka S, Aozasa K: Epidemiology and pathologic features of Hodgkin lymphoma. *Int J Hematol* 2006, 83:391–397.

2. World Health Organization Classification of Tumours: *Pathology and Genetics: Tumors of Haematopoietic and Lymphoid Tissues*. Edited by Jaffe ES, Harris NL, Stein H, Vardimam JW. Lyon: IARC Press; 2001.

3. Marafioti T, Hummel M, Foss HD, *et al.*: Hodgkin and Reed-Sternberg cells represent an expansion of a single clone originating from a germinal center B-cell with functional immunoglobulin gene rearrangements but defective immunoglobulin transcription. *Blood* 2000, 95:1443–1450.

4. Kanzler H, Kuppers R, Hansmann ML, Rajewsky K: Hodgkin and Reed-Sternberg cells in Hodgkin's disease represent the outgrowth of a dominant tumor clone derived from (crippled) germinal center B cells. *J Exp Med* 1996, 184:1495–1505.

5. Wu TC, Mann RB, Charache P, *et al.*: Detection of EBV gene expression in Reed-Sternberg cells of Hodgkin's disease. *Int J Cancer* 1990, 46:801–804.

6. Glaser SL, Lin RJ, Stewart SL, *et al.*: Epstein-Barr virus-associated Hodgkin's disease: epidemiologic characteristics in international data. *Int J Cancer* 1997, 70:375–382.

7. Keegan TH, Glaser SL, Clarke CA, *et al.*: Epstein-Barr virus as a marker of survival after Hodgkin's lymphoma: a population-based study. *J Clin Oncol* 2005, 23:7604–7613.

8. Gupta RK, Gospodarowicz MK, Lister TA: Clinical evaluation and staging of Hodgkin's disease. In *Hodgkin's Disease*. Edited by Mauch PM, Armitage JO, Diehl V. Philadelphia: Lippincott Williams & Wilkins; 1999:223–240.

9. Diehl V, Sextro M, Franklin J, *et al.*: Clinical presentation, course, and prognostic factors in lymphocyte-predominant Hodgkin's disease and lymphocyte-rich classical Hodgkin's disease: report from the European Task Force on Lymphoma Project on Lymphocyte-Predominant Hodgkin's Disease. *J Clin Oncol* 1999, 17:776–783.

10. Bodis S, Kraus MD, Pinkus G, *et al.*: Clinical presentation and outcome in lymphocyte-predominant Hodgkin's disease. *J Clin Oncol* 1997, 15:3060–3066.

11. Regula DP Jr, Hoppe RT, Weiss LM: Nodular and diffuse types of lymphocyte predominance Hodgkin's disease. *N Engl J Med* 1988, 318:214–219.

12. Hansmann ML, Stein H, Fellbaum C, *et al.*: Nodular paragranuloma can transform into high-grade malignant lymphoma of B type. *Hum Pathol* 1989, 20:1169–1175.

13. Lister TA, Crowther D, Sutcliffe SB, *et al.*: Report of a committee convened to discuss the evaluation and staging of patients with Hodgkin's disease: Cotswolds meeting. *J Clin Oncol* 1989, 7:1630–1636.

14. Biggar RJ, Jaffe ES, Goedert JJ, *et al.*: Hodgkin lymphoma and immunodeficiency in persons with HIV/AIDS. *Blood* 2006, 108:3786–3791.

15. Vassilakopoulos TP, Angelopoulou MK, Constantinou N, *et al.*: Development and validation of a clinical prediction rule for bone marrow involvement in patients with Hodgkin lymphoma. *Blood* 2005, 105:1875–1880.

16. Hasenclever D, Diehl V: A prognostic score for advanced Hodgkin's disease. International Prognostic Factors Project on Advanced Hodgkin's Disease. *N Engl J Med* 1998, 339:1506–1514.

17. Ferme C, Eghbali H, Meerwaldt JH, *et al.*: Chemotherapy plus involved-field radiation in early-stage Hodgkin's disease. *N Engl J Med* 2007, 357:1916–1927.

18. Josting A, Wolf J, Diehl V: Hodgkin disease: prognostic factors and treatment strategies. *Curr Opin Oncol* 2000, 12:403–411.

19. Meyer RM, Gospodarowicz MK, Connors JM, *et al.*: Randomized comparison of ABVD chemotherapy with a strategy that includes radiation therapy in patients with limited-stage Hodgkin's lymphoma: National Cancer Institute of Canada Clinical Trials Group and the Eastern Cooperative Oncology Group. *J Clin Oncol* 2005, 23:4634–4642.

20. Jochelson M, Mauch P, Balikian J, *et al.*: The significance of the residual mediastinal mass in treated Hodgkin's disease. *J Clin Oncol* 1985, 3:637–640.

21. Hutchings M, Loft A, Hansen M, *et al.*: FDG-PET after two cycles of chemotherapy predicts treatment failure and progression-free survival in Hodgkin lymphoma. *Blood* 2006, 107:52–59.

22. Gallamini A, Hutchings M, Rigacci L, *et al.*: Early interim 2-[18F]fluoro-2-deoxy-D-glucose positron emission tomography is prognostically superior to International Prognostic Score in advanced-stage Hodgkin's lymphoma: a report from a joint Italian-Danish study. *J Clin Oncol* 2007, 25:3746–3752.

23. Landgren O, Axdorph U, Fears TR, *et al.*: A population-based cohort study on early-stage Hodgkin lymphoma treated with radiotherapy alone: with special reference to older patients. *Ann Oncol* 2006, 17:1290–1295.

24. Noordijk EM, Carde P, Dupouy N, *et al.*: Combined-modality therapy for clinical stage I or II Hodgkin's lymphoma: long-term results of the European Organisation for Research and Treatment of Cancer H7 randomized controlled trials. *J Clin Oncol* 2006, 24:3128–3135.

25. Bonadonna G, Bonfante V, Viviani S, *et al.*: ABVD plus subtotal nodal versus involved-field radiotherapy in early-stage Hodgkin's disease: long-term results. *J Clin Oncol* 2004, 22:2835–2841.

26. Engert A, Schiller P, Josting A, *et al.*: Involved-field radiotherapy is equally effective and less toxic compared with extended-field radiotherapy after four cycles of chemotherapy in patients with early-stage unfavorable Hodgkin's lymphoma: results of the HD8 trial of the German Hodgkin's Lymphoma Study Group. *J Clin Oncol* 2003, 21:3601–3608.

27. Engert A, Franklin J, Eich HT, *et al.*: Two cycles of doxorubicin, bleomycin, vinblastine, and dacarbazine plus extended-field radiotherapy is superior to radiotherapy alone in early favorable Hodgkin's lymphoma: final results of the GHSG HD7 trial. *J Clin Oncol* 2007, 25:3495–3502.

28. Press OW, LeBlanc M, Lichter AS, *et al.*: Phase III randomized intergroup trial of subtotal lymphoid irradiation versus doxorubicin, vinblastine, and subtotal lymphoid irradiation for stage IA to IIA Hodgkin's disease. *J Clin Oncol* 2001, 19:4238–4244.

29. Eghbali H, Brice P, Creemers G, *et al.*: Comparison of three radiation dose levels after EBVP regimen in favorable supradiaphragmatic clinical stages (CS) I-II Hodgkin's lymphoma (HL): preliminary results of the EORTC-GELA H9-F trial [abstract]. *Blood* 2005, 106:abstract 814.

30. Schmitz N, Haverkamp H, Josting A, *et al.*: Long term follow up in relapsed Hodgkin's disease (HD): updated results of the HD-R1 study comparing conventional chemotherapy (cCT) to high-dose chemotherapy (HDCT) with autologous haemopoetic stem cell transplantation (ASCT) of the German Hodgkin Study Group (GHSG) and the Working Party Lymphoma of the European Group for Blood and Marrow Transplantation (EBMT) [abstract]. *J Clin Oncol* 2005, 23(16S):abstract 6508.

31. Klimm BC, Engert A, Brillant C, *et al.*: Comparison of BEACOPP and ABVD chemotherapy in intermediate stage Hodgkin's lymphoma: results of the fourth interim analysis of the HD11 trial of the GHSG [abstract]. *J Clin Oncol* 2005, 23(16S):abstract 6507.

32. Canellos GP: Chemotherapy alone for early Hodgkin's lymphoma: an emerging option. *J Clin Oncol* 2005, 23:4574–4576.

33. Yahalom J: Don't throw out the baby with the bathwater: on optimizing cure and reducing toxicity in Hodgkin's lymphoma. *J Clin Oncol* 2006, 24:544–548.

34. Laskar S, Gupta T, Vimal S, *et al.*: Consolidation radiation after complete remission in Hodgkin's disease following six cycles of doxorubicin, bleomycin, vinblastine, and dacarbazine chemotherapy: is there a need? *J Clin Oncol* 2004, 22:62–68.

35. Straus DJ, Portlock CS, Qin J, *et al.*: Results of a prospective randomized clinical trial of doxorubicin, bleomycin, vinblastine, and dacarbazine (ABVD) followed by radiation therapy (RT) versus ABVD alone for stages I, II, and IIIA nonbulky Hodgkin disease. *Blood* 2004, 104:3483–3489.

36. Duggan DB, Petroni GR, Johnson JL, *et al.*: Randomized comparison of ABVD and MOPP/ABV hybrid for the treatment of advanced Hodgkin's disease: report of an intergroup trial. *J Clin Oncol* 2003, 21:607–614.

37. Canellos GP, Anderson JR, Propert KJ, *et al.*: Chemotherapy of advanced Hodgkin's disease with MOPP, ABVD, or MOPP alternating with ABVD. *N Engl J Med* 1992, 327:1478–1484.

38. Bonadonna G, Santoro A, Gianni AM, *et al.*: Primary and salvage chemotherapy in advanced Hodgkin's disease: the Milan Cancer Institute experience. *Ann Oncol* 1991, 2(Suppl 1):9–16.

39. Somers R, Carde P, Henry-Amar M, *et al.*: A randomized study in stage IIIB and IV Hodgkin's disease comparing eight courses of MOPP versus an alteration of MOPP with ABVD: a European Organization for Research and Treatment of Cancer Lymphoma Cooperative Group and Groupe Pierre-et-Marie-Curie controlled clinical trial. *J Clin Oncol* 1994, 12:279–287.

40. Connors JM, Klimo P, Adams G, *et al.*: Treatment of advanced Hodgkin's disease with chemotherapy—comparison of MOPP/ABV hybrid regimen with alternating courses of MOPP and ABVD: a report from the National Cancer Institute of Canada Clinical Trials group. *J Clin Oncol* 1997, 15:1638–1645.

41. Horning SJ, Hoppe RT, Breslin S, *et al.*: Stanford V and radiotherapy for locally extensive and advanced Hodgkin's disease: mature results of a prospective clinical trial. *J Clin Oncol* 2002, 20:630–637.

42. Gobbi PG, Levis A, Chisesi T, *et al.*: ABVD versus modified Stanford V versus MOPPEBVCAD with optional and limited radiotherapy in intermediate- and advanced-stage Hodgkin's lymphoma: final results of a multicenter randomized trial by the Intergruppo Italiano Linfomi. *J Clin Oncol* 2005, 23:9198–9207.

43. Diehl V, Franklin J, Pfreundschuh M, *et al.*: Standard and increased-dose BEACOPP chemotherapy compared with COPP-ABVD for advanced Hodgkin's disease. *N Engl J Med* 2003, 348:2386–2395.

44. Sieniawski M, Reineke T, Nogova L, *et al.*: Fertility in male patients with advanced Hodgkin lymphoma treated with BEACOPP: a report of the German Hodgkin Study Group (GHSG). *Blood* 2008, 111:71–76.

45. Diehl V, Franklin J, Pfistner B, Engert A: Ten-year results of a German Hodgkin Study Group randomized trial of standard and increased dose BEACOPP chemotherapy for advanced Hodgkin's lymphoma (HD9) [abstract]. *J Clin Oncol* 2007, 25(18S):abstrat LBA8015.

46. Aleman BM, Raemaekers JM, Tirelli U, *et al.*: Involved-field radiotherapy for advanced Hodgkin's lymphoma. *N Engl J Med* 2003, 348:2396–2406.

47. Loeffler M, Brosteanu O, Hasenclever D, *et al.*: Meta-analysis of chemotherapy versus combined modality treatment trials in Hodgkin's disease. International Database on Hodgkin's Disease Overview Study Group. *J Clin Oncol* 1998, 16:818–829.

48. Fabian CJ, Mansfield CM, Dahlberg S, *et al.*: Low-dose involved field radiation after chemotherapy in advanced Hodgkin disease. A Southwest Oncology Group randomized study. *Ann Intern Med* 1994, 120:903–912.

49. Diehl V, Brillant C, Franklin J, *et al.*: BEACOPP chemotherapy for advanced Hodgkin's disease: results of further analyses of the HD9- and HD12- trials of the German Hodgkin Study Group (GHSG) [abstract]. *Blood* 2004, 104:abstract 307.

50. Cheson BD, Pfistner B, Juweid ME, *et al.*: Revised response criteria for malignant lymphoma. *J Clin Oncol* 2007, 25:579–586.

51. Federico M, Bellei M, Brice P, *et al.*: High-dose therapy and autologous stem-cell transplantation versus conventional therapy for patients with advanced Hodgkin's lymphoma responding to front-line therapy. *J Clin Oncol* 2003, 21:2320–2325.

52. Akpek G, Ambinder RF, Piantadosi S, *et al.*: Long-term results of blood and marrow transplantation for Hodgkin's lymphoma. *J Clin Oncol* 2001, 19:4314–4321.

53. Schmitz N, Pfistner B, Sextro M, *et al.*: Aggressive conventional chemotherapy compared with high-dose chemotherapy with autologous haemopoietic stem-cell transplantation for relapsed chemosensitive Hodgkin's disease: a randomised trial. *Lancet* 2002, 359:2065–2071.

54. Wadehra N, Farag S, Bolwell B, *et al.*: Long-term outcome of Hodgkin disease patients following high-dose busulfan, etoposide, cyclophosphamide, and autologous stem cell transplantation. *Biol Blood Marrow Transplant* 2006, 12:1343–1349.

55. Yuen AR, Rosenberg SA, Hoppe RT, *et al.*: Comparison between conventional salvage therapy and high-dose therapy with autografting for recurrent or refractory Hodgkin's disease. *Blood* 1997, 89:814–822.

56. Bartlett NL, Niedzwiecki D, Johnson JL, *et al.*: Gemcitabine, vinorelbine, and pegylated liposomal doxorubicin (GVD), a salvage regimen in relapsed Hodgkin's lymphoma: CALGB 59804. *Ann Oncol* 2007, 18:1071–1079.

57. Alvarez I, Sureda A, Caballero MD, *et al.*: Nonmyeloablative stem cell transplantation is an effective therapy for refractory or relapsed Hodgkin lymphoma: results of a Spanish Prospective Cooperative Protocol. *Biol Blood Marrow Transplant* 2006, 12:172–183.

58. Burroughs L, O'Donnell P, Sandmaier BM, *et al.*: Comparison of allogeneic hematopoietic cell transplantation (HCT) after nonmyeloablative conditioning with HLA-matched related (MRD), unrelated (URD), and related haploidentical (Haplo) donors for relapsed or refractory Hodgkin's lymphoma (HL) [abstract]. *Blood* 2007, 110:abstract 173.

59. Majhail NS, Weisdorf DJ, Wagner JE, *et al.*: Comparable results of umbilical cord blood and HLA-matched sibling donor hematopoietic stem cell transplantation after reduced-intensity preparative regimen for advanced Hodgkin lymphoma. *Blood* 2006, 107:3804–3807.

60. Younes A, Romaguera J, Hagemeister F, *et al.*: A pilot study of rituximab in patients with recurrent, classic Hodgkin disease. *Cancer* 2003, 98:310–314.

61. Oki Y, Pro B, Fayad LE, *et al.*: Phase 2 study of gemcitabine in combination with rituximab in patients with recurrent or refractory Hodgkin lymphoma. *Cancer* 2008, 112:831–836.

62. Younes A, McLaughlin P, Fayad LE, *et al.*: Six weekly doses of rituximab plus ABVD for newly diagnosed patients with classical Hodgkin lymphoma: depletion of reactive B-cells from the microenvironment by rituximab [abstract]. *Blood* 2005, 106:abstract 1499.

63. Leonard JP, Younes A, Rosenblatt JD, *et al.*: Targeting CD30 as therapy for Hodgkin's disease. Phase II results with the monoclonal antibody SGN-30 [abstract]. *J Clin Oncol* 2005, 23(16S):abstract 2553.

64. Ansell SM, Horwitz SM, Engert A, *et al.*: Phase I/II study of an anti-CD30 monoclonal antibody (MDX-060) in Hodgkin's lymphoma and anaplastic large-cell lymphoma. *J Clin Oncol* 2007, 25:2764–2769.

65. Schnell R, Dietlein M, Staak JO, *et al.*: Treatment of refractory Hodgkin's lymphoma patients with an iodine-131-labeled murine anti-CD30 monoclonal antibody. *J Clin Oncol* 2005, 23:4669–4678.

66. Blum KA, Johnson JL, Niedzwiecki D, *et al.*: Single agent bortezomib in the treatment of relapsed and refractory Hodgkin lymphoma: Cancer and Leukemia Group B protocol 50206. *Leuk Lymphoma* 2007, 48:1313–1319.

67. Bollard CM, Straathof KC, Huls MH, *et al.*: The generation and characterization of LMP2-specific CTLs for use as adoptive transfer from patients with relapsed EBV-positive Hodgkin disease. *J Immunother* 2004, 27:317–327.

68. Bollard CM, Gottschalk S, Leen AM, *et al.*: Complete responses of relapsed lymphoma following genetic modification of tumor-antigen presenting cells and T-lymphocyte transfer. *Blood* 2007, 110:2838–2845.

69. Haque T, Wilkie GM, Jones MM, *et al.*: Allogeneic cytotoxic T-cell therapy for EBV-positive posttransplantation lymphoproliferative disease: results of a phase 2 multicenter clinical trial. *Blood* 2007, 110:1123–1131.

70. Ekstrand BC, Horning SJ: Lymphocyte predominant Hodgkin's disease. *Curr Oncol Rep* 2002, 4:424–433.

71. Schlembach PJ, Wilder RB, Jones D, *et al.*: Radiotherapy alone for lymphocyte-predominant Hodgkin's disease. *Cancer J* 2002, 8:377–383.

72. Schulz H, Rehwald U, Morschhauser F, *et al.*: Rituximab in relapsed lymphocyte-predominant Hodgkin lymphoma: long-term results of a phase-II trial of the German Hodgkin Lymphoma Study Group (GHSG). *Blood* 2008, 111:109–111.

73. Ekstrand BC, Lucas JB, Horwitz SM, *et al.*: Rituximab in lymphocyte-predominant Hodgkin disease: results of a phase 2 trial. *Blood* 2003, 101:4285–4289.

74. Sleijfer S: Bleomycin-induced pneumonitis. *Chest* 2001, 120:617–624.

75. Martin WG, Ristow KM, Habermann TM, *et al.*: Bleomycin pulmonary toxicity has a negative impact on the outcome of patients with Hodgkin's lymphoma. *J Clin Oncol* 2005, 23:7614–7620.

76. Azoulay E, Herigault S, Levame M, *et al.*: Effect of granulocyte colony-stimulating factor on bleomycin-induced acute lung injury and pulmonary fibrosis. *Crit Care Med* 2003, 31:1442–1448.

77. Canellos GP, Duggan D, Johnson J, Niedzwiecki D: How important is bleomycin in the Adriamycin + bleomycin + vinblastine + dacarbazine regimen? *J Clin Oncol* 2004, 22:1532–1533.

78. Aleman BM, van den Belt-Dusebout AW, Klokman WJ, *et al.*: Long-term cause-specific mortality of patients treated for Hodgkin's disease. *J Clin Oncol* 2003, 21:3431–3439.

79. Travis LB, Hill D, Dores GM, *et al.*: Cumulative absolute breast cancer risk for young women treated for Hodgkin lymphoma. *J Natl Cancer Inst* 2005, 97:1428–1437.

80. Ng AK, Bernardo MV, Weller E, *et al.*: Second malignancy after Hodgkin disease treated with radiation therapy with or without chemotherapy: long-term risks and risk factors. *Blood* 2002, 100:1989–1996.

81. Josting A, Wiedenmann S, Franklin J, *et al.*: Secondary myeloid leukemia and myelodysplastic syndromes in patients treated for Hodgkin's disease: a report from the German Hodgkin's Lymphoma Study Group. *J Clin Oncol* 2003, 21:3440–3446.

82. Schonfeld SJ, Gilbert ES, Dores GM, *et al.*: Acute myeloid leukemia following Hodgkin lymphoma: a population-based study of 35,511 patients. *J Natl Cancer Inst* 2006, 98:215–218.

83. Swerdlow AJ, Higgins CD, Smith P, *et al.*: Myocardial infarction mortality risk after treatment for Hodgkin disease: a collaborative British cohort study. *J Natl Cancer Inst* 2007, 99:206–214.

84. Aleman BM, van den Belt-Dusebout AW, De Bruin ML, *et al.*: Late cardiotoxicity after treatment for Hodgkin lymphoma. *Blood* 2007, 109:1878–1886.

85. Hancock SL, Cox RS, McDougall IR: Thyroid diseases after treatment of Hodgkin's disease. *N Engl J Med* 1991, 325:599–605.

86. Hodgson DC, Koh ES, Tran TH, *et al.*: Individualized estimates of second cancer risks after contemporary radiation therapy for Hodgkin lymphoma. *Cancer* 2007, 110:2576–2586.

87. Johnson PW, Radford JA, Cullen MH, *et al.*: Comparison of ABVD and alternating or hybrid multidrug regimens for the treatment of advanced Hodgkin's lymphoma: results of the United Kingdom Lymphoma Group LY09 Trial (ISRCTN97144519). *J Clin Oncol* 2005, 23:9208–9218.

Non-Hodgkin's Lymphoma

Lode J. Swinnen

19

Non-Hodgkin's lymphomas (NHL) are a heterogeneous group of lymphoid malignancies defined by characteristic lymph node patterns and histology. Most NHLs are B cell in origin, with fewer of the T-cell phenotype. Each histologic entity of NHL has a distinct clinical presentation, natural history, and survival pattern [1]. Several classification schema have previously been used to organize the different histologic entities of NHL. The International Working Formulation [2] recognizes three prognostic categories, including those with low-, intermediate-, and high-grade histologies. Newer schemas like the Revised European American Lymphoma (REAL) [3] and World Health Organization (WHO) classifications [4] use morphology, immunophenotyping, and genetic and clinical features to characterize subtypes of NHL. The proposed WHO classification categorizes lymphoid neoplasms into B-cell and T-cell/natural killer (NK) cell neoplasms [4,5].

ETIOLOGY AND RISK FACTORS

Specific causes for the majority of NHLs remain unknown. Immunodeficiency states such as organ transplantation and HIV infection predispose to Epstein-Barr virus (EBV)–associated lymphoproliferations. Mucosa-associated lymphoid tissue (MALT) lymphomas are associated with *Helicobacter pylori* infection [6]. Extranodal marginal zone lymphomas have been associated with hepatitis C, and an association between ocular adnexal marginal zone lymphomas and the organism *Chlamydia psitacci* may exist [7–9]. The human T-cell lymphotrophic virus (HTLV-1) retrovirus is associated with adult T-cell leukemia/lymphoma, a form of peripheral T-cell lymphoma.

DIAGNOSIS

Diagnosis of NHL requires histopathology review in conjunction with immunophenotyping and molecular studies. The architectural pattern, either follicular or diffuse, is generally evaluated on lymph node rather than extranodal specimens. Immunohistochemical stains or flow cytometry are used to characterize cell surface markers. Demonstration of B-cell clonality may be performed on fixed tissue using immunoperoxidase methods, by Southern blot analysis, or by polymerase chain reaction (PCR) analysis. Identification of T-cell clonality is performed using molecular studies of fresh tissue for the T-cell receptor gene rearrangement. Specific immunophenotypic patterns may help distinguish histologic subtypes, which appear morphologically similar, such as mantle cell lymphoma and small lymphocytic lymphoma/chronic lymphocytic leukemia (CLL).

STAGING

After the diagnosis of NHL has been established by pathology review, a staging evaluation is performed to determine the extent of disease involvement. The Ann Arbor staging classification for Hodgkin's disease is often applied to NHL, with some modifications. Standard staging studies for NHL are provided in Table 19-1. Diagnostic staging studies include a complete blood profile and lactate dehydrogenase (LDH), CT scans, and bone marrow biopsy. Positron emission tomography (PET) now has an established role for staging. Its use for response assessment during treatment is under investigation [10,11].

INDOLENT LYMPHOMAS

FOLLICULAR LYMPHOMA (GRADES 1 AND 2), SMALL LYMPHOCYTIC LYMPHOMA, AND MARGINAL ZONE LYMPHOMA

In the REAL and WHO classifications, several histologic subtypes correspond to the low-grade histologies defined in the International Working Formulation. Small lymphocytic lymphoma is further subclassified into CLL-type small lymphocytic lymphoma, lymphoplasmacytic lymphoma, and marginal zone lymphoma (nodal, splenic, or MALT types). It is now recognized that small lymphocytic lymphoma and CLL represent different clinical presentations of the same disease. Lymphoplasmacytic lymphoma

is also considered a small lymphocytic lymphoma with plasmacytic differentiation and association with a IgM paraproteinemia [4].

Follicular lymphomas are subclassified into three histologic grades (grades 1, 2, and 3) according to the number of large cells present [4,12]. Follicular lymphomas grades 1 and 2 are thought to be closely related to each other, and generally follow an indolent course of disease. Follicular lymphoma grade 3 behaves more aggressively and is often treated like large cell lymphoma. The reciprocal t(14;18) translocation is identified in most cases of follicular lymphoma. This chromosomal aberration causes dysregulation and overexpression of *BCL-2*, an antiapoptosis oncogene.

Indolent lymphomas are generally considered incurable and follow a continual pattern of relapse despite good response to treatment [13]. They typically present in advanced stage with generalized adenopathy with or without bone marrow involvement. Hepatosplenomegaly or extranodal involvement (gastrointestinal [GI] tract, lung, skin, bone, or epidural) may also occur. GI tract involvement is particularly common in MALT lymphomas, which are associated with *Helicobacter pylori* infection in many but not all cases. Despite frequent bone marrow disease, meningeal involvement rarely occurs. Peripheral blood lymphocytosis is fairly common, as is the presence of a monoclonal gammopathy. Approximately 30% to 40% of patients with indolent lymphoma will eventually undergo histologic transformation to an aggressive NHL morphology [14,15].

Few patients with indolent lymphomas present with limited-stage disease, defined as clinical stage I or II. Patients with limited sites of disease in the periphery are candidates for regional radiation therapy alone. Treatment outcome is generally excellent, but long-term outcome is uncertain, and late complications of radiation can be a concern [16] (Table 19-2).

Most affected patients present with advanced-stage disease, defined as intra-abdominal stage II, III, or IV. Initial delay of chemotherapy does not decrease overall survival of patients with indolent NHL [17,18]. Multiple studies have demonstrated that it is feasible to observe patients without directed therapy if there is no indication for treatment. Specific indications

---

Table 19-1. Diagnostic and Staging Evaluation for Non-Hodgkin's Lymphoma

Physical examination

Examine peripheral lymph nodes, tonsils, spleen, and liver

Blood work

Complete blood count and differential, peripheral blood smear, lactate dehydrogenase, renal and liver function

Radiographic imaging

CT scans of chest, abdomen, pelvis

Positron emission tomography scan

Selected studies of the CNS, GI tract, or bone depending on symptoms

Histopathology

Lymph node biopsy

Hematopathology review; classification according to REAL or WHO

Immunophenotyping by immunohistochemistry or flow cytometry

Bone marrow biopsy

Cerebrospinal fluid cytology in aggressive lymphomas with documented bone, bone marrow, testicular, or nasopharyngeal involvement, or multiple extranodal sites of disease

CNS—central nervous system; GI—gastrointestinal; REAL—Revised European American Lymphoma; WHO—World Health Organization.

for treatment as defined by Groupe d'Etude Lymphomes Folliculaires (GELF) criteria for "high tumor burden" include a mass greater than 7 cm, three nodal sites each greater than 3 cm, systemic symptoms, splenomegaly, or end-organ compromise [19].

Many therapeutic options exist for patients with advanced-stage disease. Criteria for selection among them remain controversial because curative treatment has not been established [20]. Standard chemotherapy programs for indolent lymphomas include single agents such as fludarabine or chlorambucil, or combination regimens like CVP (cyclophosphamide, vincristine, prednisone) or CHOP (cyclophosphamide, doxorubicin, vincristine, prednisone). Fludarabine has been shown to be superior to other single agents, with response rates of 65% in follicular lymphomas, but may cause significant bone marrow suppression [21,22].

Although capable of producing remissions, the use of such chemotherapy regimens is not believed to lengthen survival [23]. Immunotherapy with the monoclonal antibody rituximab has had a major impact on the management of low-grade lymphomas. Rituximab targets the CD20 antigen found on the B lymphocytes that make up most low-grade lymphomas. Toxicity is limited when compared with chemotherapy, consisting mainly of infusional reactions, usually only with the first one or two doses. Rituximab produces a 48% response rate in relapsed disease used as a single agent, and can be used again on relapse [24–26]. In combination with chemotherapy, rituximab has resulted in higher complete remission rates and longer remissions (20 vs 45 months) than achieved with the same chemotherapy alone in randomized clinical trials [27]. Longer-term follow-up is necessary to determine whether overall survival has been affected. Current treatments for low-grade lymphomas include rituximab monotherapy or rituximab combined with chemotherapy, rather than chemotherapy alone.

The use of periodic redosing with rituximab after response has been achieved, called maintenance therapy, is currently under investigation. Longer response duration can be achieved with rituximab maintenance strategies, but it is too soon to determine whether overall survival is affected [28].

Radioimmunotherapy agents are composed of radionuclides conjugated to monoclonal antibodies used to target radiation to tumor tissue. Radiolabeled monoclonal antibodies, such as ^{131}I tositumomab and ^{90}Y ibritumomab, have shown efficacy in low-grade lymphomas resistant to rituximab. Their optimal use continues to be investigated [29–31].

High-dose chemotherapy and autologous stem cell transplantation (ASCT) for low-grade lymphomas can result in very long remissions, with about half of patients remaining in remission at 12 to 15 years' follow-up in some series [32,33]. In three randomized trials, relapse-free survival was significantly better after autologous transplantation, but it is too soon to determine whether overall survival was affected [34–36].

Promising durable remissions have been reported after conventional allotransplantation of refractory indolent lymphoma [37]. Miniallogeneic bone marrow transplantation using nonmyeloablative doses of cytotoxic chemotherapy is under investigation, which appears promising with possibly less toxicity [38,39].

AGGRESSIVE LYMPHOMAS

DIFFUSE LARGE B-CELL LYMPHOMA, PERIPHERAL T-CELL LYMPHOMA, ANAPLASTIC LARGE CELL LYMPHOMA, AND FOLLICULAR LYMPHOMA (GRADE 3)

Aggressive NHLs are composed primarily of diffuse large B-cell lymphoma, but also include peripheral T-cell lymphomas, anaplastic large cell lymphomas, and

follicular lymphoma (grade 3). Primary mediastinal large B-cell lymphoma is represented as a subcategory of diffuse large B-cell lymphoma in the present schema. Peripheral T-cell lymphomas have poor overall survival compared with diffuse large B-cell lymphomas, but anaplastic large cell lymphomas that are ALK-positive have overall survival similar to diffuse large B-cell lymphoma [1].

Aggressive lymphomas share common clinical characteristics of male preponderance, presentation in middle age, rapidly enlarging adenopathy, and advanced stage. Masses are often bulky, particularly in the mediastinum or abdomen. Large masses in these sites may cause superior vena cava syndrome, tracheal compression, or ureteral compression. Extranodal sites often cause symptoms such as ulcerated GI lesions or lytic bone lesions. Lymphomatous meningitis is more likely in the presence of bone marrow, testicular or nasopharyngeal involvement, elevated LDH, or two or more extranodal sites.

The International Prognostic Index (IPI) for non-Hodgkin's lymphoma [40] describes five prognostic variables that predict outcome based on pretreatment clinical characteristics. Adverse prognostic variables include age over 60 years, elevated serum LDH, poor performance status, advanced stage, and two or more extranodal sites of disease. Patients are stratified to low, low-intermediate, high-intermediate, or high-risk categories based on the number of poor prognostic features. Patients with IPI 4 are poor risk, and have significantly shortened survival (Table 19-3).

Aggressive diffuse lymphomas are potentially curable. A curative outcome is obtained in more than half of patients after first-line therapy. CHOP plus rituximab (R-CHOP) is the standard first-line chemotherapy regimen based on several randomized trials of CHOP or CHOP-like regimens, all showing a survival advantage for the addition of rituximab [41–44]. Patients with regional disease involvement (clinical stage I or II) may be treated with combination chemotherapy with or without regional irradiation. It is feasible to give short-course chemotherapy followed by involved-field radiotherapy for regional disease (Table 19-4) [45].

ASCT as part of initial therapy has been investigated in a number of studies with conflicting results. Meta-analysis suggests that the patients at high risk for relapse may benefit from this approach [46–48].

ASCT has also been studied extensively for treatment of relapsed or refractory disease. Patients with chemosensitive disease in first or second relapse are candidates for ASCT. The Parma trial evaluated patients with chemosensitive disease and demonstrated improved responses and overall survival for patients who received transplantation rather than additional chemotherapy [49,50]. The most significant predictor of a favorable outcome from ASCT is chemosensitivity at the time of transplantation. High-dose therapy has not proven to be useful for chemorefractory disease in first or subsequent relapse [51].

Cytoreductive regimens, such as DHAP (dexamethasone, high-dose cytarabine, cisplatin) [52] or ICE (ifosfamide, carboplatin, etoposide) [53] are given—typically with rituximab—before the conditioning regimen and ASCT. Cytoreduction serves several purposes: to identify patients with chemosensitive disease, to allow a transplant to be performed with minimal disease burden, and to decrease potential contamination of the stem cell product. In addition, cytoreductive regimens together with cytokines are used to mobilize stem cells for collection.

Table 19-2. Treatment Strategy for Indolent Lymphomas

Stage	Strategy
Stages I and peripheral II	Regional radiation therapy
Stage II (intra-abdominal), III, IV	Consider observation
	Participation in a clinical trial of immune strategies
	Palliative therapy with rituximab or chemotherapy plus rituximab

Table 19-3. International Prognostic Index for Diffuse Large B-Cell Lymphomas

Adverse prognostic features	Risk group	Adverse prognostic factors	5-year survival, %
Age > 60 y	Low	0 or 1	73
Elevated serum LDH	Low–intermediate	2	51
Karnofsky performance score	High–intermediate	3	43
Advanced stage (III or IV)	High	4 or 5	26
Extranodal sites (> 1)			
LDH—lactate dehydrogenase.			

MANTLE CELL LYMPHOMA

Mantle cell lymphoma is a separately recognized histology incorporated into the REAL and WHO classifications, previously termed *diffuse small cleaved cell lymphoma* according to the International Working Formulation. Mantle cell lymphomas have aggressive disease features and often present in advanced stage with diffuse adenopathy, as well as bone marrow, peripheral blood, colonic, and splenic involvement. Extranodal disease sites are also common; diffuse GI tract involvement is referred to as lymphomatous polyposis. The typical cytogenetic aberration in mantle cell lymphoma is a reciprocal t(11;14) translocation causing dysregulation of *BCL-1* oncogene and overexpression of cyclin D1.

Mantle cell lymphomas have poor overall and failure-free survival rates [1]. No convincing evidence shows that conventional chemotherapy is curative, because there is no plateau in the overall survival curve. Investigational therapy with upfront transplantation appears promising, with durable remissions reported out to 4 years [54,55]. The HyperCVAD regimen (cyclophosphamide, vincristine, doxorubicin, dexamethasone alternated with high-dose methotrexate and cytarabine) is widely used, but long-term results remain unknown [56].

LYMPHOBLASTIC LYMPHOMA

Lymphoblastic lymphoma shares similar features with acute lymphoblastic leukemia (ALL). This disease often presents with large mediastinal masses, and with leukemic as well as central nervous system (CNS) involvement. Most lymphoblastic lymphomas are of immature T-cell origin, although some may have pre-B cell phenotypes. Lymphoblastic lymphoma is treated in the same manner as ALL, with induction, intensive consolidation, and maintenance regimens.

DIFFUSE SMALL NONCLEAVED CELL LYMPHOMAS (BURKITT'S AND BURKITT'S-LIKE)

Diffuse small noncleaved cell lymphomas (Burkitt's and non-Burkitt's) are identified as high-grade lymphomas in the International Working Formulation [2]. Small noncleaved cell lymphomas are characterized by young age, male preponderance, rapidly enlarging bulky adenopathy, and frequent bone marrow and meningeal involvement. The t(8;14) translocation identified in Burkitt's lymphoma causes dysregulation of the *c-myc* oncogene.

Small noncleaved cell lymphomas have increased incidence within concurrent HIV infection. In this setting, sites of disease may be unusual,

including the GI tract, brain, and soft tissue. Treatment of Burkitt's and Burkitt's-like lymphoma requires rapid initiation of high-dose, short-course combination chemotherapy with CNS prophylaxis [57]. When the patient is HIV positive, chemotherapy should be administered in conjunction with highly active antiretroviral therapy (HAART). Bulky disease may be associated with tumor lysis syndrome. Attention to hydration, alkalinization, prophylactic allopurinol, and monitoring of renal function, calcium, electrolytes, and phosphate balance during and after chemotherapy infusion are therefore necessary. With HIV infection, use of intensive chemotherapy may be significantly complicated by opportunistic infections. Use of HAART has decreased the incidence of opportunistic infections [58]. There have been anecdotal reports of HIV-infected patients who have achieved spontaneous regression of NHL after being treated with HAART [59].

HIV-ASSOCIATED LYMPHOMA

HIV-associated NHLs are typically aggressive in morphology and clinical behavior. Approximately 30% are of Burkitt's type; the remainder are diffuse large B-cell lymphoma. The large B-cell lymphomas are often accompanied by low CD4 counts and are frequently EBV-associated; HIV-associated primary central nervous system lymphomas are always EBV-associated. The use of HAART has coincided with a significant improvement in outcome. Aggressive regimens such as CHOP, EPOCH (etoposide, prednisone, vincristine, cyclophosphamide, doxorubicin), or CDE (cyclophosphamide, doxorubicin, etoposide), with or without rituximab, produce durable complete response rates of 50% or more [60–62].

HTLV-1–ASSOCIATED ADULT T-CELL LEUKEMIA/LYMPHOMA

HTLV-1–associated lymphomas are a subtype of mature peripheral T-cell neoplasm in the current WHO classification [4]. Many patients present clinically with the acute form, which is characterized by rapid onset, lytic bone lesions, subcutaneous nodules, hypercalcemia, and leukemic phase. The histologic subtype is typically a diffuse large cell or immunoblastic lymphoma. Prognosis for patients with aggressive presentations is poor, with only transient responses to intensive regimens. In southern Japan, where HTLV-1 incidence is endemic, a broader clinical spectrum is seen with both indolent and aggressive clinical and histologic subtypes.

Table 19-4. Treatment Strategy for Aggressive Diffuse Lymphomas

Stage	Strategy
Stages I and nonbulky stage II	Full-course R-CHOP or short-course R-CHOP with involved-field radiation therapy
Stages II, III, and IV	R-CHOP (or other doxorubicin-containing regimen plus rituximab)
	CNS prophylaxis for patients with ≥ 2 extranodal sites, involvement of bone, bone marrow, testes, or paranasal region
	Tumor lysis precautions for bulky disease
	Localized GI tract involvement may be complicated by bleeding or perforation but rarely requires surgical resection
	Consider autologous stem cell transplantation for primary refractory or relapsed disease

CNS—central nervous system; GI—gastrointestinal; R-CHOP—rituximab, cyclophosphamide, doxorubicin, vincristine, prednisone.

CVP (CYCLOPHOSPHAMIDE, VINCRISTINE, PREDNISONE)

CVP is a well-tolerated palliative regimen. Monthly cycles are repeated to maximum response plus two cycles. Randomized studies have demonstrated no response or survival advantage with the use of CVP over continuous daily alkylating agent therapy. Responses are more rapid with CVP (within 3 months), but not more durable. Toxicity is primarily hematologic with drug-induced neutropenia. Hemorrhagic cystitis may occur; hydration reduces its frequency. Vinca-associated neurologic toxicity is mild with a capped 2-mg dose. Corticosteroid toxicities are infrequent with monthly cycles.

CANDIDATES FOR TREATMENT

Patients with low-grade NHL

ALTERNATIVE THERAPIES

Single-agent chlorambucil or cyclophosphamide; CHOP

TOXICITIES

Cyclophosphamide: myelosuppression with platelet sparing, nausea and vomiting, alopecia, darkening of skin and nails, mucositis (rare), hemorrhagic or sterile cystitis (5%–10% of patients, usually reversible, but can lead to fibrosis and bladder cancer), immunosuppression, syndrome of inappropriate antidiuretic hormone (SIADH), infertility; **Vincristine:** severe local inflammation possible if extravasated, alopecia, peripheral neuropathies, ileus; **Prednisone:** acne, thrush, thinning of the skin and striae, suppression of the adrenal–pituitary axis, hypokalemia, loss of muscle mass, increased appetite, myopathy, osteoporosis, cushingoid appearance, gastritis, peptic ulcer disease, euphoria, depression, psychosis, increased risk of infections and cataracts

DRUG INTERACTIONS

Cyclophosphamide: allopurinol, drugs that induce or block hepatic microsomal enzymes, sulfhydryl agents (*eg*, mesna); **Vincristine:** cisplatin, paclitaxel, and other drugs that affect peripheral nervous system

NURSING INTERVENTIONS

Give cyclophosphamide in the morning; administer vincristine as slow intravenous (IV) push to avoid extravasation; evaluate for neurologic deficit before each vincristine dose; maintain high fluid intake and encourage frequent voiding, stool softeners, and bulk diet

PATIENT INFORMATION

The most common side effects reported are leukopenia, hyperglycemia, weight gain, insomnia, alopecia, sensory neuropathy

DOSAGE AND SCHEDULING

Cyclophosphamide 400 mg/m^2 orally once daily × 5 d

Vincristine 1.4 mg/m^2 IV on d 1 (maximum 2 mg)

Prednisone 100 mg/m^2 orally once daily × 5 d

• Repeat cycle every 28 d

EXPERIENCES AND RESPONSE RATES

Study	Evaluable patients, *n*	Complete response, %	Median survival, *y*
Hoppe *et al.* [63]	40	85	7.5
Anderson *et al.* [64]	49	67	7

CHOP (CYCLOPHOSPHAMIDE, DOXORUBICIN, VINCRISTINE, PREDNISONE)

CHOP is a potentially curative regimen for aggressive diffuse lymphomas. It may also be used in indolent lymphomas, particularly with evidence of histologic transformation. Responses are prompt (complete responses generally obtained in less than 4 months). CHOP chemotherapy is continued for two additional cycles beyond maximal response or for a minimum of six cycles. Complete remission is achieved in 60% to 75% of patients.

Prospective comparisons with more intensive second- and third-generation regimens have shown no significant difference in the response rates or survival outcomes of patients with aggressive diffuse lymphomas. CHOP remains the standard drug regimen in this setting. Toxicity is moderate and reasonably well tolerated even in older patients. Adverse effects are similar to those outlined for CVP regimen. Potential cardiac toxicity from doxorubicin should be monitored closely; doses greater than 450 mg/m^2 should be avoided.

CANDIDATES FOR TREATMENT

Patients with indolent or aggressive diffuse NHL

SPECIAL PRECAUTIONS

Patients with hepatic dysfunction; patients with impaired cardiac function (contraindicated)

ALTERNATIVE THERAPIES

ProMACE-CytaBOM, CEPP, C-MOPP, m-BACOD, MACOP-B

TOXICITIES

Prednisone: acne, thrush, thinning of the skin and striae, suppression of the adrenal–pituitary axis, hypokalemia, loss of muscle mass, increased appetite, myopathy, osteoporosis, cushingoid appearance, gastritis, peptic ulcer disease, euphoria, depression, psychosis, increased risk of infections and cataracts; **Cyclophosphamide:** myelosuppression with platelet sparing, nausea and vomiting, alopecia, darkening of skin and nails, mucositis (rare), hemorrhagic or sterile cystitis, immunosuppression, SIADH, infertility; **Vincristine:** severe local inflammation possible if extravasated, alopecia, peripheral neuropathies, ileus; **Doxorubicin:** myelosuppression (leukocytes and platelets), nausea and vomiting, mucositis, alopecia, radiation recall, local tissue damage progressing to necrosis if extravasated, hyperpigmentation, phlebitis, irreversible congestive heart failure (dose-dependent), acute arrhythmias

DRUG INTERACTIONS

Cyclophosphamide: allopurinol, drugs that induce or block hepatic microsomal enzymes, sulfhydryl agents (*eg*, mesna); **Vincristine:** cisplatin, paclitaxel, and other drugs that affect peripheral nervous system; **Doxorubicin:** heparin, mediastinal radiation, interferon

NURSING INTERVENTIONS

Give cyclophosphamide in the morning; administer vincristine and doxorubicin as slow IV push to avoid extravasation; evaluate for neurologic deficit before each vincristine dose; maintain high fluid intake and encourage frequent voiding, stool softeners, and bulk diet

PATIENT INFORMATION

The most common side effects reported are leukopenia, alopecia, nausea, vomiting, hyperglycemia, sensory neuropathy, insomnia

DOSAGE AND SCHEDULING

Cyclophosphamide 750 mg/m^2 IV on d 1

Doxorubicin 50 mg/m^2 IV on d 1

Vincristine 1.4 mg/m^2 IV on d 1 (maximum 2 mg)

Prednisone 100 mg orally once daily × 5 d

• Repeat cycle every 21 d

EXPERIENCES AND RESPONSE RATES

Study	Regimen	Evaluable patients, *n*	Complete response, %	Median survival, %
Armitage *et al.* [65]	CHOP	75	51	31 (at 4–9 y)
Gams *et al.* [66]	CHOP	90	54	35 (at 6 y)
Coltman *et al.* [67]	CHOP	412	53	30 (at 12 y)
Feugier *et al.* [42]	R-CHOP	399	75	58 (overall survival at 5 y)

RITUXIMAB

Rituximab is an unlabeled chimeric monoclonal antibody targeting CD20 antigen on B lymphocytes. It is used as a single agent or in combination with chemotherapy for indolent lymphomas and in combination with CHOP chemotherapy for large B-cell lymphoma.

CANDIDATES FOR TREATMENT

Low-grade or follicular B-cell NHL; large B-cell lymphoma in combination with CHOP

SPECIAL PRECAUTIONS

Patients with peripheral blood lymphocytosis as in CLL or mantle cell lymphoma may develop a cytokine-release syndrome; patients with underlying cardiovascular or pulmonary disease are at risk for developing infusion-related syndrome. Do not administer live vaccines during treatment

ALTERNATIVE THERAPIES

CHOP, CVP, fludarabine

TOXICITIES

Infusion-related symptoms include fevers, chills, headache, rigors, asthenia, throat irritation, abdominal pain, neutropenia, leukopenia, or thrombocytopenia; risk of infections due to decreased serum immunoglobulins or to leukopenia. Hypersensitivity reactions related to the infusion including hypotension, bronchospasm, or angioedema. Severe infusion-related reactions (usually with the first infusion) occur rarely and are characterized by hypoxia, pulmonary infiltrates, adult respiratory distress syndrome, ventricular fibrillation, or cardiogenic shock. Rare events possibly associated with rituximab include fulminant hepatitis due to reactivation of hepatitis B, severe mucocutaneous reactions, progressive multifocal leukoencephalopathy

DRUG INTERACTIONS

No specific drug–drug interactions. Contraindicated in patients with known type I hypersensitivity or anaphylactic reactions to murine proteins or to a component of rituximab

NURSING INTERVENTIONS

Careful monitoring is required during the first infusion with frequent blood pressure and heart rate monitoring within the first 2 hours of infusion. Supportive care measures include IV saline infusion and premedications with acetaminophen and diphenhydramine as needed to minimize infusion-related adverse effects. Keep meperidine on hand for infusion-related rigors. Rituximab infusion should be interrupted if significant side effects occur and resumed at a reduced rate only if side effects have resolved. Medications for treatment of hypersensitivity reactions such as epinephrine, antihistamines, and corticosteroids should be kept on hand in the event of a reaction

PATIENT INFORMATION

Most side effects are related to the infusion, such as fevers, chills, and rigors. Patients do not experience alopecia

DOSAGE AND SCHEDULING (SINGLE-AGENT REGIMEN)

Rituximab 375 mg/m^2 IV over 3–4 h (titrated slowly as tolerated)

• Once per week × 4 wk

EXPERIENCES AND RESPONSE RATES

Study	Evaluable patients, *n*	Overall response rate, %
McLaughlin *et al.* [24]	166	48

DHAP (DEXAMETHASONE, CYTARABINE, CISPLATIN)

DHAP is a second-line salvage regimen for patients with intermediate-grade or immunoblastic NHL who have not attained a complete remission from upfront therapy or who have relapsed. Because only 45% to 50% of patients are cured with their initial chemotherapy treatment program, many patients need to receive salvage chemotherapy. Depending on the patient's age, comorbidity, and performance status, the goals of second-line therapy vary. Transplant-eligible patients require only cytoreduction, whereas in transplant-ineligible patients, a complete remission is desired.

DHAP is a treatment program that has reported efficacy in this setting. In the original report, 90 patients with progressive recurrent lymphoma were treated: 28 patients achieved a complete remission and 22 a partial remission for an overall response rate 56%. Vigorous hydration with mannitol-induced diuresis was given in all patients. The acute tumor lysis syndrome was observed in five patients, emphasizing the need for frequent monitoring of electrolytes. Toxicity was severe with neutropenia, thrombocytopenia, renal, cerebellar, and GI dysfunction common [52].

TOXICITIES

Profound myelosuppression with marked neutropenia and thrombocytopenia, especially in patients with lymphomatous involvement of the bone marrow or previous pelvic irradiation. Documented infections were seen in 30% of patients with a mortality of 33% in these patients. Tumor lysis syndrome occurred in 5% of patients. Renal insufficiency is seen in 20% and can be irreversible. Acute cerebellar dysfunction and tinnitus has been reported. Neutropenia can be shortened by growth factor support (granulocyte colony-stimulating factor [G-CSF] or granulocyte-macrophage colony-stimulating factor [GM-CSF]).

CANDIDATES FOR TREATMENT

Patients with refractory or relapsed intermediate-grade or immunoblastic NHL

SPECIAL PRECAUTIONS

Patients who are elderly; patients with renal or neurological dysfunction; patients with compromised bone marrow reserve

ALTERNATIVE THERAPIES

Ifosfamide and etoposide alone or with cisplatin or carboplatin, C-MOPP

DRUG INTERACTIONS

Aminoglycoside antibiotics should be avoided; any drugs that have renal or ototoxicity must be used with caution

NURSING INTERVENTIONS

Monitor renal function and obtain blood urea nitrogen, creatinine, and 12-h urine collection for creatinine clearance; provide proper antiemetics, hydrate well; observe for signs of infection; neutropenia is expected; severe thrombocytopenia occurs, and signs for bleeding should be monitored

PATIENT INFORMATION

The most common side effect include fever when the blood counts are low, nausea, vomiting, and alopecia

DOSAGE AND SCHEDULING

Cisplatin 100 mg/m^2 IV as continuous infusion for 24 h on d 1 or 50 mg/m^2 as 1-h infusion twice daily

Cytarabine 2 g/m^2 IV every 12 h (each infusion over 3 h) on d 2*

Dexamethasone 40 mg IV or orally daily on d 1–4

- Hydration with normal saline at 150–250 mL/h is administered for 36-h period; after first 6 h of hydration, cisplatin can be given

- Repeat every 3–4 wk for a maximum of 4 cycles after maximal tumor response

*Patients older than 70 years receive cytarabine 1 g/m^2.

ICE (IFOSFAMIDE, CARBOPLATIN, ETOPOSIDE)

This salvage combination chemotherapy regimen for aggressive large cell NHLs is often used for cytoreduction and for stem cell mobilization in transplant-eligible patients with relapsed or refractory NHL. This regimen causes less renal toxicity than DHAP, and is fairly well tolerated except for significant myelosuppression.

CANDIDATES FOR TREATMENT

Relapsed or refractory aggressive diffuse lymphomas as salvage therapy or as cytoreduction prior to ASCT

SPECIAL PRECAUTIONS

Patients who are older or with marginal performance status; patients with renal or neurologic dysfunction; patients with poor bone marrow reserve. Ifosfamide should be given with mesna at similar dosages to prevent hemorrhagic cystitis

ALTERNATIVE THERAPIES

DHAP, ESHAP, ifosfamide and etoposide without carboplatin, C-MOPP, or CEPP

TOXICITIES

Ifosfamide: myelosuppression, nausea and vomiting, alopecia, hemorrhagic cystitis, CNS toxicity, infertility, renal impairment; **Carboplatin:** myelosuppression, nausea and vomiting, renal dysfunction, liver function abnormalities, electrolyte disturbances, peripheral neuropathy; **Etoposide:** myelosuppression, nausea, vomiting, alopecia, mucositis

DRUG INTERACTIONS

Ifosfamide: warfarin; **Carboplatin:** aminoglycoside antibiotics, phenytoin; **Etoposide:** cytarabine, methotrexate, cisplatin, calcium channel blockers, warfarin, cyclosporine, tamoxifen

NURSING INTERVENTIONS

Supportive care during infusion includes adequate IV hydration and pretreatment antiemetics. Renal function, electrolytes, blood counts, and signs of bleeding should all be monitored

PATIENT INFORMATION

Common side effects include fevers when blood counts are low, alopecia, nausea, and vomiting. Low platelet counts as a consequence of treatment will increase the risk of bleeding, which may require platelet transfusions depending on severity

DOSAGE AND SCHEDULING

Ifosfamide 5 g/m^2 IV on d 2

Carboplatin AUC 5 IV on d 2

Etoposide 100 mg/m^2 on d 1, 2, and 3

Mesna 5 g/m^2 IV as continuous infusion over 24 h on d 2 with ifosfamide

Filgrastim is given midcycle

EXPERIENCES AND RESPONSE RATES

Study	Evaluable patients, n	Overall response, %
Moskowitz *et al.* [53]	163	66.3

CODOX-M (CYCLOPHOSPHAMIDE, VINCRISTINE, DOXORUBICIN, METHOTREXATE) AND IVAC (IFOSFAMIDE, ETOPOSIDE, CYTARABINE)

Diffuse small noncleaved cell lymphomas, both Burkitt's and non-Burkitt's, are considered high-grade lymphomas. These subtypes are commonly detected in the setting of HIV infection. Small noncleaved cell lymphomas not related to HIV infection are curable with high-dose, short-course chemotherapy. CNS prophylaxis is an essential component of the treatment regimens. Because tumor lysis syndrome may occur after the initiation of therapy, it is important to include IV hydration, alkalinization of the urine, and administration of allopurinol. Frequent monitoring of electrolytes, renal function, serum calcium, and phosphate is also necessary. Although adverse effects such as myelosuppression and neutropenic fevers are common, the treatment schedule should be maintained because these are rapidly growing tumors.

Patients with favorable small noncleaved cell lymphoma defined as nonbulky stage I or II disease may be treated with three cycles of CODOX-M regimen [51]. Patients with unfavorable small noncleaved cell lymphoma may be treated with CODOX-M alternating with IVAC regimen for a total of four treatment cycles. Patients with meningeal disease at presentation received additional intrathecal therapy.

CANDIDATES FOR TREATMENT

Patients with diffuse small noncleaved cell NHL

SPECIAL PRECAUTIONS

Patients with renal dysfunction

ALTERNATIVE THERAPIES

Vanderbilt regimen

TOXICITIES

Cyclophosphamide: myelosuppression, nausea and vomiting, alopecia, mucositis (rare), hemorrhagic or sterile cystitis, SIADH, infertility; **Doxorubicin:** myelosuppression, nausea and vomiting, mucositis, alopecia, radiation recall, local tissue damage if extravasated, phlebitis, congestive heart failure, arrhythmias; **Vincristine:** local inflammation if extravasated, alopecia, peripheral neuropathy, ileus; **Methotrexate:** myelosuppression, nausea and vomiting, severe mucositis with ulceration and bloody diarrhea, cirrhosis (rare), pneumonitis, alopecia, renal tubular necrosis; **Cytarabine:** nausea, vomiting, neuropathy, neurotoxicity, rash myelosuppression; ocular toxicity; **Ifosfamide:** myelosuppression, nausea and vomiting, alopecia, hemorrhagic cystitis, CNS toxicity, infertility, renal impairment; **Etoposide:** myelosuppression, nausea, vomiting, alopecia, mucositis

DRUG INTERACTIONS

Cyclophosphamide: allopurinol, drugs that induce or inhibit hepatic microsomal enzymes, sulfhydryl agents (*ie*, mesna); **Doxorubicin:** heparin, mediastinal irradiation, interferon; **Vincristine:** cisplatin, paclitaxel, other drugs that affect the peripheral nervous system; **Cytarabine:** possibly flucytosine; **Ifosfamide:** warfarin; **Etoposide:** cytarabine, methotrexate, cisplatin, calcium channel antagonists, warfarin, cyclosporine, tamoxifen; **Methotrexate:** aspirin, nonsteroidal anti-inflammatory drugs, alcohol, 5-fluorouracil, L-asparaginase, penicillin

NURSING INTERVENTIONS

Mix intrathecal methotrexate with buffered nonbacteriostatic solution; monitor methotrexate levels if renal dysfunction develops; administer leucovorin every 6 h until methotrexate levels are nontherapeutic

PATIENT INFORMATION

The most common side effects are pancytopenia, predisposition to infections, alopecia, bleeding, mucositis, peripheral neuropathy

DOSAGE AND SCHEDULING: CODOX-M REGIMEN

Cyclophosphamide 800 mg/m^2 IV on d 1, then 200 mg/m2 IV on d 2–5

Doxorubicin 40 mg/m^2 IV on d 1

Vincristine 1.5 mg/m^2 IV on d 1 and 8 (cycle 1) and on d 1, 8, and 15 (cycle 3)

Methotrexate 1200 mg/m^2 IV over 1 h then 240 mg/m^2/h continuous infusion over next 23 h, starting on d 10

Leucovorin begins 36 h after starting high-dose methotrexate; 192 mg/m^2 IV at h 36, then 12 mg/m^2 every 6 h until serum methotrexate level decreases to nontoxic level

Intrathecal cytarabine 70 mg on d 1 and 3

Intrathecal methotrexate 12 mg on d 15

DOSAGE AND SCHEDULING: IVAC REGIMEN

Cytarabine 2 g/m^2 IV every 12 h on d 1 and 2 (total 4 doses)

Ifosfamide 1500 mg/m^2 IV on d 1–5 with mesna

Etoposide 60 mg/m^2 IV on d 1–5

Intrathecal methotrexate 12 mgon d 5

EXPERIENCES AND RESPONSE RATES

Study	Patients, *n*	Event-free survival at 2 y, %
Magrath *et al.* [57]	72 (39 adults)	56 (CODOX-M); 92 (IVAC)

REFERENCES

1. Armitage JO, Weisenburger DD: New approach to classifying non-Hodgkin's lymphomas: clinical features of the major histologic subtypes. Non-Hodgkin's Lymphoma Classification Project. *J Clin Oncol* 1998, 16:2780–2795.

2. National Cancer Institute: Summary and description of a working formulation for clinical usage: the Non-Hodgkin's Lymphoma Pathologic Classification Project. *Cancer* 1982, 49:2112–2135.

3. Harris NL, Jaffe ES, Stern H, *et al.*: A revised European-American classification of lymphoid neoplasms: a proposal from the International Lymphoma Study Group. *Blood* 1994, 84:1361–1392.

4. Jaffe ES, Harris NL, Diebold J, *et al.*: World Health Organization classification of neoplastic diseases of the hematopoietic and lymphoid tissues: report of the Clinical Advisory Committee Meeting. Airlie House, Virginia, November 1997. *J Clin Oncol* 1997, 17:3835–3849.

5. Harris NL, Jaffe ES, Diebold J, *et al.*: Lymphoma classification: from controversy to consensus: the REAL and WHO classification of lymphoid neoplasms. *Ann Oncol* 2000, 11(Suppl 1):S3–S10.

6. Parsonnet J, Hansen S, Rodriguez L, *et al.*: Helicobacter pylori infection and gastric lymphoma. *N Engl J Med* 1997, 330:1267–1271.

7. Spinelli JJ, Lai AS, Krajden M, *et al.*: Hepatitis C virus and risk of non-Hodgkin lymphoma in British Columbia, Canada. *Int J Cancer* 2008, 122:630–633.

8. Husain A, Roberts D, Pro B, *et al.*: Meta-analyses of the association between Chlamydia psittaci and ocular adnexal lymphoma and the response of ocular adnexal lymphoma to antibiotics. *Cancer* 2007, 110:809–815.

9. Swinnen LJ: Organ transplant-related lymphoma. *Curr Treat Options Oncol* 2001, 2:301–308.

10. Cheson BD, Pfistner B, Juweid ME, *et al.*; the International Harmonization Project on Lymphoma: revised response criteria for malignant lymphoma. *J Clin Oncol* 2007, 25:579–586.

11. Kasamon YL, Wahl RL, Swinnen LJ: FDG PET and high-dose therapy for aggressive lymphomas: toward a risk-adapted strategy. *Curr Opin Oncol* 2004, 16:100–105.

12. Mann R, Berard C: Criteria for the cytologic subclassification of follicular lymphomas: a proposed alternative method. *Hematol Oncol* 1982, 1:187–192.

13. Horning SJ, Rosenberg SA: The natural history of initially untreated low-grade non-Hodgkin's lymphomas. *N Engl J Med* 1994, 311:1471–1475.

14. Yuen AR, Kamel OW, Halpern J, Horning SJ: Long-term survival after histologic transformation of low-grade follicular lymphoma. *J Clin Oncol* 1995, 13:1726–1733.

15. Bastion Y, Sebban C, Berger F, *et al.*: Incidence, predictive factors, and outcome of lymphoma transformation in follicular lymphoma patients. *J Clin Oncol* 1997, 15:1587–1594.

16. McManus MP, Hoppe RT: Is radiotherapy curative for stage I and II low-grade follicular lymphoma? Results of a long-term follow-up study of patients treated at Stanford University. *J Clin Oncol* 1996, 14:1282–1290.

17. Portlock CS, Rosenberg SA: No initial therapy for stage III and IV non-Hodgkin's lymphomas of favorable histologic types. *Ann Intern Med* 1979, 90:10–13.

18. Young RC, Longo DL, Glatstein E, *et al.*: The treatment of indolent lymphomas: watchful waiting vs. aggressive combined modality treatment. *Semin Hematol* 1988, 25:11–16.

19. Brice P, Bastion Y, Lepage E, *et al.*: Comparison in low-tumor burden follicular lymphomas between an initial no-treatment policy, predmustine, or interferon alfa: a randomized study from the Groupe d'Etude des Lymphomes Folliculaires. *J Clin Oncol* 1997, 15:1110–1117.

20. Horning SJ: Treatment approaches to low-grade lymphomas. *N Engl J Med* 1988, 83:881–884.

21. Redman JR, Cabanillas F, Velasquez WS, *et al.*: Phase II trial of fludarabine phosphate in lymphoma: an effective new agent in low-grade lymphoma. *J Clin Oncol* 1992, 10:790–794.

22. Solal-Celigny P, Brice P, Brousse N, *et al.*: Phase II trial of fludarabine monophosphate as first-line treatment in patients with advanced follicular lymphoma: a multicenter study by the Groupe d'Etude des Lymphomes de l'Adulte. *J Clin Oncol* 1996, 14:514–519.

23. Horning SJ: Natural history of and therapy for the indolent non-Hodgkin's lymphomas. *Semin Oncol* 1993, 20(Suppl 5):5–88.

24. McLaughlin P, Grillo-Lopez AJ, Link BK, *et al.*: Rituximab chimeric anti-CD20 monoclonal antibody therapy for relapsed indolent lymphoma: half of patients respond to a four dose treatment program. *J Clin Oncol* 1998, 16:2825–2833.

25. Maloney DG, Grillo-Lopez AJ, White CA, *et al.*: IDEC-C2B8 (rituximab) anti-CD20 monoclonal antibody therapy in patients with relapsed low-grade non-Hodgkin's lymphoma. *Blood* 1997, 90:2188–2195.

26. Davis TA, Grillo-Lopez AJ, White CA, *et al.*: Rituximab anti-CD20 monoclonal antibody therapy in non-Hodgkin's lymphoma: safety and efficacy of re-treatment. *J Clin Oncol* 2000, 18:3135–3143.

27. Cunningham D, Flores E, Catalano J, *et al.*: CVP chemotherapy plus rituximab compared with CVP as first-line treatment for advanced follicular lymphoma. *Blood* 2005, 105:1417–1423.

28. Cartron G, Solal-Celigny P: Maintenance therapy for low-grade lymphomas: has the time come? *Curr Opin Oncol* 2007, 19:425–432.

29. Kaminski MS, Zasadny KR, Francis IR, *et al.*: Radioimmunotherapy of B-cell lymphoma with 131-I anti-B1 [anti-CD20] antibody. *N Engl J Med* 1993, 329:459–465.

30. Witzig TE, White CA, Wiseman GA, *et al.*: Phase I/II of IDEC-Y2B8 radioimmunotherapy for treatment of relapsed or refractory CD20 positive B-cell non-Hodgkin's lymphoma. *J Clin Oncol* 1999, 17:3793–3803.

31. Park SI, Press OW: Radioimmunotherapy for treatment of B-cell lymphomas and other hematologic malignancies. *Curr Opin Hematol* 2007, 14:632–638.

32. Brown JR, Feng Y, Gribben JG, *et al.*: Long-term survival after autologous bone marrow transplantation for follicular lymphoma in first remission. *Biol Blood Marrow Transplant* 2007, 13:1057–1065.

33. Sabloff M, Atkins HL, Bence-Bruckler I, *et al.*: A 15-year analysis of early and late autologous hematopoietic stem cell transplant in relapsed, aggressive, transformed, and nontransformed follicular lymphoma. *Biol Blood Marrow Transplant* 2007, 13:956–964.

34. Lenz G, Dreyling M, Schiegnitz E, *et al.*: Myeloablative radiochemotherapy followed by autologous stem cell transplantation in first remission prolongs progression-free survival in follicular lymphoma: results of a prospective, randomized trial of the German Low-Grade Lymphoma Study Group. *Blood* 2004, 104:2667–2674.

35. Deconinck E, Foussard C, Milpied N, *et al.*: High-dose therapy followed by autologous purged stem-cell transplantation and doxorubicin-based chemotherapy in patients with advanced follicular lymphoma: a randomized multicenter study by GOELAMS. *Blood* 2005, 105:3817–3823.

36. Sebban C, Mounier N, Brousse N, *et al.*: Standard chemotherapy with interferon compared with CHOP followed by high-dose therapy with autologous stem cell transplantation in untreated patients with advanced follicular lymphoma: the GELF-94 randomized study from the Groupe d'Etudes des Lymphomes de l'Adulte (GELA). *Blood* 2006, 108:2540–2544.

37. van Besien K, Khouri I, Champlin R, *et al.*: Allogeneic transplantation for low-grade lymphoma: long-term follow-up. *J Clin Oncol* 2000, 18:702–703.

38. Khouri IF, Keating M, Korbling M, *et al.*: Transplant-lite: induction of graft-versus malignancy using fludarabine based non-ablative chemotherapy and allogeneic blood progenitor cell transplantation as treatment for lymphoid malignancies. *J Clin Oncol* 1998, 16:2817–2824.

39. Shimomi A, Giralt S, Khouri I, *et al.*: Allogeneic hematopoietic transplantation for acute and chronic myeloid leukemia: non-myeloablative preparative regimens and induction of the graft-versus-leukemia effect. *Curr Oncol Rep* 2000, 2:132–139.

40. Shipp M, Harrington D, Anderson J, *et al.*: A predictive model for aggressive non-Hodgkin's lymphoma: the International Non-Hodgkin's Lymphoma Prognostic Factors Project. *N Engl J Med* 1993, 329:987–994.

41. Coiffier B, Lepage E, Briere J, *et al.*: CHOP chemotherapy plus rituximab compared with CHOP alone in elderly patients with diffuse large B-cell lymphoma. *N Engl J Med* 2002, 346:235–242.

42. Feugier P, Van Hoof A, Sebban C, *et al.*: Long-term results of the R-CHOP study in the treatment of elderly patients with diffuse large B-cell lymphoma: a study by the Groupe d'Etude des Lymphomes de l'Adulte. *J Clin Oncol* 2005, 23:4117–4126.

43. Habermann TM, Weller EA, Morrison VA, *et al.*: Rituximab-CHOP versus CHOP alone or with maintenance rituximab in older patients with diffuse large B-cell lymphoma. *J Clin Oncol* 2006, 24:3121–3127.

44. Pfreundschuh M, Trumper L, Osterborg A, *et al.*: CHOP-like chemotherapy plus rituximab versus CHOP-like chemotherapy alone in younger patients with good-prognosis diffuse large B-cell lymphoma: a randomised controlled trial by the MabThera International Trial (MInT) Group. *Lancet Oncol* 2006, 7:379–391.

45. Miller TP, Dahlberg S, Cassady JR, *et al.*: Chemotherapy alone compared with chemotherapy plus radiotherapy for localized intermediate- and high-grade non-Hodgkin's lymphoma. *N Engl J Med* 1998, 339:21–26.

46. Milpied N, Deconinck E, Gaillard F, *et al.*: Initial treatment of aggressive lymphoma with high-dose chemotherapy and autologous stem-cell support. *N Engl J Med* 2004, 350:1287–1295.

47. Strehl J, Mey U, Glasmacher A, *et al.*: High-dose chemotherapy followed by autologous stem cell transplantation as first-line therapy in aggressive non-Hodgkin's lymphoma: a meta-analysis. *Haematologica* 2003, 88:1304–1315.

48. Greb A, Bohlius J, Trelle S, *et al.*: High-dose chemotherapy with autologous stem cell support in first-line treatment of aggressive non-Hodgkin lymphoma: results of a comprehensive meta-analysis. *Cancer Treat Rev* 2007, 33:338–346.

49. Philip T, Guglielmi C, Hagenbeek A, *et al.*: Autologous bone marrow transplantation as compared with salvage chemotherapy in relapses of chemotherapy-sensitive non-Hodgkin's lymphoma. *N Engl J Med* 1995, 333:1540–1545.

50. Philip T, Armitage JO, Spitzer G, *et al.*: High-dose chemotherapy and autologous bone marrow transplantation after failure of conventional chemotherapy in adults with intermediate grade or high grade non-Hodgkin's lymphoma. *N Engl J Med* 1987, 316:1493–1498.

51. Shipp MA, Abeloff MD, Antman KH, *et al.*: International consensus conference on high-dose therapy with hematopoietic stem cell transplantation in aggressive non-Hodgkin's lymphomas: report of the jury. *J Clin Oncol* 1999, 17:423–429.

52. Velasquez WS, Cabanillas F, Salvador P, *et al.*: Effective salvage therapy for lymphoma with cisplatin in combination with high dose ara-C and dexamethasone (DHAP). *Blood* 1998, 71:117–122.

53. Moskowitz CH, Bertino JR, Glassman JR, *et al.*: Ifosfamide, carboplatin, and etoposide: a highly effective cytoreduction and peripheral-blood progenitor-cell mobilization regimen for transplant eligible patients with non-Hodgkin's lymphoma. *J Clin Oncol* 1999, 17:3776–3785.

54. Khouri IF, Romajuera J, Kantarjian H, *et al.*: Hyper-CVAD and high-dose methotrexate/cytarabine followed by stem-cell transplantation: an active regimen for aggressive mantle cell lymphoma. *J Clin Oncol* 1988, 16:3803–3809.

55. Khouri I, Romajuera J, Kantarjian H, *et al.*: Update of the hyper-CVAD regimen followed by stem cell transplantation (SCT) in mantle cell lymphoma [abstract]. *Blood* 1994, 94:2713.

56. Goy A: New directions in the treatment of mantle cell lymphoma: an overview. *Clin Lymphoma Myeloma* 2006, 7(Suppl 1):S24–S32.

57. Magrath I, Adde M, Shad A, *et al.*: Adults and children with small non-cleaved cell lymphoma have a similar excellent outcome when treated with the same chemotherapy regimen. *J Clin Oncol* 1996, 14:925–934.

58. Levine AM: Acquired immunodeficiency syndrome-related lymphoma: clinical aspects. *Semin Oncol* 2000, 27:442–453.

59. Fatkenheuer G, Hell K, Roers A, *et al.*: Spontaneous regression of HIV-associated T-cell non-Hodgkin's lymphoma with highly active antiretroviral therapy. *Eur J Med Res* 2000, 5:236–240.

60. Little RF, Pittaluga S, Grant N, *et al.*: Highly effective treatment of acquired immunodeficiency syndrome-related lymphoma with dose-adjusted EPOCH: impact of antiretroviral therapy suspension and tumor biology. *Blood* 2003, 101:4653–4659.

61. Behler CM, Kaplan LD: Advances in the management of HIV-related non-Hodgkin lymphoma. *Curr Opin Oncol* 2006, 18:437–443.

62. Kaplan LD, Lee JY, Ambinder RF, *et al.*: Rituximab does not improve clinical outcome in a randomized phase 3 trial of CHOP with or without rituximab in patients with HIV-associated non-Hodgkin lymphoma: AIDS-Malignancies Consortium Trial 010. *Blood* 2005, 106:1538–1543.

63. Hoppe RT, Kushlan P, Kaplan HS, *et al.*: The treatment of advanced stage favorable histology non-Hodgkin's lymphoma: a preliminary report of a randomized trial comparing single agent chemotherapy, combination chemotherapy, and whole body irradiation. *Blood* 1981, 58:592–598.

64. Anderson T, Bender RA, Fisher RI, *et al.*: Combination chemotherapy in non-Hodgkin's lymphoma: results of a long-term followup. *Cancer Treat Rep* 1977, 61:1057–1066.

65. Armitage JO, Fyfe MA, Lewis J: Long-term remission durability and functional status of patients treated for diffuse histiocytic lymphoma with the CHOP regimen. *J Clin Oncol* 1984, 2:898–902.

66. Gams RA, Rainey M, Dandy M, *et al.*: Phase III study of BCOP v CHOP in unfavorable categories of malignant lymphoma: a Southeastern Cancer Study Group trial. *J Clin Oncol* 1985, 3:1188–1195.

67. Coltman CA, Dahlberg S, Jones SE, *et al.*: CHOP is curative in thirty percent of patients with large cell lymphoma. A twelve year Southwest Oncology Group follow up [abstract]. *Proc Am Soc Clin Oncol* 1986, 5:197.

INCIDENCE AND ETIOLOGY

Multiple myeloma is the second most common hematologic malignancy in the United States, with an annual incidence of approximately 17,000 cases. It accounts for 1% of all malignant disease and more than 10% of hematologic malignancies. The occurrence of myeloma is more common in men than in women and more common in African American than in white individuals (Table 20-1). It most commonly presents in the seventh decade of life, with fewer than 2% of patients younger than 40 years of age.

The cause of multiple myeloma remains unknown, although monoclonal gammopathy of undetermined significance (MGUS) may offer some clues to its pathogenesis [1]. More than 33% of patients with apparent benign monoclonal gammopathy will develop myeloma, another lymphoplasmacellular malignancy, or progression of their monoclonal gammopathy. The incidence of myeloma in patients with MGUS is 25% after 20 to 35 years of follow-up. These observations implicate MGUS as a premalignant clonal disorder that, on further transforming damage to the clone, can give rise to multiple myeloma. Genetic predisposition, radiation exposure, chronic antigenic stimulation, and various environmental or occupational conditions have been observed as predisposing factors. However, these account for only a small percentage of all myeloma.

DIAGNOSIS AND STAGING

The diagnosis of multiple myeloma is made based on the presence of malignant plasma cells, either in the bone marrow (usually > 10%) or by biopsy proof of a plasmacytoma, with protein evidence of myeloma (a monoclonal serum or urine protein) or characteristic osteolytic lesions. For the past 30 years, the most commonly used staging system has been that proposed by Durie and Salmon (Table 20-2). This system correlates tumor burden with the presence or absence of anemia, hypercalcemia, skeletal disease, and the amount of monoclonal protein detected in serum or urine [2]. More recently, a simplified staging system (International Staging System [ISS]) based on serum β-2 microglobulin and albumin was proposed by Greipp *et al.* [3] (Table 20-3). This system was developed and validated using a retrospective analysis of more than 10,000 patients. It divides patients into three stages, with stage I patients having a median survival of 62 months and stage III patients having a median survival of 29 months. Results of conventional cytogenetics and fluorescent in situ hybridization (FISH) were only available for a small subset of the patients and, thus, could not be incorporated into the model. Both the Durie-Salmon and ISS systems demonstrate that clinical stage appears predictive of survival. Stage I patients generally survive more than 5 years, whereas the median survival for stage II and III patients is 3 to 4 years and 2 to 3 years, respectively. The presence of renal failure has an important negative prognostic significance in myeloma. Additional studies have demonstrated that an elevated plasma β-2 microglobulin and elevated plasma cell labeling index are also impor-

tant adverse prognostic signs that may at times override the significance of clinical stage [4]. Although renal dysfunction will result in elevated serum β-2 microglobulin levels, this protein is an independent prognostic factor in myeloma [5]. Conversely, the presence of both low plasma β-2 microglobulin and a low plasma cell labeling index appears to be a strong predictor of long-term survival in patients with myeloma [4].

Other factors relating to patient differences, tumor burden, and tumor biology that have prognostic importance in myeloma are summarized in Table 20-4.

Characteristic patterns of chromosomal abnormalities occur in many patients with myeloma and have prognostic significance. Abnormalities can be detected by conventional cytogenetics in 15% to 20% of patients and by

Table 20-1. Risk Factors for the Development of Multiple Myeloma

African American race

Male gender

Advanced age

Monoclonal gammopathy of undetermined significance

Chronic immune stimulation

Exposure to ionizing radiation

Occupational exposure to pesticides, paints, and solvents

Genetic predisposition

Table 20-2. Durie-Salmon Clinical Staging System for Myeloma

Stage	Criteria	Myeloma cell mass, *cells/m²*
I	All of the following: Hemoglobin > 10 g/dL Serum calcium value normal (≤ 12 mg/100 mL) On x-ray, normal bone structure or solitary bone plasmocytoma only Low M-component production rates • IgG value < 5 g/100 mL • IgA value < 3 g/100 mL • Urine light chain M-component on electrophoresis < 4 g/24 h	< 0.6 × 10¹² (low)
II	Fitting neither stage I or III	0.6–1.2 × 10¹² (intermediate)
III	One or more of the following: Hemoglobin < 8.5 g/100 mL Serum calcium value > 12 mg/100 mL Advanced lytic bone lesions High M-component production rates • IgG value > 7 g/100 mL • IgA value > 5 g/100 mL • Urine light chain M-component on electrophoresis > 12 g/24 h	1.2 × 10¹² (high)
Subclass A	Serum creatinine < 2 mg/100 mL	
Subclass B	Serum creatinine ≥ 2 mg/100 mL	

(*Adapted from* Durie and Salmon [2].)

Table 20-3. International Staging System for Myeloma

Stage	Criteria	Survival (median), *mo*
I	Albumin ≥ 3.5 and β-2 microglobulin < 3.5	62
II	Neither I or III	44
III	β-2 microglobulin > 5.5	29

(*Adapted from* Greipp *et al.* [3].)

FISH in up to 70% of patients with myeloma. These changes include duplications, translocations, and deletions of portions of or entire chromosomes [6]. The chromosomes most commonly affected include 1, 3, 4, 7, 9, 11, 13, 14, 16, and 17. Extra chromosomes are acquired in some patients, leading to a hyperdiploid state. Characteristic translocations occur between the IgH region on chromosome 11 and partner chromosomes 4, 14, and 16. In general, patients with hyperdiploidy or a t(11;14) have a better prognosis than patients with a normal karyotype, whereas patients with t(4;14), t(4;16), or del17p tend to have a worse prognosis [7]. Although initial data suggested a poor outcome for patients with deletion of chromosome 13, recent studies suggest that the majority of these patients also have t(4;14) and it is the t(4;14) that accounts for the adverse prognosis [6,7]. Gene expression profiling and FISH studies have also identified amplifications of 1q in a subset of patients with particularly poor-prognosis myeloma [8,9].

PRIMARY DISEASE THERAPY

Because myeloma remains incurable, in most cases, the goal of treatment is to maximally extend survival while maintaining each patient's ability to lead an active life for as long as possible. Most often, this is achieved through objective disease regression with its attendant relief of pain and other disease-related symptoms.

For many years, use of the single alkylating agent melphalan or a combination of melphalan and prednisone (MP) was considered the standard of care for patients with myeloma (Fig. 20-1). When this treatment is used, objective responses, documented by a 50% or greater decrease in serum M-protein and control of other major manifestations of disease, are seen in 50% of patients. Unfortunately, response duration is generally less than 2 years, with a median overall survival of 30 months, and fewer than 20% of patients live longer than 5 years. In an effort to improve these statistics, numerous combination chemotherapy regimens have been developed. Most randomized trials and meta-analyses suggest that these more aggressive combination chemotherapy regimens may improve response rates, but with their added toxicity, they have not had a significant impact on overall survival [10]. However, with the introduction of bortezomib, thalidomide, and lenalidomide, this may be changing. These drugs—as well as combinations including them—have led to better quality and higher response rates in patients with newly diagnosed and relapsed myeloma. Trials incorporating these agents have also shown survival benefits in both newly diagnosed and relapsed myeloma. Unfortunately, despite these modest improvements in event-free and overall survival, to date, there is no clear evidence of prolonged remissions.

Table 20-4. Prognostic Factors

Patient factors

Age

Performance status

Concomitant illness

Renal function

Serum albumin

Factors reflecting tumor burden

Clinical stage (*see* Tables 20-2 and 20-3), including component factors hemoglobin, M-component concentration, serum calcium, osteolytic lesions

β-2 microglobulin

Tumor biology

Plasma cell labeling index

C-reactive protein

Lactic dehydrogenase

Plasmablastic subtype

Circulating tumor cells

Chromosomal abnormalities

The first of these agents to be approved for upfront therapy was thalidomide; approval was based on two multicenter phase 3 trials by Rajkumar *et al.* [12]. In these trials, the combination of thalidomide and dexamethasone was superior to dexamethasone alone in newly diagnosed patients [12]. The initial study, done by the Eastern Cooperative Oncology Group (ECOG), was designed to look at best response and toxicity after four cycles and concluded that patients receiving thalidomide and dexamethasone had higher rates and better quality of responses than those receiving dexamethasone alone, although with greater toxicity. This ECOG trial was not designed nor powered to look for differences in survival between the two arms. Although the subsequent multicenter trial (MM003) [12] was powered to look for differences in survival, the median overall survival has not been reached for the thalidomide/dexamethasone arm and thus this end point cannot yet be assessed.

Subsequent to this trial, Rajkumar *et al.* [13] sought to assess the effect of high (standard) dose (40 mg/d on days 1–4, 9–12, and 17–20 every 28 days) versus low-dose dexamethasone (40 mg once a week) in conjunction with lenalidomide. All patients received lenalidomide 25 mg/d (for 21 of 28 days) and were randomized to receive high- or low-dose dexamethasone. The trial was stopped early due to superior overall survival in the low-dose dexamethasone arm (96% vs 86% at 1 year; *P* = 0.015). Toxicity

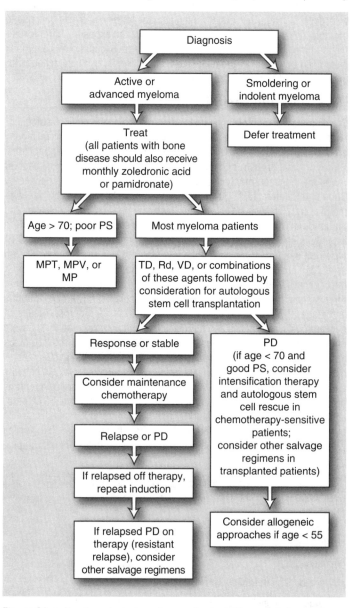

Figure 20-1. Treatment strategy for myeloma. MP—melphalan and prednisone; MPT—melphalan, prednisone, thalidomide; MPV—melphalan, prednisone, bortezomib; PD—progressive disease; PS—performance status; Rd—lenalidomide and dexamethasone; TD—thalidomide and dexamethasone.

was also lower with lower-dose dexamethasone. Analysis of response data is ongoing and results will be forthcoming. The findings from this trial are encouraging given the lower morbidity and mortality seen with low-dose dexamethasone. This almost certainly represents a quality-of-life improvement for most patients receiving dexamethasone.

In determining what type of therapy to initiate in the newly diagnosed patient, it is important to consider the extent of disease, other clinical conditions, and whether the patient is a candidate for high-dose therapy regimens. For example, several small, randomized trials have demonstrated no benefit to treating asymptomatic early-stage patients with chemotherapy. A "watch and wait" approach is warranted in this group until more effective therapies become available. In patients who are candidates for high-dose therapy followed by autologous hematopoietic support, regimens without alkylating agents are preferable because of the difficulty in collecting adequate stem cells in patients exposed to these agents prior to stem cell mobilization. In elderly patients or in persons unable to tolerate more aggressive chemotherapy, oral dexamethasone alone or MP may be considered. Recent data suggest that response rates [14] and overall survival [15] are higher in patients receiving MPT (melphalan, prednisone, and thalidomide) or MPV (melphalan, prednisone, and bortezomib) as compared with MP. Thus, strong consideration should be given to MPT or MPV over MP or dexamethasone alone if patients can tolerate more aggressive treatment approaches.

Initial chemotherapy is generally given for 4 to 12 months. Responding patients usually demonstrate a reduction in tumor mass as reflected by decreases in paraprotein levels. Until recently, complete responses were rarely seen. With the introduction of combinations that include bortezomib, thalidomide, or lenalidomide, complete response rates ranging from 3% to 20% are being reported. Responding patients who are eligible may elect to proceed with stem cell transplantation or to store autologous stem cells for future use. This is usually done after 4 to 6 months of induction therapy. Alternatively, patients may elect to continue therapy until they enter a plateau phase, at which point the monoclonal protein level remains constant despite continued chemotherapy and consideration is given to discontinuing treatment followed by watchful waiting. Some investigators are giving this even stronger consideration given the absence of long-term disease-free survival with autologous transplantation and consistent reports of complete remissions in a subset of patients with myeloma using newer agents. In a retrospective analysis, Wang *et al.* [16] found that patients achieving a complete remission lived significantly longer than patients who did not. Further, it did not appear to matter whether complete remission followed standard therapy or an autologous transplantation. Additional studies and longer follow-up are needed to determine whether this finding persists in prospective trials.

HIGH-DOSE THERAPY

Based on the higher response rates achieved with more aggressive combinations of alkylating agents, studies of high-dose chemotherapy with or without hematopoietic support were initiated. Over the past 25 years, the use of high-dose chemotherapy has evolved from melphalan in doses of 70 mg/m^2 without stem cell support in refractory relapsed patients to one or two courses of melphalan 200 mg/m^2 followed by autologous stem cell support given to patients in first remission. In a randomized French study [17] of 200 untreated patients with intermediate- to high-stage multiple myeloma, patients assigned to high-dose chemotherapy and autologous bone marrow transplantation achieved higher overall response rates and better progression-free and overall survival than that achieved by patients continued on conventional chemotherapy. Because of the encouraging results from this trial, additional studies were done comparing various regimens of standard-dose to high-dose chemotherapy. Three of these trials [17–19] showed a survival benefit of 12 to 18 months for patients receiving high-dose therapy whereas six [15,20–24] trials found no difference between the two treatments. Further, a recent meta-analysis of the randomized trials also failed to show a survival benefit for patients receiving high-dose therapy [25]. Nevertheless, given the possibility of prolonged progression-free survival with relatively low treatment-related mortality (<

2%), high-dose chemotherapy with autologous stem cell support should be considered for patients 70 years of age or younger with intermediate- to advanced-stage multiple myeloma responsive to or stable following conventional chemotherapy.

Because several studies have shown a survival benefit for patients undergoing one course of high-dose therapy with autologous stem cell support, additional studies and randomized trials have been done comparing one to two courses of high-dose melphalan and autologous stem cell support. To date, several of these trials have shown higher response rates, but only the French Intergroup trial [26] has shown an improvement in overall survival in patients receiving two courses of high-dose therapy.

Allogeneic bone marrow transplantation has also been used in myeloma. Its potential advantages include the complete absence of malignant cells in the infused product as well as a potential therapeutic form of adoptive immunotherapy or graft-versus-tumor effect mediated by the allogeneic bone marrow. Although early results from the largest study of allogeneic transplants from the European Bone Marrow Transplant Registry were encouraging [27–29], the morbidity and mortality related to the procedure were significant. Subsequent studies from several centers reported lower rates of mortality [30–32]; nevertheless, most patients do not achieve long-term disease-free survival. Additional efforts to reduce the morbidity and mortality of allogeneic transplantation in myeloma have included the use of reduced-intensity conditioning regimens [33] and tandem autologous/allogeneic transplantation using reduced-intensity conditioning regimens [34,35]. To date, the results of allogeneic transplantation in myeloma have been disappointing, with a median event-free survival of less than 3 years. Thus, allogeneic transplantation is a treatment option for patients with myeloma and, when employed, is best done in the context of a clinical trial.

THERAPY FOR REFRACTORY OR RELAPSED DISEASE

Thirty percent to 50% of multiple myeloma patients will have progressive disease despite conventional therapy and have a particularly poor prognosis. Even in patients who do achieve an initial response, nearly all will ultimately relapse and develop disease unresponsive to initial therapy. When patients relapse, repeat use of the original induction regimen may achieve remissions, especially in patients with a long duration of their initial remission. Selection of the optimal treatment for patients with relapsed or refractory disease is based in part on the initial therapy used, the response to this regimen, and any preexisting comorbid conditions.

The initial trials demonstrating antimyeloma activity of thalidomide, bortezomib, and lenalidomide were performed in the setting of relapsed refractory myeloma. Each of these agents has single-agent activity in 20% to 30% of patients, while combinations with dexamethasone or other chemotherapeutic agents lead to somewhat higher response rates. In a population of heavily pretreated patients, thalidomide led to an overall response rate of 27% [36]. In a large phase 3 trial, bortezomib was shown to be superior to dexamethasone, with a 38% overall response rate and an improvement in overall and event-free survival [37,38].

When compared with dexamethasone alone, lenalidomide led to a higher overall response rate in patients with relapsed or refractory myeloma, thus leading to US Food and Drug Administration (FDA) approval of this agent in patients who have received at least one prior therapy. High-dose glucocorticosteroids (*eg*, prednisone 200 mg every other day [or pulse 60 mg/m^2 daily for 5 days every 8 days] or dexamethasone 40 mg daily for 4 days repeated every 8–14 days) may produce excellent responses even in refractory patients. However, the duration of response is usually less than 1 year and has been largely supplanted by the aforementioned novel agents. Toxicities include insomnia, hyperglycemia, mental status changes, and increased risk of infections. VAD (vincristine, doxorubicin, and dexamethasone) may be used in patients who initially failed MP, but its efficacy in patients who previously failed high-dose dexamethasone therapy alone is less impressive.

Intravenous cyclophosphamide alone may also produce responses in patients with resistant myeloma [39].

A French study suggests that high-dose therapy may be equally effective when done at the time of first relapse as when done as part of the patient's initial treatment [21]. Thus, this is an option in patients who have relapsed following conventional therapy. However, induction of disease stabilization or response with conventional chemotherapy should be achieved prior to attempting a high-dose program; otherwise the outcome is extremely poor. In patients relapsing following high-dose therapy, another high-dose treatment regimen may be used if the initial therapy resulted in a relatively long remission following the first transplant. Alternatively, in patients who previously underwent autologous transplantation, allogeneic support may be considered, but the higher risk of treatment-related mortality must be considered in any decision regarding this form of treatment.

MAINTENANCE THERAPY

Several large, randomized trials have demonstrated that the continued use of chemotherapy during plateau phase does not improve overall survival. In fact, continuation of cytotoxic therapy leads to a permanent reduction in bone marrow reserve and increases the risk of secondary leukemia. There have been many attempts to prolong the duration of response in patients with myeloma, but most studies have failed to demonstrate a clinical benefit. A single trial performed by the Southwest Oncology Group (SWOG) demonstrated an improvement in progression-free and overall survival in patients receiving alternate-day prednisone 50 mg as compared with no maintenance following a response to VAD induction chemotherapy [40]. More than 30 randomized trials have been published looking at the role of interferon 2-α as maintenance therapy in myeloma. These trials have failed to show any consistent clinical benefit [41]. At present, there is no standard maintenance therapy in myeloma.

More recent efforts have studied the role of maintenance therapy following autologous transplantation. In particular, these studies have focused on the use of thalidomide, lenalidomide, and/or bisphosphonates in patients following autologous transplantation. In most of these trials, the starting thalidomide dose ranged from 200 to 400 mg/d with dose reductions allowed. In the first trial to demonstrate a survival benefit, Attal *et al.* [42] found that patients receiving 100 mg of thalidomide lived longer than patients who did not.

BONE DISEASE

Bone disease is a major cause of morbidity in multiple myeloma, resulting from stimulation of osteoclasts by bone-resorbing cytokines (tumor necrosis factor, interleukin [IL]-1b, and IL-6), which are overabundant in the myeloma bone marrow. Osteolytic lesions and generalized osteoporosis may lead to severe pain, pathologic fractures, and spinal cord compression or vertebral body collapse. These complications often require radiation therapy to relieve pain or to treat actual or impending pathologic fractures or spinal cord compression. Plasma cell tumors are relatively responsive to radiation treatment. Responses typically occur rapidly; most lesions are treated with approximately 3000 cGy. It is important to avoid unnecessary radiotherapy as its myelosuppressive effect may limit the ability to deliver cytotoxic doses of systemic chemotherapy. Often the latter treatment alone will be effective for relieving skeletal pain. High doses of analgesics may be necessary until pain control is achieved with radiation or chemotherapy. Surgery may be necessary to treat actual fractures or to prevent large lytic lesions from developing fractures. The placement of intramedullary rods is usually the surgical procedure of choice. Spinal disease may require surgical decompression and/or stabilization of the spine, including use of kyphoplasty or vertebroplasty. Prior attempts to reduce the development of these skeletal complications with calcium,

sodium fluoride, androgenic steroids, or combinations of the three have been unsuccessful.

Bisphosphonates inhibit osteoclastic activity and are effective in the treatment of hypercalcemia associated with myeloma. Previous attempts to use relatively weak first-generation bisphosphonates (etidronate or clodronate) orally as an adjunct to chemotherapy had no significant effect on the development of skeletal complications in myeloma patients. Subsequent randomized trials demonstrated the superiority of pamidronate over placebo in patients with lytic bone lesions receiving chemotherapy, reducing the risk of skeletal events by 40% per year of treatment [43,44]. These findings were confirmed in a randomized trial when pamidronate was compared with zoledronic acid, a more potent amino-bisphosphonate [45,46]. With continued used of bisphosphonates came the recognition of a potentially serious side effect known as osteonecrosis [47]. The exact incidence of this is not known, but appears to occur in less than 10% of patients. Risk factors include longer duration of bisphosphonate use, invasive dental procedures, older age, and, in some series, the type of bisphosphonate used [48]. The optimal duration of treatment is not known. Many groups recommend 2 years of treatment followed by consideration of reduced treatment frequency or discontinuation in patients with stable disease or better [49,50].

NEW THERAPY APPROACHES

A number of new therapeutic strategies for myeloma are now in clinical development. Several of these strategies seek to target not only the myeloma plasma cells but also the bone marrow microenvironment by targeting molecular pathways that are necessary for myeloma cell growth and survival or cell surface molecules that characterize these cells.

Ongoing studies are looking at inhibitors of the PI3K/Akt/mTOR pathway, as well as heat shock protein (HSP), histone deactylase (HDAC), and vascular endothelial growth factor (VEGF) inhibitors. Each of these pathways appears to be important in the maintenance and proliferation of myeloma. Akt1 has been shown to inhibit apoptosis. IL-6 and insulin-like growth factor-1 (IGF-1) are upstream activators of the PI3K/Akt/mTOR pathway. Perifosine is an alkylphospholipid with Akt1 inhibitory activity. It blocks the proliferative effects of IL-6 and IGF-1 by inhibiting Akt phosphorylation. It is currently in phase 2 trials in patients with myeloma. Several HDAC inhibitors are currently under investigation in patients with myeloma with promising preclinical activity alone and in combination with bortezomib [51]. These agents include vorinostat, LBH-589, depsipeptide, valproic acid, and PXD101.

Additional studies are ongoing studying new immunomodulatory inhibitors, proteosome inhibitors, and combinations of these and other agents. Other studies are ongoing that seek to enhance the immunologic attack on myeloma cells using vaccine-based approaches and efforts to harness an immunologic antimyeloma effect. Finally, studies at our institution are ongoing that seek to target the purported myeloma stem cell population [52–54].

In summary, many regimens will produce responses in patients with myeloma, but long-term disease control is uncommon. To date, high-dose therapy with peripheral blood stem cell support seems to offer both longer progression-free and overall survival than conventional treatment but is not curative in the vast majority of patients. It is unclear if this benefit will persist with the advent of new agents leading to better quality responses; studies are being designed to address this question. Use of intravenous bisphosphonates reduces the bony complications while improving the quality of life of patients with lytic bone disease. Many novel strategies are under investigation and the identification of additional agents and combined modality approaches are needed to improve the outcomes for patients with myeloma.

MP (MELPHALAN AND PREDNISONE)

Melphalan and prednisone is the prototype regimen in the single alkylating agent therapy for multiple myeloma. The high-dose, intermittent schedule has proved a simple, relatively safe way to administer melphalan. A 1972 study reported that prednisone doubled the response rate to melphalan and that it produced modest improvement in survival. MP became, and remains, the standard chemotherapy for multiple myeloma. Treatment is generally administered in cycles of 3- to 6-week duration and is continued for 1 to 2 years, although it sometimes has been continued until disease progression. An important problem with this protocol is the erratic absorption of oral melphalan, which sometimes leads to inadequate bioavailability in some patients who take apparently adequate oral doses.

DOSAGE MODIFICATIONS

After the first cycle, the melphalan dose for depressed blood counts is as follows: absolute neutrophil count (ANC) 1000–2000/mcL, give 75%; ANC 750–1000/mcL or platelets 50,000–100,000/mcL, give 50%; ANC < 750/mcL or platelets < 50,000/mcL, delay treatment.

CANDIDATES FOR TREATMENT

Patients with active or advanced myeloma, particularly those who are elderly and frail

SPECIAL PRECAUTIONS

Risk for infection is greater during early cycles (use allopurinol to prevent hyperuricemia during early months); treatment-associated myelodysplastic syndrome and acute leukemia occur in some

ALTERNATIVE THERAPIES

Melphalan alone, VMCP (vincristine, melphalan, cyclophosphamide, prednisone)/VBAP (vincristine, carmustine, doxorubicin, prednisone), ABCM (doxorubicin, carmustine, cyclophosphamide, melphalan)

TOXICITIES

Melphalan: bone marrow suppression leading to neutropenia with increased risk for infection, thrombocytopenia with risk for bleeding, erythroid hypoplasia with risk for symptomatic anemia, long-term toxicity, testicular atrophy, amenorrhea, risk for treatment-induced leukemia; **Prednisone:** immunosuppression, infection, edema, exacerbation of diabetes, weight gain, menstrual abnormalities, mental status dysfunction (especially in elderly)

DRUG INTERACTIONS

None

NURSING INTERVENTIONS

Instruct patients to seek medical attention if fever or other specific or subjective symptoms develop that could represent infection; monitor blood glucose if patient is diabetic; antacid therapy may be used

PATIENT INFORMATION

Patient should take melphalan on empty stomach and prednisone after meals; anticipate possibility of mood and appetite changes or fluid retention; be alert to early signs of bleeding or infection

Dosage and Scheduling

Melphalan 8 mg/m^2 orally on d 1–4

Prednisone 60 mg/m^2 orally on d 1–4

Complete blood count and serum creatinine on d 1 and 14

• Cycle duration 4 wk; treatment duration 6–18 mo

Experiences and Response Rates

Study	Evaluable patients, *n*	Dosage and scheduling	Objective response, %	Median survival, *mo*
Alexanian *et al.* [55]	77	Melphalan 0.25 mg/kg orally on d 1–4 + prednisone 2 mg/kg orally on d 1–4; cycle duration 6 wk	47*	24
Abramson *et al.* [56]	72	Melphalan 8 mg/m^2 orally on d 1–4 + prednisone 75 mg orally on d 1–7; cycle duration 4 wk	43†	25
Oken *et al.* [57]	217	Melphalan 8 mg/m^2 orally on d 1–4 + prednisone 60 mg/m^2 orally on d 1–4	51‡	30
Bergsagel *et al.* [58]	125	Melphalan 9 mg/m^2 orally on d 1–4 + prednisone 100 mg orally on d 1–4; cycle duration 4 wk	40*	28

*Response requires ≥ 75% decrease in M-protein production.
†Response evaluated at 6 mo only.
‡Response requires ≥ 50% decrease in M-protein value.

MPV (MELPHALAN, PREDNISONE, BORTEZOMIB)

Treatment with melphalan, prednisone, and bortezomib leads to a survival advantage over melphalan and prednisone alone. Treatment is generally administered in 4–6 week cycles and is continued for 12 months.

DOSAGE MODIFICATIONS

None

CANDIDATES FOR TREATMENT

Patients with newly diagnosed or relapsed myeloma who are older than 65 years of age or are not candidates for autologous stem cell transplantation and are in need of treatment

ALTERNATIVE THERAPIES

MP, MPT, TD, Rd, bortezomib with or without liposomal doxorubicin or dexamethasone, dexamethasone alone

SPECIAL PRECAUTIONS

Varicella zoster prophylaxis

TOXICITIES

Bortezomib: Diarrhea, constipation, peripheral neuropathy, thrombocytopenia, neutropenia, nausea, infection including varicella zoster reactivation, fatigue, asthenia; **Melphalan:** bone marrow suppression leading to neutropenia with increased risk of infection, thrombocytopenia with risk of bleeding, erythroid hypoplasia with risk of symptomatic anemia, long-term toxicity, testicular atrophy, amenorrhea, risk of treatment-induced acute leukemia, nausea, alopecia; **Prednisone:** mood swings, cognitive dysfunction (especially elderly), edema, weight gain, gastritis, peptic ulcer disease, diabetes, immunosuppression, infection, proximal muscle weakness, moon facies, hypertension, cataracts

DRUG INTERACTIONS

None

NURSING INTERVENTIONS

Instruct patient to seek medical attention for any signs or symptoms of peripheral neuropathy as well as signs or symptoms of infection; monitor blood glucose if diabetic; antacid therapy may be used

PATIENT INFORMATION

Anticipate the possibility of mood or appetite changes, fluid retention, gastrointestinal irritation including diarrhea and constipation; be alert to signs of varicella zoster reactivation, bleeding, infection.

Dosage and Administration

Bortezomib 1.3 mg/m^2 twice weekly (wk 1, 2, 4, and 5) for four 6-wk cycles (8 doses per cycle) followed by once weekly (wk 1, 2, 4, and 5) for five 6-wk cycles (4 doses per cycle)

Melphalan 9 mg/m^2 orally on d 1–4 of each cycle

Prednisone 60 mg/m^2 once daily on d 1–4 of each cycle

Complete blood count and serum creatinine continuous

• Cycle duration 4 wk; treatment duration 6 cycles

Experiences and Response Rates

Study	Evaluable patients, n	Dosage and scheduling	Objective response*, %	Overall survival, %
Mateos *et al.* [59,60]	60	Melphalan 9 mg/m^2 on d 1–4 + prednisone 60 mg/m^2 on d 1–7 + bortezomib 1.3 mg/m^2 on d 1, 4, 8, 11, 22, 25, 29, and 32	89	85 (2 y)
San Miguel *et al.* [61]	344	Melphalan 9 mg/m^2 on d 1–4 + prednisone 60 mg/m^2 on d 1–4 + bortezomib 1.3 mg/m^2 on d 1, 4, 8, 11, 22, 25, 29, and 32 (cycles 1–4) and d 1, 8, 15, and 22 (cycles 5–9) every 6 wk for 9 cycles	82	83 (2 y)

*Requires ≥ 50% decrease in M-protein.

MPT (MELPHALAN, PREDNISONE, THALIDOMIDE)

Treatment with melphalan, prednisone, and thalidomide leads to a survival advantage over melphalan and prednisone alone. Treatment is generally administered in 4-week cycles and is continued for 6 to 12 months.

DOSAGE MODIFICATIONS

None

CANDIDATES FOR TREATMENT

Patients with newly diagnosed or relapsed myeloma who are older than 65 years of age or are not candidates for autologous stem cell transplantation and are in need of treatment

SPECIAL PRECAUTIONS

Deep vein thrombosis (DVT) occurs in 17% to 20% of patients receiving thalidomide and dexamethasone combination therapy. DVT prophylaxis should be used unless contraindicated. Optimal treatment is with low molecular weight heparin or full-dose warfarin. Other less effective approaches include prophylactic doses of warfarin or aspirin 325 mg/d

ALTERNATIVE THERAPIES

MP, MPV, thalidomide/dexamethasone, lenalidomide/dexamethasone, bortezomib with or without liposomal doxorubicin or dexamethasone, dexamethasone alone

TOXICITIES

Thalidomide: Congenital anomalies including phocomelia, somnolence, constipation, peripheral neuropathy, DVT (when used in conjunction with corticosteroids), rash, toxic epidermal necrolysis, bradycardia, nausea, leukopenia, confusion, tremor; **Melphalan:** bone marrow suppression leading to neutropenia with increased risk of infection, thrombocytopenia with risk of bleeding, erythroid hypoplasia with risk of symptomatic anemia, long-term toxicity, testicular atrophy, amenorrhea, risk of treatment-induced acute leukemia, nausea, alopecia; **Prednisone:** mood swings, cognitive dysfunction (especially elderly), edema, weight gain, gastritis, peptic ulcer disease, diabetes, immunosuppression, infection, proximal muscle weakness, moon facies, hypertension, cataracts

DRUG INTERACTIONS

None

NURSING INTERVENTIONS

Instruct patient to seek medical attention for any signs or symptoms of DVT or pulmonary embolism as well as signs or symptoms of infection; monitor blood glucose if patient is diabetic; antacid therapy may be used

PATIENT INFORMATION

Patients must use two forms of birth control if the patient or female sexual partner or partners is capable of bearing children. This must continue until 4 weeks after thalidomide therapy is discontinued. Anticipate the possibility of mood or appetite changes, fluid retention, gastrointestinal irritation including gastritis and constipation; be alert to signs of DVT, bleeding, infection, rash

Dosage and Scheduling
Melphalan 4 mg/m^2 on d 1–7
Prednisone 40 mg/m^2 on d 1–7
Thalidomide 100 mg orally daily
DVT prophylaxis continuous
Complete blood count and serum creatinine
• Cycle duration 4 wk; treatment duration 6 cycles

Experiences and Response Rates				
Study	Evaluable patients, *n*	Dosage and scheduling	Objective response, %*	Overall survival
Palumbo *et al.* [14]	129	Melphalan 4 mg/m^2 on d 1–7 + prednisone 40 mg/m^2 on d 1–7 + thalidomide 100 mg every evening	76	80% (3 y)
Facon *et al.* [15]	125	Melphalan 0.25 mg/kg on d 1–4 + prednisone 2 mg/kg on d 1–4 + thalidomide 200–400 mg every evening; every 6 wk for 12 cycles	81	53.6 mo (median)

*Requires ≥ 50% decrease in M-protein.

TD (THALIDOMIDE AND DEXAMETHASONE)

DOSAGE MODIFICATIONS

Reduce thalidomide dosing for the development of grade 2 painful sensory neuropathy. For higher grades of peripheral neuropathy, hold thalidomide until resolution to grade 2 or lower and resume at lower dose. Temporary or permanent discontinuation should be considered for patients who develop motor neuropathies

CANDIDATES FOR TREATMENT

Patients with newly diagnosed or relapsed myeloma

SPECIAL PRECAUTIONS

DVT occurs in 17% to 20% of patients receiving thalidomide and dexamethasone combination therapy. DVT prophylaxis should be used unless contraindicated. Optimal treatment is with low molecular weight heparin or full-dose warfarin. Other less effective approaches include prophylactic doses of warfarin or aspirin 325 mg/d

ALTERNATIVE THERAPIES

MP, MPT, MPV, lenalidomide/dexamethasone, bortezomib with or without liposomal doxorubicin or dexamethasone, dexamethasone alone

TOXICITIES

Thalidomide: Congenital anomalies including phocomelia, somnolence, constipation, peripheral neuropathy, DVT (when used in conjunction with corticosteroids), rash, toxic epidermal necrolysis, bradycardia, nausea, leukopenia, confusion, tremor; **Dexamethasone:** mood swings, cognitive dysfunction (especially elderly), edema, weight gain, gastritis, peptic ulcer disease, diabetes, immunosuppression, infection, proximal muscle weakness, moon facies, hypertension, cataracts

DRUG INTERACTIONS

None

NURSING INTERVENTIONS

Instruct patient to seek medical attention for any signs or symptoms of DVT or pulmonary embolism as well as signs or symptoms of infection; monitor blood glucose if diabetic; antacid therapy may be used

PATIENT INFORMATION

Patients must use two forms of birth control if the patient or female sexual partner or partners is capable of bearing children. This must continue until 4 weeks after therapy with thalidomide is discontinued. Anticipate the possibility of mood or appetite changes, fluid retention, gastrointestinal irritation including gastritis and constipation; be alert to signs of DVT, bleeding, infection, rash

Dosage and Scheduling

Thalidomide 100–200 mg orally daily

Dexamethasone 40 mg on d 1–4, 9–12, and 17–20 (cycles 1–4) then on d 1–4 (subsequent cycles)

DVT prophylaxis continuous on d -28 to d 8

• Cycle duration 4 wk; treatment duration 6 mo to progressive disease

Experiences and Response Rates			
Study	Evaluable patients, *n*	Dosage and scheduling	Objective response, %*
Rajkumar *et al.* [11]	99	Thalidomide 200 mg every evening + dexamethasone 40 mg orally on d 1–4, 9–12, and 17–20 every 28 d	72
Rajkumar *et al.* [62]	50	Thalidomide 200–800 mg every evening + dexamethasone 40 mg orally on d 1–4, 9–12, and 17–20 every 28 d	77
Weber *et al.* [63]	40	Thalidomide 100–400 mg every evening + dexamethasone 20 mg/m² orally on d 1–4, 9–12, and 17–20 every 28 d	72

*Requires ≥ 50% decrease in M-protein.

R_D (LENALIDOMIDE AND DEXAMETHASONE)

DOSAGE MODIFICATIONS

The following lenalidomide dose modifications are for renal insufficiency and cytopenias (neutropenia and thrombocytopenia). **Moderate renal dysfunction (creatinine clearance [Ccr] 30 mL/min to 50 mL/min):** lenalidomide dose 10 mg once daily (may increase to 15 mg once daily if no response after two cycles); **Severe renal dysfunction (Ccr < 30 mL/min):** lenalidomide dose 15 mg every other day; **Renal dysfunction on dialysis:** lenalidomide 15 mg 3 times per week after dialysis. If ANC falls to < 1000/mcL, stop lenalidomide, begin granulocyte-colony stimulating factor (G-CSF), monitor complete blood counts (CBC) weekly, and resume at same dose if neutropenia is the only toxicity. If ANC < 1000/mcL on reinstitution of lenalidomide, stop lenalidomide, begin G-CSF, monitor CBC weekly, and resume at 15 mg/d when ANC > 1000/mcL. With each subsequent decline in ANC < 1000/mcL, lenalidomide dosing should be reduced by 5 mg when it is resumed (minimum dose, 5 mg/d). If platelets < 30,000/mcL, stop lenalidomide, monitor CBC weekly, and resume at 15 mg/d when platelets > 30,000/mcL. With each subsequent decline in platelets below 30,000/mcL, lenalidomide should be held until platelets > 30,000/mcL and the dose of lenalidomide should be reduced by 5 mg when it is resumed (minimum dose, 5 mg/d).

CANDIDATES FOR TREATMENT

Patients with newly diagnosed or relapsed myeloma in need of treatment

SPECIAL PRECAUTIONS

DVT occurs in 10% to 20% of patients receiving lenalidomide and dexamethasone combination therapy and is higher with higher doses of dexamethasone. DVT prophylaxis should be used unless contraindicated. Optimal treatment is with low molecular weight heparin or full-dose warfarin. Other less effective approaches include prophylactic doses of warfarin or aspirin 81–325 mg/d

ALTERNATIVE THERAPIES

TD, MP, MPT, MPV, bortezomib with or without liposomal doxorubicin or dexamethasone, dexamethasone alone

TOXICITIES

Lenalidomide: Neutropenia, thrombocytopenia, edema, pruritus, rash, nausea, constipation, diarrhea, dizziness, headache, fatigue, asthenia, insomnia, dyspnea, potential for congenital anomalies; **Dexamethasone:** mood swings, cognitive dysfunction (especially elderly), edema, weight gain, gastritis, peptic ulcer disease, diabetes, immunosuppression, infection, proximal muscle weakness, moon facies, hypertension, cataracts

DRUG INTERACTIONS

None

NURSING INTERVENTIONS

Monitor CBC and differential at least biweekly for the first two cycles and monthly thereafter. If neutropenia or thrombocytopenia occurs, CBC and differential should be done weekly. Instruct patient to seek medical attention for any signs or symptoms of DVT or pulmonary embolism as well as signs or symptoms of infection; monitor blood glucose if patient is diabetic; antacid therapy may be used

PATIENT INFORMATION

Patients must use two forms of birth control if the patient or female sexual partner or partners is capable of bearing children. This must continue until 4 weeks after therapy with lenalidomide is discontinued. Anticipate the possibility of mood or appetite changes, fluid retention, fatigue, gastrointestinal irritation including gastritis, nausea, constipation, and diarrhea; be alert to signs of DVT, bleeding, infection, and rash

Dosage and Scheduling

Lenalidomide 25 mg orally daily on d 1–21

Dexamethasone 40 mg once weekly

DVT prophylaxis continuous

Complete blood count and differential on d 1 and 15 of cycles 1–2 and on d 1 of cycles 3+

Creatinine on d 1

• Cycle duration 4 wk; treatment duration 6 mo to progressive disease

Experiences and Response Rates

Study	Evaluable patients, *n*	Dosage and scheduling	Objective response, %*	Overall survival, %
Lacy *et al.* [64]	34	Lenalidomide 25 mg every evening on d 1–21 every 28 d + dexamethasone 40 mg orally on d 1–4, 9–12, and 17–20 every 28 d	91	85 (3 y)
Rajkumar *et al.* [65]	207	Lenalidomide 25 mg every evening + dexamethasone 40 mg orally on d 1, 8, 15, and 22 every 28 d	NA	88 (2 y)

*Requires ≥ 50% decrease in M-protein.
NA—not applicable.

REFERENCES

1. Kyle RA, Rajkumar SV: Monoclonal gammopathy of undetermined significance. *Br J Haematol* 2006, 134:573–589.

2. Durie BG, Salmon SE: A clinical staging system for multiple myeloma. Correlation of measured myeloma cell mass with presenting clinical features, response to treatment, and survival. *Cancer* 1975, 36:842–854.

3. Greipp PR, San Miguel J, Durie BG, *et al.*: International staging system for multiple myeloma. *J Clin Oncol* 2005, 23:3412–3420.

4. Greipp PR, Lust JA, O'Fallon WM, *et al.*: Plasma cell labeling index and beta 2-microglobulin predict survival independent of thymidine kinase and C-reactive protein in multiple myeloma. *Blood* 1993, 81:3382–3387.

5. Durie BG, Stock-Novack D, Salmon SE, *et al.*: Prognostic value of pretreatment serum beta 2 microglobulin in myeloma: a Southwest Oncology Group Study. *Blood* 1990, 75:823–830.

6. Stewart AK, Fonseca R: Prognostic and therapeutic significance of myeloma genetics and gene expression profiling. *J Clin Oncol* 2005, 23:6339–6344.

7. Dewald GW, Therneau T, Larson D, *et al.*: Relationship of patient survival and chromosome anomalies detected in metaphase and/or interphase cells at diagnosis of myeloma. *Blood* 2005, 106:3553–3558.

8. Hanamura I, Stewart JP, Huang Y, *et al.*: Frequent gain of chromosome band 1q21 in plasma-cell dyscrasias detected by fluorescence in situ hybridization: incidence increases from MGUS to relapsed myeloma and is related to prognosis and disease progression following tandem stem-cell transplantation. *Blood* 2006, 108:1724–1732.

9. Fonseca R, Van Wier SA, Chang WJ, *et al.*: Prognostic value of chromosome 1q21 gain by fluorescent in situ hybridization and increase CKS1B expression in myeloma. *Leukemia* 2006, 20:2034–2040.

10. Combination chemotherapy versus melphalan plus prednisone as treatment for multiple myeloma: an overview of 6,633 patients from 27 randomized trials. Myeloma Trialists' Collaborative Group. *J Clin Oncol* 1998, 16:3832–3842.

11. Rajkumar SV, Blood E, Vesole D, *et al.*: Phase III clinical trial of thalidomide plus dexamethasone compared with dexamethasone alone in newly diagnosed multiple myeloma: a clinical trial coordinated by the Eastern Cooperative Oncology Group. *J Clin Oncol* 2006, 24:431–436.

12. Rajkumar SV, Rosiñol L, Hussein M, *et al.*: Multicenter, randomized, double-blind, placebo-controlled study of thalidomide plus dexamethasone compared with dexamethasone as initial therapy for newly diagnosed multiple myeloma. *J Clin Oncol* 2008, 26:2171–2177.

13. Rajkumar SV, Jacobus S, Callendar N, *et al.*: Phase III trial of lenalidomide plus high-dose dexamethasone compared to lenalidomide plus low-dose dexamethasone in newly diagnosed multiple myeloma (E4A03): a trial coordinated by the Eastern Cooperative Oncology Group [abstract]. *J Clin Oncol* 2007, 25:447s.

14. Palumbo A, Bringhen S, Caravita T, *et al.*: Oral melphalan and prednisone chemotherapy plus thalidomide compared with melphalan and prednisone alone in elderly patients with multiple myeloma: randomised controlled trial. *Lancet* 2006, 367:825–831.

15. Facon T, Mary JY, Hulin C, *et al.*: Melphalan and prednisone plus thalidomide versus melphalan and prednisone alone or reduced-intensity autologous stem cell transplantation in elderly patients with multiple myeloma (IFM 99-06): a randomised trial. *Lancet* 2007, 370:1209–1218.

16. Wang M, Delasalle K, Thomas S, *et al.*: Complete remission represents the major surrogate marker of long survival in multiple myeloma [abstract]. *Blood* 2007, 108:123a.

17. Attal M, Harousseau JL, Stoppa AM, *et al.*: A prospective, randomized trial of autologous bone marrow transplantation and chemotherapy in multiple myeloma. Intergroupe Francais du Myelome. *N Engl J Med* 1996, 335:91–97.

18. Palumbo A, Bringhen S, Petrucci MT, *et al.*: Intermediate-dose melphalan improves survival of myeloma patients aged 50 to 70: results of a randomized controlled trial. *Blood* 2004, 104:3052–3057.

19. Child JA, Morgan GJ, Davies FE, *et al.*: High-dose chemotherapy with hematopoietic stem-cell rescue for multiple myeloma. *N Engl J Med* 2003, 348:1875–1883.

20. Barlogie B, Kyle RA, Anderson KC, *et al.*: Standard chemotherapy compared with high-dose chemoradiotherapy for multiple myeloma: final results of phase III US Intergroup Trial S9321. *J Clin Oncol* 2006, 24:929–936.

21. Fermand JP, Ravaud P, Chevret S, *et al.*: High-dose therapy and autologous peripheral blood stem cell transplantation in multiple myeloma: up-front or rescue treatment? Results of a multicenter sequential randomized clinical trial. *Blood* 1998, 92:3131–3136.

22. Fermand JP, Katsahian S, Divine M, *et al.*: High-dose therapy and autologous blood stem-cell transplantation compared with conventional treatment in myeloma patients aged 55 to 65 years: long-term results of a randomized control trial from the Group Myelome-Autogreffe. *J Clin Oncol* 2005, 23:9227–9233.

23. Lenhoff S, Hjorth M, Holmberg E, *et al.*: Impact on survival of high-dose therapy with autologous stem cell support in patients younger than 60 years with newly diagnosed multiple myeloma: a population-based study. Nordic Myeloma Study Group. *Blood* 2000, 95:7–11.

24. Blade J, Rosinol L, Sureda A, *et al.*: High-dose therapy intensification compared with continued standard chemotherapy in multiple myeloma patients responding to the initial chemotherapy: long-term results from a prospective randomized trial from the Spanish cooperative group PETHEMA. *Blood* 2005, 106:3755–3759.

25. Koreth J, Cutler CS, Djulbegovic B, *et al.*: High-dose therapy with single autologous transplantation versus chemotherapy for newly diagnosed multiple myeloma: a systematic review and meta-analysis of randomized controlled trials. *Biol Blood Marrow Transplant* 2007, 13:183–196.

26. Attal M, Harousseau JL, Facon T, *et al.*: Single versus double autologous stem-cell transplantation for multiple myeloma. *N Engl J Med* 2003, 349:2495–2502.

27. Gahrton G, Tura S, Ljungman P, *et al.*: Allogeneic bone marrow transplantation in multiple myeloma. *N Engl J Med* 1991, 325:1267–1272.

28. Gahrton G: Allogeneic bone marrow transplantation in multiple myeloma. *Pathol Biol (Paris)* 1999, 47:188–191.

29. Gahrton G, Tura S, Ljungman P, *et al.*: An update of prognostic factors for allogeneic bone marrow transplantation in multiple myeloma using matched sibling donors. European Group for Blood and Marrow Transplantation. *Stem Cells* 1995, 13(Suppl 2):122–125.

30. Alyea E, Weller E, Schlossman R, *et al.*: T-cell-depleted allogeneic bone marrow transplantation followed by donor lymphocyte infusion in patients with multiple myeloma: induction of graft-versus-myeloma effect. *Blood* 2001, 98:934–939.

31. Huff CA, Fuchs EJ, Noga SJ, *et al.*: Long-term follow-up of T cell-depleted allogeneic bone marrow transplantation in refractory multiple myeloma: importance of allogeneic T cells. *Biol Blood Marrow Transplant* 2003, 9:312–319.

32. Gahrton G, Svensson H, Cavo M, *et al.*: Progress in allogeneic bone marrow and peripheral blood stem cell transplantation for multiple myeloma: a comparison between transplants performed 1983–93 and 1994–98 at European Group for Blood and Marrow Transplantation centres. *Br J Haematol* 2001, 113:209–216.

33. Badros A, Barlogie B, Siegel E, *et al.*: Improved outcome of allogeneic transplantation in high-risk multiple myeloma patients after nonmyeloablative conditioning. *J Clin Oncol* 2002, 20:1295–1303.

34. Bruno B, Rotta M, Patriarca F, *et al.*: A comparison of allografting with autografting for newly diagnosed myeloma. *N Engl J Med* 2007, 356:1110–1120.

35. Garban F, Attal M, Michallet M, *et al.*: Prospective comparison of autologous stem cell transplantation followed by dose-reduced allograft (IFM99-03 trial) with tandem autologous stem cell transplantation (IFM99-04 trial) in high-risk de novo multiple myeloma. *Blood* 2006, 107:3474–3480.

36. Singhal S, Mehta J, Desikan R, *et al.*: Antitumor activity of thalidomide in refractory multiple myeloma [see comments] [published erratum appears in *N Engl J Med* 2000, 342:364]. *N Engl J Med* 1999, 341:1565–1571.

37. Richardson PG, Sonneveld P, Schuster MW, *et al.*: Bortezomib or high-dose dexamethasone for relapsed multiple myeloma. *N Engl J Med* 2005, 352:2487–2498.

38. Richardson PG, Sonneveld P, Schuster M, *et al.*: Extended follow-up of a phase 3 trial in relapsed multiple myeloma: final time-to-event results of the APEX trial. *Blood* 2007, 110:3557–3560.

39. Lenhard RE Jr, Oken MM, Barnes JM, *et al.*: High-dose cyclophospha-mide. An effective treatment for advanced refractory multiple myeloma. *Cancer* 1984, 53:1456–1460.

40. Berenson JR, Crowley JJ, Grogan TM, *et al.*: Maintenance therapy with alternate-day prednisone improves survival in multiple myeloma patients. *Blood* 2002, 99:3163–3168.

41. Interferon as therapy for multiple myeloma: an individual patient data overview of 24 randomized trials and 4012 patients. *Br J Haematol* 2001, 113:1020–1034.

42. Attal M, Harousseau JL, Leyvraz S, *et al.*: Maintenance therapy with thalidomide improves survival in patients with multiple myeloma. *Blood* 2006, 108:3289–3294.

43. Berenson JR, Lichtenstein A, Porter L, *et al.*: Efficacy of pamidronate in reducing skeletal events in patients with advanced multiple myeloma. Myeloma Aredia Study Group. *N Engl J Med* 1996, 334:488–493.

44. Berenson JR, Lichtenstein A, Porter L, *et al.*: Long-term pamidronate treatment of advanced multiple myeloma patients reduces skeletal events. Myeloma Aredia Study Group. *J Clin Oncol* 1998, 16:593–602.

45. Rosen LS, Gordon D, Kaminski M, *et al.*: Long-term efficacy and safety of zoledronic acid compared with pamidronate disodium in the treatment of skeletal complications in patients with advanced multiple myeloma or breast carcinoma: a randomized, double-blind, multicenter, comparative trial. *Cancer* 2003, 98:1735–1744.

46. Rosen LS, Gordon D, Kaminski M, *et al.*: Zoledronic acid versus pamidro-nate in the treatment of skeletal metastases in patients with breast cancer or osteolytic lesions of multiple myeloma: a phase III, double-blind, comparative trial. *Cancer J* 2001, 7:377–387.

47. Ruggiero SL, Mehrotra B, Rosenberg TJ, Engroff SL: Osteonecrosis of the jaws associated with the use of bisphosphonates: a review of 63 cases. *J Oral Maxillofac Surg* 2004, 62:527–534.

48. Badros A, Weikel D, Salama A, *et al.*: Osteonecrosis of the jaw in multiple myeloma patients: clinical features and risk factors. *J Clin Oncol* 2006, 24:945–952.

49. Lacy MQ, Dispenzieri A, Gertz MA, *et al.*: Mayo Clinic consensus state-ment for the use of bisphosphonates in multiple myeloma. *Mayo Clin Proc* 2006, 81:1047–1053.

50. Kyle RA, Yee GC, Somerfield MR, *et al.*: American Society of Clinical Oncology 2007 clinical practice guideline update on the role of bisphos-phonates in multiple myeloma. *J Clin Oncol* 2007, 25:2464–2472.

51. Catley L, Weisberg E, Kiziltepe T, *et al.*: Aggresome induction by protea-some inhibitor bortezomib and alpha-tubulin hyperacetylation by tubulin deacetylase (TDAC) inhibitor LBH589 are synergistic in myeloma cells. *Blood* 2006, 108:3441–3449.

52. Matsui W, Huff CA, Wang Q, *et al.*: Characterization of clonogenic multiple myeloma cells. *Blood* 2004, 103:2332–2336.

53. Matsui WH, Huff CA, Wang Q, *et al.*: Multiple myeloma (MM) stem cells arise from post-germinal center B cells and are inhibited by rituximab in vitro [abstract]. *Blood* 2003, 102:931a.

54. Matsui WH, Huff CA, Wang Q, *et al.*: Multiple myeloma stem cells and plasma cells display distinct drug sensitivities [abstract]. *Blood* 2004, 104:679a.

55. Alexanian R, Bonnet J, Gehan E, *et al.*: Combination chemotherapy for multiple myeloma. *Cancer* 1972, 30:382–389.

56. Abramson N, Lurie P, Mietlowski WL, *et al.*: Phase III study of intermittent carmustine (BCNU), cyclophosphamide, and prednisone versus inter-mittent melphalan and prednisone in myeloma. *Cancer Treat Rep* 1982, 66:1273–1277.

57. Oken MM, Tsiatis A, Abramson N, *et al.*: Evaluation of intensive (VBMCP) vs standard (MP) therapy for multiple myeloma. *Proc Am Soc Clin Oncol* 1987, 6:203.

58. Bergsagel DE, Bailey AJ, Langley GR, *et al.*: The chemotherapy on plasma-cell myeloma and the incidence of acute leukemia. *N Engl J Med* 1979, 301:743–748.

59. Mateos MV, Hernández JM, Hernández MT, *et al.*: Bortezomib plus mel-phalan and prednisone in elderly untreated patients with multiple myelo-ma: results of a multicenter phase 1/2 study. *Blood* 2006, 108:2165–2172.

60. Mateos MV, Hernández JM, Hernández MT, *et al.*: Bortezomib plus melphalan and prednisone in elderly untreated patients with multiple myeloma: updated time-to-events results and prognostic factors for time to progression. *Haematologica* 2008, 93:560–565.

61. San Miguel JF, Schlag R, Khuageva N, *et al.*: MMY-3002: a phase 3 study comparing bortezomib-melphalan-prednisone (VMP) with melphalan-prednisone (MP) in newly diagnosed multiple myeloma [abstract]. *Blood* 2007, 11:31a.

62. Rajkumar SV, Hayman S, Gertz MA, *et al.*: Combination therapy with tha-lidomide plus dexamethasone for newly diagnosed myeloma. *J Clin Oncol* 2002, 20:4319–4323.

63. Weber D, Rankin K, Gavino M, *et al.*: Thalidomide alone or with dexa-methasone for previously untreated multiple myeloma. *J Clin Oncol* 2003, 21:16–19.

64. Lacy MQ, Gertz MA, Dispenzieri A, *et al.*: Long-term results of response to therapy, time to progression, and survival with lenalidomide plus dexamethasone in newly diagnosed melanoma. *Mayo Clin Proc* 2007, 82:1179–1184.

65. Rajkumar SV, Jacobus S, Callander N, *et al.*: Randomized trial of lenalidomide plus high-dose dexamethasone versus lenalidomide plus low-dose dexamethasone in newly diagnosed myeloma (E4A03): a trial coordinated by the Eastern Cooperative Oncology Group—analysis of response, survival, and outcome [abstract]. *J Clin Oncol* 2008, 26: abstract 8504.

Malignant Effusions in the Chest
Malcolm V. Brock

Under normal physiologic conditions, the pleural space contains approximately 7 to 16 mL of fluid [1]. In patients with malignancy, both the pleural and pericardial space may accumulate fluid that can manifest as dyspnea, chest pain, and exercise intolerance. In dyspnea, this is due to a compromise of pulmonary reserve, whereas reduced cardiac output is the main problem in exercise intolerance. Table 21-1 outlines the common and uncommon presenting signs and symptoms of both of these effusions [2,3].

CLINICAL PRESENTATION

Dyspnea, especially on exertion, is commonly the presenting symptom for pleural effusions observed in about 50% of patients [4]. As the size of the pleural effusion increases, there is a linear and rather predictable progression of associated signs and symptoms. In general, the patient's breathing becomes more rapid, shallow, and restrictive in nature. About 25% of the time, incidental pleural effusions are found radiographically, but patients remain clinically asymptomatic [5]. In contrast to primary pleural tumors, bulky, metastatic, pleural implants are rarely present without a pleural effusion [6].

With pericardial effusions, symptoms such as dyspnea occur in the patient mainly due to the speed of fluid accumulation, the amount of fluid present, and the premorbid condition of the patient's underlying myocardium [2]. More rapidly accumulating pericardial effusions are also more likely to have hemodynamic instability than those forming more gradually. In most cases, malignant pericardial effusions develop over a prolonged period, and large amounts of pericardial fluid can develop in the pericardial space. We often suspect the presence of a pericardial effusion when dyspnea, which was presumed to be related to a pleural effusion, persists after the pleural fluid is drained. In addition, hiccups may be present due to vagal or phrenic nerve irritation, and symptoms such as palpitations, tachycardia, chest discomfort, light-headedness, and even syncope may occur [7].

PATHOPHYSIOLOGY

In any body cavity, fluid accumulates as a result of a disruption in homeostasis between production and clearance of the fluid through the respective space. In benign disease, a large variety of mechanisms are responsible for this disruption, including elevated hydrostatic pressure gradients (transudation) and increased fluid extravasation from vasculature (exudation) [6,8]. On the other hand, malignant pleural and pericardial effusions are not primarily due to an overproduction of fluid, but result mainly from the obstruction and disruption of lymphatic channels caused by myriad malig-

nant cells on the parietal pleura and pericardium, respectively [9]. This is often exacerbated by a reduction in oncotic pressure due to hypoproteinemia in the patient. However, a partial role is played by the increased production of growth factors, which can increase vascular permeability of the diseased pleura and pericardium and result in effusion formation [10,11]. Finally, cancer therapy, such as radiation and chemotherapy, may occasionally cause pleural effusions. A comprehensive list of drugs associated with pleural fluid accumulation can be found at http://www.pneumotox.com [1].

Dyspnea from pleural fluid is due to a restrictive pulmonary physiology mainly because of compressive atelectasis and the fluid's effect on limiting chest wall excursion. The resulting reductions in vital capacity, shunting, and ventilation/perfusion mismatching cause gas-exchange abnormalities [12]. Larger fluid accumulations can even contribute to dyspnea by shifting the mediastinum and inciting a reflex stimulation of the chest wall and lung from altered compliance [12]. Because other contributory causes of dyspnea, such as coexisting pneumonia, compressive atelectasis, pulmonary thromboemboli, adenopathy compressing adjacent pulmonary vasculature, presence of concomitant chylothorax, superior vena cava syndrome, and chest wall inflammation, can all be obscured by large amounts of pleural fluid in the chest, in our practice we emphasize the importance of draining as much fluid as possible during any initial therapeutic thoracentesis to gain insight into these comorbidities (see below).

Similarly, in pericardial fluid accumulations, dyspnea can result from compressive effects on the heart that cause impaired ventricular filling in diastole. This is especially true on the relatively thin-walled, low-pressure right ventricle [13]. This can occur even in the absence of perceptible hemodynamic effects or cardiac tamponade physiology. A normal pericardial space holds about 50 mL of fluid that serves primarily to lubricate the visceral and parietal pericardial surfaces [14]. The stiff parietal pericardium, however, is not elastic enough to accommodate rapid accumulations of small amounts of pericardial fluid and, usually at volumes close to 200 mL, hemodynamic effects are inevitable. However, when pericardial fluid builds gradually, with concomitant stretching of the pericardium, volumes of 1000 to 2000 mL are able to be accommodated [14]. Pericardial effusions may also obscure other associated findings such as ventricular dysfunction, congestive heart failure, or constrictive pericarditic changes.

DIAGNOSTIC ALGORITHMS

As a practical issue, the importance of a detailed history and physical examination is often underappreciated. Patients can provide critical clues not only to the etiology of the fluid, but also the timing of accumulation [15,16]. This gives the clinician reasonable insight regarding possible effective therapeutic modalities before ordering any diagnostic tests. Figures 21-1 and 21-2 outline the recommended diagnostic and treatment algorithms for malignant pleural effusions and malignant pericardial effusions, respectively. These algorithms assume that the patient in question has either a pleural or malignant effusion that is highly suspicious for malignancy and are not meant for patients with a wider differential of benign medical diagnoses.

A plain chest radiograph is often the initial modality for diagnosing malignant pleural effusions and can detect as little as 200 mL of fluid [1]. Often posteroanterior and lateral chest x-rays are supplemented by decubitus chest films to show free-flowing fluid. Other often-used modalities that complement plain films are ultrasound, computed tomography (CT), and magnetic resonance imaging. Ultrasound is very sensitive and can detect very little fluid accumulation. It is most useful, however, in delineating loculated effusions that may not drain adequately through a simple needle aspiration. CT scans are the best modality to view the pleural space diagnostically, especially when more detailed information is needed [17]. A contrast-enhanced CT image of the parietal pleura, for example, may prove useful in differentiating exudative and transudative pleural effusions [18].

Table 21-1. Signs and Symptoms of Malignant Effusions in the Chest

Frequency	Pleural	Pericardial
Common	Dyspnea (exertion)	Dyspnea (exertion)
	Dyspnea (rest)	Dyspnea (rest)
	Cough	Jugular venous distension
	Dullness to percussion	Distant heart sounds
	Egophony	
Uncommon	Cyanosis	Cyanosis
	Anorexia	Peripheral vasoconstriction
	Chest pain	Pulsus paradoxus
		Narrow pulse pressure (Kussmaul's sign)
		Electrical alternans

An echocardiogram is recommended as the best diagnostic modality to view the pericardial space because it not only establishes the presence of fluid, but also detects poor diastolic filling. In our practice, we also rely heavily on the high sensitivity of the CT scan, especially in patients with a large tumor burden around the pericardium and in helping to plan therapeutic approaches. Unlike pleural biopsies, pericardial biopsies to document malignancy in the pericardial space are rarely performed. Surprisingly, many cancer patients who present with pericardial effusions have a nonmalignant cause; the percentage in breast cancer patients is as high as 50% in some series [19].

TUMOR MARKERS

Cytologic analysis using a microscope to distinguish the distinct morphology of malignant cells from a background of large numbers of reactive mesothelial cells and macrophage populations is still the gold standard for diagnosing a malignant pleural effusion. Yet, reactive hyperactive meso-

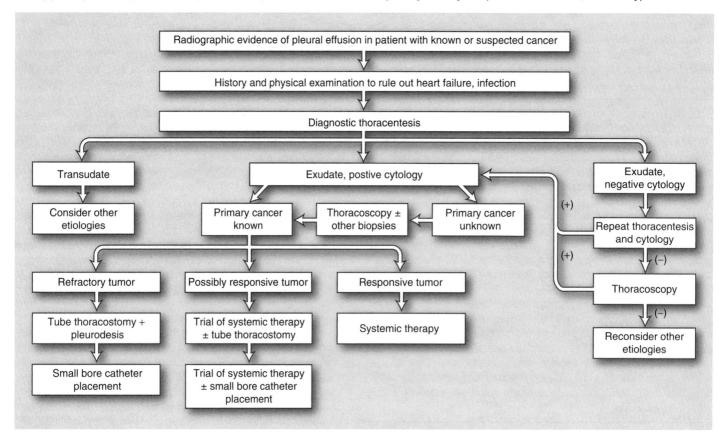

Figure 21-1. Approach to the diagnosis and therapy of malignant pleural effusion. (*Adapted from* Ruckdeschel [74].)

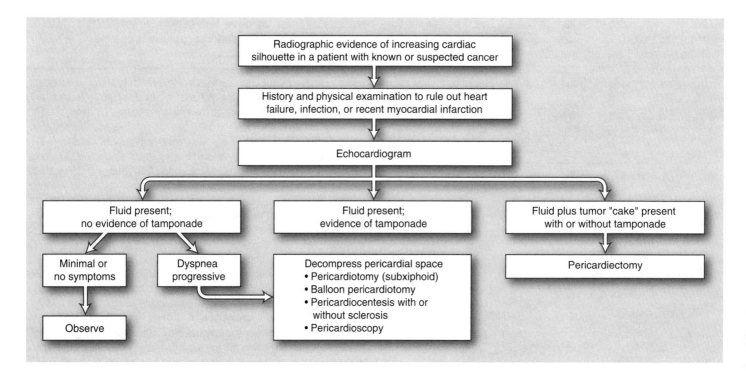

Figure 21-2. Approach to the diagnosis of malignant pericardial effusion.

thelial cells may undergo cytologic alterations and mimic neoplastic cells, especially after treatment with drugs, chemotherapy, or radiation [20–23]. In fact, the diagnostic yield of pleural fluid cytology depends on the tumor type, tumor burden, and number of needle aspirations performed [12]. A good rule-of-thumb is that after the first thoracentesis, cytology is positive 60% of the time; this increases to 90%, and then the sensitivity abruptly plateaus after the second aspiration procedure [4,6,24,25]. Debates regarding removing larger volumes of fluid to augment the sensitivity of cytology are still unresolved, and little is known about any sensitivity differences between cytologically examining less than 50 mL or more than 1 L of fluid [26].

Many ancillary modalities aimed at improving cytologic analyses using various tumor markers have been described. As a practical issue, no method of molecular detection is being used routinely to augment the sensitivity of cytology because of cost. On a case-by-case basis, immunohistochemistry is perhaps the most commonly used ancillary study to cytologic analysis of malignant pleural effusions. Although this topic is comprehensively reviewed elsewhere [27,28], it is sufficient to say that challenges still include optimizing cytology specimen processing, standardizing not only the procedure but also the interpretation of the results, and improving current antibody panels to discriminate between benign and malignant disease. There is no doubt that with continued technological innovations and new antigen validation, the reliability and reproducibility of immunohistochemistry will constantly be enhanced. Other techniques looking at protein have used fluorescent in situ hybridization (FISH) to document aneuploidy [29,30] and gene-specific probes to enhance the FISH analysis to detect gene amplification [28].

Because cytologic analysis is theoretically futile in cell-free pleural fluid, investigators have also probed the fluid for DNA markers. Early work using flow cytometry failed to enhance the sensitivity and specificity of traditional approaches [25,31], and microsatellite markers have been equivocal in their ability to distinguish reliably between benign and malignant effusions [32,33].

Recently, epigenetic markers have been used to discriminate between benign and malignant disease [34–38]. Although these studies have had somewhat limited success diagnostically to discriminate malignancy, epigenetic analysis of pleural fluid has been less effective as a prognostic tool to predict survival outcome in these patients [39]. In addition to DNA, RNA is also a potential substrate. Studies using reverse transcription-polymerase chain reaction have similarly found that this substrate may have some potential as an ancillary method to discriminate between benign and malignant pleural effusions [40–42]. In contrast to DNA, the lack of stability of RNA makes it imperative that there be strict standardization of tissue handling, biospecimen processing, and timely specimen acquisition. At present, these remain considerable challenges even at large academic medical centers.

THERAPY

Best practice guidelines have been produced for the management of malignant pleural effusions [43]. As a general principle, these guidelines advocate:

1. Intervention for malignant pleural effusions mainly after the development of symptoms such as dyspnea, exercise intolerance and/or chest pain.
2. Observation of patients with asymptomatic pleural effusions.
3. Choice of the type of therapeutic modality based on the patient's performance status, expected survival, and probable response of the known primary tumor to systemic treatment.
4. In patients with good performance status and reasonable expected survival (usually > 6 months is our usual practice guideline at our institution), the use of aggressive, often invasive therapies to obliterate the pleural space and thus prevent recurrence of the effusions.
5. In patients with poor performance status and limited expected survival, less invasive therapies aimed at avoiding long hospitalizations and prolonged iatrogenic pain.

Using these guidelines, most thoracic surgeons and pulmonologists have employed a wide range of conventional standard therapeutic modali-

ties from simple repetitive aspiration of the effusion for those patients who are moribund to pleuroperitoneal shunting, the instillation of sclerosing agents via thoracostomy or thoracoscopy, and pleurectomy.

SIMPLE THORACENTESIS

As illustrated in Figure 21-1, in our practice with rare exception, we employ thoracentesis as not only an important part in diagnosis, but also the first step in the treatment of almost all malignant pleural effusions. Because the pleural space is not obliterated by this procedure, the mean recurrence interval is within 4.2 days, and the overall recurrence rate is 98% within 30 days [44]. Our intent in performing these procedures is to ascertain vital information for surgical decision-making during this initial simple but critical procedure. Thoracentesis not only gives the patient a brief respite from the symptoms of pleural effusions, but also confirms the etiology of the effusion, ascertains whether there is free fluid, loculated fluid, or gelatinous material in the pleural space, and provides information about the ability of the lung to reexpand completely after fluid evacuation. If the pleural space is totally obscured by fluid or other debris, noninvasive radiologic exams such as chest CT scans or ultrasound are limited in their ability to provide this information. We therefore strongly advocate drainage of as much as 1 to 1.5 L at the initial thoracentesis, which then allows subsequent radiographic examinations to reveal information pertinent for further decisions about therapy. It is not uncommon in our practice to perform a thoracentesis followed almost immediately by a chest CT to document the heretofore obscured chest pathology. On nonsurgical services, however, many physicians only aspirate 200 to 300 mL at best, in a so-called "diagnostic thoracentesis." This is done presumably to avoid the sudden onset of pulmonary edema due to rapid lung reexpansion. Although unilateral reexpansion pulmonary edema is associated with rapid evacuation of more than 1.5 L of pleural fluid surrounding a chronically collapsed lung [45], this complication is uncommon [46,47]. We instead perform a "therapeutic thoracentesis," and avoid reexpansion pulmonary edema by aspirating the first liter of fluid slowly then continuing with any further evacuation of fluid from the chest after a brief pause of 20 to 30 minutes. If the patient exhibits any excessive coughing or pleuritic chest pain, the procedure is immediately terminated, oxygen is administered, the patient is placed on a monitor, and a chest radiograph is obtained. Residual fluid can always be aspirated at a later date.

In moribund patients such as those with acute life-threatening problems and with poor performance status such as a Karnofsky score below 30% [48], repeated thoracentesis is often advocated. However, repeated thoracentesis has substantial risks, including hypoproteinemia, empyema, pneumothorax, and bronchopleural fistula; it can also produce intrathoracic loculations of pleural fluid. Finally, thoracentesis can have the added advantage of being a modality through which chemical pleurodesis can be administered, although generally this is thought to be more effective when done with tube thoracostomy.

TUBE THORACOSTOMY

In terms of invasiveness, the next step in therapeutic management has conventionally been the use of a large-bore tube thoracostomy, either at the bedside under intravenous sedation with local analgesic infiltration or in the operating room [28–32]. As with simple thoracentesis, in our practice we are mindful of the potential for reexpansion pulmonary edema, and clamp the tube after 1.0 L of fluid has been evacuated, wait for 20 to 30 minutes, and then gradually drain any residual fluid. We place the chest tube to wall suction for at least 24 hours, obtain serial chest radiographs to document the underlying chest pathology, and keep a careful record of all chest drainage.

BEDSIDE PLEURODESIS WITH A SCLEROSING AGENT

Performance of a therapeutic aspiration or complete drainage of the chest with a large-bore catheter and then careful review of a chest radiograph is critical to ensure the success of chemical pleurodesis. This is because a completely reexpanded lung assumes that the parietal and visceral pleura can fully appose, which is essential for chemical pleurodesis to work. If the lung expands but the chest tube drainage persists over 200 mL per 24 hours, then this fluid may also impede pleural-to-pleural apposition. Therefore, we perform chemical pleurodesis when the chest tube output is less than 200 mL per 24 hours; usually talc is the preferred sclerosing agent. Median hospitalization for patients with tube thoracostomy and successful pleurodesis is approximately 6 days [15,49,50]. Tube thoracostomy without chemical pleurodesis almost invariably fails, with a recurrence rate of 60% to 100% [51].

CHOICE OF SCLEROSING AGENT

Sclerosants primarily act by acutely injuring the pleura, with resulting pleural inflammation, fibrosis, and ultimately pleurodesis. Many sclerosants as well as cytotoxic agents are available to scar the pleura, including antibiotics such as bleomycin, doxycycline, and tetracycline. However, talc is the agent of choice due to its efficacy (> 90% success rate), low cost, and availability [52]. It is convenient to use as it can be administered as a suspension (talc slurry) at the bedside or insufflated during thoracoscopy. However, talc has many adverse effects, including respiratory failure, acute respiratory distress syndrome, and even death [52,53]. A large, randomized controlled trial of talc insufflation versus talc poudrage documented incidences of respiratory failure of 4% and 8%, respectively [54].

PLEURECTOMY

Today, pleurectomy is largely anachronistic. Its high operative morbidity and mortality cannot be justified as a palliative measure since alternative modern therapies have much lower morbidity and mortality rates. Our preferred indication was in a patient who had excellent performance status, a long expected survival, and a diagnosis of trapped lungs.

SMALL-BORE TUNNELED PLEURAL CATHETER SYSTEMS

The recent development and more widespread use of tunneled pleural catheter systems, which allow intermittent home drainage, is establishing new practice patterns and treatment variations [15]. Standard chest tubes limit patient mobility, and the associated pain can be so debilitating that routine intravenous patient-controlled narcotic analgesia is recommended for as long as the chest tubes remain in place. In the few prospective and retrospective studies available, the smaller catheters (10–20 Fr) seem to be less painful and thus better tolerated, have fewer short- or long-term complications, and show no substantial differences in patient outcomes [55–64]. In the United States, the most commonly used small-bore catheter is the Pleurx catheter (Denver Biomedical, Inc., Golden, CO), a 24-inch long, 15.5-Fr silicone tube. It has an innovative one-way valve to allow vacuum drainage and a polyester cuff that allows tunneling under the skin before the catheter enters the pleural space to reduce infection. In addition, the patient directs his or her own therapy as an outpatient at home, draining the effusion via the catheter whenever he/she becomes symptomatic. The involvement of the patient's family and caregivers with the logistics of the pleural drainage has also been viewed as a benefit in these terminally ill patients [65].

The Pleurx catheter was initially used as a second-line therapy in patients with recurrent or recalcitrant pleural effusions or in patients too debilitated for talc. However, continued accumulating data from published series as well as positive patient reviews of the catheters are changing the practice of many pulmonologists and thoracic surgeons. A perceptible shift is now occurring in many clinical practices so that these small-bore catheters are being offered as first-line therapy for the definitive treatment of malignant pleural effusions. Although there are currently no published, randomized clinical trials comparing the gold standard of talc slurry/talc insufflation with tunneled pleural catheters, there is a burgeoning opinion that the two treatment modalities—especially vis-a-vis symptom control rates in patients—are at least comparable [64]. For the time being, the most constructive opinion is probably to view these two therapies (talc pleurodesis and tunneled catheter placement) as complementary modalities rather than competing therapies [66]. In general, the chronic, small-bore indwelling pleural catheters require no sclerosant infusion and its attendant respiratory failure, allow patients to leave the hospital within a median of 24 hours

of insertion, and are very well tolerated by patients at home. In addition, local inflammatory changes caused by the tumor or the catheter itself are sufficient to cause autopleurodesis without sclerosant. Rates of spontaneous pleurodesis in patients with these catheters are approximately 40% in most series at about 1 month after discharge [55,56,64]. Patients achieving autopleurodesis have a need for repeat ipsilateral procedures only about 9% of the time [64]. Most patient difficulties are relatively minor and mainly involve skin cellulites and frequent changes of the drainage bottles. Empyema is the most severe complication; however, it is relatively infrequent (~ 3.2% incidence) [63,64]. Relative contraindications of these small-bore catheter systems include insertions in patients who are immunoincompetent, in patients who lack the needed financial sources to secure the necessary outpatient vacuum supplies, and in patients who lack a strong social support network, such as the homeless.

PATIENTS WITH TRAPPED LUNG

If the effusion is longstanding, loculated as a result of inflammation or infection, or is encased by extensive tumor involvement, the lung can become trapped (defined as > 25% of the chest cavity with pleural dead space). Trapped lung cannot expand, and thus there is no pleural-to-pleura apposition. This leaves pleural dead space that will rapidly reaccumulate fluid and thwart attempts at pleurodesis with any sclerosant. In fact, trapped lung occurs in about 30% of patients with malignant pleural effusions [54]. Conventionally, pleuroperitoneal shunts, such as the Denver shunt (Codman and Shurtleff, Randolph, MA), were placed as an alternative [67]. These shunts are placed both in the pleural and peritoneal spaces, and work by actively pumping a subcutaneous pumping chamber, often up to 25 times every 4 hours. In addition to patient compliance being an important issue [68], there was always the concomitant risk of the shunt occluding from fibrin or blood [69]. Patients with a trapped lung are often difficult management problems, but increasingly small-bore tunneled catheters are being used to handle these loculated effusions [54,63,70].

THORACOSCOPY

A more invasive approach used primarily as a therapeutic tool, and preferred in our practice in patients with good performance status with an expected survival of more than 6 months, is thoracoscopy. Good performance status is a requirement because in addition to general anesthesia, these patients are all subjected to selective one-lung ventilation [71]. With modern optics intraoperatively, thoracoscopy is an excellent diagnostic modality. It provides magnified, panoramic views of the hemithorax, allowing the surgeon to collect copious pleural fluid for cytologic examination, obtain an adequate pleural biopsy to document malignancy, and determine the extent of pleural metastases as well as the degree of encasement of the lung by tumor. Therapeutically, it also allows various options for management, including decortication, pleurectomy, mechanical and chemical pleurodesis, and visual positioning of drainage tubes [52]. Again, the abiding surgical principles are to relieve the lung from adhesions and loculations so that complete lung reexpansion is possible and to ensure that visceral pleura to parietal pleural apposition is the operative end result. Almost invariably, the final act in the procedure involves instillation of talc or more rarely mechanical abrasion. We prefer to handle bilateral effusions during the same operative procedure, performing each side sequentially. The operative mortality for thoracoscopy and pleurodesis in patients with malignant pleural effusions is approximately 5% [71–73].

PERICARDIAL EFFUSIONS

In our practice, we do not routinely treat asymptomatic patients even if the pericardial fluid is thought highly suspicious for cancer. A "watchful waiting" approach is advocated, which involves monitoring the patient's symptoms in an effort to avert cardiac tamponade physiology. Like pleural effusions, management of pericardial effusions is often initiated with a simple needle aspiration of fluid. This should be done in a cardiac catheterization laboratory environment with the appropriate fluoroscopic, electrocardiographic, and echocardiographic guidance. A multi-holed pericardial drain is also inserted during this procedure and removed once drainage has tapered to less than 25 mL over a 24-hour period [13]. Simple drainage in this manner can be effective in a majority of patients [69]. Further treatment primarily involves sclerotherapy or creating a pericardial window either by thoracoscopy or by balloon pericardiotomy.

In summary, both pleural and pericardial effusions in malignancy are signs of terminal disease. The clinician should make every effort to substantiate the diagnosis of malignancy as the etiology of fluid accumulation, and choose a timely treatment that is palliative, suitable for the particular patient, and preventive of fluid reaccumulation. Finally, the clinician must at all times be sensitive to the balance needed between subjecting these patients to the rigors of palliative care while preserving the quality of their remaining days.

REFERENCES

1. Froudarakis ME: Diagnostic work-up of pleural effusions. *Respiration* 2008, 75:4–13.

2. Mills AS, Graeber GM, Nelson MG: Therapy of malignant tumors involving the heart and pericardium. In *Thoracic Oncology,* edn 2. Edited by Roth J, Ruckdeschel J, Weisenburger T. Philadelphia: WB Saunders; 1995:492–513.

3. Moores D, Ruckdeschel J: Pleural effusions in patients with malignancy. In *Thoracic Oncology,* edn 2. Edited by Roth J, Ruckdeschel J, Weisenburger T. Philadelphia: WB Saunders; 1995:556–566.

4. Antony VB, Loddenkemper R, Astoul P, *et al.*: Management of malignant pleural effusions. *Eur Respir J* 2001, 18:402–419.

5. Qureshi NR, Gleeson FV: Imaging of pleural disease. *Clin Chest Med* 2006, 27:193–213.

6. Sahn S: Malignant pleural effusion. In *Fishman's Pulmonary Diseases and Disorders,* edn 3. Edited by Fishman AP, Elias JA, Fishman JA, *et al.* New York: McGraw-Hill; 1998:1429–1438.

7. Spodick D: Pericardial diseases. In *Braunwald's Heart Disease: A Textbook of Cardiovascular Medicine,* edn 6. Edited by Braunwald E, Zipes DP, Libby P. Philadelphia: WB Saunders; 2001.

8. Miserocchi G: Physiology and pathophysiology of pleural fluid turnover. *Eur Respir J* 1997, 10:219–225.

9. Antunes G, Neville E: Management of malignant pleural effusions. *Thorax* 2000, 55:981–983.

10. Cheng D, Rodriguez RM, Perkett EA, *et al.*: Vascular endothelial growth factor in pleural fluid. *Chest* 1999, 116:760–765.

11. Kraft A, Weindel K, Ochs A, *et al.*: Vascular endothelial growth factor in the sera and effusions of patients with malignant and nonmalignant disease. *Cancer* 1999, 85:178–187.

12. Yung RC, Brock MV: Diagnosis and management of pleural metastases in breast cancer. In *The Breast: Comprehensive Management of Benign and Malignant Disorders,* vol 2. Edited by Bland KI, Copeland EM. Saint Louis: WB Saunders; 2004:1395–1406.

13. Aversano T: Management of pericardial metastases in breast cancer. In *The Breast: Comprehensive Management of Benign and Malignant Disorders,* vol 2. Edited by Bland KI, Copeland EM. Saint Louis: WB Saunders; 2004:1425–1431.

14. Karam N, Patel P, de Filippi C: Diagnosis and management of chronic pericardial effusions. *Am J Med Sci* 2001, 322:79–87.

15. Lee YC, Baumann MH, Maskell NA, *et al.*: Pleurodesis practice for malignant pleural effusions in five English-speaking countries: survey of pulmonologists. *Chest* 2003, 124:2229–2238.

16. Rahman NM, Chapman SJ, Davies RJ: Pleural effusion: a structured approach to care. *Br Med Bull* 2004, 72:31–47.

17. McLoud TC, Flower CD: Imaging the pleura: sonography, CT, and MR imaging. *AJR Am J Roentgenol* 1991, 156:1145–1153.

18. Aquino SL, Webb WR, Gushiken BJ: Pleural exudates and transudates: diagnosis with contrast-enhanced CT. *Radiology* 1994, 192:803–808.

19. Buck M, Ingle JN, Giuliani ER, *et al.*: Pericardial effusion in women with breast cancer. *Cancer* 1987, 60:263–269.

20. Koss L: Effusions. In *Diagnostic Cytology and its Histopathologic Bases.* Philadelphia: JB Lippincott; 1961:272–302.

21. Kho-Duffin J, Tao LC, Cramer H, *et al.*: Cytologic diagnosis of malignant mesothelioma, with particular emphasis on the epithelial noncohesive cell type. *Diagn Cytopathol* 1999, 20:57–62.

22. Bibbo M: Pleural, peritoneal, and pericardial fluids. In *Comprehensive Cytopathology.* Edited by Naylor B. Philadelphia: WB Saunders; 1997:551–621.

23. Tao LC: *Cytopathology of Malignant Effusions.* Chicago: ASCP Press; 1996.

24. Fenton KN, Richardson JD: Diagnosis and management of malignant pleural effusions. *Am J Surg* 1995, 170:69–74.

25. Joseph MG, Banerjee D, Harris P, *et al.*: Multiparameter flow cytometric DNA analysis of effusions: a prospective study of 36 cases compared with routine cytology and immunohistochemistry. *Mod Pathol* 1995, 8:686–693.

26. Sallach SM, Sallach JA, Vasquez E, *et al.*: Volume of pleural fluid required for diagnosis of pleural malignancy. *Chest* 2002, 122:1913–1917.

27. Fetsch PA, Abati A: Immunocytochemistry in effusion cytology: a contemporary review. *Cancer* 2001, 93:293–308.

28. Davidson B, Risberg B, Reich R, Berner A: Effusion cytology in ovarian cancer: new molecular methods as aids to diagnosis and prognosis. *Clin Lab Med* 2003, 23:729–754, viii.

29. Roka S, Fiegl M, Zojer N, *et al.*: Aneuploidy of chromosome 8 as detected by interphase fluorescence in situ hybridization is a recurrent finding in primary and metastatic breast cancer. *Breast Cancer Res Treat* 1998, 48:125–133.

30. Zojer N, Fiegl M, Mullauer L, *et al.*: Chromosomal imbalances in primary and metastatic pancreatic carcinoma as detected by interphase cytogenetics: basic findings and clinical aspects. *Br J Cancer* 1998, 77:1337–1342.

31. Frierson HF Jr, Mills SE, Legier JF: Flow cytometric analysis of ploidy in immunohistochemically confirmed examples of malignant epithelial mesothelioma. *Am J Clin Pathol* 1988, 90:240–243.

32. Woenckhaus M, Grepmeier U, Werner B, *et al.*: Microsatellite analysis of pleural supernatants could increase sensitivity of pleural fluid cytology. *J Mol Diagn* 2005, 7:517–524.

33. Economidou F, Tzortzaki EG, Schiza S, *et al.*: Microsatellite DNA analysis does not distinguish malignant from benign pleural effusions. *Oncol Rep* 2007, 18:1507–1512.

34. Ahrendt SA, Yang SC, Wu L, *et al.*: Molecular assessment of lymph nodes in patients with resected stage I non-small cell lung cancer: preliminary results of a prospective study. *J Thorac Cardiovasc Surg* 2002, 123:466–473; discussion 473–474.

35. Gibson M, Brock MV, Montgomery E, *et al.*: Pathologic downstaging with taxane-based neoadjuvant chemotherapy correlates with increased survival in patients with locally advanced esophageal cancer [ASCO abstract]. *J Clin Oncol* 2005, 23(16S):4039.

36. Katayama H, Hiraki A, Aoe K, *et al.*: Aberrant promoter methylation in pleural fluid DNA for diagnosis of malignant pleural effusion. *Int J Cancer* 2007, 120:2191–2195.

37. Benlloch S, Galbis-Caravajal JM, Martin C, *et al.*: Potential diagnostic value of methylation profile in pleural fluid and serum from cancer patients with pleural effusion. *Cancer* 2006, 107:1859–1865.

38. Chen ML, Chang JH, Yeh KT, *et al.*: Epigenetic changes in tumor suppressor genes, P15, P16, APC-3 and E-cadherin in body fluid. *Kaohsiung J Med Sci* 2007, 23:498–503.

39. Katayama H, Hiraki A, Fujiwara K, *et al.*: Aberrant promoter methylation profile in pleural fluid DNA and clinicopathological factors in patients with non-small cell lung cancer. *Asian Pac J Cancer Prev* 2007, 8:221–224.

40. Saito T, Kobayashi M, Harada R, *et al.*: Sensitive detection of small cell lung carcinoma cells by reverse transcriptase-polymerase chain reaction for prepro-gastrin-releasing peptide mRNA. *Cancer* 2003, 97:2504–2511.

41. Grunewald K, Haun M, Fiegl M, *et al.*: Mammaglobin expression in gynecologic malignancies and malignant effusions detected by nested reverse transcriptase-polymerase chain reaction. *Lab Invest* 2002, 82:1147–1153.

42. Yu CJ, Shew JY, Liaw YS, *et al.*: Application of mucin quantitative competitive reverse transcription polymerase chain reaction in assisting the diagnosis of malignant pleural effusion. *Am J Respir Crit Care Med* 2001, 164:1312–1318.

43. Antunes G, Neville E, Duffy J, Ali N: BTS guidelines for the management of malignant pleural effusions. *Thorax* 2003, 58(Suppl 2):ii29–ii38.

44. Whittle J, Steinberg EP, Anderson GF, Herbert R: Use of Medicare claims data to evaluate outcomes in elderly patients undergoing lung resection for lung cancer. *Chest* 1991, 100:729–734.

45. Ratliff JL, Chavez CM, Jamchuk A, *et al.*: Re-expansion pulmonary edema. *Chest* 1973, 64:654–656.

46. Tarver RD, Broderick LS, Conces DJ Jr: Reexpansion pulmonary edema. *J Thorac Imaging* 1996, 11:198–209.

47. Mahfood S, Hix WR, Aaron BL, *et al.*: Reexpansion pulmonary edema. *Ann Thorac Surg* 1988, 45:340–345.

48. Karnofsky DA, Burchenal JH: The clinical evaluation of chemotherapeutic agents in cancer. In *Evaluation of Chemotherapeutic Agents.* Edited by MacLeod CM. New York: Columbia University Press; 1949:191–205.

49. Zimmer PW, Hill M, Casey K, *et al.*: Prospective randomized trial of talc slurry vs bleomycin in pleurodesis for symptomatic malignant pleural effusions. *Chest* 1997, 112:430–434.

50. Yim AP, Chan AT, Lee TW, *et al.*: Thoracoscopic talc insufflation versus talc slurry for symptomatic malignant pleural effusion. *Ann Thorac Surg* 1996, 62:1655–1658.

51. Izbicki R, Weyhing BT III, Baker L, *et al.*: Pleural effusion in cancer patients. A prospective randomized study of pleural drainage with the addition of radioactive phosphorus to the pleural space vs. pleural drainage alone. *Cancer* 1975, 36:1511–1518.

52. Yim AP, Chung SS, Lee TW, *et al.*: Thoracoscopic management of malignant pleural effusions. *Chest* 1996, 109:1234–1238.

53. Bouchama A, Chastre J, Gaudichet A, *et al.*: Acute pneumonitis with bilateral pleural effusion after talc pleurodesis. *Chest* 1984, 86:795–797.

54. Dresler CM, Olak J, Herndon JE II, *et al.*: Phase III Intergroup study of talc poudrage vs talc slurry sclerosis for malignant pleural effusion. *Chest* 2005, 127:909–915.

55. Putnam JB Jr, Light RW, Rodriguez RM, *et al.*: A randomized comparison of indwelling pleural catheter and doxycycline pleurodesis in the management of malignant pleural effusions. *Cancer* 1999, 86:1992–1999.

56. Putnam JB Jr, Walsh GL, Swisher SG, *et al.*: Outpatient management of malignant pleural effusion by a chronic indwelling pleural catheter. *Ann Thorac Surg* 2000, 69:369–375.

57. Reinhold C, Illescas FF, Atri M, Bret PM: Treatment of pleural effusions and pneumothorax with catheters placed percutaneously under imaging guidance. *AJR Am J Roentgenol* 1989, 152:1189–1191.

58. Morrison MC, Mueller PR, Lee MJ, *et al.*: Sclerotherapy of malignant pleural effusion through sonographically placed small-bore catheters. *AJR Am J Roentgenol* 1992, 158:41–43.

59. Parker LA, Charnock GC, Delany DJ: Small bore catheter drainage and sclerotherapy for malignant pleural effusions. *Cancer* 1989, 64:1218–1221.

60. Clementsen P, Evald T, Grode G, *et al.*: Treatment of malignant pleural effusion: pleurodesis using a small percutaneous catheter. A prospective randomized study. *Respir Med* 1998, 92:593–596.

61. Sahin U, Unlu M, Akkaya A, Ornek Z: The value of small-bore catheter thoracostomy in the treatment of malignant pleural effusions. *Respiration* 2001, 68:501–505.

62. Parulekar W, Di Primio G, Matzinger F, *et al.*: Use of small-bore vs large-bore chest tubes for treatment of malignant pleural effusions. *Chest* 2001, 120:19–25.

63. Tremblay A, Michaud G: Single-center experience with 250 tunnelled pleural catheter insertions for malignant pleural effusion. *Chest* 2006, 129:362–368.

64. Stather DR, Tremblay A: Use of tunneled pleural catheters for outpatient treatment of malignant pleural effusions. *Curr Opin Pulm Med* 2007, 13:328–333.

65. Warren W: Talc pleurodesis for malignant pleural effusions is preferred over the Pleurx catheter (contrary position). *Ann Surg Oncol* 2007, 14:2700–2701.

66. Antevil JL, Putnam JB Jr: Talc pleurodesis for malignant effusions is preferred over the Pleurx catheter (pro position). *Ann Surg Oncol* 2007, 14:2698–2699.

67. Lee KA, Harvey JC, Reich H, Beattie EJ: Management of malignant pleural effusions with pleuroperitoneal shunting. *J Am Coll Surg* 1994, 178:586–588.

68. Rusch VW: Pleural effusion: benign and malignant. In *Thoracic Surgery,* edn 2. Edited by Pearson FG, Cooper JD, Deslauriers J, *et al.* Philadelphia: Churchill Livingstone; 2002:1157–1170.

69. Tsang TS, Seward JB, Barnes ME, *et al.*: Outcomes of primary and secondary treatment of pericardial effusion in patients with malignancy. *Mayo Clin Proc* 2000, 75:248–253.

70. Pien GW, Gant MJ, Washam CL, Sterman DH: Use of an implantable pleural catheter for trapped lung syndrome in patients with malignant pleural effusion. *Chest* 2001, 119:1641–1646.

71. Keller SM: Current and future therapy for malignant pleural effusion. *Chest* 1993, 103:63S–67S.

72. Ohri SK, Oswal SK, Townsend ER, Fountain SW: Early and late outcome after diagnostic thoracoscopy and talc pleurodesis. *Ann Thorac Surg* 1992, 53:1038–1041.

73. Schulze M, Boehle AS, Kurdow R, *et al.*: Effective treatment of malignant pleural effusion by minimal invasive thoracic surgery: thoracoscopic talc pleurodesis and pleuroperitoneal shunts in 101 patients. *Ann Thorac Surg* 2001, 71:1809–1812.

74. RuckdeschelJC: Management of malignant pleural effusion: an overview. *Semin Oncol* 1988, 15(Suppl):24–28.

Despite the sophisticated diagnostic tools available to establish the diagnosis of human neoplasia, oncologists frequently are asked to evaluate and treat a subset of patients with metastatic cancer in whom detailed investigations fail to identify a primary anatomic site. In patients who are diagnosed with cancer, the reported prevalence of carcinoma of unknown primary (CUP) varies from 0.5% to 9% depending upon the practice setting and the definition used [1,2]. In 2007, an estimated 32,100 cases of CUP were diagnosed in the United States [3]. Because identification of the primary has formed the basis for predicting the expected behavior and assigning appropriate therapy of malignant diseases, the absence of a primary poses a major challenge. The inability to identify a primary generates anxiety for the patient, who may believe that the physician's evaluation has been inadequate or that the prognosis would be improved if a primary could be established.

The definition of CUP has not been standardized, varying in published reports primarily with regard to the extent of evaluation required to accept this diagnosis. A recent definition identifies patients with CUP as those who have a biopsy-proven malignancy for which the anatomic origin remains unidentified after the following have been performed: history and physical examination, including breast palpation and pelvic examination in women and testicular and prostate examination in men; laboratory studies, including liver and renal function tests; hemogram; Hemoccult (Beckman Coulter, Inc., Fullerton, CA) fecal occult blood test; chest radiograph; computed tomography (CT) of the abdomen and pelvis; and mammography in women. Only positive findings on this initial evaluation are then investigated in detail [4,5]. Depending on the clinical situation, additional studies might include sputum cytology, CT of the chest, breast ultrasonography, or gastrointestinal endoscopy.

In practice, however, considerable controversy surrounds the evaluation of patients with CUP. It is clear that despite understanding their limitations, unnecessary studies are often carried out because treatment planning is based on both the anatomic origin and the histologic type of the malignancy. The arguments for an exhaustive versus directed evaluation of patients with CUP have been outlined by many authors [6–16]. The most effective strategy takes into account the projected natural history and duration of survival and provides a reasonable probability of locating the primary anatomic site without compromising quality of life with difficult and time-consuming diagnostic studies. The overall goal is to identify the treatable patient subsets or occult primaries through a rapid, rational, and calculated approach.

Several studies have evaluated whether [18F]fluoro-2-deoxy-D-glucose (FDG) positron emission tomography (PET) contributes to the diagnostic evaluation of CUP. The question is whether PET scanning would result in a more efficient, less costly, and potentially less invasive work-up that would increase the likelihood of identifying the primary tumor or tumors in a timely manner. The series were small (15–53 patients) and focused primarily on patients with cervical or supraclavicular lymphadenopathy. Because patients with metastatic lymph nodes in these regions often are treated empirically with extensive radiotherapy for a primary head and neck tumor, or conversely may be eligible for radical neck resection, this subset in particular may benefit from additional testing to identify the primary.

In general, PET was able to consistently visualize known metastatic lesions and demonstrated true positive primary tumor identification rates of 45% [17], 37.8% [18], and 47% [19]. False-positive rates were as high as 20%. Another study of 13 patients showed no improved rate of identification of squamous carcinomas of the neck compared with panendoscopy [20]. Recent studies using PET/CT scans for detection of CUP reported identification of the primary tumor in 33% to 57% of patients [21–23]. There is great variability in tissue-specific tracer uptake rates as well as interpatient glucose metabolism, which may contribute to test variability. Further, although PET/CT are promising diagnostic modalities, it is not clear whether identification of the primary and, thus, potentially more directed therapy, will lead to improved survival in patients with CUP.

BIOLOGIC ASPECTS

Carcinomas of unknown primary are heterogeneous and composed of numerous underlying primary cancers that remain occult during observation of the patient. This concept is supported by studies showing that a detailed postmortem anatomic investigation frequently establishes a primary in patients [6,24]. However, even after postmortem examinations, the primary tumor is not identified in 20% to 50% of patients [25–27]. Detailed clinical and biochemical study of CUP cells, although heterogeneous in their origins, may represent a valuable resource for understanding fundamental aspects of the metastatic phenotype [28–31]. As is the case for the specific, well-defined primary neoplasms discussed elsewhere in this book, it is the phenomenon of metastasis, as purely exemplified by the patient with CUP, that causes the majority of cancer deaths.

The fact that numerous occult anatomic sites can give rise to carcinomas that present with only metastatic disease supports the possibility that specific interactions of genetic and environmental insults could give rise to genomic and biochemical changes that lead to the early development of the metastatic phenotype without the associated changes supporting local growth in the organ of origin [32]. Although this concept must be considered highly speculative, it is a hypothesis that can be tested through analysis of available biomarkers, such as oncogenes and tumor suppressor genes, which have been characterized for cancers with known anatomic origins, such as lung, pancreatic, breast, and colorectal carcinomas. The absence of genetic changes typical for malignancies with established primaries, or the presence of unusual variants of known genetic alterations supports this hypothesis.

Whether the biology of CUP is fundamentally different from known primary carcinoma with systemic metastases remains controversial. Nystrom *et al.* [33] have argued that the distribution of metastatic sites in patients with CUP in which the primary subsequently is found is sufficiently different from known primary carcinoma to support the hypothesis that CUP is biologically unique. A preliminary analysis of a consecutive series of CUP patients showed that there are no significant differences in the patterns of metastases [34], although overall survival for CUP patients was inferior to patients in whom the primary was found [5]. Continued study of CUP patients is necessary to resolve this controversy. The reason the primary organ site cannot be diagnosed remains unknown. Previous investigators have speculated that the tumor may remain below the limits of clinical or radiographic detection or that it spontaneously regressed [32]. Another possibility is that a clinically detectable primary never develops because of the development of specific genetic changes that support metastatic over local growth.

PATHOLOGY

An early, accurate pathologic assessment of biopsy material is essential in the initial evaluation of the patient with suspected CUP. In this context, the pathologist usually is able to confirm that the lesion is neoplastic and may be able to judge if the lesion is primary or metastatic. In some situations, however, it may be impossible to determine if the tumor has arisen from the biopsied organ site. This problem often complicates the cytologic evaluation of fine-needle aspirate specimens and emphasizes the need for close communication between the clinician and the pathologist.

The initial pathologic assessment of the biopsied material usually is initiated by light microscopic examination of paraffin sections stained with hematoxylin and eosin. Based on established cytologic criteria [35], the pathologist usually can place the tumor into broad groups, such as carcinoma, sarcoma, or lymphoma. Additionally, many carcinomas are immediately recognized as manifesting at least some glandular differentiation (adenocarcinoma). When glandular differentiation is absent, patients with CUP frequently are diagnosed with poorly differentiated or undifferentiated carcinoma. Other specimens lack any cytologically distinguishing features, in which case a diagnosis of an undifferentiated malignancy is reported. In these groups with poorly differentiated carcinoma, undifferentiated carcinoma, or undifferentiated malignancy, additional pathologic studies, including histochemistry, immunohistochemistry, and electron microscopy, are employed most frequently and productively. A vast array of tissue markers is available; however, in practice, regular use is limited to a few [36]. Emphasis should be placed on the identification of patients with lymphoma because these neoplasms are curable with therapy. Increasingly, pathologists are using cytokeratin immunohistochemical stains to distinguish between neoplasms of epithelial origin as discussed in detail by Lagendijk *et al.* [37].

Some other immunohistochemical studies that are useful in identifying a primary tumor include thyroid transcription factor (TTF-1), gross cystic disease fibrous protein (GCDFP), and uroplakin III (URO III) [38,39]. TTF-1 staining is positive in lung and thyroid carcinomas; URO III staining is positive in urothelial carcinoma.

Because special studies usually are not performed routinely unless there is a reasonable suspicion that they will be contributory, direct discussions between the pathologist and clinician are critical to ensure the most focused pathologic characterization possible. Random use of large numbers of tissue markers is rarely helpful for establishing a diagnosis or planning therapy.

CLINICAL CHARACTERISTICS AND NATURAL HISTORY

The clinical presentations of CUP are extremely varied. Historically, patients have been characterized according to whether they have disease above or below the diaphragm [40]. Given the heterogeneity and widespread metastases that characterize this disease, however, this arbitrary division is of doubtful value. Other investigators have begun to subclassify patients based largely on clinicopathologic criteria of histology, involved organ sites, and responsiveness to therapy. This approach has led to the definition of well-characterized patient subsets, which are discussed subsequently. Despite these efforts at subclassification, the majority of patients present with solitary or multiple areas of involvement in a variety of visceral sites. In most cases, the presenting symptoms and physical signs simply reflect the neoplastic involvement of these organ sites.

The demographics of the CUP patient population mirror those of the general population of patients referred to a large cancer center, except for an excess of men among the CUP patients [2]. The median age is approximately 60 years. The family history frequently identifies additional cancers with established origins in other family members; however, no clearly familial instances of CUP have been reported. Table 22-1 shows the distribution of metastatic sites and histologic classification of 1196 CUP patients from one series. These data remained unchanged as compared with the original series reported in 1994 [2].

Table 22-1. Histologic Diagnoses and Major Sites of Tumor Involvement in 1196 Patients with Carcinoma of Unknown Primary

	Patients, *n*	%
Histologic diagnosis		
Adenocarcinoma	706	59.0
Carcinoma	335	28.0
Squamous carcinoma	75	6.3
Neuroendocrine carcinoma	54	4.5
Unknown/other*	26	2.2
Major metastatic sites		
Lymph nodes	519	43.4
Liver	404	33.8
Bone	334	27.9
Lung	315	26.3
Pleura and pleural space	129	10.8
Peritoneum	118	9.9
Brain	84	7.0
Adrenal	71	5.9
Skin	41	3.4

*Includes malignant neoplasm (5) and unknown (21).
(*Adapted from* Abbruzzese *et al.* [2].)

Table 22-2. Univariate and Multivariate Survival Analyses

Variable	*P* value*	Effect on survival	Relative risk†
Univariate survival analysis			
Age, *y*‡	0.43	None	–
Sex (male, female)	0.002	Decreased survival for men	–
Race (white, other)	0.86	None	–
Number of organ sites (1, 2, 3+)	0.002	Decreased survival with more organ sites	–
Involved organ sites			
Lung	0.0014	Deleterious	–
Bone	0.0005	Deleterious	–
Liver	0.0050	Deleterious	–
Pleura	0.002	Deleterious	–
Brain	0.014	Deleterious	–
Lymph nodes	< 0.0001	Advantageous	–
Axillary	0.0003	Advantageous	–
Supraclavicular	0.44	None	–
Peritoneum	0.59	None	–
Skin	0.69	None	–
Histology			
Adenocarcinoma	< 0.0001	Deleterious	–
Carcinoma	0.006	Advantageous	–
Squamous carcinoma	0.058	Advantageous	–
Neuroendocrine carcinoma	0.001	Advantageous	–
Multivariate survival analysis			
Male sex	0.001	Deleterious	1.39
Increasing number of organ sites	< 0.0001	Deleterious	1.23
Involved organ sites			
Liver	0.006	Deleterious	1.33
Lymph nodes	< 0.0001	Advantageous	0.46
Supraclavicular	0.013	Deleterious	1.56
Peritoneum	0.010	Advantageous	0.59
Histology			
Adenocarcinoma	0.0001	Deleterious	1.46
Neuroendocrine carcinoma	0.001	Advantageous	0.30

*Log-rank test.
†Calculated from the Cox proportional hazards regression.
‡Age grouping: 20–39 y, 40–49 y, 50–59 y, 60–69 y, 70+ y.
(*Adapted from* Abbruzzese *et al.* [2].)

The clinical features outlined have been analyzed to determine their effect on survival. There are considerable differences in survival for the four most frequently encountered pathologic subtypes of CUP. The median survival was 13 months for patients with squamous carcinoma (exclusive of patients with mid-high cervical adenopathy), 6 months for adenocarcinoma, 11 months for carcinoma, and 27 months for neuroendocrine carcinoma. The state of differentiation or mucin production does not significantly influence the poor survival of patients with adenocarcinoma. The influence of other clinicopathologic features of CUP on survival has been assessed using univariate and multivariate analyses. These data are summarized in Table 22-2. Other studies have documented similar results [41].

THERAPEUTIC APPROACH AND RESPONSE TO THERAPY

Carcinomas of unknown primary are a heterogeneous group of tumors with widely varying natural histories; therefore, in discussing treatment and survival, it is imperative to understand the patient population studied. When all patients are considered, CUP is a highly aggressive neoplasm with an overall median survival of 3 to 4 months according to older series [7,33]. More recent studies have documented median survivals of 9 to 12 months [42–44]. In a series of 657 consecutive patients, the median survival was

11 months [2]; this number remained consistent in the expanded series that included 1196 patients.

The treatment of CUP continues to evolve. Although the majority of patients are treated with systemic chemotherapy, the careful integration of surgery, radiation therapy, and even periods of observation is important in the overall management of these patients [13]. Observation is particularly important for patients with single sites of disease that have received adequate local therapy.

The most common problem is treatment of the patient with progressive metastatic carcinoma or adenocarcinoma involving two or more organ sites [45–69]. Table 22-3 outlines the results from 13 trials. Hainsworth *et al.* [70] reported that a combination of carboplatin, paclitaxel, and etoposide was effective for some patients with CUP. Use of a chemosensitivity assay may help guide the selection of the optimal combination [71]. Treatment of these patients remains suboptimal and awaits discovery of novel strategies applicable to other highly resistant adenocarcinomas, such as those originating in the lung or gastrointestinal tract. This situation is contrasted with the management of the favorable subsets described. These patients have been grouped together primarily on the basis of their responsiveness to therapy or favorable natural histories. The number of patients who fall into these groups is small; however, they are important to recognize because specific treatment may significantly extend survival.

Table 22-3. Selected Chemotherapeutic Trials in Carcinoma of Unknown Primary

Study	Histology	Regimen	Patients, *n*	Response, %	Median survival, *mo*
Pasterz *et al.* [41]	Adenocarcinoma, undifferentiated carcinoma	5-FU/doxorubicin/ cyclophosphamide/cisplatin	44	28	NS
Greco *et al.* [42]	PDA, PDC	Cisplatin/vinblastine/ bleomycin ± doxorubicin	68	56 (22 CR)	18*
Moertel *et al.* [45]	Adenocarcinoma	5-FU	88	16	NS
Woods *et al.* [48]	Adenocarcinoma, undifferentiated carcinoma	Doxorubicin/mitomycin C	25	36	4.5
Raber *et al.* [55]	Adenocarcinoma, undifferentiated carcinoma	Cisplatin/etoposide/5-FU	36	22	NS
Lenzi *et al.* [57]	Adenocarcinoma, PDC	Cisplatin/5-FU/folinic acid	31	30	18
Hainsworth *et al.* [58]	PDC	Cisplatin/etoposide	32	60 (32 CR)	NS
Hainsworth *et al.* [70]	Adenocarcinoma, PDA, PDC	Paclitaxel/carboplatin/etoposide	55	47	13.4
Greco *et al.* [101]	PDA, PDC, neuroendocrine small cell carcinoma	Group 1: docetaxel/cisplatin	26	26	8
		Group 2: docetaxel/carboplatin	47	22	12
Culine *et al.* [102]	WDA, PDC, PDA, poorly differentiated neuroendocrine carcinoma	Group A: high-dose doxorubicin/ cyclophosphamide, etoposide/ carboplatin, PBSC support	20	42	11
		Group B: doxorubicin/cyclophosphamide, etoposide/cisplatin	40	39	8
Briasoulis *et al.* [103][†]	PDA, PDC, MDA, WDA	Carboplatin/epirubicin/etoposide	62	37	8 (visceral); 10 (nodal)
Briasoulis *et al.* [104][‡]	PDA, PDC	Carboplatin/paclitaxel	77	47.8 (nodal); 68.4 (PC); 15.1 (visceral)	13 (nodal); 15 (PC); 10 (visceral)
Greco *et al.* [105]	WDA, PDA	Paclitaxel/carboplatin/oral etoposide followed by gemcitabine/irinotecan	131	30	9.1
Schneider *et al.* [106]	WDA, MDA, PDA, PDC, squamous cell carcinoma	Gemcitabine/carboplatin/ capecitabine	33	39.4	7.6

*Calculated from data presented.
[†]This study provided survival data for two patient groups: 1) predominantly nodal disease or midline involvement, and 2) predominantly splanchnic involvement.
[‡]This study provided response rates and survival data for three patient groups: 1) predominantly nodal/pleural disease, 2) peritoneal carcinomatosis, and 3) visceral or disseminated metastases.
CR—complete response; 5-FU—5-fluorouracil; MDA—moderately differentiated adenocarcinoma; NS—not stated; PBSC—peripheral blood stem cell; PC—peritoneal carcinomatosis; PDA—poorly differentiated adenocarcinoma; PDC—poorly differentiated carcinoma; WDA—well-differentiated adenocarcinoma.

SQUAMOUS CARCINOMA INVOLVING MID-HIGH CERVICAL LYMPH NODES

High cervical adenopathy with squamous carcinoma is an important clinical subset because of its well-defined natural history and responsiveness to therapy [72–75]. With appropriate evaluation, including direct visualization of the hypopharynx, nasopharynx, larynx, and upper esophagus, an occult primary lesion will be frequently identified. When no primary is found, aggressive local therapy is applied to the involved neck [74–76]. Thirty percent to 50% of 5-year survivals have been reported with radical neck surgery, high-dose radiotherapy, or a combination of both modalities. A potential advantage of radiation therapy is that the suspected primary anatomic sites (nasopharynx, oropharynx, and hypopharynx) can be included in the radiation port [74,75]. Studies suggest that the eventual emergence of the primary site adversely affects the prognosis [77]. The role of chemotherapy in these patients is unclear. One randomized study, however, suggested that chemotherapy with cisplatin and 5-fluorouracil (5-FU) improved the response rate and median survival relative to radiation alone [78].

Patients with adenocarcinoma involving mid-high cervical nodes and patients with lower cervical or supraclavicular adenopathy of all histologies have a much poorer prognosis [79]. These patients are managed with local measures (usually radiation therapy) or may be candidates for systemic chemotherapy protocols.

RECOMMENDED THERAPY

Low N stage (NX, N1, N2A): surgery followed by radiation therapy (> 50 Gy) or radiation therapy alone (minimum 50 Gy) to ipsilateral neck with or without naso-oropharynx.

High N stage (N2B, N3A, N3B) or poorly differentiated tumors: cisplatin 100 mg/m^2 on d 1, 22, and 43 with concurrent radiation therapy, or cisplatin 100 mg/m^2 on d 1 plus 5-FU 1000 mg/m^2/d by continuous infusion on d 1–5. Repeat courses of cisplatin and 5-FU every 3–4 wk for three courses followed by radiation therapy.

WOMEN WITH ISOLATED AXILLARY ADENOPATHY

Isolated axillary adenopathy secondary to metastatic adenocarcinoma usually occurs in women and has unique clinical features. Many of these women have occult breast primaries, which can be identified in 40% to 70% of these patients who undergo mastectomy [80,81]. In this setting, rebiopsy of involved axillary nodes for estrogen and progesterone levels should be considered in view of the influence of this information on diagnosis and management. Breast magnetic resonance imaging has been shown to provide significant diagnostic accuracy in identifying occult breast carcinoma in women with axillary lymphadenopathy [82]. This may aid substantially in treatment planning for those patients considering surgery versus whole breast irradiation; however, it would not change the need for systemic chemotherapy in these women. Management is based on the treatment of stage II breast cancer, and this should include both local and systemic therapies. Prognosis following treatment is comparable to women with stage II breast cancer [82,83]. Older series have advocated modified radical mastectomy and axillary dissection for primary treatment [80,81,84]. A series of 42 patients suggested that survival was superior in patients receiving systemic chemotherapy, and local control was improved by irradiating the breast and the axilla [83]. The actuarial disease-free survival in this study was 71% at 5 years and 65% at 10 years.

Patients with axillary adenopathy and involvement of additional sites (usually liver or bone) or with nonadenocarcinoma histology constitute a much more heterogeneous group composed of equal numbers of men and women as well as a broader histologic spectrum, with poorly differentiated carcinoma and neuroendocrine carcinomas represented in addition to adenocarcinoma. The survival of patients with axillary adenopathy and other involved organ sites is intermediate between that of the overall CUP population and women with isolated axillary adenopathy [34].

The management of patients with involvement of the axilla as well as other sites or nonadenocarcinoma histology is less certain. These patients generally are approached using a combination of local and systemic modalities and, again, may be good candidates for novel systemic chemotherapy protocols.

RECOMMENDED THERAPY

General principles are based on the management of women with stage II breast cancer. Tamoxifen or an aromatase inhibitor (anastrozole, letrozole) is added to the systemic therapy of patients with estrogen receptor–positive neoplasms.

Modified radical mastectomy with axillary nodal dissection followed by systemic chemotherapy with FAC (5-FU, doxorubicin, cyclophosphamide), AC (doxorubicin, cyclophosphamide) with sequential paclitaxel, or similar regimen for six to eight courses, or chemotherapy with FAC, FEC (5-FU, epirubicin, cyclophosphamide), AC, or similar regimen for six to eight courses followed by radiation therapy to the ipsilateral breast and axillary nodes. (Axillary dissection can be considered before chemotherapy to assess receptor status and complete nodal staging but increases the risk of arm edema following radiation therapy.)

PERITONEAL CARCINOMATOSIS

Women with diffuse peritoneal carcinomatosis with adenocarcinoma constitute another recently recognized CUP subset. These patients form a distinctive subset because of their clinical similarities to typical ovarian carcinoma. Often, papillary histology and elevations in cancer antigen (CA)-125 are found, but exploratory laparotomy fails to document a primary [85,86]. Other researchers have also recognized this patient subset, terming this syndrome *peritoneal papillary serous carcinoma* or *multifocal extraovarian serous carcinoma*. These patients frequently respond to platinum-based chemotherapy [86–88]. Many patients in these series also underwent exploratory laparotomy with surgical debulking followed by chemotherapy. Median survivals are reported to be 16 months to 2 years.

The natural histories of men with isolated peritoneal carcinomatosis or patients with histologies inconsistent with ovarian carcinoma (*eg*, mucin-positive adenocarcinoma) or additional metastatic sites are much more poorly characterized, but overall survival, even with therapy, is poor.

RECOMMENDED THERAPY

Papillary serous carcinoma of the peritoneum: surgical debulking followed by systemic chemotherapy with carboplatin AUC-6 (area under the curve 6 mg/mL/min) IV on d 1 plus paclitaxel 175 mg/m^2 IV on d 1, repeated every 3–4 wk.

Adenocarcinoma of the peritoneum: systemic chemotherapy using cisplatin 75 mg/m^2 IV on d 1; folinic acid 500 mg/m^2 in 200 mL normal saline IV over 2 h on d 1–5; 5-FU 375 mg/m^2 IV after 1 h of folinic acid on d 1–5; carboplatin AUC-6 IV on d 1 plus paclitaxel 175 mg/m^2 on d 1, repeated every 3–4 wk; or a similar regimen.

POORLY DIFFERENTIATED AND UNDIFFERENTIATED CARCINOMA

Approximately one third of patients with CUP are defined as having this histologic picture. In this subset, detailed histochemical or immunohistochemical studies are most likely to identify highly treatment-responsive patients with lymphoma (leukocyte common antigen), germ cell (β-HCG, AFP), or neuroendocrine (neuron-specific enolase, chromogranin) neoplasms [36]. Additionally, Greco *et al.* [42] have identified a group of patients with poorly differentiated carcinoma or poorly differentiated adenocarcinoma who are responsive to platinum-based chemotherapy. Other investigators, however, conclude that these highly responsive patients are infrequently encountered in a consecutive series of CUP patients [89,90]. Most of these patients had clinical features (young age, mediastinal and retroperitoneal involvement, and rapid growth) of the extragonadal germ cell syndrome [91–94]. Many of these patients are male and have elevated β-HCG or AFP, although the usefulness of these serum tumor markers in predicting response is in question [89,95]. Motzer *et al.* [28] identified abnormalities in chromosome 12 specific for germ cell neoplasms in a group of male patients with poorly differentiated carcinoma involving midline structures, confirming the germ cell origin of these tumors.

Combination chemotherapy regimens specific for germ cell carcinoma of testicular origin have usually been employed in the treatment of these patients [42,96]. These regimens have produced documented complete responses and an actual 10-year disease-free survival of 16% [96].

RECOMMENDED THERAPY

Cisplatin 20 mg/m^2 daily for 5 d plus etoposide 100 mg/m^2 daily for 3–5 d with or without bleomycin 30 U/wk. Assess response after two courses of therapy; total of four to six courses for responding patients. Alternative approaches include carboplatin AUC-6 plus paclitaxel 200 mg/m^2 by 1-h infusion plus oral etoposide 50 mg/m^2 in 200 mL normal saline IV over 2 h on d 1–5; or 5-FU 375 mg/m^2 IV after 1 h of folinic acid on d 1–5.

POORLY DIFFERENTIATED NEUROENDOCRINE CARCINOMA

Poorly differentiated (anaplastic) neuroendocrine carcinoma is an emerging clinicopathologic entity recognized primarily for its responsiveness to therapy. There is probably considerable overlap with extrapulmonary small cell carcinomas, anaplastic carcinoid, anaplastic islet cell tumors, Merkel's cell tumors, and paragangliomas. Histologically, these tumors are poorly differentiated, but histochemical stains are positive for chromogranin or neuron-specific enolase. These patients often present with diffuse hepatic or bone metastases but do not have the indolent histologic or clinical features of typical carcinoid tumors, islet cell tumors, or paragangliomas, and thus observation may not be appropriate. These tumors are also highly responsive to platinum-based chemotherapy [97–99].

RECOMMENDED THERAPY

Etoposide 130 mg/m^2 daily for 3 d plus cisplatin 45 mg/m^2 on d 2 and 3; courses repeated every 4 wk

PATIENTS WITH ADENOCARCINOMA OR CARCINOMA OF UNKNOWN ORIGIN

The optimistic results for the favorable patients described previously do not apply to the vast majority of patients with CUP. Two thirds of CUP patients have metastatic adenocarcinoma with involvement of two or more visceral sites, usually some combination of liver, lung, lymph nodes, or bone. In addition, many men and women with poorly differentiated carcinoma or poorly differentiated adenocarcinoma have none of the clinical features outlined and respond poorly to chemotherapy [89]. Even in series showing optimistic results for selected patients with poorly differentiated carcinoma or poorly differentiated adenocarcinoma, the overall median survival remains poor at 12 months [96].

For unselected patients, numerous empiric chemotherapy combinations have been reported. Many have been based on doxorubicin, 5-FU, or cisplatin. A recent report using carboplatin, paclitaxel, and etoposide reported that 47% (25 of 53 patients) had objective responses [70]. In this series, seven patients (13%) experienced complete responses. The actuarial median survival for the entire group, however, was 13.4 months. The disappointing aspect of this survival statistic is that it is not substantially different from the 11-month median survival reported in large consecutive series of CUP patients [2,100]. There is little information on the use of biologic agents alone or with chemotherapy. Response rates generally range from 20% to 30%; however, most responses are partial and brief, resulting in little or no impact on median survival. Newer regimens continue to be tested; however, there has been no substantial progress in the treatment of these patients to date (*see* Table 22-3).

RECOMMENDED THERAPY

Cisplatin 20 mg/m^2 for 5 d plus etoposide 100 mg/m^2 for 3–5 d or cisplatin 100 mg/m^2 plus etoposide 100 mg/m^2 for 3 d (courses repeated every 3–4 wk); paclitaxel 200 mg/m^2 by 1-h IV infusion on d 1 plus carboplatin AUC-6 IV on d 1, plus oral etoposide 50 mg alternated with 100 mg/m^2 on d 1–10 (courses repeated every 21 d); or cisplatin 75 mg/m^2 IV on d 1 plus folinic acid 500 mg/m^2 in 200 mL normal saline IV over 2 h on d 1–5; or 5-FU 375 mg/m^2 IV after 1 h of folinic acid 1–5; or similar regimen (courses repeated every 28 d).

REFERENCES

1. Greco FA, Hainsworth JD: Cancer of unknown primary site. In *Cancer: Principles and Practice of Oncology*, edn 6. Edited by De Vita VT Jr, Hellman S, Rosenberg SA. Philadelphia: JB Lippincott; 2001:2537–2560.

2. Abbruzzese JL, Abbruzzese MC, Hess KR, *et al.*: Unknown primary carcinoma: natural history and prognostic factors in 657 consecutive patients. *J Clin Oncol* 1994, 12:1272–1280.

3. Jemal A, Siegel R, Ward E, *et al.*: Cancer statistics 2007. *CA Cancer J Clin* 2007, 57:43–66.

4. Abbruzzese JL: An effective strategy for the evaluation of unknown primary tumors. *Cancer Bull* 1989, 41:157–161.

5. Abbruzzese JL, Abbruzzese MC, Lenzi R, *et al.*: Analysis of a diagnostic strategy for patients with suspected tumors of unknown origin. *J Clin Oncol* 1995, 13:2094–2103.

6. Nystrom JS, Weiner JM, Wolf RM, *et al.*: Identifying the primary site in metastatic cancer of unknown origin: inadequacy of roentgenographic procedures. *JAMA* 1979, 241:381–383.

7. Neumann KH, Nystrom JS: Metastatic cancer of unknown origin: nonsquamous cell type. *Semin Oncol* 1982, 9:427–434.

8. Stewart JF, Tattersall MH, Woods RL, Fox RM: Unknown primary adenocarcinoma: incidence of over investigation and natural history. *Br Med J* 1979, 1:1530–1533.

9. Karsell PR, Sheedy PF II, O'Connell MJ: Computed tomography in search of cancer of unknown origin. *JAMA* 1982, 248:340–343.

10. Didolkar MS, Fanous N, Elias EG, Moore RH: Metastatic carcinoma from occult primary tumors: a study of 254 patients. *Ann Surg* 1977, 186:625–630.

11. McMillan JH, Levine E, Stephens RH: Computed tomography in the evaluation of metastatic adenocarcinoma from an unknown primary site. *Radiology* 1982, 143:143–146.

12. Walsh JW, Rosenfield AT, Jaffe CC, *et al.*: Prospective comparison of ultrasound and computed tomography in the evaluation of gynecologic pelvic masses. *AJR Am J Roentgenol* 1978, 131:955–960.

13. Raber MN, Abbruzzese JL, Frost P: Unknown primary tumors. *Curr Opin Oncol* 1992, 4:3–9.

14. Shahangian S, Fritsche HA: Serum tumor markers as diagnostic aids in patients with unknown primary tumors. *Cancer Bull* 1989, 41:152.

15. Koch M, McPherson TA: Carcinoembryonic antigen levels as an indicator of the primary site in metastatic disease of unknown origin. *Cancer* 1981, 48:1242–1244.

16. Abbruzzese J, Raber M, Frost P: The role of CA-125 in patients with unknown primary tumors [abstract]. *Proc Am Soc Clin Oncol* 1990, 9:118.

17. Lassen U, Daugaard G, Eigtved A, *et al.*: 18F-FDG whole body positron emission tomography (PET) in patients with unknown primary tumors (UPT). *Eur J Cancer* 1999, 35:1076–1082.

18. Bohuslavizki KH, Klutmann S, Kroger S, *et al.*: FDG PET detection of unknown primary tumors. *J Nucl Med* 2000, 41:816–822.

19. Aassar OS, Fischbein NJ, Caputo JR, *et al.*: Metastatic head and neck cancer: role and usefulness of FDG PET in locating occult primary tumors. *Radiology* 1999, 210:177–181.

20. Greven KM, Keyes JW Jr, Williams DW III, *et al.*: Occult primary tumors of the head and neck: lack of benefit from positron emission tomography imaging with 2-[F18]fluoro-2-deoxy-d-glucose. *Cancer* 1999, 86:114–118.

21. Gutzeit A, Antoch G, Kuhe H, *et al.*: Unknown primary tumors: detection with dual-modality PET/CT. Initial experience. *Radiology* 2005, 234:227–234.

22. Pelosi E, Pennone M, Deandreis D, *et al.*: Role of whole body positron emission tomography/computed tomography scan with 18F-fluorodeoxyglucose in patients with biopsy proven tumor metastases from unknown primary site. *Euro J Nucl Med Mol Imaging* 2006, 50:15–22.

23. Nanni C, Rubello D, Castellucci P, *et al.*: Role of 18F-FDG PET/CT imaging for the detection of an unknown primary tumor: preliminary results in 21 patients. *Euro J Nucl Med Mol Imaging* 2005, 32:589–592.

24. Le Cesne A, Le Chevalier T, Caille P, *et al.*: Metastases from cancers of unknown primary site: data from 302 autopsies. *Pesse Med* 1991, 20:1369–1373.

25. Hillen HF: Unknown primary tumors. *Postgrad Med J* 2000, 76:690–693.

26. Bugat R, Bataillard A, Lesimple T, *et al.*: Summary of the standards, options and recommendations for the management of patients with carcinoma of unknown primary site (2002). *Br J Cancer* 2003, 89(Suppl 1):S51–S66.

27. Blasz KH, Hartmann A, Bjorsson J: Cancer of unknown primary: clinicopathologic correlations. *APMIS* 2003, 111:1089–1094.

28. Motzer RJ, Rodriguez E, Reuter VE, *et al.*: Genetic analysis of an aid in diagnostic for patients with midline carcinomas of uncertain histologies. *J Natl Cancer Inst* 1991, 83:341–346.

29. Ilson DH, Motzer RJ, Rodriguez F, *et al.*: Genetic analysis in the diagnosis of neoplasms of unknown primary site. *Semin Oncol* 1992, 20:229–237.

30. Motzer RJ, Rodriguez E, Reuter VE, *et al.*: Molecular and cytogenetic studies in the diagnosis of patients with poorly differentiated carcinomas of unknown primary site. *J Clin Oncol* 1995, 13:274–282.

31. Bar-Eli M, Abbruzzese JL, Lee-Jackson D, *et al.*: p53 mutation spectrum in human unknown primary tumors. *Anticancer Res* 1993, 13:1619–1624.

32. Frost P, Raber M, Abbruzzese J: Unknown primary tumors: are they a unique subgroup of neoplastic disease? *Cancer Bull* 1987, 39:216–218.

33. Nystrom JS, Weiner JM, Heffelfinger-Juttner J, Irwin LE: Metastatic and histologic presentations in unknown primary cancer. *Semin Oncol* 1977, 4:53–58.

34. Abbruzzese JL, Raber MN: Unknown primary carcinoma. In *Clinical Oncology*. Edited by Abeloff MD, Armitage JO, Lichter AS, Niederhuber JE. New York: Churchill Livingstone; 1995:1822–1845.

35. Mackay B, Ordoñez NG: The role of the pathologist in the evaluation of poorly differentiated tumors and metastatic tumors of unknown origin. In *Poorly Differentiated Neoplasms and Tumors of Unknown Origin*. Edited by Fer MF, Greco AF, Oldham RK. Orlando: Grune & Stratton; 1986:3.

36. Hainsworth JD, Wright EP, Johnson DH, *et al.*: Poorly differentiated carcinoma of unknown primary site: clinical usefulness of immunoperoxidase staining. *J Clin Oncol* 1991, 9:1931–1938.

37. Lagendijk JH, Mullink H, Van Diest PJ, *et al.*: Tracing the origin of adenocarcinomas with unknown primary using immunohistochemistry: differential diagnosis between colonic and ovarian carcinomas as primary sites. *Hum Pathol* 1998, 29:491–497.

38. Chu PG, Weiss LM: Keratin expression in human tissues and neoplasms. *Histopathology* 2002, 40:403–439.

39. Varadhachary GR, Abbruzzese J, Lenzi R: Diagnostic strategies for unknown primary cancer. *Cancer* 2004, 100:1776–1785.

40. Ultmann JE, Phillips TL: Cancer of unknown primary site. In *Cancer: Principles and Practice of Oncology*. Edited by DeVita VT Jr, Hellman S, Rosenberg SA. Philadelphia: JB Lippincott; 1989:1941–1950.

41. Pasterz R, Savaraj N, Burgess M: Prognostic factors in metastatic carcinoma of unknown primary. *J Clin Oncol* 1986, 4:1652–1657.

42. Greco FA, Vaughn WK, Hainsworth JD: Advanced poorly differentiated carcinoma of unknown primary site: recognition of a treatable syndrome. *Ann Intern Med* 1986, 104:547–553.

43. Sporn JR, Greenberg BR: Empiric chemotherapy in patients with carcinoma of unknown primary site. *Am J Med* 1990, 88:49–55.

44. Kambhu SA, Kelsen D, Fiore J, *et al.*: Metastatic adenocarcinomas of unknown primary site. *Am J Clin Oncol* 1990, 13:55–60.

45. Moertel CG, Reitmeier RJ, Schutt AJ, *et al.*: Treatment of patient with adenocarcinomas of unknown origin. *Cancer* 1972, 30:1469–1472.

46. McKeen E, Smith F, Haidak D, *et al.*: Fluorouracil (F), Adriamycin (A), and mitomycin (M), FAM for adenocarcinoma of unknown origin [abstract]. *Proc Am Assoc Cancer Res* 1980, 21:358.

47. Rudnick S, Tremont S, Staab E, *et al.*: Evaluation and therapy for adenocarcinoma of unknown primary (ACUP) [abstract]. *Proc Am Assoc Cancer Res* 1981, 22:379.

48. Woods RL, Fox RM, Tattersall MH, *et al.*: Metastatic adenocarcinomas of unknown primary site. *N Engl J Med* 1980, 303:87–89.

49. Valentine J, Rosenthal S, Arseneau JC: Combination chemotherapy for adenocarcinoma of unknown primary origin. *Cancer Clin Trials* 1979, 2:265–268.

50. Bedikian AY, Bodey GP, Valdevieso M, Burgess MA: Sequential chemotherapy for adenocarcinoma of unknown primary. *Am J Clin Oncol* 1983, 6:219–224.

51. Goldberg RM, Smith FP, Ueno W, *et al.*: 5-fluorouracil, Adriamycin, and mitomycin in the treatment of adenocarcinoma of unknown primary. *J Clin Oncol* 1986, 4:395–399.

52. Walach N: Treatment of adenocarcinoma of unknown origin with cyclophosphamide (C), Oncovin (O), methotrexate (M), and 5-fluorouracil (F), (COMF) [abstract]. *Proc Am Soc Clin Oncol* 1986, 5:125.

53. Shildt RA, Kennedy PS, Chen TT, *et al.*: Management of patients with metastatic adenocarcinoma of unknown origin: a Southwest Oncology Group study. *Cancer Treat Rep* 1983, 67:77–79.

54. Anderson H, Thatcher N, Rankin E, *et al.*: VAC (Vincristine, Adriamycin, Cyclophosphamide) chemotherapy for metastatic carcinoma from an unknown site. *Eur J Cancer Clin Oncol* 1983, 19:49–52.

55. Raber MN, Faintuch J, Abbruzzese JL, *et al.*: Continuous infusion 5-fluorouracil, etoposide and cis-diamminedichloroplatinum in patients with metastatic carcinoma of unknown primary origin. *Ann Oncol* 1991, 2:519–520.

56. LeChevalier T, Tremblay J, Rouesse J, *et al.*: Phase II trial of methotrexate-FAM in adenocarcinoma of unknown primary [abstract]. *Proc Am Soc Clin Oncol* 1987, 6:130.

57. Lenzi R, Raber MN, Frost P, *et al.*: Phase II study of cisplatin, 5FU, and folinic acid in patients with tumors of unknown primary origin. *Eur J Cancer* 1993, 29A:1634.

58. Hainsworth JD, Johnson DH, Greco FA: The role of etoposide in the treatment of poorly differentiated carcinoma of unknown primary site. *Cancer* 1991, 67(Suppl):310–314.

59. Lenzi R, Raber MN, Gravel D, *et al.*: Phase I and II trials of a laboratory derived synergistic combination of cisplatin and 29-deoxy-5-azacytidine. *Int J Oncol* 1995, 6:447–450.

60. Kelsen D, Martin DS, Coloriore J, *et al.*: A phase II trial of biochemical modulation using N-phosphonacetyl-L-aspartate, high-dose methotrexate, high-dose 5-fluorouracil, and leucovorin in patients with adenocarcinoma of unknown primary site. *Cancer* 1992, 70:1988–1992.

61. Gill I, Guaglianone P, Gruneberg SM, *et al.*: High dose intensity of cisplatin and etoposide in adenocarcinoma of unknown primary. *Anticancer Res* 1991, 11:1231–1235.

62. Porta C, Moroni M, Nastasi G, *et al.*: COMF combination chemotherapy for the treatment of adenocarcinoma of unknown primary origin. *Ann Oncol* 1992, 3(Suppl):48.

63. Trudeau M, Thirlwell MP, Boos G, *et al.*: Cancer of unknown primary syndrome (CUPS): predictive value of CA-125 in patients treated with 5-fluorouracil, doxorubicin and cisplatin (FAP) [abstract]. *Proc Am Soc Clin Oncol* 1993, 12:399.

64. Ahlgren JD, Bern M, Booth B, *et al.*: Protracted infusional 5FU (PIF): an active, well-tolerated regimen in metastatic adenocarcinoma of undetermined primary (AUP): a mid-Atlantic Oncology Program (MOAP) study [abstract]. *Proc Am Soc Clin Oncol* 1993, 12:401.

65. Nole F, Colleoni M, Buzzoni R, Bajetta E: Fluorouracil plus folinic acid in metastatic adenocarcinoma of unknown primary site suggestive of a gastrointestinal primary. *Tumori* 1993, 79:116–118.

66. van der Gaast A, Henzen-Logmans SC, Planting AS, *et al.*: Phase II study of oral administration of etoposide for patients with well- and moderately-differentiated adenocarcinomas of unknown primary site. *Ann Oncol* 1993, 4:789–790.

67. de Campos ES, Menasce LP, Radford J, *et al.*: Metastatic carcinoma of uncertain primary site: a retrospective review of 57 patients treated with vincristine, doxorubicin, cyclophosphamide (VAC) or VAC alternating with cisplatin and etoposide (VAC/PE). *Cancer* 1994, 73:470–475.

68. Akerley W, Thomas A, Miller M, *et al.*: Phase II trial of oral etoposide for carcinoma of unknown primary (CUP) [abstract]. *Proc Am Soc Clin Oncol* 1994, 13:406.

69. Merrouche Y, Lasset C, Trillet-Lenoir V, *et al.*: Phase II study of cisplatin and etoposide in a subgroup of patients with carcinoma of unknown primary [abstract]. *Proc Am Soc Clin Oncol* 1994, 13:401.

70. Hainsworth JD, Erland JB, Kalman LA, *et al.*: Carcinoma of unknown primary site: treatment with 1-hour paclitaxel, carboplatin, and extended-schedule etoposide. *J Clin Oncol* 1997, 15:2385–2393.

71. Hanauske AR, Clark GM, Von Hoff DD: Adenocarcinoma of unknown primary: retrospective analysis of chemosensitivity of 313 freshly explanted tumors in a tumor cloning system. *Invest New Drugs* 1995, 13:43–49.

72. Jesse RH, Perez CA, Fletcher GH: Cervical lymph node metastases: unknown primary cancer. *Cancer* 1973, 31:854–859.

73. Wang RC, Goepfert H, Barber AE, Wolf P: Unknown primary squamous cell carcinoma metastatic to the neck. *Arch Otolaryngol Head Neck Surg* 1990, 116:1388–1393.

74. Weir L, Keane T, Cummings B, *et al.*: Radiation treatment of cervical lymph node metastases from an unknown primary: an analysis of outcome by treatment volume and other prognostic factors. *Radiother Oncol* 1995, 35:206–211.

75. Marcial-Vega VA, Cardenes H, Perez CA, *et al.*: Cervical metastases from unknown primaries: radiotherapeutic management and appearance of subsequent primaries. *Int J Radiat Oncol Biol Phys* 1990, 19:919–928.

76. Carlson LS, Fletcher GH, Oswald MJ: Guidelines for the radiotherapeutic techniques for cervical metastases from an unknown primary. *Int J Radiat Oncol Biol Phys* 1986, 12:2101–2110.

77. Talmi YP, Wolf GT, Hazuka M, *et al.*: Unknown primary of the head and neck. *J Laryngol Otol* 1996, 110:353–356.

78. de Braud F, Heilbrun LK, Ahmed K, *et al.*: Metastatic squamous cell carcinoma of an unknown primary localized to the neck: advantages of an aggressive treatment. *Cancer* 1989, 64:510–515.

79. Lee NK, Byers RM, Abbruzzese JL, Wolf P: Metastatic adenocarcinoma to the neck from an unknown primary. *Am J Surg* 1991, 162:306–309.

80. Patel J, Nemoto T, Rosner D, *et al.*: Axillary lymph node metastasis from an occult breast cancer. *Cancer* 1981, 47:2923–2927.

81. Ashikari R, Rosen PP, Urban JA, Senoo T: Breast cancer presenting as an axillary mass. *Ann Surg* 1976, 183:415–417.

82. Henry-Tillman RS, Harms SE, Westbrook KC, *et al.*: Role of breast magnetic resonance imaging in determining breast as a source of unknown metastatic lymphadenopathy. *Am J Surg* 1999, 178:496–500.

83. Ellerbroek N, Holmes F, Singletary E, *et al.*: Treatment of patients with isolated axillary nodal metastases from an occult primary carcinoma consistent with breast origin. *Cancer* 1990, 66:1461–1467.

84. Jackson B, Scott-Conner C, Moulder J: Axillary metastasis from occult breast carcinoma: diagnosis and management. *Am Surg* 1995, 61:431–434.

85. August CZ, Murad TM, Newton M: Multiple focal extraovarian serous carcinoma. *Int J Gynecol Pathol* 1985, 4:11–23.

86. Dalrymple JC, Bannatyne P, Russell P, *et al.*: Extraovarian peritoneal serous papillary carcinoma: a clinicopathologic study of 31 cases. *Cancer* 1989, 64:110–115.

87. Strnad CM, Grosh WW, Baxter J, *et al.*: Peritoneal carcinomatosis of unknown primary site in women. A distinctive subset of adenocarcinoma. *Ann Intern Med* 1989, 111:213–217.

88. Ransom DT, Patel SR, Keeney GL, *et al.*: Papillary serous carcinoma of the peritoneum: a review of 33 cases treated with platin-based chemotherapy. *Cancer* 1990, 66:1091–1094.

89. Lenzi R, Hess KR, Abbruzzese MC, *et al.*: Poorly differentiated carcinoma and poorly differentiated adenocarcinoma of unknown origin: favorable subsets of patients with unknown primary carcinoma? *J Clin Oncol* 1997, 15:2056–2066.

90. Farrugia DC, Norman AR, Nicolson MC, *et al.*: Unknown primary carcinoma: randomised studies are needed to identify optimal treatments and their benefits. *Eur J Cancer* 1996, 32A:2256–2261.

91. van der Gaast A, Verweij J, Henzen-Logmans SC, *et al.*: Carcinoma of unknown primary: identification of a treatable subset? *Ann Oncol* 1990, 1:119–122.

92. Jones A, Farrow G, Richardson FL: The extragonadal germ cell cancer syndrome: the Mayo Clinic experience. In *Poorly Differentiated Neoplasms and Tumors of Unknown Origin.* Edited by Fer MF, Greco FA, Oldham RK. Orlando: Grune & Stratton; 1986:203.

93. Richardson RL, Schoumacher RA, Fer MF, *et al.*: The unrecognized extragonadal germ cell cancer syndrome. *Ann Intern Med* 1981, 94:181–186.

94. Fox RM, Woods RL, Tattersall MH, McGovern VJ: Undifferentiated carcinoma in young men: the atypical teratoma syndrome. *Lancet* 1979, 1:1316–1318.

95. Currow DC, Findlay M, Cox K, *et al.*: Elevated germ cell markers in carcinoma of uncertain primary site do not predict response to platinum-based chemotherapy. *Eur J Cancer* 1996, 32A:2357–2359.

96. Hainsworth JD, Johnson DH, Greco FA: Cisplatin-based combination chemotherapy in the treatment of poorly differentiated carcinoma and poorly differentiated adenocarcinoma of unknown primary site: results of a 12-year experience. *J Clin Oncol* 1992, 10:912–922.

97. Hainsworth JD, Johnson DH, Greco FA: Poorly differentiated neuroendocrine carcinoma of unknown primary site. A newly recognized clinicopathologic entity. *Ann Intern Med* 1988, 109:364–371.

98. Moertel CG, Kvols LK, O'Connell MJ, Rubin J: Treatment of neuroendocrine carcinomas with combined etoposide and cisplatin: evidence of major therapeutic activity in the anaplastic variants of these neoplasms. *Cancer* 1991, 68:227–232.

99. Hainsworth JD, Spigel DR, Litchy S, Greco FA: Phase II trial of paclitaxel, carboplatin and etoposide in advanced poorly differentiated neuroendocrine carcinoma: a Minnie Pearl Cancer Research Network study. *J Clin Oncol* 2006, 24:3548–3553.

100. Hess K, Abbruzzese MC, Lenzi R, *et al.*: Classification and regression tree analysis of 1000 consecutive patients with unknown primary carcinoma [abstract]. *Proc Am Soc Clin Oncol* 1996, 15:452.

101. Greco FA, Erland JB, Morrissey LH, *et al.*: Carcinoma of unknown primary site: phase II trials with docetaxel plus cisplatin or carboplatin. *Ann Oncol* 2000, 11:211–215.

102. Culine S, Fabbro M, Ychou M, *et al.*: Chemotherapy in carcinomas of unknown primary site: a high-dose intensity policy. *Ann Oncol* 1999, 10:569–575.

103. Briasoulis E, Tsavaris N, Fountzilas G, *et al.*: Combination regimen with carboplatin, epirubicin and etoposide in metastatic carcinomas of unknown primary site: a Hellenic Co-Operative Oncology Group Phase II study. *Oncology* 1998, 55:426–430.

104. Briasoulis E, Kalofonos H, Bafaloukos D, *et al.*: Carboplatin plus paclitaxel in unknown primary carcinoma: a phase II Hellenic Cooperative Oncology Group study. *J Clin Oncol* 2000, 18:3101–3107.

105. Greco FA, Rodriguez GI, Shaffer DW, *et al.*: Carcinoma of unknown primary site: sequential treatment with paclitaxel/carboplatin/etoposide and gemcitabine/irinotecan: a Minnie Pearl Cancer Research Network phase II trial. *Oncologist* 2004, 9:644–652.

106. Schneider BJ, El-Rayes JH, Philip PA, *et al.*: Phase II trial of carboplatin, gemcitabine and capecitabine in patients with carcinoma of unknown primary. *Cancer* 2007, 110:770–775.

HIV is the fourth leading cause of death worldwide, with an annual death rate reaching nearly 3 million [1]. In North America, approximately 1.4 million people are currently infected and almost half a million have died since the beginning of the epidemic. HIV is associated with a wide spectrum of disease, ranging from asymptomatic patients to those who are profoundly immunosuppressed. HIV RNA levels are important predictors of the rate of progression, whereas CD4+ T-cell counts are markers of immunologic status. Even in the absence of opportunistic infections or malignancy, constitutional signs and symptoms, including fevers, weight loss, anorexia, nausea, and vomiting, are quite common. Antiretroviral therapy further complicates interpretation of these symptoms because many of the drugs cause similar side effects. Nonetheless, persistent fever always requires a search for opportunistic infections. Common infections in HIV-infected patients include pneumocystic pneumonia (caused by *Pneumocystis jiroveci*), chronic sinusitis, oral and esophageal candidiasis, herpes simplex infections, shingles, cytomegalovirus retinitis, and enterocolitis associated with various bacteria and protozoans. A variety of infections, including toxoplasmosis, progressive multifocal leukoencephalopathy, and cryptococcal meningitis, manifest in the central nervous system. Skin infections with molloscum contagiosum and dermatophytic fungi are also common. With appropriate prophylaxis, several of these infections can be prevented.

Highly active antiretroviral therapy (HAART) is generally recommended for patients with any of the following: acute HIV infection (or within the first 6 months after seroconversion), symptomatic AIDS, thrush, unexplained fever, or CD4+ T-cell counts below 200/mm³ [2–4]. In an international study comparing the continuous use of HAART with episodic treatment, based on CD4 T-cell levels, opportunistic infections and deaths were increased in the arm with treatment interruptions [5]. Interestingly, the AIDS-defining malignancy rate per 1000 person-years was higher in the drug conservation arm (3.0 vs 0.5), providing further evidence against interruptions in antiretroviral therapy [6].

AIDS-related mortality has dramatically declined in patients with access to antiretroviral therapy. In a population-based cohort analysis of AIDS patients, the rate of decline of deaths was significantly higher for HIV-related deaths compared with non–HIV-related deaths, which accounted for one fourth of all deaths [7]. Twenty percent of these deaths were attributable to non–HIV-related cancers. Cancer risk is increased among individuals infected with HIV. In the United States, Kaposi's sarcoma (KS), non-Hodgkin's lymphoma (NHL), and invasive cervical cancer are currently considered AIDS-defining malignancies by the Centers for Disease Control and Prevention.

As patients with HIV continue to live longer, oncologists face the challenge of dealing with the neoplastic complications of HIV. While the approach to treatment may not always differ from that of the non–HIV-infected population, recognition of the special infectious risks associated with HIV and concomitant chemotherapy is important. This chapter focuses on the epidemiology, diagnostic methods, and management of Kaposi's sarcoma and NHL. In addition, key aspects of other non–AIDS-defining cancers will be briefly reviewed.

KAPOSI'S SARCOMA

EPIDEMIOLOGY

KS is an AIDS-defining cancer, accounting for nearly one third of all cases of cancer among people with AIDS in the United States [8] (Fig. 23-1). The use of antiretroviral therapy has considerably diminished the incidence of KS [9]. The KS herpesvirus (KSHV), also referred to as HHV-8, is a required cofactor [10]. Men who have sex with men are at especially high risk for KSHV infection, although the precise mode of sexual transmission remains poorly understood. Opportunistic infections often precede the presentation or exacerbation of KS. Among individuals who are both seropositive for HIV and KSHV, the sequence of exposure appears to be an important risk factor for KS development, with a higher risk for KS when KSHV seroconversion follows HIV seroconversion [11], thus suggesting an underlying impaired immune status.

DIAGNOSTIC METHODS

KS lesions typically arise on the skin or mucous membranes. They are often symmetrically distributed and follow Langer's lines (Fig. 23-2). The legs, face (especially the nose and ears), and the hard palate are common locations for lesions. KS can have visceral involvement but virtually never involves the brain parenchyma. The distinctive flat, deep-purple plaques may progress to form nodules. KS lesions are generally not pruritic or painful, except when involving the plantar foot. The problems associated with KS vary as a function of the location of the lesions. Lower extremity lesions often lead to lymphatic obstruction with painful edema. Pulmonary lesions may be associated with dyspnea; however, hemoptysis occurs rarely. Gastrointestinal lesions may be asymptomatic or may cause symptoms such as diarrhea, cramping, pain, and bleeding.

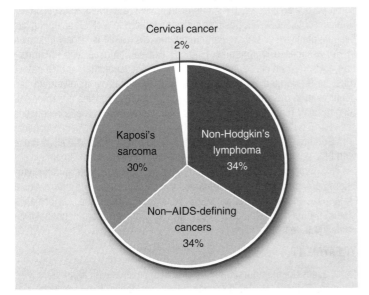

Figure 23-1. Risk of cancer among people with AIDS in the United States, 1996–2002. (*Adapted from* Engels *et al.* [8].)

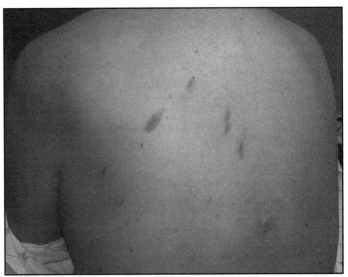

Figure 23-2. Cutaneous Kaposi's sarcoma lesions.

Evaluation of KS involves determination of the CD4+ T-cell count and HIV viral load. The diagnosis is confirmed by biopsy. This is most commonly a punch biopsy of a skin lesion, although lymph node, transbronchial, pleural, or gastrointestinal endoscopic biopsies are occasionally required. Computed tomography (CT) scans of the chest and abdomen are typically obtained, and a gastrointestinal endoscopy is performed if clinically indicated.

Standard TNM (tumor, node, metastasis) staging has not proved particularly useful for KS, partly because KS is a multicentric disease but also because the status of HIV disease is of overriding importance, with several reports of KS remission with suppression of HIV replication [12,13]. The AIDS Clinical Trials Group (ACTG) designed a staging system taking into consideration these unique KS features in HIV-infected individuals [14]. Patients are classified as "good risk" or "poor risk" based on the extent of tumor, CD4+ T-cell count, and evidence of HIV-associated systemic symptoms. When the ACTG staging system was reevaluated in patients receiving HAART, immune status was no longer associated with an increased risk of death, even when lowering the CD4 from the previously established cut point of 200/mm^3 or less to 100/mm^3 or less [15].

TREATMENT

The impact of HAART has profoundly impacted the survival of patients with KS. Prior to HAART, KS was associated with a 90% mortality rate; since then, for patients treated with HAART, the mortality rate has nearly halved [16]. In fact, treatment with antiretroviral therapy is sometimes associated with remission of KS [12,17]; thus, therapy begins with ensuring that the antiretroviral regimen has been optimized. It is often appropriate to withhold KS-directed systemic treatment for several months to assess the full impact of HAART. Rapidly progressive disease, defined by more than 10 new lesions in the past months, lymphedema, or symptomatic visceral or cosmetically disfiguring disease, is the exception. In these patients, systemic treatment should not be delayed.

SYSTEMIC THERAPY

Single-agent therapy with a liposomal anthracycline or with paclitaxel is now the standard of care. In phase 3 trials, liposomal doxorubicin has been shown to be at least as effective and less toxic than combination regimens including nonliposomal anthracyclines [18,19]. Low-dose paclitaxel administered every 2 weeks is associated with an overall response rate of 70% in treatment-naive patients and a 53% response among poor-prognosis patients, with a median CD4+ T-cell count of 5/mm^3 [20].

Several other agents have been tested and appear to have promising results. Interferon-α is active in a subset of patients, and when effective, responses are often long-lasting [21,22]. However, the delayed response of 8 to 12 weeks precludes its use in patients with very symptomatic or aggressive disease. Oral therapies, including thalidomide, imatinib, rapamycin, and alitretinoin (9-cis-retinoic acid) have also been reported to be active against KS in small series [23–26].

LOCAL THERAPY

Local therapies are appropriate for patients with few lesions and slowly progressive disease. Treatments include alitretinoin topical gel, intralesional vinblastine, interferon, sodium tetradecyl sulfate, liquid nitrogen, and radiation therapy [27].

LYMPHOMA

EPIDEMIOLOGY

Both NHL and Hodgkin's lymphomas are increased in incidence in patients with HIV infection, although the increase in NHL is much greater and only aggressive B-cell NHLs have been formally recognized as AIDS-defining illnesses. In contrast to KS, lymphomas occur in all HIV populations and show no marked predilection for men who have sex with men. Evaluation of cancer and AIDS registries demonstrates a much more dramatic increase in particular types of lymphoma, with brain, immunoblastic, and Burkitt's lymphomas having 1020-fold, 60-fold, and 50-fold higher incidences in comparison with the general population, respectively [8]. With HAART, the overall incidence of lymphoma is decreasing, with the most marked decrease occurring in primary brain lymphoma [28–30]. The length of time

with HIV infection prior to diagnosis of lymphomas is increasing, as is the CD4+ T-cell count at the time of diagnosis. The incidence of Hodgkin's lymphoma, which is 10- to 20-fold higher than the general population, has temporally increased with the availability of HAART over the past decade [8,31,32]. Hodgkin's lymphoma typically develops in HIV patients with relatively high CD4 counts maintained over several years. HIV-associated Hodgkin's lymphoma is characterized by a predominance of unfavorable subtypes, with mixed cellularity being most common followed by lymphocyte depletion [33,34].

The Epstein-Barr virus (EBV) genome is detectable in nearly half of the lymphomas arising in HIV-infected individuals. Particular anatomic sites and histologic types are especially likely to be EBV associated. Primary brain lymphomas and lymphomas with central nervous system involvement are virtually always EBV positive. The histologies that are frequently associated with EBV include primary effusion lymphomas, plasmablastic oral lymphomas, and Hodgkin's lymphoma. Interestingly, AIDS-associated Burkitt's lymphoma is infrequently associated with EBV, despite the near 100% association of EBV with endemic African Burkitt's lymphoma.

DIAGNOSTIC METHODS

Patients frequently present with advanced stage, extranodal disease, and constitutional symptoms. In 20% to 30% of patients, the disease is entirely extranodal, with nearly 90% of patients having some extranodal involvement. Unusual sites, not typically involved by lymphoma, have been reported, including heart, common bile duct, skin, and many others. The gastrointestinal tract is a common extranodal site in patients with HIV.

With the possible exception of primary brain lymphoma, a biopsy is required to diagnose lymphoma. Benign hyperplasia is often encountered in individuals with HIV; therefore, several lymph node biopsies may be required prior to establishing a diagnosis. Lymph nodes are best assessed by excisional biopsy, which allows for assessment of architectural patterns. However, lesions devoid of lymphoid tissue are adequately assessed by needle biopsy.

Because brain biopsy is a risky endeavor, attempts are made to avoid the procedure if possible [35]. Toxoplasmosis is the most common intracranial mass lesion in the HIV setting [36], and the typical presentation—ring-enhancing lesions—is often indistinguishable from primary brain lymphoma. Instead of biopsying suspicious lesions, seropositive patients are empirically treated, and biopsy is relegated only for those individuals who fail to respond to toxoplasmosis therapy or for those with evidence of progression over a 2-week therapeutic trial. Another diagnostic approach involves evaluating for EBV DNA by polymerase chain reaction in cerebrospinal fluid, which is fairly specific [37,38].

Staging lymphoma is not unlike that in the non-HIV population, with some particular caveats. CT scans of the chest, abdomen, and pelvis are routinely obtained. While positron emission tomography (PET) scanning has become standard in staging lymphoma, the role of PET is largely unknown in HIV-associated lymphomas. Findings can be confused with inflammation, infection, or persistent generalized lymphadenopathy, and therefore must be interpreted with caution [39,40]. Bone marrow involvement can occur even in the absence of cytopenias; therefore, biopsies are standard. Staging also requires imaging of the brain either by magnetic resonance scans or CT. Diagnostic lumbar punctures should be performed in patients with Burkitt's, Burkitt-like, and immunoblastic lymphomas, as well as those with EBV-positive tumors and those with bone marrow involvement.

The response to antiviral therapy is a key factor in determining lymphoma outcome [28]. Lymphoma-associated factors (ie, the International Prognostic Index, age, tumor stage, lactate dehydrogenase, performance status, number of extranodal sites) have also proven prognostic in AIDS-related NHL [41,42].

TREATMENT

Rapid assessment and treatment is critical in patients with aggressive lymphomas. Patients should be monitored for evidence of tumor lysis syndrome and treatment with aggressive hydration and allopurinol should be initiated when the staging evaluation is still under way.

Infusional regimens are well tolerated and have yielded impressive results in HIV patients. In a multi-institutional study, CDE (cyclophosphamide, doxorubicin, etoposide) administered as a 96-hour infusion yielded a failure-free survival rate of 36% at 2 years [43]. The addition of rituximab appears to improve response rates, although it may be associated with an increased risk of life-threatening infections [44]. A National Cancer Institute trial evaluating EPOCH (infusional etoposide, prednisone, vincristine, cyclophosphamide, doxorubicin) yielded a 92% disease-free survival at 53 months [45]. These excellent results have yet to be duplicated. In a randomized trial evaluating CHOP (cyclophosphamide, doxorubicin, vincristine, prednisone) chemotherapy with or without rituximab, rituximab did not improve outcome and was associated with more infectious complications [46]. In a recent French study evaluating rituximab plus CHOP, the estimated 2-year overall survival rate was 75% and the infectious concerns related to rituximab were not borne out [47]. While many clinicians now routinely incorporate rituximab in chemotherapy regimens for HIV patients, caution is still advised. Pneumocystis prophylaxis should be administered to all patients undergoing intensive chemotherapy regardless of CD4+ T-cell count. In addition, patients should receive antifungal and antiherpes viral prophylaxis as well as hematopoietic growth factors. Intrathecal prophylaxis should be administered for individuals with bone marrow involvement, Burkitt or Burkitt-like histology, or EBV-positive tumors. Typically, five treatments with either cytarabine or methotrexate interspersed throughout the chemotherapy course are given.

Patients with HIV and Hodgkin's lymphoma often present with advanced-stage disease. Combination chemotherapy is thus the mainstay of therapy. ABVD (doxorubicin, bleomycin, vinblastine, and dacarbazine) and Stanford V [48] have both been studied [49–51]. In a phase 2 study of Stanford V in 59 patients with Hodgkin's lymphoma receiving concomitant HAART, the estimated 3-year disease-free and overall survival rates were 51% and 68%, respectively [51]. Randomized controlled trials are lacking [52].

For relapsed or refractory disease, salvage therapies often have disappointing results. ESHAP (etoposide, methylprednisolone, cisplatin, and high-dose cytarabine) is the best studied regimen [53]. High-dose therapy with autologous peripheral stem cell transplantation is an appropriate salvage for patients with either NHL or Hodgkin's lymphoma and chemotherapy-sensitive disease [54,55].

Radiation therapy remains the mainstay treatment for primary brain lymphomas. Retrospective studies demonstrate tumor responses and improved quality of life, but long-term survivals are rare.

OTHER CANCERS IN HIV-POSITIVE PATIENTS

The spectrum of malignancies in patients with HIV continues to evolve. While cervical cancer is recognized by the Centers for Disease Control and Prevention as an AIDS-defining illness, an excess of cervical cancer directly attributable to HIV remains to be conclusively demonstrated. Non–AIDS-defining cancers, including those most common in the general population (lung, colon, and skin cancer) as well as multiple myeloma and anal cancer, are on the rise. While lung and colon cancers are indistinguishable from the general population, plasma cell dyscrasias are quite distinctive. They often present with visceral or leukemic involvement and are EBV associated. Anal cancer occurs with a 20-fold excess in people with HIV compared with the general population [8]. Receptive anal intercourse is a well-established risk factor for anal cancer and the relative contribution of HIV remains ill-defined. The approach to treatment of these disorders is not different from that in the non–HIV-infected population, although recognition of the increased risk for potential infectious complications is imperative. The higher rates of cancer seen in the HIV population, coupled with higher life expectancies, highlight the need for more intensive prevention and screening efforts.

CONCLUSIONS

For an increasing number of patients, HIV infection is most appropriately viewed as a chronic illness. AIDS-related mortality has dramatically declined for those with access to antiretroviral therapy. The improved prognosis for patients with HIV infection has prompted a paradigm shift, with a new focus on the neoplastic complications of HIV. The widespread use of HAART in developed countries has greatly impacted chemotherapy tolerance and overall survival. In general, patients with HIV-associated malignancies are being treated with standard or only slightly modified chemotherapy regimens. Great strides have been made in the treatment of NHL, with response rates encroaching upon those of lymphoma patients without HIV. Large, randomized controlled trials are ultimately needed to determine the optimal treatment regimens for both NHL and KS.

LIPOSOMAL ANTHRACYCLINES

In animal models and early clinical trials in human patients, liposomal formulations (microscopic phospholipid spheres) of some anthracyclines (doxorubicin [Doxil, OrthoBiotech, Raritan, NJ] and daunorubicin [DaunoXome, Gilead Sciences, Inc., Foster City, CA]) have been shown to improve the therapeutic index when compared with the native anthracycline preparation, with less toxicity and comparable and/or improved efficacy in patients with AIDS-related KS. Pharmacokinetic advantages of these formulations include a several-fold increase in plasma half-life with resultant prolonged circulation time, reduced clearance, a small volume of distribution, and markedly increased area under the curve. A putative advantage of the pegylated liposomal formulation (*eg*, liposomal doxorubicin) over the simple liposomal formulations is that the pegylated liposome reduces liposome opsonization and inhibits uptake by the reticuloendothelial system. The clinical significance of this remains to be determined; to date, there are no comparative data of the two liposomal formulations of doxorubicin and daunorubicin. It is advisable for the clinician to become familiar and knowledgeable with one of the two agents. In the trial data outlined below, both formulations were compared with an ABV regimen (doxorubicin, bleomycin, vincristine); however, for liposomal daunorubicin, the ABV regimen was dose-modified when compared with the traditional regimen.

Liposomal doxorubicin was investigated in an early phase 2 setting in patients with advanced KS [56]. All 34 patients had poor prognostic disease as judged by ACTG criteria. Patients were treated with liposomal doxorubicin 20 mg/m^2 IV every 3 wk on an outpatient basis. Nineteen of 34 patients had received prior chemotherapy for KS, although no patient had received prior anthracyclines. An overall response rate of 73.5% was observed, with a complete response rate of 5.8%. In patients who had received previous chemotherapy, the response rate was 68.4%. Median duration of response was 9 wk. The major toxicity was neutropenia. Liposomal doxorubicin has also been investigated in patients with advanced KS who failed standard chemotherapy [57]. While receiving standard ABV or BV (bleomycin and vincristine) chemotherapy, 53 patients who experienced disease progression or intolerable toxicity received liposomal doxorubicin at a dose of 20 mg/m^2 IV every 3 wk. Nineteen patients (36%) had a partial response and one had a clinical complete response. The most common adverse effect was leukopenia, which occurred in 40% of patients.

In a large, randomized phase 3 clinical trial of liposomal doxorubicin versus ABV in 258 AIDS-related KS patients, liposomal doxorubicin was superior both in terms of toxicity and response rates [19]. In this study, the liposomal doxorubicin yielded a superior response rate of 45.9% versus 24.8% (a much lower response rate than previously reported for the ABV regimen). The toxicity profile also favored the liposomal doxorubicin formulation, with 1) less alopecia, nausea/vomiting, and peripheral neuropathy; 2) comparable leukopenia; and 3) more stomatitis/mucositis.

Liposomal daunorubicin has also been investigated in a prospective, randomized phase 3 trial. In this study, 232 patients were randomized to receive liposomal daunorubicin (40 mg/m^2) or an ABV regimen (doxorubicin 10 mg/m^2, bleomycin 15 U, vincristine 1 mg [reduced vs standard ABV]) both given IV every 2 wk. The overall response rate for liposomal daunorubicin was 25%, similar to the 28% in the ABV group. There was significantly less alopecia and peripheral neuropathy but significantly more grade 4 neutropenia in patients treated on the liposomal daunorubicin arm [58].

CANDIDATES FOR TREATMENT

Patients with rapidly progressive disease, extensive disease with edema, or pulmonary involvement should be treated aggressively; liposomal anthracyclines may be used in this setting; clinicians should be alert to opportunistic infections; all patients should receive prophylaxis for *P. jiroveci* pneumonia

ALTERNATIVE THERAPY

Single-agent paclitaxel 100 mg/m^2 IV administered every 2 or 3 wk

SPECIAL PRECAUTIONS

Experience with liposomal anthracyclines is limited in patients with cardiac disease or risk factors; until further experience is recorded with these agents, the recommended total cumulative dose of liposomal doxorubicin is identical to that reported for doxorubicin. Liposomal daunorubicin is perhaps less cardiotoxic; with appropriate monitoring of left ventricular function, liposomal daunorubicin dosage can be escalated. The pharmacokinetics of the liposomal anthracyclines have not been studied in patients with hepatic impairment and renal insufficiency and dose modifications are recommended in these settings.

NURSING INTERVENTIONS

Both agents are not as likely as either native drug to cause severe extravasation; however, caution is advised in administering and monitoring infusions to avoid extravasation

TOXICITIES

When compared with ABV regimens, the liposomal formulations appear to be characterized by 1) significantly less alopecia, neurotoxicity, and gastrointestinal toxicity, 2) more stomatitis/mucositis, and 3) comparable myelosuppression, especially neutropenia. Principal clinical toxicities include myelosuppression (60% risk of leukopenia) and ~ 10% chance of thrombocytopenia and cardiotoxicity. Infusion reactions occurring with the first cycle of therapy are not uncommon with liposomal doxorubicin (6.8%); these are characterized by flushing, shortness of breath, facial swelling, headache, chest tightness, and back pain. The reactions generally do not recur with later cycles; palmar-plantar erythrodysesthesia occurs in 3.4% of patients receiving liposomal doxorubicin and is characterized by swelling, pain, erythema, and, in some circumstances, desquamation of the skin of the hands and feet. The incidence may be increased with higher dosage or more frequent administration. Similarly, a triad of back pain, flushing, and chest tightness has been reported in 13.8% of patients receiving liposomal daunorubicin; this usually occurs during the first 5 minutes of the infusion and subsides with interruption of the infusion. In both situations, reduction of the infusion rate may be helpful, and these reactions do not preclude further therapy.

Continued on the next page

LIPOSOMAL ANTHRACYCLINES *(CONTINUED)*

DRUG INTERACTIONS

No formal drug interaction studies have been conducted with liposomal anthracyclines; until specific compatibility data are available, it is not recommended that liposomal anthracyclines be mixed with other drugs. Liposomal anthracyclines may interact with drugs known to interact with the conventional formulation of doxorubicin or daunorubicin

PATIENT INFORMATION

Compared with ABV regimens, the liposomal anthracycline formulations caused significantly less alopecia in controlled clinical trials; this is likely an important consideration for many patients

Dosage and Scheduling

Liposomal doxorubicin 20 mg/m^2 IV over 30 min every 2–3 wk

or

Liposomal daunorubicin 40 mg/m^2 IV over 1 h every 2 wk

Experiences and Response Rates

Study	Evaluable patients, *n*	Drug	Dosage schedule	Response rate, %
Northfelt *et al.* [19]	133	Liposomal doxorubicin	20 mg/m^2 every 2 wk	45.9
Harrison *et al.* [56]	34	Liposomal doxorubicin	20 mg/m^2 every 3 wk	73.5
Northfelt *et al.* [57]	53	Liposomal doxorubicin	20 mg/m^2 every 3 wk	38.0
Gill *et al.* [58]	116	Liposomal daunorubicin	40 mg/m^2 every 2 wk	25.0

INFUSIONAL CDE (CYCLOPHOSPHAMIDE, DOXORUBICIN, ETOPOSIDE)

Investigators at Albert Einstein initially reported this regimen in a pilot study with 12 patients. The regimen consists of a continuous 96-h infusion of cyclophosphamide, doxorubicin, and etoposide. Patients with small, non–cleaved cell lymphoma and those with bone marrow involvement received central nervous system prophylaxis consisting of intrathecal chemotherapy and whole brain radiotherapy. This study and subsequent reports demonstrated a response rate of 58%–93%. The initial study had a long median survival of 17.4 mo. Therapy was generally well tolerated and was given on an outpatient basis using a portable infusion pump [59]. The Eastern Cooperative Oncology Group conducted a phase 2 pilot study of infusional CDE coupled with dideoxyinosine and granulocyte-macrophage colony-stimulating factor and reported a 44% complete response rate with a 43% 2-year overall survival [43]. The addition of rituximab to the CDE infusional regimen was associated with an improved complete response rate of 70% and a 2-year overall survival rate of 64%. Regardless of CD4 count, all patients should receive prophylaxis for *P. jiroveci* pneumonia during treatment.

ALTERNATIVE THERAPY
EPOCH or CHOP

TOXICITIES
Opportunistic infection is of primary concern, especially if CD4 lymphocyte counts are below 25/μL; concomitant steroid use increases this risk; the combination of this regimen and dideoxyinosine is associated with significantly less neutropenia and thrombocytopenia and fewer erythrocyte and platelet transfusions; CDE results in a significant decrease in CD4 and CD8 lymphocytes, an effect not abrogated by coadministration with dideoxyinosine; nonhematologic toxicity consists of nausea and vomiting (72%) and stomatitis (56%); one patient developed heart failure due to this regimen.

PATIENT INFORMATION
This regimen requires placement of a central venous access device and patients will likely have to be hospitalized for 4 d in the absence of appropriate home care support or if the clinician is not familiar with the regimen. This regimen has resulted in the longest survival reported for patients with AIDS-related lymphoma.

Dosage and Scheduling

Cyclophosphamide 200 mg/m^2/d as 96-h continuous infusion every 4 wk

Doxorubicin 12.5 mg/m^2/d as 96-h continuous infusion every 4 wk

Etoposide 60 mg/m^2/d as 96-h continuous infusion every 4 wk

Granulocyte colony-stimulating factor 5 μg/kg subcutaneously on d 6 until absolute neutrophil count > 10,000/μL

CNS prophylaxis*

  Cytarabine 50 mg intrathecally on d 1 and 4 for cycles 1 and 2

• Two cycles beyond achieving complete response for minimum of 4 and maximum of 8 cycles

*In select patients.

Experiences and Response Rates

Study	Evaluable patients, *n*	Median CD4 count/mm^3	Response rate, %	Median survival, *mo*
Sparano *et al.* [43]	98	160	57	12.8
Spina *et al.* [44]	74	161	75	Not reached at 23-mo follow-up

REFERENCES

1. United Nations Programme on HIV/AIDS and World Health Organization: AIDS epidemic update, 2006. http://data.unaids.org/pub/EpiReport/2006/2006_EpiUpdate_en.pdf. UNAIDS/WHO; 2006.

2. Dybul M, Fauci AS, Bartlett JG, et al.: Guidelines for using antiretroviral agents among HIV-infected adults and adolescents. *Ann Intern Med* 2002, 137:381–433.

3. Trotta MP, Ammassari A, Melzi S, et al.: Treatment-related factors and highly active antiretroviral therapy adherence. *J Acquir Immune Defic Syndr* 2002, 31(Suppl 3):S128–S131.

4. Thorner A, Rosenberg E: Early versus delayed antiretroviral therapy in patients with HIV infection: a review of the current guidelines from an immunological perspective. *Drugs* 2003, 63:1325–1337.

5. El-Sadr WM, Lundgren JD, Neaton JD, et al.: CD4+ count-guided interruption of antiretroviral treatment. *N Engl J Med* 2006, 355:2283–2296.

6. Silverberg MJ, Neuhaus J, Bower M, et al.: Risk of cancers during interrupted antiretroviral therapy in the SMART study. *AIDS* 2007, 21:1957–1963.

7. Sackoff JE, Hanna DB, Pfeiffer MR, et al.: Causes of death among persons with AIDS in the era of highly active antiretroviral therapy: New York City. *Ann Intern Med* 2006, 145:397–406.

8. Engels EA, Pfeiffer RM, Goedert JJ, et al.: Trends in cancer risk among people with AIDS in the United States 1980–2002. *AIDS* 2006, 20:1645–1654.

9. Carrieri MP, Pradier C, Piselli P, et al.: Reduced incidence of Kaposi's sarcoma and of systemic non-Hodgkin's lymphoma in HIV-infected individuals treated with highly active antiretroviral therapy. *Int J Cancer* 2003, 103:142–144.

10. Moore PS: The emergence of Kaposi's sarcoma-associated herpesvirus (human herpesvirus 8). *N Engl J Med* 2000, 343:1411–1413.

11. Jacobson LP, Jenkins FJ, Springer G, et al.: Interaction of human immunodeficiency virus type 1 and human herpesvirus type 8 infections on the incidence of Kaposi's sarcoma. *J Infect Dis* 2000, 181:1940–1949.

12. Gill J, Bourboulia D, Wilkinson J, et al.: Prospective study of the effects of antiretroviral therapy on Kaposi sarcoma–associated herpesvirus infection in patients with and without Kaposi sarcoma. *J Acquir Immune Defic Syndr* 2002, 31:384–390.

13. Martinez V, Caumes E, Gambotti L, et al.: Remission from Kaposi's sarcoma on HAART is associated with suppression of HIV replication and is independent of protease inhibitor therapy. *Br J Cancer* 2006, 94:1000–1006.

14. Krown SE, Testa MA, Huang J: AIDS-related Kaposi's sarcoma: prospective validation of the AIDS Clinical Trials Group staging classification. AIDS Clinical Trials Group Oncology Committee. *J Clin Oncol* 1997, 15:3085–3092.

15. Nasti G, Talamini R, Antinori A, et al.: AIDS-related Kaposi's sarcoma: evaluation of potential new prognostic factors and assessment of the AIDS Clinical Trial Group Staging System in the Haart Era—the Italian Cooperative Group on AIDS and Tumors and the Italian Cohort of Patients Naive From Antiretrovirals. *J Clin Oncol* 2003, 21:2876–2882.

16. Holkova B, Takeshita K, Cheng DM, et al.: Effect of highly active antiretroviral therapy on survival in patients with AIDS-associated pulmonary Kaposi's sarcoma treated with chemotherapy. *J Clin Oncol* 2001, 19:3848–3851.

17. Tam HK, Zhang ZF, Jacobson LP, et al.: Effect of highly active antiretroviral therapy on survival among HIV-infected men with Kaposi sarcoma or non-Hodgkin lymphoma. *Int J Cancer* 2002, 98:916–922.

18. Stewart S, Jablonowski H, Goebel FD, et al.: Randomized comparative trial of pegylated liposomal doxorubicin versus bleomycin and vincristine in the treatment of AIDS-related Kaposi's sarcoma. International Pegylated Liposomal Doxorubicin Study Group. *J Clin Oncol* 1998, 16:683–691.

19. Northfelt DW, Dezube BJ, Thommes JA, et al.: Pegylated-liposomal doxorubicin versus doxorubicin, bleomycin, and vincristine in the treatment of AIDS-related Kaposi's sarcoma: results of a randomized phase III clinical trial. *J Clin Oncol* 1998, 16:2445–2451.

20. Tulpule A, Groopman J, Saville MW, et al.: Multicenter trial of low-dose paclitaxel in patients with advanced AIDS-related Kaposi sarcoma. *Cancer* 2002, 95:147–154.

21. Krown SE, Li P, Von Roenn JH, et al.: Efficacy of low-dose interferon with antiretroviral therapy in Kaposi's sarcoma: a randomized phase II AIDS clinical trials group study. *J Interferon Cytokine Res* 2002, 22:295–303.

22. Krown SE, Lee JY, Lin L, et al.: Interferon-alpha2b with protease inhibitor-based antiretroviral therapy in patients with AIDS-associated Kaposi sarcoma: an AIDS malignancy consortium phase I trial. *J Acquir Immune Defic Syndr* 2006, 41:149–153.

23. Little RF, Wyvill KM, Pluda JM, et al.: Activity of thalidomide in AIDS-related Kaposi's sarcoma. *J Clin Oncol* 2000, 18:2593–2602.

24. Koon HB, Bubley GJ, Pantanowitz L, et al.: Imatinib-induced regression of AIDS-related Kaposi's sarcoma. *J Clin Oncol* 2005, 23:982–989.

25. Stallone G, Schena A, Infante B, et al.: Sirolimus for Kaposi's sarcoma in renal-transplant recipients. *N Engl J Med* 2005, 352:1317–1323.

26. Miles SA, Dezube BJ, Lee JY, et al.: Antitumor activity of oral 9-cis-retinoic acid in HIV-associated Kaposi's sarcoma. *AIDS* 2002, 16:421–429.

27. Ramirez-Amador V, Esquivel-Pedraza L, Lozada-Nur F, et al.: Intralesional vinblastine vs. 3% sodium tetradecyl sulfate for the treatment of oral Kaposi's sarcoma. A double blind randomized clinical trial. *Oral Oncol* 2002, 38:460–467.

28. Hoffmann C, Wolf E, Fatkenheuer G, et al.: Response to highly active antiretroviral therapy strongly predicts outcome in patients with AIDS-related lymphoma. *AIDS* 2003, 17:1521–1529.

29. Kirk O, Pedersen C, Cozzi-Lepri A, et al.: Non-Hodgkin lymphoma in HIV-infected patients in the era of highly active antiretroviral therapy. *Blood* 2001, 98:3406–3412.

30. Besson C, Goubar A, Gabarre J, et al.: Changes in AIDS-related lymphoma since the era of highly active antiretroviral therapy. *Blood* 2001, 98:2339–2344.

31. Herida M, Mary-Krause M, Kaphan R, et al.: Incidence of non-AIDS-defining cancers before and during the highly active antiretroviral therapy era in a cohort of human immunodeficiency virus-infected patients. *J Clin Oncol* 2003, 21:3447–3453.

32. Biggar RJ, Jaffe ES, Goedert JJ, et al.: Hodgkin lymphoma and immunodeficiency in persons with HIV/AIDS. *Blood* 2006, 108:3786–3791.

33. Tirelli U, Spina M, Gaidano G, et al.: Epidemiological, biological and clinical features of HIV-related lymphomas in the era of highly active antiretroviral therapy. *AIDS* 2000, 14:1675–1688.

34. Spina M, Vaccher E, Nasti G, et al.: Human immunodeficiency virus-associated Hodgkin's disease. *Semin Oncol* 2000, 27:480–488.

35. Skolasky RL, Dal Pan GJ, Olivi A, et al.: HIV-associated primary CNS lymorbidity and utility of brain biopsy. *J Neurol Sci* 1999, 163:32–38.

36. Sacktor N, Lyles RH, Skolasky R, et al.: HIV-associated neurologic disease incidence changes: Multicenter AIDS Cohort Study, 1990–1998. *Neurology* 2001, 56:257–260.

37. Cingolani A, De Luca A, Larocca LM, et al.: Minimally invasive diagnosis of acquired immunodeficiency syndrome-related primary central nervous system lymphoma. *J Natl Cancer Inst* 1998, 90:364–369.

38. Bossolasco S, Cinque P, Ponzoni M, et al.: Epstein-Barr virus DNA load in cerebrospinal fluid and plasma of patients with AIDS-related lymphoma. *J Neurovirol* 2002, 8:432–438.

39. O'Doherty MJ, Barrington SF, Campbell M, et al.: PET scanning and the human immunodeficiency virus-positive patient. *J Nucl Med* 1997, 38:1575–1583.

40. Bhargava P, Chang CW, Glickman B, et al.: Persistent generalized lymphadenopathy (PGL) mimicking lymphoma on whole-body FDG PET/CT imaging. *Clin Nucl Med* 2006, 31:398–400.

41. Bower M, Gazzard B, Mandalia S, et al.: A prognostic index for systemic AIDS-related non-Hodgkin lymphoma treated in the era of highly active antiretroviral therapy. *Ann Intern Med* 2005, 143:265–273.

42. Lim ST, Karim R, Tulpule A, et al.: Prognostic factors in HIV-related diffuse large-cell lymphoma: before versus after highly active antiretroviral therapy. *J Clin Oncol* 2005, 23:8477–8482.

43. Sparano JA, Lee S, Chen MG, *et al.*: Phase II trial of infusional cyclophosphamide, doxorubicin, and etoposide in patients with HIV-associated non-Hodgkin's lymphoma: an Eastern Cooperative Oncology Group Trial (E1494). *J Clin Oncol* 2004, 22:1491–1500.

44. Spina M, Jaeger U, Sparano JA, *et al.*: Rituximab plus infusional cyclophosphamide, doxorubicin, and etoposide in HIV-associated non-Hodgkin lymphoma: pooled results from 3 phase 2 trials. *Blood* 2005, 105:1891–1897.

45. Little RF, Pittaluga S, Grant N, *et al.*: Highly effective treatment of acquired immunodeficiency syndrome-related lymphoma with dose-adjusted EPOCH: impact of antiretroviral therapy suspension and tumor biology. *Blood* 2003, 101:4653–4659.

46. Kaplan LD, Lee JY, Ambinder RF, *et al.*: Rituximab does not improve clinical outcome in a randomized phase 3 trial of CHOP with or without rituximab in patients with HIV-associated non-Hodgkin lymphoma: AIDS-Malignancies Consortium Trial 010. *Blood* 2005, 106:1538–1543.

47. Boue F, Gabarre J, Gisselbrecht C, *et al.*: Phase II trial of CHOP plus rituximab in patients with HIV-associated non-Hodgkin's lymphoma. *J Clin Oncol* 2006, 24:4123–4128.

48. Bartlett NL, Rosenberg SA, Hoppe RT, *et al.*: Brief chemotherapy, Stanford V, and adjuvant radiotherapy for bulky or advanced-stage Hodgkin's disease: a preliminary report. *J Clin Oncol* 1995, 13:1080–1088.

49. Levine AM, Li P, Cheung T, *et al.*: Chemotherapy consisting of doxorubicin, bleomycin, vinblastine, and dacarbazine with granulocyte-colony-stimulating factor in HIV-infected patients with newly diagnosed Hodgkin's disease: a prospective, multi-institutional AIDS clinical trials group study (ACTG 149). *J Acquir Immune Defic Syndr* 2000, 24:444–450.

50. Xicoy B, Ribera JM, Romeu J, *et al.*: Response to highly active antiretroviral therapy as the only therapy in an HIV-infected patient with interfollicular Hodgkin's lymphoma. *Leuk Lymphoma* 2007, 48:2058–2059.

51. Spina M, Gabarre J, Rossi G, *et al.*: Stanford V regimen and concomitant HAART in 59 patients with Hodgkin disease and HIV infection. *Blood* 2002, 100:1984–1988.

52. Marti-Carvajal AJ, Cardona AF, Rodriguez ML: Interventions for treating AIDS-associated Hodgkin s lymphoma in treatment-naive adults. *Cochrane Database Syst Rev* 2007:CD006149.

53. Bi J, Espina BM, Tulpule A, *et al.*: High-dose cytosine-arabinoside and cisplatin regimens as salvage therapy for refractory or relapsed AIDS-related non-Hodgkin's lymphoma. *J Acquir Immune Defic Syndr* 2001, 28:416–421.

54. Re A, Cattaneo C, Michieli M, *et al.*: High-dose therapy and autologous peripheral-blood stem-cell transplantation as salvage treatment for HIV-associated lymphoma in patients receiving highly active antiretroviral therapy. *J Clin Oncol* 2003, 21:4423–4427.

55. Krishnan A, Molina A, Zaia J, *et al.*: Durable remissions with autologous stem cell transplantation for high-risk HIV-associated lymphomas. *Blood* 2005, 105:874–878.

56. Harrison M, Tomlinson D, Stewart S: Liposomal-entrapped doxorubicin: an active agent in AIDS-related Kaposi's sarcoma. *J Clin Oncol* 1995, 13:914–920.

57. Northfelt DW, Dezube BJ, Thommes JA, *et al.*: Efficacy of pegylated-liposomal doxorubicin in the treatment of AIDS-related Kaposi's sarcoma after failure of standard chemotherapy. *J Clin Oncol* 1996, 15:653–659.

58. Gill PS, Wenrz J, Scadden DT, *et al.*: Randomized phase II trial of liposomal daunorubicin versus doxorubicin, bleomycin, and vincristine in AIDS-related Kaposi's sarcoma. *J Clin Oncol* 1996, 14:2353–2364.

59. Sparano JA, Wiernik PH, Hu X, *et al.*: Pilot trial of infusional cyclophosphamide, doxorubicin, and etoposide plus didanosine and filgrastim in patients with human immunodeficiency virus-associated non-Hodgkin's lymphoma. *J Clin Oncol* 1996, 14:3026–3035.

Palliative care is comprehensive care for serious illnesses, including cancer, with the goal of preventing and relieving suffering and maximizing quality of life for patients and their families [1]. Palliative care can be provided concurrently with life-prolonging or curative cancer care, or can become the main focus of care. It is most often given by the primary team, which includes oncologists, surgeons, radiation oncologists, nurses, social workers, and chaplains, but can be supplemented by specialty interdisciplinary palliative care teams or pain specialists. Palliative care includes the provision of hospice services, but can be given at any time during a patient's illness. It is especially important during times of transition, including the time of diagnosis, when an assessment of palliative care domains can help identify issues such as sources of suffering and information and caregiving needs. It is also essential when there are issues with treatment (eg, lack of efficacy or complications), when there is disease progression, and when the focus of care switches from cure or life prolongation to quality of life.

The assessment and provision of palliative care includes the domains of physical symptoms and complications of the disease and treatment; psychological and psychiatric issues, including grief and bereavement; social issues, including caregiving and family needs; spiritual, religious, and existential aspects of care; culture-specific patient and family needs; care at the end of life; and discussion of and respect for goals, preferences, and choices [1]. A palliative care assessment also includes evaluating the patient's current medical situation and prognosis, the benefits and burdens of current and potential treatment options, and determining the patient's and family's understanding of these issues and needs and preferences for information.

This chapter concentrates on a number of issues related to the delivery of good palliative care. In particular, focus is placed on issues related to management of pain and other distressing physical symptoms. Other relevant topics covered are the patient's final hours of life, decision making, care planning, and hospice care.

PAIN

Nearly one third of newly diagnosed cancer patients and two thirds of patients with advanced disease suffer from pain. Oncologists tend to underestimate the severity of cancer patients' pain, which has led to major disparities in appropriate pain management [2]. Furthermore, patients and caregivers alike are fearful of the potential for opioid addiction, while in actuality the risk of iatrogenic addiction is exceedingly small [3]. Nonetheless, underprescribing continues to be a barrier in achieving adequate analgesia, thus underscoring the need for enhanced awareness among oncologists.

ASSESSMENT

The first step in establishing effective pain management requires a comprehensive assessment. Assessing the pain descriptively is important for the diagnosis, and quantifying the pain is essential for choosing the initial treatment and monitoring an intervention's success. Patients may not have physical findings or clear anatomic explanations for their pain. Determining the pain's etiology is helpful for proper management, but should not delay appropriate treatment. Taking an appropriate pain history should include the key elements of "PQRST": palliating/provocative/psychosocial features, quality, radiation, severity, and treatment history. Physical examination and assessment for coexisting causes of suffering (eg, depression) should further direct treatment. These issues should be addressed as part of the whole palliative care patient evaluation.

Communication with patients and families is also a key component in pain assessment, as pain is subjective and defined by the patient's reports. Screening methods include numeric pain scores (rating from 0–10), visual analogue scales, and behavioral screening tools. A systematic review of cancer pain quality measures and supporting evidence reveals that routine pain assessments are key in quality improvement interventions [4].

PHARMACOLOGIC MEASURES

Competency with analgesics is imperative for the oncologist. Numerous resources, including the National Comprehensive Cancer Network's Clinical Practice Guidelines in Oncology (available at http://www.nccn.org), are available to help direct oncologists in achieving adequate analgesia for their patients. The World Health Organization "analgesic ladder," developed in 1987, provides a standard approach to managing pain based on pain severity and prior analgesic use. Pain medications are divided into three levels: nonopioids, opioids for mild to moderate pain, and opioids for moderate to severe pain. The initial treatment of pain in advanced or terminal illness should be based on pain severity, as detailed in Table 24-1 [5]. When pain is constant, pain medications should be given around the clock rather than on demand. For constant, moderate to severe pain, starting on a low dose of a long-acting opioid can be an effective approach. Using more than two to three breakthrough doses in a 24-hour period is an indication that either

Table 24-1. Treatment Recommendations According to Pain Intensity		
Pain intensity	**Initial treatment**	**Treatment details**
7–10 (severe or pain emergency)	Rapidly titrate short-acting opioids	Administer 5–10 mg of oral morphine or equivalent and reassess at 60 min
		If pain score is unchanged, repeat or give double the original dose
		If pain score is decreased < 50%, repeat same dose
		Once pain score has decreased > 50%, consider this the effective dose and administer every 4 h with breakthrough dose available
		For patients already on opioids, consider increasing dose 50%–100%
4–6 (moderate)	Titrate short-acting opioid	Administer 5–10 mg of oral morphine or equivalent and reassess at 4 h
		If pain score is decreased < 50%, increase dose 25%–50%
		If pain score is decreased > 50%, consider this the effective dose and administer every 4 h
		For patients already on opioids, consider increasing dose 25%–50%
1–3 (mild)	Consider adjuvant treatment or short-acting opioid	Consider nonsteroidal anti-inflammatory drug or acetaminophen
		Can also consider titrating short-acting opioid (see "moderate" dosing above)
		For patients already on opioids, consider increasing dose 25%

a long-acting opioid should be started or that the current dose should be increased. An increase of at least 25% is typically needed to have an appreciable effect. A safe approach is to add up the total opioid dosage in the previous 24-hour period and convert it to a long-acting opioid. The breakthrough dose should be approximately 10% to 20% of the 24-hour total opioid dose. For equianalgesic calculations, one can refer to the Hopkins Opioid Program, which can be downloaded to a handheld computer [6]. It is important to remember that equianalgesic conversions are approximate and vary among individuals. Therefore, if pain is well controlled, it is usually recommended to decrease the starting dose of the new opioid by approximately 25% with rapid titration and provision of adequate amounts of breakthrough medications. For patients with poorly controlled pain, doses should not be reduced. Newer formulations of opioids, such as oral transmucosal fentanyl citrate, have recently become available and allow for enhanced absorption and rapid onset of action [7].

Specific pain problems may not be responsive to opioids despite appropriate titration. Adjuvant analgesics may be particularly helpful in these scenarios (Table 24-2). Acetaminophen or nonsteroidal anti-inflammatory drugs (NSAIDs) may be indicated if the pain is bone-related or has an inflammatory component. In a recent double-blind, randomized controlled trial, the addition of acetaminophen improved pain scores in patients already on strong opioid regimens [8]. However, it is important to beware of masking fevers with acetaminophen and NSAIDs during chemotherapy, especially during count nadirs. Glucocorticoids can also prove useful in some types of inflammatory or bony pain. In particular, neuropathic pain responds well to adjuvant analgesics. Antidepressants such as amitriptyline and nortriptyline can be effective. Nortriptyline is preferred in the elderly due to a lower incidence of anticholinergic side effects [9]. Anticonvulsants such as gabapentin can also treat neuropathic pain and may be more effective when used in conjunction with opioids [10,11]. Because adjuvant therapies for neuropathic pain can take weeks to be titrated to full effect and may be ineffective in some patients, those with moderate to severe neuropathic pain should be treated with opioids as needed while doses are being escalated. Opioid doses can always be reduced later if adjuvant agents are effective. Pregabalin is a newer neuromodulator, and while only approved for neuropathic pain associated with diabetic nephropathy, it likely has broader therapeutic indications [12].

MANAGEMENT OF OPIOID-INDUCED SIDE EFFECTS

Adverse effects of opioids are common but can usually be effectively managed. A history of adverse effects to opioids often contributes to a patient's reluctance to take them again. Because patients may tolerate one class of opioid over another, whenever possible, the same opioid should be used for long-lasting and breakthrough dosing. For elderly patients, those with a history of adverse reactions, and patients afraid of adverse effects, consider starting opioids at a lower dose. When continuous dosing is needed, long-acting opioids will achieve constant blood levels and may be associated with fewer adverse consequences. Adverse effects of other medications, disease, and comorbidities may mimic opioid adverse effects and need to be considered and managed accordingly.

Table 24-2. Summary of Adjuvant Therapies

Type of pain	Adjuvant therapy
Pain associated with inflammation	Nonsteroidal anti-inflammatory drugs, glucocorticoids
Bone pain without oncologic emergency	Bisphosphonates, radiation, radiopharmaceuticals
Neuropathic pain	Antidepressants (ie, nortriptyline 10–100 mg/d*)
	Anticonvulsants (ie, gabapentin 100–1200 mg 3 times daily*)
	Topical agents (eg, capsaicin, ketamine) or specialty consultations may be helpful

*Start at low dose and increase every 3–5 d.

Common opioid-induced side effects include constipation, nausea, and vomiting. Patients should be started on scheduled stool softeners and stimulant laxatives to prevent constipation. Other preventative measures include ensuring adequate hydration, dietary fiber intake, and exercise. Rotation of opioids may also reduce symptoms [13]. If constipation occurs, impaction and obstruction need to be ruled out first. Stimulants can be titrated to maximal dose and osmotic laxatives, suppositories, or enemas can be added to effect. Methylnaltrexone is a peripheral opioid antagonist that has shown promise in the treatment of refractory constipation [14]. Nausea and vomiting can be prevented with prophylactic antiemetics and a gradual titration of the opioid. Unlike constipation—in which tolerance does not occur—tolerance usually develops rapidly for nausea and vomiting. Other etiologies need to be ruled out, specifically constipation or impaction, other emetogenic drugs, central nervous system pathology, and hypercalcemia. Treatment options include phenothiazines, antihistamines, dopamine antagonists, and serotonin antagonists. If the nausea/vomiting persists for longer than 1 week despite interventions, consider switching to an alternate opioid.

Cognitive impairments, such as sedation and delirium, frequently occur with either initiation or titration of opioids. Again, it is important to rule out other etiologies and also to evaluate for polypharmacy. Patients are often severely sleep-deprived from prior pain; therefore, this must be considered when evaluating sedation. Fortunately, tolerance to sedation develops quickly. In addition to reducing sedating medications and rotating opioids, psychostimulants may have a role in reversing sedation. Modafinil, a nonamphetamine psychostimulant, is approved for narcolepsy and shift work sleep disorder. In a small, retrospective study, modafinil appeared effective [15], although widespread adoption of this drug should be withheld until prospective clinical trials are conducted. Delirium is more frequently associated with the intravenous route and with highly lipophilic drugs. Dose reductions of opioids can be effective. Haloperidol is the first-line therapy when dose reduction alone is not effective. Haloperidol is highly effective and has a low incidence of cardiovascular and anticholinergic side effects.

The mechanisms for myoclonus and hyperalgesia, which can occasionally be seen with opioids, are poorly described. Opioid rotation and/or reduction may be helpful. Treatments with anticonvulsants, benzodiazepines, and muscle relaxants have also been attempted with some success. Pruritus occurs in approximately 2% to 10% of patients on opioids. It is associated with histamine release and can be treated with antihistamines.

Respiratory depression is one of the most feared side effects of opioids. All opioids affect the medullary respiratory center and at equianalgesic doses, pure opioid agonists are equally implicated in producing dose-dependent respiratory depression to the point of apnea. Respiratory depression is unusual in opioid-tolerant individuals. A number of medications to prevent respiratory depression have been evaluated but none is widely adopted [16–18]. To prevent systemic withdrawal, opioid antagonists should only be used if the respiratory rate is less than 8 breaths per minute or if the patient is symptomatic. The elimination half-life of naloxone is 30 to 80 minutes; therefore, doses may need to be repeated as necessary.

Most of the commonly encountered opioid-induced side effects are preventable or at least manageable. Early recognition of these side effects will greatly improve success in cancer pain management.

NONPHARMACOLOGIC MEASURES

Acknowledging the emotional reactions to pain and providing the necessary psychosocial support requires a multidisciplinary approach. The acquisition of adaptive coping skills and education enhance pain relief and a sense of control [19,20]. Cognitive and physical modalities, including distraction, guided imagery, massage, and acupuncture, have proven helpful in the treatment of cancer related pain [21,22].

INTERVENTIONAL STRATEGIES

Several invasive procedure options are available for patients who do not achieve adequate analgesia despite optimal pharmacologic measures. Intrathecal and epidural opioid infusions are indicated when adequate analgesia cannot be achieved without intolerable side effects [23]. Regional plexus blocks are performed in many tumor types, most commonly described in pancreatic cancer [24,25]. Percutaneous vertebroplasty provides significant analgesic effect for patients with symptomatic vertebral metastases [26]. Radiopharmaceuticals such as samarium-153 and strontium-89 are palliative options for patients with multiple sites of metastatic bone disease [27,28].

Inadequately treated pain has many potential consequences, including reduced quality of life and functional status, social, familial, and financial difficulties, and even requests for physician-assisted suicide. It is essential that we educate patients/families to overcome the societal barriers that preclude adequate pain management (Table 24-3). Successfully treating the pain of a cancer patient can be one of the most rewarding experiences for an oncologist.

DYSPNEA

More than half of cancer patients, and up to 90% at the end of life, experience dyspnea, with increased prevalence in lung cancer and metastatic lung disease [4,29]. Dyspnea can be very distressing to patients and families, and can impact quality of life and provoke anxiety [30]. In urgent settings, patients and families may choose intubation because of lack of adequate symptomatic treatment of the dyspnea or lack of awareness that it can be effectively palliated. Like many cancer-related symptoms, subjective dyspnea correlates poorly with physiologic parameters, such as pulse oximetry. Therefore, the need for and effectiveness of treatments should be measured by patients' self-reports, such as whether the dyspnea is mild, moderate, or severe [1].

Dyspnea may be due to direct lung or upper airway involvement (*eg*, pleural effusions or obstruction of the bronchi or trachea) or to complications from cancer or its treatment (*eg*, pneumonia or anemia). Particularly in lung cancer, dyspnea is frequently related to comorbidities such as chronic obstructive pulmonary disease. Breathing abnormalities are also common in the dying process. Primary causes should be assessed and treated if the potential benefits outweigh the risks and discomfort, in light of the patient's prognosis and goals. In particular, malignant pleural effusions are common in many types of cancer, particularly lung and breast, and are associated with dyspnea in approximately half of patients [30]. They are also an indicator of advanced disease and poor prognosis. Thoracentesis, pleurodesis, and pleural drainage catheters may all be effective, but are associated with substantial risks and discomforts that should be weighed against the anticipated benefits [30].

Several nonpharmacologic treatments have been shown to be effective. These include relaxation and breathing exercises; treating psychosocial causes of anxiety or distress; reducing room temperature, humidifying the air, or using fans; and raising the head of the bed [31]. A trial of oxygen therapy may be useful even in patients without significant hypoxemia [32]. In a patient without other treatable causes (or in whom treatment does not completely relieve symptoms), opioids and/or benzodiazepines may be helpful. The same principles in opioid management for pain can be applied to dyspnea, although starting with low doses and titrating judiciously are of paramount importance in this setting. A meta-analysis of nine randomized controlled trials supports the effectiveness of oral or parenteral (but not nebulized) opioids. Although adverse effects were uncommon, there were no significant respiratory effects [33]. An additional randomized controlled trial in terminal cancer patients supports a potential additive effect of benzodiazepines when added to opioid therapy [34].

FATIGUE AND WEAKNESS

Three quarters of patients with solid malignancies report fatigue at some point in their illness, and 80% to 99% of cancer patients who undergo chemotherapy, radiotherapy, or both report fatigue [35]. Fatigue often impairs patients' participation in social activities, employment, and performance of typical cognitive tasks, and affects the burdens and employment of caregivers [35]. In most cancer patients, fatigue is related to the cancer or its complications. Treatable conditions may also contribute to fatigue, including anemia, treatment or medication side effects, and poor oral intake. Fatigue can be related to other symptoms, including sleep disturbances, pain, and depression, and treatment of these symptoms may improve fatigue [36,37]. Although there are numerous small, uncontrolled pilot studies of various drugs for primary treatment of fatigue, the only randomized controlled trials—of paroxetine and methylphenidate—did not show evidence for benefit. The use of erythropoietin-stimulating agents for symptomatic anemia in this setting remains controversial.

Multiple qualitative reviews and meta-analyses have summarized the extensive randomized controlled trial evidence for exercise for fatigue in patients with solid tumors, mostly during active treatment [37]. The meta-analyses did not find a significant impact for fatigue or other symptoms, but there was a statistically significant effect on physical function [36]. Education about fatigue, including counseling about energy conservation, may be helpful in patients with more advanced disease. One randomized controlled trial showed a small but statistically significant benefit for energy conservation and management [36]. Families may focus on the lack of activity as a cause for decline in a dying patient rather than as a symptom of advanced disease; therefore, education about the natural course of illness may be helpful. Adapting activities of daily living, assistive devices, and prioritizing activities and periods of rest may help to improve quality of life.

ANOREXIA AND CACHEXIA

The anorexia-cachexia syndrome varies in prevalence with different studies and cancers (between 6%–74%) and tends to be more common in gastrointestinal malignancies or advanced disease. As with fatigue, anorexia and cachexia can be distressing to caregivers, who become concerned that lack of eating is contributing to the patient's decline. In most situations, anorexia and weight loss result from the underlying cancer or the dying process and are not affected by nutritional interventions, although they can be due to treatable factors or other untreated symptoms, such as pain or depression. In patients in whom chemotherapy, radiation, or tumor involvement (*eg*, head and neck cancer) affects nutritional intake directly, nutritional interventions may be beneficial. Two of three randomized controlled

Table 24-3. Potential Solutions for Overcoming Barriers to Adequate Pain Control	
Common barriers to pain management	**Potential solutions**
Fear of becoming addicted	Explain difference between tolerance and addiction and the palliative intent of opioids
Fear that use of pain medicine now means it will not be available for use later in disease	Educate that there are not upper limits on opioids and that doses can be increased if opioids lose their efficacy
Fear of adverse effects	Educate about tolerance to adverse effects such as sedation, management of constipation, and availability of alternate opioids
Fear that taking pain medications means illness is getting worse	Address fears about progressive illness as appropriate
Dislike of taking medications	Discuss how untreated pain can adversely affect patient functioning; discuss pain management in terms of functional goals
Feeling that pain is a retribution by God for past sins that must therefore be suffered	Address spiritual concerns; consider involving a chaplain, pastoral services, or a social worker
Fear of distracting from the care/cure of underlying disease	Discuss how management of pain is part of the treatment plan and will not interfere with other treatment modalities

trials addressing the impact of nutritional counseling and supplements in patients with gastrointestinal malignancies undergoing treatment found a significant impact [38–40].

Enteral or parenteral nutrition can also be beneficial in patients unable to sustain sufficient oral intake. However, evidence does not support its routine use for quality of life or survival in patients receiving active treatment, weight-losing patients who are able to eat, or patients with a survival prognosis of less than 3 months [41]. Gastrostomy tube placement and parenteral nutrition are associated with significant discomfort and risks of complications in patients with advanced disease [41]; therefore, intravenous hydration may provide a better benefit-risk ratio in alert patients unable to eat with a prognosis limited to weeks.

Education on the natural course of anorexia and cachexia is appropriate in advanced disease. Often times, the patient will not experience hunger or any associated discomfort, but the lack of dietary intake and associated weight loss can nonetheless be distressing to the patient and family. Counseling family members on how best to provide food to maximize quality of life, including discontinuation of preexisting dietary restrictions (such as for tight diabetes control), meeting food preferences, reduction of portion sizes, providing a positive eating environment, and reducing pressure to eat may all be helpful. Evidence does not support the use of nutritional supplements. For patients in whom lack of appetite is affecting quality of life, meta-analyses of randomized controlled trials have shown strong evidence of the effectiveness of progestins (megestrol acetate and medroxyprogesterone) and corticosteroids for increasing appetite. However, effects may be time-limited, there is no evidence for impact on survival, and these medications can have significant side effects and may be contraindicated in particular tumor types [42,43]. In a European randomized controlled trial evaluating the effects of whole plant cannabis extract, delta-9-tetrahydrocannabinol, or placebo on cancer cachexia, no difference in appetite or quality of life was noted between the arms and the trial was stopped early [44].

OBSTRUCTING GASTROINTESTINAL AND GYNECOLOGIC MALIGNANCIES

Bowel obstruction from malignancy is common in gastrointestinal malignancies and advanced cancer; an estimated 30% of patients with ovarian cancer and 10% to 20% of patients with colorectal cancer will develop obstruction. Intraluminal or extrinsic compression is involved, sometimes at multiple sites. Dysmotility due to tumor involvement of autonomic nerves or drugs, as well as constipation, edema, or adhesions, may also be contributing factors. Surgical intervention is often appropriate in patients with a reversible cause, good performance status, and lack of complicating factors [45]. Stents are also an appropriate alternative in many situations [46], although both have significant risks and rates of recurrence in advanced disease. Obstruction may reverse spontaneously or with medical treatment, and a trial of supportive care is sometimes warranted before more invasive treatment is initiated or in patients at high surgical risk.

Numerous case series describe relief of symptoms with decompression percutaneous endoscopic gastrostomy tube placement [47], and decompression colostomy or ileostomy can also relieve symptoms when appropriate. Anticholinergic agents, such as hyoscine, may also be effective. In particular, three randomized controlled trials showed reductions in nausea and vomiting with the use of octreotide [48], although the evidence did not support the use of steroids [49].

DELIRIUM

Delirium is common in cancer patients, with a prevalence of 38% in elderly cancer patients admitted to the hospital [50]. More mild cognitive impairment is also common in patients with cancer. In one study of patients receiving chemotherapy, radiotherapy, or both, self-assessed symptoms were present throughout the course but were at their worst during treatment: 48% of patients before treatment (5% severe), 67% during treatment (18% severe), and 58% after treatment (8% severe) reported difficulty with concentration, with similar percentages reporting difficulty with memory [51]. Terminal restlessness, a syndrome of agitated delirium in dying patients, was present in 28% to 42% of patients in one study of admissions to a palliative care unit [52]. Many aspects of delirium, such as cognitive and behavioral difficulties or disturbance of the sleep-wake cycle, can be distressing for patients and families; mental alertness is one of the most highly valued goals at the end of life [52,53]. Delirium is often missed without screening—because patients may be able to answer routine questions appropriately—or it is frequently misdiagnosed as dementia, depression, or another symptom [54]. Assessing for delirium may be particularly important before communicating complex information or making important decisions about treatment. A number of tools can be used to screen for delirium [55], including two simple scales with four to five items [56,57].

Delirium may be due to a variety of treatable causes, such as brain metastases, infections, hypercalcemia, impaired renal function, and other uncontrolled symptoms. Many medications commonly used in cancer and palliative care can also precipitate or worsen delirium. In ill patients, delirium is often multifactorial, and in patients with advanced disease, the risk-benefit ratio should be considered when evaluating for or treating specific causes or weighing the potential contribution of opioids. Although multicomponent interventions have not been evaluated in cancer patients, a randomized controlled trial of hospitalized geriatric patients including comprehensive assessment, environmental adjustments (eg, addressing the sleep-wake cycle and providing a more familiar environment), neuroleptics as needed, and other geriatric interventions showed significantly more rapid improvement in the intensity and symptoms of delirium [58]. Several randomized controlled trials have supported the use of neuroleptics for the treatment of delirium and terminal restlessness, although these trials were performed without placebo controls and generally not in cancer patients [55,59].

FINAL HOURS

The last days of a patient's life are critical not only for the individual's comfort, but for the family who will live with the memory of how their loved one died. Preparation and education of the family on the dying process are critical. Palliating symptoms, answering questions, and providing for the family's comfort allows for the important work of saying goodbye, rituals, spiritual comfort, grief, and bereavement.

The dying process can take days to weeks, or death can occur suddenly from complications such as pulmonary emboli or cardiac events. When patients or families ask about prognosis, it is always important to emphasize uncertainty and the importance of not delaying preparation and meeting goals, such as making financial arrangements or saying important things to loved ones.

Dying is a clinical diagnosis, and may sometimes be difficult to determine when patients are on life-sustaining interventions. The early stage is characterized by increasing time in bed, loss of interest and ability to drink and eat, and cognitive changes, usually hypoactive (but sometimes hyperactive) delirium. In the mid-stage there is a further decline in mental status to the state of obtundation; the "death rattle," caused by pooled oral secretions that are not cleared due to loss of swallowing reflex, may occur. In the late stage, there is coma and cool extremities and mottling may occur. In addition, breathing changes may occur, including tachypnea, Cheynes-Stokes breathing, deep respirations, and periods of apnea.

As cardiac output and intravascular volume decrease, there will be evidence of diminished perfusion. Tachycardia, hypotension, peripheral cooling, peripheral (nail bed) and central cyanosis, and mottling of the skin (livedo reticularis) (usually starting in lower extremities) are normal. Urine output falls as kidney perfusion diminishes. Oliguria or anuria is normal and parenteral fluids will generally not reverse this circulatory shut-down, but instead cause leakage into peripheral tissues or the pleural space, and may therefore provide more burden than benefit.

COMMUNICATION, DECISION-MAKING, AND CARE PLANNING

Communication and decision-making about difficult issues are essential to good palliative care. Similar techniques can be helpful in patients who are terminal and those with chronic, serious illness who are continuing treatment [60]. First, it is important to start with open-ended questions, such as "What have you been told about your illness?" and "How is treatment going for you?" to ensure patients' understanding and allow them to express concerns. When patients share emotions, it is important to respond with validating statements rather than to change the topic or retreat into technical discussions. The next step is to elicit patients' goals, hopes, and values. Conversations about specific clinical decisions will be easier when this information is known [60]. Oncologists have an important role in providing information to their patients about dying, and ideally these conversations should take place early in the course of the patient's disease. These discussions will help the patient and family members to prepare for death.

Although advance directives are an important part of this process, learning about the patient's quality of life, goals, and values are also important because preferences for care may often change as the disease worsens. In patients in whom significant life-prolonging therapy is no longer an option, or in whom the risks and suffering may outweigh the benefits, it is often appropriate to discuss providing more palliative and comfort care and less aggressive care. Although issues pertaining to resuscitation and artificial ventilation may be an important part of this discussion, determining the overall goal of care will help to address the appropriateness of other current or potential treatments. Chemotherapy, invasive tests or surgeries, and dialysis may all be less valuable to patients at this point than making sure that pain and symptoms are well controlled and meeting life goals such as spending time at home with family.

Determining prognosis is an important part of knowing when to emphasize palliative care and providing information to patients. In general, patients with metastatic solid tumors (except breast and prostate) who are not eligible for chemotherapy have a prognosis of less than 6 months. Other helpful factors in determining a 6-month prognosis are progressive loss of functional status (in bed > 50% of the time or dependent in three activities of daily living) and unintentional, progressive weight loss (> 10% over the past 6 months) due to the terminal illness. Serious complications such as pleural effusions, spinal cord compression, multiple brain metastases, and leptomeningeal disease are all also signs of a likely limited prognosis.

The benefits of palliative chemotherapy have been reported repeatedly for several tumor types [61–64]. Given the positive outcomes on quality of life and symptom control, other trials assessing palliative chemotherapy are currently under way. The decision to prescribe palliative chemotherapy is individualized for each patient and is largely based on the patient's wishes and functional status and the likelihood that the treatment will provide an improvement in quality of life. Treatment goals should be clearly outlined with the patient at the time of initiation and readdressed on a routine basis. The toxicities and overall burden related to the chemotherapy must be carefully balanced with the potential benefits. Palliative radiotherapy is a proven modality for relieving pain related to symptomatic bone metastases; however, balancing the potential benefit with the burden of daily radiation visits must be considered.

HOSPICE

Hospice is an insurance-covered program that provides comprehensive, multidisciplinary care for patients at the end of life and their families. Eligibility under the Medicare Hospice Benefit requires a physician-certified expected prognosis of less than 6 months and prior treatment oriented toward quality of life [65]. Patients who prefer not to go to the hospital are appropriate candidates for hospice care, and a do-not-resuscitate order is helpful, although not necessary. Patients do not need 24-hour care if they are safe while unsupervised at the time of hospice referral. Most hospice care is provided at home, although it can also be delivered in the nursing home setting when long-term care is needed. Inpatient hospices are available in many communities for patients who are actively dying or have acute symptom management needs.

Patients continue to be followed and seen, if appropriate, by their oncologist or other primary physician. Hospice provides intensive care management, including nursing visits one to three times per week as needed and 24-hour on-call for nursing advice or emergency home visits. In order to provide help with bathing and personal care, home health aide services are available 1 to 2 hours a day up to 6 days/week. Also included are social workers, who help with advance care and financial planning, family conflict, and social support; pastoral counseling and chaplains; and volunteers to provide companionship and respite for caregivers [66]. Hospice covers all medications and equipment related to the hospice diagnosis, as well as monthly short respite stays and inpatient hospice admissions if needed for symptom management. Hospice does not provide 24-hour care giving; families can sometimes hire paid caregivers, or long-term-care placement is sometimes necessary.

When considering hospice, it is helpful to review all current interventions to minimize family caregiving burden while maximizing the benefit-risk ratio of current treatments—usually those focused on symptoms and quality of life. Hospice routinely provides patient-controlled analgesia and enteral feeding when indicated, but the availability of hospice care concurrent with complex interventions not always oriented to quality of life, such as total parenteral nutrition, chemotherapy, dialysis, or blood products, may depend on insurance coverage, the capacity of the local hospice provider, and the specific patient circumstances.

REFERENCES

1. Dyspnea. Mechanisms, assessment, and management: a consensus statement. American Thoracic Society. *Am J Respir Crit Care Med* 1999, 159:321–340.

2. Pargeon KL, Hailey BJ: Barriers to effective cancer pain management: a review of the literature. *J Pain Symptom Manage* 1999, 18:358–368.

3. Hojsted J, Sjogren P: Addiction to opioids in chronic pain patients: a literature review. *Eur J Pain* 2007, 11:490–518.

4. Lorenz KA, Lynn J, Dy S, et al.: Quality measures for symptoms and advance care planning in cancer: a systematic review. *J Clin Oncol* 2006, 24:4933–4938.

5. National Comprehensive Cancer Network: Cancer Pain Practice Guideline. http://www.nccn.org/professionals/physician_gls/PDF/pain.pdf. Accessed October 14, 2007.

6. Hopkins Opioid Program. http://www.hopweb.org. Accessed October 14, 2007.

7. Slatkin NE, Xie F, Messina J, et al.: Fentanyl buccal tablet for relief of breakthrough pain in opioid-tolerant patients with cancer-related chronic pain. *J Support Oncol* 2007, 5:327–334.

8. Stockler M, Vardy J, Pillai A, et al.: Acetaminophen (paracetamol) improves pain and well-being in people with advanced cancer already receiving a strong opioid regimen: a randomized, double-blind, placebo-controlled cross-over trial. *J Clin Oncol* 2004, 22:3389–3394.

9. Collins SL, Moore RA, McQuay HJ, et al.: Antidepressants and anticonvulsants for diabetic neuropathy and postherpetic neuralgia: a quantitative systematic review. *J Pain Symptom Manage* 2000, 20:449–458.

10. Caraceni A, Zecca E, Bonezzi C, et al.: Gabapentin for neuropathic cancer pain: a randomized controlled trial from the Gabapentin Cancer Pain Study Group. *J Clin Oncol* 2004, 22:2909–2917.

11. Gilron I, Bailey JM, Tu D, et al.: Morphine, gabapentin, or their combination for neuropathic pain. *N Engl J Med* 2005, 352:1324–1334.

12. Shneker BF, McAuley JW: Pregabalin: a new neuromodulator with broad therapeutic indications. *Ann Pharmacother* 2005, 39:2029–2037.

13. Radbruch L, Sabatowski R, Loick G, et al.: Constipation and the use of laxatives: a comparison between transdermal fentanyl and oral morphine. *Palliat Med* 2000, 14:111–119.

14. Yuan CS, Israel RJ: Methylnaltrexone, a novel peripheral opioid receptor antagonist for the treatment of opioid side effects. *Expert Opin Investig Drugs* 2006, 15:541–552.

15. Webster L, Andrews M, Stoddard G: Modafinil treatment of opioid-induced sedation. *Pain Med* 2003, 4:135–140.

16. Mildh L, Taittonen M, Leino K, et al.: The effect of low-dose ketamine on fentanyl-induced respiratory depression. *Anaesthesia* 1998, 53:965–970.

17. Vaupel DB, Lange WR, London ED: Effects of verapamil on morphine-induced euphoria, analgesia and respiratory depression in humans. *J Pharmacol Exp Ther* 1993, 267:1386–1394.

18. Vedrenne JB, Esteve M, Guillaume A: Prevention by naloxone of adverse effects of epidural morphine analgesia for cancer pain. *Ann Fr Anesth Reanim* 1991, 10:98–103.

19. Allard P, Maunsell E, Labbe J, *et al.*: Educational interventions to improve cancer pain control: a systematic review. *J Palliat Med* 2001, 4:191–203.

20. Devine EC: Meta-analysis of the effect of psychoeducational interventions on pain in adults with cancer. *Oncol Nurs Forum* 2003, 30:75–89.

21. Mehling WE, Jacobs B, Acree M, *et al.*: Symptom management with massage and acupuncture in postoperative cancer patients: a randomized controlled trial. *J Pain Symptom Manage* 2007, 33:258–266.

22. Bardia A, Barton DL, Prokop LJ, *et al.*: Efficacy of complementary and alternative medicine therapies in relieving cancer pain: a systematic review. *J Clin Oncol* 2006, 24:5457–5464.

23. Smith TJ, Staats PS, Deer T, *et al.*: Randomized clinical trial of an implantable drug delivery system compared with comprehensive medical management for refractory cancer pain: impact on pain, drug-related toxicity, and survival. *J Clin Oncol* 2002, 20:4040–4049.

24. Lillemoe KD, Cameron JL, Kaufman HS, *et al.*: Chemical splanchnicectomy in patients with unresectable pancreatic cancer. A prospective randomized trial. *Ann Surg* 1993, 217:447–455; discussion 456–447.

25. Wong GY, Schroeder DR, Carns PE, *et al.*: Effect of neurolytic celiac plexus block on pain relief, quality of life, and survival in patients with unresectable pancreatic cancer: a randomized controlled trial. *JAMA* 2004, 291:1092–1099.

26. Calmels V, Vallee JN, Rose M, *et al.*: Osteoblastic and mixed spinal metastases: evaluation of the analgesic efficacy of percutaneous vertebroplasty. *AJNR Am J Neuroradiol* 2007, 28:570–574.

27. Bauman G, Charette M, Reid R, *et al.*: Radiopharmaceuticals for the palliation of painful bone metastasis: a systemic review. *Radiother Oncol* 2005, 75:258–270.

28. Finlay IG, Mason MD, Shelley M: Radioisotopes for the palliation of metastatic bone cancer: a systematic review. *Lancet Oncol* 2005, 6:392–400.

29. Claessens MT, Lynn J, Zhong Z, *et al.*: Dying with lung cancer or chronic obstructive pulmonary disease: insights from SUPPORT. Study to Understand Prognoses and Preferences for Outcomes and Risks of Treatments. *J Am Geriatr Soc* 2000, 48:S146–S153.

30. Kvale PA SM, Prakash UB, Lorenz K, *et al.*: End-of-life care and outcomes. *Evidence Report. Technology Assessment*, No. 110. Vol. 05-E004-2: AHRQ Publication; 2004.

31. Bredin M, Corner J, Krishnasamy M, *et al.*: Multicentre randomised controlled trial of nursing intervention for breathlessness in patients with lung cancer. *BMJ* 1999, 318:901–904.

32. Lorenz K, Lynn J, Dy S, *et al.*: Cancer care quality measures: symptoms and end-of-life care. *Evid Rep Technol Assess (Full Rep)* 2006, 1:1–77.

33. Jennings AL, Davies AN, Higgins JP, *et al.*: A systematic review of the use of opioids in the management of dyspnoea. *Thorax* 2002, 57:939–944.

34. Navigante AH, Cerchietti LC, Castro MA, *et al.*: Midazolam as adjunct therapy to morphine in the alleviation of severe dyspnea perception in patients with advanced cancer. *J Pain Symptom Manage* 2006, 31:38–47.

35. Curt GA, Breitbart W, Cella D, *et al.*: Impact of cancer-related fatigue on the lives of patients: new findings from the Fatigue Coalition. *Oncologist* 2000, 5:353–360.

36. Mitchell SA, Berger AM: Cancer-related fatigue: the evidence base for assessment and management. *Cancer J* 2006, 12:374–387.

37. National Comprehensive Cancer Network (NCCN): Cancer-related fatigue. http://www.nccn.org/professionals/physican_gls/PDF/fatigue.pdf. Accessed December 4, 2006.

38. Ravasco P, Monteiro-Grillo I, Vidal PM, *et al.*: Dietary counseling improves patient outcomes: a prospective, randomized, controlled trial in colorectal cancer patients undergoing radiotherapy. *J Clin Oncol* 2005, 23:1431–1438.

39. Isenring EA, Capra S, Bauer JD: Nutrition intervention is beneficial in oncology outpatients receiving radiotherapy to the gastrointestinal or head and neck area. *Br J Cancer* 2004, 91:447–452.

40. Persson CR, Johansson BB, Sjoden PO, *et al.*: A randomized study of nutritional support in patients with colorectal and gastric cancer. *Nutr Cancer* 2002, 42:48–58.

41. Dy SM: Enteral and parenteral nutrition in terminally ill cancer patients: a review of the literature. *Am J Hosp Palliat Care* 2006, 23:369–377.

42. Yavuzsen T, Davis MP, Walsh D, *et al.*: Systematic review of the treatment of cancer-associated anorexia and weight loss. *J Clin Oncol* 2005, 23:8500–8511.

43. Berenstein EG, Ortiz Z: Megestrol acetate for the treatment of anorexia-cachexia syndrome. *Cochrane Database Syst Rev* 2005:CD004310.

44. Strasser F, Luftner D, Possinger K, *et al.*: Comparison of orally administered cannabis extract and delta-9-tetrahydrocannabinol in treating patients with cancer-related anorexia-cachexia syndrome: a multicenter, phase III, randomized, double-blind, placebo-controlled clinical trial from the Cannabis-In-Cachexia-Study-Group. *J Clin Oncol* 2006, 24:3394–3400.

45. Feuer DJ, Broadley KE, Shepherd JH, *et al.*: Systematic review of surgery in malignant bowel obstruction in advanced gynecological and gastrointestinal cancer. The Systematic Review Steering Committee. *Gynecol Oncol* 1999, 75:313–322.

46. Dormann A, Meisner S, Verin N, *et al.*: Self-expanding metal stents for gastroduodenal malignancies: systematic review of their clinical effectiveness. *Endoscopy* 2004, 36:543–550.

47. Ripamonti C, Twycross R, Baines M, *et al.*: Clinical-practice recommendations for the management of bowel obstruction in patients with end-stage cancer. *Support Care Cancer* 2001, 9:223–233.

48. Mercadante S, Casuccio A, Mangione S: Medical treatment for inoperable malignant bowel obstruction: a qualitative systematic review. *J Pain Symptom Manage* 2007, 33:217–223.

49. Feuer DJ, Broadley KE: Corticosteroids for the resolution of malignant bowel obstruction in advanced gynaecological and gastrointestinal cancer. *Cochrane Database Syst Rev* 2000:CD001219.

50. Bond SM, Neelon VJ, Belyea MJ: Delirium in hospitalized older patients with cancer. *Oncol Nurs Forum* 2006, 33:1075–1083.

51. Kohli S GJ, Roscoe JA, Jean-Pierre P, *et al.*: Self-reported cognitive impairment in patients with cancer. *J Oncol Pract* 2007, 3:54–59.

52. Lawlor PG, Gagnon B, Mancini IL, *et al.*: Occurrence, causes, and outcome of delirium in patients with advanced cancer: a prospective study. *Arch Intern Med* 2000, 160:786–794.

53. Caraceni A, Nanni O, Maltoni M, *et al.*: Impact of delirium on the short term prognosis of advanced cancer patients. Italian Multicenter Study Group on Palliative Care. *Cancer* 2000, 89:1145–1149.

54. Lawlor PG, Bruera ED: Delirium in patients with advanced cancer. *Hematol Oncol Clin North Am* 2002, 16:701–714.

55. Lacasse H, Perreault MM, Williamson DR: Systematic review of antipsychotics for the treatment of hospital-associated delirium in medically or surgically ill patients. *Ann Pharmacother* 2006, 40:1966–1973.

56. Fayers PM, Hjermstad MJ, Ranhoff AH, *et al.*: Which mini-mental state exam items can be used to screen for delirium and cognitive impairment? *J Pain Symptom Manage* 2005, 30:41–50.

57. Gaudreau JD, Gagnon P, Harel F, *et al.*: Fast, systematic, and continuous delirium assessment in hospitalized patients: the nursing delirium screening scale. *J Pain Symptom Manage* 2005, 29:368–375.

58. Pitkala KH, Laurila JV, Strandberg TE, *et al.*: Multicomponent geriatric intervention for elderly inpatients with delirium: a randomized, controlled trial. *J Gerontol A Biol Sci Med Sci* 2006, 61:176–181.

59. Kehl KA: Treatment of terminal restlessness: a review of the evidence. *J Pain Palliat Care Pharmacother* 2004, 18:5–30.

60. Lo B, Quill T, Tulsky J: Discussing palliative care with patients. ACP-ASIM End-of-Life Care Consensus Panel. American College of Physicians-American Society of Internal Medicine. *Ann Intern Med* 1999, 130:744–749.

61. Ranson M, Davidson N, Nicolson M, *et al.*: Randomized trial of paclitaxel plus supportive care versus supportive care for patients with advanced non-small-cell lung cancer. *J Natl Cancer Inst* 2000, 92:1074–1080.

62. Osoba D, Tannock IF, Ernst DS, *et al.*: Health-related quality of life in men with metastatic prostate cancer treated with prednisone alone or mitoxantrone and prednisone. *J Clin Oncol* 1999, 17:1654–1663.

63. Henry B, Becouarn Y, Aussage P: Clinical benefits of stabilisation with second line chemotherapy in patients with metastatic colorectal cancer. *Crit Rev Oncol Hematol* 1999, 32:145–154.

64. el-Kamar FG, Grossbard ML, Kozuch PS: Metastatic pancreatic cancer: emerging strategies in chemotherapy and palliative care. *Oncologist* 2003, 8:18–34.

65. Gazelle G: Understanding hospice: an underutilized option for life's final chapter. *N Engl J Med* 2007, 357:321–324.

66. Dy SM RE, McHale J, Clayton T, *et al.*: Caring for patients in an inner-city home hospice: Challenges and rewards. *Home Health Care Manage Pract* 2003, 15:291–299.

Patients receiving chemotherapy or radiation therapy experience certain side effects. Some (*eg*, acute nausea and vomiting) occur acutely and are managed with medications or intravenous fluids designed to counteract these effects. Other side effects (*eg*, alopecia)—although uncomfortable and perhaps damaging in terms of patient self-image—are not dangerous and resolve at the conclusion of therapy. Among all side effects seen, those associated with the effects of anticancer therapy on the bone marrow represent a potentially dangerous and even life-threatening circumstance [1]. Because most anticancer treatments affect rapidly dividing cells preferentially, bone marrow is an ideal target for these effects. This is the primary reason that myelosuppression is among the complications most frequently seen in the cancer patient population.

Temporary damage to bone marrow can result in decreases in all three major strains of peripheral blood, although effects on leukocytes and especially the myeloid series tend to dominate, given that they have the shortest survival of all bone marrow–derived cells (Table 25-1). This results in a drop in the infection-fighting neutrophil series, with an associated increased risk of infection. Although patients are at increased risk for both bacterial and fungal forms of infection, the former tends to be more commonly seen. Generally, only patients with long-term severely low absolute neutrophil counts (ANC, < 250 cells/µL) for lengthy periods experience mycotic infections. Bodey *et al.* [2] reviewed the experience at the National Institutes of Health leukemia service, which defined that both the depth and duration of neutropenia play roles in the risk of developing systemic infectious complications. Because in most cases neutropenia is of short duration, the average risk of infection with standard chemotherapy is relatively low. Among the remaining lineages, anemia is most often cumulative in nature. A current controversy disputes what level of anemia represents a sufficiently significant drop to warrant medical therapy intervention even though transfusion therapy continues to be the mainstay of this side effect's management. Anemia most often lowers patients' quality of life by fatiguing them.

Finally, a small percentage of patients develop clinically significant thrombocytopenia from cancer therapy. The risk of clinically severe bleeding in patients with thrombocytopenia is low and occurs primarily when the platelet count falls to dangerously low levels. Overall, development of myelosuppression as a complication of cancer therapy can be related to a range of variables (Table 25-2); the development of other complications such as disseminated intravascular coagulopathy (DIC) or other underlying illness can complicate this issue.

PATHOPHYSIOLOGY

Production of blood cells by bone marrow is an orderly process controlled by positive and negative regulators known as hematopoietic growth factors and cytokines [2]. These include early-acting stem cell factors (primarily interleukin [IL]-1, IL-3, and IL-6, as well as stem cell factors) and the lineage-specific colony-stimulating factors (*eg*, granulocyte colony-stimulating factors [G-CSF], granulocyte-macrophage colony-stimulating factors [GM-CSF], and erythropoietin). These biologic agents control the proliferation, differentiation, and maturation of multipotential precursor cells that can be directed to various lineages based on the relative expression of specific factors in a bone marrow microenvironment. Hematologic

lineages are regulated by a series of feedback loops such as those of the renal tubules, which control erythropoietin expression in response to hematocrit. Blood cell production begins with the multipotential stem cell, which has the ability to self-replicate and thereby ensure that adequate precursor cells are always available. The exhaustion of this stem cell supply, although theoretical, could lead to severe bone marrow aplasia and hypoproduction of all blood cells. However, bone marrow aplasia as a result of cancer therapy is rare; it generally only happens with the most intensive chemotherapy regimens.

In general, the environment in which the stem cells exist must be conducive to their growth and development. Severe fibrosis from diseases, such as the myeloproliferative disorders, or chronic changes as a result of radiation therapy tends to make bone marrow space inhospitable to blood cell production. This can contribute significantly to the development of myelosuppression.

Kinetically, the myelosuppressive effects of cancer therapy tend to be related to the stage of development damaged by the agent in question. Neutrophils, which usually survive 7 hours in circulation, are most sensitive to treatment effects. Similarly, platelets that last 7 to 10 days are more commonly affected than erythrocytes, which last 120 days in circulation. The progression of hematopoietic development is similar for all lineages, taking approximately 7 days to progress from stem cell to committed progenitor and another 7 to 10 days to progress from committed progenitor to mature cell, ready for release into the circulation. It is this latter 7- to 10-day period that can be compressed by the available colony-stimulating factors to accelerate blood cell production rapidly.

CAUSES

The principal forms of cancer therapy that cause myelosuppression are chemotherapy and radiation therapy. In the case of radiation, the damaging effect is not limited to the hematopoietic compartment but to the marrow microenvironment itself. Not uncommonly, it can take up to several years for recovery of a previously irradiated area. In contrast to these two therapies, biologic therapy or targeted therapies (*eg*, antibody therapies, tyrosine kinase inhibitors) may cause myelosuppression by inducing a peripheral consumptive state related to hypersplenism or some similar mechanism, direct destruction of peripheral blood cells, or indirect inhibition of normal progenitor cells [3]. The former effect most commonly resolves quickly following discontinuation of these agents.

CHEMOTHERAPY

Chemotherapy affects hematologic cells in much the same way it does cancer cells. Chemotherapy drugs can be classified into categories based on

Table 25-1. Categories of Cytopenias

Lineage	Approximate survival (in circulation)	Deficiency
Myeloid	7 h	Neutropenia
Erythroid	120 d	Anemia
Megakaryocyte	7–10 d	Thrombocytopenia

Table 25-2. Factors Associated With Myelosuppression

Therapy

Choice of chemotherapy agents and dose intensity

Radiation therapy including total dose and volume radiated

Bone marrow reserve

Patient's age and nutritional status

Prior therapy

Bone marrow involvement with malignancy or other process

Bone marrow involvement with cancer or other process

Comorbid conditions such as autoimmune processes

Drug-related effects (nonchemotherapy)

Infection-related complications (*ie*, disseminated intravascular coagulation)

mechanism of action. Alkylating agents typically bind to nucleotide bases of DNA and thereby inhibit protein synthesis and replication. This effect is similar to that of the antitumor antibiotics (*eg*, doxorubicin or daunorubicin), which intercalate into DNA strands, thus preventing DNA synthesis. Vinca alkaloids (vincristine or vinblastine) and the taxanes (paclitaxel and docetaxel) inhibit microtubular synthesis that inhibits spindle formation, preventing cells from actively undergoing mitosis. Finally, antimetabolites frequently substitute themselves for purine or pyrimidine nucleotides, thereby blocking DNA or RNA synthesis. These latter agents may also block specific enzymes required for nucleotide synthesis. Bone marrow cells take up these chemotherapy drugs in much the same way as cancer cells. Hence, bone marrow, because of its rapidly proliferating state, often tends to be more sensitive to the effects of chemotherapy because unlike cancer cells, these progenitors often lack mechanisms of resistance to the chemotherapy. Several agents such as vincristine, low-dose methotrexate, L-asparaginase, and oral cyclophosphamide generally do not cause significant myelosuppression. Conversely, agents such as the nitrosoureas and mitomycin C frequently induce delayed and prolonged myelosuppression because of their relative effects on the stem cell population.

IMMUNOTHERAPY

Biologic agents can be divided into two specific groups with regard to their effects on the hematologic system. The first group, which includes the interferons (α, β, and γ), can exert a direct suppressive effect on bone marrow. Although this group is not specifically myelotoxic, it is certainly not myelosuppressive. The impact on blood counts is typically relatively rapidly reversible after the drug has been discontinued. In contrast, lymphopenia and neutropenia associated with IL-2 appear to be predominantly related to peripheral consumption by immunostimulated cells or by vascular margination of pools of cells. Both these side effects are rapidly reversible, appear to be dose related, and generally are not associated with infectious complications. In addition to the IL-2–mediated neutropenia, IL-2 has the ability to induce neutrophil dysfunction, which lasts longer than quantitative neutropenia and may be associated with increased infectious risk.

TARGETED THERAPIES

Humanized antibodies are playing a larger role in our anticancer armamentarium. Although these agents are "targeted," they can result in hematologic toxicity, especially when they are paired with cytotoxic chemotherapies. In some cases, these therapies can cause a pancytopenia or bone marrow hypoplasia, and may also lead to autoimmune thrombocytopenias or hemolytic anemias. Hematologic toxicities have been observed with alemtuzumab, cetuximab, gemtuzumab, ibritumomab, and rituximab [3].

RADIATION THERAPY

Radiation therapy induces cell death by causing lethal double-stranded DNA breaks. These DNA breaks result in cell death and apoptosis when the cell enters the cell cycle. For this reason, cells in G0 tend to be more sensitive to DNA damage than those in G1 or S-phase, which tend to be more resistant due to their ability to correct damage enzymatically. Hence, myelosuppression associated with radiation therapy is often related to the volume of bone marrow irradiated, the total radiation dose, and the patient's overall bone marrow reserve (which may be compromised by either prior therapy or bone marrow involvement with cancer).

DIAGNOSIS

The first evidence of myelosuppression is often a defined drop in the number of peripherally circulating blood cells. Because of the kinetics and life span of blood cells, leukopenia and neutropenia are typically the first deficiencies noted. This drop, which may be mild, is frequently found 7 to 10 days following the completion of therapy, although more intensive treatments may accelerate the process. In the case of moderately to severely intensive regimens, thrombocytopenia may be noted at or around the same time. As a side effect of therapy, anemia is more commonly cumulative and develops over time or a series of cycles. In typical situations, response to the development of cytopenias is an increase in bone marrow production

of blood cells. This generally corrects mild leukopenia or thrombocytopenia in a short time (7 to 14 days). In some cases, in which more severe or prolonged myelosuppression occurs, further investigation may be necessary.

PERIPHERAL BLOOD SMEAR

Evaluation of a peripheral blood smear is the easiest form of tissue biopsy available. Comprehensive review of a peripheral blood smear can provide significant insight—both before and after chemotherapy—as to the risk and complications of chemotherapy administration. In addition to being able to evaluate leukocytes, erythrocytes, and platelets quantitatively, a peripheral blood smear allows qualitative evaluation. Prechemotherapy evaluation may demonstrate important findings such as that of a leukoerythroblastic picture (elevated numbers of early leukocytes and nucleated erythrocytes) consistent with bone marrow involvement with tumor or fibrosis. Both these situations may increase the risk of more severe myelosuppression. After therapy has been administered, a review of the peripheral blood smear will allow a differential count to be performed on the peripheral blood leukocytes and a calculation of the ANC, which is the total number of leukocytes multiplied by the percentage of segmented neutrophils plus band forms. The ANC is a critical calculation on which treatment of patients with fever during leukopenia is based. Early bone marrow recovery is typically heralded by a peripheral blood monocytosis. Monocytes, a more primitive type of anti-infectious cell, tend to increase in number transiently before granulocytosis.

In addition to quantitative evaluation of blood cells, qualitative analysis of the peripheral blood smear is critical. Complications such as infection with DIC may be identified on the smear based on the features of fragmented erythrocytes and deficient platelets. Furthermore, patients with prolonged leukopenia who are at risk for secondary malignancies following chemotherapy with or without radiation may demonstrate signs of an underlying myelodysplastic syndrome. Evidence in support of this diagnosis may include pseudo-Pelger-Huet neutrophils (unilobed or bilobed segmented neutrophils), hypogranularity of the myeloid series, or long-standing peripheral blood monocytosis with erythrocyte macrocytosis.

BONE MARROW EVALUATION

In some settings, bone marrow evaluation may be necessary to explore etiologies for relative or absolute cytopenias. Examples of such diagnoses include those performed on superimposed autoimmune cytopenias. Such diagnosis is conducted through bone marrow aspiration and biopsy, typically on the posterior iliac spine unless the pelvis has been previously irradiated. In that case, a sternal bone marrow aspirate alone is appropriate. A sternal bone marrow aspirate is performed in the region approximately 2 to 3 cm below the sternomanubrial joint in the midline. The key feature of a successful bone marrow aspirate is the presence of spicules, which represent small bony particles around which hematopoietic precursors develop. Occasionally, it may be impossible to attain an adequate aspirate due to the lack of spicules (as may be the case in severely aplastic marrows) or because of a "dry tap," which may occur due to scarring or fibrosis in the bone marrow space. In these situations, a bone marrow biopsy is critical to adequately evaluate the bone marrow pathophysiology. Magnetic resonance imaging (MRI) to investigate bone marrow cellularity using the difference in water content between hypocellular bone marrow (high-fat content) and hypercellular bone marrow is being investigated. Abnormal signal in the bone marrow may also be seen on MRI, which may indicate involvement of the bone marrow space with malignant tumor.

HEMATOLOGIC TOXICITY

NEUTROPENIA

As noted previously, neutropenia is one of the first findings consistent with myelosuppression. It is of potential value in terms of monitoring the effect of orally administered chemotherapy, in which variable absorption may play a role in drug activity. Such is the case for oral melphalan in the setting of multiple myeloma, in which serial blood counts demonstrating development of mild to moderate neutropenia indicates adequate drug absorption. Neutropenia is a deficiency of the number of circulating neutrophilic granulocytes. As the primary bacterial infection–fighting cell of the body, it is responsible for preventing overwhelming pyogenic infections. A pool of neutrophils exists in a marginated state and some patients, particularly those of African descent, have a relative neutropenia that responds to the administration of low doses of epinephrine, which redistributes the marginated pool. This is more of a pseudoneutropenia and is not associated with an increased risk of infection. ANC levels below 500 cells/µL are associated with increased risk of infection. This is common in instances in which patients are receiving combination chemotherapy. Incidence of infection is directly related to the depth of the neutropenia as well as its absolute duration (how low and for how long) [4]. As previously noted, recovery of ANC to normal levels may take approximately 2 weeks following administration of standard-dose chemotherapy. During the period in which patients are effectively neutropenic, close monitoring for signs or symptoms of infection must take place. Any clinically significant fever must be met with a thorough investigation of potential sources of infection, including infection risk related to indwelling central venous catheters. After a patient with neutropenia has been determined to have a fever (temperature ≥ 38.5°C), appropriate antibiotic coverage is indicated. Monotherapy with broad-spectrum antibiotics has replaced the classic combination therapy. Empiric coverage with glycopeptides is no longer recommended without documentation of a gram-positive infection. Newly developed risk stratification models (Table 25-3) can identify patients who can be safely treated as outpatients or discharged early from the hospital [5,6].

The use of antibiotic prophylaxis in neutropenic patients remains controversial. The benefits of prophylactic antibiotics include a reduction in all infection-related events; however, these benefits must be balanced against a lack of a clear survival benefit and the risks of antibiotic resistance. Current evidence supports the use of prophylactic fluoroquinolones in acute leukemia and high-dose chemotherapy patients. Current practice guidelines advise against routine use of prophylactic antibiotics in other neutropenic patients [7].

The two hematopoietic colony-stimulating factors (G-CSF, GM-CSF) entered into clinical use in the early 1980s. Approved several years later, G-CSF has demonstrated the ability to reduce the depth and duration of chemotherapy-induced neutropenia associated with combination chemotherapy [8]. As a result of this effect, it also significantly decreases incidence of febrile neutropenia. Although GM-CSF has similar biologic activities, its benefits are seen in the setting of bone marrow transplantation, in which it accelerates recovery of neutrophils and hastens patient discharge from the hospital [9].

A recent meta-analysis of randomized controlled trials of prophylactic G-CSF has demonstrated a significant reduction in febrile neutropenia. Furthermore, prophylactic G-CSF has been shown to reduce the risk of early death, including infection-related mortality, while increasing relative dose intensity. There are still no conclusive data on the impact on disease-free and overall survival with G-CSF prophylaxis [10].

ANEMIA

The past several years have seen more and more attention focused on the impact of anemia on patient's chemotherapy tolerance and overall quality of life. Anemia is defined as a drop in the hemoglobin or hematocrit to a level below the lower limit of normal. In most institutions, this is represented by a hemoglobin fall below 12 g/dL or a hematocrit level of 36%. Although most patients at this level are minimally symptomatic in terms of fatigue, new studies suggest that mild anemia may contribute to slowing of the mental processes with decision making. This so-called "executive function" is a critical new end point in anemia research. Evaluation for contributing factors such as nutritional deficiencies (folic acid or vitamin B_{12}) or a destructive process must be completed.

Declines in hematocrit levels tend to be cumulative; patients progressively develop more symptoms, which include fatigue, exercise intolerance, tachycardia, dyspnea on exertion, and, in extreme cases, exacerbation of preexisting cardiopulmonary disease. Most of these symptoms can be alleviated by the transfusion of packed erythrocytes, although transfusions are expensive and not without risks (*eg*, viral infections). As an alternative to

transfusions, use of recombinant human erythropoietin has been explored [11,12]. Recently, the US Food and Drug Administration (FDA) published new guidelines on the use of erythropoietin-stimulating agents (ESAs) [13]. They determined that:

- A higher chance of death and an increased rate of tumor growth were reported in patients with advanced head and neck cancer receiving radiation therapy and in patients with metastatic breast cancer receiving chemotherapy when ESAs were given to maintain hemoglobin levels of more than 12 g/dL.
- A higher chance of death was reported and no fewer blood transfusions were received when ESAs were given to patients with cancer and anemia not receiving chemotherapy.
- A higher chance of death was reported and increased numbers of blood clots, strokes, heart failure, and heart attacks were reported in patients with chronic kidney failure when ESAs were given to maintain hemoglobin levels of more than 12 g/dL.
- A higher chance of blood clots was reported in patients who were scheduled for major surgery and given ESAs.

Furthermore, the FDA urged physicians to:

- Understand that ESAs are given to decrease the need for red blood cell transfusions;
- Consider both the risks of transfusions and those of ESAs when deciding to prescribe an ESA;
- Adjust the dose of ESA to maintain the lowest hemoglobin level necessary to avoid the need for transfusions.
- Monitor patients' hemoglobin levels to ensure they do not exceed 12 g/dL;
- Understand that ESAs have not been shown to improve the outcomes of chemotherapy treatment (*eg*, better tumor shrinkage, delay in tumor growth, or longer time for survival); and
- Understand that in patients with cancer whose anemia is caused by chemotherapy and in patients with HIV whose anemia is caused by zidovudine, there are no data to support claims of improvement in health-related quality of life, including effects on fatigue, energy, or strength.

THROMBOCYTOPENIA

Thrombocytopenia represents a deficiency in the number of circulating platelets, which normally circulate at levels between 150 and 400,000/µL. Levels of 50,000/µL and higher are generally adequate for hemostasis to allow minor or major surgical procedures. The degree to which patients develop thrombocytopenia is directly related to the incidence of bleeding complications. Spontaneous minor bleeding episodes increase in frequency when the platelet count falls below 20,000/µL. Major bleeding complications occur in the setting of more severe thrombocytopenia (platelet counts < 10,000/µL). With the use of more intensive regimens, newer drugs,

Table 25-3. MASCC Risk Scoring Index for Identification of Low-Risk Febrile Neutropenic Patients at Presentation

Characteristic	Score
No symptoms	5
Mild symptoms	5
Moderate symptoms	3
No hypotension	5
No chronic obstructive pulmonary disease	4
Solid tumor or no fungal infection	4
No dehydration	3
Outpatient at onset of fever	3
Age < 60 years	2

*A risk index score of ≥ 21 indicates a low risk for complications and morbidity.
MASCC—Multinational Association of Supportive Care in Cancer.
(*Adapted from* Klastersky *et al.* [16].)

and patients' receiving overall more chemotherapy, thrombocytopenia is becoming more common.

Increased risk of bleeding can be seen in patients with coagulation disorders contributing to their thrombocytopenia. In these cases, processes such as DIC, which can be associated with metastatic cancer as well as infection, can increase risk of bleeding. In addition, this risk can also be affected by drugs that affect platelet function (*eg*, aspirin or other nonsteroidal anti-inflammatory agents) or coagulation function (*eg*, heparins or warfarin).

Recent studies have validated an acceptable threshold of 10,000/µL for platelet transfusion and have recognized single-donor or pooled random-donor platelets as reasonable options for transfusion. This lower threshold has the potential not only to limit viral infection exposure and potentially reduce the development of alloimmunization, but also to reduce costs related to transfusion support. Advances in the field of hematopoietic growth factors have resulted in the approval of IL-11 (Neumega [oprelvekin]; Wyeth Pharmaceuticals, Inc., Philadelphia, PA) for prevention of severe chemotherapy-induced thrombocytopenia [14]. These data support its use in settings in which the risk of severe thrombocytopenia and the likelihood of the need for transfusion are high. There are also a growing number of thrombopoetin peptide and nonpeptide agonists currently in clinical trials. Some of these small molecules appear promising; however, additional clinical evaluation is needed prior to their approval for clinical use [15].

NEUTROPENIA

Neutropenia is defined as a deficiency in the number of functional neutrophils granulocytes. The criterion for neutropenia is an ANC less than 1000/μL. Patients with neutropenia are at greatest risk of developing infections, particularly if they are undergoing dose-intensified or prolonged chemotherapy.

INTERVENTIONS

1. Prevention
   a. Avoid concurrent myelosuppressive agents and radiation therapy
   b. Chemotherapy dose reduction, if appropriate, while maintaining schedule
   c. Delay interval between treatment cycles until neutrophils recovery
   d. Interrupt radiation therapy until neutrophils recovery
   e. Hematopoietic growth factor support (G-CSF, GM-CSF)
   f. Nutritional support
2. Prevention and treatment of sequelae
   a. Avoid exposure to infection and reverse isolation
   b. Meticulous personal hygiene
   c. Early antimicrobial treatment for associated fevers (broad-spectrum antibiotics with staphylococcal and gram-negative coverage; biliary tree–enteric anaerobe; bowel–enteric anaerobe)
   d. Transfusion of neutrophils
   e. Prophylactic antibiotics

DOSAGE AND ADMINISTRATION

G-CSF or filgrastim: 5 μg/kg/d subcutaneously or IV to begin ≥ 24 h after chemotherapy

GM-CSF or sargramostim: 250 μg/m^2/d for 21 d by 2-h IV infusion beginning 2–4 after autologous stem cell transplantation; discontinue therapy when neutrophils count is > 20,000/mm^3

INDICATIONS

G-CSF or filgrastim: patients with malignancies receiving myelosuppressive chemotherapy associated with a significant (minimal 40%) incidence of severe neutropenia and fever

GM-CSF or sargramostim: patients with non-Hodgkin's lymphoma, acute lymphocytic leukemia, and Hodgkin's disease undergoing high-dose chemotherapy with progenitor cell support and elderly patients with acute myeloid leukemia receiving chemotherapy

CONTRAINDICATIONS

G-CSF or filgrastim: patients with known hypersensitivity to *Escherichia coli*–derived proteins

GM-CSF or sargramostim: patients with known hypersensitivity to GM-CSF, yeast-derived products, or any components of the product

LABORATORY MONITORING

G-CSF or filgrastim: initial baseline complete blood count (CBC) and platelet counts; biweekly thereafter

GM-CSF or sargramostim: if blast cells appear, discontinue therapy; biweekly monitoring of renal and hepatic function and CBC with differential

ADVERSE REACTIONS

G-CSF or filgrastim: medullary bone pain; increased uric acid, alkaline phosphatase, and lactic dehydrogenase; transient decreased blood pressure (rare)

GM-CSF or sargramostim: > 5% incidence over placebo; diarrhea, exacerbation of preexisting asthma, renal or hepatic dysfunction, rash, exacerbation of arrhythmia, malaise, fever, headache, bone pain, hives, myalgia, dyspnea, peripheral edema

CAUSATIVE FACTORS

Primary: benign; chronic (severe, congenital, cyclic, idiopathic); **Secondary:** neoplastic (hematologic malignancy, metastatic tumor); non-neoplastic (autoimmune, drug-related [chemotherapy, antibiotics, anticonvulsants, antidepressants]); infection (bacterial, viral, mycobacterial); radiation; hematologic disease (aplastic anemia, myelofibrosis, paroxysmal nocturnal hemoglobinuria, T-γ syndrome); organomegaly; nutritional deficiency

PATHOLOGIC PROCESS

Many unknown, possibly overproduction of cytokine suppressors or loss of growth factor receptors on progenitors, inhibition of nucleic acid and protein syntheses, maturation arrest, overproduction of hematopoietic inhibitors, antibody-induced destruction, drug-induced destruction, replacement of bone marrow by tumor or fibrosis, defective folate metabolism

PATIENT ASSESSMENT

Leukocyte count and differential; review of smear for morphology; bone marrow aspiration and biopsy; karyotype; culture bone marrow; special bone marrow stains, including reticulin and acid-fast bacilli; serum B$_{12}$ and folate levels; analysis of T-cell receptor gene rearrangement; review of medication

	Toxicity Grading				
Parameter	**0**	**1**	**2**	**3**	**4**
White blood cells × 10^3	> 4.5	3.0– < 4.5	2.0– < 3.0	1.0– < 2.0	< 1.0
Neutrophils × 10^3	> 1.9	1.5– < 1.9	1.0– < 1.5	0.5– < 1.0	< 0.5

THROMBOCYTOPENIA

Thrombocytopenia is a shortage of functional platelets due to decreased production, increased consumption, defective function, or splenic pooling. The condition is often exacerbated by cancer therapy and can place the patient at risk of hemorrhage.

INTERVENTIONS

1. Prevention
   a. Avoid antiplatelet agents (*eg*, aspirin)
   b. Chemotherapy dose adjustment, maintaining schedule
2. Prevention and treatment of sequelae
   a. Avoid invasive procedures (intramuscular injection, rectal suppositories)
   b. Use progesterones to prevent menses
   c. Gastrointestinal tract prophylaxis (*ie*, antacids, stool softeners)
   d. Platelet transfusion (see below)

DOSAGE AND ADMINISTRATION

Platelet transfusion: 6 U (random donor) or 1 bag (single donor) IV infusion. Count should increase 5000–10,000/uL per random donor bag. A poor response in platelet increment may be due to splenomegaly, fever, sepsis, DIC, or alloimmunization (1-h increment < 50% of expected suggests alloimmunization)

IL-11: 50 µg/kg/d subcutaneously to begin following chemotherapy (no sooner than 6 h after chemotherapy) and continued until a postnadir platelet count of 50,000/µL is achieved or for a maximum of 21 d (do not round to vial size)

INDICATIONS

Platelet transfusion: prophylaxis for patients with platelet counts < 10,000–20,000/mm³; prophylaxis for surgery if counts < 50,000/mm³; treatment of hemorrhage if < 50,000–100,000/mm³; signs and symptoms indicating need for transfusion (*ie*, bruisability, petechiae, mucous membrane bleeding)

IL-11: patients with nonmyeloid malignancies receiving dose-intensive chemotherapy and at a high risk for the development of severe chemotherapy-induced thrombocytopenia

PREPARATIONS

Platelet transfusion: all are ABO compatible and may be leukocyte depleted at the bedside; from whole blood (random donor), ≥ 5.5 × 10¹⁰/bag; apheresis (single donor), > 3 × 10¹¹/bag; leukocyte poor and single donor delay development of alloimmunization; human leukocyte antigen (HLA) matched for patients already alloimmunized

CONTRAINDICATIONS

IL-11: patients with known hypersensitivity to *E. coli*–derived products

LABORATORY MONITORING

IL-11: Twice weekly CBC and platelet counts

ADVERSE REACTIONS

Platelet transfusion: immune (fever, allergic reaction, graft-versus-host reaction); nonimmune (volume overload, transmission of infection)
IL-11: asthenia, edema, dyspnea, rare incidence of atrial arrhythmias

CAUSATIVE FACTORS

Quantitative: decreased production—congenital, acquired (alcoholism, drug-related [chemotherapy and radiation, diuretics, H_2 blockers], infections [viral]), nutritional deficiency, tumor involvement of bone marrow, myelofibrosis, primary hematologic disorder; increased consumption—autoimmune (immune and thrombotic thrombocytopenic purpura, hematologic malignancy), DIC, drug-related (heparin, antibiotics), infection; **Qualitative:** drug-related (nonsteroidal anti-inflammatory drugs, antimicrobials, psychiatric drugs, alcohol); concomitant illness (uremia, chronic liver disease, myeloproliferative disorders)

PATHOLOGIC PROCESS

Clot formation, antibody-induced destruction, inhibition of nucleic acid synthesis, bone marrow replacement with tumor or fibrosis, sequestration in enlarged spleen, defective maturation, drug-induced acetylation of platelet cyclooxygenase

PATIENT ASSESSMENT

CBC, peripheral blood smear, mean platelet volume, bone marrow aspiration or biopsy, karyotype, platelet aggregation studies, bleeding time (if platelet count adequate)

Toxicity Grading					
Parameter	**0**	**1**	**2**	**3**	**4**
Platelets × 10³	> 130	90– < 130	50– < 90	25– < 50	< 25

ANEMIA

The patient with anemia has an abnormally low concentration of erythrocytes and hemoglobin. The potential risks of anemia are less serious than those of neutropenia and thrombocytopenia; however, with the trend toward intensified therapy doses and bone marrow transplant, the incidence and severity of anemia are increasing. Transfusion continues to be the conventional method of support.

INTERVENTIONS

1. Prevention: erythropoietin support
2. Prevention and treatment of sequelae; transfusion of erythrocytes; management of fatigue

DOSAGE AND ADMINISTRATION

Transfusion of erythrocytes: dose based on severity. In otherwise healthy patients, transfuse to hemoglobin ≥ 8 g/dL. In patient with cardiac disease, frequently transfuse to hemoglobin ≥ 10 g/dL. Infuse over 4 h via IV catheter with normal saline for flushing

Erythropoietin: for chronic renal failure, 50–100 U/kg IV three times per week. Reduce dose if target hematocrit is reached or if it increases > 4% in 2 wk; increase dose if target not reached or no increase of 5%–6% in 8 wk; maintenance dose is individualized. For chemotherapy, 150 U/kg IV or subcutaneously three times per week with an increase to 300 U/kg three times per week if no response after 8 wk; alternatively, weekly dosing can be used with 40,000 U subcutaneously per week

INDICATIONS

Transfusion of erythrocytes: patients with symptomatic anemia requiring increased red cell mass and improved oxygen-carrying capacity. Symptoms may include tachycardia, dyspnea, angina, decreased mentation, transient ischemic attacks, syncope, postural hypotension, inability to maintain reasonable level of daily activity

Erythropoietin: patients with chronic renal failure, patients with anemia due to chemotherapy

PREPARATIONS

Transfusion of erythrocytes: for all ABO-compatible and cross-matched, packed red blood cells is blood component of choice; majority of plasma removed, 50–75 mL remain in each unit, preservative solution added; hematocrit 70%–80%; 1 U increases hemoglobin in 70-kg adult by 1–1.5 g/dL. Leukocyte-poor erythrocytes are used to prevent febrile transfusion reactions and alloimmunization to leukocyte; antigen and platelet transfusion. Washed erythrocytes are for patients with history of transfusion-related allergic reactions (usually due to plasma proteins); hematocrit 50%–70%

CONTRAINDICATIONS

Transfusion of erythrocytes: asymptomatic patients with vitamin-responsive anemia, iron-responsive anemia, erythropoietin-responsive anemias

Erythropoietin: patients with uncontrolled hypertension or hypersensitivity to mammalian cell–derived products of human albumin

LABORATORY MONITORING

Erythropoietin: blood pressure, hematocrit 1–2 times per week during dose adjustment, iron and iron-binding capacity

ADVERSE REACTIONS

Transfusion of erythrocytes: nonimmune—volume overload, iron overload, transmission of infections (hepatitis [1–2:100 transfusions], cytomegalovirus, HIV, HTLV-1, Epstein-Barr, bacterial infections [rare], Lyme disease, babesiosis, Chagas disease, *Brucella*, malaria, possibly tuberculosis); immune—acute or delayed hemolysis, fever (most common), allergic (urticaria, wheezing, angioedema), graft-versus-host (prevented by radiation therapy of blood product with 1500–3000 cGy)

Erythropoietin: chronic renal failure patients—hypertension, thrombotic events, headache, shortness of breath, tachycardia, hypercalcemia, nausea and vomiting, diarrhea (most frequent); flu-like symptoms, rash, urticaria, seizures (rare); patients receiving chemotherapy—diarrhea, edema (frequent); fever, shortness of breath, paresthesia, upper respiratory infection (less frequent)

CAUSATIVE FACTORS

Blood loss, chemotherapy and radiation, chronic disease—tumor, infection, drug-related (zidovudine); hemolysis—autoimmune (tumor [chronic lymphocytic leukemia, lymphoma]), drug-related; mechanical—chemotherapy (mitomycin C), DIC (tumor- or infection-related); nutritional deficiency—poor nutrition, postsurgery of gastrointestinal tract; bone marrow involvement (hematologic malignancy, metastatic tumor, myelofibrosis); concomitant illness (renal insufficiency, endocrine deficiencies)

PATHOLOGIC PROCESS

Defective hemoglobin production, glucolysis, DNA synthesis, iron and B_{12} absorption, purine and pyrimidine synthesis; blockade in folate metabolism; erythrocyte parasites; bacterial toxins; antibody-induced destruction; erythropoietin deficiency; production of cytokines that inhibit hematopoiesis; replacement of bone marrow by tumor or fibrosis

PATIENT ASSESSMENT

Erythrocyte count, hemoglobin concentration, hematocrit, mean corpuscular hemoglobin concentration, reticulocyte count, erythrocyte morphology, additional tests based on clinical evaluation (total and fractionated bilirubin, serum iron, total iron-binding capacity, stool hematocrit, serum vitamin B_{12}, red cell folate, hemoglobin electrophoresis, direct and indirect Coombs test, bone marrow aspiration and biopsy, thyroid function tests)

Toxicity Grading				
Parameter	0	1	2	3
Hemoglobin, *g/dL*	> 11	9.5–10.9	< 9.5	Transfusion required
Hematocrit, %	> 32	28–31.9	< 28	Transfusion required

REFERENCES

1. De Vita V Jr: Principles of cancer management: chemotherapy. In *Cancer: Principles and Practice of Oncology.* Edited by De Vita V Jr, Hellman S, Rosenberg S. Philadelphia: Lippincott-Raven; 1997:333–348.

2. Bodey G, Buckley M, Sathe Y, *et al.*: Quantitative relationships between circulating leukocytes and infection in patients with acute leukemia. *Ann Intern Med* 1966, 64:328–340.

3. Klastersky J: Adverse effects of the humanized antibodies used as cancer therapeutics. *Curr Opin Oncol* 2006, 18:316–320.

4. Bagby G Jr, Segal G: Growth factors and the control of hematopoiesis. In *Hematology: Basic Principles and Practice.* Edited by Hoffman R, Benz EJ Jr, Shattil SJ, *et al.* New York: Churchill Livingstone; 1995:207–241.

5. Ziglam HM, Gelly K, Olver W: A survey of the management of neutropenic fevers in oncology units in the UK. *Int J Antimicrob Agents* 2007, 29:430–433.

6. Sipsas NV, Bodey G, Kontoyiannis D: Perspectives for the management of febrile neutropenic patients with cancer in the 21st century. *Cancer* 2005, 103:1103–1113.

7. Lo N, Cullen M: Antibiotic prophylaxis in chemotherapy-induced neutropenia: time to reconsider. *Hematol Oncol* 2006, 24:120–125.

8. Crawford J, Ozer H, Stoller R, *et al.*: Reduction by granulocyte colony-stimulating factor of fever and neutropenia by chemotherapy in patients with small-cell lung cancer. *N Engl J Med* 1991, 325:164–170.

9. Nemunaitis J, Rabinowe S, Singer J, *et al.*: Recombinant granulocyte-macrophage colony-stimulating factor after autologous bone marrow transplantation for lymphoid cancer. *N Engl J Med* 1991, 324:1773–1778.

10. Kuderer N, Dale D, Crawford J, Lyman G: Impact of primary prophylaxis with granulocyte colony stimulating factor on febrile neutropenia and mortality in adult cancer patients receiving chemotherapy: a systematic review. *J Clin Oncol* 2007, 25:3158–3167.

11. Glaspy J, Bukowski R, Steinberg D, *et al.*: Impact of therapy with epoetin alfa on clinical outcomes in patients with nonmyeloid malignancies during cancer chemotherapy in community oncology practice. Procrit Study Group. *J Clin Oncol* 1997, 15:1218–1234.

12. Demetri G, Kris M, Wade J, *et al.*: Quality-of-life benefit in chemotherapy patients treated with epoetin alfa is independent of disease response or tumor type: results from a prospective community oncology study. Procrit Study Group. *J Clin Oncol* 1998, 16:3412–3425.

13. FDA public health advisory: erythropoiesis-stimulating agents, March 9, 2007. Available at http://www.fda.gov/CDER/DRUG/advisory/RHE2007.htm. Accessed July 15, 2008.

14. Tepler I, Elias L, Smith JI, *et al.*: A randomized, placebo-controlled, trial of recombinant human interleukin-11 in cancer patients with severe thrombocytopenia due to chemotherapy. *Blood* 1996, 87:3607–3614.

15. Ciurea S, Hoffman R: Cytokines for the treatment of thrombocytopenia. *Semin Hematol* 2007, 44:166–182.

16. Klastersky J, Paesmans M, Rubenstein EB, *et al.*: The Multinational Association for Supportive Care in Cancer Risk Index: a multinational scoring system for identifying low-risk febrile neutropenic cancer patients. *J Clin Oncol* 2000, 18:3038–3051.

A classification of cancer-associated renal and metabolic abnormalities is shown in Table 26-1. Acute and chronic renal failure, proteinuria (the hallmark of glomerular involvement), hemorrhagic cystitis, fluid and electrolyte disorders (including hypercalcemia, hyponatremia, and syndrome of inappropriate antidiuresis [SIAD]), and ectopic adrenocorticotropic hormone (ACTH) syndrome may all be associated with cancer, the treatment of malignant diseases, or both. This chapter highlights these renal and metabolic abnormalities, focusing on their clinical features, causes, and treatment.

ACUTE RENAL FAILURE

PRERENAL ACUTE FAILURE

Cancer-associated acute renal failure affects the clinical management of patients and has an impact on patient morbidity and mortality. Acute renal failure can be classified into prerenal, postrenal, and intrarenal causes of renal dysfunction (Table 26-1). This classification serves as a framework for diagnostic and therapeutic management.

Anorexia, vomiting, and diarrhea associated with either tumor involvement or chemotherapy may cause volume depletion resulting in prerenal azotemia. Clues to the development of acute renal failure due to volume depletion include a history suggesting volume loss, signs of volume depletion on physical examination, an elevated blood urea nitrogen (BUN)-to-creatinine ratio (> 20:1), and a low urinary sodium value and fractional excretion of sodium (< 20 mEq/L and < 1%, respectively). Patients with cardiomyopathy that causes decreased renal perfusion and those with a reduced effective circulating volume (as in cirrhosis, nephrotic syndrome, or sepsis with vasodilation) may also develop prerenal acute renal failure characterized by an elevated BUN-to-creatinine ratio and low urinary sodium. Nonsteroidal anti-inflammatory drugs may potentiate acute renal failure in individuals with reduced effective circulating volume and should be avoided in such patients. The treatment of prerenal acute renal failure is volume repletion or correction of the reduced renal perfusion (*ie*, improving cardiac function).

POSTRENAL ACUTE FAILURE

Obstruction may occur at any site along the urinary tract and cause postrenal acute renal failure. Common malignancies associated with postrenal acute renal failure include cervical and testicular (particularly seminoma) carcinomas that cause ureteral obstruction, lymphomas with periaortic lymphadenopathy causing ureteral obstruction, and prostate and bladder carcinomas, which may cause bladder outlet obstruction. Malignant infiltration of the retroperitoneal space or the ureters can also result in obstruction [1]. A history of urinary urgency, frequency, and reduced urine output with physical findings of a distended bladder and abdominal or pelvic mass are suggestive of obstruction of the lower urinary tract. The acute onset of flank pain may occur with rapid dilation of the renal pelvis and ureter proximal to an obstruction. More often, however, obstruction is diagnosed serendipitously by routine radiographic studies done for tumor monitoring, or noted following investigation for asymptomatic azotemia (*ie*, bone scan, computed tomography [CT] scan).

In obstructive acute renal failure, the BUN-to-creatinine ratio is usually elevated. Obstruction is confirmed by the demonstration of hydronephrosis on renal ultrasound. In rare occasions, postrenal acute renal failure may result from ureteral encasement. In such cases, obstruction may occur without hydronephrosis. A clinical suspicion of obstruction requires prompt urologic investigation, usually by retrograde pyelography. Relief of obstruction can be accomplished by placement of either ureteral stent(s) or nephrostomy tube(s). Renal recovery depends upon prompt recognition and resolution of obstruction. In patients for whom the obstruction cannot be resolved or in those who do not recover renal function following the correction of obstruction, uremia may develop and aggressive intervention (dialysis) must be discussed candidly in light of the long-term prognosis.

INTRARENAL ACUTE FAILURE

Once prerenal and postrenal causes for acute renal failure are excluded in the azotemic patient with cancer, intrinsic causes of acute renal failure must be considered (Table 26-1). Intrinsic acute renal failure is characterized by a preserved BUN-to-creatinine ratio (10–20:1) and can be caused by thrombosis or infarction of the renal vessels (a rare cause for acute renal failure), interstitial inflammation (acute allergic interstitial nephritis or lymphomatous infiltration), glomerulonephritis (characterized by proteinuria), or acute tubular necrosis (ATN) caused by ischemia or nephrotoxins [1]. ATN due to either ischemic (prolonged prerenal failure or sepsis) or nephrotoxic (aminoglycoside or contrast agent) causes are the most common form of acute renal failure. Certain

Table 26-1. Cancer-Associated Renal and Metabolic Abnormalities

Acute renal failure

Prerenal

Postrenal

  Urethral

    Bladder neck: prostatic or bladder cancer

    Bilateral ureteral: cervical or testicular cancer

Intrarenal

  Vascular (thrombosis/infarction of renal vessels)

  Interstitial nephritis (allergic interstitial nephritis; tumor infiltration and radiation nephritis)

  Bone marrow transplantation–associated renal failure

  Glomerulonephritis

  Acute tubular necrosis

    Nephrotoxic

      • Endogenous: uric acid, myoglobin, immmunoglobulins, hypercalcemia

      • Exogenous: contrast, antibiotics, analgesics, antineoplastic agents

    Ischemic (sepsis, prolonged prerenal)

Chronic renal failure

Prolonged obstruction (prostate, cervical, uterine, testicular, primary renal cancers, or retroperitoneal lymphoma; stones)

Nephrotoxic (antineoplastic agents and radiation)

Glomerulonephropathies (proteinuria)

With Hodgkin's disease (minimal change GN)

With solid tumors (membranous GN)

With antineoplastic agents

Urologic complications

Hemorrhagic cystitis

Metabolic complications

Tumor lysis syndrome

Hyponatremia and SIAD

Hypercalcemia

Ectopic ACTH syndrome

ACTH—adrenocorticotropic hormone; GN—glomerulonephritis; SIAD—syndrome of inappropriate antidiuresis.

types of intrinsic acute renal failure are more common in patients with cancer and are discussed briefly.

TUMOR INFILTRATION AND RADIATION NEPHRITIS

Tumor and lymphomatous infiltration of the kidneys rarely cause renal failure but should be considered in cases of unexplained acute renal failure in predisposed patients [2]. Renal biopsy may be required to make the diagnosis. Treatment of the underlying malignancy may improve renal function [2]. Radiation to the renal bed can cause a spectrum of renal problems, including malignant hypertension as well as acute and chronic renal failure. Radiation-induced chronic renal failure occurs with exposure to more than 2500 rads and is characterized by hypertension, anemia, fatigue, and proteinuria (usually > 1 g per 24 hours) [3]. Histologically, interstitial nephritis accompanied by widespread glomerular sclerosis, tubular atrophy, and arteriolar fibrinoid necrosis is seen [3]. The recognition of radiation nephritis as a clinical entity has resulted in an emphasis on limiting renal exposure to radiation. Improved radiation delivery techniques and awareness of its potential impact on the kidney has resulted in a decline in the incidence of radiation nephritis.

BONE MARROW TRANSPLANTATION–ASSOCIATED RENAL FAILURE

Renal failure that occurs in the setting of bone marrow transplantation may be caused by entities unique to this patient population. The timing of the development of acute renal failure following bone marrow transplantation may be important in defining the causative events and subsequent treatment related to the renal failure. In addition to prerenal azotemia and ATN, bone marrow transplant recipients may develop acute renal failure as a result of tumor lysis and stored marrow infusion, a hepatorenal-like acute renal failure associated with hepatic venoocclusive disease or hemolytic uremic syndrome as a result of cytoreductive therapy and/or with use of cyclosporine or tacrolimus [4]. The hepatorenal-like form of acute renal failure typically occurs 10 to 21 days following transplant and is often associated with amphotericin therapy and sepsis. Recently, nephrotic syndrome has been described as a manifestation of chronic graft-versus-host disease in bone marrow transplant recipients [5]. This is the most common unique form of acute renal failure in the bone marrow transplant patient. Diagnosis of this syndrome can be difficult, and dialysis is often needed. Despite such supportive measures, mortality remains high in those patients with chronic graft-versus-host disease.

ACUTE TUBULAR NECROSIS

ATN can be characterized etiologically as ischemic or nephrotoxic. The classic finding in either type of ATN is dirty brown casts on urinalysis. Decreased tubular sodium reabsorption is a hallmark of ATN and is caused by renal tubular dysfunction. Thus, urinary sodium concentration and fractional excretion of sodium are high. The endogenous toxins associated with intrinsic acute renal failure include hypercalcemia, free myoglobin (seen in cases of rhabdomyolysis), uric acid (as in the tumor lysis syndrome), and immunoglobulin (as in multiple myeloma and amyloidosis, in which light chains, for unexplained reasons, are nephrotoxic). Acute renal failure associated with hypercalcemia is likely multifactorial in origin but includes a direct effect of hypercalcemia that reduces glomerular filtration and volume depletion as a result of hypercalcemia's natriuretic effect [1]. Serum calcium reductions and correction of volume deficits generally reverse the acute renal failure. Nontraumatic rhabdomyolysis may occur in the cancer patient in a variety of settings, including electrolyte disorders (hypokalemia and hypophosphatemia) and prolonged immobilization [1]. Appropriate treatment includes urinary alkalinization and maintenance of urinary output with mannitol and/or diuretics.

Exposure to exogenous renal toxins is perhaps the most common cause of acute renal failure in oncology patients. The widespread use of intravenous (IV) contrast agents, aminoglycoside antibiotics, amphotericin, and nephrotoxic antineoplastic agents frequently contributes to the development of ATN. The elderly are at increased risk for ATN due to nephron loss with age, which is frequently underestimated because these patients may have normal creatinine levels. Additionally, patients with baseline renal dysfunction from any cause, particularly those with multiple myeloma, are at particular risk for ATN with contrast agent or aminoglycoside exposure. Appropriate dosing of medications, hydration, and administration of N-acetylcysteine prior to IV contrast may reduce the potential for nephrotoxic ATN.

NEPHROTOXICITY AND ANTINEOPLASTIC AGENTS

The nephrotoxicity of antineoplastic agents is shown in Table 26-2. Acute renal failure is the most common nephrotoxic complication of antineoplastic agents. Cases of chronic renal failure occurring distant to chemotherapy exposure have been seen in a dose-related fashion with the nitrosoureas and cisplatin. Cisplatin and high-dose methotrexate are notorious for causing acute renal failure. Biologic response modifiers, particularly interleukin, may also cause acute renal failure through a variety of mechanisms, including prerenal factors and glomerular and interstitial involvement [1] (Table 26-2).

Brief discussions of the specific antineoplastic agents known to cause nephrotoxicity follow.

ALKYLATING AGENTS

CISPLATIN AND CARBOPLATIN

Cisplatin (cis-diamminedichloroplatinum II) is among the most widely used chemotherapeutic agents, with efficacy against a wide variety of cancer types [1]. Nephrotoxicity is the limiting factor in the use of cisplatin and undoubtedly is related to renal excretion of the drug [1,6]. Reduced glomerular filtration rate, polyuria, and hypomagnesemia caused by renal magnesium wasting are frequently seen with cisplatin administration [1,6]. The risk of cisplatin-induced acute renal failure can be reduced by administration of large volumes of normal saline hydration [1,6,7]. Careful attention to baseline renal function before treatment with cisplatin is required for appropriate dosing (Table 26-3). Because the renal effects of cisplatin are cumulative, clinical practice has been to discontinue cisplatin once the serum creatinine is greater than 1.5 mg/dL. Amifostine (a phosphorylated aminothiol prodrug) can reduce the frequency of cumulative cisplatin damage to the kidney without decreasing its antitumor efficacy and is sometimes used, although the considerable nausea and vomiting associated with its use are often prohibitive [8]. Carboplatin appears to be less nephrotoxic than cisplatin but can also cause acute renal failure and requires careful monitoring of renal function with appropriate predosage adjustment for renal insufficiency in addition to pretreatment hydration [9].

CYCLOPHOSPHAMIDE

Cyclophosphamide and ifosfamide have been used for many years to treat hematologic malignancies, lymphomas, and a variety of solid tumors. The primary renal toxicities from these agents are hemorrhagic cystitis and impaired water excretion after high-dose (> 50 mg/kg body weight) therapy [1]. A sustained diuresis after high-dose cyclophosphamide therapy is needed to avoid hemorrhagic cystitis. In general, patients are treated with large-volume normal saline infusion in combination with mesna following high-dose therapy. Mesna is a uroprotective agent that acts by binding the urotoxic metabolites (ie, acrolein) of cyclophosphamide. Because of the risk of hyponatremia secondary to cyclophosphamide-induced water retention, half-normal saline infusion before and throughout cyclophosphamide administration is recommended in patients with a history of renal dysfunction and in the elderly [1]. Ifosfamide (isomeric with cyclophosphamide and activated via the same metabolic pathway) is now widely used because some studies have shown superior results. However, ifosfamide can cause proximal tubular atrophy resulting in Fanconi's syndrome, which has not been seen with cyclophosphamide. In one study, 5% of patients developed Fanconi's syndrome, with 15% developing subclinical tubular atrophy. Risk factors include a high cumulative dose, unilateral nephrectomy, and therapy with platinum derivatives [10,11]. The pathophysiology of ifosfamide-induced Fanconi's syndrome is unknown and mesna does not prevent Fanconi's syndromes [12].

NITROSOUREAS

Streptozocin is unique among the nitrosoureas for its effects on the proximal tubule and the development of Fanconi's syndrome [1,13]. Monitoring of proteinuria is required when streptozocin is given, as in oncologic treatment of islet cell carcinoma of the pancreas and carcinoid tumor [13]. Discontinuation of the drug is recommended when proteinuria develops to avoid permanent renal dysfunction [1,13]. Hypophosphatemia may be an initial manifestation of renal tubular dysfunction caused by streptozocin [1,13], and hyperuricosuria without hyperuricemia has been postulated as a causative event in streptozocin-induced renal failure [14].

Table 26-2. Possible Nephrotoxicity of Antineoplastic Agents

Drug	High	Intermediate	Low	Renal effects
Alkylating agents				
Carboplatin			X	ARF
Cisplatin	X			ARF: decreased risk with aggressive hydration
Cyclophosphamide			X	Doses > 50 mg/kg associated with hemorrhagic cystitis
Ifosfamide	X			ARF, CRF, Fanconi's syndrome
Nitrosoureas				
Streptozocin	X			Fanconi's syndrome, may cause CRF
Carmustine			X	CRF: delayed effects, dose related
Lomustine			X	CRF: delayed effects, dose related
Semustine			X	CRF: delayed effects with cumulative doses > 1200 mg/m²
Antimetabolites				
High-dose methotrexate	X			ARF
Cytosine arabinoside			X	ARF
Gemcitabine			X	Hemolytic uremic syndrome
5-Fluorouracil*			X	ARF
5-Azacytidine			X	ARF; proximal and distal tubular dysfunction
6-Thioguanine			X	ARF
Vincristine, vinblastine			X	Impaired water excretion
Antitumor antibiotics				
Mitomycin			X	Hemolytic uremic syndrome
Mithromycin	X			ARF: dose related
Doxorubicin			X	ARF: case reports
Biologic agents				
Interferon-α			X	ARF: interstitial nephritis; proteinuria (minimal-change disease)
Interferon-γ		X		ARF; acute tubular necrosis; proteinuria
Interleukin-2		X		ARF: prerenal azotemia with low FeNA
Bevacizumab		X		Proteinuria, hypertension

*When given with mitomycin C.
ARF—acute renal failure; CRF—chronic renal failure; FeNA—[(urine sodium × plasma creatinine)/(plasma sodium × urine creatinine)] × 100.
(*Adapted from* Weber *et al.* [104].

Table 26-3. Dosing of Antineoplastic Agents in Patients With Renal Failure

Drug	Excreted unchanged, %	Half-life (normal/ESRD), h	Normal renal function dose	GFR > 50	GFR 10–50	GFR < 10
Bleomycin	60	9/20	10–20 U/m²	NR	NR	NR
Carboplatin	50–70	6/increased	3660 mg/m²	100	75	50
Cisplatin	27–45	0.3–0.5/unknown	20–50 mg/m²/d	100	50	25
Cyclophosphamide	10–15	4–7.5/10	1.5 mg/kg/d	100	75	50
Hydroxyurea	Substantial	Unknown	20–30 mg/kg/d	100	100	75
Melphalan	12	1.1–1.4/4–6	6 mg/d	100	50	20
Methotrexate	80–90	8–12/increased	15 mg/d–12 g/m²	100	75	50
Mitomycin C	Unknown	0.5–1/unknown	20 mg/m² every 6–8 wk	100	50	Avoid
Nitrosoureas	Substantial	Short/unknown	—	100	100	75
Prototype semustine	—	Metabolites with variable half-life	Irreversible toxicity with doses > 1500 mg/m²	100	75	25–50
Streptozocin	None	0.25/unknown	500 mg/m²/d	100	75	50

ESRD—end-stage renal disease; GFR—glomerular filtration rate (mg/mL/1.73 m²); NR—not reported.
(*Adapted from* Bennett *et al.* [105].)

Chronic renal failure is the primary manifestation of nephrotoxicity of the other nitrosoureas (carmustine [BCNU], lomustine [CCNU], semustine [methyl-CCNU]), which vary in their potential for renal dysfunction, with semustine (methyl-CCNU) most commonly causing renal failure (Table 26-2). Cumulative doses of nitrosoureas totaling more than 1200 to 1400 mg/m² are associated with irreversible renal failure that can progress to end-stage renal disease and the need for dialysis [15,16]. Such cases of renal failure may present months to years after the completion of treatment with nitrosoureas, particularly with semustine, and often in the absence of underlying or transient acute renal failure [15,16].

ANTIMETABOLITES

HIGH-DOSE METHOTREXATE

Although conventional-dose methotrexate rarely causes nephrotoxicity, high-dose methotrexate (25–50 mg/kg to 1–7 g/m²) has been associated with nonoliguric acute renal failure [1]. Because methotrexate is primarily renally excreted, any alteration in renal function directly affects plasma methotrexate levels and the rate of methotrexate elimination. With prolonged elevation of plasma methotrexate levels, bone marrow and gastrointestinal toxicity may occur [17]. Maintaining a high urinary volume and pH by alkalinization of the urine reduces the nephrotoxicity of high-dose methotrexate [18] and is integral to therapy with this agent. Methotrexate is poorly dialyzed [19], making management of patients with elevated methotrexate levels and renal insufficiency challenging and emphasizing the need for careful dosing of methotrexate in patients with renal dysfunction (Table 26-3). Previously, all patients who received high-dose methotrexate were first subjected to a 24-hour urine collection to determine the creatinine clearance. Recently, a retrospective analysis compared measured versus calculated creatinine clearance for 25 patients undergoing a total of 287 treatments with high-dose methotrexate for primary central nervous system (CNS) lymphoma. This analysis found significant correlation between the measured and the calculated creatinine clearance using the Cockcroft-Gault equation and determined that calculated creatinine clearance was a reasonable alternative to a 24-hour urine collection in calculating the appropriate methotrexate dose [20].

OTHER ANTIMETABOLITES

Table 26-2 shows other antimetabolites capable of causing nephrotoxicity; renal dysfunction is much less common with these agents than with high-dose methotrexate. 5-Fluorouracil has been reported to cause acute renal failure as a result of hemolytic uremic syndrome but only when given in combination with mitomycin [1]. Gemcitabine is effective against pancreatic cancer as well as non–small cell lung cancer, advanced ovarian cancer, and other malignancies. There have been case reports of acute renal failure from hemolyticuremic syndrome associated with the use of gemcitabine [21]. Abnormalities of both proximal and distal tubular function may occur with 5-azacytidine. These are manifested by hypophosphatemia, hypokalemia, low serum bicarbonate, polyuria or glucosuria, and renal salt wasting, which can result in volume depletion with hypotension and mild azotemia [22]. Supportive therapy with replacement of the lost electrolytes and minerals is required. Resolution of the acquired defects of tubular function occurs with discontinuation of 5-azacytidine [22]. Fludarabine is a purine analogue frequently used in the treatment of lymphoid malignancies and as a part of low-intensity conditioning regimens in bone marrow transplant. Case reports of transient, reversible acute renal failure appear in the literature [23]. Although rare, cladribine, another purine analogue principally used for the treatment of hairy cell leukemia, may also have renal toxicity.

ANTITUMOR ANTIBIOTICS

MITOMYCIN

Two patterns of mitomycin C–associated renal failure occur: a relatively uncommon dose-related acute renal failure seen with administration of mitomycin C alone [24] and a hemolytic-uremic type of renal failure seen when a combination of mitomycin C and 5-fluorouracil is given [1,25]. The latter is characterized by a microangiopathic hemolytic anemia and thrombocytopenia with acute renal failure, with microthrombi on renal biopsy [1,25]. Renal failure may persist and result in end-stage renal disease; fatal cases are not unusual [25]. Plasma exchange may be useful in some cases [26]. The renal failure seen with high-dose mitomycin C alone is characteristically less fulminant and related to cumulative drug dosage [1,25]. Microangiopathic hemolytic anemia is less frequent with this type of mitomycin C–induced renal dysfunction, but renal biopsy shows similar changes [25]. Mortality with this type of renal failure is high, usually occurring within 3 to 8 months [25].

MITHRAMYCIN

Nonrenal toxicity generally limits the use of high-dose (25–50 mg/kg daily for 5 days) mithramycin [1]. Nephrotoxicity, defined as a BUN more than 25 mg/dL or a reduction in creatinine clearance, was noted in 22 of 54 patients (40%) given high-dose mithramycin for a variety of tumors [27]. Qualitative proteinuria (1+ on urine dipstick) was noted in 78% of the patients. Underlying renal insufficiency and higher cumulative doses of mithramycin increased the risk of nephrotoxicity [27]. Histopathologic examination of renal tissue was consistent with ATN. Currently, low-dose mithramycin (25 mg/kg) is more commonly used to treat hypercalcemia [1]. Renal failure is less likely with this dosage regimen, although case reports of renal failure associated with single doses of mithramycin used for this indication do exist [28]. When giving mithramycin, renal function should be monitored carefully, particularly in those with underlying renal impairment.

ANTHRACYCLINES

Despite the development of specific renal lesions (glomerular vacuolation) in animals given anthracycline antibiotics, such as doxorubicin and daunomycin [29], nephrotoxicity rarely occurs in humans. A single case report suggested that doxorubicin causes renal toxicity [30], but there are no confirming data. Cardiac toxicity is the dose-limiting factor for doxorubicin administration and may occur at lower cumulative doses than the nephrotoxicity, thereby limiting the development of renal toxicity [1].

BIOLOGIC AGENTS

INTERFERONS

The literature on interferon-α–induced nephrotoxicity consists primarily of case reports documenting proteinuria and renal failure [31–33] or immune complex membranoproliferative glomerulonephritis [34]. Proteinuria and renal failure with focal segmental glomerulosclerosis and ATN on renal biopsy have been reported in a child treated with interferon-γ [35]. In addition, one of the cases of interferon-α nephrotoxicity described acute interstitial nephritis with minimally changed nephropathy on biopsy [33]. Interferons are unique in that glomerular involvement is a common feature of their nephrotoxicity. Immune complex glomerulonephritis in an HIV-positive patient treated with interferon-α has been reported [36]. The authors suggested that a disruption in immunoregulation at the renal tissue level may underlie the observed pathologic responses seen with interferon therapy [36]. Additional study of the renal effects of interferons is needed.

Interleukin-2, with or without lymphokine-activated killer cells, can cause prerenal azotemia characterized by oliguria, hypotension, and a low fractional excretion of sodium [37]. Fluid retention with edema formation also occurs, suggesting a leaky capillary syndrome associated with renal hypoperfusion [1]. The rapid development and resolution of the renal failure in most patients suggests a hemodynamic cause [38]. Patients particularly at risk for interleukin-2–induced acute renal failure are those with underlying renal insufficiency; the degree of renal failure was greater and the duration of renal impairment was longer in such patients [37]. Prompt recognition of the syndrome and appropriate fluid resuscitation are required. Nephrotoxicity is less likely with continuous infusion therapy [39].

BEVACIZUMAB

A humanized monoclonal antibody against vascular endothelial growth factor (VEGF), bevacizumab has become a routine part of therapy for colon and renal cell cancer and is also frequently being used in breast and lung cancers. Bevacizumab therapy has been associated with the development of largely asymptomatic proteinuria in 23% to 38% of patients with colon cancer and up to 64% of patients with renal cell cancer [40,41]. Therapy with this agent is also associated with the development of hypertension, which may contribute to renal dysfunction. The mechanism for the development of proteinuria with bevacizumab is unknown, but it can be severe in some patients, leading to development of nephrotic-range protein excretion [42]. Therapy discontinuation may be necessary in patients who develop symptomatic nephrotic syndrome or uncontrollable hypertension.

CHRONIC RENAL FAILURE

As previously noted, chronic renal failure in the oncology patient may result from nephrotoxin exposure, notably from radiation and certain antineoplastic agents, particularly the nitrosoureas and cisplatin (Table 26-2). However, it is more likely to be caused by obstruction. As with acute renal failure, chronic renal insufficiency from obstruction is most frequently caused by cervical, testicular, bladder, and prostate cancers. The extent and duration of the obstruction are the primary factors affecting the degree of renal recovery. As with obstruction-induced acute renal failure, diagnosis is usually made by renal ultrasound, which demonstrates hydronephrosis. Treatment is aimed at relief of the obstruction.

GLOMERULONEPHROPATHIES

The nephrotic syndrome can occur as a paraneoplastic manifestation in patients with solid tumors and lymphomas. Proteinuria is the cardinal finding, and the nephrotic syndrome (> 3.5 g protein in 24-hour urine collection, hypoalbuminemia, edema) confirms glomerular involvement. The type of glomerulopathy tends to be related to the cancer: membranous glomerulopathy is often seen in patients with solid tumors (*ie,* colon and lung cancer), and minimal-change glomerulopathy occurs in patients with Hodgkin's lymphoma [43,44]. Nephrotic syndrome has also been reported in patients with non-Hodgkin's lymphomas but occurs less commonly [43,45] and is often associated with more extensive glomerular involvement and renal failure in this population [46]. This syndrome has also been reported in patients with chronic lymphocytic leukemia [45]. The nephrotic syndrome may precede, occur concurrently with, or follow the diagnosis of cancer or lymphoma and is unrelated to the stage of the disease [45]. There is some evidence for tumor-related antigens as pathogenetic triggers in the glomerulopathies of cancer, but the precise mechanisms for the development of these syndromes are not understood [43]. Frequently, tumor remission results in resolution of proteinuria and tumor recurrence is accompanied by its reappearance [43,45].

As noted above, some antineoplastic agents have been associated with the development of proteinuria (Table 26-2), the most notable of these being anti-VEGF therapy. The interferons have also been associated with the development of proteinuria. The single case report of glomerulonephritis in a patient given doxorubicin has not been confirmed by additional reports.

UROLOGIC COMPLICATIONS

HEMORRHAGIC CYSTITIS

Uncontrolled urinary tract hemorrhage in the cancer patient is less common today because of improvements in radiation therapy dosing and the use of reducing agents such as mesna, which is given in conjunction with cyclophosphamide or ifosfamide therapy [47]. With both alkylating agents and radiation therapy, urothelial damage is the initiating event resulting in hemorrhagic cystitis. An underlying bleeding diathesis or the concomitant use of anticoagulants may potentiate urothelial damage and exacerbate medication-induced or radiation-induced genitourinary bleeding. Other antineoplastic agents implicated in the development of hemorrhagic cystitis include L-asparaginase, dactinomycin, mitomycin C, mithramycin, and 6-mercaptopurine [47]. The management of hemorrhagic cystitis from cancer therapy includes bladder catheterization for drainage and continuous irrigation. Intravesical cauterization and surgical intervention may also be required in refractory cases [47]. Hemorrhagic cystitis is also a frequent late (> 2 weeks) complication of allogeneic bone marrow transplant, with 5% to 40% of patients developing symptoms. This condition is frequently associated with BK viruria, although this alone is not sufficient to cause cystic bleeding. One recent study demonstrated increased risk for hemorrhagic cystitis associated with myeloablative conditioning regimens, high-titer BK viruria, and unrelated donor source [48].

METABOLIC COMPLICATIONS

TUMOR LYSIS SYNDROME

Tumor lysis syndrome (TLS) is a metabolic disorder characteristic of a variety of tumors. It is a true oncologic emergency and prompt recognition and therapy can have a profound impact on outcome. This disorder may occur spontaneously in rapidly proliferating hematologic malignancies, including acute lymphoblastic leukemia, lymphoma, and acute myeloid leukemia, but is also seen in a range of solid and hematologic tumors following chemotherapy, most notably small cell lung cancer. Patients at highest risk for the syndrome are those with a large, rapidly proliferative tumor burden or patients with underlying renal dysfunction. Appropriate management and diagnosis depend upon a high clinical suspicion and adequate serial monitoring for the development of characteristic electrolyte abnormalities.

PHYSIOLOGY

TLS is characterized by hyperkalemia, hyperphosphatemia, hypocalcemia, and hyperuricemia. Patients will almost always also have an elevated lactate dehydrogenase level, reflecting the volume of tumor burden. These electrolyte abnormalities are the result of rapid tumor cell turnover, which results in the release of normally sequestered intracellular contents into the circulation. These include potassium, phosphate, nucleic acid, and lactate dehydrogenase. Symptoms of TLS are largely related to the resulting electrolyte abnormalities from this cellular breakdown. The purine nucleotides released in this manner are principally metabolized by the liver and converted by the enzyme xanthine oxidase into uric acid [49]. During acute TLS, the uric acid produced in this manner can precipitate in the distal nephron, resulting in urate nephropathy and acute renal failure. This dreaded TLS complication can exacerbate the already significant electrolyte abnormalities described previously.

CLINICAL SYMPTOMS

The electrolyte and renal abnormalities described above usually result in the typical clinical symptoms of TLS. Significant hyperkalemia can ultimately result in cardiac arrhythmias, but also manifest as fatigue, muscle cramping, anorexia, paresthesias, and irritability. Hyperkalemia is defined as a serum potassium level of more than 6.0 mEq/L. Hyperkalemia may be exacerbated by metabolic acidosis, renal insufficiency, and potassium-sparing diuretics.

Hyperphosphatemia and hypocalcemia are also characteristic of TLS. The former is defined as a serum phosphate of greater than 4.5 mg/dL and the latter by serum calcium less than 7.0 mg/dL. Impaired glomerular handling of calcium and phosphate can exacerbate the hyperphosphatemia and hypocalcemia that result from massive tumor breakdown. Calcium phosphate precipitation can occur when the calcium phosphate product exceeds a critical threshold, resulting in progressive hypocalcemia and calcium deposition–related organ dysfunction, particularly nephrocalcinosis. Hypocalcemia will ultimately result in muscle cramping, tetany, and seizure activity as well as prolongation of the QT interval and decreased cardiac contractility.

Hyperuricemia is defined as a serum uric acid level of greater than 8.0 mg/dL, and although urate accumulation is independently benign, uric acid deposition within the kidney due to crystallization of urate at a pH below 5.5 frequently results in renal dysfunction.

MANAGEMENT

Management of TLS is largely dependent on prevention of urate nephropathy, hyperphosphatemia, and dehydration. Patients at high risk for TLS or who present with hallmarks suggestive of early TLS should immediately be treated with IV hydration to achieve a urine flow rate of more that 100 mL/m^2/h. Although urinary alkalinization can decrease the risk of urate nephropathy, it carries an increased risk of calcium phosphate precipitation, and thus alkaline IV hydration is not recommended. Patients should routinely be started on a phosphate binder (*ie,* sevelamer) to control hyperphosphatemia. Nephrotoxins should be studiously avoided in patients who are at high risk of TLS and medications recognized to interfere with renal potassium handling should be discontinued (*ie,* angiotensin-converting enzyme I, angiotensin II receptor blockers, and potassium-sparing diuretics).

Several agents exist that are used to decrease systemic uric acid levels to avoid urate nephropathy. The oldest and most well known of these is allopurinol, an irreversible xanthine oxidase inhibitor that has long been the mainstay of uric acid management. This agent prevents the conversion of xanthine to uric acid. Xanthine, which does not crystallize, is then filtered freely at the glomerulus and excreted through the kidney. Although effective, allopurinol does not address the burden of circulating uric acid and usually requires several days to be efficacious. For patients with a high tumor burden for whom the risk of tumor lysis is high, it is appropriate to start allopurinol several days prior to initiation of chemotherapy.

A relatively new addition to the armamentarium for TLS treatment is rasuricase, a urate oxidase originally purified from *Aspergillus flavus*. This enzyme catalyzes the conversion of uric acid to allantoin, which is 5 to 10 times more soluble than urate and is thus freely filtered and excreted by the kidney. The final results of the North American trial using this agent reported on the treatment of 1069 patients with a variety of hematologic and solid malignancies who manifested symptoms of TLS. In this study, patients were treated with rasuricase at a dose of 0.2 mg/kg, and could receive therapy for 1 to 7 days every 12 hours as their physician deemed appropriate. The average number of doses was three. Grade 3 or 4 adverse events were reported in only 1.2% of patients. This study confirmed that rasuricase was well tolerated and safe and suggested that treatment with rasuricase could decrease the need for renal replacement therapy in patients with TLS [50].

In patients who develop worsening azotemia, refractory electrolyte abnormalities, or those in whom volume overload becomes a problem, early initiation of renal replacement therapy is appropriate. Intermittent hemodialysis and continuous venovenous hemodialysis are both appropriate management strategies and renal function will usually recover [51].

SYNDROME OF INAPPROPRIATE ANTIDIURETIC HORMONE (SIADH)

Although there are many causes for the syndrome of inappropriate antidiuretic hormone (SIADH), the most common cause remains malignancy, particularly small cell carcinoma of the lung. In 1957, Schwartz *et al.* [52] described two patients with bronchogenic cancer who manifested hyponatremia and continued urinary loss of sodium and postulated that this syndrome might be caused by inappropriate secretion of an antidiuretic substance. In several instances, inappropriately high circulating levels of antidiuretic hormone (ADH) have been reported, hence the term SIADH. Because in some cases ADH may not be the causative agent, the syndrome is best referred to as SIAD (syndrome of antidiuresis).

The diagnosis requires the presence of hyponatremia, hypoosmolality, an inappropriately concentrated urine, and exclusion of other conditions that can cause hyponatremia, including renal, adrenal, thyroid, cardiac, and hepatic abnormalities, as well as volume depletion, congestive heart failure, and diuretic use. Other characteristic features include low serum urea and uric acid and continued renal excretion of sodium [53].

PHYSIOLOGY OF ANTIDIURETIC HORMONE SECRETION

ADH, also called arginine vasopressin, is a peptide synthesized within the hypothalamus and stored in the posterior lobe of the pituitary gland. ADH release is regulated by hypothalamic osmoreceptors. Increased plasma osmolality triggers release of ADH, which acts at the distal tubule and collecting duct to promote retention of free water and restore normal plasma osmolality. Conversely, a decrease in plasma osmolality suppresses ADH release [54].

Volume stimuli also regulate ADH release. A decrease in plasma volume as a result of hemorrhage, peripheral vasodilation, sustained quiet standing, or positive pressure ventilation can all stimulate the release of ADH by decreasing baroreceptor signaling in the atria. This compensatory mechanism restores plasma volume. By contrast, increases in plasma volume inhibit ADH release by increasing baroreceptor signaling. In the absence of ADH, diuresis occurs. Other conditions that inhibit ADH release include negative pressure ventilation, recumbency, lack of gravity, submersion in water, and exposure to cold. Volume stimulation will override osmotic stimuli.

In addition to volume and osmotic stimuli, pharmacologic agents can stimulate ADH release, including the chemotherapeutic agents cyclophosphamide [55], vinblastine [56], and vincristine [57]. ADH release can also be triggered by nausea, pain, and surgery [54].

PATHOPHYSIOLOGY OF SIAD

The hallmark of SIAD is the inability to dilute the urine maximally in the presence of hyponatremia. Urinary osmolality in SIAD is typically higher than plasma osmolality. This phenomenon may also occur in the absence of abnormalities in ADH secretion, as in elderly patients, those with renal disease, and those using diuretics; therefore, these conditions must be excluded before making the diagnosis. Assessment of volume status is critical to differentiate volume contraction from SIAD. Patients with SIAD are euvolemic. In volume-contracted patients, the decrease in effective blood volume provides a nonosmotic, volume-responsive stimulus for ADH

release. As a result of ADH release, hyponatremia can occur, and the urine can become inappropriately concentrated; however, these patients will respond to volume resuscitation.

Ingestion of water in patients with SIAD leads to a prompt natriuresis [58]. Although it was originally thought that the natriuresis was the result of aldosterone suppression by expansion of the extracellular volume [52], it has subsequently been shown that circulating levels of aldosterone are normal and respond normally to stimuli [59,60]. Atrial natriuretic peptide levels, which increase with modest volume expansion following acute water ingestion and correlate with the prompt increase in sodium excretion [61], may cause natriuresis in this syndrome. Patients with SIAD who have low sodium intake or who develop extracellular volume contraction are able to conserve sodium. In these instances, patients with SIAD may have low urinary sodium concentrations. Once the volume contraction is corrected, urinary sodium excretion increases.

Patients with SIAD will only develop hyponatremia if water intake is excessive. Although they rarely report excessive thirst, the continued ingestion of water during hypo-osmolality observed in these patients is considered inappropriate. Although ADH itself is not dipsogenic, the factors responsible for continued ingestion of water in this syndrome have not yet been identified.

In some cases of SIAD, especially in patients with cancer who develop this syndrome, frank hyponatremia may not develop. In these instances, water intake appears to be more appropriate for the degree of hyponatremia. Why this should occur more often in cancer-related than other causes of SIAD remains unknown.

SYNTHESIS AND SECRETION OF ADH IN CANCERS

Peptide and messenger RNA for ADH have been identified in the tumors of several patients with clinical SIAD, and circulating plasma levels of ADH are frequently increased. ADH is synthesized and processed in these tumors in a manner similar to its synthesis in the hypothalamus [62,63]. Although small cell (oat cell) carcinomas are most frequently associated with SIAD [63], a variety of carcinomas from many different tissues have also been associated with this syndrome. It should also be remembered that SIAD may also result from other stimuli including nausea, pain, drugs, and chemotherapeutic agents.

TREATMENT

Because elevated levels of ADH lead to hyponatremia only if water intake exceeds its excretion, restriction of water intake is the cornerstone of therapy. To achieve a negative water balance, fluid intake should be restricted to approximately 800 mL/d. Correction of hyponatremia should be done slowly. Overzealous correction can lead to the rare but disabling condition known as central pontine myelinolysis [64,65]. Patients are at risk for this disorder if serum sodium is corrected at a rate more rapidly than 2 mEq/L/ h, particularly if the hyponatremia is chronic. A more rapid correction can take place if the development of hyponatremia has been acute. The correction of hyponatremia with isotonic (0.9%) saline is usually ineffective because the sodium is excreted and the water is retained, which results in a paradoxical lowering of the serum sodium. Saline should be used only when given together with a loop diuretic, which impairs urine-concentrating ability by facilitating free water excretion. The use of hypertonic (3%) saline should be reserved for emergencies in which neurologic symptoms such as seizures or coma occur or if the sodium level is below 110 mEq/L.

The following are a list of guidelines for therapy. First, hyponatremia can be corrected at a rate of 0.5 mEq/L/h when not emergent. Second, in emergent situations, the rate of correction should not exceed 2 mEq/L/h. Third, once the serum sodium is above 120 mEq/L, the rate of correction can be slowed. During correction, the serum sodium must be monitored frequently.

Outpatient long-term treatment is directed at fluid restriction, but in instances of noncompliance or if impractical because of obligate fluid requirements, long-term daily furosemide with sodium chloride tablets to compensate for sodium loss can be used [66]. An alternate approach is to use an agent such as demeclocycline in doses of 600 to 1200 mg/d, which produces ADH-resistant nephrogenic diabetes insipidus, which is fully reversible on withdrawal of the medication [67]. Nonsteroidal antiinflammatory agents should also be discontinued because they potentiate the effect of ADH by blocking prostaglandin synthesis.

Other therapies are directed at decreasing tumor synthesis and secretion of ADH by reducing tumor burden with surgery, radiotherapy, or chemotherapy. Because several of the chemotherapeutic agents may promote ADH release, careful attention to fluid management is necessary.

HYPERCALCEMIA ASSOCIATED WITH MALIGNANCY

CLINICAL FEATURES

Hypercalcemia is the most common life-threatening metabolic disorder associated with malignancy and typically results in neuromuscular, renal, and gastrointestinal symptoms as well as impaired cognitive function. Marked dehydration and severe mental status changes accompany greater degrees of hypercalcemia. Hypercalcemic crisis with dehydration, renal insufficiency, and obtundation may be the first clinical manifestation of malignancy, although it is more often a late complication of disease. The symptoms of hypercalcemia may mimic those of the underlying malignancy, and include anorexia, weight loss, muscle weakness, and altered mental status. The severity of these symptoms is often correlated with the degree of hypercalcemia.

CAUSES

Hypercalcemia of malignancy can be caused by local osteolytic hypercalcemia or humoral hypercalcemia of malignancy. In some patients, both of these mechanisms may occur.

Humoral hypercalcemia of malignancy (HHM) is associated with tumor production of a factor termed parathyroid hormone (PTH)–related peptide (PTHrP) [68–71]. PTHrP is secreted into the circulation [68–73] and leads to osteoclastic bone resorption. The clinical HHM syndrome is characterized by hypercalcemia, hypercalciuria, hypophosphatemia, reduced levels of PTH, increased nephrogenous cyclic AMP, reduced plasma 1,25-vitamin D levels, and increased levels of PTHrP. Skeletal biopsy reveals a marked increase in osteoclastic bone resorption with a marked reduction in osteoblastic activity [74,75]. This dissociation of osteoclastic and osteoblastic activities contrasts with the bone morphology in primary hyperparathyroidism, in which osteoclastic and osteoblastic activities are increased in a coupled fashion. The tumors most frequently associated with HHM include squamous cell carcinomas of all subtypes, renal, breast, bladder, ovarian, and endometrial carcinomas, and human T-cell lymphotropic virus-1 lymphomas [76]. By contrast, adenocarcinomas of the prostate, colon, stomach, and pancreas are rarely associated with phenomena.

The absence of PTHrP in the sera of some patients with hypercalcemia of malignancy coupled with the observations that tumors are capable of making many factors that increase osteoclastic resorption of bone indicates that PTHrP is not the sole mediator of hypercalcemia of malignancy [77–79]. Several growth factors have been proposed as osteoclast-activating factors, including interleukins 1 and 2, tumor necrosis factor-α, transforming growth factors, and prostaglandins [80–83]. A number of these factors may lead to local bone resorption in local osteolytic hypercalcemia.

TREATMENT

Treatment of hypercalcemia is summarized in Table 26-4. Severe hypercalcemia requires emergent treatment with aggressive intravascular volume repletion and forced saline diuresis [84,85]. Loop diuretics should not be used until intravascular volume has been restored. Loop diuretics given before volume restoration may worsen dehydration and increase serum calcium due to enhanced proximal sodium and calcium resorption. Because the mechanism of hypercalcemia of malignancy is increased bone resorption, the mainstay for long-term control of hypercalcemia is an antiresorptive agent, such as a bisphosphonate. However, the most effective treatment for this disorder is management of the underlying disease.

Bisphosphonates are analogues of pyrophosphate that bind to bone hydroxyapatite. The compounds are taken up by osteoclasts and inhibit osteoclast action [86,87]. Several of these agents are clinically available. The two most frequently used agents are zoledronic acid, which should be given as a single 4 mg IV dose over 15 minutes, and pamidronate which is given as a single 45 to 60 mg IV dose over 24 hours. Both agents are equally effective and safe, but renal function should be monitored with long-term use [88–90]. Serum calcium levels will gradually decline beginning 24 to 48 hours after the dose and may remain normal for weeks, although serum calcium levels should be monitored serially after treatment. The duration of effects appears to be shorter in patients with HHM than in patients with local osteolytic hypercalcemia [89,91]. Side effects from these agents include hypocalcemia and hypomagnesemia in 10%, hypophosphatemia in 10% to 30%, and transient fever or flu-like symptoms [87,90].

Calcitonin therapy has its greatest utility within the first 24 to 36 hours in the treatment of severe hypercalcemia and should be used in conjunction with the more potent, slower-acting bisphosphonate therapy [84,85]. Calcitonin is given as a dose of 4 U/kg body weight intramuscularly or subcutaneously every 12 hours. Tachyphylaxis often develops with calcitonin therapy. Calcitonin is considered only as an adjunctive therapy because calcium will usually fall by only 2 mg/dL.

Glucocorticoids have their greatest efficacy in patients with glucocorticoid-responsive diseases, such as myeloma or lymphoma, or in patients whose hypercalcemia is associated with increased 1,25-vitamin D absorption of calcium and resorption of bone. A dose of 200 mg of hydrocortisone or its equivalent is given IV for 3 to 5 days [84,85].

ADRENOCORTICOTROPIC HORMONE

Cushing's syndrome resulting from the ectopic production and secretion of ACTH by a tumor accounts for about 10% of all patients diagnosed with the disease [92]. As a result of the excess secretion of ACTH by the nonpituitary source, the adrenal gland becomes hyperplastic, and overproduction of cortisol ensues. Cortisol inhibits the biosynthesis and secretion of hypothalamic corticotropin-releasing factor (CRF) and pituitary ACTH in a classic fashion that exemplifies the negative feedback of hormones. However, the secretion of ACTH by the nonpituitary tumor is usually not suppressed by the excess cortisol. This feature of nonsuppressibility of ACTH by the tumor is useful to differentiate ACTH secretion from a pituitary source, which is suppressible. ACTH in the normal pituitary as well as in nonpituitary tumors is derived from processing of the proopiomelanocortin (*POMC*) gene. Ectopic secretion of ACTH likely results from abnormal gene expression [93].

CLINICAL FEATURES

The clinical presentation of patients with this disorder is varied and appears to reflect the tumor type and the rapidity and severity of the

Table 26-4. Treatment of Hypercalcemia

Treatment	Onset of action	Duration of action	Normalization, %	Advantages	Disadvantages
Saline	Hours	During infusion	10	Rehydration	Cardiac compromise, intensive monitoring, hypokalemia, hypomagnesemia
Saline and loop diuretic	Hours	During infusion	10	Enhanced renal calcium excretion	Cardiac compromise, intensive monitoring, hypokalemia, hypomagnesemia
Calcitonin	Hours	2–3 d	10–20	Nontoxic, rapid onset of action in life-threatening hypercalcemia	Only lowers calcium by 2 mg/dL, tachyphylaxis
Pamidronate	24–48 h	10–14 d	70–100	Potent, relatively nontoxic	Fever, hypophosphatemia, hypomagnesemia, hypocalcemia
Zoledronic acid	24–48 h	32–43 d	70–100	Potent, relatively nontoxic	Flu-like symptoms, hypophosphatemia, hypomagnesemia, hypocalcemia

hypercortisolism. The acute syndrome consists of rapid onset of hypertension, hypokalemia, edema, and glucose intolerance, and is most often associated with small cell lung carcinoma, which accounts for about three fourths of all cases of ectopic ACTH secretion [94,95]. Chronic ACTH overproduction due to malignancy is indistinguishable from Cushing's syndrome and is associated with indolent tumors, most frequently bronchial carcinoids but also pancreatic or thymic carcinoid, medullary carcinoma of the thyroid, pheochromocytoma, and other neuroendocrine tumors [96].

BIOCHEMICAL AND RADIOLOGIC DIAGNOSIS

Diagnosis requires the demonstration of hypercortisolism by elevated 24-hour urinary free cortisol excretion and failure of cortisol suppression following a standard low-dose dexamethasone suppression test. Additional tests are required to distinguish ectopic ACTH production from other forms of Cushing's syndrome. Distinguishing ACTH-dependent from non–ACTH dependent causes of Cushing's syndrome is easily done by determination of serum ACTH and cortisol levels. In ACTH-dependent causes, like ectopic ACTH syndrome, serum levels of ACTH are normal or elevated, whereas in the latter, ACTH levels are suppressed.

It is necessary to distinguish pituitary-dependent Cushing's syndrome from the ectopic ACTH syndrome. Patients with rapidly progressive ectopic ACTH syndrome are usually easy to diagnose. Those with more indolent nonpituitary tumors can present a diagnostic challenge. Differentiation of these two entities requires the use of dynamic tests based on the assumption that pituitary-dependent disease will demonstrate responsiveness to cortisol feedback, whereas ectopic ACTH production will not.

The dynamic tests used include cortisol response to high-dose dexamethasone suppression, ACTH response to CRF during inferior petrosal sinus sampling, and cortisol response to metyrapone. Although malignant ectopic ACTH-secreting neoplasms, like small cell lung carcinoma, will usually fail to suppress with high-dose dexamethasone, the more indolent ectopic ACTH-secreting tumors, like bronchial carcinoid, will frequently demonstrate suppression [93,97].

Inferior petrosal sinus sampling can help to distinguish these indolent tumors. Cannulae are placed in the bilateral inferior petrosal sinuses that drain the pituitary gland and ACTH levels before and after corticotropin-releasing hormone stimulation are evaluated in both the petrosal veins and at a distant peripheral site. A ratio of basal petrosal to peripheral ACTH of more than two is highly predictive (> 95%) of pituitary-dependent disease [94].

Once a diagnosis of ectopic ACTH syndrome has been considered, radiographic studies, including chest radiograph, and CT or magnetic resonance imaging (MRI) of the chest are indicated. Small cell carcinoma of the lung is usually apparent on plain film or CT scan; however, bronchial carcinoids can be quite small and may require MRI. Ectopic ACTH-secreting tumors may not become clinically apparent for many years after the diagnosis of Cushing's syndrome has been established.

TREATMENT

Management of this syndrome must be determined by the severity of the illness and the long-term prognosis due to the underlying malignancy. It is directed at both the ACTH-secreting tumor and the hypercortisolism. Surgical and medical interventions have been used to control the hypercortisolism associated with inoperable ectopic ACTH production. Bilateral adrenalectomy is of questionable benefit in patients whose life expectancy is measured in months from the time of diagnosis. The prognosis of small cell carcinoma of the lung also appears to be worse when it is associated with the ectopic ACTH syndrome, possibly due to the complications of hypercortisolism (*ie*, weakness, hypokalemia, secondary infection).

Medical therapy for hypercortisolism involves use of both inhibitors of steroid biosynthesis (ketoconazole, metyrapone, aminoglutethimide) and adrenolytic (mitotane) agents. Ketoconazole, an antifungal agent that inhibits the P-450 enzymes involved, cortisol, aldosterone, and sex steroids biosynthesis has been used with variable results [98].

In general, mild hypercortisolism is easier to control than severe disease. Metyrapone can also block steroidogenesis, but is associated with gastrointestinal side effects and allergic reactions. Aminoglutethimide is also associated with skin rash, sedation, dizziness, ataxia, and gastrointestinal irritation. Mitotane, an adrenolytic, has been reported to result in biochemical and clinical improvement in a few cases, but has a slow onset of action and a myriad of side effects. Octreotide, a long-acting somatostatin analogue, has also been tried in a few patients, but results have been highly variable [99–102]. Glucocorticoid receptor antagonists, like RU486, offer a method of alleviating excessive glucocorticoid action but their efficacy in this syndrome has not been determined [103].

URINARY TRACT OBSTRUCTION

Retroperitoneal tumors causing ureteral obstruction can occur with any solid neoplasm. Urologic and gynecologic cancers, together with lymphomas, are the most common causes of obstruction. The effects of obstruction on kidney function result in an early inability to concentrate the urine maximally. Renal blood flow is also markedly diminished, particularly in the setting of unilateral obstruction. Regardless of the precipitating neoplasm, the presenting clinical manifestation is usually excruciating pain.

MANAGEMENT OR INTERVENTION

1. Establish histologic diagnosis of the underlying neoplasm
2. Introduce appropriate therapeutic modalities based on primary disease and obstruction:
   a. For prostate cancer causing bilateral obstruction, consider urethral catheterization, suprapubic cystostomy, immediate bilateral orchiectomy, or other endocrine therapeutic approaches
   b. For lymphomas causing retroperitoneal obstruction, radiation therapy or combination chemotherapy can be employed
   c. For isolated metastases, localized radiation therapy can be effective
   d. For retroperitoneal metastases or lymphoma with loss of renal function, if the neoplasm has not been controlled, immediate percutaneous nephrotomy with placement of antegrade or retrograde stents in the immediate future should be considered
   e. For sensitive neoplasms and testicular cancer, the presence of renal function abnormalities mandates consideration of temporary percutaneous nephrotomies
3. Inhibit xanthine oxidase with allopurinol to prevent a surge of uric acid, which could compromise renal function during systemic treatment
4. Minimize likelihood of infectious complications during manipulation of the obstructed urinary tract
5. Carefully manage postobstructive diuresis and natriuresis with intensive metabolic monitoring

CAUSATIVE FACTORS

Retroperitoneal tumors; urologic cancers, gynecologic cancers, and lymphomas causing lymphadenopathy in the para-aortic, paracaval, and periureteral locations; prostate and advanced cervical cancers commonly causing distal urinary tract obstruction; testicular cancers, especially seminoma, capable of obstructing both ureters simultaneously; metastatic neoplasms forming a plaque-like sheet of tumor

PATHOLOGIC PROCESS

Dilatation of proximal anatomic regions due to obstruction; kidney increases in weight and size and gradually atrophies; inability to concentrate urine maximally and marked diminution of renal blood flow

DIFFERENTIAL DIAGNOSES

Retroperitoneal fibrosis, ureteral metastases, bladder neck obstruction, lymphadenopathy, kidney stones

PATIENT ASSESSMENT

Ultrasonography (method of choice); radionuclide studies; bone scans with technetium concentration to quantify renal blood flow; on occasion, retrograde and antegrade pyelography; cystoscopy and other interventional approaches for staging purposes; FeNA to determine duration of obstruction

TOXICITY GRADING FOR RENAL IMPAIRMENT

Parameter	Grade 0	Grade 1	Grade 2	Grade 3	Grade 4
BUN or serum creatinine	$\leq 1.25 \times$ ULN	1.26–$2.53 \times$ ULN	2.6–$5 \times$ ULN	5.1–$10 \times$ ULN	$> 10 \times$ ULN
Proteinuria	None	1+ or < 0.3 mg/dL	2–3+ or 0.3–1.0 mg/dL	4+ or > 1.0 mg/dL	Nephrotic syndrome
Hematuria	None	Microscopic	Gross	Gross + clots	Obstructive uropathy

BUN—blood urea nitrogen; ULN—upper limit of normal value of population under study.

GENITOURINARY HEMORRHAGE

Hemorrhage into the genitourinary tract is a problem often seen with certain malignancies. It requires vigilant anticipation and specialized care. Specific antineoplastic agents, such as cyclophosphamide and ifosfamide, are associated with this complication. Management differs according to the site of the process, tumor involvement, and status of the patient.

MANAGEMENT OR INTERVENTION

Hemorrhagic cystitis: catheter drainage and continuous irrigation; intravesical cautery; intravesical therapy with formalin

Refractory bleeding: cystotomy with instillation of phenol and ligation of the bladder vessels. In severe cases, urinary diversion and removal of the organ to stop life-threatening bleeding are necessary.

CAUSATIVE FACTORS

Cyclophosphamide, ifosfamide, L-asparaginase, actinomycin D, mitomycin C, mithramycin, 6-mercaptopurine, anticoagulants

PATHOLOGIC PROCESS

Toxic metabolites of certain chemotherapeutic agents have direct effect on urethral surface; high concentrations of these metabolites can cause erosion of the bladder mucosal system, leading to microscopic and gross bladder hemorrhage

DIFFERENTIAL DIAGNOSES

Chemotherapeutic agents, tumor involvement, prostate disorders

PATIENT ASSESSMENT

Clinical examination, urinalysis, cystoscopy, urinary irrigation and drainage

TOXICITY GRADING

Parameter	Grade 0	Grade 1	Grade 2	Grade 3	Grade 4
Hematuria	None	Microscopic	Gross	Gross + clots	Obstructive uropathy

REFERENCES

1. Rieselbach RE, Garnick MB: Renal diseases induced by antineoplastic agents. In *Diseases of the Kidney*, edn 3. Edited by Schrier RW, Gottschalk CW. Boston: Little Brown & Co.; 1993:1165–1186.

2. Kanfer A, Vandewalle A, Morel-Maroger L, *et al.*: Acute renal insufficiency due to lymphomatous infiltration of the kidneys: report of six cases. *Cancer* 1976, 38:2588–2592.

3. Luxton RW: Radiation nephritis: a long-term study of 54 patients. *Lancet* 1961, 2:1221–1223.

4. Zager RA: Acute renal failure in the setting of bone marrow transplantation. *Kidney Int* 1994, 46:1443–1458.

5. Oliveira JS, Bahia D, Franco M, *et al.*: Nephrotic syndrome as a clinical manifestation of graft-versus-host disease (GVHD) in a marrow transplant recipient after cyclosporine withdrawal. *Bone Marrow Transplant* 1999, 23:99–101.

6. Safirstein R, Winston J, Goldstein M, *et al.*: Cisplatin nephrotoxicity. *Am J Kidney Dis* 1986, 8:356–367.

7. Santoso JT, Lucci JA, Coleman RL *et al.*: Saline, mannitol, and furosemide hydration in acute cisplatin nephrotoxicity: a randomized trial. *Cancer Chemother Pharmacol* 2003, 52:13–18.

8. Capizzi R: Amifostine reduces the incidence of cumulative nephrotoxicity from cisplatin: laboratory and clinical aspects. *Semin Oncol* 1999, 26:72–81.

9. Reed E, Jacob J: Carboplatin and renal dysfunction. *Ann Intern Med* 1989, 110:409.

10. Rossi R, Godde A, Klreinebrand A, *et al.*: Unilateral nephrectomy and cisplatin as risk factors of ifosfamide-induced nephrotoxicity: analysis of 120 patients. *J Clin Oncol* 1994, 12:159–165.

11. Rossi R, Kleta R, Ehrich JH: Renal involvement in children with malignancies. *Pediatr Nephrol* 1999, 13:153–162.

12. Sangster G, Kaye SB, Calman KC, *et al.*: Failure of 2-mercaptoethane (mesna) to protect against ifosfamide nephrotoxicity. *Eur J Cancer* 1984, 20:435–436.

13. Weiss RB: Streptozotocin: a review of its pharmacology, efficacy, and toxicity. *Cancer Treat Rep* 1982, 66:427–438.

14. Hricik DE, Goldsmith GH: Uric acid nephrolithiasis and acute renal failure secondary to streptozotocin nephrotoxicity. *Am J Med* 1988, 84:153–156.

15. Schacht RG, Feiner HD, Gallo GR, *et al.*: Nephrotoxicity of nitrosoureas. *Cancer* 1981, 48:1328–1334.

16. Micetich KC, Jensen-Akula M, Mandard JC, Risher RI: Nephrotoxicity of semustine (methyl-CCNU) in patients with malignant melanoma receiving adjuvant chemotherapy. *Am J Med* 1981, 71:967–972.

17. Pitman SW, Parker LM, Tattersall MH, *et al.*: Clinical trial of high-dose methotrexate (NSC-740) with citrovorum factor (NSC-3590): toxicologic and therapeutic observations. *Cancer Chemother Rep* 1975, 6:43–49.

18. Pitman SW, Frei E III: Weekly methotrexate-calcium leucovorin rescue: effect of alkalinization on nephrotoxicity; pharmacokinetics in the CNS; and use in CNS non-Hodgkin's lymphoma. *Cancer Treat Rep* 1977, 61:695–701.

19. Thierry FX, Vernier I, Dueymes JM, *et al.*: Acute renal failure after high-dose methotrexate therapy: role of hemodialysis and plasma exchange in methotrexate removal. *Nephrology* 1985, 51:416–417.

20. Gerber DE, Grossman SA, Batchelor T, *et al.*: Calculated versus measured creatinine clearance for dosing methotrexate in the treatment of primary central nervous system lymphoma. *Cancer Chemother Pharmacol* 2007, 59:817–823.

21. Flombaum CD, Mouradian JA, Ephraim SC, *et al.*: Thrombotic microangiopathy as a complication of long-term therapy with gemcitabine. *Am J Kidney Dis* 1999, 33:555–562.

22. Peterson BA, Collins AJ, Vogelzang NJ, Bloomfield CD: 5-Azacytidine and renal tubular dysfunction. *Blood* 1981, 57:182–185.

23. Nunes R, Passos-Coelho JL, Miranda N, *et al.*: Reversible acute renal failure following single administration of fludarabine. *Bone Marrow Transplant* 2004, 33:671.

24. Hamner RW, Verani R, Weinman EJ: Mitomycin-associated renal failure: case report and review. *Arch Intern Med* 1983, 143:803–807.

25. Hanna WT, Krauss S, Regester RF, Murphey WM: Renal disease after mitomycin C therapy. *Cancer* 1981, 48:2583–2588.

26. Price TM, Murgo AJ, Keveney JJ, *et al.*: Renal failure and hemolytic anemia associated with mitomycin C: a case report. *Cancer* 1985, 55:51–56.

27. Kennedy B: Metabolic and toxic effects of mithramycin during tumor therapy. *Am J Med* 1970, 49:494–503.

28. Benedetti RG, Heilman KJ, Gabow PA: Nephrotoxicity following single-dose mithramycin therapy. *Am J Nephrol* 1983, 3:277–278.

29. Fajardo LF, Eltringham JR, Stewart JR, Klauber MR: Adriamycin nephrotoxicity. *Lab Invest* 1980, 43:242–253.

30. Burke JF, Laucins JF, Brodovsky HS, Soriano RZ: Doxorubicin hydrochloride associated renal failure. *Arch Intern Med* 1977, 137:385–388.

31. Selby P, Kohn J, Raymond J, Judson I: Nephrotic syndrome during treatment with interferon. *Br Med J (Clin Res Ed)* 1985, 290:1180.

32. Lederer E, Truong L: Unusual glomerular lesion in a patient receiving long-term interferon alpha. *Am J Kidney Dis* 1992, 20:516–518.

33. Averbuch SD, Austin HA, Sherwin SA, *et al.*: Acute interstitial nephritis with the nephrotic syndrome following recombinant leukocyte A interferon therapy for mycosis fungoides. *N Engl J Med* 1984, 310:32–35.

34. Hermann J, Gabriel F: Membranoproliferative glomerulonephritis in a patient with hairy-cell leukemia treated with alpha II interferon. *N Engl J Med* 1987, 316:112–113.

35. Ault BH, Stapleton FB, Gaber L, *et al.*: Acute renal failure during therapy with recombinant human gamma interferon. *N Engl J Med* 1988, 319:1397–1400.

36. Kimmel PL, Abraham AA, Phillips TM: Membranoproliferative glomerulonephritis in a patient treated with interferon-alpha for human immunodeficiency virus infection. *Am J Kidney Dis* 1994, 24:858–863.

37. Bellegrun A, Webb DE, Austin HA, *et al.*: Effects of interleukin-2 on renal function in patients receiving immunotherapy for advanced cancer. *Ann Intern Med* 1987, 106:817–822.

38. Textor SC, Margolin K, Blayney D, *et al.*: Renal, volume, and hormonal changes during therapeutic administration of recombinant interleukin-2 in man. *Am J Med* 1987, 83:1055–1061.

39. West WH, Tauer KN, Yannelli JR, *et al.*: Constant infusion recombinant interleukin-2 in adoptive immunotherapy of advanced cancer. *N Engl J Med* 1987, 316:898–905.

40. Gordon MS, Cunningham D: Managing patients treated with bevacizumab combination therapy. *Oncology* 2005, 69(Suppl):S25–S33.

41. Yang JC, Haworth L, Sherry RM, *et al.*: A randomized trial of bevacizumab, an anti-vascular endothelial growth factor antibody, for metastatic renal cancer. *N Engl J Med* 2003, 349:427–434.

42. Zhu X, Wu S, Dahut WL, *et al.*: Risks of proteinuria and hypertension with bevacizumab, an antibody against vascular endothelial growth factor: systematic review and meta-analysis. *Am J Kidney Dis* 2007, 49:186–193.

43. Martinez-Maldonado M, Benabe JE: Nonrenal neoplasms and the kidney. In *Diseases of the Kidney*, edn 5. Edited by Schrier RW, Gottschalk CW. Boston: Little Brown & Co.; 1993:2265–2285.

44. Dabbs DJ, Morel-Maroger L, Mignon F, Striker G: Glomerular lesions in lymphomas and leukemias. *Am J Med* 1986, 80:63–70.

45. Zimmerman SW, Vishnu-Moorthy A, Burkholder PM, *et al.*: Glomerulopathies associated with neoplastic disease. In *Cancer and the Kidney*. Edited by Rieselbach RE, Garnick MB. Philadelphia: Lea & Febiger; 1982:306–378.

46. Rault R, Holley JL, Banner BF, El-Shawy M: Glomerulonephritis and non-Hodgkin's lymphoma: a report of two cases and review of the literature. *Am J Kidney Dis* 1992, 20:84–89.

47. Garnick MB: Renal and metabolic complications. In *Current Cancer Therapeutics*, edn 3. Edited by Kirkwood JM, Lotze MT, Yasko JM. Philadelphia: Current Medicine; 1994:264–269.

48. Giraud G, Bogdanovic G, Priftakis P, *et al.*: The incidence of hemorrhagic cystitis and BK-viruria in allogeneic hematopoietic stem cell recipients according to intensity of the conditioning regimen. *Haematologica* 2006, 91:401–404.

49. Tiu RV, Mountantonakis SE, Dunbar AJ, Schreiber MJ Jr: Tumor lysis syndrome. *Semin Thromb Hemost* 2007, 33:397–407.

50. Jeha S, Kantarjian H, Irwin D, *et al.*: Efficacy and safety of rasburicase, a recombinant urate oxidase (Elitek), in the management of malignancy-associated hyperuricemia in pediatric and adult patients: final results of a multicenter compassionate use trial. *Leukemia* 2005, 19:34–38.

51. Briglia AE: The current state of nonuremic applications for extracorporeal blood purification. *Semin Dial* 2005, 18:380–390.

52. Schwartz WB, Bennett W, Curelop S, *et al.*: A syndrome of renal sodium loss and hyponatremia probably resulting from inappropriate secretion of antidiuretic hormone. *Am J Med* 1957, 23:529–542.

53. Beck LH: Hypouricemia in the syndrome of inappropriate secretion of antidiuretic hormone. *N Engl J Med* 1979, 301:528–530.

54. Reeves BW, Andreoli TE: The posterior pituitary and water metabolism. In *Williams Textbook of Endocrinology*. Edited by Wilson JD, Foster DW. Philadelphia: WB Sanders; 1992:311–356.

55. DeFronzo RA, Braine H, Colvin OM, *et al.*: Water intoxication in man after cyclophosphamide therapy: time course and relation to drug activation. *Ann Intern Med* 1973, 78:861–869.

56. Stahel RA, Oelz O: Syndrome of inappropriate ADH secretion secondary to vinblastine. *Cancer Chemother Pharmacol* 1982, 8:253–254.

57. Stuart MJ, Cuaso C, Miller M, *et al.*: Syndrome of recurrent increased secretion of antidiuretic hormone following multiple doses of vincristine. *Blood* 1975, 45:315–320.

58. Goldberg M: Hyponatremia and the inappropriate secretion of antidiuretic hormone. *Am J Med* 1963, 35:293–298.

59. Bartter FC, Schwartz WB: The syndrome of inappropriate secretion of antidiuretic hormone. *Am J Med* 1967, 42:790–806.

60. Fichman MP, Michaelakis AM, Horton R: Regulation of aldosterone in the syndrome of inappropriate antidiuretic hormone secretion (SIADH). *J Clin Endocrinol Metab* 1974, 39:136–144.

61. Cogan E, DeBieve MF, Pepersack T, *et al.*: Natriuresis and atrial natriuretic factor secretion during inappropriate antidiuresis. *Am J Med* 1988, 84:409–418.

62. North WG, Ware J, Chahinian AP, *et al.*: Clinical evaluation of the neurophysins as tumor markers in small cell lung cancer. *Recent Res Cancer Res* 1985, 99:187–193.

63. Sorensen JB, Anderson MK, Hansen HH: Syndrome of inappropriate secretion of antidiuretic hormone (SIADH) in malignant disease. *J Intern Med* 1995, 238:97–110.

64. Sterns RH, Riggs JE, Schochet SS: Osmotic demyelination syndrome following correction on hyponatremia. *N Engl J Med* 1986, 314:1535–1542.

65. Ayus JC, Krothapalli RK, Arieff AI: Treatment of symptomatic hyponatremia and its relation to brain damage: a prospective study. *N Engl J Med* 1987, 317:1190–1195.

66. Decaux G, Waterlot Y, Genette F, *et al.*: Treatment of the syndrome of inappropriate secretion of antidiuretic hormone with furosemide. *N Engl J Med* 1981, 304:329–330.

67. Cherril DA, Stote RM, Birge JR, *et al.*: Demeclocycline treatment in the syndrome of inappropriate antidiuretic hormone secretion. *Ann Intern Med* 1975, 83:654–656.

68. Heath DA, Senior PV, Varley VM, *et al.*: Parathyroid hormone–related protein in tumors associated with hypercalcemia. *Lancet* 1990, 335:66–69.

69. Ratcliff WA, Hutchesson AC, Bundred NJ, *et al.*: Role of assays for parathyroid-hormone-related protein in investigation of hypercalcemia. *Lancet* 1992, 339:164–167.

70. Burtis WJ, Brady TG, Orloff JJ, *et al.*: Immunochemical characterization of circulating parathyroid hormone–related protein in patients with humoral hypercalcemia of malignancy. *N Engl J Med* 1990, 32:1106–1112.

71. Goltzman D, Henderson JE: Parathyroid hormone-related peptide and hypercalcemia of malignancy. *Cancer Treat Res* 1997, 89:193–215.

72. Rankin W, Grill V, Mardin JJ: Parathyroid hormone-related protein and hypercalcemia. *Cancer* 1997, 80(Suppl):1564–1571.

73. Guise TA: Parathyroid hormone-related protein and bone metastases. *Cancer* 1997, 80(Suppl):1572–1580.

74. Stewart AF, Vignery A, Silverglate A, *et al.*: Quantitative bone histomorphometry in humoral hypercalcemia of malignancy: uncoupling of bone cell activity. *J Clin Endocrinol Metab* 1982, 55:219–227.

75. Nakayama K, Fukumoto S, Takeda S, *et al.*: Differences in bone and vitamin D metabolism between primary hyperparathyroidism and malignancy-associated hypercalcemia. *J Clin Endocrinol Metab* 1996, 81:607–611.

76. Stewart AF, Horst R, Deftos LJ, *et al.*: Biochemical evaluation of patients with cancer associated hypercalcemia: evidence for humoral and nonhumoral groups. *N Engl J Med* 1980, 303:1377–1383.

77. Mundy GR: Malignancy and the skeleton. *Horm Metab Res* 1997, 29:120–127.

78. Roodman GD: Mechanisms of bone lesions in multiple myeloma and lymphoma. *Cancer* 1997, 80:1557–1563.

79. Mundy GR: Mechanisms of bone metastasis. *Cancer* 1997, 80:1546–1556.

80. Bertolini DR, Nedwin GE, Bringman TS, *et al.*: Stimulation of bone resorption and inhibition of bone formation in vitro by human tumor necrosis factor. *Nature* 1986, 319:516–518.

81. Black KS, Mundy GR, Garrett IR: Interleukin-6 causes hypercalcemia in vivo and enhances the bone resorbing potency of interleukin-1 and tumor necrosis factor by two orders of magnitude in vitro. *J Bone Min Res* 1990, 5(Suppl):S271.

82. Mundy GR: Hypercalcemic factors other than parathyroid hormone–related protein. *Endocrinol Metab Clin North Am* 1989, 18:795–806.

83. Sato K, Fujii Y, Kasono K, *et al.*: Parathyroid hormone–related protein and interleukin 1b synergistically stimulate bone resorption in vitro and increase serum calcium concentration in mice in vivo. *Endocrinology* 1989, 24:2172–2178.

84. Bilezikian JP: Management of acute hypercalcemia. *N Engl J Med* 1992, 326:1196–1203.

85. Chisholm MA, Mulloy AL, Taylor AT: Acute management of cancer-related hypercalcemia. *Ann Pharmacother* 1996, 30:507–513.

86. Canfield RE: Rationale for diphosphonate therapy in hypercalcemia of malignancy. *Am J Med* 1987, 82(Suppl):1–5.

87. Merlini G, Turesson I: Utility of bisphosphonates in treating bone metastases. *Med Oncol* 1996, 13:215–221.

88. Vinholes J, Guo CY, Purohit OP, *et al.*: Evaluation of new bone resorption markers in a randomized comparison of pamidronate or clodronate for hypercalcemia of malignancy. *J Clin Oncol* 1997, 15:131–138.

89. Dodwell DJ, Abbas SK, Morton AR, et al.: Parathyroid hormone–related protein and response to pamidronate therapy for tumor-induced hypercalcemia. *Eur J Cancer* 1991, 27:1629–1633.

90. Lipton A: The safety of zoledronic acid. *Expert Opin Drug Saf* 2007, 6:305–313.

91. Gurney H, Kefford R, Stuart-Haarris R: Renal phosphate threshold and response to pamidronate in humoral hypercalcemia of malignancy. *Lancet* 1989, 2:241–244.

92. Findling JW, Tyrrell JB: Occult ectopic secretion of corticotropin. *Arch Intern Med* 1986, 146:929–933.

93. DeKeyzer Y, Bertagna X, Lenne F, *et al.*: Altered proopiomelanocortin gene expression in adrenocorticotropin-producing nonpituitary tumors: comparative studies with corticotropic adenomas and normal pituitaries. *J Clin Invest* 1985, 76:1892–1898.

94. Tsigos C, Chrousos GP: Differential diagnosis and management of Cushing's syndrome. *Annu Rev Med* 1996, 47:443–461.

95. Gizza G, Chrousos GP: Adrenocorticotropic hormone-dependent Cushing's syndrome. *Cancer Treat Res* 1997, 89:25–40.

96. Orth DN: Ectopic hormone production. In *Endocrinology and Metabolism*, edn 2. Edited by Felig P, Baxter JD, Broadus AE, Frohman LA. New York: McGraw-Hill; 1987:1692–1735.

97. Malchoff CD, Orth DN, Abboud C, *et al.*: Ectopic ACTH syndrome caused by a bronchial carcinoid tumor responsive to dexamethasone, metyrapone, and corticotropin-releasing tumor. *Am J Med* 1988, 84:760–764.

98. Farwell AP, Devlin JT, Stewart JA: Total suppression of cortisol excretion by ketoconazole in the therapy of the ectopic adrenocorticotropic hormone syndrome. *Am J Med* 1988, 84:1063–1066.

99. Woodhouse NJ, Dagog-Jack S, Ahmed M, *et al.*: Acute and long-term effects of octreotide in patients with ACTH-dependent Cushing's syndrome. *Am J Med* 1993, 95:305–308.

100. de Herder WW, Lamberts SW: Is there a role for somatostatin and its analogues in Cushing's syndrome? *Metabolism* 1996, 45:830.

101. Vignati F, Loli P: Additive effect of ketoconazole and octreotide in the treatment of severe adrenocorticotropin-dependent hypercortisolism. *J Clin Endocrinol Metab* 1996, 81:2885.

102. Christin-Maitre S, Bouchard P: Use of somatostatin analog for localization and treatment of ACTH secreting bronchial carcinoid tumor. *Chest* 1996, 109:845–846.

103. Sartor O, Cutler GB Jr: Mifepristone: treatment of Cushing's syndrome. *Clin Obstet Gynecol* 1996, 39:506–510.

104. Weber B, Gasnick MB, Rieselbach R: Nephropathies due to antineoplastic agents. In *Textbook of Nephrology*, edn 2. Edited by Massry SC, Glassock RJ. Baltimore: Williams & Wilkins; 1989.

105. Bennett WM, Aronoff GR, Golpher TA: *Drug Prescribing in Renal Failure: Dosing Guidelines for Adults*, edn 3. Philadelphia: American College of Physicians; 1994.

PULMONARY COMPLICATIONS OF CYTOTOXIC THERAPY

Pulmonary complications arising from antineoplastic drugs can range from asymptomatic, mild abnormalities (detected by chest radiograph or pulmonary function tests) to fatal pulmonary fibrosis. The number of antineoplastic drugs with possible pulmonary toxicity is growing steadily. The severity of pulmonary complication ranges from subclinical findings (detected on chest imaging or pulmonary function tests) to fatal respiratory failure. While the mechanisms leading to pulmonary damage are mostly poorly understood, the clinical effects can be classified by the affected lung compartment and the histopathologic picture: 1) parenchymal lung disease, which can be further subdivided into hypersensitivity pneumonitis, interstitial pneumonia/pulmonary fibrosis, noncardiogenic pulmonary edema/diffuse alveolar damage, and cryptogenic organizing pneumonia (formerly referred to as "bronchiolitis obliterans organizing pneumonia" [BOOP]); 2) airway disease; and 3) disease of the pulmonary vasculature, which includes pulmonary hemorrhage/hemoptysis, pulmonary arterial hypertension, and thromboembolic complications. Figure 27-1 shows characteristic radiologic appearance of common pulmonary complications. Cancer therapy predisposes to a number of typical and opportunistic infectious complications that will not be discussed in this chapter.

HYPERSENSITIVITY PNEUMONITIS

Hypersensitivity pneumonitis can be caused by almost any drug. The most commonly associated antineoplastic drugs are methotrexate, bleomycin, fludarabine, busulfan, nitrogen mustard, and procarbazine. More recently, an increasing number of case reports have implicated the taxanes docetaxel and paclitaxel as causing hypersensitivity pneumonitis. The clinical picture is often characterized by Loeffler's syndrome, consisting of cough, fever, myalgias, rash, peripheral eosinophilia, and fleeting pulmonary infiltrates; however, eosinophilia is absent in about 50% of all cases and more subacute presentations can occur. The diagnosis requires a high degree of clinical suspicion, especially in the absence of peripheral blood eosinophilia. Bronchoscopy with bronchoalveolar lavage (BAL) characteristically reveals a lymphocyte-predominant infiltrate. Histologically, a mononuclear cell and eosinophilic infiltrate involving airspaces and interstitium is characteristic. Treatment strategies involve withdrawal of the offending agent and the use of systemic corticosteroids. Symptoms usually respond rapidly. Progression to pulmonary fibrosis is estimated to occur in less than 10% of cases. The mortality of hypersensitivity pneumonitis is estimated to be less than 10%.

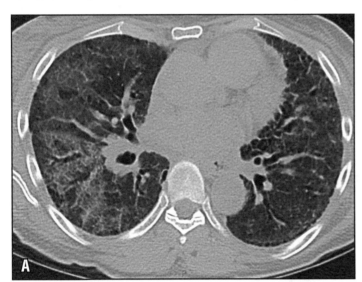
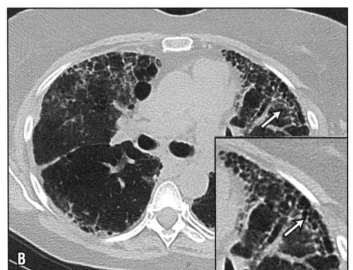
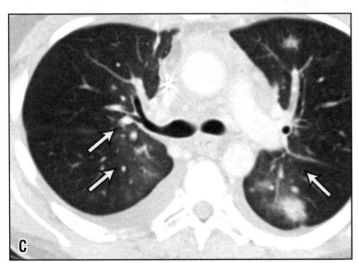
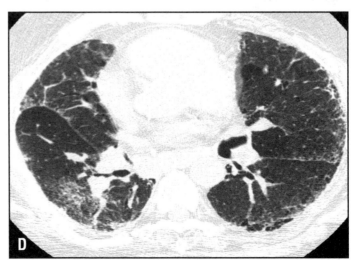

Figure 27-1. **A**, Cryptogenic organizing pneumonia. The CT shows bilateral ground-glass infiltrates, interstitial thickening and areas of consolidation. **B**, Pulmonary fibrosis. End-stage fibrotic lung disease is characterized by interstitial thickening and subpleural honeycombing (*arrows*). **C**, Radiation pneumonitis. Classic acute radiation pneumonitis shows ground-glass infiltrates that are strictly delineated according to the radiation port (*arrows*). **D**, Hypersensitivity pneumonitis. Characteristic diffuse ground-glass infiltrates are shown.

NONCARDIOGENIC PULMONARY EDEMA

Patients with noncardiogenic pulmonary edema typically present with acute onset of dyspnea and cough, occasionally with frothy sputum, which might rapidly progress to respiratory failure. The physical examination reveals diffuse crackles, and diffuse alveolar infiltrates will be seen on chest x-ray. Computed tomography (CT) scans will reveal ground-glass infiltrates in the early stages and alveolar filling in more advanced stages. Histopathologically, a picture consistent with diffuse alveolar damage is frequently seen. The etiology of noncardiac pulmonary edema is not exactly understood. Alterations of the capillary membrane either by direct drug effects or by indirect effects via the central nervous system resulting in neurogenic pulmonary edema have been postulated.

INTERSTITIAL PNEUMONITIS/PULMONARY FIBROSIS

A large number of chemotherapeutic drugs have been associated with interstitial pneumonitis and pulmonary fibrosis. The best established example is bleomycin, but multiple agents have been implicated (Table 27-1). For bleomycin, the incidence of pulmonary fibrosis is dose dependent; for other agents, this is less well established. Recently, the small molecule inhibitors of the epidermal growth factor receptor (EGFR) erlotinib and gefitinib have been implicated. Patients usually have an insidious onset of symptoms with slowly progressing dyspnea and dry cough. Systemic symptoms such as fever and malaise are usually absent. Physical examination reveals bibasilar crackles and possibly clubbing. Radiograph and CT imaging will typically reveal reticular infiltrates and possibly honeycombing at later stages. On biopsy, a various degree of an interstitial mononuclear cell infiltrate and interstitial fibrosis is typically seen. Chemotherapy-induced pulmonary fibrosis might be characterized by the presence of abnormal type II pneumocytes that are larger, more frequent than usual, and have an abnormal chromatin pattern. Avoidance of drug combinations with synergistic pulmonary toxicity, monitoring of the cumulative dose (for bleomycin), and a high level of suspicion in patients with otherwise unexplained pulmonary symptoms are important strategies to reduce the incidence of this complication. Administration of systemic corticosteroids often for a total duration of weeks to months is the mainstay of therapy.

CRYPTOGENIC ORGANIZING PNEUMONIA

Patients with cryptogenic organizing pneumonia may present with similar symptoms as those with interstitial pneumonitis. Dyspnea and dry cough are most prominent and fever is usually absent. The physical examination typically also reveals crackles and often inspiratory squeaks. Radiographs show patchy ground-glass infiltrates. Because cryptogenic organizing pneumonia can have many other etiologies, open lung biopsies are usually required to establish a firm diagnosis. The mainstay of treatment is withdrawal of the offending agent and administration of corticosteroids.

BRONCHOSPASM

Chemotherapy-induced bronchospasm is relatively rare. Patients typically develop wheezing, dyspnea, and cough during or shortly after administration of the offending drug. Agents most frequently associated with bronchospasm are methotrexate, vinblastine (especially in combination with mitomycin), and paclitaxel, especially before premedication with corticosteroids became standard practice. Bronchospasm is also frequently observed with biologic therapies such as interleukin-2 (IL-2).

PULMONARY HEMORRHAGE/HEMOPTYSIS

Pulmonary hemorrhage almost always requires the presence of abnormal pulmonary or bronchial vasculature. The most frequent cause of hemoptysis in all patients is chronic bronchitis. In cancer patients with either a primary chest malignancy or metastasis to the chest, hemoptysis is frequently caused by endobronchial metastasis or erosion of the tumor into bronchial or pulmonary arteries. The anti–vascular endothelial growth factor (VEGF) drugs have led to a significant increase of major pulmonary hemorrhage in some patients, usually those with malignancies involving the central airways and most often lung cancer patients with squamous cell histology that may enlarge or cavitate. First-line treatment is bronchial artery embolization of the tumor vasculature. If not successful, surgery can be considered.

PULMONARY VASCULAR DISEASE

Pulmonary arterial hypertension is a rare complication of cancer chemotherapy and has been described for IL-2 and mitomycin. The major symptom is dyspnea on exertion and, at later stages, the development of right

Table 27-1. Pulmonary Complications of Cancer Therapies

Agent	Pulmonary effect
Bleomycin	Interstitial pneumonitis/fibrosis, hypersensitivity pneumonitis, bronchospasm, pleural effusion, pulmonary veno-occlusive disease
Mitomycin	Interstitial pneumonitis/fibrosis, hypersensitivity pneumonitis, bronchospasm, diffuse alveolar damage
Methotrexate	Hypersensitivity pneumonitis, pulmonary fibrosis
Cyclophosphamide	Interstitial pneumonitis/pulmonary fibrosis
Nitrosoureas	Interstitial pneumonitis/pulmonary fibrosis
Busulfan	Interstitial pneumonitis/pulmonary fibrosis
Cytarabine	Noncardiogenic pulmonary edema, pleural effusions
Gemcitabine	Noncardiogenic pulmonary edema, ARDS, interstitial pneumonitis/fibrosis
Fludarabine	Interstitial pneumonitis
Taxanes	Hypersensitivity pneumonitis
EGFR TKI	Interstitial pneumonitis/pulmonary fibrosis
VEGF inhibitors	Pulmonary hemorrhage, tracheo-esophageal fistula with radiation therapy in small cell lung cancer with bevacizumab, venous thromboembolism
Vinca alkaloids	Mostly in combination with mitomycin: bronchospasm, diffuse alveolar damage
Interleukin-2	Pleural effusion, pulmonary hypertension, capillary leak, ARDS
Procarbazine	Pulmonary fibrosis
Etoposide	Rarely diffuse alveolar damage
Rituximab	Interstitial pneumonitis

ARDS—acute respiratory distress syndrome; EGFR—endothelial growth factor receptor; TKI—tyrosine kinase inhibitor; VEGF—vascular endothelial growth factor.

heart failure with peripheral edema, hepatomegaly, and syncope. Pulmonary veno-occlusive disease is a rare but serious complication and has been reported in conjunction with busulfan. Symptoms are usually those observed with pulmonary hypertension of other etiologies. Radiographs may show Kerley B lines in the absence of cardiomegaly. Pleural effusions are common in pulmonary veno-occlusive disease. Thromboembolic disease is common in cancer patients. Antiangiogenic drugs and thalidomide are associated with venous thromboembolism.

PULMONARY COMPLICATIONS OF CHEMOTHERAPY AGENTS

BLEOMYCIN

The pulmonary toxicity of bleomycin has been well established. Clinically significant toxicity is seen in about 4% of patients [1]; subclinical changes such as changes in the diffusing capacity (DL_{CO}) occur in about 25% of patients. Most often, bleomycin causes pulmonary fibrosis; however, hypersensitivity pneumonitis and bronchospasm have also been described. In some cases, development of exudative pleural effusions has been ascribed to treatment with bleomycin. The fundamental insult appears to be oxidant damage to pulmonary endothelial cells and type I pneumocytes, resulting in an inflammatory exudate within the alveoli and a subsequent fibrotic reaction that may permanently impair DL_{CO} and reduce lung volumes. The onset of symptoms is usually insidious. Patients typically present with dyspnea and, occasionally, a nonproductive cough. Dry rales and a pleural friction rub may be present on examination, and low-grade fever may be present. Chest radiograph typically reveals diffuse interstitial infiltrates but may be normal and, rarely, may show pulmonary nodules that can cavitate and be mistaken for metastases. On pulmonary function tests, the earliest change is a decrease in DL_{CO} followed by a loss of lung volumes consistent with a restrictive pattern. Mild subclinical toxicity may not predict for the development of clinically significant fibrosis, and loss of lung function may occur suddenly long after treatment has been discontinued. Therefore, the usefulness of serial DL_{CO} measurements is limited. Although the routine use of DL_{CO} to detect subclinical toxicity is controversial, it is important to recognize early clinical signs and symptoms of bleomycin toxicity (*eg*, dyspnea, dry cough, fine rales, and the development of subtle reticulonodular infiltrates on chest radiograph). Bleomycin should be discontinued when any of these signs or symptoms is present until drug toxicity can be reasonably excluded as a cause of the finding. Risk factors for pulmonary toxicity from bleomycin are well recognized and include the following: 1) cumulative dose greater than 400 IU, which increases the incidence of pulmonary fibrosis to greater than 10%; 2) supplemental oxygen (even exposure after a long hiatus from bleomycin exposure); 3) age greater than 70 years; 4) prior or concurrent radiotherapy to the chest; and 5) concurrent use of other drugs with potential pulmonary toxicity (Table 27-2). There is ongoing discussion regarding whether hematopoietic growth factors contribute to bleomycin-related pulmonary toxicity. Small case series in patients with non-Hodgkin's disease treated with BACOP (bleomycin, doxorubicin, cyclophosphamide, vincristine, and prednisone) suggest a slightly increased incidence of pulmonary toxicity [2], whereas this has not been found in patients with testicular cancer who received bleomycin and granulocyte colony-stimulating factor [3]. The mainstay of therapy is discontinuation of the offending drug, avoidance of supplemental oxygen and other pulmonary toxins, and treatment with corticosteroids. The prognosis is poor, with permanent pulmonary compromise in about 30% to 50% of all cases with severe pneumonitis.

MITOMYCIN C

The pulmonary toxicity of mitomycin C follows several patterns. It can cause interstitial fibrosis with a clinical and histologic pattern that strongly resembles bleomycin lung toxicity. There is a dose-dependent relationship; this complication seems to be rare under a cumulative dose of 30 mg/m². In addition, the combination of mitomycin C with vinca alkaloids has been shown to frequently produce bronchospasm and acute interstitial pneumonia and diffuse alveolar damage with high rates of chronic respiratory failure [4]. Mitomycin C has also been associated with the hemolytic uremic syndrome [5] and acute lung injury

in the setting of this systemic disease has occurred. Treatment consists of withdrawal of the drug and administration of corticosteroids [6].

NITROSOUREAS

Carmustine (BCNU) is associated with dose-dependent pulmonary fibrosis that occurs in 20% to 30% of patients and that may become clinically evident many years after treatment. Toxicity is rare in patients who receive less than 960 mg/m² but is seen in 30% to 50% of patients when the cumulative dose is greater than 1500 mg/m² [7].

Symptoms include dyspnea, dry cough, and bibasilar rales. Histologically, fibrosis predominates, and the inflammatory picture seen in early bleomycin toxicity is usually absent. Mortality is reported to be 24% to 90%. Steroids may be beneficial. Pulmonary toxicity resulting from other nitrosoureas—lomustine (CCNU) and semustine (methyl-CCNU)—has rarely been reported.

ALKYLATING AGENTS

Pulmonary toxicity occurs with several alkylating agents but is most often associated with busulfan, occurring in approximately 4% of patients [8]. The onset of the typical symptoms of dyspnea, cough, and a low-grade fever may occur up to 10 years after the administration of busulfan. Although a clear dose-response curve has not been demonstrated, a threshold for toxicity may exist at a cumulative dose of approximately 500 mg. Steroids administered concurrently with busulfan do not appear to decrease the risk of fibrosis and are minimally effective in halting its progression. Mortality is approximately 50%. Cyclophosphamide-associated pulmonary toxicity is rare and has been reported in about 1% of patients. Two distinct clinical presentations of interstitial lung disease have been reported [9]. Early-onset interstitial pneumonitis is radiographically characterized by increased reticular changes and the presence of ground-glass infiltrates. Histologically, interstitial inflammation is observed. This presentation usually starts within 6 months after cyclophosphamide administration and responds well to corticosteroids. The late-onset interstitial pneumonitis typically develops in patients who took cyclophosphamide at low doses for a long period of time [9]. This form is histologically characterized more by fibrosis than by interstitial inflammation and is usually relentlessly progressive without response to corticosteroids. Case reports of pulmonary toxicity resulting from melphalan or chlorambucil are rare.

METHOTREXATE

Methotrexate causes a wide spectrum of pulmonary complications, most frequently acute hypersensitivity pneumonitis. The incidence of pulmonary complications depends on the schedule of administration. Some regimens, especially those that employ more frequent administration at lower doses carry an incidence of about 8%. Withdrawal of the drug and the administration of steroids may produce rapid resolution of symptoms, and the overall prognosis is good, although approximately 10% of patients may develop pulmonary fibrosis. In rarer instances, methotrexate can cause noncardiogenic pulmonary edema, pleuritis, and pulmonary fibrosis that were not preceded by hypersensitivity pneumonitis.

Table 27-2. Risk Factors for Pulmonary Toxicity from Bleomycin

Increased cumulative dose (10% incidence of fibrosis with doses > 400 U)

Increased age (especially > 70 y)

Supplemental oxygen

Prior or concurrent radiotherapy to the chest

Renal dysfunction (concurrent cisplatin administration)

Concurrent administration of other drugs with pulmonary toxicity

Administration of hematopoietic growth factors or other cytokines (controversial, under investigation)

Bolus administration (some evidence that continuous infusion schedules result in less pulmonary toxicity but data are limited and inconsistent)

TAXANES

The pulmonary complications of the taxanes docetaxel and paclitaxel can be divided into two groups: 1) anaphylactic reactions, and 2) type IV hypersensitivity reactions. Allergic reactions were very common in early trials with paclitaxel and manifested as bronchospasm, urticaria, rash, and possibly hypotension [10]. After obligatory premedication with steroids became standard practice, the incidence decreased dramatically from around 30% to 1% to 3% [11]. Hypersensitivity pneumonitis has been reported in small case series both for paclitaxel [12] as well as docetaxel [13,14]. Patients typically presented with subacute to acute-onset dyspnea, fever, and bilateral infiltrates. The response of taxanes-induced hypersensitivity pneumonitis to corticosteroids seems to be poor. Long-term respiratory failure and fatalities have been reported. Cross-reactivity between docetaxel and paclitaxel in the induction of hypersensitivity pneumonitis has been reported in one case [15].

PYRIMIDINE ANALOGUES

The pyrimidine analogues gemcitabine and cytarabine can cause pulmonary toxicity. High-dose cytarabine, given as consolidation treatment for a variety of hematologic malignancies (usually 3.0 g/m^2 every 12 hours for 8–12 doses), may result in noncardiogenic pulmonary edema. Patients present with dyspnea and physical and radiographic signs of pulmonary edema, but they lack other signs of heart failure. Treatment is supportive; close attention to volume status and the judicious use of diuretics and supplemental oxygen are mainstays of management. The prognosis is generally good. Gemcitabine, a drug with close structural relationship to cytarabine, has been associated with a variety of pulmonary complications. The overall incidence of grade 3 and 4 pulmonary toxicity is 1.4% [16]. Most commonly seen are noncardiogenic pulmonary edema and hypersensitivity pneumonitis. Cases of acute respiratory distress syndrome, interstitial pneumonitis, and pulmonary fibrosis have all been described. Gemcitabine-related pulmonary toxicity generally responds to corticosteroids and in most cases, the prognosis is good; however, fatalities have been described [17].

PURINE ANALOGUES

Fludarabine, pentostatin, and cladribine are approved purine analogue antimetabolites with activity in various hematologic malignancies. Clofarabine is currently under investigation for its role in refractory myeloid leukemia. Pulmonary toxicity of fludarabine is a well-recognized phenomenon that occurs in 8.6% of all cases [18]. Patients with chronic lymphocytic leukemia appear to have a higher risk than patients with other hematologic malignancies. Clinically, most patients presented with fever and dyspnea. Interstitial or interstitial and alveolar infiltrates are the most common radiographic findings and on histology an interstitial process with various degrees of fibrosis can be observed. Fludarabine-associated pulmonary toxicity can respond to steroids [19], but fatalities have been reported. Combination chemotherapy with pentostatin and fludarabine has led to severe or fatal pulmonary toxicity in four of six patients and is therefore contraindicated [20]. Pentostatin itself can induce bronchospasm and laryngeal edema. Cladribine has not been shown to have pulmonary toxicity. In pediatric patients, one study reported respiratory distress in 14% of patients treated with clofarabine and the development of pleural effusions in 10% [21].

EGFR TYROSINE KINASE INHIBITORS

The EGFR tyrosine kinase inhibitors erlotinib and gefitinib are important agents in the treatment of non–small cell lung cancer and pancreatic cancer. Interstitial pneumonitis leading to pulmonary fibrosis has been described for both drugs. The incidence of pulmonary toxicity has been repeatedly found to be higher in Japan [22], raising the possibility that a racial predisposition to pulmonary toxicity exists. Other predisposing factors are male sex, smoking history, and most importantly history of interstitial lung disease prior to treatment. Both, erlotinib (B21 trial) and gefitinib (Iressa Survival Evaluation in Lung Cancer [ISEL] trial) were evaluated in placebo-controlled trials. The incidence of interstitial lung disease for erlotinib was 0.7% in both the placebo as well as in the treatment arm [23]. For gefitinib, the incidence of interstitial lung disease was 3% in the treatment arm versus 4% in the

placebo arm [24]. The ISEL trial was a multinational trial with sites also in Asia. Asian patients had a higher incidence of interstitial lung disease with gefitinib in this trial. In a randomized trial of erlotinib plus gemcitabine versus gemcitabine alone, the incidence of interstitial lung disease was 2.4% versus 0.4% [25]. Data from the United States Expanded Access Program for gefitinib suggest an incidence of interstitial lung disease in 0.3% of the American population. Despite the fact that a higher risk of interstitial lung disease has not been proven for non-Asian patients treated with an EGFR tyrosine kinase inhibitor, physicians are urged to maintain a high level of suspicion if new pulmonary symptoms develop in their patients. If in doubt, it is recommended to stop the drug. Empiric corticosteroids should be given, although their effectiveness has not been clearly established. Cetuximab, a monoclonal antibody against EGFR, is frequently associated with cough and dyspnea that are in direct timely relationship with the infusion of the drug. Interstitial lung disease is rare, but has been reported in about 0.5% of patients treated with cetuximab [26]. Similar data are available for the fully humanized anti-EGFR antibody panitumumab [27].

VEGF INHIBITORS

Bevacizumab is a monoclonal antibody against VEGF, whereas sorafenib and sunitinib are multitargeted tyrosine kinase inhibitors whose activity also includes blocking the signaling of the VEGF receptor 2. VEGF inhibition has been linked to thromboembolic complications as well as to pulmonary hemorrhage. In the initial phase 2 evaluation of bevacizumab in combination with carboplatin and paclitaxel, life-threatening or fatal hemoptysis was observed in about 9% of patients. This was highly associated with squamous histology (31% of patients with squamous cell carcinoma developed major hemoptysis), location in the central airways, and cavitation of the primary tumor [28]. Patients with squamous cell lung cancer were excluded from the subsequent phase 3 trial. The incidence of fatal hemoptysis in this trial was 1.2% for the bevacizumab/carboplatin/paclitaxel arm versus 0% in the control arm of carboplatin and paclitaxel [29]. In limited-stage small cell lung cancer, bevacizumab in combination with other chemotherapeutic drugs and also with radiation in some but not all cases has been linked to the development of tracheoesophageal fistulas.

IRINOTECAN

Irinotecan is a topoisomerase I inhibitor. Several case reports exist about irinotecan-associated pulmonary complications. The clinical picture ranges from hypersensitivity pneumonitis with a good response to corticosteroids [30] to refractory or relapsing interstitial pneumonitis with poor prognosis [31,32]. These complications have not been described with another inhibitor of the topoisomerase I. Etoposide is an inhibitor of the topoisomerase II. Pulmonary complications with this drug are uncommon.

OXALIPLATIN

Oxaliplatin has been associated with interstitial pneumonitis and pulmonary fibrosis in less than 1% of patients, which may be fatal [33]. Careful attention should be paid to unexplained respiratory symptoms in patients who are undergoing chemotherapy with oxaliplatin.

BIOLOGIC RESPONSE MODIFIERS

Biologic agents can induce a wide range of potential pulmonary complications, which are very much dependent on the nature of the drug. IL-2 has a role in the treatment of metastatic renal cell carcinoma and metastatic melanoma. The mechanism of action is presumably T-cell activation. Treatment side effects are frequently indistinguishable from a systemic inflammatory response syndrome. Fluid retention, capillary leak, and hypotension are frequently observed. Bronchospasm, pleural effusions, and pulmonary edema commonly lead to respiratory compromise. Therapy with interferon-α can lead to dyspnea and cough in about 7.5% and 10% of cancer patients treated with this drug, respectively. Case reports of interstitial pneumonia have been described. All-trans-retinoic acid and arsenic are common drugs in the treatment of acute promyelocytic leukemia (APL). Neither of these agents is cytotoxic. Rather, they help overcome the block in differentiation that arrests the differentiation of the malignant clone at the level of the promyelocyte. Typically, an increase in the total white blood cell count is seen with initiation of therapy. The APL differentiation syndrome is clinically characterized by fever, bilateral alveolar infiltrates, and hypoxemia. It typically responds well to withdrawal of the offending drug and therapy with high doses of corticosteroids.

PULMONARY COMPLICATIONS OF ALLOGENEIC BONE MARROW TRANSPLANTATION

There is a myriad of potential pulmonary complications from allogenic bone marrow transplantation that can be divided into several groups: 1) infectious complications, 2) direct drug and radiation effects, and 3) immunologic effects such as idiopathic pneumonia syndrome and graft-versus-host disease. A detailed discussion of these complications is beyond the scope of this chapter.

PULMONARY COMPLICATIONS OF RADIOTHERAPY

Pulmonary complications relating to radiotherapy can be categorized into acute and chronic forms. In the acute form, pneumonitis dominates the clinical picture, whereas pulmonary fibrosis is the hallmark of the chronic form. The diagnosis of radiation pneumonitis can be challenging because confounding clinical conditions such as infection or tumor progression are frequent and need to be ruled out. Many studies have evaluated the pathogenesis of radiation-induced lung injury. Ionizing radiation in an oxygen-rich environment generates free radicals, leading to DNA double-strand breaks. Mouse models prove that oxidative stress is indeed a major contributor to radiation-induced lung injury and that it can be prevented by overexpression of the scavenging enzyme manganese superoxide dismutase [34] The initial insult leads to an inflammatory response with overexpression of multiple cytokines such as transforming growth factor (TGF)-β, tumor necrosis factor (TNF)-α, IL-1-α, platelet-derived growth factor, and basic fibroblast growth factor, forming the molecular basis for the eventual development of radiation fibrosis. Major risk factors for the development of radiation-induced lung injury are the cumulative dose, the volume of irradiated lung, and the fractionation [35]. Other risk factors include the use of oxygen or concurrent chemotherapy as radiosensitizer, poor lung function, smoking status, young age, the presence of atelectasis, and female gender (Table 27-3). The relationship between total radiation dose and irradiated lung volume is best expressed by calculation of the V_{20}, which determines the percentage of the total lung volume that is exposed to more than 20 Gy [36]. For a V_{20} of less than 22%, pulmonary complications from radiation are rare, while unacceptably high rates of radiation pneumonitis including fatalities were observed for V_{20} greater than 35%. The use of amifostine, a prodrug whose active form can function as a scavenger for free radicals and which has been approved for the prevention of radiation-induced xerostomia, might serve as a radioprotectant for the prevention of pneumonitis [37].

ACUTE RADIATION PNEUMONITIS

The incidence of radiation pneumonitis largely depends on the specifics of the radiation protocol used and the clinical indication. Generally, radiographic evidence of radiation-induced lung injury is more frequent than clinical symptoms. Clinically, the incidence is about 0% to 10% in breast cancer and 5% to 15% in lung cancer, while radiographic findings are present in up to 40% of breast and 66% of lung cancer patients undergoing radiotherapy [38].Clinically, acute radiation pneumonitis manifests as dyspnea, nonpro-

ductive cough, low-grade fever, and malaise. The onset of symptoms is typically 2 to 3 months after the completion of radiotherapy. Initially, the physical examination is usually nonspecific and frequently normal. In some cases, crackles and a pleural friction rub may be heard. Early radiographic signs are the development of perivascular ground-glass infiltrates in the irradiated area, which might later progress to patchy alveolar infiltrates. Frequently, the infiltrates are demarcated by a straight line that outlines the radiation field. If present, this is virtually a diagnostic sign. Pulmonary function tests typically show a restrictive pattern with a decrease in DL_{CO}. Histologically, sloughing of endothelial and epithelial cells and abnormalities of type II pneumocytes are observed. Surfactant is reduced and alveoli are filled with exudative material. Hyaline membranes may be present. In rare instances, patients may develop a hyperacute response to radiation therapy that is typical of a hypersensitivity pneumonitis with bilateral infiltrates that do not correspond to the radiation field [39], peripheral blood eosinophilia, fever, dyspnea, and lymphocytosis on BAL. Corticosteroids are the mainstay of treatment for acute radiation pneumonitis. No controlled clinical trials have been conducted to document their efficacy, but animal data and nonrandomized series suggest a benefit. Although steroids may clearly produce symptomatic improvement, it is unclear whether their use during acute radiation pneumonitis reduces the severity of subsequent fibrosis. It is common practice to begin prednisone, 1 mg/kg/d, once the diagnosis of radiation pneumonitis is reasonably certain. Prednisone is administered at this dose for 2 to 3 weeks and then tapered very slowly over several additional weeks. Tapering too rapidly may cause relapse of symptoms.

RADIATION FIBROSIS

Radiologic evidence of fibrosis is seen in most patients who received chest radiation regardless of whether they experienced acute radiation pneumonitis. Radiation changes (linear streaking in mild cases; frank consolidation with air bronchograms and bronchiectatic airway changes in more severe cases) are usually confined to the area irradiated but may be more extensive. It is sometimes difficult to determine whether the radiographic abnormality represents fibrotic changes or recurrent malignancy, and biopsy may be necessary to answer the question. Corticosteroids appear to be of no benefit once fibrosis has developed, and treatment is supportive. In severe cases, the development of cor pulmonale and heart failure are consequences that may result in significant morbidity and mortality.

RADIATION RECALL PNEUMONITIS

The radiation recall phenomenon is characterized by an inflammatory reaction in a previously irradiated area following the administration of certain systemic chemotherapies. Usually a dermatologic complication, it has also been described for internal organs including the occurrence of pneumonitis. The exact pathophysiology is unknown. Radiation recall has been described mostly with anthracycline, taxanes, and gemcitabine chemotherapy [40]. However, case reports implicating other chemotherapeutic drugs such as carmustine and nonantineoplastic drugs such as isoniazid, simvastatin, and tamoxifen also exist. The treatment approach is withdrawal of the inciting agent and therapy with corticosteroids.

CARDIAC COMPLICATIONS OF CANCER THERAPY

The use of chemotherapy in the cancer patient produces a wide range of direct and indirect cardiovascular effects. The risk for complications is significantly higher in the elderly population and in patients with cardiovascular

Table 27-3. Factors Influencing the Development of Radiation Pneumonitis and Fibrosis

Factor	Influence
Total dose	In whole lung irradiation, there is a threshold and a steep dose-response curve once the threshold is met
Volume irradiated	The higher the volume irradiated, the greater the risk
Fractionation and rate	Increased rate of irradiation and decreased fractionation increases risk
Chemotherapy	Concurrent or prior chemotherapy, especially with drugs with established pulmonary toxicity increases risk
Supplemental oxygen	Increases pulmonary toxicity

risk factors or known cardiac diseases. These should be considered by the treating physician. Cardiovascular complications of chemotherapy fall into the following major categories: general cardiovascular concerns, cardiomyopathies, anginal syndromes, arrhythmias, and pericardial disease (Table 27-4). Cancer chemotherapy frequently leads to changes in volume status, electrolyte balance, and anemia, and can directly or indirectly cause arterial hypertension or hypotension. Patients with underlying coronary artery disease, congestive heart failure, valvular disease, or arrhythmias are particularly prone to the development of potentially serious complications in these contexts. Guidelines for the management for chemotherapy-induced anemia exist [41]. Based on symptoms and the risk for the development of symptomatic anemia, patients should receive either blood products, therapy with erythropoiesis-stimulating agents, or observation. Side effects of erythropoiesis-stimulating agents include increased risk for deep venous thrombosis, rarely pure-red cell aplasia, and also rarely hypotension and seizures. It is important to point out that erythropoiesis-stimulating agents have been approved for the management of chemotherapy- and radiotherapy-related anemia. When used for cancer-related anemia in general, two studies demonstrated a possibly inferior survival of patients treated with erythropoiesis-stimulating agents compared with controls [42,43].

ANTHRACYCLINES

Cardiac toxicity from anthracyclines is a well-known complication. Mechanistically, it is related to free-radical formation and lipid oxygenation. This in turn, leads to release of Fe^{3+} ions, which form complexes with the anthracycline, potentiating the release of free radicals [44]. The cardiac toxicity of anthracyclines is dose dependent. The major risk factor for the development of a cardiomyopathy is the cumulative anthracycline dose. Studies have identified 550 mg/m^2 of doxorubicin [45] and 900 mg/m^2 of epirubicin [46] as the recommended maximal cumulative dose. At this dose, the incidence of doxorubicin-induced clinically overt cardiomyopathy was 8%. However, more recent studies suggest that this might be an underestimation of the true incidence. In these studies, the incidence of clinically manifest congestive heart failure at this dose was 20% to 25% and approximately 35%, when objective measures of a reduction in left ventricular ejection fraction (LVEF) were used [47]. Pathologically, the process shows characteristic changes on electron microscopy such as microfibrillar loss and vacuolization (Table 27-5) [48]. Further risk factors for the development of anthracycline-induced cardiomyopathy are advanced age, underlying cardiac disease, concomitant treatment with cyclooxygensase-2 (COX-2) inhibitors, and concurrent administration of other potentially cardiotoxic chemotherapy agents or prior radiation therapy. It has been shown that chemotherapy with paclitaxel before administration of an anthracycline leads to impaired secretion of the anthracycline and its metabolites and increased cardiotoxicity [49]. This effect is highly dependent on the time interval between the drugs and the sequence of their administration [50]. To avoid excess cardiac toxicity, doxorubicin should be administered before paclitaxel, and a waiting period of 15 minutes between the completion of doxorubicin and the initiation of paclitaxel should be observed. Conversely, docetaxel, another taxane, does not appear to interfere with doxorubicin pharmacokinetics and coadministration of the drugs does not increase cardiac toxicity [51]. Another example of an unexpected high rate of congestive heart failure was when an anthracycline (doxorubicin or epirubicin) was administered with trastuzumab, a humanized monoclonal antibody targeting the HER2 receptor in advanced breast cancer. Although the combination of trastuzumab and an anthracycline demonstrated a greater antitumor effect than an anthracycline alone in a randomized trial, 28% of patients who received combination therapy developed cardiac toxicity (including 19% with New York Heart Association [NYHA] class III or IV congestive heart failure), compared with only 7% of patients who received anthracycline alone. Strategies at reducing cardiac toxicity from anthracyclines include careful monitoring, coadministration

Table 27-4. Cardiac Complications of Anticancer Drugs

Agent	Cardiac effect
Chemotherapeutics	
Amsacrine	Arrhythmias
Anthracyclines	Arrhythmias, congestive cardiomyopathy, pericardial effusion
Anthrapyrazoles	Congestive cardiomyopathy
Bleomycin	Raynaud's phenomenon
Cyclophosphamide	Acute congestive heart failure, hemorrhagic myocarditis, pericardial effusions
5-Fluorouracil	Myocardial ischemia, arrhythmias
Mitoxantrone	Congestive cardiomyopathy
Paclitaxel	Arrhythmias (bradycardia), electrocardiogram changes, ischemia, increased cardiomyopathy
Vinca alkaloids	Angina, Raynaud's phenomenon
Biologic response modifiers	
Interferon-α	Hypotension, tachycardia
Interferon-β	Hypotension
Interferon-γ	Hypotension
Interleukin-1α	Hypotension
Interleukin-2	Congestive heart failure, hypotension, arrhythmias, ischemia
Interleukin-4	Congestive heart failure
Tumor necrosis factor	Hypotension, ischemia
GM-CSF	Hypotension, pericardial effusion
Trastuzumab	Congestive heart failure (in combination)
Radiation therapy	Congestive heart failure, coronary artery disease, pericarditis/effusion
Small molecule inhibitors	
Imatinib	Congestive cardiomyopathy, fluid retention
Sorafenib	Slightly increased rate of myocardial infarction
Sunitinib	Cardiomyopathy
Erlotinib	Possibly slightly increased rate of myocardial ischemia
Antibodies	
Bevacizumab	Arterial thromboembolism, hypertension, left ventricular dysfunction
Alemtuzumab	Hypotension during infusion

GM-CSF—granulocyte-macrophage colony-stimulating factor.
(*Adapted from* Speyer and Freeberg [84].)

Table 27-5. Histopathologic Scale of Doxorubicin Cardiomyopathy

Grade	Description
0	Within normal limits
1	Less than 5% of cells with early changes (myofibrillar loss and distended sarcoplasmic reticulum)
1.5	Small groups of cells (5%–15%) involved with definitive changes (marked myofibrillar loss and/or vacuolization)
2	Groups of cells (16%–25%) involved with definitive changes (marked myofibrillar loss and/or vacuolization)
2.5	Groups of cells (26%–35%) involved with definitive changes (marked myofibrillar loss and/or vacuolization)
3	Diffuse cell damage (> 35%) with marked change, including degeneration of organelles, mitochondria, and nucleus and loss of contractile elements

of dexrazoxane, prolonged infusion of doxorubicin, structural variations of doxorubicin, liposome encapsulation, and possibly the coadministration of angiotensin-converting enzyme (ACE) inhibitors or β-blockers. Guidelines for careful cardiac monitoring using objective measurements of the LVEF have been established (Table 27-6) [52]. One study demonstrated that by adherence to these guidelines, the incidence of clinically significant heart failure in a high-risk cohort could be reduced to 3% as compared with 21% in patients in whom the guidelines were not followed strictly. In this study, radionuclide angiography was used to determine the LVEF. Echocardiography is an acceptable alternative. Both tests detect only changes in systolic function. Exercise ventriculography could detect diastolic dysfunction as an earlier sign of anthracycline-related cardiotoxicity [53], but the clinical implications of such a finding are not clear. Dexrazoxane is an EDTA-like chelator and is believed to decrease oxidative stress by chelating intramyocardiac Fe^{3+} ions, which play an integral role in myocyte damage. The effectiveness of dexrazoxane in decreasing anthracycline-induced cardiac toxicity has been demonstrated in multiple trials when it was started with the first dose or after a cumulative dose of 300 mg/m^2 had been reached [54,55]. In combination with dexrazoxane, cumulative doses of doxorubicin in excess of 1000 mg/m^2 were achieved without significant cardiotoxicity. However, one trial raised the possibility that dexrazoxane might decrease the effectiveness of anthracycline chemotherapy [55], a finding that was not confirmed by other studies. Guidelines for the use of dexrazoxane were initially published by the American Society for Clinical Oncology in 1999 and revised in 2002 [56]. The major recommendations are that dexrazoxane can be considered for patients with metastatic cancer who have received a cumulative dose of 300 mg/m^2 of doxorubicin or an equivalent dose of epirubicin. Because there is potentially a reduction in efficacy, dexrazoxane is not recommended outside of clinical trials in the adjuvant setting or in the treatment of children. It has been shown that prolonged infusion of doxorubicin has a lesser risk of cardiotoxicity [57], but these findings have not found widespread clinical application. Epirubicin is structurally related to doxorubicin and has been shown to be less cardiotoxic at equal concentrations. However, it is also less active, suggesting the possibility that the dose-response curve is merely shifted to the right. Mitoxantrone, an anthraquinone, was developed with the goal of achieving less cardiotoxicity. The mechanism of myocardial damage is different from anthracyclines, but congestive heart failure occurs in about 5% of patients after a cumulative dose of 140 mg/m^2 has been reached [58]. Liposome-encapsulated formulations of doxorubicin and daunorubicin are available and have significantly less cardiotoxicity than conventional anthracyclines, allowing the administration of higher doses [59]. However, data on long-term cardiac effects are not yet available. Finally, small studies have suggested a possible benefit of prophylactic therapy with carvedilol [60] or an ACE inhibitor [61] but larger trials are needed to confirm those data. The prognosis of anthracycline-induced cardiomyopathy depends on the severity of symptoms and cardiac dysfunction when congestive heart failure is first diagnosed. In initial series, the mortality rate was close to 60%. With improved cardiomyopathy management including ACE inhibitors and β-blockers, significant improvements in symptoms and ejection fraction are common.

HER-2 ANTAGONISTS

Trastuzumab, a monoclonal antibody against HER-2, was discovered to be a cardiotoxin when administered in combination with anthracyclines. The incidence of congestive heart failure in these early trials was 26% for

the combination therapy as discussed above. The mechanism of trastuzumab-induced cardiomyopathy is not entirely clear, but it seems that HER-2 plays a role in embryonal cardiac development and in the maintenance of normal myocyte function. Mice in which myocardial expression of HER-2 was knocked-out developed a dilated cardiomyopathy [62]. The trastuzumab-induced cardiomyopathy differs ultrastructurally from the anthracycline-induced cardiomyopathy, suggesting a different etiologic mechanism. Clinically, the cardiomyopathy most often presents as asymptomatic decrease in LVEF and less frequently in overt congestive heart failure. Trastuzumab cardiotoxicity in the metastatic setting was assessed in a meta-analysis of seven phase 2 and 3 trials involving 1219 patients [63]. With trastuzumab monotherapy, the incidence of cardiac dysfunction was 7%, rising to 13% in combination with paclitaxel. Three trials examined the effects of 1-year long adjuvant therapy with trastuzumab [64,65]. In the National Surgical Adjuvant Breast and Bowel Project (NSABP) B31 trial, treatment with trastuzumab was stopped in 18% of participants due to cardiac complications. Four percent of the patients had symptomatic heart failure, and the remaining 14% had asymptomatic decrease in ejection fraction. The cardiomyopathy improved in all but one patient after 6 months of follow-up. In the Intergroup trial N-9831, 18% of patients stopped trastuzumab because of reduction in the ejection fraction, 2.8% patients had grade 3, 4, or 5 cardiomyopathy, and one treatment-related death was reported. In the HERA (Herceptin in Adjuvant Breast Cancer) trial, the incidence of trastuzumab-related cardiac problems was slightly lower, necessitating a discontinuation of the drug in 4% of patients. In total, 0.54% of patients had grade 3 and 4 cardiotoxicity [66]. Trastuzumab-induced cardiomyopathy typically responds to standard heart failure regimens and frequently improves after discontinuation of therapy [67]. Small studies suggest that it might be safe to rechallenge patients with trastuzumab after the cardiac dysfunction has resolved. However, this will require a careful risk-benefit analysis by the treating physician. Lapatinib is a small molecule dual tyrosine kinase inhibitor with activity against HER-2 and EGFR. Studies so far suggest a smaller risk of cardiac toxicity than with trastuzumab [68] but more data and longer follow-up are clearly needed.

5-FLUOROURACIL AND CAPECITABINE

5-Fluorouracil (5-FU) is the chemotherapy drug associated with the highest reported incidence of myocardial ischemia. The proposed mechanism is by direct induction of coronary artery spasm. Clinically, 5-FU produces angina with typical symptoms, electrocardiogram changes, and response to nitroglycerin, although some patients studied have had normal coronary angiograms [69]. Moreover, there have been reports of patients who, after experiencing an anginal syndrome during 5-FU, have successfully been reexposed at lower doses without significant subsequent toxicity [70]. Preexisting coronary artery disease is a risk factor. In a review of 1000 patients receiving 5-FU, a 4.5% incidence of cardiac ischemia or arrhythmia was noted in patients with a history of coronary artery disease versus a 1.1% incidence of cardiac toxicity in those patients with no previous cardiac history. This association is more striking in those patients who receive a continuous infusion of 5-FU and in those patients who receive concomitant cisplatin [71]. Akhtar *et al.* [72] noted an 8% incidence of cardiac side effects in patients without cardiac history who were treated with 96-hour 5-FU infusion in combination with mitomycin C or cisplatin. There was no relationship between cardiotoxicity and age, sex, tumor, or drug combination. The cardiac side effects of capecitabine, an oral prodrug for 5-FU, are

Table 27-6. Guidelines for Cardiac Monitoring Using LVEF Measurements

	Baseline MUGA before start of chemotherapy	
Initial result	LVEF ≥ 50%	LVEF < 50%
Follow-up study	At 250–300 mg/m^2 then at 400 mg/m^2 in the presence of risk factors* or 450 mg/m^2 without risk factors	For LVEF between 30%–50%, before each new dose
Criteria for discontinuation	Decline in LVEF by > 10% or below 50%	Decline in LVEF by > 10% or below 30%

*Risk factors include mediastinal radiation, preexisting cardiomyopathy, and concurrent use of cyclophosphamide.
LVEF—left ventricular ejection fraction; MUGA—multiple uptake gated acquisition scan.

very similar and were reported to occur in about 7% [73]. In addition to direct cardiac effects, both 5-FU and capecitabine can have indirect effect on the cardiovascular system by causing profound diarrhea, potentially leading to significant electrolyte abnormalities and dehydration.

VEGF ANTAGONISTS

Bevacizumab has been associated with an increased risk of arterial thromboembolism including myocardial infarction. The overall incidence is 4.4%; however, patients older than 65 years are at increased risk with an overall incidence of 8% [74]. In addition, bevacizumab has been shown to cause left ventricular dysfunction in about 2% of patients. A significant percentage of patients (30%) develop arterial hypertension (grade 3/4 hypertension in 10%). Most cases respond to antihypertensive therapy. Treatment with the multitargeted tyrosine kinase inhibitor sorafenib is associated with a slightly increased risk of myocardial infarction (1%) [26].

CYCLOPHOSPHAMIDE

High doses of cyclophosphamide (> 100 mg/kg) as used in conditioning regimes for bone marrow transplants and ifosfamide (> 1000 mg/m^2) can cause an acute hemorrhagic myopericarditis that is frequently fatal [75]. The exact incidence and the exact mechanism of this complication are unknown. It is usually seen about 2 weeks after the administration of chemotherapy. Loss of voltage of the QRS complex can be an early warning sign, but the positive predictive power of this finding is poor.

PACLITAXEL

Intravenous infusion of paclitaxel was initially associated with a high incidence of bradyarrhythmias [76]. As a result, initial National Cancer Institute (NCI)–sponsored studies eliminated all patients with cardiac risk factors and required cardiac monitoring. With these precautions, a reassessment of the 3400 patients in the NCI database demonstrated only a 0.29% incidence of grade 4 or 5 cardiac toxicity, including heart block (four patients), atrial arrhythmias (three patients), ventricular tachycardia (nine patients), and myocardial infarction within 14 days of paclitaxel infusion (seven patients) [77]. Ten of these patients had prior cardiac risk factors. At present, routine cardiac monitoring for paclitaxel administration is not recommended, although it may be considered for patients with known cardiac conditions.

CISPLATIN

Cisplatin induces renal tubular dysfunction, resulting in urinary magnesium and potassium loss. These electrolyte abnormalities may result in prolongation of the QT interval and subsequent ventricular arrhythmia. Oral supplementation with both magnesium and potassium salts may be necessary chronically.

CYTOKINES

Almost all patients treated with IL-2 develop a capillary leak syndrome that is clinically indistinguishable from sepsis. Direct cardiac effects of IL-2 can be present as well. Arrhythmias and myocardial infarction have been reported [78], mostly in patients with underlying coronary artery disease. Denileukin diftitox is a fusion protein linking the diphtheria toxin to an antibody against the α chain of the IL-2 receptor. Capillary leak syndromes, arrhythmias, and myocardial infarction as well as severe hypersensitivity reactions have been reported [79]. Like IL-2, interferon-α has also been linked to arrhythmias

and myocardial infarctions. Supraventricular tachycardias are frequent and can occur in 20% of cases. Long-time administration of interferon-α can cause a cardiomyopathy, which is reversible in a subset of cases after cessation of therapy [80]. The pathogenetic mechanism is unclear.

DIFFERENTIATING AGENTS

Both all-trans-retinoic acid and arsenic trioxide are used as differentiating agents in the treatment of APL. Both agents can cause the APL differentiation syndrome, which can lead to the rapid development of large pericardial effusions and tamponade (see the section on pulmonary complications). Emergent pericardiocentesis should be performed for clinical signs of tamponade. Otherwise, high-dose steroids might be beneficial. Arsenic trioxide can lead to QT prolongation and to complete heart block. Electrocardiogram monitoring before therapy and weekly during therapy is recommended. Careful monitoring of serum electrolytes is critical.

IMATINIB

Imatinib is an oral tyrosine kinase inhibitor that was initially designed to inhibit the BCR-ABL tyrosine kinase, but also inhibits c-kit and platelet-derived growth factor receptor signaling. To date, 10 cases of severe cardiomyopathy that developed in patients with normal cardiac function prior to treatment with imatinib have been reported. It is speculated that inhibition of the c-ABL tyrosine kinase in these patients activated the endoplasmatic stress response, ultimately leading to collapse of the mitochondrial membrane potential and cell death. Edema is a common side effect of the treatment with imatinib [81]. It is observed in 70% to 80% of patients. Grade 3/4 edema occurs in approximately 7% of patients and pleural effusions are observed in about 2%. Pericardial effusions are relatively rare and evidence of active pericarditis is found in less than 0.1%.

CYTARABINE

Multiple case reports of cytarabine-induced pericarditis that might progress to pericardial tamponade exist [82,83]. Treatment with corticosteroids is felt to be beneficial.

CONCLUSIONS

In summary, both cardiac and pulmonary complications of cancer therapy are common. Mechanisms of toxicity have been elucidated especially for the drugs that are frequently associated with cardiac toxicity. Guidelines for cumulative dose and prevention of cardiac toxicity have been developed for some of these agents, such as the anthracyclines. Recent years have brought the realization that most antineoplastic agents can lead to pulmonary toxicity. The underlying mechanisms have been much less well defined. Avoidance and early recognition of cardiac or pulmonary complications is of major importance. In this regard, the use of combination regimens with a synergistic toxicity profile should be discouraged especially in patients with limited cardiopulmonary reserve. The treating physicians should also maintain a high degree of suspicion in cases of unexplained cardiopulmonary symptoms. The prognosis for both cardiac and pulmonary complications largely depends on the inciting agent. Management for pulmonary complications consists of a trial of corticosteroids, which frequently have to be given for an extended period of time and otherwise supportive care. A treatment-related cardiomyopathy will be managed with standard congestive heart failure regimens.

REFERENCES

1. Crooke ST, Bradner WT: Bleomycin, a review. *J Med* 1976, 7:333–428.

2. Lei KI, Leung WT, Johnson PJ: Serious pulmonary complications in patients receiving recombinant granulocyte colony-stimulating factor during BACOP chemotherapy for aggressive non-Hodgkin's lymphoma. *Br J Cancer* 1994, 70:1009–1013.

3. Saxman SB, Nichols CR, Einhorn LH: Pulmonary toxicity in patients with advanced-stage germ cell tumors receiving bleomycin with and without granulocyte colony stimulating factor. *Chest* 1997, 111:657–660.

4. Rivera MP, Kris MG, Gralla RJ, *et al.*: Syndrome of acute dyspnea related to combined mitomycin plus vinca alkaloid chemotherapy. *Am J Clin Oncol* 1995, 18:245–250.

5. Sheldon R, Slaughter D: A syndrome of microangiopathic hemolytic anemia, renal impairment, and pulmonary edema in chemotherapy-treated patients with adenocarcinoma. *Cancer* 1986, 58:1428–1436.

6. Chang AY, Kuebler JP, Pandya KJ, *et al.*: Pulmonary toxicity induced by mitomycin C is highly responsive to glucocorticoids. *Cancer* 1986, 57:2285–2290.

7. Weinstein AS, Diener-West M, Nelson DF, *et al.*: Pulmonary toxicity of carmustine in patients treated for malignant glioma. *Cancer Treat Rep* 1986, 70:943–946.

8. Ginsberg SJ, Comis RL: The pulmonary toxicity of antineoplastic agents. *Semin Oncol* 1982, 9:34–51.

9. Malik SW, Myers JL, DeRemee RA, *et al.*: Lung toxicity associated with cyclophosphamide use. Two distinct patterns. *Am J Respir Crit Care Med* 1996, 154:1851–1856.

10. Weiss RB, Donehower RC, Wiernik PH, *et al.*: Hypersensitivity reactions from Taxol. *J Clin Oncol* 1990, 8:1263–1268.

11. Bookman MA, Kloth DD, Kover PE, *et al.*: Short-course intravenous prophylaxis for paclitaxel-related hypersensitivity reactions. *Ann Oncol* 1997, 8:611–614.

12. Goldberg HL, Vannice SB: Pneumonitis related to treatment with paclitaxel. *J Clin Oncol* 1995, 13:534–535.

13. Read WL, Mortimer JE, Picus J: Severe interstitial pneumonitis associated with docetaxel administration. *Cancer* 2002, 94:847–853.

14. Wang GS, Yang KY, Perng RP: Life-threatening hypersensitivity pneumonitis induced by docetaxel (Taxotere). *Br J Cancer* 2001, 85:1247–1250.

15. Denman JP, Gilbar PJ, Abdi EA: Hypersensitivity reaction (HSR) to docetaxel after a previous HSR to paclitaxel. *J Clin Oncol* 2002, 20:2760–2761.

16. Aapro MS, Martin C, Hatty S: Gemcitabine: a safety review. *Anticancer Drugs* 1998, 9:191–201.

17. Pavlakis N, Bell DR, Millward MJ, *et al.*: Fatal pulmonary toxicity resulting from treatment with gemcitabine. *Cancer* 1997, 80:286–291.

18. Helman DL Jr, Byrd JC, Ales NC, *et al.*: Fludarabine-related pulmonary toxicity: a distinct clinical entity in chronic lymphoproliferative syndromes. *Chest* 2002, 122:785–790.

19. Stoica GS, Greenberg HE, Rossoff LJ: Corticosteroid responsive fludarabine pulmonary toxicity. *Am J Clin Oncol* 2002, 25:340–341.

20. *Fludara* [package insert]. Wayne, NJ: Bayer HealthCare; November 2007. Available at http://www.fludara.com/hcp/index.html. Accessed August 4, 2008.

21. *Clolar* [package insert]. Cambridge, MA: Genzyme Corp.; February 2008. Available at http://www.clolar.com/hcp/pi/cl_hc_pi_overview.asp. Accessed August 4, 2008.

22. Takano T, Ohe Y, Kusumoto M, *et al.*: Risk factors for interstitial lung disease and predictive factors for tumor response in patients with advanced non-small cell lung cancer treated with gefitinib. *Lung Cancer* 2004, 45:93–104.

23. Shepherd FA, Rodrigues Pereira J, Ciuleanu T, *et al.*: Erlotinib in previously treated non-small-cell lung cancer. *N Engl J Med* 2005, 353:123–132.

24. Thatcher N, Chang A, Parikh P, *et al.*: Gefitinib plus best supportive care in previously treated patients with refractory advanced non-small-cell lung cancer: results from a randomised, placebo-controlled, multicentre study (Iressa Survival Evaluation in Lung Cancer). *Lancet* 2005, 366:1527–1537.

25. Moore MJ, Goldstein D, Hamm J, *et al.*: Erlotinib plus gemcitabine compared with gemcitabine alone in patients with advanced pancreatic cancer: a phase III trial of the national Cancer Institute of Canada clinical trials group. *J Clin Oncol* 2007, 25:1960–1966.

26. *Nexavar* [package insert]. Wayne, NJ and Emeryville, CA: Bayer HealthCare and Onyx Pharmaceuticals; 2008. Available at http://www.nexavar.com. Accessed August 4, 2008.

27. *Vectibix* [package insert]. Thousand Oaks, CA: Amgen Inc.; 2008. Available at http://www.vectibix.com. Accessed August 4, 2008.

28. Johnson DH, Fehrenbacher L, Novotny WF, *et al.*: Randomized phase II trial comparing bevacizumab plus carboplatin and paclitaxel with carboplatin and paclitaxel alone in previously untreated locally advanced or metastatic non-small-cell lung cancer. *J Clin Oncol* 2004, 22:2184–2191.

29. Sandler A, Gray R, Perry MC, *et al.*: Paclitaxel-carboplatin alone or with bevacizumab for non-small-cell lung cancer. *N Engl J Med* 2006, 355:2542–2550.

30. Inoue KI, Hiraoka N, Kasamatsu Y, *et al.*: A case of irinotecan induced pneumonitis. *Jap J Lung Cancer* 2000, 40:219–221.

31. Nayak L, Malik K, Seidl E, *et al.*: Irinotecan associated interstitial pneumonitis [abstract]. *Proc Am Soc Clin Oncol* 2003, 22:abstract 3090.

32. Madarnas Y, Webster P, Shorter AM, *et al.*: Irinotecan-associated pulmonary toxicity. *Anticancer Drugs* 2000, 11:709–713.

33. *Eloxatin* [package insert]. Bridgewater, NJ: Sanofi-Aventis US LLC; 2008. Available at http://www.eloxatin.com. Accessed August 4, 2008.

34. Epperly M, Bray J, Kraeger S, *et al.*: Prevention of late effects of irradiation lung damage by manganese superoxide dismutase gene therapy. *Gene Ther* 1998, 5:196–208.

35. Roach M III , Gandara DR, Yuo HS, *et al.*: Radiation pneumonitis following combined modality therapy for lung cancer: Analysis of prognostic factors. *J Clin Oncol* 1995, 13:2606–2612.

36. Graham MV, Purdy JA, Emami B, *et al.*: Clinical dose-volume histogram analysis for pneumonitis after 3D treatment for non-small cell lung cancer (NSCLC). *Int J Radiat Oncol Biol Phys* 1999, 45:323–329.

37. Antonadou D: Radiotherapy or chemotherapy followed by radiotherapy with or without amifostine in locally advanced lung cancer. *Semin Radiat Oncol* 2002, 12:50–58.

38. McDonald S, Rubin P, Phillips TL, *et al.*: Injury to the lung from cancer therapy: Clinical syndromes, measurable endpoints, and potential scoring systems. *Int J Radiat Oncol Biol Phys* 1995, 31:1187–1203.

39. Martin C, Romero S, Sanchez-Paya J, *et al.*: Bilateral lymphocytic alveolitis: a common reaction after unilateral thoracic irradiation. *Eur Respir J* 1999, 13:727–732.

40. Schwarte S, Wagner K, Karstens JH, *et al.*: Radiation recall pneumonitis induced by gemcitabine. *Strahlenther Onkol* 2007, 183:215–217.

41. National Comprehensive Cancer Network: NCCN clinical practice guidelines in oncology: cancer and treatment related anemia. V.1.2009. Available at http://www.nccn.org/professionals/physician_gls/PDF/anemia.pdf. Accessed August 4, 2008.

42. Henke M, Laszig R, Rube C, *et al.*: Erythropoietin to treat head and neck cancer patients with anaemia undergoing radiotherapy: Randomised, double-blind, placebo-controlled trial. *Lancet* 2003, 362:1255–1260.

43. Leyland-Jones B, BEST Investigators and Study Group: Breast cancer trial with erythropoietin terminated unexpectedly. *Lancet Oncol* 2003, 4:459–460.

44. Gianni L, Zweier JL, Levy A, *et al.*: Characterization of the cycle of iron-mediated electron transfer from adriamycin to molecular oxygen. *J Biol Chem* 1985, 260:6820–6826.

45. Von Hoff DD, Rozencweig M, Layard M, *et al.*: Daunomycin-induced cardiotoxicity in children and adults. A review of 110 cases. *Am J Med* 1977, 62:200–208.

46. Ryberg M, Nielsen D, Skovsgaard T, *et al.*: Epirubicin cardiotoxicity: an analysis of 469 patients with metastatic breast cancer. *J Clin Oncol* 1998, 16:3502–3508.

47. Swain SM, Whaley FS, Ewer MS: Congestive heart failure in patients treated with doxorubicin: a retrospective analysis of three trials. *Cancer* 2003, 97:2869–2879.

48. Billingham ME, Mason JW, Bristow MR, *et al.*: Anthracycline cardiomyopathy monitored by morphologic changes. *Cancer Treat Rep* 1978, 62:865–872.

49. Gianni L, Vigano L, Locatelli A, *et al.*: Human pharmacokinetic characterization and in vitro study of the interaction between doxorubicin and paclitaxel in patients with breast cancer. *J Clin Oncol* 1997, 15:1906–1915.

50. Holmes FA, Madden T, Newman RA, *et al.*: Sequence-dependent alteration of doxorubicin pharmacokinetics by paclitaxel in a phase I study of paclitaxel and doxorubicin in patients with metastatic breast cancer. *J Clin Oncol* 1996, 14:2713–2721.

51. Sparano JA: Doxorubicin/taxane combinations: cardiac toxicity and pharmacokinetics. *Semin Oncol* 1999, 26:14–19.

52. Schwartz RG, McKenzie WB, Alexander J, *et al.*: Congestive heart failure and left ventricular dysfunction complicating doxorubicin therapy. Seven-year experience using serial radionuclide angiocardiography. *Am J Med* 1987, 82:1109–1118.

53. Palmeri ST, Bonow RO, Myers CE, *et al.*: Prospective evaluation of doxorubicin cardiotoxicity by rest and exercise radionuclide angiography. *Am J Cardiol* 1986, 58:607–613.

54. Swain SM, Whaley FS, Gerber MC, *et al.*: Delayed administration of dexrazoxane provides cardioprotection for patients with advanced breast cancer treated with doxorubicin-containing therapy. *J Clin Oncol* 1997, 15:1333–1340.

55. Swain SM, Whaley FS, Gerber MC, *et al.*: Cardioprotection with dexrazoxane for doxorubicin-containing therapy in advanced breast cancer. *J Clin Oncol* 1997, 15:1318–1332.

56. Schuchter LM, Hensley ML, Meropol NJ, *et al.*: 2002 update of recommendations for the use of chemotherapy and radiotherapy protectants: Clinical practice guidelines of the American Society of Clinical Oncology. *J Clin Oncol* 2002, 20:2895–2903.

57. Legha SS, Benjamin RS, Mackay B, *et al.*: Reduction of doxorubicin cardiotoxicity by prolonged continuous intravenous infusion. *Ann Intern Med* 1982, 96:133–139.

58. Saletan S: Mitoxantrone: an active, new antitumor agent with an improved therapeutic index. *Cancer Treat Rev* 1987, 14:297–303.

59. Berry G, Billingham M, Alderman E, *et al.*: The use of cardiac biopsy to demonstrate reduced cardiotoxicity in AIDS Kaposi's sarcoma patients treated with pegylated liposomal doxorubicin. *Ann Oncol* 1998, 9:711–716.

60. Kalay N, Basar E, Ozdogru I, *et al.*: Protective effects of carvedilol against anthracycline-induced cardiomyopathy. *J Am Coll Cardiol* 2006, 48:2258–2262.

61. Cardinale D, Colombo A, Sandri MT, *et al.*: Prevention of high-dose chemotherapy-induced cardiotoxicity in high-risk patients by angiotensin-converting enzyme inhibition. *Circulation* 2006, 114:2474–2481.

62. Crone SA, Zhao YY, Fan L, *et al.*: ErbB2 is essential in the prevention of dilated cardiomyopathy. *Nat Med* 2002, 8:459–465.

63. Seidman A, Hudis C, Pierri MK, *et al.*: Cardiac dysfunction in the trastuzumab clinical trials experience. *J Clin Oncol* 2002, 20:1215–1221.

64. Romond EH, Perez EA, Bryant J, *et al.*: Trastuzumab plus adjuvant chemotherapy for operable HER2-positive breast cancer. *N Engl J Med* 2005, 353:1673–1684.

65. Piccart-Gebhart MJ, Procter M, Leyland-Jones B, *et al.*: Trastuzumab after adjuvant chemotherapy in HER2-positive breast cancer. *N Engl J Med* 353: 2005, 1659–1672.

66. Smith I, Procter M, Gelber RD, *et al.*: 2-year follow-up of trastuzumab after adjuvant chemotherapy in HER2-positive breast cancer: A randomised controlled trial. *Lancet* 2007, 369:29–36.

67. Ewer MS, Vooletich MT, Durand JB, *et al.*: Reversibility of trastuzumab-related cardiotoxicity: new insights based on clinical course and response to medical treatment. *J Clin Oncol* 2005, 23:7820–7826.

68. Geyer CE, Forster J, Lindquist D, *et al.*: Lapatinib plus capecitabine for HER2-positive advanced breast cancer. *N Engl J Med* 2006, 355:2733–2743.

69. Freeman NJ, Costanza ME: 5-fluorouracil-associated cardiotoxicity. *Cancer* 1988, 61:36–45.

70. Weidmann B, Teipel A, Niederle N: The syndrome of 5-fluorouracil cardiotoxicity: an elusive cardiopathy. *Cancer* 1994, 73:2001–2002.

71. de Forni M, Malet-Martino MC, Jaillais P, *et al.*: Cardiotoxicity of high-dose continuous infusion fluorouracil: A prospective clinical study. *J Clin Oncol* 1992, 10:1795–1801.

72. Akhtar SS, Salim KP, Bano ZA: Symptomatic cardiotoxicity with high-dose 5-fluorouracil infusion: a prospective study. *Oncology* 1993, 50:441–444.

73. Ng M, Cunningham D, Norman AR: The frequency and pattern of cardiotoxicity observed with capecitabine used in conjunction with oxaliplatin in patients treated for advanced colorectal cancer (CRC). *Eur J Cancer* 2005, 41:1542–1546.

74. *Avastin* [package insert]. South San Francisco, CA: Genentech, Inc.; March 2008. Available at http://www.avastin.com. Accessed August 4, 2008.

75. Appelbaum F, Strauchen JA, Graw RG Jr, *et al.*: Acute lethal carditis caused by high-dose combination chemotherapy. A unique clinical and pathological entity. *Lancet* 1976, 1:58–62.

76. Rowinsky EK, McGuire WP, Guarnieri T, *et al.*: Cardiac disturbances during the administration of Taxol. *J Clin Oncol* 1991, 9:1704–1712.

77. Arbuck SG, Strauss H, Rowinsky E, *et al.*: A reassessment of cardiac toxicity associated with Taxol. *J Natl Cancer Inst Monogr* 1993, 15:117–130.

78. Margolin KA, Rayner AA, Hawkins MJ, *et al.*: Interleukin-2 and lymphokine-activated killer cell therapy of solid tumors: Analysis of toxicity and management guidelines. *J Clin Oncol* 1989, 7:486–498.

79. Foss F: Clinical experience with denileukin diftitox (ONTAK). *Semin Oncol* 2006, 33:S11–S6.

80. Sonnenblick M, Rosin A: Cardiotoxicity of interferon. A review of 44 cases. *Chest* 1991, 99:557–561.

81. Kerkela R, Grazette L, Yacobi R, *et al.*: Cardiotoxicity of the cancer therapeutic agent imatinib mesylate. *Nat Med* 2006, 12:908–916.

82. Reykdal S, Sham R, Kouides P: Cytarabine-induced pericarditis: a case report and review of the literature of the cardio-pulmonary complications of cytarabine therapy. *Leuk Res* 1995, 19:141–144.

83. Hermans C, Straetmans N, Michaux JL, *et al.*: Pericarditis induced by high-dose cytosine arabinoside chemotherapy. *Ann Hematol* 1997, 75:55–57.

84. Speyer J, Freedberg R: *Clinical Oncology*. New York: Churchill Livingstone, Inc.; 1995.

Neurologic signs and symptoms, which are common in cancer patients, have several potential etiologies, including metastatic involvement of the central nervous system (CNS) or peripheral nervous system (PNS), paraneoplastic disorders, and treatment-related neurotoxicity. Treatment-related neurotoxicity is common with many chemotherapy regimens and may be severe and dose-limiting. Strategies such as bone marrow transplantation and growth factor supplements have overcome many dosing limitations caused by bone marrow toxicity; however, as increasingly higher doses of chemotherapy are permitted, the risk of neurotoxicity increases. In addition, many novel targeted therapies have neurotoxicities that are only recently being described.

One major limitation in addressing chemotherapy-induced neurotoxicity has been the inability to reliably quantify the spectrum of neurologic disease associated with a given agent. Peripheral neuropathy has been the most widely investigated neurotoxicity and is traditionally scored based on definitions in the National Cancer Institute Common Toxicity Criteria for Adverse Events and the World Health Organization Toxicity Criteria for Peripheral Neuropathy. These scales define neuropathy broadly and differently from one another [1]. In dedicated studies of neuropathy, a cohort of patients is often studied using subjective reports of severity paired with "objective" measures such as vibratory perception thresholds (VPT) or nerve conduction studies. Such subjective reports often result in two problems: 1) the true incidence of neuropathy may not be captured, and 2) it is difficult to compare trial results in the absence of standardized, validated measures. Therapeutic trials for chemotherapy-related neuropathy have similarly used a variety of assessment tools; hence, it is difficult to compare results. Despite data from more than 30 clinical trials for agents used to treat chemotherapy-related neuropathy, a standard therapy does not yet exist.

A promising trend is the incorporation of specific measures to assess neuropathy early in large clinical trials [2,3]. In addition, rating scales such as the Total Neuropathy Score are being used with increasing frequency. The Total Neuropathy Score has been validated as accurate for detecting and describing neuropathy across patients with various underlying malignancies who have been exposed to various chemotherapies [4,5]. Our hope is that more uniform use of such assessment scales will contribute to the identification of effective strategies for preventing or treating chemotherapy-induced neuropathy.

Common agents resulting in PNS and CNS neurotoxicities are reviewed in this chapter. An overview of common chemotherapeutic agents causing neurotoxicity is provided in Table 28-1.

PERIPHERAL NEUROPATHIES

Neuropathy is one of the most common forms of chemotherapy-related neurotoxicity. Peripheral neuropathy is a disease of the nerves outside of the CNS. The most common symptoms are numbness, pain, and tingling (paresthesias) in the hands and feet. Loss of sensory function can result in clumsiness and inability to perform fine motor movements, such as closing buttons and writing, as well as difficulty walking. When motor nerves are involved, there may be overt muscle weakness. On examination, common findings are a length-dependent (feet and hands dominant) alteration in sensation, loss of deep tendon reflexes, and possibly loss of position sense or impaired coordination. Symptoms often progress proximally with continued exposure. Neuropathy results from either injury to the sensory and motor nerves (axonopathy) or the neurons from which they arise (neuronopathy). The three classes of antineoplastic drugs most commonly associated with peripheral neuropathy are the vinca alkaloids, platinum analogues, and taxanes. All these agents are in wide clinical use for multiple cancers and therefore their impact on the incidence of treated-related neuropathy is high.

VINCA ALKALOIDS

The vinca alkaloids arrest cell division by inhibiting microtubule formation in the mitotic spindle. There are natural alkaloids (vincristine and vinblastine) and semisynthetic compounds (vindesine and vinorelbine). The precise mechanism for vinca alkaloid–induced neuropathy is not known; however, disruption of axonal transport due to breakdown of microtubules, eventually leading to axonal degeneration, is a likely explanation [6,7].

Vincristine is widely recognized for causing an often dose-limiting sensory neuropathy. The most common signs are length-dependent loss of ankle reflexes, paresthesias, and numbness, with paresthesias occurring in up to 60% of patients [8–10]. Motor neuropathy can also develop and commonly involves finger and wrist extensor muscles first, progressing to dorsiflexors of the toes and ankles [8]. Painful sensory neuropathy and progressive motor neuropathy are indications for dose reduction or cessation of vincristine therapy.

Electrophysiologic studies show distal axonal neuropathic changes with decreased amplitude of distal motor and sensory nerve action potentials. Slight reductions of motor and sensory nerve conduction velocities may also be found [9]. Sural nerve histology shows primarily axonal degeneration, with some associated demyelination [11].

In addition to length-dependent sensorimotor neuropathy, mononeuropathies may occur [12]. Cranial nerve palsies, including vocal cord paresis, diplopia, ophthalmoplegia, ptosis, facial palsy, loss of corneal reflexes, and paroxysmal jaw pain, have all been reported with vincristine [13–15]. Autonomic neuropathy may also occur. Troublesome constipation was reported in one third of patients with a higher frequency, greater severity, and earlier onset after high-dose vincristine. Other reported autonomic side effects include bladder atony with urinary retention, impotence, and orthostatic hypotension. Cranial nerve and autonomic manifestations generally occur only with high doses.

CNS toxicities with vincristine are rare, possibly due to poor penetration of vincristine across the blood-brain barrier. Decreased alertness, agitation, insomnia, confusion, hallucinations, transient cortical blindness, ataxia, syndrome of inappropriate antidiuretic hormone secretion, seizures, and coma have all been reported in a small number of patients, but often in combination with other chemotherapies or with high-dose vincristine. Accidental massive overdoses of intravenous (IV) vincristine caused pronounced PNS and CNS toxicity, resulting in death in three of five reported patients [16] in the few cases in which vincristine has been erroneously infused into the intrathecal space. There have been universally severe adverse events ranging from paralysis to death [17–19].

Vinblastine produces a similar clinical spectrum of neurotoxicity but, unlike vincristine, it also produces a severe degree of bone marrow suppression that usually precedes neurotoxicity as the dose-limiting toxicity. Vindesine and vinorelbine normally produce mild neurotoxicity, mainly consisting of a dose-dependent loss of deep tendon reflexes.

Neurotoxicity of the vinca alkaloids is enhanced in the setting of underlying neuropathic disease including inherited diseases like Charcot-Marie-Tooth syndrome or more common neuropathic diseases such as diabetic nephropathy [20,21]. In addition, concomitant administration of agents that alter the metabolism of vincristine, such as isoniazid or L-asparaginase, can substantially exaggerate the neurotoxicities of vincristine [22].

Vincristine-induced neuropathy generally recovers to some extent after drug discontinuation [23]. Improvement of paresthesias is the first sign of recovery. Cranial nerve palsies resolve within months in most patients, although visual changes and hearing loss may persist. Several attempts have been pursued to ameliorate or prevent vincristine-induced neurotoxicity. In general, neurotoxicity is less severe with lower doses and longer intervals between doses. Both gangliosides and glutamic acid have reduced vincristine neurotoxicity in preclinical models [24,25]. The adrenocorticotropic hormone (ACTH) analogue Org 2766 modulated vincristine-induced neurotoxicity in an experimental snail model and appeared to be protective in a pilot clinical trial [26,27]. However, in a larger, randomized controlled study, there was no neuroprotective effect when Org 2766 was given before and after each dose of vincristine [28].

PLATINUM ANALOGUES

The platinum analogue class includes three widely used chemotherapies: cisplatin, carboplatin, and oxaliplatin. These agents work by binding DNA and forming interstrand and intrastrand crosslinks. Platinum compounds are widely applied to solid and hematologic malignancies and are first-line therapy for the most common malignancies such as lung and breast cancer.

Mild neurotoxicity is common with standard dosing of cisplatin (50–100 mg/m^2/cycle), but occasionally the neuropathy is severe with pronounced sensory loss that may be irreversible [29]. The exact mechanism of cisplatin neurotoxicity remains unclear but may be related to damage of the sensory neuron within the dorsal root ganglia [30]. Pathologic studies suggest platinum is tightly bound within nerve tissue, leading to dorsal root ganglia neurotoxicity [31,32]. Although peripheral nerve histopathology shows axonal degeneration of distal more than proximal nerves and secondary myelin breakdown, a recent study demonstrated electrophysiologic findings most consistent with a primary neuronopathy [30].

Sensory symptoms are the most common manifestation. Length-dependent paresthesias and numbness are common initial symptoms. The symptoms worsen with increasing cumulative doses, spread proximally, and can become disabling. Impaired proprioception may lead to ataxia, clumsiness of fine movements, and gait disturbances. On neurologic examination, decreased VPT and loss of ankle reflexes are early signs of neuropathy. A positive Lhermitte's sign has been reported, presumably due to involvement of ascending posterior spinal cord tracts. Symptoms of autonomic neuropathy are relatively infrequent. A striking characteristic of cisplatin-induced neuropathy is continued neurologic deterioration after cessation of therapy. This deterioration, referred to as "coasting," may continue for several months after therapy is stopped.

The incidence of sensory neuropathy following cisplatin largely depends on the cumulative dose, with symptoms generally presenting after 300 to 400 mg/m^2. After completion of a standard regimen (commonly a total dose of 600 mg/m^2), up to 90% of patients may have clinical signs and symptoms [33]. Both cumulative-dose and single-dose regimens are relevant for development of neuropathy [34]. Combination therapy with other drugs known to cause neurotoxicities results in greater subjective and objective evidence of neuropathy [35]. This contributes to a treatment dilemma, as combined use of neurotoxic therapies results in improved survival but comes at the cost of higher incidence of often irreversible neuropathy [2].

Table 28-1. Peripheral and Central Neurotoxicities Caused by Chemotherapeutic Agents

Drug	PNS neurotoxicity	CNS neurotoxicity	Comments
Cytarabine	Sensory neuropathy, plexopathy	Cerebellar dysfunction, atrophy, confusion, lethargy, somnolence	Meningitis, seizures, myelopathy after intrathecal administration
Etoposide	Sensory neuropathy	Headache, seizures, and somnolence at high dose	
Ifosfamide	Painful neuropathy	Encephalopathy, cerebellar dysfunction, seizures, delirium, coma	Neuropathy only sporadic with high doses
Immunomodulators (*eg*, cyclosporine, (interferon-α, tacrolimus)	Motor and sensory neuropathy, auditory impairment, plexopathy, cranial nerve palsy	Encephalopathy, anxiety, tremor, akathisia, depression, confusion, seizures, headache	Sporadic reversible posterior leukoencephalopathy syndrome
Methotrexate	Radiculopathy (rare)	Encephalopathy, seizures, aseptic meningitis, leukoencephalopathy	Depending on dose, route of administration, relation with RT
Platinum analogues			
Carboplatin	Peripheral neuropathy (high dose)	Cortical blindness, focal deficit	
Cisplatin	Sensory, autonomic, and cranial neuropathy; plexopathy; ototoxicity	Headache, cortical blindness, encephalopathy, seizures, focal deficit	Frequent off-therapy worsening; often residual symptoms/signs; dose dependency
Oxaliplatin	Highest risk with cold exposure		
Procarbazine	Sensory or sensorimotor neuropathy	Encephalopathy, optic neuroretinitis	
Purine analogues (*eg*, cladribine, fludarabine, pentostatin)	Motor and sensory neuropathy	Encephalopathy, dementia, coma, cortical blindness, progressive multifocal leukoencephalopathy	Dose dependency
Taxanes			
Docetaxel	Predominantly sensory neuropathy; proximal extremity weakness at high dose		Sometimes off-therapy worsening; dose dependency
Paclitaxel	Predominantly sensory neuropathy; sensorimotor neuropathy (high doses); cranial neuropathy	Seizures, encephalopathy	Dose dependency; usually partial recovery; CNS toxicity only with high doses
Vinca alkaloids (*eg*, vinblastine, vincristine, vindesine, vinorelbine)	Sensorimotor, autonomic, cranial, and mononeuropathy	Agitation, somnolence, seizures, coma, SIADH	Usually favorable outcome; dose dependency; vindesine and vinorelbine have much less neurotoxicity compared with vincristine

CNS—central nervous system; PNS—peripheral nervous system; RT—radiotherapy; SIADH—syndrome of inappropriate antidiuretic hormone.

Cranial nerve impairment has been observed in patients who received intra-arterial or intracarotid cisplatin for head and neck or CNS tumors, in rare cases resulting in permanent optic toxicity [36,37]. Ototoxicity is a well-described complication of both systemic and locally delivered cisplatin. Plexopathies have also been observed after intra-arterial cisplatin administration [38]. Although CNS toxicity is rare with cisplatin monotherapy— likely reflecting poor penetration across the blood-brain barrier—headache, transient cortical blindness, optic neuritis, encephalopathy, and stroke have been reported with combination regimens [39–42].

Because cisplatin is a key agent in multiple chemotherapeutic regimens, strategies have been applied to try to reduce, delay, and treat the associated neurotoxicity. Amifostine is a prodrug that is activated by dephosphorylation and acts as a scavenger of oxygen-free radicals. A randomized controlled trial of amifostine with cyclophosphamide and cisplatin showed significant reduction in the severity of cisplatin-induced neuropathy in patients pretreated with amifostine [43]. However, a single-arm trial of amifostine plus cisplatin showed a 52% incidence of neuropathy with no apparent benefit from amifostine [44]. Similarly, a single-arm trial of amifostine, cisplatin, and paclitaxel was negative [45]. These discrepancies may be due to the timing of the amifostine relative to the chemotherapy, assessment of neuropathy, or the use of concomitant neurotoxic agents. In addition to unclear efficacy, amifostine use is limited by its associated side effects of hypotension and nausea.

Glutathione is an endogenous protein that has prevented cisplatin-related neuropathy in a rat model [46]. In clinical trials to date, cisplatin appears to decrease platinum-related neurotoxicity across a variety of tumor types [47,48]. The ACTH-(4-9) analogue Org 2766 has also been tested against cisplatin-induced neuropathy in two randomized, blinded, placebo-controlled studies. Patients reported fewer subjective symptoms of neuropathy, but there was no improvement in the VPT in both studies [49,50]. In fact, there was some evidence to suggest that Org 2766 enhanced the development of neuropathy. To date, no agent has shown proven benefit in cisplatin-induced neuropathy.

Carboplatin is a cisplatin analogue that is associated with more myelosuppression and less neuropathy than cisplatin. However, severe neuropathy has been described in patients treated with high-dose carboplatin [51]. Moreover, there appears to be enhanced neurotoxicity when carboplatin is combined with other neurotoxic therapies. Other neurologic side effects that have been rarely reported are blindness and thrombotic microangiopathy with multiple cerebrovascular infarcts [52,53]. Finally, carboplatin has been associated with myalgias and muscle weakness [54].

Oxaliplatin is a new-generation platinum analogue that has unique sites and mechanisms of action. It has been shown to significantly improve survival in colorectal cancer and is under investigation for several other solid tumors. One of the most common side effects of oxaliplatin is a peripheral sensory neuropathy [55]. The neuropathy is unique in that it is severely exacerbated by exposure to cold and often resolves completely with the cessation of oxaliplatin. However, the full spectrum of neurotoxicity related to oxaliplatin is not yet known as it is a relatively new agent. A recent phase 1 study in children with refractory solid tumors reported sensory neuropathy, pharyngolaryngeal dysesthesia, and ataxia [56]. Although reversible, the sensory neuropathy associated with oxaliplatin is often disabling and represents the dose-limiting toxicity in many studies. For this reason, multiple neuroprotective agents have been tried to prevent the oxaliplatin neurotoxicity including alpha-lipoic acid, amifostine, calcium and magnesium supplements, carbamazepine, and glutathione [57]. All these agents have shown some degree of protection; however, the significant methodologic inconsistencies across studies preclude comparison.

TAXANES

The two taxanes widely used in cancer therapy are paclitaxel and docetaxel. Paclitaxel induces polymerization and stabilization of microtubules, subsequently preventing the cell from completing cell division and leading to cell death. Paclitaxel is widely used in the management of lung, breast, ovarian, and head and neck cancers. Docetaxel is a semisynthetic analogue of paclitaxel that is also used for lung and ovarian cancer. The mechanism by which taxanes causes neuropathy is not known, but it may be via disruption of axonal transport via impaired microtubule function, similar to vincristine. However, it is unclear if the primary site of toxicity is the cell body (neuronopathy) or the axon (axonopathy). In experimental models, paclitaxel accumulates preferentially in the dorsal root ganglia and fast axonal transport is blocked, suggesting contributions from both mechanisms [58,59].

Neuropathy is one of the most common side effects of paclitaxel. The neuropathy is predominantly sensory and can develop as early as 48 hours after treatment. Initial symptoms are length-dependent paresthesias with impaired VPT. Motor signs are mild, but with higher doses per cycle (250 mg/m^2), patients may develop decreased hand grip strength and thumb weakness. High doses are also associated with loss of deep tendon reflexes. Myalgia and arthralgia occur temporarily after therapy, especially with higher doses, possibly due to motor neuropathy [60,61]. A clear correlation exists between neuropathic signs and symptoms and cumulative dose or dose intensity per course. Neuropathy is the major dose-limiting toxicity with 250 to 300 mg/m^2 per course or after a cumulative dose of 1400 mg/m^2 [62]. Infusion time may also influence side effects, with rapid infusions more likely to result in neurotoxicity.

Electrophysiologic studies show reduction of sensory nerve action potentials in large fibers more than small fibers in a symmetric, distal, length-dependent fashion. Sural sensory nerve action potentials are nearly always reduced or absent in symptomatic patients. Abnormal peroneal motor action potentials, median and ulnar nerve conduction velocities, tibial motor nerve conduction velocity, and denervation on needle examination have all been described [60]. A sural nerve biopsy in a symptomatic patient revealed fiber loss, lack of axonal sprouting, and axonal atrophy associated with secondary demyelination and remyelination [63].

Autonomic neuropathy has also been observed with doses above 170 to 250 mg/m^2 [64]. Perioral numbness and optic nerve toxicity have been reported with dosages between 175 and 225 mg/m^2 and high-dose paclitaxel can result in bilateral facial nerve palsy [65]. Paclitaxel toxicity rarely involves the CNS; however, seizures and acute encephalopathy have been reported after high-dose infusions [66].

After discontinuation of therapy, neuropathic signs usually resolve; however, this may take months and permanent neuropathy has been reported. In some patients, neuropathy may progress for 1 to 3 weeks after the end of treatment. Several agents have been tested to reduce paclitaxel-induced neuropathy, including recombinant human leukemia inhibitory factor (rhu-LIF), acetyl-L-carnitine, amifostine, glutamine, and vitamin E [67–71]. Amifostine showed benefit in two different randomized controlled trials, but did not in another two [57]. There were encouraging results with acetyl-L-carnitine with improvement in sensory and motor measures; however, this was a nonrandomized small trial that needs to be confirmed [69].

Like paclitaxel, docetaxel is a potent inhibitor of cell replication via disruption of microtubule assembly. Neuropathy resulting from docetaxel is generally mild to moderate presenting with paresthesias, loss of deep tendon reflexes, and decreased VPT after high doses. However, it can be a dose-limiting toxicity [72]. Docetaxel-related neuropathy is more likely to occur if patients have been previously exposed to neuropathic chemotherapies or receive a high cumulative dose, a single high dose, or rapid infusion. Hilkens *et al.* [73] reported a predominantly sensory neuropathy in half the patients treated with a 1-hour infusion of docetaxel 100 mg/m^2 once every 21 days. Paresthesias, pain, numbness, unsteady gait, positive Lhermitte's sign, and loss of both ankle and patellar reflexes were found. Patients can become symptomatic over a wide range of cumulative doses (50–720 mg/m^2) and dose levels (10–115 mg/m^2); however, more severe clinical and electrophysiologic abnormalities were noted at cumulative doses greater than 400 mg/m^2 [74].

The most common abnormalities on electrophysiologic examination are low-amplitude motor and sensory potentials, moderately slow motor conduction velocities (peroneal and tibial), and absent sural sensory nerve potentials. A superficial peroneal nerve biopsy showed loss of large myelinated fibers and occasional axonal degeneration. The neuropathy generally improves once therapy is stopped; however, off-therapy deterioration has been observed [73].

ADDITIONAL AGENTS COMMONLY ASSOCIATED WITH PNS TOXICITY

Procarbazine is an alkylating agent commonly used for hematologic malignancies and some primary brain cancers. Peripheral neuropathy presenting as paresthesias and decreased tendon reflexes occurs in 10% to 20% of patients. Ataxia, orthostatic hypotension, and weakness of intrinsic hand muscles are additional recognized findings. Procarbazine is also associated with CNS side effects such as encephalopathy that may range from mild drowsiness to confusion to stupor [75]. Finally, optic neuroretinitis has been reported [76].

Cytarabine (cytosine arabinoside, Ara-C) is an antimetabolite used most frequently in the treatment of leukemia and non-Hodgkin's lymphoma. It has been associated with sporadic cases of painful sensory peripheral neuropathy, particularly when used in combination therapy [77]. Although relatively rare, cytarabine neuropathy can be irreversible. In a case of severe neuropathy, axonal degeneration and scattered destruction of myelin was observed [78]. Brachial plexus neuropathy and Horner's syndrome have also been associated with cytarabine therapy [79].

High-dose cytarabine is most commonly associated with CNS toxicities such as severe ataxia and encephalopathy [80,81]. This often correlates with cerebellar atrophy and white matter abnormalities on computed tomography (CT) or magnetic resonance imaging (MRI). In at least one case of acute cerebellar toxicity from cytarabine, flushing of the cerebrospinal fluid resulted in clinical improvement, implicating high CNS concentrations after systemic dosing [82]. Intrathecal cytarabine is used for leptomeningeal carcinomatosis. In this setting, aseptic meningitis and myelopathy may occur. Less often, intrathecal cytarabine can result in seizures or subacute encephalopathy.

Nelarabine is a recently approved purine nucleoside that is a pro-drug to arabinosylguanine (ara-G). It induces cell arrest in the S phase, leading to apoptosis, and is used predominantly to treat relapsed acute T-cell lymphoblastic leukemias and lymphomas. In the trials considered for regulatory approval, neurologic toxicity (both CNS and PNS) was the dose-limiting toxicity in both adults and children [83]. Although there is relatively little experience with this agent to date, it appears to have multiple neurotoxicities, including peripheral neuropathy, headache, seizures, and encephalopathy. Roughly 21% of adult patients and 16% of pediatric patients develop a dose-limiting PNS toxicity, most commonly length-dependent paresthesias. Nelarabine is also associated with proximal muscle weakness. Moreover, the neuropathic symptoms may not resolve after discontinuation of the drug [84]. At high doses, a fulminant neurologic presentation including ascending paralysis, myoclonus, and seizures has been reported [84]. A related agent, gemcitabine, is also associated with peripheral neuropathy in roughly 20% of patients [85]. However, gemcitabine is often combined with other neurotoxic agents such as cisplatin and paclitaxel; hence, it may be difficult to capture the true incidence of gemcitabine-specific neurotoxicity.

Etoposide (VP-16) is a semisynthetic derivative of podophyllotoxin with established antineoplastic activity. Sensory neuropathy has been recognized in patients receiving intensive therapy with etoposide and melphalan in roughly 1% to 2% of patients [86]. When etoposide is administered at higher doses, headache, seizures, and somnolence can occur. A related compound, teniposide (VM-26), has not been clearly associated with either PNS or CNS neurotoxicity.

CYTOSTATIC AND TARGETED THERAPIES

Bortezomib is a proteosome inhibitor that has recently been approved for recurrent multiple myeloma. Although clinical experience with this agent is limited, it has been associated with sensory neuropathy in up to 56% of patients and thus far is the drug's dose-limiting toxicity [87]. Moreover, in 30% of those patients, the neuropathy appears to be irreversible.

Thalidomide is an immunomodulatory drug that was approved for multiple myeloma in 2006. It is also increasingly being investigated in combination regimens for solid tumors based on its antiangiogenic properties. Thalidomide is associated with a sensory more than motor neuropathy and presents most commonly with painful paresthesias that can be severe and are a common reason for stopping therapy [88]. This may occur in as many

as 25% to 81% of patients and there is a clear association between dose and severity of neuropathy [89]. Duration of therapy also predicts development of neuropathy. Sural nerve biopsies show loss of myelinated fibers and evidence of Wallerian degeneration [88]. Upon discontinuation of the drug, the neuropathy tends to improve; however, it can be chronic.

CENTRAL NERVOUS SYSTEM TOXICITIES

CNS toxicity can manifest as a broad complex of symptoms ranging from headache to overt leukoencephalopathy (white matter disease presenting with altered mental status and focal neurologic deficits). Some chemotherapeutic agents, such as methotrexate, ifosfamide, and cytarabine, have been specifically linked with short-term and-long term CNS toxicity. However, many agents in current use can cause acute CNS disease [90]. In addition to acute CNS toxicity, there is growing recognition of the subtle and often long-term impact of various chemotherapy regimens on cognition both in adults and children.

ACUTE CNS TOXICITY

Methotrexate is an antimetabolite in wide use for both hematologic malignancies and solid tumors. It is known for its CNS neurotoxic effects, which are categorized into immediate, acute, subacute, and chronic neurologic syndromes. The route, schedule, and dose of methotrexate as well as concomitant therapies appear to affect the severity of neurologic manifestations. However, great variability exists. For example, high-dose systemic methotrexate given with or after brain radiation is associated with subacute to chronic disseminated leukoencephalopathy that can have areas of necrosis (necrotizing leukoencephalopathy), manifested by symptoms of a progressive dementia and focal neurologic deficits [91,92]. In contrast, high-dose systemic methotrexate monotherapy has far less frequent associations with leukoencephalopathy [93]. However, encephalopathy with somnolence, confusion, and focal neurologic deficits has been reported after a single IV dose of methotrexate [94,95].

Neurologic deficits that occur in the first 10 to 14 days may be due to a white matter edematous process similar to that seen with re versible posterior leukoencephalopathy syndrome (RPLS) or to stroke-like episodes with evidence of restricted diffusion on diffusion-weighted MRI [96,97]. However, immediate and acute methotrexate-related toxicity may be asymptomatic and noted on imaging only. For example, up to 40% of children receiving IV and intrathecal methotrexate have radiographically defined leukoencephalopathy (diffuse white matter changes); however, long-term clinical neurologic injury is far less common [98,99] The highest risk for long-term encephalopathy is associated with multiple intrathecal or high-dose IV methotrexate infusions, increased age, and the combination of radiotherapy and subsequent methotrexate therapy. Imaging features include predominantly deep white matter hyperintensities, but may have contrast-enhancing areas consistent with necrosis [100].

The exact mechanism of methotrexate-induced encephalopathy is not known. Animal models investigating systemically delivered methotrexate have shown preferential toxicity to the Alzheimer type II astrocytes, which may be reversible with limited exposure but permanent with high-dose repeated therapy [101]. After intrathecal delivery of methotrexate in cats, there is targeted injury to the axons as well as fibrin deposition in vessels [102]. Therapeutic interventions with IV leucovorin, high-dose steroids, and cerebrospinal fluid flushing have had mixed results and there is no definitive therapy to date [103]. Autopsy studies in adults with clinical evidence of leukoencephalopathy given high-dose methotrexate for primary CNS lymphoma showed no evidence of active lymphoma, but gliosis, spongiosis, and both myelin and axonal injury [104]. Interestingly, fibrinoid necrosis of vessels as well as notable atherosclerosis of the major intracranial vessels was also seen, supporting the observations in animal studies and suggesting at least a partial vascular etiology.

Intrathecal methotrexate is often used in pediatric and adult patients for CNS prophylaxis in acute hematologic malignancies and occasionally in the management of leptomeningeal carcinomatosis. Intrathecal methotrexate has been associated with aseptic meningitis and acute encephalopathy with stroke-like episodes; rarely, paraplegia with spinal cord necrosis or anterior lumbosacral radiculopathy has been described [105–107]. Finally, a rare but notable complication of methotrexate therapy occurs with inadvertent intraparenchymal delivery. In select cases in which the catheter tip from an Ommaya reservoir is misplaced to the parenchyma, there can be focal leukoencephalopathy associated with mass effect and contrast enhancement on imaging associated with focal neurologic deficits and increased intracranial pressure [108,109].

Ifosfamide may cause acute (but usually reversible) encephalopathy with cerebellar dysfunction, extrapyramidal signs, hallucinations, seizures, delirium, and coma. These effects may begin within hours of administration or may be delayed up to 6 days after treatment. Severe painful axonal peripheral neuropathy associated with high-dose ifosfamide has also been described [110].

Interferon is used most often in the treatment of hairy cell leukemia; however, it has more recently been applied to a variety of solid tumors such as melanoma and renal cell carcinoma. It is associated with both CNS and PNS toxicities, although the CNS toxicities are most prevalent. A broad range of CNS toxicities has been reported including headache, anxiety and depression, extreme fatigue, tremor, akathisia, confusion, and somnolence [111–113]. There may also be transient brain lesions manifesting on MRI as distinct hyperintensities [114]. PNS toxicities include polyneuropathy, neuralgic amyotrophy, myalgia, and bilateral oculomotor nerve paralysis. Auditory impairment (tinnitus, hearing loss, or both) was found in 45% of patients receiving long-term treatment with interferon. Audiometry-documented sensorineural hearing loss was found in approximately one third of patients.

Three purine analogues—fludarabine, cladribine, and pentostatin—can produce severe, predominantly CNS toxicity with high-dose therapy (delayed progressive encephalopathy with cortical blindness, dementia, coma). Even with standard therapy, there may be transient CNS toxicity with altered mental status as well as peripheral neuropathy [115]. Fludarabine has also been associated with progressive multifocal leukoencephalopathy [116,117].

The immunosuppressants cyclosporine and tacrolimus (FK 506) are most notable for their association with RPLS, discussed below in greater detail. Cyclosporine has also been reported to cause tremor, seizures, ataxia, paraparesis, quadriparesis, and psychological disorders in addition to leukoencephalopathy. There has also been a case of recurrent acute inflammatory demyelinating polyradiculopathy, possibly related to cyclosporine therapy. All of these agents have potential to cause both motor and sensorimotor neuropathy.

Histone deacetylase inhibitors such as valproic acid and novel agents such as MS-275 are under increasing clinical investigation for a variety of hematologic and solid tumors. With both of these agents, CNS toxicity manifests predominantly as confusion, mood alteration, and somnolence [118,119].

REVERSIBLE POSTERIOR LEUKOENCEPHALOPATHY SYNDROME

RPLS is defined as a syndrome of headache, visual abnormalities, variable degrees of altered mental status, and seizures. It has characteristic features on MRI including symmetric T2 hyperintensity generally limited to the white matter in bilateral occipital and parietal lobes [120]. As the name implies, it is often reversible with removal of the offending agent and supportive care; however, this is not always the case [121]. Agents that have been associated with RPLS include cisplatin, gemcitabine, cyclosporine and tacrolimus, cytarabine, rituximab, bevacizumab, and sorafenib as well as supportive medications such as granulocyte colony-stimulating factor and erythropoietin [90,122–127]. The exact pathophysiology of RPLS is not known; however, it is presumed to be due to vasculopathy and endothelial dysfunction. Aggressive management of blood pressure is an important intervention as is management of seizures and prompt discontinuation of any suspected agents. Although this syndrome is relatively rare, it is important to recognize it early as appropriate management can result in complete resolution of neurologic symptoms.

CHEMOTHERAPY AND GENERALIZED COGNITIVE DYSFUNCTION

There is increasing concern both by patients and their oncologists about the subtle and possibly long-term cognitive effects of chemotherapy. This condition has been nicknamed "chemo-brain" in the popular press and is characterized by a wide array of neurocognitive difficulties such as impaired concentration, short-term memory, and executive function [128]. The condition was first recognized in breast cancer patients who were found to have a frequency of cognitive dysfunction ranging from 25% to 40% with formal neuropsychiatric testing [129–131]. Neither a standard phenotype of cognitive dysfunction nor the exact etiology has been defined. Early studies did not include prechemotherapy assessments and did not uniformly account for confounding variables such as depression or concomitant therapies.

More recent studies have prospectively evaluated breast cancer patients from the time of diagnosis through acute therapy and then follow-up. Initial results suggest that some degree of cognitive dysfunction at baseline exists that is often exacerbated by various chemotherapies but possibly improves with treatment of the cancer. The chronic effects of chemotherapy on cognition are increasingly recognized and currently under investigation [130]. As therapies become increasingly successful in providing long-term survival, the neurologic injury related to these agents may become more apparent and strategies for minimizing such injury will need to be developed.

REFERENCES

1. Postma TJ, Heimans JJ, Muller MJ, *et al.*: Pitfalls in grading severity of chemotherapy-induced peripheral neuropathy. *Ann Oncol* 1998, 9:739–744.

2. Fleming GF, Brunetto VL, Cella D, *et al.*: Phase III trial of doxorubicin plus cisplatin with or without paclitaxel plus filgrastim in advanced endometrial carcinoma: a Gynecologic Oncology Group Study. *J Clin Oncol* 2004, 22:2159–2166.

3. Baas P, Boogerd W, Dalesio O, *et al.*: Thalidomide in patients with malignant pleural mesothelioma. *Lung Cancer* 2005, 48:291–296.

4. Cavaletti G, Bogliun G, Marzorati L, *et al.*: Grading of chemotherapy-induced peripheral neurotoxicity using the Total Neuropathy Scale. *Neurology* 2003, 61:1297–1300.

5. Cavaletti G, Jann S, Pace A, *et al.*: Multi-center assessment of the Total Neuropathy Score for chemotherapy-induced peripheral neurotoxicity. *J Peripher Nerv Syst* 2006, 11:135–141.

6. Sahenk Z, Brady ST, Mendell JR: Studies on the pathogenesis of vincristine-induced neuropathy. *Muscle Nerve* 1987, 10:80–84.

7. Tanner KD, Levine JD, Topp KS: Microtubule disorientation and axonal swelling in unmyelinated sensory axons during vincristine-induced painful neuropathy in rat. *J Comp Neurol* 1998, 395:481–492.

8. Casey EB, Jellife AM, Le Quesne PM, Millett YL: Vincristine neuropathy. Clinical and electrophysiological observations. *Brain* 1973, 96:69–86.

9. Pal PK: Clinical and electrophysiological studies in vincristine induced neuropathy. *Electromyogr Clin Neurophysiol* 1999, 39:323–330.

10. Verstappen CC, Koeppen S, Heimans JJ, *et al.*: Dose-related vincristine-induced peripheral neuropathy with unexpected off-therapy worsening. *Neurology* 2005, 64:1076–1077.

11. Ja'afer FM, Hamdan FB, Mohammed FH: Vincristine-induced neuropathy in rat: electrophysiological and histological study. *Exp Brain Res* 2006, 17:334–345.

12. Levitt LP, Prager D: Mononeuropathy due to vincristine toxicity. *Neurology* 1975, 25:894–895.

13. Toker E, Yenice O, Ogut MS: Isolated abducens nerve palsy induced by vincristine therapy. *J AAPOS* 2004, 8:69–71.

14. Ozyurek H, Turker H, Akbalik M, *et al.*: Pyridoxine and pyridostigmine treatment in vincristine-induced neuropathy. *Pediatr Hematol Oncol* 2007, 24:447–452.

15. Weisfeld-Adams JD, Dutton GN, Murphy DM: Vincristine sulfate as a possible cause of optic neuropathy. *Pediatr Blood Cancer* 2007 48:238–240.

16. Kaufman IA, Kung FH, Koenig HM, Giammona ST: Overdosage with vincristine. *J Pediatr* 1976, 89:671–674.

17. Dettmeyer R, Driever F, Becker A, *et al.*: Fatal myeloencephalopathy due to accidental intrathecal vincristine administration: a report of two cases. *Forensic Sci Int* 2001, 122:60–64.

18. Alcaraz A, Rey C, Concha A, Medina A: Intrathecal vincristine: fatal myeloencephalopathy despite cerebrospinal fluid perfusion. *J Toxicol Clin Toxicol* 2002, 40:557–561.

19. Qweider M, Gilsbach JM, Rohde V: Inadvertent intrathecal vincristine administration: a neurosurgical emergency. Case report. *J Neurosurg Spine* 2007, 6:280–283.

20. Hildebrandt G, Holler E, Woenkhaus M, *et al.*: Acute deterioration of Charcot-Marie-Tooth disease IA (CMT IA) following 2 mg of vincristine chemotherapy. *Ann Oncol* 2000, 11:743–747.

21. Chauvenet AR, Shashi V, Selsky C, *et al.*: Vincristine-induced neuropathy as the initial presentation of Charcot-Marie-Tooth disease in acute lymphoblastic leukemia: a Pediatric Oncology Group study. *J Pediatr Hematol Oncol* 2003, 25:316–320.

22. Bermudez M, Fuster JL, Llinares E, *et al.*: Itraconazole-related increased vincristine neurotoxicity: case report and review of literature. *J Pediatr Hematol Oncol* 2005, 27:389–392.

23. Postma TJ, Benard BA, Huijgens PC, *et al.*: Long-term effects of vincristine on the peripheral nervous system. *J Neurooncol* 1993, 15:23–27.

24. Di Gregorio F, Favaro G, Panozzo C, Fiori MG: Efficacy of ganglioside treatment in reducing functional alterations induced by vincristine in rabbit peripheral nerves. *Cancer Chemother Pharmacol* 1990, 26:31–36.

25. Boyle FM, Wheeler HR, Shenfield GM: Glutamate ameliorates experimental vincristine neuropathy. *J Pharmacol Exp Ther* 1996, 279:410–415.

26. Kiburg B, Moorer-van Delft C, Heimans JJ, *et al.*: In vivo modulation of vincristine-induced neurotoxicity in Lymnaea stagnalis, by the ACTH(4-9) analogue Org 2766. *J Neurooncol* 1996, 30:173–180.

27. van Kooten B, van Diemen HA, Groenhout KM, *et al.*: A pilot study on the influence of a corticotropin (4-9) analogue on vinca alkaloid-induced neuropathy. *Arch Neurol* 1992, 49:1027–1031.

28. Koeppen S, Verstappen CC, Korte R, *et al.*: Lack of neuroprotection by an ACTH (4-9) analogue. A randomized trial in patients treated with vincristine for Hodgkin's or non-Hodgkin's lymphoma. *J Cancer Res Clin Oncol* 2004, 130:153–160.

29. Willemse PH, van Lith J, Mulder NH, *et al.*: Risks and benefits of cisplatin in ovarian cancer: a quality-adjusted survival analysis. *Eur J Cancer* 1990, 26:345–352.

30. Krarup-Hansen A, Helweg-Larsen S, Schmalbruch H, *et al.*: Neuronal involvement in cisplatin neuropathy: prospective clinical and neurophysiological studies. *Brain* 2007, 130:1076–1088.

31. Gregg RW, Molepo JM, Monpetit VJA, *et al.*: Cisplatin neurotoxicity: the relationship between dosage, time, and platinum concentration in neurologic tissues, and morphologic evidence of toxicity. *J Clin Oncol* 1992, 10:795–803.

32. Meijer C, de Vries EG, Marmiroli P, *et al.*: Cisplatin-induced DNA-platination in experimental dorsal root ganglia neuronopathy. *Neurotoxicology* 1999, 20:883–887.

33. Visovsky C: Chemotherapy-induced peripheral neuropathy. *Cancer Invest* 2003, 21:439–451.

34. Cavaletti G, Marzorati L, Bogliun G, *et al.*: Cisplatin-induced peripheral neurotoxicity is dependent on total-dose intensity and single-dose intensity. *Cancer* 1992, 69:203–207.

35. Bacon M, James K, Zee B: A comparison of the incidence, duration, and degree of the neurologic toxicities of cisplatin-paclitaxel (PT) and cisplatin-cyclophosphamide (PC). *Int J Gynecol Cancer* 2003, 13:428–434.

36. Pomes A, Frustaci S, Cattaino G, *et al.*: Local neurotoxicity of cisplatin after intra-arterial chemotherapy. *Acta Neurol Scand* 1986, 73:302–303.

37. Dropcho EJ, Rosenfeld SS, Vitek J, *et al.*: Phase II study of intracarotid or selective intracerebral infusion of cisplatin for treatment of recurrent anaplastic gliomas. *J Neurooncol* 1998, 36:191–198.

38. Kahn CE Jr, Messersmith RN, Samuels BL: Brachial plexopathy as a complication of intraarterial cisplatin chemotherapy. *Cardiovasc Intervent Radiol* 1989, 12:47–49.

39. Verschraegen C, Conrad CA, Hong WK: Subacute encephalopathic toxicity of cisplatin. *Lung Cancer* 1995, 13:305–309.

40. Gonzalez F, Menendez D, Gomez-Ulla F: Monocular visual loss in a patient undergoing cisplatin chemotherapy. *Int Ophthalmol* 2001, 24:301–304.

41. Dietrich J, Marienhagen J, Schalke B, *et al.*: Vascular neurotoxicity following chemotherapy with cisplatin, ifosfamide, and etoposide. *Ann Pharmacother* 2004, 38:242–246.

42. Manchana T, Sirisabya N, Lertkhachonsuk R, Tresukosol D: Transient cortical blindness during chemotherapy (PVB) for ovarian germ cell tumor. *J Med Assoc Thai* 2006, 89:1265–1268.

43. Kemp G, Rose P, Lurain J, *et al.*: Amifostine pretreatment for protection against cyclophosphamide-induced and cisplatin-induced toxicities: results of a randomized control trial in patients with advanced ovarian cancer. *J Clin Oncol* 1996, 14:2101–2112.

44. Gradishar WJ, Stephenson P, Glover DJ, *et al.*: A phase II trial of cisplatin plus WR-2721 (amifostine) for metastatic breast carcinoma: an Eastern Cooperative Oncology Group Study (E8188). *Cancer* 2001, 92:2517–2522.

45. Moore DH, Donnelly J, McGuire WP, *et al.*: Limited access trial using amifostine for protection against cisplatin- and three-hour paclitaxel-induced neurotoxicity: a phase II study of the Gynecologic Oncology Group. *J Clin Oncol* 2003, 21:4207–4213.

46. Tredici G, Cavaletti G, Petruccioli MG, *et al.*: Low-dose glutathione administration in the prevention of cisplatin-induced peripheral neuropathy in rats. *Neurotoxicology* 1994, 15:701–704.

47. Cascinu S, Cordella L, Del Ferro E, *et al.*: Neuroprotective effect of reduced glutathione on cisplatin-based chemotherapy in advanced gastric cancer: a randomized double-blind placebo-controlled trial. *J Clin Oncol* 1995, 13:26–32.

48. Bogliun G, Marzorati L, Marzola M, *et al.*: Neurotoxicity of cisplatin +/- reduced glutathione in the first-line treatment of advanced ovarian cancer. *Int J Gynecol Cancer* 1996, 6:415–419.

49. van der Hoop RG, Vecht CJ, van der Burg ME, *et al.*: Prevention of cisplatin neurotoxicity with an ACTH(4-9) analogue in patients with ovarian cancer. *N Engl J Med* 1990, 322:89–94.

50. Roberts JA, Jenison EL, Kim K, *et al.*: A randomized, multicenter, double-blind, placebo-controlled, dose-finding study of ORG 2766 in the prevention or delay of cisplatin-induced neuropathies in women with ovarian cancer. *Gynecol Oncol* 1997, 67:172–177.

51. Heinzlef O, Lotz J-P, Roullet E: Severe neuropathy after high dose carboplatin in three patients receiving multidrug chemotherapy. *J Neurol Neurosurg Psychiatry* 1998, 64:667–669.

52. Walker RW, Rosenblum MK, Kempin SJ, Christian MC: Carboplatin-associated thrombotic microangiopathic hemolytic anemia. *Cancer* 1989, 64:1017–1020.

53. Watanabe W, Kuwabara R, Nakahara T, *et al.*: Severe ocular and orbital toxicity after intracarotid injection of carboplatin for recurrent glioblastomas. *Graefes Arch Clin Exp Ophthalmol* 2002, 240:1033–1035.

54. Downs LS Jr, Judson PL, Argenta PA, *et al.*: A phase I study of ifosfamide, paclitaxel, and carboplatin in advanced and recurrent cervical cancer. *Gynecol Oncol* 2004, 95:347–351.

55. Grothey A: Oxaliplatin-safety profile: neurotoxicity. *Semin Oncol* 2003, 30:5–13.

56. Spunt SL, Freeman BB, Billups CA, *et al.*: Phase I clinical trial of oxaliplatin in children and adolescents with refractory solid tumors. *J Clin Oncol* 2007, 25:2274–2280.

57. Wilkes G: Peripheral neuropathy related to chemotherapy. *Semin Oncol Nurs* 2007, 23:162–173.

58. Nakata T, Yorifuji H: Morphological evidence of the inhibitory effect of Taxol on the fast axonal transport. *Neurosci Res* 1999, 35:113–122.

59. Cavaletti G, Cavalletti E, Oggioni N, *et al.*: Distribution of paclitaxel within the nervous system of the rat after repeated intravenous administration. *Neurotoxicology* 2000, 21:389–393.

60. Chaudhry V, Rowinsky EK, Sartorius SE, *et al.*: Peripheral neuropathy from Taxol and cisplatin combination chemotherapy: clinical and electrophysiological studies. *Ann Neurol* 1994, 35:304–311.

61. Freilich RJ, Balmaceda C, Seidman AD, *et al.*: Motor neuropathy due to docetaxel and paclitaxel. *Neurology* 1996, 47:115–118.

62. Postma TJ, Vermorken JB, Liefting AJ, *et al.*: Paclitaxel-induced neuropathy. *Ann Oncol* 1995, 6:489–494.

63. Sahenk Z, Barohn R, New P, Mendell JR: Taxol neuropathy. Electrodiagnostic and sural nerve biopsy findings. *Arch Neurol* 1994, 51:726–729.

64. Jerian SM, Sarosy GA, Link CJ, *et al.*: Incapacitating autonomic neuropathy precipitated by Taxol. *Gynecol Oncol* 1993, 51:277–280.

65. Lee RT, Oster MW, Balmaceda C, *et al.*: Bilateral facial nerve palsy secondary to the administration of high-dose paclitaxel. *Ann Oncol* 1999, 10:1245–1247.

66. Nieto Y, Cagnoni PJ, Bearman SI, *et al.*: Acute encephalopathy: a new toxicity associated with high-dose paclitaxel. *Clin Cancer Res* 1999, 5:501–506.

67. Vahdat L, Papadopoulos K, Lange D, *et al.*: Reduction of paclitaxel-induced peripheral neuropathy with glutamine. *Clin Cancer Res* 2001, 7:1192–1197.

68. Argyriou AA, Polychronopoulos P, Iconomou G, *et al.*: Paclitaxel plus carboplatin-induced peripheral neuropathy. A prospective clinical and electrophysiological study in patients suffering from solid malignancies. *J Neurol* 2005, 252:1459–1464.

69. Bianchi G, Vitali G, Caraceni A, *et al.*: Symptomatic and neurophysiological responses of paclitaxel- or cisplatin-induced neuropathy to oral acetyl-L-carnitine. *Eur J Cancer* 2005, 41:1746–1750.

70. Davis ID, Kiers L, MacGregor L, *et al.*: A randomized, double-blinded, placebo-controlled phase II trial of recombinant human leukemia inhibitory factor (rhuLIF, emfilermin, AM424) to prevent chemotherapy-induced peripheral neuropathy. *Clin Cancer Res* 2005, 11:1890–1898.

71. Hilpert F, Stahle A, Tome O, *et al.*: Neuroprotection with amifostine in the first-line treatment of advanced ovarian cancer with carboplatin/paclitaxel-based chemotherapy--a double-blind, placebo-controlled, randomized phase II study from the Arbeitsgemeinschaft Gynakologische Onkologoie (AGO) Ovarian Cancer Study Group. *Support Care Cancer* 2005, 13:797–805.

72. Zwerdling T, Krailo M, Monteleone P, *et al.*: Phase II investigation of docetaxel in pediatric patients with recurrent solid tumors: a report from the Children's Oncology Group. *Cancer* 2006, 106:1821–1828.

73. Hilkens PH, Verweij J, Stoter G, *et al.*: Peripheral neurotoxicity induced by docetaxel. *Neurology* 1996, 46:104–108.

74. New PZ, Jackson CE, Rinaldi D, *et al.*: Peripheral neuropathy secondary to docetaxel (Taxotere). *Neurology* 1996, 46:108–111.

75. Postma TJ, van Groeningen CJ, Witjes RJ, *et al.*: Neurotoxicity of combination chemotherapy with procarbazine, CCNU and vincristine (PCV) for recurrent glioma. *J Neurooncol* 1998, 38:69–75.

76. Lennan RM, Taylor HR: Optic neuroretinitis in association with BCNU and procarbazine therapy. *Med Pediatr Oncol* 1978, 4:43–48.

77. Powell BL, Capizzi RL, Lyerly ES, Cooper MR: Peripheral neuropathy after high-dose cytosine arabinoside, daunorubicin, and asparaginase consolidation for acute nonlymphocytic leukemia. *J Clin Oncol* 1986, 4:95–97.

78. Borgeat A, De Muralt B, Stalder M: Peripheral neuropathy associated with high-dose Ara-C therapy. *Cancer* 1986, 58:852–854.

79. Nevill TJ, Benstead TJ, McCormick CW, Hayne OA: Horner's syndrome and demyelinating peripheral neuropathy caused by high-dose cytosine arabinoside. *Am J Hematol* 1989, 32:314–315.

80. Lazarus HM, Herzig RH, Herzig GP, *et al.*: Central nervous system toxicity of high-dose systemic cytosine arabinoside. *Cancer* 1981, 48:2577–2582.

81. Herzig RH, Herzig GP, Wolff SN, *et al.*: Central nervous system effects of high-dose cytosine arabinoside. *Semin Oncol* 1987, 14:21–24.

82. Pellier I, Leboucher B, Rachieru P, *et al.*: Flushing out of cerebrospinal fluid as a therapy for acute cerebellar dysfunction caused by high dose of cytosine arabinoside: a case report. *J Pediatr Hematol Oncol* 2006, 28:837–839.

83. Cohen MH, Johnson JR, Massie T, *et al.*: Approval summary: nelarabine for the treatment of T-cell lymphoblastic leukemia/lymphoma. *Clin Cancer Res* 2006, 12:5329–5335.

84. Kurtzberg J, Ernst TJ, Keating MJ, *et al.*: Phase I study of 506U78 administered on a consecutive 5-day schedule in children and adults with refractory hematologic malignancies. *J Clin Oncol* 2005, 23:3396–3403.

85. Masters GA, Declerck L, Blanke C, *et al.*: Phase II trial of gemcitabine in refractory or relapsed small-cell lung cancer: Eastern Cooperative Oncology Group Trial 1597. *J Clin Oncol* 2003, 21:1550–1555.

86. Imrie KR, Couture F, Turner CC, *et al.*: Peripheral neuropathy following high-dose etoposide and autologous bone marrow transplantation. *Bone Marrow Transplant* 1994, 13:77–79.

87. Badros A, Goloubeva O, Dalal JS, *et al.*: Neurotoxicity of bortezomib therapy in multiple myeloma: a single-center experience and review of the literature. *Cancer* 2007, 110:1042–1049.

88. Chaudhry V, Cornblath DR, Corse A, *et al.*: Thalidomide-induced neuropathy. *Neurology* 2002, 59:1872–1875.

89. Mileshkin L, Stark R, Day B, *et al.*: Development of neuropathy in patients with myeloma treated with thalidomide: patterns of occurrence and the role of electrophysiologic monitoring. *J Clin Oncol* 2006, 24:4507–4514.

90. Norden AD, Batchelor TT: Reversible posterior leukoencephalopathy syndrome. *Onkologie* 2007, 30:90–91.

91. Sakamaki H, Onozawa Y, Yano Y, *et al.*: Disseminated necrotizing leukoencephalopathy following irradiation and methotrexate therapy for central nervous system infiltration of leukemia and lymphoma. *Radiat Med* 1993, 11:146–153.

92. Fernandez-Bouzas A, Ramirez Jiminez H, Vazquez Zamudio J, *et al.*: Brain calcifications and dementia in children treated with radiotherapy and intrathecal methotrexate. *J Neurosurg Sci* 1992, 36:211–214.

93. Batchelor T, Loeffler JS: Primary CNS lymphoma. *J Clin Oncol* 2006, 24:1281–1288.

94. Kubo M, Azuma E, Arai S, *et al.*: Transient encephalopathy following a single exposure of high-dose methotrexate in a child with acute lymphoblastic leukemia. *Pediatr Hematol Oncol* 1992, 9:157–165.

95. Valik D, Sterba J, Bajciova V, Demlova R: Severe encephalopathy induced by the first but not the second course of high-dose methotrexate mirrored by plasma homocysteine elevations and preceded by extreme differences in pretreatment plasma folate. *Oncology* 2005, 69:269–272.

96. Rollins N, Winick N, Bash R, Booth T: Acute methotrexate neurotoxicity: findings on diffusion-weighted imaging and correlation with clinical outcome. *AJNR Am J Neuroradiol* 2004, 25:1688–1695.

97. Eichler AF, Batchelor TT, Henson JW: Diffusion and perfusion imaging in subacute neurotoxicity following high-dose intravenous methotrexate. *Neuro Oncol* 2007, 9:373–377.

98. Asato R, Akiyama Y, Ito M, *et al.*: Nuclear magnetic resonance abnormalities of the cerebral white matter in children with acute lymphoblastic leukemia and malignant lymphoma during and after central nervous system prophylactic treatment with intrathecal methotrexate. *Cancer* 1992, 70:1997–2004.

99. Shuper A, Stark B, Kornreich L, *et al.*: Methotrexate-related neurotoxicity in the treatment of childhood acute lymphoblastic leukemia. *Isr Med Assoc J* 2002, 4:1050–1053.

100. Ziereisen F, Dan B, Azzi N, *et al.*: Reversible acute methotrexate leukoencephalopathy: atypical brain MR imaging features. *Pediatr Radiol* 2006, 36:205–212.

101. Gregorios JB, Gregorios AB, Mora J, *et al.*: Morphologic alterations in rat brain following systemic and intraventricular methotrexate injection: light and electron microscopic studies. *J Neuropathol Exp Neurol* 1989, 48:33–47.

102. Shibutani M, Okeda R: Experimental study on subacute neurotoxicity of methotrexate in cats. *Acta Neuropathol (Berl)* 1989, 78:291–300.

103. Jaksic W, Veljkovic D, Pozza C, Lewis I: Methotrexate-induced leukoencephalopathy reversed by aminophylline and high-dose folinic acid. *Acta Haematol* 2004, 111:230–232.

104. Lai R, Abrey LE, Rosenblum MK, DeAngelis LM: Treatment-induced leukoencephalopathy in primary CNS lymphoma: a clinical and autopsy study. *Neurology* 2004, 62:451–456.

105. Koh S, Nelson MD Jr, Kovanlikaya A, Chen LS: Anterior lumbosacral radiculopathy after intrathecal methotrexate treatment. *Pediatr Neurol* 1999, 21:576–578.

106. Counsel P, Khangure M: Myelopathy due to intrathecal chemotherapy: magnetic resonance imaging findings. *Clin Radiol* 2007, 62:172–176.

107. Watterson J, Toogood I, Nieder M, et al.: Excessive spinal cord toxicity from intensive central nervous system-directed therapies. *Cancer* 1994, 74:3034–3041.

108. Colamaria V, Caraballo R, Borgna-Pignatti C, et al.: Transient focal leuko-encephalopathy following intraventricular methotrexate and cytarabine. A complication of the Ommaya reservoir: case report and review of the literature. *Childs Nerv Syst* 1990, 6:231–235.

109. de Waal R, Algra PR, Heimans JJ, et al.: Methotrexate induced brain necrosis and severe leukoencephalopathy due to disconnection of an Ommaya device. *J Neurooncol* 1993, 15:269–273.

110. Patel SR, Vadhan-Raj S, Papadopolous N, et al.: High-dose ifosfamide in bone and soft tissue sarcomas: results of phase II and pilot studies: dose-response and schedule dependence. *J Clin Oncol* 1997, 15:2378–2384.

111. Caraceni A, Gangeri L, Martini C, et al.: Neurotoxicity of interferon-alpha in melanoma therapy: results from a randomized controlled trial. *Cancer* 1998, 83:482–489.

112. Kirkwood JM, Bender C, Agarwala S, et al.: Mechanisms and manage-ment of toxicities associated with high-dose interferon alfa-2b therapy. *J Clin Oncol* 2002, 20:3703–3718.

113. Majhail NS, Hussein M, Olencki TE, et al.: Phase I trial of continuous infusion recombinant human interleukin-4 in patients with cancer. *Invest New Drugs* 2004, 22:421–426.

114. Wada Y, Kuwahara T, Uyama E, et al.: Neurologic toxicity associated with interferon alpha therapy for renal cell carcinoma. *Int J Urol* 2006, 13:811–813.

115. Cheson BD, Vena DA, Foss FM, Sorensen JM: Neurotoxicity of purine analogs: a review. *J Clin Oncol* 1994, 12:2216–2228.

116. Saumoy M, Castells G, Escoda L, et al.: Progressive multifocal leuko-encephalopathy in chronic lymphocytic leukemia after treatment with fludarabine. *Leuk Lymphoma* 2002, 43:433–436.

117. Vidarsson B, Mosher DF, Salamat MS, et al.: Progressive multifocal leukoencephalopathy after fludarabine therapy for low-grade lymphopro-liferative disease. *Am J Hematol* 2002, 70:51–54.

118. Gojo I, Jiemjit A, Trepel JB, et al.: Phase 1 and pharmacologic study of MS-275, a histone deacetylase inhibitor, in adults with refractory and relapsed acute leukemias. *Blood* 2007, 109:2781–2790.

119. Bug G, Ritter M, Wassmann B, et al.: Clinical trial of valproic acid and all-trans retinoic acid in patients with poor-risk acute myeloid leukemia. *Cancer* 2005, 104:2717–2725.

120. Mukherjee P, McKinstry RC: Reversible posterior leukoencephalopathy syndrome: evaluation with diffusion-tensor MR imaging. *Radiology* 2001, 219:756–765.

121. Ay H, Buonanno FS, Schaefer PW, et al.: Posterior leukoencephalopathy without severe hypertension: utility of diffusion-weighted MRI. *Neurol-ogy* 1998, 51:1369–1376.

122. Connolly RM, Doherty CP, Beddy P, O'Byrne K: Chemotherapy induced reversible posterior leukoencephalopathy syndrome. *Lung Cancer* 2007, 56:459–463.

123. Allen JA, Adlakha A, Bergethon PR: Reversible posterior leukoencepha-lopathy syndrome after bevacizumab/FOLFIRI regimen for metastatic colon cancer. *Arch Neurol* 2006, 63:1475–1478.

124. Govindarajan R, Adusumilli J, Baxter DL, et al.: Reversible posterior leukoencephalopathy syndrome induced by RAF kinase inhibitor BAY 43-9006. *J Clin Oncol* 2006, 24:e48.

125. Haefner MD, Siciliano RD, Widmer LA, et al.: Reversible posterior leukoencephalopathy syndrome after treatment of diffuse large B-cell lymphoma. *Onkologie* 2007, 30:138–140.

126. Ozcan C, Wong SJ, Hari P: Reversible posterior leukoencephalopathy syndrome and bevacizumab. *N Engl J Med* 2006, 354:980–982.

127. Kastrup O, Diener HC: Granulocyte-stimulating factor filgrastim and molgramostim induced recurring encephalopathy and focal status epilep-ticus. *J Neurol* 1997, 244:274–275.

128. Burstein HJ: Cognitive side-effects of adjuvant treatments. *Breast* 2007, 16(Suppl):S166–S168.

129. Ahles TA, Saykin AJ: Breast cancer chemotherapy-related cognitive dysfunction. *Clin Breast Cancer* 2002, 3:S84–S90.

130. Ahles TA, Saykin AJ, Furstenberg CT, et al.: Neuropsychologic impact of standard-dose systemic chemotherapy in long-term survivors of breast cancer and lymphoma. *J Clin Oncol* 2002, 20:485–493.

131. Schagen SB, van Dam FS, Muller MJ, et al.: Cognitive deficits after post-operative adjuvant chemotherapy for breast carcinoma. *Cancer* 1999, 85:640–650.

The impact of disease and the rigors of treatment are of utmost importance to cancer patients. Until recently, the focus of clinical trials was predominantly on biologic outcomes. Indirect measures of a patient's physical function or quality of life (QoL) were offered by the clinician, often providing an inaccurate and incomplete assessment of a patient's direct experience with his or her disease. A greater appreciation for the impact of disease and intervention on a patient's QoL has evolved as a result of a better understanding of the pathophysiology of cancer, improved treatments for the disease, prolonged survival, and a broader application of the biopsychosocial model of health. Patient-reported QoL outcomes are now included as end points in many clinical trials to provide information about the patient's experience with the disease process independent of and in synergy with traditional biologic end points. This chapter focuses primarily on the measurement and application of QoL end points in clinical trials.

WHAT IS HEALTH-RELATED QUALITY OF LIFE?

Health status, QoL, and health-related QoL (HrQoL) are descriptive terms that fall along a continuum of personal experience from the global to the specific. *Health* can be defined as "a state of complete physical, mental, and social well-being" [1] or as homeostasis, a state in which the body sustains effective balance in the setting of multiple stressors [2]. *QoL* is a self-reported measure of health in the context of one's daily activities, societal and cultural standards, and internal values [3]. Thus, QoL is inherently a subjective, summary measure. When these same domains are impacted by a medical condition and its treatment, QoL is shifted along an experience continuum and manifests as *HrQoL*. HrQoL, in essence, is health status from an individual's perspective and experience. It is both informative, measuring a respondent's perceived status (rating of pain), and evaluative (how does pain affect your job performance?). In general, HrQoL is a multidimensional (multiple domains) concept, whereas patient-reported QoL outcomes may be unidimensional or multidimensional. Thus, the measurement of HrQoL may be quite complex, multifaceted, and both subjective and objective.

HISTORICAL BACKGROUND FOR QUALITY-OF-LIFE MEASURES IN CLINICAL TRIALS

The traditional emphasis of clinical trials has been on the assessment of the biophysical end points of survival and morbidity [4]. However, as early as 1948, there was awareness that some measure of QoL should be included when assessing a patient in the context of disease and treatment. Karnofsky *et al.* [5] introduced a clinician-reported scale (Karnofsky Performance Status [KPS]) to quantify a patient's physical function from death (0%) to normal function (100%) along an 11-point scale. As a measure of QoL, interpretation of the KPS score assumes that the physician can accurately interpret the patient's experience. However, it often correlates poorly with patient-reported QoL outcomes and although it has been widely applied, it has never been validated [3].

In the 1970s, a transition away from paternalism and toward patient-involved decision-making occurred, leading to incorporation of patients' direct experiences into evaluable outcome measures. In 1975, Burge *et al.* [6] assessed the benefit of aggressive chemotherapy for acute myeloid leukemia on the quantity and quality of life. An independent observer graded the patients' QoL based on symptoms and their impact on function. Although this was an indirect measure of QoL, it generated a greater interest in QoL assessment in the inpatient and clinical arenas. In the late 1970s, the value of QoL measures in breast cancer management was acknowledged. Priestman and Baum [7] applied a linear analog scale [8] to measure the subjective benefits of chemotherapy in women with advanced breast cancer, demonstrating reliable correlation between the measured patient-reported QoL outcomes and the patients' clinical status. In woman with stage II breast cancer, the psychosocial effects of adjuvant chemotherapy were pervasive across the physical, emotional, and social domains of HrQoL [9], and yet these women would recommend treatment to other breast cancer patients at a very high rate. The juxtaposition between apparent impaired QoL and unfaltering decision-making helped to inform other patients about the risks and benefits of treatment. The benefit of therapy for refractory pancreatic cancer was measured in terms of clinical benefit response (level of pain, use of pain medication, weight change, and activity level) and not solely on survival [10]. The US Food and Drug Administration (FDA) approved gemcitabine for the treatment of pancreatic cancer based on this QoL endpoint. Collectively, the acknowledgement of the importance of QoL as a dynamic measure of the cancer experience led to institutional endorsements of the application of patient-reported QoL outcomes in clinical trials.

Institutionally, the evolution of QoL measurement began in earnest in 1985 when the FDA recognized the need to humanize medicine and embrace cancer as a chronic disease, and incorporated "favorable effects on survival and/or QoL" into its approval criteria for anticancer agents [4]. Similarly, the National Cancer Institute's (NCI) Cancer Therapy Evaluation Program revised its mission statement to reflect the incorporation of elements of the biopsychosocial model of medicine "improved survival and QoL (were deemed to be of) highest priority" [4,11]. Other NCI-supported committees declared new initiatives to improve and unify the design, execution, analysis, reporting, and interpretation of QoL measures [11,12]. In 2006, the FDA once again set precedent by recommending inclusion of trial end points demonstrating a longer or better quality of life [11]. Recently, PRO-ACT (Patient-Reported Outcomes Assessment in Clinical Trials) and PRO-MIS (Patient-Reported Outcomes Measurement Information System) were established to refine the current infrastructure and organization of ongoing and future trials, and to provide standardization of measurement, collection, and analysis of patient-reported QoL outcomes [13,14]. The rapid evolution of outcomes research and these recent initiatives have led to a better understanding and appreciation of the application of QoL measures in research settings and clinical practice.

WHY MEASURE QUALITY OF LIFE?

Traditional biophysical measures are meaningful in the global scientific context of medical advances and in clinical application, but may have secondary import to an individual patient or caregiver. Psychosocial measures broaden the profile of effectiveness of treatment and address questions pertinent to the patient. Evaluation of QoL may provide additional prognostic data [3,15–18], improve decision-making capacity for patient and physician, generate hypotheses for future research trials, address patients' preference for discussing QoL concerns [15], and provide a context for cost assessment and policy generation [18].

INSTRUMENTS

Prior to choosing an appropriate QoL instrument for a clinical trial, one must first consider whether or not QoL outcomes should be included as an end point for a given trial. Presently, QoL measures are chosen as primary and secondary end points in phase 3 clinical trials and longitudinal studies, occasionally in phase 1 and 2 clinical trials, and increasingly in clinical practice [19]. QoL measures in phase 2 trials are limited to trial designs that evaluate response to treatment when there is no measurable disease, where tumor response is not an adequate surrogate for patient benefit, when measuring directly the impact of toxic therapies on HrQoL, or that test the feasibility, applicability, and validity of a measure in a specific population prior to inclusion in phase 3 trials [19]. Overall, inclusion of QoL end points in a clinical trial should be considered when 1) biomedical outcomes are expected to be equivalent or demonstrate a small difference between study arms, 2) interventions are expected to be equivalent but the toxicity profiles may be vastly different, 3) interventions differ in short-term efficacy but overall benefit is limited, 4) overall survival advantage and long-term impact of an intervention are unknown, 5) comparing palliative interventions, or 6) evaluating benefit of psychosocial interventions [11,17,18]. When a QoL end point is pertinent to a trial design or a clinical practice paradigm, the appropriateness, not the availability, of a given instrument for a given trial is of key concern. When selecting an instrument, Gelber and Gelber [20] suggest considering the five "Ps": Purpose, population, protocol, profile, and pragmatism (Table 29-1). In other words, choice of instrument should be based on the research objective which in turn, defines the QoL domain of interest.

INSTRUMENT TYPES

QoL instruments can be characterized as generic or specific questionnaires. Generic questionnaires, such as the Medical Outcomes Study 36-Item Short-Form Survey (SF-36) [21], are used to assess the general health status of individuals across different populations, health states, and medical conditions [18]. Generic tools may be limited by their inherent design, rendering them insensitive to changes in individuals or small populations and specific situations [22]. General cancer instruments, such as the Functional Assessment of Cancer Therapy – General (FACT-G) [23], assess the respondent's experience over a broad range of cancer-related events independent of tumor type but within the context of the disease. Targeted instruments, designed to measure QoL for a given tumor type or disease-related condition, are likely to be more sensitive to changes in QoL for an individual or a specified group of patients. Generic and specific instruments are often combined into a hybrid questionnaire to provide greater breadth of application. Hybrid questionnaires include a core generic questionnaire (FACT-G) to address issues related to a diverse population with multiple disease states, and supplemental modules to address specific disease-based (FACT-Lung), intervention-related (FACT-bone marrow transplant [BMT]), and symptom-associated (FACT-Nausea) issues. Hybrid tools are useful in large, multisite clinical trials [11,18]. Examples of QoL instruments are listed in Table 29-2.

Quality of life instruments may be further classified as non–preference-based or preference-based measures. Non–preference-based or health profile measures address the core QoL domains of physical, emotional, social, and functional well-being and general health status based on psychometric properties of the items and scale. Likert or linear analog self-assessment (LASA) scales are applied per item [3] to quantify the outcome. The Likert scale has discrete categories to rate the intensity or frequency of a given item and the LASA scale is a continuum anchored by extremes (none or all). Questionnaires using these formats have been shown to be valid, reliable, and reproducible [3]. Questionnaires are scored by item and domain, and a summary score is often calculated based on total response, and for ease of application and comparison across studies.

Preference-based or utility measures focus on an individual's preference for a given health state, ranging from "0" (death) to "1" (life) [17,22,31]. Utility is often measured to account for differences in survivorship by combining morbidity and mortality into one measurement [32], for ease of comparisons across different populations, to develop medical decision-making models based on probability of occurrence and patient preference (32), and in cost-effectiveness trials [33]. Methods for calculating a utility score include the standard gamble [34] and time trade-off [35] approaches that require patient interview. Both techniques ask respondents about their current health and health states that they may or may not have experienced. The Standard Gamble approach offers the patient a choice between a chronic health state with certainty (cancer) or an uncertain state related to an intervention that results in either death (1-p) or perfect health (p). The probability of either state is varied until the interviewed subject is indifferent between the two uncertain states. This indifference or probability is the utility score. The Time Trade-off method offers a "trade-off" between life in perfect health for a limited period of time and life in current health state for a longer period of time. The length of time in perfect health is varied until indifference between the two states is noted. The ratio of the time in each state is the utility score. Although these methods are effective, they are time-consuming and cumbersome. Utility scores, which are single summary scores, may lack sensitivity to changes over time [22], be subject to variability based on the method used in calculation, be less responsive than descriptive measures, and are likely to reflect an internal standard that may not be directly altered by a time-limited intervention (*eg*, treatment) or a situation (*eg*, cancer).

BARRIERS TO APPLICATION OF QUALITY-OF-LIFE MEASURES IN CLINICAL TRIALS

There are multiple barriers to the application of QoL end points in clinical trials and practice. These barriers include, but are not limited to cost, burden, and general skepticism about the statistical and clinical value of QoL measures [14]. Funding for purchase of copyrighted instruments and statistical preparation and analysis of measures is of major concern. The NCI's commitment to prioritizing funding will address collection and analysis costs [11]. Burden is related to the patient and administrative burden of repeated measures, data collection, and management [22]. PROMIS and item banking may help to diffuse costs and develop more precise and generalizable tools [14].

Unlike the barriers of cost and burden, skepticism arises from the concern regarding statistical robustness and usefulness of a subjective measure. To overcome some of these concerns, development and selection of a QoL instrument should meet several rigorous statistical and epidemiologic criteria (Table 29-3) as outlined by the Medical Outcomes Trust (MOT) [36,37].

The Minimum Standard Checklist for Evaluating HrQoL Outcomes in Cancer Clinical Trials assesses the essential determinants of a high-quality, reli-

Table 29-1. Guidelines for Instrument Selection

Purpose	Establish an a priori hypothesis regarding importance of QoL measures
Protocol	Model and accurately address QoL issues pertinent to the hypothesis
	Define clearly the intervention and the primary and seconary goals
	Outline the intended analyses
Population	Define inclusion and exclusion criteria for the population
Profile	Assess known or presumed benefits, side effects, and toxicities of an intervention
	Select specific QoL domains based on criteria such as hypothesis, prior experience
Pragmatism	Consider issues of funding, patient compliance, time limitations

QoL—quality of life.

Table 29-2. Quality-of-Life Measurement Instruments

Type	Instrument
Generic	
Non-preference based	Sickness Impact Profile [24]
	Medical Outcomes 36-Item Short-Form Health Survey (SF-36) [21]
Preference based	Health Utilities Index (HUI) [25]
	Spitzer's Quality of Life Index (QLI) [26]
Cancer specific	Functional Living Index – Cancer (FLIC) [27]
	Cancer Rehabilitation Evaluation System (CARES) [28]
Hybrid	European Organisation for Research and Treatment of Cancer Scale (EORTC-QLQ30) with disease and symptom-specific modules [29]
	Functional Cancer Therapy – General (FACT-G) with disease and symptom-specific modules [23,30]

able randomized clinical trial that studies and reports HrQoL data [38,39]. The checklist is comprised of 11 criteria addressing issues of modeling, measurement, methodology, and interpretation of HrQoL in clinical trials; studies that meet 8 of 11 criteria are considered high-quality HrQoL trials. Among a panel of HrQoL researchers, the criteria of reporting compliance and missing data as well as demonstrating psychometric properties of the instruments and outcomes were of greatest priority when applying the checklist. When the checklist was applied to 24 randomized clinical trials of treatment for prostate cancer (which included HrQoL measures), 33% of the trials met criteria for high-quality trials. Most trials were lacking in modeling (no statement of a priori hypothesis) and interpretation (lack of discussion of clinical significance of data). Application of the MOT criteria and the Checklist to randomized clinical trial design and execution should improve interpretability and applicability of HrQoL outcomes across trials and in clinical practice.

To address validity, reliability, and responsiveness of instruments across items and trials, two approaches have been adopted by the NCI: Application of hybrid instruments and development of an "item bank" via item response theory (IRT) [13,31,40]. PROMIS' goal to develop a set of "publicly available, standardized instruments for self-reported QOL domains" [14] will improve validity by making outcomes comparable across populations and items. Under IRT, "each item within a domain is calibrated with a set of statistical properties to allow researchers to select any set of items from the bank to match the characteristics of the study population" [13]. This item-trait relationship allows for items from multiple instruments to be used simultaneously, thus, broadening the application of any given measure, generating more precise instruments, and increasing the reliability and validity of the generated instrument via universal comparison [22, 31].

FREQUENCY OF MEASURES

The frequency and timing of QoL measurements in a clinical trial are dependent on the hypothesis and objectives of the trial, the natural course of the disease, the specific intervention protocol, and the anticipated onset and duration of the benefit, toxicity, or outcome related to the intervention [17,18,41]. Frequent collection of data is desirable; however, it may add unnecessary cost and burden to a given study design. Baseline measurements should be made, preferably prior to randomization, to assess pretreatment differences in QoL between and within individuals in each study arm and to establish a data set from which to make future comparisons. Baseline measurements may also provide prognostic information on survival and treatment response [3,18,42]. QoL data should also be measured at the completion of a study (or specific intervention) to allow for calculation of "change scores" from baseline, and assessment of treatment benefit and toxicity. In order to assess the impact of an intervention and its toxicity during the recovery phase, additional HrQoL data should be collected at a predetermined interval after completion of a trial. Intervals may be shorter for studies assessing palliative regimens, end-of-life-care or acute events, and longer for studies assessing early-stage disease and survivorship [17]. Other assessments may be performed during or after the trial based on a specified time interval (weeks, months, years) or event occurrence (number of cycles, scheduled imaging); these intervals should be the same across study arms. To minimize burden and cost, improve compliance, and limit missing data, collection should occur during scheduled appointments based on protocol design, and be kept at a necessary minimum.

STATISTICAL ANALYSIS

Statistical analysis of QoL data should be performed with the same statistical rigor as for biologic end points. However, these analyses are often complicated by the multidimensionality of the construct, the longitudinal design of most assessments, missing data, survival data, and conceptualization of clinical significance of the outcome [43]. As with traditional end points, proper sample size and power calculations should be performed during protocol development. Computation should include estimates of variation and correlation. Sensitivity of a QoL instrument related to an established clinical reference can aide in choosing an effect size for calculation [43]. However, the subjective nature of the collected QoL measures and the issues related to multiple measures and missing data complicate these calculations. As

with biologic end points, analysis should begin with descriptive statistics. Application of nonparametric tests may be useful for analysis of QoL data that are often skewed by "ceiling and floor" effects [18]. To address multiple items and domains and repeated measures in QoL data, the following should be considered when performing univariate analyses: Simplify analysis by using summary scores when applicable, limit the false-positive rate by restricting analysis to a few primary and secondary QoL outcomes, use a more conservative P value ($P < 0.01$), apply a BonFerroni correction, or perform repeated measures analyses when appropriate [18,41,43]. Multivariate analyses, such as analysis of covariance (ANCOVA) and multivariate analysis of covariance (MANCOVA), allow for time × interaction modeling and an estimation of within- and between-subject variation over time. However, data are often incomplete and the repeated measures are not independent, underestimating the standard error. Application of the Random or Mixed Effects model or Generalized Estimating Equation model [44] may overcome this bias in analyses with repeated measures by accounting for correlations within data. Nonparametric methods such as ranking may also be used to account for incomplete data.

Missing data is an issue that plagues the data integrity of QoL studies, especially in trials assessing palliative therapy, supportive interventions, or survivorship. Data may be missing as a result of missing items or missing forms. Missing-ness may be "ignorable" (not related to respondent's QoL), or "not ignorable." Missing items within a questionnaire are less serious but missing questionnaires can lead to biased results and a loss of power [18]. Attention should be paid to documenting the number of missing items and questionnaires at each collection point, and the presumed reason for their "missing-ness." To minimize missing data, QoL data collection should be directly integrated into the study protocol to ensure baseline measurements of QoL [8,41,45]. Further collection of QoL end points should coincide with measurement of traditional end points or required protocol visits [17,41]. Standard operating procedures for administering questionnaires, entering data, and monitoring visits should be developed [40]. For trials of advanced disease or palliative care, proxy and patient data should be collected from baseline to reduce missing data over time and allow for assessment of concordance between patient and proxy [41]. Accounts of missing data should be reported for all clinical trials. To adjust results for missing-ness, several techniques may be employed: imputation, subgroup analyses, selected data assessment. or data modeling [19].

Missing data may also be a result from group differences in mortality. To account for differential survival when estimating changes in QoL, summary preference-based measures, which account for an individual's survival weighted by the QoL experienced, are often employed. These quality-adjusted end points allow comparison of interventions that differ in their QoL effects and survival, and are particularly pertinent in treatments that impact survival at the cost of increased toxicity. QALYs adjust for differences in life expectancy by accounting for different levels of HrQoL experienced

Table 29-3. The Medical Outcomes Trust's Attributes of Quality-of-Life Instruments

Attribute	Description
Conceptual model	Rationale for measure and assessment of aggregation and scoring
Validity	Whether an instrument measures what it claims to measure
Reliability	Internal consistency and reproducibility
Responsiveness	Ability to detect changes over time; sensitivity to detect differences at a given time point
Interpretability	Meaning associated with a quantitative score
Burden	Time, effort, and other similar factors associated with delivery and assessment of measure
Adaptability	Equivalence across languages and populations

(*Adapted from* Lipscomb *et al.* [36] and Lohr *et al.* [37].)

or to be experienced during a given time period [33]. Unfortunately, QALYs may bias the outcome since they make value-laden assumptions about the worthiness of life [15,32]. The quality-adjusted time without symptoms or toxicity (Q-TwiST) method measures the "trade-off" between intervention-related toxicity and decrements in the time-dependent outcome of QoL [41]. The Q-TwiST analysis is a three-step process: 1) definition of health states as toxicity experienced during treatment (TOX), state of no toxicity during treatment (TWIST), and state at time of relapse (PROG); 2) partitioning of overall survival for each state (mean duration of each health state is estimated by Kaplan-Meier curves); and 3) comparison of treatments using a weighted sum of mean duration in each health state [43]. The "effect" can be measured by calculating the difference in QTwiST between or among groups. QTwiST is calculated as $(U_{TOX} \times TOX) + TWIST + (U_{PROG} \times PROG)$, with "U" being the derived utility coefficient that is invariant with respect to QoL experienced [46]. Both QALY and QTwiST evaluate therapy in the context of the quantity and quality of life.

INTERPRETING THE DATA

Statistical significance is the standard of reporting data in clinical trials; however, it may not provide information on clinical significance, the arena in which QoL end points may have most impact. Determination of clinical significance may be based on (historical) experience with a given intervention, convergent evidence across trials, or the predictive validity of prior outcomes. To improve the interpretability of QoL outcomes from a clinical significance standpoint, two methods are employed in QoL analyses: the anchor-based method and the distribution-based method. The anchor-based method uses an anchor, an independent, quantifiable, interpretable measure that is associated with the QoL end point, to define the minimum important difference (MID) [17,18,31,47]. The MID is " the smallest difference in score in the domain of interest that patients perceive as important… which leads the clinician to consider a change in the patient's management" [18]. Defining the MID via an anchor-based method confirms construct validity evaluates responsiveness of an instrument and allows for more precise power and sample size calculations [18,48].

In the distribution-based method, the data are interpreted in terms of the relation between an individual's or group's effect and its variability from an assumed underlying distribution of results [17,18]. Estimates of variability by effect size or standard deviation (SD) are vulnerable to the heterogeneity of different study populations. The effect size is sample dependent and can be measured as the difference in mean QoL scores divided by the SD in QoL baseline scores. Meaningful effect size has been defined by Cohen as 0.2 (small), 0.5 (medium), and 0.8 (large) [48]. Application of the standard error of the mean (SEM), which is the variability between an observed score and the true score, may correct for this heterogeneity [18]; it is a fixed characteristic of a measure regardless of the sample size unless the sample is skewed by ceiling or floor effects [48]. It is expressed in score units, reflecting the instrument's metric [43]. SEM, like the t-test and effect size, provides information on the relative degree of change (within person variability over time) in a QoL measure for an observed study [41]. It can be calculated as the baseline SD multiplied by the square root of the (1-reliability) coefficient of QoL measure [49]. There is apparent congruence between

the anchor- and distribution-based methods of assessing meaningfulness of changes in QoL scores.

In order to fully assess the responsiveness of an outcome over time, methods for addressing "response shift" should be applied. Response shift is a change in "internal standards, values or the conceptualization of QoL during a disease (and recovery) trajectory" as a result of (non)adaptation to a change in health status [41,31]. These shifts may render outcomes at different time points noncomparable. These shifts are most likely to have an impact when changes in health status during a trial are acute and intense [41]. Preference-based measures can overcome response shift by relating one's current state to one's conception of perfect health. To improve comparability across trials, Rasch analysis method can be used to identify and study anomalies in data and estimate independence of sample and questions. This method is based on a "probalistic model between the level of the latent trait and the item used for measurement" [50], which assumes that the outcome measured is independent of the measurement tool used [51].

REPORTING

Data reporting in scientific journals often focuses on the biologic end points of clinical trials and their statistical significance; patient-reported QoL outcomes data are often overshadowed by the more familiar and traditional end points, and frequently not reported in the same journals as biologic outcomes. Patient-reported QoL outcomes data are often relegated to method-based or other niche journals. To overcome reporting discrepancies between traditional and patient-reported QoL outcomes data, Lipscomb *et al.* [13] suggest that each result set be published in the same journal, and preferably the same issue of the journal, as separate articles that complement each other. Results may also be published in separate journals that are pertinent to the clinical research and practice community. Lipscomb *et al.* [13] also recommend that patient-reported QoL outcomes data should be presented in an evidence-based manner, applying statistical and clinical terms that allow for direct and equal comparison with standard trial results.

CONCLUSIONS

Quality of life is a subjective measure that has gained momentum in oncology clinical trials. Cancer is often associated with a high rate of anxiety, morbidity, and mortality in spite of advances in the etiology, diagnosis, and treatment of the disease. When addressing the needs of patients with an acute or chronic disease, the issues of quantity—life expectancy and burden (toxicities of intervention, economic costs, and caregiver issues)—and quality—impact of process on an individual and society—must be considered. Biomedical outcomes are necessary but not sufficient to describe the patient's personal experience with his or her cancer and benefit or harm from its treatment. Patient-reported QoL outcomes in general and HrQoL measures specifically provide additional information on the burden of cancer and the effectiveness of treatment [11]. Both quantity and quality are measurable concepts but the subjective nature of a qualitative assessment renders it prone to speculation about its accuracy and validity. Proper assessment, analysis, and interpretation of quality (of life) measures provide information about the impact of disease processes and treatment on the patient independent of and in synergy with traditional biologic end points.

REFERENCES

1. World Health Organization: Preamble to the Constitution of the World Health Organization as adopted by the International Health Conference, New York, 19–22 June, 1946; signed on 22 July 1946 by the representatives of 61 States (Official Records of the World Health Organization, no. 2, p. 100) and entered into force on 7 April 1948. http://www.who.int/about/definition/en/print.html. Accessed July 16, 2008.

2. Medical Dictionary: Health. http://www.medical-dictionary.com. Accessed July 16, 2008.

3. Michael M, Tannock IF: Measuring health-related quality of life in clinical trials that evaluate the role of chemotherapy in cancer treatment. *CMAJ* 1998, 158:1727–1734.

4. Bruner DW, Bryan CJ, Aaronson N, *et al.*: Issues and challenges with integrating patient-reported outcomes in clinical trials supported by the National Cancer Institute-sponsored clinical trials network. *J Clin Oncol* 2007, 25:5051–5057.

5. Karnofsky DA, Abelmann WH, Craver LF, Burchenal JH: The use of nitrogen mustards in the palliative treatment of carcinoma. *Cancer* 1948, 1:634.

6. Burge PS, Richards JDM, Thompson DS, *et al.*: Quality and quantity of survival in acute myeloid leukaemia. *Lancet* 1975, 4:621–624.

7. Priestman TJ, Baum M: Evaluation of quality of life in patients receiving treatment for advanced breast cancer. *Lancet* 1976, 1:899–900.

8. Sutherland HJ, Dunn V, Boyd NF: Measurement of values for states of health with linear analog scales. *Med Decis Making* 1983, 3:477–487.

9. Meyerowitz BE, Sparks FC, Spears IK: Adjuvant chemotherapy for breast carcinoma: psychosocial implications. *Cancer* 1979, 43:1613–1618.

10. Rothenberg ML, Moore MJ, Cripps MC, *et al.*: A phase II trial of gemcitabine in patients with 5-FU refractory pancreas cancer. *Ann Oncol* 1996, 7:347–353.

11. Lipscomb J, Gotay CC, Snyder CF: Patient-reported outcomes in cancer: a review of recent research and policy initiatives. *CA Cancer J Clin* 2007, 57:278–300.

12. Clauser SB, Ganz PA, Lipscomb J, Reeve BB: Patient-reported outcomes assessment in cancer trials: evaluating and enhancing the payoff to decision making. *J Clin Oncol* 2007, 25:5049–5062.

13. Lipscomb J, Reeve BB, Clauser SB, *et al.*: Patient-reported outcomes assessment in cancer trials: taking stock, moving forward. *J Clin Oncol* 2007, 25:5133–5140.

14. Garcia SF, Cella D, Clauser SB, *et al.*: Standardizing patient-reported outcomes assessment in cancer clinical trials: a patient-reported outcomes measurement information system initiative. *J Clin Oncol* 2007, 25:5106–5112.

15. Fallowfield L: Quality of life: a new perspective for cancer patients. *Nat Rev Cancer* 2002, 2:873–879.

16. Gotay CC: Assessing cancer-related quality of life across a spectrum of applications. *J Natl Cancer Inst Monographs* 2004, 33:126–133.

17. Movsas B: Quality of life in oncology trials: a clinical guide. *Semin Radiat Oncol* 2003, 13:235–247.

18. Siddiqui F, Kachnic LA, Movsas B: Quality-of-life outcomes in oncology. *Hematol Oncol Clin North Am* 2006, 20:165–185.

19. Wagner LI, Wenzel L, Shaw E, Cella D: Patient-reported outcomes in phase II cancer clinical trials: lessons learned and future directions. *J Clin Oncol* 2007, 25:5058–5062.

20. Gelber RD, Gelber S: Quality-of-life assessment in clinical trials. *Cancer Treat Res* 1995, 75:225–246.

21. Ware JE, Sherbourne CD: The MOS 36-item short-form health survey (SF-36). Conceptual framework and item selection. *Med Care* 1992, 30:473–483.

22. Cella D, Chang CH, Lai JS, Webster K: Advances in quality of life measurements in oncology patients. Semin Oncol 2002, 29:60–68.

23. Cella D, Tulsky D, Gray G, *et al.*: The functional assessment of cancer therapy scale: development and validation of the general measure. *J Clin Oncol* 1993, 11:570–579.

24. Gilson BS, Gilson JS, Bergner M, *et al.*: The sickness impact profile. Development of an outcome measure of health care. *Am J Public Health* 1975, 65:1304–1310.

25. Feeny D, Furlong W, Boyle M, Torrance GW: Multi-attribute health status classification systems: Health Utilities Index. *Pharmacoeconomics* 1995, 7:490–502.

26. Spitzer WO, Dobson AJ, Hall J, *et al.*: Measuring the quality of life of cancer patients: a concise QL-index for use by physicians. *J Chronic Dis* 1981, 34:583–597.

27. Schipper H, Clinch J, McMurray A, *et al.*: Measuring the quality of life of cancer patients: the Functional Living Index–cancer: development and validation. *J Clin Oncol* 1984, 2:272–283.

28. Schag CA, Ganz PA, Heinrich RL: Cancer Rehabilitation Evaluation System–short form (CARES-SF). A cancer specific rehabilitation and quality of life instrument. *Cancer* 1991, 68:1406–1413.

29. Aaronson NK, Ahmedzai S, Bergman B, *et al.*: The European Organization for Research and Treatment of Cancer QLQ-C30: a quality-of-life instrument for use in international clinical trials in oncology. *J Natl Cancer Inst* 1993, 85:365–376.

30. Webster K, Cella D, Yost K: The functional assessment of chronic illness therapy (FACIT) measurement system: properties, applications, and interpretation. *Health Qual Life Outcomes* 2003, 1:79.

31. Lipscomb J, Donaldson MS, Arora NK, *et al.*: Cancer outcomes research. *J Natl Cancer Inst Monographs* 2004, 33:178–197.

32. Bennett KJ, Torrance GW: Measuring health care preferences and utilities: rating scale, time trade-off and standard gamble techniques. In *Quality of Life and Pharmacoeconomics in Clinical Trials*, edn 2. Edited by Spilker B. New York: Raven Press; 1996:253–265.

33. Sassi F: Calculating QALYs, comparing QALY and DALY calculations. *Health Policy Plan* 2006, 21:402–408.

34. Perez DJ, McGee R, Campbell AV, Christensen EA: A comparison of time trade-off and quality of life measures in patients with advanced cancer. *Qual Life Res* 1997, 6:133–138.

35. Morimoto T, Fukui T: Utilities measured by rating scale, time trade-off and standard gamble: review and reference for health care professionals: *J Epidemiol* 2002, 12:160–178.

36. Lipscomb J, Snyder CF, Gotay CC: Cancer outcomes measurement: through the lens of the Medical Outcomes Trust framework. *Qual Life Res* 2007, 16:143–164.

37. Lohr KN, Aaronson NK, Alonso J, *et al.*: Evaluating quality of life and health status instruments: development of scientific review criteria. *Clin Ther* 1996, 18:979–992.

38. Efficace F, Bottomley A, Osoba D, *et al.*: Beyond the development of health-related quality-of-life measures: a checklist for evaluating HRQOL outcomes in cancer clinical trials–does HRQOL evaluation in prostate cancer research inform clinical decision making?. *J Clin Oncol* 2003, 21:3502–3511.

39. Wedding U, Pientka L, Hoffken K: Quality-of-life in elderly patients with cancer: a short review. *Eur J Cancer* 2007, 43:2203–2210.

40. Osoba D: What has been learned from measuring health-related quality of life in clinical oncology? *Eur J Cancer* 1999, 35:1565–1570.

41. Sprangers MA, Moinpour CM, Moynihan TJ, *et al.*: Clinical Significance Consensus Meeting Group: assessing meaningful change in quality of life over time: a users' guide for clinicians. *Mayo Clinic Proc* 2002, 77:561–571.

42. Stephens R: Quality of life. *Hematol Oncol Clin North Am* 2004, 18:483–497.

43. Fairclough DL, Gelber RD: Quality of life: statistical issues and analysis. In *Quality of Life and Pharmacoeconomics in Clinical Trials*, edn 2. Edited by Spilker B. New York: Raven Press, 1996:427–435.

44. Zeger SL, Liang KY: Longitudinal data analysis for discrete and continuous outcomes. *Biometrics* 1986, 42:121–130.

45. Smith KW, Avis NE, Assmann SF: Distinguishing between quality of life and health status in quality of life research: a meta-analysis. *Qual Life Res* 1999, 8:447–459.

46. Billingham LJ, Abrams KR, Jones DR: Methods for the analysis of quality of life and survival in health technology assessment. *Health Technol Assess* 1993, 3:1–149.

47. Guyatt GH, Osoba D, Wu AW, *et al.*: Clinical Significance Consensus Meeting Group. Methods to explain the clinical significance of health status measures. *Mayo Clinic Proc* 2002, 77:371–383.

48. Wyrwich KW, Bullinger M, Aaronson N, *et al.*: Estimating clinically significant difference in quality of life outcomes. *Qual Life Res* 2005, 14:285–295.

49. Wyrwich KW, Nienaber NA, Tierney WM, Wolinsky FA: Linking clinical relevance and statistical significance in evaluating intra-individual changes in HrQoL. *Med Care* 1999, 37:469–478.

50. Smith AB, Wright P, Selby PJ, Velikova G: A Rasch and factor analysis of FACT-G. *Health Qual Life Outcomes* 2007; 5:19–29.

51. Rasch Analysis. http://www.rasch-analysis.com. RUMMLaboratory Pty Ltd.; 2005–2006. Accessed July 18, 2008.

For most patients with cancer, clinical features are directly attributable to the local effects of the primary tumor or metastases. However, in about 5% to 10% of patients, certain systemic and organ-specific manifestations cannot be directly attributed to the underlying cancer. These systemic effects, or paraneoplastic syndromes, are mediated by a variety of mechanisms, including atypical hormone secretion, inflammatory mediators such as cytokines, interleukin, or growth factors, and immune processes mediated by antibodies and T lymphocytes.

Because paraneoplastic syndromes can be an early manifestation of an underlying cancer, their diagnosis should prompt a search for the malignancy to allow early diagnosis and treatment. Many of these syndromes improve with the treatment of the underlying malignancy, although temporalizing measures may have to be initiated to control the symptoms. The paraneoplastic syndromes may also act as a marker of disease activity and provide interesting insights into tumor biology and immunology.

Paraneoplastic syndromes generally fulfill the following criteria:

1. Direct association between the syndrome and the presence of cancer;
2. Presence of an identifiable mediator in the circulation or within tumor cells (effective treatment of the tumor should lead to a reduction in this mediator); and
3. Clinical improvement of the paraneoplastic effects following treatment of the primary malignancy, although this is not often the case.

The systemic effects of cancer are often multifactorial and significant physiologic or systemic effects can occur even in the absence of a well-defined syndrome. This chapter summarizes the clinical features, mechanisms, and management of the main systemic and paraneoplastic manifestations of cancer.

SYSTEMIC SYNDROMES

CACHEXIA AND ANOREXIA SYNDROME

Cachexia and anorexia represent the most common systemic syndrome seen in patients with malignancy. It has been estimated that approximately one fourth of patients suffer from either weight loss, anorexia, or both at the time of diagnosis; these are almost universal in the presence of widely metastatic disease.

The importance of these syndromes lies in their effect on survival and their influence on the quality of life of cancer patients and their families. Furthermore, prognosis and ability to tolerate treatment are both often influenced by nutritional status. Malnutrition is a significant cause of mortality, contributing to about 20% of deaths not caused by direct tumor effects [1]. Loss of lean body mass (as distinct from adipose tissue), which is the predominant effect of starvation, has been demonstrated to be an important predictor of early mortality.

Cachexia may be caused by multiple factors:

1. Nutrition may be reduced due to the direct effects of tumor (eg, head and neck or gastrointestinal tumors) or treatment (nausea, vomiting, anorexia, and altered taste sensation commonly accompany chemotherapy and radiotherapy).
2. Metabolic abnormalities often occur secondary to cancer. These can include glucose intolerance and increases in hepatic gluconeogenesis, protein breakdown, and lipolysis. Whole body protein turnover is increased, resulting in muscle catabolism. Hyperlipidemia may result from elevated lipoprotein lipase levels.
3. Metabolic requirements in patients with cancer, in contrast to those seen in starving patients, are higher than in healthy subjects.
4. Cytokines. Under normal circumstances, the production of these glycoprotein regulators of cell and tissue function, such as growth and differentiation, wound repair, immune responses, and angiogenesis, is regulated by a variety of tightly controlled mechanisms. Increasingly, cytokines have been recognized as key mediators of many

systemic manifestations of cancer. No single cytokine is consistently elevated in the blood of cancer patients; however, clinically detectable levels are not required for these molecules to have an effect because much of their activity occurs at a local tissue level. Common syndromes such as cachexia, anorexia, and asthenia are likely to be caused, at least in part, by the actions of various cytokines.

The host's production of inflammatory cytokines in response to the tumor mediates a series of complex interrelated steps that can lead to a chronic state of wasting, malnutrition, and death. Tumor necrosis factor (TNF), a macrophage-derived cytokine, is the best understood of these, and has a clear role in cachexia associated with malignant and also nonmalignant disease. Other cytokines implicated include interleukins (IL)-6 and -1 and interferon-γ. In various studies, both have been shown to be associated with the signs of cancer cachexia and elevated in patients with cancer.

TNF-α, also known as cachectin, has a role in cancer cachexia and anorexia as well as the weight loss associated with chronic infection. Administration of TNF to experimental animals stimulates changes associated with cancer cachexia, which can be blocked by antisera [1]. Experimental infusion of TNF into the third ventricle of rats results in the suppression of glucose-sensitive neurons in the lateral hypothalamus and suppressed food intake [2]. TNF-neutralizing antibodies are able to reverse weight loss in mice with tumors, suggesting an important pathophysiologic role for TNF-α [3].

IL-1 has similarly been associated with anorexia. Intracerebroventricular administration of IL-1 in rats suppressed food intake via an effect on neurons in the lateral hypothalamus [2]. Schwarz et al. [4] postulated that IL-1 impairs appetite by increasing hypothalamic corticotropin-releasing hormone (CRH) production as well as suppressing neuropeptide Y, which has a stimulating effect on appetite. A rise in IL-1 levels detected in patients undergoing radiotherapy was associated with increased fatigue [5].

IL-6 also appears to play a role in the production of anorexia-cachexia. Administration of IL-6 to humans can be associated with weight loss, nausea, and anorexia [6]. In a small study, the administration of anti–IL-6 monoclonal antibody to patients with HIV and lymphoma resulted in weight gain for eight of 11 patients [7]. Oral medroxyprogesterone reduced IL-6 levels in breast cancer patients, and those with more significant reductions in IL-6 levels were more likely to achieve weight gain and increased appetite [8]. A potential mechanism for this effect is once again via the hypothalamus. IL-6 has been shown to stimulate release of cortisol, adrenocorticotropic hormone (ACTH), and antidiuretic hormone (ADH), suggesting activation of the hypothalamic-pituitary-adrenal axis [9].

MANAGEMENT

Attempts to delay or stop the weight loss associated with cancer are often futile due to altered metabolism caused by the neoplasm. Efforts have focused on reversing the cachexia and anorexia seen in cancer patients. Classes of agents used include orexigenic (appetite stimulants), anticatabolic, and antimetabolic (primarily hormonal). Corticosteroids, such as dexamethasone, have been found to stimulate appetite and cause weight gain in cancer patients but do not prolong survival. Megestrol acetate in doses of between 240 and 1600 mg/d has proven to be effective as well; it increases appetite and causes weight gain by downregulating the synthesis and release of cytokines [10]. Dronabinol, a cannabinoid, has been found to ease chemotherapy-associated nausea but does not reverse weight loss. Cyproheptadine, a serotonin antagonist, is similarly not effective in cancer cachexia [11].

ASTHENIA

From the Greek words for "absence of strength," asthenia involves three distinct symptom complexes: 1) fatigue or lassitude (easy tiring and decreased ability to maintain performance); 2) generalized weakness defined as the anticipatory sensation of difficulty in initiating a certain activity; and 3) mental fatigue (including impaired concentration, memory loss, and emotional lability) [12].

Asthenia is a common feature of advanced malignancy. However, it may occur with less advanced disease and has been reported in more than 80% of patients receiving chemotherapy [13]. Other estimates have ranged from 40% to 75%, the variation likely due in part to the population studied and the definition of asthenia used.

In general, the specific mechanism of asthenia is not well understood. Cytokine production, such as TNF or IL-1, either by the tumor itself or as part of a host response to the tumor, may play a role in the development of asthenia via alterations in intermediary metabolism.

It has been suggested that impaired muscle function may play a major role in producing asthenia [14], and abnormalities in both function and structure have been documented in cancer patients. Atrophy of type 2 muscle fibers, reductions in maximum strength, decreased reaction velocity, and increased fatigue have all been recorded. It is also common to see loss of muscle mass in cancer patients, particularly those with anorexia-cachexia. Bolus injections of TNF are associated with evidence of muscle catabolism in human subjects [15].

Several potentially reversible factors may contribute to asthenia in an individual patient:

1. Infection. Chronic infections may induce common cytokines. Such infections may complicate the disease or its treatment.
2. Psychologic distress. The incidence of depression in cancer patients has been found to be in the order of 25% [16]. Asthenia can be a feature of a major depressive episode or of an adjustment disorder.
3. Treatment side effects. Antineoplastic treatment, particularly radiotherapy and chemotherapy, can cause asthenia, although the means by which it does this is not well understood. Biologic therapies such as IL-2 and interferon-α predictably cause asthenia, especially at higher doses. Other medications such as opioids or benzodiazepines also commonly cause sedation and asthenia.
4. Anemia. In many cases, the correction of anemia does not result in improvement in asthenia. The exception may be when the hemoglobin has fallen rapidly or is extremely low.
5. Endocrine/metabolic abnormalities. Diabetes, Addison's syndrome, hypercalcemia, hyponatremia, hypokalemia, and hypomagnesemia should be identified and treated appropriately.
6. Overexertion. This factor may be important in patients undergoing treatment and attempting to continue social and work commitments.
7. Paraneoplastic neurologic syndromes. Although less common, syndromes such as myasthenia gravis, Guillain-Barré, and Lambert-Eaton are important to identify as they may respond to specific intervention or treatment of the primary tumor. Cachexia-related loss of muscle mass or muscle dysfunction and renal or hepatic failure are among contributing causes that are not easily reversed.

MANAGEMENT

Reversible causes should be identified and treated appropriately. Unfortunately, in many patients, no specific cause for asthenia is identified. In others, there are multiple contributing factors; therefore, treatment should be individualized.

Nonpharmacologic interventions are important in all patients and will often involve members of the multidisciplinary team. Occupational therapists offer advice about energy-conserving strategies and can provide assistive devices. Physiotherapy interventions may include an individualized program of exercise that aims to avoid deconditioning.

Education is a crucial factor in managing asthenia. Ensuring that the patient and caregivers are aware of the causes of asthenia, the presence or absence of therapeutic interventions, and what to expect in the future will assist in the

Table 30-1. Possible Causes of Fever in Patients With Cancer

Infection

Drug related

Transfusion

Tumor related (cytokines)

Necrotic tumor mass

establishment of realistic goals. Practical suggestions (*eg*, delegating household tasks or scheduling regular rest periods) can be particularly valuable.

In a randomized trial, methylprednisolone (31 mg/d) was demonstrated to improve activity levels in cancer patients, albeit for a limited period [17]. Most responders noted a benefit within 72 hours; therefore, it is reasonable to initiate a short trial of steroids and to cease treatment if no improvement is noted after 3 days. Because of the immunosuppressive and metabolic effects of corticosteroids, such treatment is best reserved for the latter stages of the patient's life. Dexamethasone is commonly used for this indication, with doses of 1 to 4 mg daily.

No definitive trials have directly examined the effect of amphetamines on asthenia in cancer patients. Methylphenidate may have a role in the management of asthenia in patients on high doses of opioids.

FEVER

Fever is common in patients with cancer and may be due to a variety of causes (Table 30-1). It is important to look for and exclude infection. The neutrophil count is important: in neutropenic patients, infection is responsible for more than two thirds of fevers, whereas only 20% of fevers in nonneutropenic patients are caused by infection. Malignancies classically associated with fever include renal cell carcinoma, hepatoma, metastases involving the liver, lymphoma, acute leukemia, myxoma, and osteogenic sarcoma. The mechanism of fever may relate to the action of cytokines TNF, IL-1, and IL-6 on the hypothalamus, stimulating release of prostaglandin E2 [18].

MANAGEMENT

It is paramount to first exclude an infectious etiology to the fever. Only then can one attribute the fever to the underlying malignancy and use nonsteroidal anti-inflammatory drugs (NSAIDs), which can be useful, for example indomethacin 25 mg three times daily or naproxen sodium 250 mg three times daily. The NSAIDs are thought to abate the fever by resetting the "thermostat" in the anterior hypothalamus, which is elevated in inflammatory fevers. Steroids and acetaminophen are reasonable alternatives if NSAIDs proved unsuccessful or are contraindicated. Effective treatment of the underlying malignancy remains the definitive treatment. Nonpharmacologic measures (fans, sponging) are useful adjuncts.

METABOLIC AND ENDOCRINE SYNDROMES

HYPERCALCEMIA

Hypercalcemia is a potentially life-threatening metabolic disorder commonly seen in cancer. It is seen in up to 30% of patients [19], most commonly in breast cancer, squamous cell carcinoma of the lung, and multiple myeloma. It is due to an increase in bone resorption and release of calcium from the mineralized bone matrix, either by osteolytic or humoral pathways.

The normal range for corrected calcium is 8.8 to 10.3 mg/dL (2.2–2.6 mmol/L). In hypoalbuminemic patients, the serum calcium must be corrected according to the following formula:

Corrected calcium = serum calcium (mg/dL) + 0.83 (40 serum albumin [g/L]).

Three major mechanisms are involved:

1. Tumor secretion of parathyroid hormone–related peptide (PTHrP). The tumor secretion of PTHrP is the most common mechanism involved in the syndrome of hypercalcemia of malignancy. PTHrP shares 80% homology with the first 13 amino acids of parathyroid hormone (PTH), which in turn is responsible for binding to the same skeletal and renal receptors as PTH, and therefore has the same effect on calcium and phosphorus metabolism (see below).
2. Osteolytic metastases with local release of cytokines. Osteolytic metastases release several growth factors and cytokines, including TNF and IL-1, which stimulate differentiation of osteoclasts, thereby increasing bone resorption.
3. Tumor secretion of calcitriol. This mechanism is rare. It is seen in Hodgkin's and non-Hodgkin's lymphomas.

NORMAL CALCIUM HOMEOSTASIS

PTH controls calcium levels in the short term. Release of PTH is stimulated by hypocalcemia. It acts to increase calcium levels by several mechanisms, including 1) increasing the efficacy of renal tubular calcium resorption, 2) increasing calcium resorption from bone, 3) converting vitamin D to its active form (calcitriol), which increases intestinal absorption of both calcium and phosphorus, and 4) in hypercalcemia (whether caused by PTH or PTHrP), sodium and water resorption is decreased, leading to dehydration as dilute urine is excreted. Nephrocalcinosis, the precipitation of calcium in the tubules, can lead to irreversible renal compromise.

CLINICAL PRESENTATION

Malaise, fatigue, and altered conscious state are among the most common symptoms reported by patients. Other symptoms are anorexia, nausea, and vomiting accompanied by polyuria and bony pain. Neurologic signs reflect a decrease in neuronal excitability. Weakness, hyporeflexia, delirium, and cognitive decline may be seen.

Signs of dehydration include dry mucous membranes, altered skin turgor, postural hypotension and tachycardia, and decreased jugular venous pressure. Cardiovascular events relate to irritability and increased contractility seen in the heart. Slowed conduction results in electrocardiogram changes, such as increased PR interval and QRS prolongation, which can ultimately progress to bradycardia, bundle branch block, asystole, and cardiac arrest. Depression of the autonomic nervous system leads to smooth muscle hypertonicity in the gastrointestinal tract, causing anorexia, nausea and vomiting, and abdominal pain.

MANAGEMENT

Patients at risk of hypercalcemia due to their underlying malignancy, immobility, dehydration, nausea, or vomiting must be educated about the symptoms and prevention of hypercalcemia. Advice should include encouraging fluid intake to 3 L/d if tolerated, increased mobility, and seeking early medical advice if symptoms appear. Thiazide diuretics should be ceased and calcium supplements and antacids avoided.

Treatment of hypercalcemia entails several approaches:

1. Increase urinary calcium excretion. Proximal tubule resorption of calcium is inhibited by volume expansion with intravenous (IV) saline. Monitoring of serum electrolytes and calcium should be carried out regularly. The volume infused and the speed at which it is administered will depend on volume depletion and comorbidities such as congestive cardiac failure. After euvolemia has been established, gentle use of a loop diuretic such as furosemide (*eg*, 20 mg orally twice daily) may be used if needed to prevent or treat fluid overload while hydration continues. Loop diuretics inhibit calcium resorption in the ascending limb of the loop of Henle. Thiazide diuretics are contraindicated as they enhance calcium resorption. In mild cases of hypercalcemia, hydration alone may suffice.

2. Decrease bone resorption. Bisphosphonates are the treatment of choice and act by binding to hydroxyapatite in calcified bone. They decrease the number of osteoclasts in sites undergoing resorption and may prevent osteoclast differentiation, therefore decreasing bone resorption. Pamidronate is more effective than etidronate [20], reducing calcium in 90% of patients [21], and has fewer side effects [22]. Bisphosphonates have also been proven to reduce skeletal complications of malignant disease when used prophylactically. Pamidronate (90 mg IV monthly) has been shown to decrease skeletal complications in patients with metastatic breast cancer or multiple myeloma with skeletal involvement. Corticosteroids (*eg*, dexamethasone 16 mg/d in divided doses) may be useful in sensitive tumors, particularly hematologic malignancies. Calcitonin (4 IU/kg subcutaneously twice daily) is safe but expensive and only effective in 60% to 70% of cases, with many patients swiftly developing tachyphylaxis, rendering it ineffective. Mithramycin (25 µg/kg IV) is rarely used due to its toxicity. However, it is reliable and effective, and doses can be repeated. Gallium (200 mg/m^2 per 24 hours) is effective, but requires infusion over 5 days, and is nephrotoxic.

The mortality in malignancy-associated hypercalcemia is as high as 75% at 3 months despite treatment, reflecting the poor prognosis of the underlying malignancy [23]. Other poor prognostic factors identified include older age and lower serum albumin and serum calcium levels after treatment. Treatment of the hypercalcemia enhances survival if systemic treatment for the malignancy is available. In others, the aim of treatment should be symptom control [24].

HYPONATREMIA

Hyponatremia (serum sodium < 135 mmol/L) is a common electrolyte disturbance in patients with cancer and may have a variety of causes, including conditions unrelated to the tumor (Table 30-2). The syndrome of inappropriate antidiuretic hormone (SIADH) secretion is the most common cause of hyponatremia in cancer patients.

Defining the cause of hyponatremia can be challenging. The first step is to assess the volume of extracellular fluid (ECF) as increased, decreased, or normal on the basis of history, physical examination, and plasma creatinine and urea. (ECF comprises plasma volume [25%] and interstitial fluid [75%].) Serum osmolality (normal is 280–296 mOsmol/L of water) and urinary sodium are also useful.

Reduced ECF causes decreased tissue turgor, dry mucous membranes with or without hypotension, tachycardia, and elevated serum urea. In this condition, hyponatremia is associated with dehydration. Low urinary sodium suggests extrarenal losses, whereas levels above 20 mmol/L occur with diuretics, hyperglycemia, and hypoaldosteronism.

Increased ECF causes peripheral edema and ascites with or without raised jugular venous pressure. In this condition, hyponatremia occurs in association with edema and may be due to hepatic failure, congestive cardiac failure, or renal disease.

The main causes of hyponatremia with normal ECF include SIADH, renal disease, and endocrine causes (adrenal failure, hypothyroidism). In SIADH, the serum osmolality is low, with inappropriately high urine sodium excretion (< 20 mmol/L) and osmolality.

CLINICAL PRESENTATION

Many patients are asymptomatic and hyponatremia is detected on routine blood tests. Symptoms usually appear at sodium levels less than 125 mmol/L and the rate of decline is equally important. Fatigue, anorexia, nausea, and confusion occur initially and can progress to coma, seizures, and eventually death if untreated.

MANAGEMENT

The treatment initiated will depend on the rate of decline in sodium levels, the severity of hyponatremia, and the presence of symptoms. In most cases, fluid restriction (500–1000 mL/d, depending on severity) is a useful initial strategy. Treatment of the underlying cause is the most effective way of correcting hyponatremia and chemotherapy for small cell lung cancer (SCLC) is generally effective treatment for SIADH. Drugs that may be responsible should be ceased.

In symptomatic patients or those with a rapid onset, hypertonic saline (3%) with or without IV furosemide should be used to increase the serum sodium by a rate not exceeding 12 mmol/L/d or 1 mmol/L/h. More rapid correction can result in central pontine myelinolysis [14].

When these measures are unsuccessful or undesirable, pharmacologic therapy may be instituted. Demeclocycline is a tetracycline analogue that acts by blocking the effect of ADH on the distal tubule, thereby causing nephrogenic diabetes insipidus. The usual regimen is 600 to 1200 mg/d in divided doses. Side effects include photosensitivity, gastrointestinal disturbance, and hypersensitivity reactions. Lithium has also been used and acts in a similar manner but has greater potential for toxicity.

Table 30-2. Causes of Hyponatremia

Cause	Description
SIADH	CNS origin (infection, vasculitis, stroke, head injury, tumor, psychologic stress); pulmonary origin (infection, tumor, asthenia, COPD, pneumothorax); drug related (carbamazepine, chlorpropamide, tolbutamide, haloperidol, amitriptyline, vincristine, morphine)
Organ failure	Adrenal insufficiency, hepatic dysfunction, cardiac failure, renal disease, hypothyroidism
GI losses	Vomiting, diarrhea, fistulas
Other drugs	Diuretics, cisplatin

CNS—central nervous system; COPD—chronic obstructive pulmonary disease; GI—gastrointestinal; SIADH—syndrome of inappropriate antidiuretic hormone.

CUSHING'S SYNDROME

In its classic form, Cushing's syndrome is easily recognized. However, in the setting of neoplasia, the clinical appearance may be confounded by other features of cancer such as weight loss. A high index of suspicion is required. The most common cancer associated with Cushing's syndrome is SCLC (about 50% of cases), with carcinoid tumors, neural crest tumors, and bronchial carcinoid also contributing significant numbers. Tumors may be occult at presentation.

CLINICAL PRESENTATION

Clinical features include hypertension, hirsutism, and myopathy with muscle weakness and wasting. Hyperpigmentation is more common than in Cushing's disease (adrenal overproduction of cortisol). Truncal obesity may occur but is often hidden by weight loss. Severe hypokalemic alkalosis can occur. The molecules involved in the syndrome in the setting of malignancy are precursors of ACTH, arising from the pro-opiomelanocortin (*POMC*) gene on the short arm of chromosome 23. These include pro-ACTH, endorphins, and melanocyte-stimulating hormone.

DIAGNOSIS

A stepwise approach to diagnosis is helpful:

1. Establish the presence of hypercortisolism. Screening tests for cortisol overproduction are 24-hour urinary free cortisol and a low-dose dexamethasone test (2 mg dexamethasone at 2300 h and measure cortisol at 0800 h; morning cortisol is suppressed in normal people).

2. Distinguish between primary adrenal pathology and ACTH-dependent disease. Measure ACTH levels: in primary adrenal disease, ACTH will be suppressed compared with normal or elevated levels in pituitary disease or ectopic ACTH production.

3. Distinguish between pituitary disease and ectopic ACTH. Failure of cortisol suppression with the high-dose dexamethasone suppression test (8 mg at 2300 h and measure cortisol at 0800 h) suggests ectopic ACTH production, as cortisol will be suppressed in pituitary disease. Because the sensitivity and specificity of this test are not perfect, other investigations may include CRH stimulation, metyrapone stimulation, and inferior petrosal sinus sampling.

4. Localize site of ectopic ACTH production. Imaging of the chest with plain x-rays and CT scanning will detect the majority of lung carcinoma and bronchial carcinoid. Octreotide receptor scintigraphy has also been used for localizing ACTH-producing tumors [25].

MANAGEMENT

Where possible, treatment of the underlying tumor should be undertaken. Resection is preferred if feasible, otherwise standard treatment should be offered. In SCLC, chemotherapy or radiotherapy may be associated with a decline in ACTH levels, although high levels may persist in long-term survivors.

Medical therapy revolves around the inhibition of adrenal steroid synthesis. Ketoconazole inhibits cytochrome P-450–dependent steroid hydroxylases and can be used in doses of 400 to 1200 mg/d. Side effects include nausea, headache, rash, and hepatic dysfunction. There are several important drug interactions, and hepatic impairment is a contraindication to its use.

Aminoglutethimide is an aromatase inhibitor, which at high doses (500–2000 mg/d) inhibits production of glucocorticoids, mineralocorticoids, and androgens. Side effects are significant at this dose.

Metyrapone (250–750 mg four times daily) acts by inhibiting the final step in cortisol synthesis. Toxicity is predominantly gastrointestinal and it may not be effective when levels of ACTH are very high.

Combining low doses of metyrapone (250 mg four times daily) and aminoglutethimide (250 mg twice daily) may be an effective treatment that minimizes the toxicities of the two agents. Replacement therapy with fludrocortisone and prednisolone may be required.

Suppression of ACTH production may be achieved with octreotide. Surgical adrenalectomy is also an effective palliative procedure.

NEUROLOGIC SYNDROMES

It is not uncommon for cancer patients to develop neurologic symptoms. The symptoms can be attributed to the direct effects of the disease (*eg,* tumor compression), chemotherapy-related toxicity, or malnutrition. Neurologic paraneoplastic syndromes are uncommon, occurring in about 3% of patients with cancer. Almost any part of the nervous system can be affected and their management remains challenging.

Nerve-specific autoantibodies mediate a number of these syndromes and are associated with specific cancer types. Lymphocytic infiltration is often found in the affected nervous tissues, further suggesting an immune-mediated mechanism. Table 30-3 shows the neurologic syndromes with the respective autoantibodies.

PARANEOPLASTIC ENCEPHALOMYELITIS

Paraneoplastic encephalomyelitis (PEM) is an inflammatory disorder that can affect the central nervous system at a number of different anatomic sites. The term *encephalomyelitis with carcinoma* was first coined by Henson *et al.* in 1965 [26]; since then a number of other terms such as *limbic encephalitis, subacute encephalomyelitis,* or *subacute cortical cerebellar degeneration* have been used. It has since become apparent that all of these conditions describe a similar pathologic process, irrespective of site, that can affect a number of different cell types.

Paraneoplastic limbic encephalitis usually presents with memory loss, confusion, hallucinations, and seizures and can occur as a distinct clinical entity or as part of the PEM syndrome. Temporal lobe changes are often seen on electroencephalogram and MRI. There are extensive neuronal loss and perivascular lymphocyte cuffing in the affected nervous tissues, reflecting multifocal inflammatory changes.

PEM involving the brainstem usually presents with opsoclonus, vertigo, and hearing loss, and central respiratory failure may ensue. The most common presentation is a disabling sensory neuropathy due to involvement of the dorsal root ganglia. Autonomic nervous system can also be affected and patients can present with postural hypotension, intestinal pseudo-obstruction, and urinary retention.

There is a strong association of PEM with an underlying autoimmune process. High titers of anti-Hu antibodies were identified in cerebrospinal fluid of SCLC patients who develop PEM. These antibodies are polyclonal

Table 30-3. Antineuronal Antibodies in Paraneoplastic Neurologic Syndromes

Antibody	Target cell	Main tumor association	Neurologic syndrome
Anti-Hu	All CNS neurons	SCLC, breast	PEM, PCD, peripheral neuropathy
Anti-Yo	Purkinje cells	Ovarian, Hodgkin's disease	PCD
Anti-Ri	All CNS neurons	SCLC, breast	Opsoclonus-myoclonus
Anti-retinal	Retinal photoreceptor cells	SCLC, melanoma	Cancer-associated retinopathy
Anti-MAG	Myelin	Paraproteinemias (MGUS, multiple myeloma, Waldenström's)	Peripheral neuropathy
Anti-VGCC	Presynaptic neuromuscular junction	SCLC	Lambert-Eaton myasthenic syndrome
Anti-Tr	Purkinje cells	Hodgkin's disease	PCD

CNS—central nervous system; MGUS—monoclonal gammopathy of undetermined significance; PCD—paraneoplastic cerebellar degeneration; PEM—paraneoplastic encephalomyelitis; SCLC—small cell lung cancer.

IgG$_1$ antineuronal antibodies (ANNA-1) that react against a number of RNA-binding proteins found on both neurones and SCLC cells. In a study of PEM in neuroblastomas and SCLC, patients with these antibodies appeared to have a longer survival than the seronegative patients, suggesting an underlying antitumor immune response [27]. Both neuroblastoma and SCLC are neuroectodermal in origin and express a high level of Hu antigen on their cell surfaces. Interestingly, PEM did not develop in patients with Hu antigen–expressing tumors but undetectable level of these antibodies. Moreover, attempts to transfuse anti-Hu antigens into animals failed to cause PEM, suggesting an immune-mediated process, rather than a primary antigenic effect, as the cause of PEM.

Neurologic symptoms often predate the diagnosis of cancer by an average of 6 months. Most patients progress onto widespread encephalomyelopathy, although spontaneous remissions had been reported. The median survival after onset of neurologic symptoms is about 1 year.

The treatment options include corticosteroids, IV immunoglobulin (IVIG), and plasmapheresis, although with little success [28]. Patients tend to die from respiratory and cardiac complications related to autonomic dysfunction rather than directly from their malignancy.

PARANEOPLASTIC CEREBELLAR DEGENERATION

Paraneoplastic cerebellar degeneration (PCD) is the most common paraneoplastic neurologic syndrome affecting the central nervous system. The process is usually associated with SCLC, breast cancer, ovarian cancer, and Hodgkin's disease.

The onset of symptoms is usually abrupt, with severe truncal ataxia, dysarthria, dysphagia, and nystagmus that develop within days. The rare disorder is found in about 1% of cancer patients, and conversely, approximately 50% of patients who develop subacute pancerebellar degeneration will eventually be diagnosed with an underlying cancer.

Several autoantibodies have been identified in patients with PCD (Table 30-4). Anti-Yo is a cytoplasmic antibody directed against Purkinje cells and often found in women with breast and gynecologic malignancies. In a large reported series, seropositivity for anti-Yo antibodies was found in 26 of 55 patients with ovarian cancer, 13 with breast cancer, and seven with other gynecologic malignancies [29]. Patients with high titers of anti-Hu antibodies tend to have PCD associated with PEM. Other autoantibodies associated with PCD alone include anti-Tr, which is usually found with Hodgkin's disease.

PCD usually presents prior to the diagnosis of cancer and almost always independent of the primary tumor. However, it is important to note that events unrelated to PCD, such as metastatic disease and chemotherapy toxicity, are still the more common causes of cerebellar dysfunction in cancer patients [30,31]. It has been recommended that women presenting with pancerebellar degeneration should be tested for anti-Yo antibodies, and if positive, be investigated for breast and gynecologic malignancies. Men with anti-Yo antibodies and PCD are extremely rare.

The patients with anti-Yo antibody tend to have an abrupt and rapidly progressive course compared with seronegative patients, although the differences are not noticeable when the disease progresses. Treatment with

corticosteroids, immunosuppressive drugs (*eg*, azathioprine), and plasma exchange have been largely unsuccessful to date.

OPSOCLONUS-MYOCLONUS

Opsoclonus, a form of ocular dyskinesia, is a result of the loss of inhibitory neural control and presents with involuntary, high-amplitude, chaotic saccadic eye movements. This is often accompanied by irritability, ataxia, and myoclonus of the extremities and trunk.

Nonmalignant causes, such as viral infections and trauma, are more common in children with opsoclonus. Paraneoplastic opsoclonus is most commonly associated with neuroblastomas in children. In adults, it is associated with a number of tumor types, particularly SCLC and breast and ovarian cancer. Paraneoplastic opsoclonus typically presents acutely and can predate the diagnosis of cancer by up to a year.

The diagnosis is largely clinical. A mild lymphocytic pleocytosis on cerebrospinal fluid examination is common. Neuroimaging studies are usually normal. Like other paraneoplastic neurologic syndromes, an autoimmune etiology is suspected and anti-Ri and anti-Hu antibodies had been identified in a few cases in cancer patients with opsoclonus. However, no specific antibody has yet been associated with paraneoplastic opsoclonus.

Corticosteroids are often used to treat symptoms, with occasional initial responses. Symptoms may improve with regression of the tumor in some cases, and spontaneously improve in others. Unfortunately, most affected individuals are left with residual neurologic deficits.

CANCER-ASSOCIATED RETINOPATHY

Cancer-associated retinopathy is rare, often in association with SCLC, melanoma, and gynecologic tumors. It is characterized by subacute visual loss with night blindness, photosensitivity, and impaired color vision [30,31]. Visual symptoms usually predate the diagnosis of the tumor, with patients developing blurred vision, photopsias, and scotomata (often with bizarre, episodic visual defects) followed by rapidly progressive painless loss of vision.

Fundoscopic examination may reveal arterial narrowing and abnormal mottling of the retinal pigment. The electroretinogram is always abnormal, and is diagnostic. Different antiretinal antibodies have been identified; the best characterized of these is the anti-recoverin (a photoreceptor protein) antibody. Treatment with corticosteroids has led to stabilization and improvement in some patients.

PERIPHERAL NEUROPATHIES

Peripheral neuropathy is common in cancer patients. In most, the disorder is due to direct tumor effect (such as compression or leptomeningeal infiltration of the nervous system), chemotherapy-induced (with cisplatin, vincristine, and taxanes), or secondary to nutritional/metabolic causes (cancer cachexia, vitamin deficiency, uremia). Paraneoplastic peripheral neuropathy is often diagnosed after these causes have been excluded.

SENSORY NEUROPATHY

Subacute sensory neuropathy (SSN) is a rare paraneoplastic neurologic syndrome that is part of the PEM syndrome, with around 50% of patients

Table 30-4. Treatment Modalities in Paraneoplastic Neurologic Syndromes			
Paraneoplastic syndrome	Plasmapheresis	Corticosteroids	Immunosuppressive drugs
Paraneoplastic encephalomyelitis	—	—	—
Paraneoplastic cerebellar degeneration	+	—	—
Opsoclonus-myoclonus	+	+++	+
Cancer-associated retinopathy	+	+	0
Sensory neuropathy	++	+	—
Autonomic neuropathy	0	+	0
Lambert-Easton myasthenic syndrome	+++	++	++
Polymyositis/dermatomyositis	—	+++	++
— Indicates treatment not shown to be effective; 0 indicates unknown efficacy; + indicates occasional reports of efficacy; ++ indicates treatment shown to be effective; +++ indicates standard of treatment.			

having evidence of PEM elsewhere in the nervous system. Although it is much more commonly associated with Sjogren's syndrome, about 20% of affected patients have been found to have a cancer, mostly SCLC.

Clinically, patients usually present with rapidly developing sensory loss, affecting all four limbs, beginning distally and extending proximally. Associated symptoms include areflexia, pain, and a debilitating sensory ataxia. There is a strong association between SSN and anti-Hu antibodies and patients with rapid onset of SSN should be tested for anti-Hu antibodies. If positive, workup for underlying cancer should be initiated [32]. The nerve conduction studies in SSN shows markedly decreased or absent sensory potentials, while motor nerve conduction and F waves are usually completely normal.

Treatment is usually unsuccessful, although there have been reports of regression with antitumor treatment or with the use of IVIG.

MOTOR NEUROPATHIES AND MOTOR NEURON DISEASE

Subacute motor neuropathy (SMN) is a very rare condition and is the motor counterpart to SSN. It has been associated with lymphoma and SCLC. Patients can present with progressive motor weakness over weeks to months, with marked muscle atrophy and flaccid muscle weakness. Lower limbs are affected more than the upper limbs, and bulbar involvement is rare. Patients with SMN in association with SCLC often have detectable anti-Hu antibodies.

An association between cancer and motor neuron disease (MND) has been reported. In a report of 14 patients with both cancer and MND, a rapidly progressive MND was reported in a series of 14 cancer patients with detectable anti-Hu antibodies that resembled the neurologic deterioration seen in amyotrophic lateral sclerosis (ALS) [33]. There have also been reports of an increased incidence of lymphomas in patients with MND, especially those presenting with ALS. The clinical presentation is usually identical to that of ALS, although the course tends to be a relapsing/remitting one subsequently.

SENSORIMOTOR NEUROPATHIES

The most common form of paraneoplastic neuropathy is a subacute or chronic sensorimotor neuropathy, representing 30% to 50% of peripheral neuropathies. Lung cancer (usually SCLC) is the most common underlying tumor; however, carcinomas of the breast, stomach, colon, and even lymphoproliferative disorders and myelomas have been implicated.

As opposed to Guillain-Barré syndrome, pathology specimens and nerve conduction studies usually reveal an axonal neuropathy rather than a demyelinating process. Clinical presentation usually consists of mild motor weakness, hyporeflexia, and symmetrical distal sensory loss, and lower limbs are more likely to be involved. Cerebrospinal fluid examination shows elevated protein with a normal cell count. A distinct autoantibody has not been identified, and the pathogenesis is not particularly well understood. The clinical course tends to stabilize and remain chronic, although improvements have been reported with the use of immunosuppressive drugs.

Sensory neuropathy can be seen commonly in patients with monoclonal gammopathies, such as multiple myeloma, Waldenström's macroglobulinemia, B-cell lymphomas, chronic lymphocytic leukemia, and monoclonal gammopathy of undetermined significance (MGUS). Typical presentation includes symmetrical sensory and motor loss affecting all limbs, often with tremor.

Electrophysiologic studies show marked slowing of conduction velocity and conduction block with focal areas of axonal degeneration along with demyelination and remyelination on nerve biopsy. Antibody against myelin-associated glycoprotein (MAG) can be found in patients with IgM monoclonal gammopathy. Selective deposition of IgM gammaglobulin in areas of myelin where pathologic changes occurred can be demonstrated on electron microscopy. Furthermore, passive transfer of human anti-MAG IgM to animals produces a similar neurologic disorder, suggesting an antibody-mediated process.

The neuropathy may improve with treatment of the underlying malignancy. The neuropathy associated with MGUS usually responds well to plasmapheresis, IVIG, and immunosuppression.

Patients with Hodgkin's disease can present with an acute neuropathy that is indistinguishable from Guillain-Barré. Response to treatment with plasmapheresis and IVIG is similar to the nonmalignant variant.

AUTONOMIC NEUROPATHY

Paraneoplastic autonomic neuropathy can present as an isolated disorder, or part of another syndrome, such as PEM or Lambert-Eaton myasthenic syndrome. It is most frequently associated with SCLC, and can be found in lymphomas and pancreatic and stomach cancers. It may affect part or all of the autonomic nervous system and clinical presentation includes dry mouth, postural hypotension, intestinal pseudo-obstruction, esophageal dysmotility, gastroparesis, and urinary retention. The clinical course is variable and specific treatments are usually unsuccessful.

LAMBERT-EATON MYASTHENIC SYNDROME

Lambert-Eaton myasthenic syndrome (LEMS) is a myoneural disorder characterized by impaired release of acetylcholine from presynaptic nerve terminals that result in muscle weakness. An underlying malignancy is found in two thirds of patients with LEMS [34]. Most patients with LEMS have SCLC and about 1% to 3% of SCLC patients develop LEMS [35].

The disorder is characterized by varying degrees of muscle weakness and fatigability. Unlike classic myasthenia gravis, the disorder does not usually involve the bulbar or ocular/orbital muscles. Initial symptoms include weakness and aches in thigh and pelvic girdle muscles. Most patients also complain of autonomic symptoms including dry mouth, erectile dysfunction, and constipation [34].

Electrophysiologic features of LEMS are pathognomic. The amplitude of compound muscle action potential increases with repeated muscle stimulation and decreases with low frequencies of stimulation [36].

The pathogenesis of LEMS is well understood, and is thought to be mediated by antibodies against the presynaptic nerve terminal, specifically against the voltage-dependent calcium channels. This results in less acetylcholine being released in response to an action potential.

Unlike other paraneoplastic neurologic syndromes, patients with LEMS respond well to plasmapheresis or IVIG. Short-term use of steroids or immunosuppressives may also be beneficial. Agents that increase acetylcholine release, such as 3,4-diaminopyridine, may improve the symptoms. Cholinesterase inhibitors, effective in myasthenia gravis, are usually ineffective in LEMS. Treatment of the underlying malignancy may lead to neurologic response in some patients.

MUSCULOSKELETAL AND CUTANEOUS SYNDROMES

POLYMYOSITIS AND DERMATOMYOSITIS

Polymyositis (PM) and dermatomyositis (DM) are inflammatory myopathies associated with cancer. Clinical presentation includes subacute symmetrical proximal muscle weakness with or without pain and muscle tenderness. Skin changes are seen in DM in addition to myositis, and the classic heliotrope rash typically involve the eyelids, cheeks, elbows, knees, and knuckles.

The diagnosis is made based on clinical and laboratory abnormalities that include elevated muscle enzymes (creatine kinase, lactate dehydrogenase), a myopathic electromyographic finding, and biopsy-proven inflammatory muscle degeneration. Treatment of PM and DM in cancer patients is similar to noncancer patients, consisting of immunosuppressives and corticosteroids. The clinical course is often independent of the cancer itself.

The risk of cancer diagnosis with DM was reported to be about 10% [37]. The most common DM/PM-associated cancers were lung cancer in men, and ovarian and breast cancer in women. Patients older than 40 years of age presenting with DM should be investigated for possible underlying cancer. Although the details of the investigation remain controversial, it is reasonable to include chest radiography and mammography, pelvic assessment, and serum Ca-125 level in women.

MUCOCUTANEOUS PARANEOPLASTIC SYNDROMES

The spectrum of mucocutaneous paraneoplastic syndromes is wide and varied. Detailed descriptions of each disorder are beyond the scope of this chapter; a selection of the more classic syndromes is outlined in Table 30-5. As in other paraneoplastic syndromes, their manifestation may occur prior to, concurrently with, or subsequent to the diagnosis of a malignancy. Therefore, it is important to initiate a workup for underlying malignancy once one of the cutaneous paraneoplastic syndromes is suspected.

Table 30-5. Mucocutaneous Paraneoplastic Syndromes

Disease	Major features	Associated malignancies	Cancer, %	Comments
Disorders of pigmentation				
Acanthosis nigricans	Dark velvety plaques on neck and flexor areas	Adenocarcinoma, especially gastric cancer	Most	Appearance of skin condition may precede malignancy by many years
Sweet's syndrome	Fever, neutrophilia, erythematous raised plaques	AML, other hematologic malignancies	20	May precede or present concurrently with tumor; treat with corticosteroids
Paget's disease	Erythematous keratotic patch; classic Paget's cells on histopathology	Breast, anorectal	50	Malignancy usually arises in area underlying skin changes
Erythematous conditions				
Exfoliative dermatitis	Progressive erythema followed by scaling	Cutaneous T cell, Hodgkin's lymphomas	20	
Flushing	Episodic reddening of the face and neck lasting for a few minutes at a time	Carcinoid medullary thyroid carcinoma	Most	Caused by serotonin, other vasoactive peptides
Bullous lesions				
Bullous pemphigoid	Large tense bullae	Chronic lymphocytic leukemia, lymphomas	Unclear	Usually has poor prognosis
Pemphigus vulgaris	Intraepidermal bullae of skin, oral mucosa	Lymphoma, breast, Kaposi's sarcoma	Unclear	
Dermatitis herpetiformis	Lifelong gluten-sensitive skin disorder with chronic intensely itchy vesicles over elbows, knees, and lumbosacral region	Non-Hodgkin's lymphoma, especially arising in jejunum	20–30	Unclear whether gluten-free diet reduces risk of malignancy
Conditions characterized by scaling and hypertrichosis				
Acquired ichthyosis	Generalized dry cracking skin with scales on trunk and extremities	Hodgkin's disease, Kaposi's sarcoma	Unclear	Can occur in up to 30% of patients with AIDS
Other				
Clubbing and HOA	Digital clubbing and periostosis must be present for diagnosis of HOA to be made	Lung	20	10%–20% of patients with clubbing also have HOA; signs and symptoms may improve with treatment of tumor
Prorates	Most common skin condition in patients with cancer	Lymphoma (typically), leukemias, myeloma	10	Usually associated with benign disease, but failure to elicit a cause necessitates a search for underlying malignancy

AML—acute myelogenous leukemia; HOA—hypertrophic osteoarthropathy.

REFERENCES

1. Langstein HN, Norton JA: Mechanisms of cancer cachexia. *Hematol Oncol Clin North Am* 1991, 5:103–123.

2. Plata-Salaman CR, Oomura Y, Kai Y: Tumor necrosis factor and interleukin-1b: suppression of food intake by direct action in the central nervous system. *Brain Res* 1988, 448:106–114.

3. Yoneda T, Alsina MA, Chavez JB, *et al.*: Evidence that tumor necrosis factor plays a pathogenic role in the paraneoplastic syndrome of cachexia, hypercalcaemia and leukocytosis in a human tumor in nude mice. *J Clin Invest* 1991, 87:977–985.

4. Schwarz MW, Dallman MF, Woods SC: Hypothalamic response to starvation: implications for the study of wasting disorders. *Am J Physiol* 1995, 269:R949–R957.

5. Greenberg DB, Gray JL, Mannix CM, *et al.*: Treatment related fatigue and interleukin-1 levels in patients during external beam radiotherapy for prostate cancer. *J Pain Symptom Manage* 1993, 8:196–200.

6. Weber J, Gunn H, Yang Y, *et al.*: A phase 1 trial of intravenous interleukin-6 in patients with advanced cancer. *J Immunother Emphasis Tumor Immunol* 1994, 15:292–302.

7. Emilie D: Administration of an anti-interleukin-6 monoclonal antibody to patients with acquired immunodeficiency syndrome and lymphoma: effect on lymphoma growth and on B clinical symptoms. *Blood* 1994, 84:2472–2479.

8. Yamashita J, Hideshima T, Shirakusa T, Ogawa M: Medroxyprogesterone acetate treatment reduces serum interleukin-6 levels in patients with metastatic breast cancer. *Cancer* 1996, 78:2346–2352.

9. Spath-Schwalbe E, Born J, Schrezenmeier H, *et al.*: Interleukin-6 stimulates the hypothalamus-pituitary-adrenocortical axis in man. *J Clin Endocrinol Metab* 1994, 79:1212–1214.

10. Mantovani G, Maccio A, Lai P, *et al.*: Cytokine involvement in cancer anorexia/cachexia: role of megestrol acetate and medroxyprogesterone acetate on cytokine downregulation and improvement of clinical symptoms. *Crit Rev Oncog* 1998, 9:99–106.

11. Kardinal CG, Loprinzi CL, Schaid DJ, *et al.*: A controlled trial of cyproheptadine in cancer patients with anorexia and/or cachexia. *Cancer* 1990, 65:2657–2662.

12. Watanabe S, Bruera E: Anorexia and cachexia, asthenia and lethargy. *Hematol Oncol Clin North Am* 1996, 10:189–206.

13. Irvine DM, Vincent L, Bubela N, *et al.*: A critical appraisal of the research literature investigating fatigue in the individual with cancer. *Cancer Nursing* 1991, 14:188–199.

14. Neuenschwander H, Bruera E: Asthenia. In *Oxford Textbook of Palliative Medicine.* Edited by Doyle D. New York: Oxford University Press, Inc.; 1998:573–581.

15. Warren RS, Starnes HF Jr, Gabrilove JL, *et al.*: The acute metabolic effects of tumour necrosis factor administration in humans. *Arch Surg* 1987, 122:1396–1400.

16. Pirl WF, Roth A: Diagnosis and treatment of depression in cancer patients. *Oncology (Williston Park)* 1999, 9:1293–1301.

17. Bruera E, Roca E, Cedaro L, *et al.*: Action of oral methylprednisolone in terminal cancer patients: a prospective randomized double-blind study. *Cancer Treat Rep* 1985, 69:751–754.

18. Blatteis CM: Neuromodulative actions of cytokines. *Yale J Biol Med* 1990, 63:71–85.

19. Frolich A: Prevalence of hypercalcaemia in normal and hospital populations. *Dan Med Bull* 1998, 45:436–439.

20. Eloma I: Diphosphonates for osteolytic metastases. *Lancet* 1985, 8430:1155–1156.

21. Body JJ: Current and future directions in medical therapy: hypercalcaemia. *Cancer* 2000, 88:3054–3058.

22. Zoger N: Comparative tolerability of drug therapies for hypercalcaemia of malignancy. *Drug Saf* 1999, 5:389–406.

23. Ralston SH, Gallacher SJ, Patel U, *et al.*: Cancer associated hypercalcaemia: morbidity and mortality. *Ann Intern Med* 1990, 7:499–504.

24. Ling PJ: Analysis of survival following treatment of tumour-induced hypercalcaemia with intravenous pamidronate (APD). *Br J Cancer* 1995, 1:206–209.

25. de Herder WW, Krenning EP, Malchoff CD, *et al.*: Somatostatin receptor scintigraphy: its value in tumour localization in patients with Cushing's syndrome caused by ectopic corticotropin or corticotropin-releasing hormone secretion. *Am J Med* 1994, 96:305–312.

26. Henson RA, Hoffman HL, Urich H: Encephalomyelitis with carcinoma. *Brain* 1965, 88:449–464.

27. Dalmau J, Graus F, Cheung NK, *et al.*: Major histocompatibility proteins, anti-Hu antibodies, and paraneoplastic encephalomyelitis in neuroblastoma and small cell lung cancer. *Cancer* 1995, 75:99–109.

28. Voltz RD, Posner JB, Dalmau J, Graus F: Paraneoplastic encephalomyelitis: an update of the effects of the anti-Hu immune response on the nervous system and tumour. *J Neurol Neurosurg Psychiatr* 1997, 63:133–136.

29. Posner JB: Paraneoplastic syndromes. *Neurol Clin* 1991, 9:919–936.

30. Anderson NE, Rosenblum MK, Posner JB: Paraneoplastic cerebellar degeneration: clinical-immunological correlations. *Ann Neurol* 1988, 24:559–567.

31. Jacobson DM, Thirkill CE, Tipping SJ: A clinical triad to diagnose paraneoplastic retinopathy. *Ann Neurol* 1990, 28:162–167.

32. Dalmau JO, Posner JB: Paraneoplastic syndromes affecting the nervous system. *Semin Oncol* 1997, 24:318–328.

33. Forsyth PA, Dalmau J, Graus F, *et al.*: Motor neuron syndromes in cancer patients. *Ann Neurol* 1997, 41:722–730.

34. O'Neill JH, Murray NM, Newsom-Davis J: The Lambert-Eaton myasthenic syndrome: a review of 50 cases. *Brain* 1988, 111:577–596.

35. van Oosterhout AG, van de Pol M, ten Velde GP, Twijnstra A: Neurologic disorders in 203 consecutive patients with small cell lung cancer: results of a longitudinal study. *Cancer* 1996, 77:1434–1441.

36. Sanders DB: Lambert-Eaton myasthenic syndrome: clinical diagnosis, immune-mediated mechanisms, and update on therapies. *Ann Neurol* 1995, 37(Suppl):S63–S73.

37. Sigurgeirsson B, Lindelof B, Edhag O, Allander E: Risk of cancer in patients with dermatomyositis or polymyositis: a population-based study. *N Engl J Med* 1992, 326:363–367.

Cancer Cachexia
MiKaela Olsen, Joanne Finley, Keri Culton

Cancer cachexia is a complex syndrome characterized by weight loss, fatigue, early satiety, anorexia, edema, and asthenia in conjunction with progressive loss of muscle mass and adipose tissue. Numerous changes in carbohydrate, lipid, and protein metabolism have also been described. Lean body mass depletion is a sequela of cancer cachexia, involving both skeletal muscle and cardiac proteins [1]. The massive depletion of lean body mass is what differentiates cachexia from starvation. In simple starvation, the body conserves both energy and muscle mass, instead utilizing fat stores primarily for energy.

Cancer cachexia is a debilitating syndrome experienced by as many as 80% of patients with cancer [2]. It is a distressing and burdensome problem for both patients and their family members. Family members express considerable concern and feelings of helplessness when anorexia and cachexia persist. Often, persisting anorexia and cachexia can cause conflict between the patient and family. Patients often appear weak and thin, prompting family members or friends to put pressure on the patient to eat more for fear they will "waste away." During end-of-life care, convincing family members to accept the lack of nutritional intake as part of the dying process is challenging. Patient and family education is essential during this time to ensure that patient comfort is achieved and family members do not experience unnecessary guilt.

Historically, cachexia was believed to be related to enhanced energy consumption by tumors coupled with decreased energy intake by the host. Treatment was focused on the administration of parenteral or enteral nutrition to compensate for weight loss and inadequate caloric intake. These interventions were found to be ineffective in advanced cancer patients and did not yield improvements in weight gain, performance status, or quality of life [3]. In a randomized study by Evans *et al.* [3], no differences in overall survival, tolerance of treatment-related toxicities, or progression of disease were noted between patients given expanded nutritional support and those with a diet as tolerated. In a review of 11 randomized controlled trials of oral nutritional supplements in patients with cancer, body weight, body composition, and functional outcomes did not improve [4]. In addition, nutritional support in cancer patients has not yielded improvements in lean muscle mass, which is one of the desired outcomes of an intervention [5]. A more thoughtful approach to nutrition utilization is necessary to ensure that the patient gains from the intervention instead of worsening as a result of the malignancy.

The presence of cachexia is a known predictor for decreased overall survival in cancer patients [6]. It is a direct cause of death in at least 20% of this population [7]. Cancer cachexia significantly decreases performance status and quality of life, increases psychological distress, and increases morbidity and mortality. The cachexia syndrome begins prior to noticeable weight loss and thus should be an assumed and expected outcome of cancer that receives attention and early intervention. Unfortunately, cancer cachexia is often misdiagnosed and mistreated. In its advanced stages, cancer cachexia interventions are unlikely to be helpful.

Increased knowledge of the molecular physiology of cachexia in cancer patients has opened the door for clinical trials that involve targeted pharmacologic therapies. These therapies should improve lean muscle mass, functional status, and quality of life. Regardless of the goals of cancer therapies, nutritional status in the cancer patient should be assessed at the time of diagnosis to optimize treatment tolerance and outcomes and to improve quality of life. When the goal is cure, maintenance of nutrition and weight can maximize treatment response and minimize related toxicities. Cachexia is associated with a decreased response to chemotherapy and increases in treatment-related toxicities [8].

INCIDENCE

Cachexia is believed to affect between 50% and 80% of cancer patients, with higher rates seen in those with disease progression or impending death. Cachexia is more notable at the time of diagnosis in select cancers such as head and neck, pancreatic, gastrointestinal (GI), and lung. As many as 80% of patients with pancreatic cancer present with signs of cachexia upon diagnosis [9]. This syndrome is reported in as many as 59% of terminal ovarian cancer patients [10]. More than 50% of patients with gastric, lung, prostate, or colon cancer and non-Hodgkin's lymphoma suffer from cachexia during their illness.

RISK FACTORS

Cachexia is a multifactorial syndrome that requires skillful assessment of risk factors to ensure treatment is initiated in a timely manner. In addition to the tumor types previously mentioned, the very young and those older than 70 years of age are particularly vulnerable to this condition and must be screened appropriately. Paillaud *et al.* [11] studied 88 patients with advanced cancer and found that those over the age of 70 were less able to increase their energy and nutritional intake and were found to be at higher risk. Weight loss is often notable in this group despite normal nutritional intake, indicating a more complex physiologic etiology.

As a group, patients with late-stage cancer have an extremely high risk of anorexia and cachexia; therefore, the palliation of these patients is a priority. In a study of 100 patients undergoing radiotherapy for head and neck cancer, weight loss was seen in more than 50% of patients [12]. Symptoms most commonly associated with weight loss included xerostomia (59%), taste changes (28%), metallic taste (19%), loss of taste (20%), missing meals on a regular basis (22%), nausea (19%), and constipation (28%) [12]. In addition, 57% of patients in this study (mean age, 64 years) wore dentures, which was associated with difficult mastication of food and subsequent weight loss.

Anorexia, a lack of appetite, coexists with cachexia in most cases and is a contributing factor in the progression of this syndrome. More than 66% of patients experience anorexia [13]. Anorexia and cachexia may result from chronic nausea/vomiting, pain, anxiety, depression, hypogeusia, dysgeusia, taste and food aversions, xerostomia, early satiety, delayed digestion or emptying, constipation, malabsorption, infections, and production of other complex substances by tumor cells.

Treatment modalities such as chemotherapy, radiation therapy, surgery, and biotherapy also can contribute to cachexia. Interventions to minimize or eliminate symptoms of cancer treatment can have a positive impact on cachexia and allow for improved quality of life.

PATHOPHYSIOLOGY

Cachexia is a multifactorial syndrome that is not completely understood. Cachexia has been described as a complex syndrome and is a by-product of host and tumor interactions. The losses of lean muscle mass and fat stores are significant in cancer cachexia and increased nutritional intake alone cannot reverse this process. Furthermore, the extent to which patients lose weight and experience cachexia does not correlate with the size of a tumor.

Alterations in energy metabolism are known to exist in patients with cancer. Resting energy expenditure has been an area of investigation. Resting energy expenditure is the amount of calories required by the body in a 24-hour period during nonactive periods. Studies are under way to characterize resting energy expenditure in various cancer types in relation to total energy expenditure, which is often decreased due to a reduction in physical activity. Cancer causes increased energy expenditure which, coupled with decreased or even normal intake of nutrients, results in cachexia. This negative energy balance is thought to be a key component of cancer cachexia.

Numerous studies have described the presence of proteolysis-inducing factor and proinflammatory cytokines in the etiology of cancer cachexia. Proteolysis-inducing factor causes the degradation of skeletal muscle and decreased muscle protein synthesis. Proinflammatory cytokines, induced by tumor cell lines in host tissue, induce a systemic inflammatory response. These cytokines include interleukin-1 (IL-1), IL-6, interferon, tumor necrosis factor, parathyroid hormone–related peptide, and macrophage migratory inhibitory factor. The role of these cytokines in cachexia continues to be studied. It is believed that they work in conjunction with other processes to cause metabolic abnormalities that induce both anorexia and cachexia. Alterations in carbohydrate, lipid, and protein metabolism are the most common metabolic abnormalities described in cachexia [14].

Loss of body fat occurs in cachexia due to increased lipid mobilization. For patients who lose at least 30% of their weight, as much as 85% of body fat loss can be noted [7]. Neuroendocrine activation increases the stress response and contributes to cachexia. Other tumor-produced cytokines are also thought to contribute to the cachexia syndrome and require further study [15].

Any process that directly or indirectly affects a patient's ability to eat or desire to eat contributes to anorexia and cachexia. Direct involvement of the GI tract with tumor(s), such as those in head and neck malignancies, can cause obstructions, dysphagia, and other digestive problems. Chemotherapy can cause nausea and vomiting, taste alterations, alimentary mucositis, lactose intolerance, food absorption, and food aversions, which all contribute to the problem of cachexia and anorexia. Radiation therapy directed at the upper airways or anywhere in the GI tract can cause symptoms such as xerostomia, mucositis, taste changes, dysphagia, nausea/vomiting, or diarrhea. Biotherapy can cause flu-like symptoms with arthralgias, myalgias, fevers, fatigue, and lack of appetite. Targeted therapies are associated with fatigue, weakness, nausea/vomiting, diarrhea, rashes, and edema. The key to minimizing anorexia and cachexia related to treatment toxicities is to anticipate and prevent them through vigorous assessment and early intervention using evidence-based practice symptom management guidelines.

ASSESSMENT

Currently, an agreed upon standard for the assessment of nutrition in cancer patients does not exist. Patients undergoing investigational clinical trials are also not thoroughly assessed as a routine part of protocol eligibility. Examinations of weight and performance status are done prior to enrollment in a trial; however, risk factors for cachexia are not extensively screened despite cachexia's role as an important prognostic factor. Baseline and ongoing weight measurement is an essential part of the cancer patient's physical assessment. Concern for cachexia should be prompted if weight loss is more than 5%

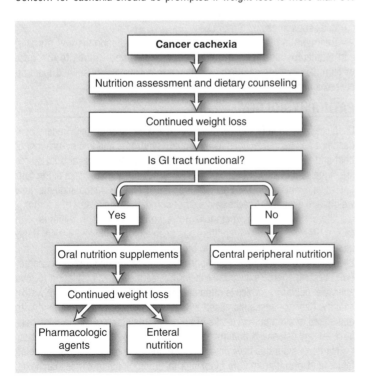

Figure 31-1. Supportive treatment algorithm for cancer cachexia patients.

of baseline within a 6-month period [5]. In obese patients, a weight loss of more than 10% is indicative of cachexia and should trigger increased monitoring and potential intervention. A body mass index measurement should be obtained upon presentation and on a regular basis. A decreased weight is associated with decreased performance status and is correlated with the number of metastatic sites present [16]. Weight loss has been associated with decreased median survival in cancer patients [16].

One of the most frequently used laboratory tests for detection of nutritional problems in cancer patients is serum albumin. Protein albumin is a major component of plasma and an index of nutritional status. A low protein albumin level is a predictor of health and a poor outcome. Albumin can also be decreased with increased inflammation, liver disease, and shock. A false high protein albumin level can be noted if an individual is dehydrated. Other laboratory tests used for the detection of cachexia include prealbumin, transferrin, total body nitrogen, total peripheral lymphocytes, and urinary creatinine clearance [17].

Anthropometry is the study of the measurement of the body in terms of bone, muscle, and adipose tissue. Anthropometric indices include measurements of triceps skinfold and arm muscle circumference.

In cancer patients, weight gain alone cannot be used as a measure of improved nutrition. Enteral or parenteral nutrition often improves weight through the addition of body water and fat but fails to increase protein and muscle mass [18]. A combination of objective measures should be used in the assessment.

Quality-of-life and symptom assessment tools can be extremely useful when evaluating a patient for cachexia. An established tool that is both valid and reliable assists in the monitoring of treatment interventions and their outcomes. One example is the Functional Assessment of Anorexia and Cachexia Therapy (FAACT) tool, an 18-item addition to the Functional Assessment of Cancer Therapy (FACT) assessment developed in 1993. The FAACT tool has been shown to be a valid and reliable instrument that assists in the measurement of anorexia, cachexia, and quality of life [19]. Additional testing has been performed using this tool to further assess instrument reliability and to shorten the length of time it takes to complete the assessment for anorexia and cachexia [20]. Another tool, the Patient-Generated Subjective Global Assessment developed in 1994, has demonstrated reliability and validity in cancer patients and has been used in various cancer populations to assess cachexia.

A third example, the Malnutrition Screening Tool, was developed and tested in outpatients with cancer receiving radiation therapy and was found to be highly predictive of nutritional status [21]. Patients diagnosed with cancer should be thoroughly assessed and screened for nutritional problems from the onset of their disease and routinely throughout their lifetime. Nutritional issues are potentiated by advanced cancer and escalate in the terminal stages of cancer. They can be evident in cancer survivors if long-term, treatment-related toxicities exist. Patients and their families should be educated accordingly.

Assessment of anorexia and cachexia can be extremely useful when followed in conjunction with patient and family education as well as evidence-based treatment interventions. Assessment should be performed at the time of diagnosis and on a regular basis during and after treatment.

TREATMENT

Cachexia has been the focus of much research in the hope of finding effective treatments; however, the syndrome has remained elusive, likely due to its multifactorial nature. The primary treatment is to eliminate the cancer. Tumor elimination, whether by surgery, chemotherapy, or radiation, is paramount and may reverse many contributing factors related to cancer cachexia. All other treatments are supportive, including pharmacologic agents aimed at appetite stimulation and decreasing proinflammatory cytokines, nutritional support, exercise, and symptom management (Fig. 31-1).

SYMPTOM MANAGEMENT

Cancer treatment through surgery, chemotherapy, or radiation therapy may eliminate the cancer and problems such as obstruction and dysphagia. However, it may also contribute to the problem through treatment-related side effects such as nausea, vomiting, mucositis, constipation, taste alterations, and anorexia [22]. Symptoms, whether related to the tumor or the treatment, should be controlled or eliminated because they contribute to the weight loss problem. Respective chapters in this textbook discuss specific symptom management strategies.

PHARMACOLOGIC AGENTS

Most of the research on cachexia treatment centers on pharmacologic agents. Pharmacologic agents are aimed at appetite stimulation and reducing proinflammatory cytokines. Protocols using multiple agents have shown little advantage over single agents [23,24]. The two established therapies for treatment of cancer cachexia based on many randomized controlled trials are progestational agents and corticosteroids [25,26]. Current research is focused on omega-3 fatty acids, cannabinoids, thalidomide, cyclooxygenase (COX) inhibitors, anabolic steroids, melatonin, and combinations of drugs. Many other therapies have been tried with limited or no success (*eg*, hydrazine sulfate, cyproheptadine, and pentoxifylline) (Table 31-1).

MEGESTROL ACETATE

Megestrol acetate is a synthetic progestogen. The role of its mechanism of action on appetite stimulation is not well understood; however, it was found serendipitously to increase weight in breast cancer patients. Since then, many randomized controlled trials have been conducted using megestrol acetate as an appetite stimulant. The Cochrane Review included 30 trials comparing megestrol acetate with placebo or other drug treatments. Twenty-two of the trials looked at cancer patients. The medial trial duration was 12 weeks. Overall results showed an improvement in appetite and weight gain [27]; however, it is important to note that weight gain was found to consist of increase in fat mass rather than lean body mass [28]. The optimal dose was not able to be determined due to insufficient data. Maltoni *et al.* [29] reviewed 15 randomized trials and concluded that high-dose progestins increase appetite and weight; however, the researchers could not determine an optimal dose either. Prescribed doses range from 160 to 800 mg/d based on effectiveness and side effects. Although usually well tolerated, potential adverse effects include fluid retention, thrombosis, male impotence, and adrenal insufficiency [30,31]. Megestrol is available in tablet or liquid format. A newer, more concentrated formula is available at 5 mL once daily [32].

CORTICOSTEROIDS

Corticosteroids were one of the first categories of agents used for appetite stimulation. Their mechanism of action may be related to their anti-inflammatory and euphoric effects. Their duration of action is shorter than megestrol and, therefore, they are most often used for short-term use treatment. The side effect profile of corticosteroids tends to be significant, including immunosuppression, muscle wasting, and hyperglycemia [33,34]. Corticosteroids may be useful for patients at risk for thrombus, in whom megestrol is contraindicated, or for patients in need of an antiemetic in addition to an appetite stimulant. The recommended dose for dexamethasone is 3 to 6 mg/d and prednisolone 15 mg/d in divided doses after breakfast and lunch or the entire dose given with breakfast [35].

OMEGA-3 FATTY ACIDS

Eicosapentaenoic acid (EPA) is a polyunsaturated fatty acid found in some fish, such as salmon, sardines, and tuna. The routes of administration for cancer cachexia are usually fish oil capsules or liquid. EPA is a nonprescription drug that acts by inhibiting proinflammatory cytokines. Side effects include abdominal cramps, fatty stools, and nausea. EPA has been the focus of many clinical trials related to treatment of cancer cachexia due to its promising anticachectic properties. A systematic review of five randomized controlled trials by Dewey *et al.* [36] totaled 587 patients with a variety of diagnoses. There was no significant gain in weight or appetite and the authors concluded that there is not enough evidence at this time to recommend its use, although there is little evidence of harm. Jatoi [24] suggests discussing the pros and cons of fish oil with patients and allowing them to decide if they wish to try it. The cost of this and other supplements must also be part of the discussion, as it may be prohibitive.

CANNABINOIDS

Tetrahydrocannabinol (THC) is the main active ingredient in the *Cannabis sativa* plant. The only oral cannabinoid available in the United States is the

synthetic THC dronabinol. The proposed mechanism of action is prostaglandin inhibition and endorphin release [37]. Dronabinol is effective as an antiemetic at a dose of 2.5 to 5 mg; the recommended dose for appetite stimulation is 5 to 7.5 mg/d. Psychotomimetic side effects, which may or may not be distressing to the patient, include relaxation, drowsiness, and an improved sense of well being but may progress to anxiety, delusions, and hallucinations at higher doses. Physical effects include increased heart rate, decreased muscle strength, reddened conjunctiva, and cognitive deficits [38]. A recent randomized, double-blind study showed that 5 mg daily of THC was well tolerated; however, there was no difference in appetite or quality of life between THC and placebo over 6 weeks of treatment [22]. Another study comparing dronabinol with megestrol acetate found that the combination of the two was not better than megestrol acetate alone [23].

THALIDOMIDE

Thalidomide inhibits tumor necrosis factor and other proinflammatory cytokines. Originally used for cachexia treatment in AIDS and tuberculosis patients, recent studies in cancer patients have been promising. A pilot study in 11 inoperable esophageal cancer patients found that 200 mg daily of thalidomide increased weight and lean body mass [39]. A randomized controlled trial of patients with pancreatic cancer also demonstrated weight and muscle mass gain at a dose of 200 mg daily, compared with a weight loss in the placebo group. Duration of survival was longer in the thalidomide group, although not statistically significant [40]. The main adverse effects are sedation, peripheral neuropathy, rash, and myelosuppression.

COX INHIBITORS

Inhibition of the enzyme COX may result in decreased systemic inflammation—and subsequently decreased cachexia—by inhibiting prostaglandin production. In a retrospective, case-control analysis, long-term use of indomethacin resulted in total body fat preservation [41]. Patients taking ibuprofen in addition to megestrol acetate alone maintained or gained weight over 12 weeks [42]. Mantovani *et al.* [43] used celecoxib 200 mg daily as part of a combination treatment with nutritional support, fatty acids, and progestogen to show improvement in weight and lean body mass, as well as a decrease in proinflammatory cytokines in advanced cancer patients. A similar combination treatment with nutritional support, progestogen, and celecoxib showed stable weights in advanced lung cancer patients [44]. Celecoxib has less GI toxicity than the traditional nonsteroidal anti-inflammatory drugs such as indomethacin.

OTHERS

Anabolic agents, such as androgens and growth factors, have the ability to improve lean body mass. Unfortunately, there are limited studies in cancer patients to warrant their use [44]. Potential adverse effects are significant, including virilization and hepatic complications. Melatonin has been studied in cancer patients with stabilization of weight at a dose of 20 mg/d. Melatonin decreases levels of the cytokines IL-6 and tumor necrosis factor. It is relatively well tolerated and requires further study [45].

EXERCISE

Exercise has been the focus of clinical studies aimed at reducing fatigue and improving quality of life [46]. Exercise may also reduce the inflammatory response and enhance insulin sensitivity, protein synthesis, and anti-

Table 31-1.Overview of Pharmacologic Agents Used in Cancer Cachexia

Established therapies	Therapies currently under investigation	Therapies with little or no efficacy
Megestrol acetate	Omega-3 fatty acids	Hydrazine
Corticosteroids	Cannabinoids	Pentoxifylline
	Thalidomide	Cyproheptadine
	COX inhibitors	
	Melatonin	
	Anabolic agents	

COX—cyclooxygenase.

oxidant activity, thereby decreasing the effects of cancer cachexia. There is insufficient information to recommend type, frequency, and duration of activity [47]. Exercise may also decrease the loss of muscle mass seen in cancer cachexia [48].

NUTRITIONAL SUPPORT

Early nutrition assessment and intervention is associated with increased protein energy intake, improved nutritional status, and fewer declines in quality of life and physical functioning [49–51]. Cachexia and weight loss have been shown to correlate with shorter survival, as weight loss appears to be an independent consequence of cancer survival and prognosis [16].

Ravasco *et al.* [51] demonstrated improved nutritional status and quality of life for head and neck cancer patients undergoing radiation treatment. Three groups were compared: 1) nutrition counseling to meet estimated protein energy needs while consuming a regular diet, 2) counseling with addition of oral nutrition supplements, or 3) ad lib intake without nutrition counseling. Those counseled based on regular diet had greater total energy intakes; however, protein intake was higher in the group receiving oral supplements. Total energy and protein intake decreased in the ad lib group. Quality-of-life scores improved in both counseled groups; however, for those receiving oral supplements, quality of life was associated only with increased protein intake. Despite this, it can be concluded that quality of life is positively affected with nutrition intervention to assist with increasing protein and energy intake. The majority of nutrition intervention studies included oral nutrition supplements if patients could not meet estimated protein energy needs. Overall, benefit was shown with early nutrition intervention at the start of cancer treatment, weekly during treatment, and biweekly after treatment completion. Isenring *et al.* [50] found less weight loss, improved quality of life and physical functioning, and quicker radiation recovery. Other studies have found similar results, with greater protein energy intakes and positive changes in lean body mass and functional capacity [50,51].

ORAL NUTRITION SUPPLEMENTS

Use of oral nutrition supplements has become popular in the oncology community. One explanation may be that patients with cancer cachexia have increased nutrient needs and decreased protein energy intake. Oral nutrition supplements offer a convenient and concentrated source of protein, energy, vitamins, and minerals. There are a variety of oral nutrition supplements available for use. They differ in taste and content to allow for individualized needs. Varying amounts of calories, protein, and sugar can be found, as well as addition of fiber or omega-3 fatty acids. Disadvantages to recommending oral nutrition supplements include cost and limited availability and accessibility in some areas. However, addition of oral nutrition supplements can result in increased protein energy intake and weight stabilization [49,52,53].

High protein energy–dense supplements may be especially beneficial when intake is not sufficient due to treatment-related side effects. These products may be used as a meal replacement if intake is severely reduced or as a supplement consumed in between meals. Formulas may also be an addition to homemade milkshakes or smoothies to increase total calorie and protein content.

Bauer and Capra [52] compared a supplement containing omega-3 fatty acids versus a standard supplement. Results showed greater protein energy intakes and improved quality of life with the omega-3–supplemented group; however, there were no significant differences in weight maintenance, improved lean body mass, or survival [52,53]. In conclusion, more intense study of this particular nutritional supplement is needed to show a clear benefit.

SPECIALIZED NUTRITION SUPPORT

Common adverse effects of chemotherapy and radiation previously described include anorexia, emesis, diarrhea, dysgeusia, mucositis, and dysphagia to mention a few. These effects, and the fact that cancer patients have increased protein energy needs, make this group attractive to treat with specialized nutrition support. If cachexia and weight loss continue despite nutrition intervention, specialized nutrition support may be warranted. As recommended by the American Society for Parenteral and Enteral Nutrition [54], specialized nutrition support, given enterally or parenterally, should be provided for those who cannot and will not be able to consume or absorb adequate energy and nutrients to sustain nutritional status. Table 31-2 includes a list of indications and contraindications for the use of enteral and parenteral nutrition [54,55].

CENTRAL PARENTERAL NUTRITION

Central parenteral nutrition is indicated when the GI tract is not functional due to obstruction or ileus or when patients cannot absorb sufficient nutrients due to short bowel syndrome, intractable vomiting, or diarrhea. Central parenteral nutrition results in weight gain, increased fat mass, and improved nitrogen balance [56].

Shang *et al.* [55] compared changes in body weight, total caloric intake, serum albumin, and quality of life in patients with advanced cancer who received oral nutrition supplements or oral nutrition supplements plus parenteral nutrition. The group receiving parenteral nutrition in addition to oral supplements had significant increases in body weight, serum albumin, quality of life, and survival. Careful consideration must be given to the use of parenteral nutrition because greater risks and complications are associated with its use. Complications include catheter occlusion or sepsis, bloodstream infections, cholestasis, and loss of intestinal function. When compared with enteral nutrition, increased cost, infectious complications, and longer hospital length of stay have been documented with central parenteral nutrition use [57–59].

Despite increased risk of complications, providing central parenteral nutrition preoperatively for severely malnourished patients has shown benefit over enteral nutrition [58–60]. Heys *et al.* [59] also found fewer postoperative complications for significantly malnourished patients who were given central

Table 31-2. American Dietetic Association's Clinical Guide to Oncology Nutrition

Nutrition type	Indications	Contraindications
Enteral nutrition	Malnourished or unable to ingest adequate energy or nutrients during treatment	Obstruction distal to access site
		Diffuse peritonitis
		Intractable vomiting
		Paralytic ileus
		Severe gastrointestinal bleeding
		Uncorrectable diarrhea
		High-output enterocutaneous fistula > 800 mL/d
		Intestinal schemia
		Hemodynamic instability
		Patient not consistent with aggressive treatment
Parenteral nutrition	Nonfunctional gastrointestinal tract	Functional gastrointestinal tract
	Severe diarrhea or malabsorption	Inability to obtain intravenous access
	Radiation enteritis	Needed for < 5 d for persons without malnutrition
	Short bowel syndrome	
	Intractable nausea/vomiting	Short life expectancy
	Bowel obstruction	
	Ileus	
	Severe pancreatitis	
	Enterocutaneous fistula GVHD of the gut	

GVHD—graft-versus-host disease.

parenteral nutrition compared with oral intake. However, there is no evidence that any course of central parenteral nutrition shorter than 7 to 10 days has clinical efficacy. It should be noted that the use of central parenteral nutrition in mildly cachectic oncology patients may cause more harm than benefit.

ENTERAL NUTRITION

In patients with nonfunctional GI systems, the parenteral route is the only option that can be used. If the enteral route is an option, there is clear evidence that this is the preferable route. Enteral nutrition is associated with less infectious complications, lower cost, and shorter hospital length of stay [58,60]. It mimics normal eating patterns by stimulating release of bile, leading to normal digestive processes and prevention of cholestasis. Enteral nutrition can help maintain intestinal function with specialized formulas containing fiber and prebiotics such as fructo-oligosaccharides. Enteral nutrition can also provide immunologic formulas with amino acids (arginine and glutamine), nucleotides, or omega-3 fatty acids.

Enteral nutrition supplemented with arginine has been compared with standard formulas. Van Bokhorst-de Van der Schuer *et al.* [61] discovered no significant improvement in quality of life and physical functioning when an arginine-supplemented formula was used before and following surgery. Therefore, no obvious benefit with arginine-supplemented formulas can be seen at this time.

The advantage of enteral nutrition was evaluated in malnourished surgical head and neck cancer patients with more than 10% preoperative weight loss. Enteral nutrition was provided 7 to 10 days preoperatively and 14 days postoperatively. Patients had increased protein energy intake, meeting 150% of estimated caloric needs. Results revealed improved quality of life and physical and emotional functioning. It was concluded that enteral nutrition is especially beneficial for cachectic patients when provided preoperatively and postoperatively. Placement of a gastrostomy or jejunostomy tube may be necessary based on patient preference and resources available.

Nutrition intervention with a clinical dietitian is key to minimizing loss of body weight, increasing functional capacity, and improving emotional functioning. Early nutrition assessment and supplementation may not reverse cancer cachexia; however, it may hinder weight loss and improve quality of life.

REFERENCES

1. Argiles JM, Moore-Carrasco R, Fuster G, *et al.*: Cancer cachexia: the molecular mechanisms. *Int J Biochem Cell Biol* 2003, 35:405–409.

2. Ramos EJ, Suzuki S, Marks D, *et al.*: Cancer anorexia-cachexia syndrome: cytokines and neuropeptides. *Curr Opin Clin Nutr Metab Care* 2004, 7:427–434.

3. Evans WK, Nixon DW, Daly JM, *et al.*: A randomized study of oral nutritional support versus ad lib nutritional intake during chemotherapy for advanced colorectal and non-small-cell lung cancer. *J Clin Oncol* 1987, 5:113–124.

4. Stratton RJ, Elia M: A critical systematic analysis of the use of oral nutritional supplements in the community. *Clin Nutr* 1999, 18(Suppl 2):29–84.

5. Inui A: Recent development in research and management of cancer anorexia-cachexia syndrome [in Japanese]. *Gan To Kagaku Ryoho* 2005, 32:743–749.

6. Hauser CA, Stockler MR, Tattersall MH: Prognostic factors in patients with recently diagnosed incurable cancer: a systematic review. *Support Care Cancer* 2006, 14:999–1011.

7. Muscaritoli M, Bossola M, Aversa Z, *et al.*: Prevention and treatment of cancer cachexia: new insights into an old problem. *Eur J Cancer* 2006, 42:31–41.

8. Uomo G, Gallucci F, Rabitti PG: Anorexia-cachexia syndrome in pancreatic cancer: recent development in research and management. *JOP* 2006, 7:157–162.

9. Ockenga J, Valentini L: Review article: anorexia and cachexia in gastrointestinal cancer. *Aliment Pharmacol Ther* 2005, 22:583–594.

10. Sun XG, Wu M, Ma SQ, *et al.*: Study of symptoms in terminally ill patients with ovarian carcinoma [in Chinese]. *Zhonghua Fu Chan Ke Za Zhi* 2007, 42:192–195.

11. Paillaud E, Caillet P, Campillo B, Bories PN: Increased risk of alteration of nutritional status in hospitalized elderly patients with advanced cancer. *J Nutr Health Aging* 2006, 10:91–95.

12. Lees J: Incidence of weight loss in head and neck cancer patients on commencing radiotherapy treatment at a regional oncology centre. *Eur J Cancer Care (Engl)* 1999, 8:133–136.

13. Wilcock A: Anorexia: a taste of things to come? *Palliat Med* 2006, 20:43–45.

14. Tisdale MJ: Metabolic abnormalities in cachexia and anorexia. *Nutrition* 2000, 16:1013–1014.

15. Argiles JM, Busquets S, Garcia-Martinez C, Lopez-Soriano FJ: Mediators involved in the cancer anorexia-cachexia syndrome: past, present, and future. *Nutrition* 2005, 21:977–985.

16. Dewys WD, Begg C, Lavin PT, *et al.*: Prognostic effect of weight loss prior to chemotherapy in cancer patients. Eastern Cooperative Oncology Group. *Am J Med* 1980, 69:491–497.

17. Hirschfeld S: Working group session report: cancer. *J Nutr* 1999, 129(Suppl):306S–307S.

18. Cohn SH, Vartsky D, Vaswani AN, *et al.*: Changes in body composition of cancer patients following combined nutritional support. *Nutr Cancer* 1982, 4:107–119.

19. Chang VT, Xia Q, Kasimis B: The Functional Assessment of Anorexia/Cachexia Therapy (FAACT) appetite scale in veteran cancer patients. *J Support Oncol* 2005, 3:377–382.

20. Ribaudo JM, Cella D, Hahn EA, *et al.*: Re-validation and shortening of the Functional Assessment of Anorexia/Cachexia Therapy (FAACT) questionnaire. *Qual Life Res* 2000, 9:1137–1146.

21. Ferguson ML, Bauer J, Gallagher B, *et al.*: Validation of a malnutrition screening tool for patients receiving radiotherapy. *Australas Radiol* 1999, 43:325–327.

22. Strasser F: The silent symptom early satiety: a forerunner of distinct phenotypes of anorexia/cachexia syndromes. *Support Care Cancer* 2006, 14:689–692.

23. Jatoi A, Windschitl HE, Loprinzi CL, *et al.*: Dronabinol versus megestrol acetate versus combination therapy for cancer-associated anorexia: a North Central Cancer Treatment Group study. *J Clin Oncol* 2002, 20:567–573.

24. Jatoi A: Omega-3 fatty acid supplements for cancer-associated weight loss. *Nutr Clin Pract* 2005, 20:394–399.

25. Del Fabbro E, Dalal S, Bruera E: Symptom control in palliative care. Part II: cachexia/anorexia and fatigue. *J Palliat Med* 2006, 9:409–421.

26. Jatoi A: Pharmacologic therapy for the cancer anorexia/weight loss syndrome: a data-driven, practical approach. *J Support Oncol* 2006, 4:499–502.

27. Berenstein EG, Ortiz Z: Megestrol acetate for the treatment of anorexia-cachexia syndrome. *Cochrane Database Syst Rev* 2005, 2:CD004310.

28. Loprinzi CL, Jensen MD, Jiang NS, Schaid DJ: Effect of megestrol acetate on the human pituitary-adrenal axis. *Mayo Clin Proc* 1992, 67:1160–1162.

29. Maltoni M, Nanni O, Scarpi E, *et al.*: High-dose progestins for the treatment of cancer anorexia-cachexia syndrome: a systematic review of randomised clinical trials. *Ann Oncol* 2001, 12:289–300.

30. Nelson KA: The cancer anorexia-cachexia syndrome. *Semin Oncol* 2000, 27:64–68.

31. Tchekmedyian NS: Treating the anorexia/cachexia syndrome. *J Support Oncol* 2006, 4:506–507.

32. Megestrol acetate NCD oral suspension: Par Pharmaceutical—megestrol acetate nanocrystal dispersion oral suspension, PAR 100.2, PAR-100.2. *Drugs R D* 2007, 8:251–254.

33. Gagnon B, Bruera E: A review of the drug treatment of cachexia associated with cancer. *Drugs* 1998, 55:675–688.

34. Mattox TW: Treatment of unintentional weight loss in patients with cancer. *Nutr Clin Pract* 2005, 20:400–410.

35. Inui A: Cancer anorexia-cachexia syndrome: current issues in research and management. *CA Cancer J Clin* 2002, 52:72–91.

36. Dewey A, Baughan C, Dean T, *et al.*: Eicosapentaenoic acid (EPA, an omega-3 fatty acid from fish oils) for the treatment of cancer cachexia. *Cochrane Database Syst Rev* 2007, 1:CD004597.

37. Davis MP: New drugs for the anorexia-cachexia syndrome. *Curr Oncol Rep* 2002, 4:264–274.

38. Walsh D, Nelson KA, Mahmoud FA: Established and potential therapeutic applications of cannabinoids in oncology. *Support Care Cancer* 2003, 11:137–143.

39. Khan ZH, Simpson EJ, Cole AT, *et al.*: Oesophageal cancer and cachexia: the effect of short-term treatment with thalidomide on weight loss and lean body mass. *Aliment Pharmacol Ther* 2003, 17:677–682.

40. Gordon JN, Trebble TM, Ellis RD, *et al.*: Thalidomide in the treatment of cancer cachexia: a randomised placebo controlled trial. *Gut* 2005, 54:540–545.

41. Lundholm K, Daneryd P, Korner U, *et al.*: Evidence that long-term COX-treatment improves energy homeostasis and body composition in cancer patients with progressive cachexia. *Int J Oncol* 2004, 24:505–512.

42. McMillan DC, O'Gorman P, Fearon KC, McArdle CS: A pilot study of megestrol acetate and ibuprofen in the treatment of cachexia in gastrointestinal cancer patients. *Br J Cancer* 1997, 76:788–790.

43. Mantovani G, Maccio A, Massa E, Madeddu C: Managing cancer-related anorexia/cachexia. *Drugs* 2001, 61:499–514.

44. Cerchietti LC, Navigante AH, Peluffo GD, *et al.*: Effects of celecoxib, medroxyprogesterone, and dietary intervention on systemic syndromes in patients with advanced lung adenocarcinoma: a pilot study. *J Pain Symptom Manage* 2004, 27:85–95.

45. Davies M: Nutritional screening and assessment in cancer-associated malnutrition. *Eur J Oncol Nurs* 2005, 9(Suppl 2):S64–S73.

46. Dimeo FC, Stieglitz RD, Novelli-Fischer U, *et al.*: Effects of physical activity on the fatigue and psychologic status of cancer patients during chemotherapy. *Cancer* 1999, 85:2273–2277.

47. Ardies CM: Exercise, cachexia, and cancer therapy: a molecular rationale. *Nutr Cancer* 2002, 42:143–157.

48. Zinna EM, Yarasheski KE: Exercise treatment to counteract protein wasting of chronic diseases. *Curr Opin Clin Nutr Metab Care* 2003, 6:87–93.

49. Davidson W, Ash S, Capra S, Bauer J; Cancer Cachexia Study Group: Weight stabilisation is associated with improved survival duration and quality of life in unresectable pancreatic cancer. *Clin Nutr* 2004, 23:239–247.

50. Isenring EA, Capra S, Bauer JD: Nutrition intervention is beneficial in oncology outpatients receiving radiotherapy to the gastrointestinal or head and neck area. *Br J Cancer* 2004, 91:447–452.

51. Ravasco P, Monteiro-Grillo I, Marques Vidal P, Camilo ME: Impact of nutrition on outcome: a prospective randomized controlled trial in patients with head and neck cancer undergoing radiotherapy. *Head Neck* 2005, 27:659–668.

52. Bauer JD, Capra S: Nutrition intervention improves outcomes in patients with cancer cachexia receiving chemotherapy: a pilot study. *Support Care Cancer* 2005, 13:270–274.

53. Fearon KC, Von Meyenfeldt MF, Moses AG, *et al.*: Effect of a protein and energy dense N-3 fatty acid enriched oral supplement on loss of weight and lean tissue in cancer cachexia: a randomised double blind trial. *Gut* 2003, 52:1479–1486.

54. ASPEN Board of Directors and the Clinical Guidelines Task Force: Guidelines for the use of parenteral and enteral nutrition in adult and pediatric patients. *JPEN J Parenter Enter Nutr* 2002, 26(1 Suppl):1SA–138SA.

55. Shang E, Weiss C, Post S, Kaehler G: The influence of early supplementation of parenteral nutrition on quality of life and body composition in patients with advanced cancer. *JPEN J Parenter Enter Nutr* 2006, 30:222–230.

56. Elliot L, Molseed L, Davis McCallum P: *The Clinical Guide to Oncology Nutrition*, edn 2. Chicago: American Dietetic Association; 2006.

57. Huhmann MB, Cunningham RS: Importance of nutritional screening in treatment of cancer-related weight loss. *Lancet Oncol* 2005, 6:334–343.

58. Nitenberg G, Raynard B: Nutritional support of the cancer patient: issues and dilemmas. *Crit Rev Oncol Hematol* 2000, 34:137–168.

59. Heys SD, Gough DB, Eremin O: Is nutritional support in patients with cancer undergoing surgery beneficial? *Eur J Surg Oncol* 1996, 22:292–297.

60. Bozzetti F, Braga M, Gianotti L, *et al.*: Postoperative enteral versus parenteral nutrition in malnourished patients with gastrointestinal cancer: a randomised multicentre trial. *Lancet* 2001, 358:1487–1492.

61. Van Bokhorst-de Van der Schuer MA, Langendoen SI, Vondeling H, *et al.*: Perioperative enteral nutrition and quality of life of severely malnourished head and neck cancer patients: a randomized clinical trial. *Clin Nutr* 2000, 19:437–444.

Cancer is a disease of aging. The longer a person lives, the longer carcinogens and defects in internal cell regulation have to produce clinically evident cancers. Currently in the United States, 60% of all cancers and 70% of all cancer deaths occur in patients older than 65 years of age. In the next 25 years, the number of people who are 65 years of age and older will double, and the largest increases in cancer incidence will occur in those older than 80 years of age [1]. Therefore, the growing burden of cancer in the elderly will require a more comprehensive approach to their unique health needs.

Older adults with cancer often have other chronic health problems and may be taking multiple medications that can affect their cancer treatment plan. Ageism, cultural beliefs, illness, and limited access to care marginalize many individuals and present barriers to appropriate health care. In patients with multiple health and psychosocial issues, the mismatch between the disease-focused, acute care orientation of the health care system and the more holistic chronic care needs of the patient is glaringly obvious and often leads to insufficient and ineffective care.

Despite the prevalence of cancer in the elderly, we know surprisingly little about the course of cancer and its treatment in this population. Misconceptions and prejudice have excluded older patients from most clinical trials. In clinical practice, these biases cut both ways: elderly cancer patients are as often overtreated as they are undertreated.

DECISION MAKING

Deciding how aggressively to treat cancer in an elderly patient is an ethical dilemma that first requires a thorough understanding of the indications and possible outcomes of the medical intervention [2]. Adequate information is the necessary condition for informed decision making. This includes knowledge of the natural history of the cancer as well as one's life expectancy with and without the cancer. A thorough understanding of how the cancer will affect one's life and what one can expect in terms of cancer-related symptoms is also essential.

With this information, it is next appropriate to consider the treatment options and their efficacy. It is important to be clear about the goals of treatment. In addition to the traditional goals of tumor response and increased survival, elderly patients are likely to have goals related to their quality of life, especially their physical and intellectual independence. They may also have goals related to their family or friends.

Next, one must understand the patient's preferences regarding his or her goals and the treatment and—especially when these cannot be elicited—the range and degree of the patient's future prospects. If one or more of the treatment options is likely to meet the patient's goals, a thorough understanding of the potential side effects is essential.

Finally, while mindful of the established goals, the patient should weigh the burdens and benefits of the treatment options and make a decision. The discussion of treatment options should include all of the alternatives, including information about palliative care and hospice. Physicians are duty bound to help the patient and family focus on obtainable goals.

CAUSE OF DEATH: CANCER OR OLD AGE?

Will the cancer end the patient's life prematurely? To answer this important question, a thorough understanding of the interplay between age and cancer is required. The patient's chronological age and the stage-specific natural history of his or her cancer provide the context for decision making. However, chronological age is not the best surrogate for one's health status or ability to handle anticancer treatment. Even the expected behaviors of some cancers vary between young and old patients.

THE EFFECT OF AGE ON CANCER

LYMPHOMA AND LEUKEMIA

For patients with non-Hodgkin's lymphoma, age is an independent negative risk factor, and one of the key determinants of survival in the International Prognostic Index [3,4]. The biology of acute myeloid leukemia is different in younger and older patients, although the reason for these intrinsic age-related differences is not clear.

BREAST CANCER

Breast cancer characteristics and tumor biology are different in older women. As patients age, their breast tumors more frequently express hormone receptors, have lower rates of tumor cell proliferation, and have lower expression of Her-2/neu [5]. Although these more favorable tumor characteristics suggest a more indolent course for breast cancer in older women, more recent studies [6] show no major age-related differences in breast cancer survival. In fact, older women with metastases often have more aggressive disease than their younger counterparts [7]. Survival is similar in older and younger women with localized and regional stages of breast cancer; however, the very young (< 35 years of age) generally have shorter survival times.

This may be explained in part by patterns of hormone receptor expression. Tumors in young women are usually estrogen receptor (ER)-negative/progesterone receptor (PR)-negative. The proportion of ER-negative and PR-negative patients decreases with increasing age, but the number of women with PR-negative tumors begins to increase again at age 50. Older women are more often ER-positive/PR-negative and, therefore, carry a worse prognosis than those with ER-positive/PR-positive tumors [8,9]. Among elderly patients, the risk of death from breast cancer does not decrease with increasing age. This fact should be remembered when discussing primary and adjuvant treatment with breast cancer patients.

THE EFFECT OF AGE ON PATIENTS

CHRONOLOGICAL AGE

Despite advanced age, men and women who are relatively healthy often have a life expectancy that may exceed their life expectancy with cancer. The average 70-year-old woman is likely to live another 16 years. Similarly, an 85-year-old can expect to live an additional 6 years and remain functionally independent for most of that time. Even an unwell 75-year-old man will probably live 5 more years, which is long enough to experience cancer-related morbidity and mortality (Fig. 32-1) [10].

Chronological age is the traditional determinant of "old age." Worldwide, old age is defined as beginning at age 65; in the United States, Medicare uses the same codification. Balducci [11] stratifies older cancer patients into three categories: 1) young old (age 65–75); 2) old old (age 76–85); and 3) oldest old (more than 85 years of age).

Although comorbidity and functional limitations disproportionately affect older adults, especially cancer patients, advanced age alone should not be the sole determinant of how and when to use life-prolonging or palliative anticancer treatment [12,13]. By itself, age is not reliable in estimating life expectancy, functional reserve, or the risk of treatment complications [14]. Definitions that are more relevant include biological and functional changes associated with aging rather than a discrete age in cut-off years. Biological determinants of age include sarcopenia, body mass index (BMI), cytokine expression, and glomerular filtration rate (GFR).

FRAILTY

Frailty is a biological syndrome that is highly prevalent in old age. Fried *et al.* [15] define frailty as a clinical syndrome in which three or more of the following criteria are present: 1) unintentional weight loss (10 lbs or more in the past year), 2) self-reported exhaustion, 3) weakness (grip strength), 4) slow walking speed, and 5) low physical activity (Table 32-1). Frail individuals have decreased reserve and resistance to stressors, which cause vulnerability to adverse outcomes. These include a high risk for falls, disability, hospitalization, and early mortality (Table 32-2). The impact of cancer on frailty and the value of this frailty phenotype for predicting a cancer patient's treatment risk or benefit have yet to be determined. However, it does provide a useful framework in which to consider the older cancer patient.

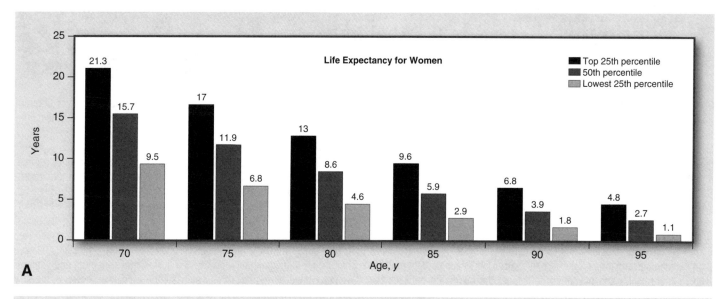

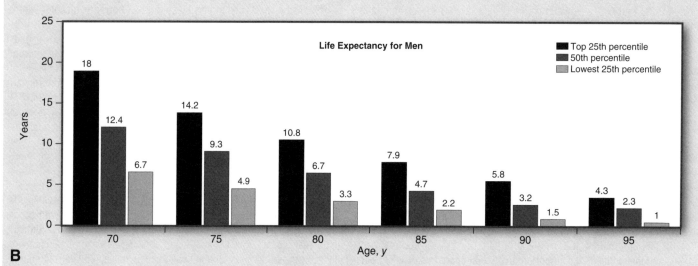

Figure 32-1. Life expectancy for older adult women (**A**) and older adult men (**B**). (*From* Walter and Covinsky [10]; with permission.)

Table 32-1. Frailty Phenotype

Parameter	Description/measurement	Frailty phenotype
Weight loss (shrinking)	Unintentional weight loss over past 12 mo	> 5% body weight
Exhaustion (fatigue)	Response to "How often in the last week do you feel like everything was an effort?"	≥ moderate (3–4 times)
Physical activity	Minnesota Leisure Time Activity Questionnaire	Men < 383 kcal/wk; women < 270 kcal/wk
Slowness (walk time)	15-ft walk stratified by height	> 6–7 sec
Strength (weakness)	Grip strength stratified by gender and body mass index	Men < 29–32; women < 17–21

(*Adapted from* Fried *et al.* [15].)

Table 32-2. Frailty and the Incidence of Adverse Outcomes

	Death rate, %		First hospitalization, %		First fall, %		ADL disability, %		Mobility disability, %	
	3 y	7 y	3 y	7 y	3 y	7 y	3 y	7 y	3 y	7 y
Not frail	3	12	33	79	15	27	8	23	23	41
Prefrail	7	23	43	83	19	33	20	41	40	58
Frail	18	43	59	96	28	41	39	63	51	71

ADL—activities of daily living.
(*Adapted from* Fried *et al.* [15].)

In the future, it may be possible to determine frailty by measuring various biological markers. Increased serum levels of inflammatory markers such as interleukin-6 correlate with the presence of the frailty phenotype determinants [16]. It may soon be possible to move patients from the "frail" to the "prefrail" or "not frail" categories by modifying these markers with pharmacologic or other interventions. Indeed, cancer patients who are currently cared for in geriatric oncology programs already experience some of these benefits, as multidisciplinary teams of oncologists, geriatricians, psychiatrists, pharmacists, physiatrists, social workers, and dieticians work together to identify and manage the stressors that can limit effective cancer treatment.

These multidisciplinary teams use some form of the Comprehensive Geriatric Assessment (CGA) to assess the older cancer patients' functional status, comorbidities, socioeconomic issues, and nutritional status, and to determine the presence of polypharmacy or geriatric syndromes (Table 32-3). Comorbidity is associated with mortality, both in general and specifically in cancer patients. This effect is independent of functional status and appears to have very little impact on the behavior of the cancer itself. Studies do show that comorbidity has a major impact on toxicity and treatment outcome [17].

Although the best form of the CGA in cancer patients remains to be defined, growing evidence demonstrates that the variables examined in a CGA can predict morbidity and mortality in older patients with cancer and uncover problems relevant to cancer care that would otherwise go unrecognized [18]. The International Society of Geriatric Oncology (SIOG) has recommended its use as an essential component for improving cancer care and possibly survival in older cancer patients [19].

THE EFFECT OF AGE ON DECISION MAKING

In conjunction with knowledge of the stage-specific natural history of a patient's cancer, the frailty phenotype provides the necessary information for deciding whether the patient's cancer will cut his or her life short, and what symptoms he/she is likely to experience as the cancer progresses. If a patient's life expectancy is so short that the cancer will not significantly affect it (*eg*, the elderly patient with early-stage chronic lymphocytic leukemia), anticancer treatment is not indicated, especially if there is a low likelihood of developing significant symptoms. On the other hand, anticancer treatment should be considered if the patient is likely to live long enough to experience cancer-related symptoms or premature cancer-related death.

UNDERSTANDING THE BENEFITS AND HARMS OF TREATMENT

THE EFFICACY OF ANTICANCER TREATMENT IN THE ELDERLY

Like all treatment decisions, the decision to use anticancer treatment in the elderly requires a careful weighing of its burdens and benefits. This assessment must take into account all the relevant factors of the impact of age. We have already discussed several examples of how age affects treatment and toxicity; however, its impact on efficacy is minimal. There is an ongoing belief that the elderly do not respond to standard treatment and/or cannot tolerate usual doses of cancer drugs; however, there is now good evidence to the contrary [20–22].

THE GOALS OF TREATMENT

A treatment may be efficacious for a class of patients, but each patient, in light of his or her own goals, must weigh these potential benefits. Given this information, rational patients may vary with regard to how they rank the harms and benefits of a suggested treatment. It is important to be clear whether the goal of treatment is cure or palliation. If the goal is palliation, all parties should be clear if the intent of palliative treatment is to extend life and/or improve the quality of life by controlling bothersome symptoms. Of course, it is also important to know the likelihood of achieving these goals and to understand the probable duration of the positive effects of treatment.

TRADE-OFFS: SURVIVAL VERSUS QUALITY OF LIFE

Contrary to the opinion of most medical professionals, many patients are willing to accept severe toxicity from treatment for the small chance of extended life [23]. Even cancer chemotherapy patients are generally unwilling to trade-off survival rate for improved quality of life [24,25]. This is particularly true of the very old [26].

Physicians usually underestimate the physical and mental abilities of elderly people and their willingness to face chronic and life-threatening conditions. Doctors frequently decide to withhold life-sustaining treatments from seriously ill patients. The Study to Understand Prognoses and Preferences for Outcomes and Risks of Treatment (SUPPORT) report [27] eloquently demonstrates how physicians' tendency to underestimate elderly patients' desire for aggressive treatments results in high rates of withholding life-sustaining treatments. Family members are no better at making these predictions [28,29]. Patients and families may consider cancer untreatable in the aged and not understand the possibilities offered by treatment.

Doctors have a moral duty to provide patients (and their families) with comprehensible, adequate information about potential treatments and alternatives. Studies clearly show that patients want this detailed information [30]. Just as when considering the benefits of treatment, this information must take into account all of the relevant factors of the impact of age on toxicity.

THE SIDE EFFECTS OF ANTICANCER TREATMENT IN THE ELDERLY

Older patients tolerate surgery, radiation therapy, and chemotherapy relatively well. However, it is important to realize that the few clinical trials that have been done, including those cited here, have included highly selected fit patients with little significant comorbidity. These studies had few "old old" patients and rarely any of the "oldest old," and many of the patients who were studied received nonstandard, low-intensity therapy. When contemplating anticancer treatment, it is critical to understand that the elderly have

Table 32-3. Elements of the Comprehensive Geriatric Assessment

Factor	Assessment*
Functional status	Lawton Instrumental Activities of Daily Living Scale
	Katz Index of Activities of Daily Living
	Eastern Cooperative Oncology Group performance status
Comorbidity	Charlson Comorbidity Index
	Cumulative Illness Rating Scale – Geriatric
Socioeconomic status	Isolation
	Caregiver
	Financial/medical insurance
	Transportation
	Type of residence/condition of living conditions
Nutritional status	Mini-Nutritional Assessment Screen
	Body mass index (height and weight)
Polypharmacy	Number of medications
	Doses of medications
Geriatric syndromes	
Depression	Geriatric Depression Scale – Short Form
Dementia, delirium	Mini-Mental Status Exam, CLOX, clinical trials
Falls	
Osteoporosis	Bone density dual-energy x-ray absorptiometry
Incontinence	
Neglect or abuse	
Failure to thrive	

*The Functional Assessment of Cancer Therapy – Geriatrics (FACT-G) is not part of the classical Comprehensive Geriatric Assessment but provides a useful assessment of the patient's quality of life.
CLOX—clock drawing task.

an increased risk of toxicity by virtue of the aging process itself, as well as due to factors related to frailty, comorbidity, or functional and socioeconomic limitations. While both types can be managed, only the latter group has potential for amelioration. Of course, the more impairments the patient has, the greater the risks. At some point, these burdens outweigh the potential benefits, and a comfort care/hospice approach is more appropriate.

The toxic effects of cancer treatment are never less burdensome in the elderly. In addition to the standard side effects of cancer treatment, there are significant age-related toxicities to consider. As we have discussed, most of these are more a function of frailty than chronological age, but even the fittest senior cannot avoid the physiologic effects of aging. These include modifications of renal, hepatic, and gastrointestinal function, and changes in body fluid and muscle-fat composition. These in turn affect the pharmacokinetic and pharmacodynamic properties of many drugs used in treating cancer. The recent report of the SIOG Chemotherapy Task Force is an excellent and thorough review of this medical literature [31].

RENAL

Physicians cannot change the decline in organ function or physiologic reserve that comes with aging, but they can measure GFR and choose drugs and drug doses accordingly. Like all organs, the kidneys become more vulnerable as one gets older. In cancer patients, they are particularly susceptible to the nephrotoxic effects of the medicines that the elderly often take, as well as the dehydration that often accompanies cancer and its treatment. Unlike the decline in renal function that accompanies aging, it may be possible to minimize these effects.

GLOMERULAR FILTRATION RATE

After 30 to 40 years of age, renal function declines approximately 1% per year, and by 70 years of age, GFR may have declined by as much as 40%. This often leads to enhanced toxicity of drugs such as cisplatin, carboplatin, topotecan, methotrexate, and ifosfamide. The SIOG Task Force on Renal Safety recommends that the dose of renally excreted chemotherapeutic agents be reduced when the estimated GFR falls below 60 mL/min [32]. In the elderly, serum creatinine is not a good indicator of GFR. All older cancer patients should have GFR assessed by creatinine clearance measurement or estimation. The SIOG has published extensive guidelines detailing the recommend dose adjustments for each chemotherapeutic agent [33].

POLYPHARMACY

Polypharmacy is quite prevalent in the geriatric oncology population. Because of comorbidities, the average elderly patient takes five different prescribed medications. Approximately 25% of these patients also use nonprescription drugs. Drug–drug interactions increase with the number of medications an individual takes [32]. Polypharmacy has ramifications on many organs, but it most commonly affects the kidneys. Nonsteroidal anti-inflammatory drugs (NSAIDs), zoledronic acid, and chemotherapeutic agents such as cisplatin can also adversely affect the kidneys.

CISPLATIN

Cisplatin should be used with caution in the elderly. Retrospective analysis of clinical trials has not reported any age-related nephrotoxicity, but the frail elderly are particularly vulnerable to cisplatin-related vomiting, dehydration, and functional decline. Hydration must be monitored carefully to prevent fluid overload, and the high incidence of age-related hearing loss should also be considered. Dehydration secondary to diarrhea or vomiting is common in elderly patients receiving chemotherapy; this in turn leads to nephrotoxicity.

LIVER

The liver also loses physiologic reserve as one gets older, but, unlike the kidney, the decrease in hepatic clearance is not uniform and, unless patients have obvious signs of liver impairment, it is not necessary to make adjustments for drugs cleared by the liver. However, physicians should be aware of the role of cytochrome P450 in drug metabolism and alert to drug interactions (*eg*, ketoconazole, phenobarbital, grapefruit juice) with chemotherapeutic agents (*eg*, paclitaxel) competing for this mechanism. If one must use paclitaxel in patients with liver dysfunction, its dose should be reduced. Although the Cancer and Leukemia Group B found some decrease in paclitaxel clearance with increasing age, it resulted in no adverse reactions [34]. They concluded that there is no basis for a dose reduction of paclitaxel based on age alone.

GASTROINTESTINAL TRACT

Age-related reductions in gastric secretions, gastric emptying, gastrointestinal motility, and splanchnic blood flow might diminish drug absorption in the elderly. Polypharmacy also has an impact on the anticancer drugs absorbed through the gastrointestinal tract. Medications like the H_2 blockers, antacids, and proton pump inhibitors can alter their absorption.

BODY FLUID/FAT COMPOSITION

As one ages, body fat increases and intracellular water decreases. These changes can affect drug distribution in older patients. Reductions in albumin concentrations affect the distribution of highly protein-bound agents like etoposide and the taxanes. For those who are malnourished, a dietician often can provide advice for nutritional support.

COMMON TREATMENT COMPLICATIONS IN THE ELDERLY

BONE MARROW TOXICITY/CYTOPENIAS

ANEMIA

Anemia is common in the elderly, especially the frail elderly [35]. It is also a well-described complication of radiation therapy and most cytotoxic regimens, regardless of age. Anemia decreases the efficacy of anticancer treatment, alters the pharmacokinetics of chemotherapeutic agents, increases morbidity (fatigue, functional and cognitive decline), and may alter tumor biology [36]. Maintaining adequate hemoglobin levels has proven quite effective in minimizing many of these side effects in elderly cancer patients. The National Comprehensive Cancer Network (NCCN) recommends treating hemoglobin levels less than 10 g/dL with erythropoietin-stimulating agents [37].

MYELOSUPPRESSION

In the elderly, only minimal stress will disrupt hematopoiesis. Thus, it is not uncommon to see declines in white blood cell counts that are more pronounced and more prolonged than those typically seen in younger patients receiving radiation or chemotherapy. Depressed neutrophil counts often lead to an increased risk of infection with significant morbidity and mortality (5%–30%). Primary prophylaxis with granulopoietic growth factors significantly decreases infections and their life-threatening complications (by as much as 50%–75%) in elderly patients receiving chemotherapy. The liberal use of these agents makes it possible for elderly patients to receive full doses of potentially curable antilymphoma or adjuvant chemotherapy for breast and colorectal cancer [38].

MUCOSITIS, DIARRHEA, AND DEHYDRATION

Mucositis is often more severe in older patients receiving chemotherapy or head and neck radiation therapy. This may be due to decreased mucosal stem cell reserve and repair. Early diagnosis and treatment are critical to prevent dehydration, malnutrition, and sepsis.

Diarrhea is another well-recognized side effect of chemotherapy and gastrointestinal radiation therapy in the elderly. It is particularly a problem in 5-fluorouracil (5-FU) and irinotecan-based regimens. Like mucositis, it can lead to profound dehydration, renal insufficiency, and electrolyte abnormalities.

Elderly patients are particularly predisposed to dehydration. In addition to their age-related diminished intracellular water, they often have inadequate fluid intake and are taking diuretic medication. In 2004, the American Society of Clinical Oncology (ASCO) published guidelines for the diagnosis and management of chemotherapy-induced diarrhea [39] and mucositis [40].

A number of studies give conflicting results as to whether 5-FU–based chemotherapy is more toxic in elderly patients with colorectal cancer. However, a meta-analysis of six randomized trials demonstrated that this was due to the different infusion schedules used [41]. Compared with younger patients, older patients had more diarrhea, mucositis, nausea, and vomiting. Older female patients had the highest incidence of nonhematologic toxicity. The data suggest no reason to reduce the dose of 5-FU unless there is severe renal dysfunction or comorbidity. It is clear that older patients tolerate the weekly 5-FU regimen better than the monthly Mayo Clinic regimen (bolus 5-FU plus leucovorin). Although infusional therapy is probably even less toxic, it is often difficult for elderly patients (especially those with mobility problems) to deal with its logistics [42].

Capecitabine is a popular drug in both breast and colon cancer. Elderly colorectal cancer patients tolerate it better than the monthly Mayo Clinic regimen. Studies of capecitabine in elderly breast cancer patients showed that the dose could probably be reduced from 1250 mg/m^2 to 1000 mg/m^2 with reduced toxicity but equal efficacy. However, the dose does need to be adjusted for renal insufficiency, and doctors must be aware that many elderly patients (especially those taking multiple medications or who are cognitively impaired) often have more difficulty managing oral medications than those given intravenously.

Adjuvant FOLFOX (oxaliplatin plus 5-FU/leucovorin) is also as efficacious in older patients with colorectal cancer as younger patients. While older age appears to be associated with a higher incidence of neutropenia and thrombocytopenia, these are manageable. Diarrhea is no more frequent than in younger patients, but, in the elderly, the resulting dehydration and debilitation can be considerable. Studies have shown that FOLFOX can be safely given with close monitoring and immediate intervention [43,44].

NEUROTOXICITY AND COGNITIVE EFFECTS

Chemotherapeutic agents exert central nervous system effects by direct injury, endothelial injury, and inflammation. These effects, referred to as "chemo-brain," can be particularly important in cognitively impaired patients. Many of the adjuncts to chemotherapy are also potential neurotoxins. Psychosis is a recognized side effect of dexamethasone, and ranitidine is associated with agitation. Diphenhydramine and some of the antiemetics can cause sedation.

Although the rate of neurotoxicity is no greater in older patients than in younger patients, older patients may have preexisting neurologic deficits that warrant caution when choosing one of the platinum compounds or the taxanes. Elderly patients with hearing loss or peripheral neuropathy (from, for example, diabetes) have decreased reserve, and are highly vulnerable to cisplatin.

Falls are one of the most common problems in the elderly. Judicious selection of chemotherapeutic agents and adjuncts is critical in those at high risk for falls. In addition to those with a history of falls or preexisting neurocognitive problems, patients at high risk for falls include those with gait or balance problems, deconditioning or diminished muscle mass, and impaired vision or mobility. Physical and occupational therapy evaluations (including home safety visits) are often quite effective at addressing these and other risk factors associated with all forms of physical decline.

FATIGUE AND DEPRESSION

Fatigue is a near universal complaint of elderly cancer patients. It is particularly a problem for those who are socially isolated or dependent upon others in activities of daily living or instrumental activities of daily living. It is not necessarily related to depression, but can be. Depression is quite common in the elderly, and the CGA serves an essential role in early diagnosis and management. With proper attention from psychiatrists, social workers, geriatricians, and physiatrists, many of these patients can safely receive anticancer treatment.

HEART

Anthracycline-related cardiomyopathy increases progressively with age after 70 years. A recent study found increased risk of congestive heart failure in older patients with hypertension, diabetes, coronary artery disease, and trastuzumab therapy. However, with careful monitoring it can been used safely in the elderly.

OSTEOPOROSIS

Five years of adjuvant hormonal therapy has been shown to decrease breast cancer recurrence and mortality by approximately one third, regardless of age. The Arimidex, Tamoxifen, Alone or in Combination (ATAC) trial showed that aromatase inhibitors were 3% to 5% more efficacious, and generally less toxic, than tamoxifen in postmenopausal women. On the other hand, they are associated with an increased risk of osteoporosis and related fractures [45]. These toxicities are of particular importance in elderly women; therefore, pre-aromatase inhibitor bone density (DEXA) scans are essential screening tools in the elderly. They should be followed regularly during the course of treatment so that the benefits of this adjuvant therapy can be weighed against any deterioration in bone health. The appropriate use of calcium and bisphosphonates are important adjuncts to the use of aromatase inhibitors.

SURGERY

In and of itself, chronological age is not a major risk for surgery [46]. Currently, the multicenter, international, cooperative Preoperative Assessment of Cancer in Elderly (PACE) trial is prospectively analyzing cancer surgery in the elderly, with the goal of clarifying risk and screening tools for the geriatric population. The SIOG Surgical Task Force reported that surgical outcomes for elderly patients were not significantly different from their younger counterparts [47].

Unfortunately, surgery is not always offered to the elderly cancer patient. For example, older woman are often undertreated and, consequently, have significantly worse outcomes than younger patients. In 2007, Bouchardy *et al.* [48] reviewed 30 studies evaluating the treatment of older women with breast cancer. All the studies (published between 1997 and 2006) reported significant numbers of elderly breast cancer patients who received substandard treatment. Compared with their younger counterparts, older women had less breast-conserving surgery, less axillary node sampling, less radiation therapy, and less adjuvant chemotherapy. Although the discrepancy was not as dramatic, they also got less adjuvant hormonal therapy. Substandard treatments increased with the age of the patient, and though there was some correlation with other factors (*eg*, race, stage, and the presence of comorbid conditions), age remained an independent risk factor for substandard therapy.

For the majority of older patients, early-stage breast cancer should be treated with standard surgical procedures. Breast surgery is a relatively low-risk operative procedure, and advanced age alone should not compromise definitive surgery. Body image is just as important to older women as younger women, and it should not be assumed that the older breast cancer patient is not interested in breast conservation or reconstruction. On the contrary, older women, with limited mobility or difficulties with transportation, may prefer mastectomy to the frequent visits to the hospital required for postlumpectomy radiation therapy.

CONCLUSIONS

Paternalistic stereotypes, not evidence, are too often the basis for the current practice of care for elderly cancer patients. Unfortunately, there is little evidence to guide the conscientious physician. Only 36% of the 29,000 patients in 55 cancer trials registered by the US Food and Drug Administration were 65 years of age or older [49].

Although organizations like the SIOG [50] the Geriatric Oncology Consortium [51], and ASCO [52] have done much to refocus the research agenda, it will take some time for clinicians to benefit from these nascent efforts. Until then, physicians must familiarize themselves with the studies that are available, and apply general principles of geriatric medicine as they extrapolate data from studies conducted in younger cancer patients.

Guidelines, such as those developed by the NCCN [53], help direct the clinician through an appropriate geriatric assessment and suggest evidence-based strategies to minimize adverse events. For breast, colon, and lung cancer, risk-benefit assessment tools like Adjuvant! Online [54] provide invaluable assistance to shared decision making, with clear graphic displays that incorporate specific tumor characteristics with age-related data and comorbidities.

When doctors help elderly patients weigh the burdens and benefits of therapy in relation to well-defined and attainable goals, good treatment decisions are possible in the older cancer patient. The patient-centric model of decision making that emphasizes patient autonomy may not always be the best model in the elderly. Elderly patients are more likely to adhere to "traditional" religious or cultural attitudes toward health issues. They may prefer to rely on their own family or community for advice, and some will go as far as to delegate major medical decisions to those individuals. Although many elderly patients may appear to prefer a doctor-centric model of decision making, most want to have control of their own destiny. While cognitively impaired patients pose a unique challenge, they are frequently capable of participating in goal setting and simple discussions about treatment side effects and logistics. Caring family members and friends are often able to share the patient's "life narrative story" so that health care workers can work with them to make good substituted or best interest judgments for those who are truly impaired.

REFERENCES

1. Yancik R, Ries LA: Aging in America: demographic and epidemiologic perspectives. *Hematol Oncol Clin North Am* 2000, 14:17–23.

2. Jonsen AR, Siegler M, Winslade WJ: *Clinical Ethics: A Practical Approach to Ethical Decisions in Clinical Medicine.* New York: McGraw-Hill/Appleton & Lange; 2002.

3. A predictive model for aggressive non-Hodgkin's lymphoma. The International non-Hodgkin's Lymphoma Prognostic Factors Project. *N Engl J Med* 1993, 329:987–994.

4. Solal-Celigny P, Roy P, Colombat P, *et al.*: Follicular lymphoma International Prognostic Index. *Blood* 2004, 104:1258–1265.

5. Diab SG, Elledge RM, Clark GM: Tumor characteristics and clinical outcome of elderly women with breast cancer. *J Natl Cancer Inst* 2000, 92:550–556.

6. Singh R, Hellman S, Heimann R: The natural history of breast carcinoma in the elderly: implications for screening and treatment. *Cancer* 2004, 100:1807–1813.

7. Ugant AM, Xie L, Morriss J, *et al.*: Survival of women with breast cancer in Ottawa, Canada: variation with age, stage, histology, grade and treatment. *Br J Cancer* 2004, 90:1138–1143.

8. Lamy PJ, Pujol P, Thezenas S, *et al.*: Progesterone receptor quantification as a strong prognostic determinant in postmenopausal breast cancer women under tamoxifen therapy. *Breast Cancer Res Treat* 2002, 76:65–71.

9. Tai P, Cserni G, Van De Steene J, *et al.*: Modeling the effect of age in T1-2 breast cancer using the SEER database. *BMC Cancer* 2005, 5:130.

10. Walter LC, Covinsky KE: Cancer screening in elderly patients. *JAMA* 2001, 285:2750–2756.

11. Balducci L: Management of cancer in the elderly. *Oncology* 2006, 20:135–152.

12. Saltzstein SL, Behling CA: 5- and 10- year survival in cancer patients aged 90 and older: a study of 37,318 patients from SEER. *J Surg Oncol* 2002, 81:113–116.

13. Yancik R, Ganz PA, Varricchio CG, Conley B: Perspectives on comorbidity and cancer in older patients: approaches to expand the knowledge base. *J Clin Oncol* 2001, 19:1147–1151.

14. Wedding U, Honecker F, Bokemeyer C, *et al.*: Tolerance to chemotherapy in elderly patients with cancer. *Cancer Control* 2007, 14:44–56.

15. Fried LP, Tangen CM, Walston J, *et al.*: Frailty in older adults: evidence for a phenotype. *J Gerontol Med Sci* 2001, 56A:M146–M156.

16. Cohen JH, Harris T, Pieper CF: Coagulation and activation of inflammatory pathways in the development of functional decline and mortality in the elderly. *Am J Med* 2003, 114:180–187.

17. Piccirillo JF: Inclusion of comorbidity in a staging system for head and neck cancer. *Oncology (Huntington)* 1995, 9:831–836.

18. Extermann M, Hurria A: Comprehensive geriatric assessment for older patients with cancer. *J Clin Oncol* 2007, 25:1824–1831.

19. Extermann M, Aapro M, Bernabei R, *et al.*: Use of comprehensive geriatric assessment in older cancer patients: recommendations from the Task Force on CGA of the International Society of Geriatric Oncology (SIOG). *Crit Rev Oncol Hematol* 2005, 55:241–255.

20. Sargent D, Goldberg R, Jacobson SD, *et al.*: A pooled analysis of adjuvant chemotherapy for resected colon cancer in elderly patients. *N Engl J Med* 2001, 345:1091–1097.

21. Coiffier B, Herbrecht R, Tilly H, *et al.*: GELA study comparing CHOP and R-CHOP in elderly patients with DLCL: 3-year median follow-up with an analysis according to comorbidity factors. *J Clin Oncol* 2003, 22(Suppl):2395.

22. Feugier P, Van Hoof A, Sebban C, *et al.*: Long-term results of R-CHOP study in the treatment of elderly patients with diffuse large B-cell lymphoma: a study by the Group d-Etude des Lymphomes De L'Adulte. *J Clin Oncol* 2005, 23:4117–4126.

23. Slevin ML: Quality of life: philosophical questions or clinical reality? *Br Med J* 1992, 305:466–469.

24. Silvestri G, Pritchard R, Welch HG: Preferences for chemotherapy in patients with advanced non-small cell lung cancer: descriptive study based on scripted interviews. *Br Med J* 1998, 317:771–775.

25. Brescia FJ: Lung cancer: a philosophical, ethical, and personal perspective. *Crit Rev Oncol Hematol* 2001, 40:139–148.

26. Tsevat J, Dawson NV, Wu AW, *et al.*: Health values of hospitalized patients 80 years or older. *JAMA* 1998, 279:371–375.

27. Hamel MB, Teno JM, Goldman L, *et al.*: Patient age and decisions to withhold life-sustaining treatments from seriously ill, hospitalized adults. *Ann Intern Med* 1999, 130:116–125.

28. Covinsky KE, Fuller JD, Yaffe K, *et al.*: Communication and decision-making in seriously ill patients: findings of the SUPPORT project. *J Am Geriatr Soc* 2000, 48:S187–S193.

29. Way J, Back AL, Curtis JR: Withdrawing life support and resolution of conflict with families. *Br Med J* 2002, 325:1342–1345.

30. Hagerty RG, Butow PN, Ellis PA, *et al.*: Cancer patient preferences for communication of prognosis in the metastatic setting. *J Clin Oncol* 2004, 22:1721–1730.

31. Lichman SM, Widiers H, Chateult E, *et al.*: International Society of Geriatric Oncology Chemotherapy Taskforce: evaluation of chemotherapy in older patients: an analysis of the medical literature. *J Clin Oncol* 2007, 25:1832–1843.

32. Aapro M, Launay-Vacher V, Lichtman S, *et al.*: International Society for Geriatric Oncology (SIOG): a report from SIOG Task Force on renal safety in the elderly. *SIOG Newsletter* 2005, 1:1. http://www.cancerworld.org/cancerworldadmin/getStaticModFile.aspx?id=893.

33. Launay-Vacher V, Chatelut E, Lichtman SM, *et al.*: Renal insufficiency in elderly cancer patients: International Society of Geriatric Oncology clinical practice recommendations. *Ann Oncol* 2007, 18:1314–1321.

34. Lichtman SM, Hollis D, Miller AA, *et al.*: Prospective evaluation of the relationship of patient age and paclitaxel clinical pharmacology: Cancer and Leukemia Group B (CALGB 9762). *J Clin Oncol* 2006, 24:1846–1851.

35. Baraldi-Junkin CA, Beck AC, Rothstein G: Hematopoiesis and cytokines. Relevance to cancer and aging. *Hematol Oncol Clin North Am* 2000, 14;45–61, viii.

36. Van Belle SJ, Cocquyt V: Impact of haemoglobin levels on the outcome of cancers treated with chemotherapy. *Crit Rev Oncol Hematol* 2003, 47:1–11.

37. Balducci L, Yates J: General guidelines for the management of older patients with cancer. *Oncology (Williston Park)* 2000, 14:221–227.

38. Dixon DO, Neilan B, Jones SE, *et al.*: Effect of age on therapeutic outcome in advanced diffuse histocytic lymphoma: the Southwest Oncology Group experience. *J Clin Oncol* 1986, 4:295–305.

39. Benson AB, Ajani JA, Catalano RB, *et al.*: Recommended guidelines for the treatment of cancer treatment-induced diarrhea. *J Clin Oncol* 2004, 22:2918–2926.

40. Rubenstein EB, Peterson DE, Schubert M, *et al.*: Clinical practice guidelines for the prevention and treatment of cancer therapy-induced oral and gastrointestinal mucositis. *Cancer* 2004, 100:2026–2046.

41. Meta-Analysis Group in Cancer: Toxicity of fluorouracil in patients with advanced colorectal cancer: effect of administration schedule and prognostic factors. *J Clin Oncol* 1998, 16:3537–3541.

42. Folprecht G, Cunningham D, Ross P, *et al.*: Efficacy of 5-fluorouracil-based chemotherapy in elderly patients with metastatic colorectal cancer: a pooled analysis of clinical trials. *Ann Oncol* 2004, 15:1330–1338.

43. Goldberg RM, Tabah-Fisch I, Bleiberg H, *et al.*: Pooled analysis of safety and efficacy of oxaliplatin plus fluorouracil-leucovorin administered bi-monthly in elderly patients with colorectal cancer. *J Clin Oncol* 2006, 24:4085–4091.

44. Haller DG, Catalano PJ, Macdonald JS, *et al.*: Phase III study of fluorouracil, leucovorin, and levamisole in high-risk stage II and III colon cancer: final report of Intergroup 0089. *J Clin Oncol* 2005, 23:8671–8878.

45. Baum M, Budzar AU, Cuzick J, *et al.*: Anastrozole alone or in combination with tamoxifen versus tamoxifen alone for adjuvant treatment of postmenopausal women with early breast cancer: first results of the ATAC randomized trial. *Lancet* 2002, 359:2131–2139.

46. Audisio RA, Zbar AP, Jaklitsch MT: Surgical management of oncogeriatric patients. *J Clin Oncol* 2007, 25:1924–1929.

47. Audisio RA, Bozzetti F, Gennari R, *et al.*: The surgical management of elderly cancer patients. Recommendations of the SIOG Surgical Task Force. *Eur J Cancer* 2004, 40:926–938.

48. Bouchardy C, Rapiti E, Blagojevic S, *et al.*: Older female cancer patients: importance, causes, and consequences of undertreatment. *J Clin Oncol* 2007, 25:1858–1869.

49. Talarico L, Chen G, Pazdur R: Enrollment of elderly patients in clinical trials for cancer drug registration: a 7-year experience by the US Food and Drug Administration. *J Clin Oncol* 2004, 22:4626–4631.

50. International Society of Geriatric Oncology. http://www.cancerworld.org/CancerWorld/home.aspx?id_stato=1&id_sito=3. Accessed May 27, 2008.

51. Geriatric Oncology Consortium. http://www.thegoc.org/. Accessed May 9, 2008.

52. American Society of Clinical Oncology: Geriatric cancer. http://geriatricsca.asco.org/. Accessed May 27, 2008.

53. National Comprehensive Cancer Network. http://www.nccn.org/default.asp. Accessed May 27, 2008.

54. Adjuvant! Online. http://www.adjuvantonline.com/. Accessed May 27, 2008.

There are many challenges associated with the use of medications in the management of disease and disease-related complications for individuals with cancer. The goal of therapy is to optimize efficacy of treatment while minimizing and/or managing toxicities of therapy. Unfortunately, antineoplastic agents are among the group of drugs with the lowest therapeutic index in clinical practice. The amount of drug producing unacceptable toxicity is often very close to the amount of drug required to produce cytotoxic effects. As outlined in previous chapters, the planning and implementation of therapy is dependent on a number of disease and individual specific factors. This chapter provides an overview of some of the important considerations for optimizing drug therapy for individuals with cancer.

DOSING OF CANCER DRUG THERAPY

Historically, most cytotoxic agents used for cancer treatment have been dosed based on weight (eg, milligram per kilogram) or body surface area (BSA; eg, milligram per square meter [mg/m²]). Drug dosing based on BSA is a method that approximates a medication dose between species, and is often used to determine a dose of drug for humans from animal studies. This dosing strategy attempts to take into consideration the concern of the narrow therapeutic window of many chemotherapy agents. Newer strategies for cancer treatment incorporate agents dosed as a fixed dose (milligram per dose), but even these medications may require dose modifications in certain clinical situations (eg, renal or liver dysfunction). Unfortunately, there is still much to be learned to determine the best method(s) to dose cancer agents and how to appropriately modify the dose regimen. The use of clinical pharmacokinetic and pharmacodynamic assessments is one strategy to help optimize the dosing of individual cancer agents; the application of drug levels for dose individualization is potentially beneficial for select patient populations (eg, older adults) or individual patients. There is a need to develop practical strategies that can be applied broadly in clinical practice for dosing of medications used for cancer treatment in order to optimize their use [1].

STANDARDIZATION BY BODY SURFACE AREA OR BODY WEIGHT

Many anticancer agents are currently dosed by weight or BSA; the rationale for this dosing strategy is based on the relationship between body size (eg, weight or surface area) and physiologic functions (eg, liver blood flow, glomerular filtration) [2]. This relationship is not always accurate.

The use of weight for dosing medications is relatively easy, if not always appropriate, as weight is easily measurable. BSA is calculated based on height and weight. Initial nomograms using an individual's weight and height to derive BSA were based on work published in the early 1900s by DuBois and DuBois [3] from nine nonobese individuals of varying age, shape, and size. In the 1970s, this formula was confirmed by Gehan and George [4], who directly measured the skin surface area of approximately 400 individuals. The method of calculation has been confirmed, although the utility of BSA for correlation of drug exposure with drug dose is not as clear. The goal of dosing per BSA or weight, as a gross method of standardization, is an attempt to produce relatively consistent systemic drug exposure after a given dose of drug. The correlation of body size to organ function is not uniform in some populations (eg, elderly, individuals with comorbidities affecting organ function). Consequently, following administration of equivalent drug doses based on BSA a wide variability in plasma drug concentrations may be seen between patients. Clinical situations that may be problematic when dosing an antineoplastic agent(s) according to BSA or weight include individuals following amputation of limb(s), those with edema, and those who are overweight or underweight [5]. There is no one appropriate method to modify the use of BSA across these clinical situations, as the method to modify dose is often agent dependent.

OBESITY

The prevalence of obesity in the Western world is dramatically rising, with many obese individuals requiring therapeutic intervention for a variety of disease states including cancer. Despite the growing prevalence of obesity there is a paucity of evidence-based information describing how drug doses should be adjusted, or indeed whether they need to be adjusted, in clinical practice. The pharmacokinetic profile of a drug in the obese individual could range from distribution of drug to clearance of drugs and metabolites [6]. For example, obese individuals have a larger absolute lean body mass and fat mass compared with nonobese individuals of the same age, gender, and size; this may impact drug distribution. Cardiac performance may be altered in the obese, which may also impact drug distribution. Information on drug hepatic metabolism in obesity has been described; activity of hepatic enzymes may be altered, which could impact the metabolism and/or activation of some drugs [6].

An important clinical question concerning pharmacokinetic changes of drugs in the obese patient is as simple as the degree of obesity. For example, in patients who are moderately obese, cardiac output and glomerular filtration rates may increase proportionally with BSA, and dose modification of drugs cleared by the kidney not is appropriate [7]. Comparatively, in the massively obese patient, infiltration of organs such as the liver may change liver function, and dosing modifications may be warranted.

The practice of dose modification of drugs in obesity is very controversial, and should be evaluated on a drug-by-drug basis. Various empiric approaches are utilized in clinical practice (Table 33-1). These methods have not been evaluated widely for all cancer drugs, drug combinations, treatment regimens, or in specific diseases. A study that evaluated treatment patterns in overweight and obese women undergoing adjuvant chemotherapy after surgery for breast cancer found that more than 50% of obese women had first-cycle dose reduction of chemotherapy. Importantly, the method of dose reduction was not consistent among those evaluated [5]. Few studies have addressed the relationship between obesity and clearance of drug or volume of distribution of the drug [8].

Underdosing of medications is of major concern for individuals with cancer who are overweight. Reports of full-dose chemotherapy in obese patients with small cell lung cancer demonstrate that obesity at the start of treatment was not associated with increased toxicity from treatment or a shortened survival [9]. The conclusion from this small study is that there is no support for empiric chemotherapy dose reductions based on ideal body weight in this population. Another study undertaken to examine toxicity in relation to BMI in women with ovarian cancer treated with carboplatin demonstrated that obese women are less likely to experience treatment-related toxicity. The authors expressed concern that obese women were receiving lower doses of drug based on underestimation of glomerular filtration based on the calculated formulas [10].

There are many descriptors of body size, but little is known about the correlation of these descriptors and the relationship between drug dose and

Table 33-1. Approaches to Dose Modification in Obesity

Arbitrary BSA capping (eg, BSA of 2 m²)

BSA calculated based on lean body mass

BSA calculated based on IBW

BSA calculated on adjusted body weight (IBW + % fat weight)

BSA calculated using weight obtained by averaging measured weight + IBW

Empiric dose reduction

BSA—body surface area; IBW—ideal body weight.

concentration in the obese patient. Actual weight, lean body weight, ideal body weight, BSA, body mass index (BMI), fat-free mass, percent ideal body weight, adjusted body weight, and predicted normal body weight are considered as potential size descriptors. Some work is ongoing to determine if the BMI should be included in consideration with BSA for dosing of antineoplastic agents for obese patients (BMI > 30 kg/m^2) [11]. There has been some suggestion that use of lean body weight may be a better way to assess body composition compared with ideal body weight [12].

Currently, there are no comprehensive recommendations for dose modifications in the obese patient with cancer. In a recently published study of eight anticancer drugs in adults, it appeared that a number of widely used empiric strategies for dose adjustments in obese patients—including a priori dose reduction—should not be routinely used [13]. The conclusion of these investigators was that the selection of alternate size descriptors for dose calculations in the obese is drug specific and sex dependent. Additionally, they encouraged further prospective studies in this very important area for individual agents.

A PRIORI DOSE DETERMINATION

The goal of dose adaptation for individual patients is to maximize the probability of producing a desired therapeutic effect while minimizing the probability of toxicity. The use of dose adaptation is an attempt to factor pretreatment patient characteristics into drug dosing. The focus has historically been to factor in those characteristics that may impact the pharmacokinetics of drug therapy. Clinically important are those factors that impact the pharmacodynamics of a drug or drug regimen. A priori adaptive dosage determination of anticancer drug dose is based on the contributions of identifiable characteristics of the individual, drug therapy, and disease state(s) that may influence plasma drug concentrations. This approach is probably best used in situations when drug clearance is dependent on a readily available patient characteristic, such as renal function.

RENAL FUNCTION

Drug dose modification is often considered in patients with renal dysfunction. Again, this may be very appropriate for some medications and unnecessary for others. Alterations in renal elimination of drug may occur for many reasons, including age-related changes in the kidney [14], drug-induced changes [15], and disease-related kidney injury. The pharmacokinetics of drugs excreted via they kidneys can be affected by altered kidney metabolic capacity, altered renal excretion because of altered blood flow to the kidney, or damage to the kidney structures [16].

In clinical practice, serum creatinine is most frequently used to estimate renal function. Although serum creatinine may offer a useful estimate of renal function, there are a number of problems with using this surrogate marker as a definitive assessment of renal function. Similarly, estimation of renal function based on calculations of creatinine clearance (CrCl) are simply guides, and not definitive. Standard nomograms estimate CrCl as a function of serum creatinine, age, and body size. In most CrCl formulas the use of serum creatinine is "normalized" with the use of age and weight. Standard nomograms do not always fit select populations including individuals with cachexia, obesity, and/or the elderly. Fortunately, the option of measuring CrCl is a relatively simple method to determine the actual renal function in certain populations (*eg*, elderly, malnourished, and obese). Methods of measurement to determine actual CrCl may be as simple as a timed urine collection for creatinine measurement or the measurement of glomerular filtration rate using the clearance of inulin or radio contrast materials.

A recent review provides some guidelines for consideration of dose modification of antineoplastic agents in the setting of renal dysfunction [16]. Additionally, the International Society of Geriatric Oncology (SIOG) published a position paper for the adjustment of medication dosing used in the treatment and management of elderly cancer patients with renal insufficiency [14].

HEPATIC FUNCTION

There are multiple mechanisms in which hepatic dysfunction impacts the pharmacokinetics and ultimately pharmacodynamic of anticancer agents.

The most obvious is the impact that changes in hepatic clearance of drugs may have on the time and extent of elimination of an agent from the site of action and the body. Additionally changes in hepatic metabolism may affect the clearance of an agent or the extent of metabolism to an active agent (*eg*, temozolomide). Unfortunately, there is not an easy in vivo method to predict hepatic drug clearance. The use of hepatic enzymes and/or serum bilirubin to estimate the ability of the liver to metabolize medications has not been shown to be a good indicator of liver functions [17,18]. Serum bilirubin level is the most frequently utilized parameter to adjust chemotherapy dosing. It is important to consider the impact of other factors on interpretation of bilirubin (*eg*, hemolysis) and evaluate the benefit of using fractionated bilirubin in the context of such clinical situations.

A recent review provides some guidelines for consideration of dose modification of antineoplastic agents in the setting of hepatic dysfunction [16,19].

PHARMACOKINETIC PROFILE

Modification of drug dose may also be based on an assessment of drug levels to determine an individual's handling of a drug. Adaptive dosage adjustments made based on drug levels during repetitive or continuous administration of a drug is common for very few drugs. This method is based on the practice of determining a target plasma concentration or area under the concentration-time curve (AUC) to use as a guide for dose modification during the cycle of chemotherapy (*eg*, high-dose busulfan in the preparative regimens prior to hematopoietic stem cell transplantation) or for subsequent cycles of therapy. Monitoring plasma concentrations is based on the following premises: 1) primary clinical end points are not easily assessed as a basis for altering drugs, 2) appropriate assays for drug measurements are available, 3) individual variations in the pharmacokinetics of the drug are the source of different drug exposure, 4) reducing the pharmacokinetic variations in a drug will result in reduction of pharmacodynamic variations of the drug, and 5) the relationship between drug concentration and drug effect is better than the relationship between drug dose and drug effect [20].

The use of this strategy is often limited by the readily available assays for drug measurements. Advances in assay developments and the evaluation of the assays give promise to the strategy of optimizing drug dosing via therapeutic drug monitoring for antineoplastic agents [21–23].

DRUG INTERACTIONS

A true challenge in optimizing the pharmacotherapy and care of an individual with cancer is determining and managing clinically important drug interactions. Drug interactions may include drug–drug, drug–food, drug–laboratory, and drug–disease interactions. Unfortunately, drug interactions are not uncommon in patients receiving cancer treatment. A survey of more than 400 individuals with solid tumors found at least one drug interaction was discovered in more than one fourth of patients in the 4 weeks prior to survey [24]. Importantly, most of the drug interactions involved noncancer agents. Not surprising, the increased risk of potential drug interactions was associated with the increasing number of drugs an individual received. A patient population that is considered at high risk for drug interactions is the older adult with cancer based on the high number of concomitant medications and comorbidities in this population [25].

Toxicities associated with adverse drug–drug interactions are a major cause of morbidity and mortality [26]. The impact of concurrent drug therapy on the efficacy of cancer treatment strategies is also an important consideration. Unfortunately, there is no simple approach to identifying and/or managing drug interactions for individuals.

Individuals with cancer have been identified as a particularly high-risk patient population for drug interactions [26]. Typically, these individuals receive a large number of drugs during the treatment of cancer, including anticancer drugs, drugs for treatment and cancer-related complications, and a variety of other chronic medications for other health issues and comorbidities. Because many of the drugs associated with cancer care are not be given chronically (*eg*, daily), it is even more challenging to estimate the potential of drug–drug interactions over the course of treatment and during the time between treatment.

The risk of drug–drug interactions increases with the number of concomitant medications taken by a patient. In one report, the incidence of drug–drug interactions with two medications was close to 6%, but as the number of medications increased to eight the chance of an interaction was about 100% [27]. This study did not specifically evaluate the impact of drugs being added for short periods (*eg*, corticosteroids as therapy in myeloma) or use of as-needed medications for symptom management (*eg*, prochlorperazine taken as needed for nausea). It is during active drug therapy that patients receiving cancer treatment are often prescribed, and take, the most medications and are the most susceptible to effects from drug–drug interactions. Additionally, for patients with cancer who have comorbidities requiring drug therapy [28], modification of these therapies may need to be considered during and after cancer treatment.

The potential for drug interactions extend beyond prescription medications. The use of nonprescription medications, herbals, dietary supplements, and complementary and/or alternative medicines (CAM) may also be a source of drug interactions. The use of over-the-counter (OTC) medications requires thorough evaluation. More and more medications are available without a prescription, and with the growing use of OTC medications for management of symptoms and health problems, there is a growing potential for drug interactions. The use of CAM continues to grow in the general population and in individuals with cancer [29]. Again, the addition of these therapies increases the complexity of drug therapy regimens. Most concerning is the potential for these drug interactions to be undetected and underevaluated by the health care team.

Drug–drug interactions may result in a variety of outcomes including increased toxicity, decreased therapeutic effect, and/or unique response that is not seen with either drug alone. Pharmacokinetic interactions occur when one drug influences the absorption, distribution, metabolism, and/or excretion of other agents. The human cytochrome P450 (CYP) system consists of enzymes responsible for metabolism of many substances including medications. It is estimated that greater than 90% of drug oxidation can be attributed to CYP1A2, CYP2C9, CYP2C19, CYP2D6, CYP2E1, and CYP

3A4. Inhibition and induction of these enzymes by a medication may impact many other drugs an individual is taking. Additionally, the timing of a drug's impact on these enzymes is not always predictable, and may vary depending on duration of therapy. A number of medications used in the care of the individual with cancer are associated with effects on these enzymes; some examples are listed in Table 33-2 [30]. This list is not inclusive, and the modification of drug therapy for individuals with cancer should be evaluated with consideration of the impact of the change on concurrent therapies.

Pharmacodynamic interactions occur when two or more drugs have mechanisms of actions that influence the same physiologic process; this may include pharmacotherapy for the management of comorbidities, health maintenance, as well as for the prevention and/or treatment of cancer and cancer-treatment toxicities. The influence of polypharmacy on the pharmacokinetics and pharmacodynamics of anticancer therapy must be considered.

A number of strategies can help to minimize the clinical impact of drug interactions. The approach to care requires careful assessment of an individual patient's risk factor(s), education of patient and caregivers concerning communication of drug therapy modification during treatment, and communication among all health care providers. Importantly, the assessment for drug interactions should occur routinely, as therapies for management of cancer and cancer complications are frequently modified.

Coordination of care is a primary goal to minimize potential drug–drug interactions. Encourage individuals to coordinate medications through a single pharmacy to assure that one pharmacist is aware of all medications. Additionally, suggest that the patient develop a professional relationship with a pharmacist, to ensure drug therapy is evaluated with each change in medication at the pharmacy. The same strategy should be used to coordinate prescribing of medication through a primary health care member and to designate one caregiver to coordinate medication administration as a resource to the patient. Because it may be difficult for a patient to recall side effects, it may be helpful to develop a tool for the patient to keep notes about drugs and drug effects (*eg*, patient log) that can be shared routinely with the health care team. Again, instruct patients to inform all members of their health care team about new medications.

It is important to be aware of the potential for interactions even if no interaction has been described. A review of drug interactions in oncology [31,32] is a good resource to assess drug interactions between cancer therapy and other medications. This review includes a table of drug–drug interactions and recommendation for management. Additionally, there are a number of Internet-based references that provide information on drug interactions; examples are listed in Table 33-3.

DRUG–FOOD INTERACTION

The impact of food on drug absorption has long been recognized. A drug–nutrient interaction is defined as an alteration of the pharmacokinetics or pharmacodynamics of a drug or nutritional element or a compromise in nutritional status as a result of the addition of a drug [33]. Classically, food–drug interactions were thought to result in changes of the absorption or bioavailability of a medication. Concern exists that decreased bioavailability of a drug can impact efficacy (*eg*, treatment failure) or that an increase in bioavailability increases the risk of toxicities. The oral absorption of poorly

Table 33-2. Selected Agents With Effects on Cytochrome P450 Enzymes

CYP3A inhibitors	CYP3A inducers	CYP2D6 inhibitors
Clarithromycin	Carbamazepine	Clomipramine
Diltiazem	Efavirenz	Fluoxetine
Erythromycin	Nevirapine	Haloperidol
Indinavir	Phenobarbital	Paroxetine
Itraconazole	Phenytoin	
Ketoconazole	Rifampin	
Ritonavir	St. John's wort	
Saquinavir		
Verapamil		

(*Data from* Goodin [30].)

Table 33-3. Web-Based References for Drug Interactions

Reference	Website
FDA Office of Food Safety and Nutrition	http://www.cfsan.fda.gov
Alternative Medicine Foundation's HerbMed	http://www.herbmed.org
Natural Medicines Comprehensive Database	http://www.naturaldatabase.com
Natural Standard	http://www.naturalstandard.com
NIH National Center for Complementary and Alternative Medicine	http://nccam.nih.gov
CAM on PubMed	http://www.nlm.nih.gov/nccam/camonpubmed.html

CAM—complementary alternative medicine; FDA—US Food and Drug Administration; NIH—National Institutes of Health.

water-soluble drugs is known to increase when they are administered after food intake [34]. The secretion of bile juice into the gastrointestinal tract, one of the main effects of food, is accelerated by food intake. Bile secretion may enhance the solubility and dissolution rate and impact absorption of drugs after oral administration.

Animal studies are carried out to detect the effect of food on oral absorption of drugs before advancing to clinical trials in humans. Unfortunately, animal studies often show large variation in results depending on the species and might result in uncertain estimation on drug absorption in humans. Similarly, studies in humans are challenged by intrapatient characteristics. The true impact of food/ nutrients on medications may be much broader than impact on absorption.

Drug–food interactions are classified based on the nature and mechanism of the interaction [35]. Type I interactions involve ex vivo inactivation of drugs by interactions caused via chemical or physical reactions. Type I interactions are most common between medications given intravenously and parenteral nutrition, but may also be seen with enteral nutrition formulations and medications given via feeding tubes. Type II food–drug interactions involve absorption; the precipitating agent may modify the function of enzymes or transport mechanisms that are responsible for the biotransformations or deactivating processes that occur in the gastrointestinal tract. The rate and/or extent of absorption may be impacted by food. Food stimulates both gastric and intestinal acids that may be important in the dissolution of drugs to facilitate absorptions. Foods with high fat content stimulate the release of bile salts and may increase the intestinal uptake of highly lipophilic drugs. Therefore, it is important to realize that the content of a meal may impact absorption of specific medications. This is important in individuals with cancer who are utilizing nutritional supplements to increase caloric intake. A type III food–drug interaction may affect the systemic disposition of a drug and occurs after the drug has been absorbed. The metabolism of orally ingested drugs prior to being absorbed into the systemic circulation impacts a drug's potency and efficacy. Liver and intestinal metabolism may play a role in drug disposition. Grapefruit juice, for example, has been shown to cause several clinically significant interactions with CYP3A [36]. The organic anion-transporting polypeptide (OATP) drug transporter was inhibited by grapefruit juice, orange juice, and apple juice [36]. Other fruit juices also interacted with drug-metabolizing enzymes and transporters in vitro, but more studies are needed to determine whether these interactions are clinically significant. Type IV interaction refer to elimination or clearance of the drug or nutrients [37].

Another important clinical drug–food interaction is the impact of medications on food choices. Many medications, both oral and parenteral, impact the sense of taste, smell, and/or willingness to eat. The impact of chemotherapy-induced nausea and vomiting certainly plays a role in a patient's appetite. Similarly, other medication toxicities such as sedation, constipation, diarrhea, bloating, taste disturbances, and anorexia may also impact types and extent of food intake.

DRUG–ENTERAL NUTRITION INTERACTIONS

The use of enteral nutrition has increased for patients in the hospital and at home due to increasing durable access. Drug interactions with enteral nutrition can create a unique challenge in the individual with cancer. Nutritional supplementation may change bioavailability of enteral medications, ultimately impacting treatment outcome.

The anatomic site of delivery and the feeding tube size must be considered when delivering medications via the enteral route [37]. Nasoenteric feeding tubes will deliver medications into the stomach or duodenal or jejunal positions. Nasogastric tubes and percutaneous gastronomies deliver into the stomach. Some feeding tubes deliver contents into the small bowel, such as nasojejunal and jejunal tubes.

Most oral medications are primarily absorbed in the small bowel, but there are aspects of drug delivery that may make other areas of the gastrointestinal tract more advantageous for drug delivery. For example, the stomach is able to tolerate more concentrated and hypertonic medications as compared with the small bowel. Some drugs are targeted for gastric delivery, and medications may be removed or rendered ineffective when drainage or frequent suctioning removes gastric contents. Another issue is when the enteral access is too far distal to the typical site of absorption.

More recently the impact of food on drug effect is being addressed in the literature [38,39]. Reviews of pharmaceuticals that interact with food can be helpful, but these lists are not inclusive of all medications and/or diets [40]. There are a number of strategies to minimize complications when administering medications concomitantly with enteral nutrition (Table 33-4) [41]. To prevent clogging of enteral access devices, liquid medicates are preferred over crushed tablets. Some medications should not be crushed if they cannot be swallowed intact [42]. Medications should be delivered via the largest tube when multiple accesses are available. Liquid medications should be drawn up in an oral syringe to prevent inadvertent parenteral administration. If the oral syringe does not securely connect to the feeding tube, a catheter tip adapter may be used. When tablets are crushed, the powder should be mixed in a minimum of 30 to 60 mL of diluent to avoid thick pastes that may clog up the tube. Medications should not be directly mixed with enteral formulations because many liquid formulations of medications are acidic and may result in denaturing of the proteins in the nutrition formulations. Additionally, the changes in enteral rates, discarding of unused bags, and the delay in administration may result in underdosing.

OVER-THE-COUNTER MEDICATIONS, DIETARY SUPPLEMENTS, AND HERBS

Herbs, dietary supplements, and OTC medications are frequently used to treat disease, manage symptoms of disease and disease treatment, and for health maintenance. With the aging population of the United States and the increasing age of the population with cancer, these medications are used for treatment of comorbidities as well as for cancer and cancer-related symptoms. It is estimated that more than half of individuals with cancer are taking CAMs. The use of herbs and dietary supplements continues to grow in the United States, and patients often take more than one of these supplements at a time. In the individual with cancer, as with the

---

Table 33-4. Guidelines for Drug Administration Via Enteral Access

Consider the type of enteral access device

Know the location of tip (*eg*, small bowel, stomach)

Use liquid formulations of medications when possible

Administer medications through the larger enteral access (gastric vs jejunal)

Do not crush or open medications without literature support

Crushing or opening of antineoplastic agent tablets should be done with caution

Flush feeding tube with 15–30 mL of water before and after each drug administration

Administer each drug separately

Administer the entire dose of medication as a bolus

Do not mix medication with enteral nutrition formulas

Teach ambulatory patient and/or caregiver how to use oral syringe for self-medication

Develop protocols to assist health care providers and patient caregivers in determining which medications to switch from the parenteral to enteral route to facilitate transistion and potenially result in faster discharge from inpatient setting

Patients, family, and/or caregivers shoud be instructed how to properly administer the medications and flushes via the feeding tubes

Teach ambulatory patient and/or cargiver to notify health care team when problems occur such as diarrhea, abdominal distention, or vomiting

(*Adapted from* Magnuson *et al.* [41].)

general population, there is a concern of drug interactions among these agents, as well as drug interactions between these products and prescription medications [43].

For the practioner, the strategy for optimizing care for individuals with cancer includes the recognition, assessment, and management of these interactions. Unfortunately many of the interactions are not known or described in the literature. Published print texts exist as resources, but the information on adverse effects, drug interactions, and/or management is not comprehensive [43]. The use of web-based references may provide more current information and are listed in Table 33-3.

ADHERENCE TO THERAPY

Adherence, often referred to as *compliance* in older literature, is defined as the extent to which a patient's behavior coincides with medical advice. Adherence to medication regimens is described as the extent to which a patient takes medications as prescribed by his or her health care providers [44]. Estimates of adherence to long-term medication regimens range from 17% to 80% [45]. The impact of nonadherence has been described in many health states, and poor adherence to medication regimens has been shown to contribute to worsening of disease and disease symptoms and health and increasing health care cost [44]. As with other medication-related issues in the individual with cancer, nonadherence extends beyond cancer therapy. Nonadherence also occurs in regard to antineoplastic agents; medications for prevention and/or management of treatment-related and/or cancer-related symptoms and complications; and medication therapies for prevention, management, or treatment of comorbidities and/or most commonly combinations of these. The use of oral agents in the management of cancer includes drugs classified as hormonal therapy, targeted therapies, and chemotherapy, and is done at home.

The issue of adherence to cancer treatment has become a major focus in recent years because of the increasing use of oral therapies for cancer [46]. Suboptimal adherence may prove one the greatest barriers to oral therapy. This risk is especially important if the health care team dose not consider the potential obstacles. Strategies to assess adherence to therapy based on experiences with parenteral therapy are often ineffective simply because parenteral therapy is traditionally done within the clinic or hospital settings. Oral therapies, whether alone or in combination with parenteral treatment, impact cancer care in a variety of ways, including the shift of antineoplastic therapy oversight to patients, family, and/or caregivers.

Individuals with cancer are generally thought to be highly motivated by the gravity of their disease, but the challenges of coordinating care are often not determined by motivation. Even the most highly motivated patient or caregiver requires sufficient education about many aspects of care including medication regimens and schedules, problem solving, resources, and coordination of care among the patient, family, and health care team. Something as straightforward as a medication regimen may be an obstacle when different medications are given on various days of the week or month. For chemotherapy that is given for limited days, followed by days off schedules, it is extremely important that the plan of care is discussed with the patient, caregiver, and all members of the health care team. For example, a patient who is admitted to a hospital for care of a chronic medical problem should communicate with the hospital team the medication, medication schedule, and the current point in therapy when seen. Additionally, the management of drug therapy side effects must be discussed and understood, and the decision to hold a cancer medication should be clear and coordinated with instructions on how to obtain additional advice when needed.

Another concern is overadherence of self-administered medication. Patients and caregivers should be instructed about concerns with modifying medication doses, such as increasing medications without the input of their health care team.

A challenge for the health care team is determining whether an individual patient is adherent to medications and drug therapy. General predictors for medication adherence are listed in Table 33-5. Predictors for nonadherence are listed in Table 33-6. For assessment in individual patients, a number of strategies may be used. Adherence behavior is not stable and may change over time. Dose observation is the most precise method to monitor adherence, but is impractical in many real life situations. Unfortunately, self-reporting has been the most commonly used method to measure patient adherence to oral therapies, and patient recall is often unreliable or inaccurate. It is not surprising that an individual is often reluctant to admit to "bad behavior" or to inability to pay for medications. Direct questioning at each visit may be an effective strategy for some patients; recommended questions are listed in Table 33-7. Pill counts, also considered unreliable, do not provide information about adherence to dosing schedules. Other strategies—using drug levels for select drugs and evaluating pharmacy and insurance records—also have limitations. One emerging strategy is

---

Table 33-5. Predictors for Medication Adherence

Less frequent dosing

Acute (versus chronic) illness

Type of medications

Severity of illness

Symptoms score

Older age of patient

Female gender

Patient belief in therapy

Positive attitude of treating health care provider

Table 33-6. Factors Associated With Poor Adherence to Oral Medications

Presence of psychological problems, particularly depression

Presence of cognitive impairment

Treatment of asymptomatic disease

Inadequate follow-up/supervision

Inadequate discharge planning

Inadequate social support

Side effects of medications

Patient's lack of belief in benefits of treatment

Patients's lack of insight into illness

Poor provider–patient relationship and/or communication

Presence of barriers to care or medications

Missed appointments

Complexity of treatment

Cost of medication, copayment, or both

Substantial behavior change required

(*Data from* Osterberg and Blaschke [44] and Weingart *et al.* [48].)

Table 33-7. Questions for Assessing Medication Adherence

Has any medication(s) been added since your last visit?

Have you started to use any new over-the-counter medications since your last visit?

Have you changed your dose of any medications?

At what times do you take medications?

Do you have any concerns about your medications?

What is the purpose of each of your medications?

What problems could occur if you choose not to take your medication?

What do you do if you forget to take your medications?

How do you pay for your medications?

the use of helpful technology to record how a patient takes medication. The microelectronic monitoring system (MEMS) involves the use of a medication container that records the time when the container cap is removed (Table 33-8).

Coordination of care among health care providers is essential. A survey of comprehensive cancer centers in the United States regarding the practice of prescribing oral chemotherapy demonstrated that there is considerable variation in prescribing practices [47]. Additionally, the distribution of oral chemotherapy is often a challenge, as prescriptions for oral chemotherapy may be limited based on the drug. The challenge of this is the fragmentation of care between drug sources. The National Comprehensive Cancer Network (NCCN) has recently published a report of a multidisciplinary task force that met to discuss the impact of the increasing use of oral chemotherapy and is a good resource for some of the issues discussed [48].

The issue of adherence for individuals with cancer extends beyond that of oral chemotherapy. There is a very real concern that the complexity of medication regimens impacts the ability of a patient to take all of his or her medications correctly. Additionally, the cost of medications escalates as the number of medications for cancer management, cancer side effects, and cancer treatment side effects increases. An important issue to assess for an individual patient is the impact these medications may have on concurrent therapy for other health-related issues.

Table 33-8. Strategies for Improving Adherence to Medications

Identify poor adherence risks
  Missed appointments
  Missed refills of medications
Offer education
  Reason for medications
  Side effects
  Instructions when to contact health care team
  How to contact health care team (including off hours)
  Importance of communicating care to other health care providers (*eg*, dentists, primary care physicians, pharmacists)
Provide simple clear instructions
  Written and oral if possible
Simplify regimens as much as possible
  Simplify schedules
  Consider more "forgiving" medication schedules (*eg*, transdermal medications)
Identify patient caregiver(s)
  Identify patient's role in medication management
  Identify family and/or caregivers involved in care (not always the family member that brings the patient to physician appointments)
Reinforce desirable behavior
Institute medication-taking systems and/or practices
  Microelectronic monitoring system (MEMS)
  Use of medication refill records

(*Adapted from* Osterberg and Blaschke [44] and Partridge *et al.* [46].)

REFERENCES

1. Canal P, Chatelut E, Guichard S: Practical treatment guide for dose individualization in cancer chemotherapy. *Drugs* 1998, 56:1019–1038.

2. Reilly JJ, Workman P: Normalization of anti-cancer drug dosage using body weight and surface area: is it worthwhile? A review of theoretical and practical considerations. *Cancer Chemother Pharmacol* 1993, 32:411–418.

3. DuBois D, DuBois EF: A formula to estimate the approximate surface area if height and weight be known. *Arch Intern Med* 1916, 17:863–871.

4. Gehan EA, George SL: Estimation of human body surface area from height and weight. *Cancer Chemother Rep* 1970, 54:225–235.

5. Griggs JJ, Sorbero ME, Lyman GH: Undertreatment of obese women receiving breast cancer chemotherapy. *Arch Intern Med* 2005, 165:1267–1273.

6. Cheymol G: Effects of obesity on pharmacokinetics. Implications for drug therapy. *Clin Pharmacokinet* 2000, 39:215–231.

7. Grochow LB, Baraldi C, Noe D: Is dose normalization to weight or body surface area useful in adults? *J Natl Cancer Inst* 1990, 82:323–325.

8. Green B, Duffull SB: What is the best size descriptor to use for pharmacokinetic studies in the obese? *Br J Clin Pharmacol* 2004, 58:119–133.

9. Georgiadis MS, Steinberg SM, Hankins LA, *et al.*: Obesity and therapy-related toxicity in patients treated for small-cell lung cancer. *J Natl Cancer Inst* 1995, 87:361–366.

10. Wright JD, Tian C, Mutch DG, *et al.*: Carboplatin dosing in obese women with ovarian cancer: a Gynecologic Oncology Group study. *Gynecol Oncol* 2008, 109:353–358.

11. Portugal RD: Obesity and dose individualization in cancer chemotherapy: the role of body surface area and body mass index. *Med Hypotheses* 2005, 65:748–751.

12. Han PY, Duffull SB, Kirkpatrick CM, Green B: Dosing in obesity: a simple solution to a big problem. *Clin Pharmacol Ther* 2007, 82:505–508.

13. Sparreboom A, Wolff AC, Mathijssen RH, *et al.*: Evaluation of alternate size descriptors for dose calculation of anticancer drugs in the obese. *J Clin Oncol* 2007, 25:4707–4713.

14. Lichtman SM, Wildiers H, Launay-Vacher V, *et al.*: International Society of Geriatric Oncology (SIOG) recommendations for the adjustment of dosing in elderly cancer patients with renal insufficiency. *Eur J Cancer* 2007, 43:14–34.

15. Pannu N, Nadim MK: An overview of drug-induced acute kidney injury. *Crit Care Med* 2008, 36(Suppl):S216–S223.

16. Superfin D, Iannucci AA, Davies AM: Commentary: oncologic drugs in patients with organ dysfunction: a summary. *Oncologist* 2007, 12:1070–1083.

17. Donelli MG, Zucchetti M, Munzone E, *et al.*: Pharmacokinetics of anticancer agents in patients with impaired liver function. *Eur J Cancer* 1998, 34:33–46.

18. Eklund JW, Trifilio S, Mulcahy MF: Chemotherapy dosing in the setting of liver dysfunction. *Oncology* 2005, 19:1057–1069.

19. Tchambaz L, Schlatter C, Jakob M, *et al.*: Dose adaptation of antineoplastic drugs in patients with liver disease. *Drug Saf* 2006, 29:509–522.

20. Grochow LB: Individualized dosing of anti-cancer drugs and the role of therapeutic monitoring. In *A Clinician's Guide to Chemotherapy Pharmacokinetics and Pharmacodynamics.* Edited by Grochow LB, Ames MM. Baltimore: Lippincott Williams & Wilkins; 1998:3–16.

21. Gamelin E, Delva R, Jacob J, *et al.*: Individual fluorouracil dose adjustment based on pharmacokinetic follow-up compared with conventional dosage: results of a multicenter randomized trial of patients with metastatic colorectal cancer. *J Clin Oncol* 2008, 26:2099–2105.

22. Di Paolo A, Lencioni M, Amatori F, *et al.*: 5-fluorouracil pharmacokinetics predicts disease-free survival in patients administered adjuvant chemotherapy for colorectal cancer. *Clin Cancer Res* 2008, 14:2749–2755.

23. Walko CM, McLeod HL: Will we ever be ready for blood level-guided therapy? *J Clin Oncol* 2008, 26:2078–2079.

24. Riechelmann RP, Tannock IF, Wang L, *et al.*: Potential drug interactions and duplicate prescriptions among cancer patients. *J Natl Cancer Inst* 2007, 99:592–600.

25. Sokol KC, Knudsen JF, Li MM: Polypharmacy in older oncology patients and the need for an interdisciplinary approach to side-effect management. *J Clin Pharm Ther* 2007, 32:169–175.

26. Blower P, de Wit R, Goodin S, Aapro M: Drug-drug interactions in oncology: why are they important and can they be minimized? *Clin Rev Oncol Hematol* 2005, 55:117–142.

27. Karas S Jr: The potential for drug interactions. *Ann Emerg Med* 1981, 10:627–630.

28. Yancik R, Ganz PA, Varricchio CG, Conley B: Perspectives in comorbidity and cancer in older patients: approaches to expand the knowledge base. *J Clin Oncol* 2001, 19:1147–1154.

29. Weneke U, Earl J, Seydel O, *et al.*: Potential health risks of complementary alternative medicines in cancer patients. *Br J Cancer* 2004, 9:408–413.

30. Goodin S: Oral chemotherapeutic agents: understanding mechanisms of action and drug interactions. *Am J Health Syst Pharm* 2007, 64(Suppl 5): S15–S24.

31. Lam MSH, Ignoffo RJ: A guide to clinically relevant drug interactions in oncology. *J Oncol Pharm Pract* 2003, 9:45–85.

32. Scripture CD, Figg WD: Drug interactions in cancer therapy. *Nat Rev Cancer* 2006, 6:546–558.

33. Genser D: Food and drug interactions: consequences for the nutrition/ health status. *Ann Nutr Metab* 2008, 52(Suppl 1):29–32.

34. Kataoka M, Masaoka Y, Sakuma S, *et al.*: Effect of food intake on oral absorption of poorly water-soluble drugs: In vitro assessment of drug dissolution and permeation assay system. *J Pharm Sci* 2006, 95:2052–2061.

35. Chan LN: Drug–nutrient interactions. In *Modern Nutrition in Health and Disease.* Edited by Shils ME, Shike M, Ross AC, *et al.* Baltimore: Lippincott Williams & Wilkins; 2006:1540–1553.

36. Farkas D, Greenblatt DJ: Influence of fruit juices on drug disposition: discrepancies between in vitro and clinical studies. *Expert Opin Drug Metab Toxicol* 2008, 4:381–393.

37. McCarthy MS, Fabling JC, Bell DE: Drug-nutrient interactions. In *Nutritional Considerations in the Intensive Care Unit.* Edited by Shikora SA, Martindale RG, Schwaitzberg SD. Dubuque, IA: Kendal Hunt Publishing Company; 2002:153–171.

38. Cheng TS: Letter to the editor: food–drug interactions. *Intern J Cardiol* 2006, 106:392–393.

39. Leibovitch ER, Deamer RL, Sanderson LA: Food-drug interactions. Careful drug selection and patient counseling can reduce the risk in older patients. *Geriatrics* 2004, 59:19–33.

40. Sorenson JM: Herb-drug, food-drug, nutrient-drug, and drug-drug interactions: mechanisms involved and their medical implications. *J Altern Complement Med* 2002, 18:293–308.

41. Magnuson BL, Clifford TM, Hoskins LA, Bernard AC: Enteral nutrition and drug administration, interactions and complications. *Nutr Clin Pract* 2005, 20:618–624.

42. Mitchell JF, Leady MA: Oral dosage forms that should not be crushed, July 2004 [chart]. *Hospital Pharmacy.* St. Louis, MO: Wolters Kluwer Health, Inc.; 2004.

43. Haller CA, Anderson IB, Kim S, Blanc P: An evaluation of selected herbal reference texts and comparison to published reports of adverse herbal events. *Adv Drug React Toxicol Rev* 2002, 21:143–150.

44. Osterberg L, Blaschke T: Drug therapy: adherence to medication. *N Engl J Med* 2005;353:487–497.

45. Krueger KP, Berger BA, Felkey B: Medication adherence and persistence: a comprehensive review. *Adv Ther* 2005, 22:313–356.

46. Partridge AH, Avorn J, Wang PS, Winer EP: Adherence to therapy with oral antineoplastic agents. *J Natl Cancer Inst* 2002, 94:652–661.

47. Weingart SN, Flug J, Brouillard D, *et al.*: Oral chemotherapy safety practices in US cancer centers: questionnaire survey. *BMJ* 2007, 334:407–409.

48. Weingart SN, Brown E, Bach PB, *et al.*: NCCN task force report: oral chemotherapy. *J Natl Compr Canc Netw* 2008, 6(Suppl 3):S1–S14.

Venous access is one of the most important considerations in the management of cancer patients. Too often, the most appropriate venous access is only seriously considered after the patient has experienced numerous peripheral intravenous (IV) devices and venipunctures for blood draws. Repeated venipunctures result in infiltrations, phlebitis, hematomas, and progressive difficulty with subsequent venous access and venipuncture. Patients experience complications and anticipatory anxiety with each attempted access. In many cases, quality of life is compromised and options for venous access device (VAD) insertion become limited. A more thoughtful, upfront approach to the continued management of venous access is a priority in the cancer patient population. Initiation of VAD algorithms available for treatment support (Fig. 34-1) can improve outcomes and increase patient satisfaction [1]. Oncology nurses play a pivotal role in the recommendation, selection, utilization, and management of all VADs.

In the United States, approximately 5 million central venous access devices (CVADs) are used annually [2]. Although some cancer patients can tolerate peripheral IV therapy, the majority will require a CVAD. Central venous access makes it possible to draw blood and infuse blood products, parenteral nutrition, and medications or fluids, including drugs classified as irritants or vesicants. CVADs have revolutionized the care of cancer patients at home. According to the Strategic Health Care Programs National Database, which included 50,470 patients receiving home infusions, there were a reported 2.83 million catheter-days per year in 2001 [3]. Oncology patients comprise a large number of the individuals discharged from hospitals annually who have CVADs and are either self-managing or returning for the care and maintenance of their device.

Over the past decade, the types of available CVADs have grown significantly; health care providers and patients now have a variety of options for central access. Careful consideration must be used in determining the most appropriate and reliable device for each individual. Patients must be included in the decision-making process to ensure compliance with CVAD

management to maximize quality of life during cancer treatments. Potential complications related to indwelling catheters must be discussed with patients so that they have a clear understanding of the risks, benefits, and self-care requirements of CVAD use.

Unfortunately, the use of CVADs is not without risk. The most significant complication of CVAD use is catheter-related infection, followed by risk of thromboembolic events, catheter occlusion, and malposition. CVADs are the major cause of health care–associated bloodstream infections, causing 250,000 to 500,000 CVAD-related bloodstream infections annually in the United States [4]. The importance of evidence-based practice guidelines for the insertion and maintenance of these lines is a priority. A commitment by health care providers to decrease CVAD complications will drastically impact the morbidity and mortality of patients with CVADs and should be a priority in settings in which CVADs are placed and managed.

CATHETER TYPES

Catheter types vary by material, size, indication, limitations, insertion technique, and complication rates. VADs are classified as peripheral or central. Peripheral devices include short IV device catheters that are changed frequently and ideally placed in the upper extremities. These devices have limited functionality and are associated with phlebitis and infiltrations. The type of infusate/medication administered through these types of lines must be carefully considered to avoid pain, burning, and possible infiltration with subsequent tissue necrosis. Table 34-1 includes a list of drugs that require assessment before use in the peripheral IV setting. Midline catheters, peripheral catheters with a longer length, are placed in the upper arm, terminating in the bicep area. Midlines provide a larger venous access; however, they should not be confused with a CVAD.

CVADs provide access to the central circulation with the tip ideally terminating in the superior vena cava and right atrial juncture. Examples of these lines include the traditional catheter type; short-term, noncuffed, non-

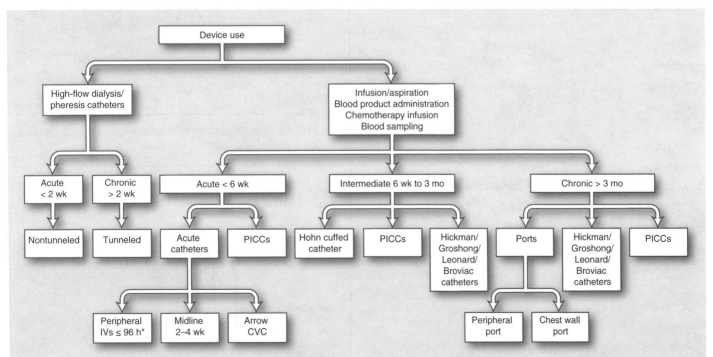

Figure 34-1. The 2007 Johns Hopkins Hospital venous access device policy. More lumen leads to a larger catheter, and thus a greater risk of infection and venous thrombosis. The *asterisk* indicates peripheral intravenous (IV) use in the adult population. In some pediatric populations, a peripheral IV may be left in for longer than 96 hours. CVC—central venous catheter; PICC—peripherally inserted central catheter. Arrow CVC (Arrow International, Inc., Reading, PA); Hohn, Hickman, Groshong, Leonard, Broviac catheters (Bard Access Systems, Salt Lake City, UT). (*Adapted from* Johns Hopkins Hospital [36].)

tunneled, double or triple lumen catheters; peripherally inserted central-line catheters (PICC); surgically implanted ports (Fig. 34-2); tunneled central venous catheters (Fig. 34-3); and tunneled or nontunneled hemodialysis/hemepheresis catheters. The recent discovery of "power" lines allows for increased catheter functionality. These lines can withstand high infusion rates of fluids or high pressures during injection of contrast media. Power lines are indicated for accurate central venous pressure monitoring. Power lines are available as peripherally inserted central lines (Fig. 34-4), ports, and tunneled and nontunneled central catheters. Each of these power catheters has unique characteristics. Recent discovery of the first saline-only, proximal-valved, power-injectable PICC line allows for the elimination of heparin when flushing.

Choosing an appropriate VAD for the administration of cancer therapies is a patient-specific process. Assessment should include quality of veins, types of therapies to be infused, length of treatment, and comorbidities. The pH and osmolality of the drug must be considered when deciding between peripheral and central venous access. Drugs known as vesicants that are associated with tissue necrosis when extravasated should generally be administered through central venous catheters unless administered by a trained and competent provider following institutional guidelines. Each patient presents unique risk factors, lifestyle considerations, and psychosocial factors that will impact catheter selection. Table 34-2 includes a list of central venous catheters and their characteristics.

COMPLICATIONS

OCCLUSION

One of the most common complications of VADs is catheter occlusion. It is estimated that as many as 50% to 90% of patients with CVADs will experience partial or complete catheter occlusions. Partial occlusions allow for infusion through the catheter; however, aspiration is not possible. Partial

Table 34-1. Irritant or Vesicant Drugs Associated With Phlebitis and Peripheral IV Restarts

Drug	Description
Acyclovir	
Amphotericin	Irritant
Calcium gluconate	Hypertonic
Ceftriaxone	Irritant/hypertonic
Cephalosporins	Hypertonic
Chemotherapy vesicants	
Ciprofloxacin	pH 3.3
Dobutamine	pH 2.5
Dopamine	pH 2.5
Doxycycline	pH 1.8
Erythromycin	Irritant
Mannitol	Hypertonic/pH 4.5
Morphine (continuous)	pH 2.5
Penicillins	pH 10
Pentamidine	pH 4.09
Peripheral parenteral nutrition	Hypertonic
Phenytoin	pH 12
Potassium (> 20 mEq)	Hypertonic
Promethazine	pH 4.0
Tobramycin	pH 3.0
Trimethoprim/sulfamethoxazole	pH 10
Vancomycin	pH 2.4

IV—intravenous.

occlusions can also include any amount of resistance with flushing, which is usually a sign of impending catheter malfunction. Complete occlusion occurs when the catheter cannot be flushed or aspirated. It is most likely the result of clot formation; however, it may also represent a drug precipitation within the lumen or a mechanical or positional problem. To rule out a positional problem, the patient should undergo a Valsalva test or cough during aspiration. If blood return is immediately noticeable, catheter position problem should be suspected. If this persists, the catheter will need to be evaluated radiographically and potentially repositioned or replaced. Complete occlusions are difficult to manage and should be avoided by ensuring consistent patency of the catheter. Occlusions can be related to drug precipitate, intraluminal clotted blood, and fibrin formation such as a fibrin sheath

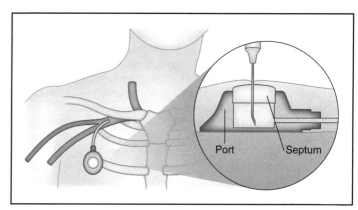

Figure 34-2. Surgically implanted port catheter system.

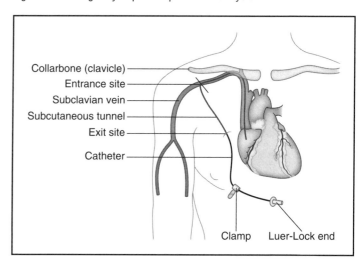

Figure 34-3. Tunneled central venous access device. Luer-Lock (Becton Dickinson, Franklin Lakes, NJ).

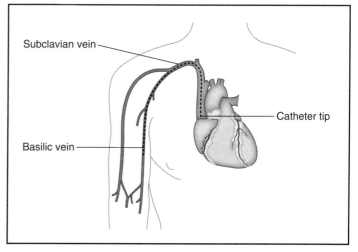

Figure 34-4. Peripherally inserted central-line catheter.

or fibrin tail (Fig. 34-5). A VAD occlusion should always be considered an abnormal finding and investigation into the etiology with prompt resolution should be initiated. Improper evaluation of an occluded catheter can result in life-threatening catheter-related bloodstream infection, delay of infusional treatments, and removal of the nonfunctional catheter. Reinsertion of a new catheter can be costly and burdensome for the patient.

Thrombotic occlusions account for approximately 60% of catheter occlusions [5]. Fibrin formation on and around a catheter begins immediately upon placement and is unavoidable. Unfortunately, fibrin isolated from catheters is frequently colonized with bacteria [6]. Remnants of blood from blood collection or administration or fibrin formation can cause thrombotic occlusions either in the lumen of catheters, around the tip of the catheter, or in a port reservoir. Intraluminal clot formation can occur because of inadequate flushing of a catheter, failure to use a positive-pressure flush technique or positive-pressure valve, or backflow of blood into the tip of the catheter caused by central venous pressure fluctuation that occurs during patient coughing or vomiting. Intraluminal clot formation can impact catheter flushing and lead to a complete occlusion. Intraluminal clots can be reduced with adequate flushing using a turbulent flushing technique—clamping during the last 2 mL of a syringe flush—to overfill the catheter. This flushing technique displaces blood away from the tip of the catheter, preventing backflow of blood and subsequent clot formation. Various flushing procedures exist and should be tailored to the type of catheter, the patient's medical and catheter history, and frequency of treatment through the VAD. Flushing using normal saline and/or heparin is necessary to ensure patency. Use of positive-pressure valves that prevent backflow of blood into the tip of the catheter when disconnecting from the catheter hub have been suggested as a solution to heparin-free flushing. Many of these valves have become available, although unfortunately some have been linked to increased rates of infection and require further study to determine the risk-benefit ratio. If a needleless valve of any type is implemented in a particular setting, close monitoring should occur to detect significant increased rates of catheter-related bloodstream infections.

A fibrin tail or flap is described as fibrin that attaches to the tip of the catheter and can flap over the distal tip when aspiration is attempted. Infusions can be normal or sluggish. This finding, noted upon flushing and aspirating, is called a *partial withdrawal occlusion*. A fibrin sheath or sleeve is described as fibrin that covers a portion of the interior or exterior catheter or the entire catheter wall. Fibrin sheath formation can cause retrograde flow of infusions, which can result in an infiltration at the catheter exit site. Serious evidence of tissue necrosis has been observed due to infiltration of vesicant therapies in this manner.

Table 34-2. Venous Access Device Types and Characteristics

Catheter type	Characteristics	Advantages	Disadvantages
Peripheral IV	Short, ½ to ¾ inch	↓ infection risk; ease of placement; ↓ cost	Replacement every 96 h; phlebitis, infiltration, extravasation, and vein damage with long-term use; contraindicated with certain drugs/solutions with high osmolality (*eg*, central parenteral nutrition); cannot be used for continuous infusion of vesicants
External jugular IV	Peripheral line placed by physician	Easy insertion; ↓ cost	Same as peripheral IV; uncomfortable position for patient; difficult to cover with dressing
Midline	Peripheral line, length ~ 3–8 cm, tip in upper arm	Useful when therapy exceeds 6 d; single or double can be used; no chest x-ray required postinsertion	Replacement required every 2–4 wk; phlebitis, infiltration, and extravasation; cannot be used for continuous infusion of vesicants or hyperosmotic solutions
PICC	Central-line catheter, tip in superior vena cava/right atrial juncture	Placement can be done at bedside; eliminates risk of insertion-related pneumothorax; ↓ infection rate related to insertion location; useful when IV therapy exceeds 6 d	Mechanical phlebitis; thrombus; care and maintenance issues related to location; requires covering during showers/bathing
Implantable port	Placed in a SC pocket in chest or arm; accessed with special Huber needle for infusions	Can be deaccessed when not in use to eliminate maintenance; less limitations in activity; single and double ports available	Placed with sedation; placement is costly; insertion and removal by surgeon required; discomfort from needle accessing; occlusion problems if not flushed properly; access and flush required at least monthly; risk of port pocket infections; risk of thrombus
Short-term CVC	Short central-line catheter placed in subclavian vein	Multilumen access; placed at bedside; easily removed at bedside; can be rewired if mechanical problems exist	Risk of pneumothorax during insertion; ↑ infection rates, especially with femoral or jugular insertion sites; exit site may be difficult to dress and uncomfortable for patient; femoral lines restrict patient activity
Nontunneled CVC	Single or double placed by surgeon (*eg*, Hohn)	Antimicrobial cuff; can be rewired	↑ complications if left in > 6 wk; not accurate for hemodynamic monitoring
Tunneled CVC	Examples include Hickman, Broviac, Groshong, Leonard	SC tunnel created to decrease risk of infection; antimicrobial cuffs in tunnel*	Costly to place in operating room by surgeon; placed with sedation; removal can be difficult; damage to catheter is sometimes difficult to repair; thrombus; requires special education for care and maintenance
Hemepheresis or dialysis	Tunneled or nontunneled	Tunneled catheters with or without antimicrobial cuffs	Large-bore catheter; ↑ risk of thrombus; placed with sedation; higher doses of heparin needed to ensure patency; ↑ risk of infection; weight of catheter can be heavy; difficult to dress and immobilize

*4–6 wk after catheter placement, a tissue ingrowth matrix forms around cuffs that provides an antimicrobial barrier and secures catheter in place.
Hohn, Hickman, Broviac, Groshong, and Leonard catheters (Bard Access Systems, Salt Lake City, UT).
CVC—central venous catheter; IV—intravenous; PICC—peripherally inserted central-line catheter; SC—subcutaneous.
(*Adapted from* Rabinowitz and Olsen [34].)

A mural thrombus is a clot that develops at the distal tip of the catheter and can result in occlusion of the vein containing the VAD, resulting in a deep vein thrombosis. Any fibrin formation increases the risk of infection in the host and serves as an ideal medium for bacterial growth. To avoid such complications, prompt recovery of a catheter with any sign of occlusion is critical. Various strategies have been studied to reduce catheter occlusion.

An additional risk factor for the development of VAD thrombus is the catheter tip location. Ideally, tip location should be visible at the superior vena cava/right atrial juncture. Catheters placed with the tip terminating in the subclavian vein or the upper superior vena cava are associated with higher rates of thrombus [7]. Catheter migration can occur with many CVADs; therefore, radiographic evaluation of the catheter tip should be performed if malfunction is noted.

VAD thrombus is a challenging problem in oncology patients who may concurrently have low platelets or coagulation alterations. Patients, caregivers, and health care providers must be educated in the care and maintenance of CVADs to prevent or minimize occlusions and thrombi. Heparin flush to prevent the formation of clots has been a traditional practice; however, it is not without risks. The emergence of heparin-induced thrombocytopenia has left health care providers to ponder the most effective and safest intervention to prevent catheter occlusion. Furthermore, the increased propensity for clotting in cancer patients makes this a difficult issue that requires further study.

The standard treatment for occluded catheters secondary to any type of clot formation is use of a thrombolytic. Other mechanical techniques for removal of clots have been studied but are considered high risk. Treatment using a thrombolytic is primarily aimed at dissolving the clot to allow for proper catheter function. A thrombolytic can be instilled in a catheter with a partial occlusion. However, in the event of a complete occlusion, a negative-pressure technique may be necessary. This technique can be used by attaching a stopcock to the hub of the catheter. A thrombolytic-containing syringe is attached to one port of the stopcock and an empty 10-mL syringe to the other port. It is important to ensure that the stopcock is off to the thrombolytic syringe and on to the empty syringe. Aspirate back to about 7 to 8 mL, creating negative pressure within the catheter. Turn the stopcock on to the thrombolytic, allowing for drug to be pulled into the catheter. These steps may need to be repeated in order to get drug into the catheter. The empty syringe must be removed with each attempt to purge air from the syringe, and care must be taken to avoid injection of air into the catheter and contamination of the hub.

The importance of evaluating and treating catheter occlusions should be underscored. Thrombosis is known to increase the risk of catheter-related bloodstream infections and is associated with a cost of approxi-

mately $5000 for catheter replacement [7]. Clot formation can lead to thrombus development in the vein where the catheter is placed. The term *mural thrombi* refers to a thrombus that blocks a vessel partially or completely [7].

Risk factors for thrombus formation consist of venous stasis, hypotension, immobilization, congestive heart failure, vessel wall trauma, and the presence of malignancy. Thrombus formation can also be the result of access difficulties during the initial CVAD placement. Multiple punctures to the vein and surrounding tissues can induce trauma and inflammation, resulting in clot formation. Catheter material can also influence thrombus formation, with certain catheter types being more thrombogenic than others. For example, catheters made with silicone are associated with a higher risk of thrombus formation. In one study of 111 CVADs, there was a 33% incidence of thrombosis in the silicone catheters and a 19% incidence in the polyurethane catheters [8]. In recent years, changes to catheter materials, design, and insertion methods have been studied in an effort to decrease thrombotic complications. More studies are need in patients with all catheter types to determine the significance of these changes in thrombosis formation.

The type of chemotherapy is also a possibly significant risk factor for thrombus formation. Sclerosing chemotherapy is related to a higher risk of catheter-related thrombus [9]. Ong *et al.* [10] also found an increased risk (7% vs 1%) of thrombus in patients with PICCs receiving chemotherapy compared with those who did not. However, the specific drugs were not characterized in this study. Further study is needed to illicit the relationship between various cancer therapies and risk of thrombus.

The clinical manifestations of a thrombus can include swelling, pain, and phlebitis. Superior vena cava syndrome can result if the thrombus exists at the catheter tip or around the catheter within the superior vena cava. Catheter-related thrombus can be present without symptoms in a portion of patients. In a prospective study of 444 cancer patients, a rate of 4.3% (0.3 per 1000 catheter-days) for symptomatic catheter-related thrombus was observed [11]. The median time to symptom development of thrombus was 30 days and the median catheter life-span was 88 days. Significant risk factors consisted of more than one insertion attempt, ovarian cancer, and previous insertion of a CVAD. Catheter types in this study consisted of PICCs (67%), port (19%), and Hickman (Bard Access Systems, Salt Lake City, UT)/apheresis (14%) [11]. PICC-related thrombi can be reduced by placing the catheter on the right side, using ultrasound technology for placement, avoiding trauma during insertion, and ensuring proper tip location in the superior vena cava/right atrial juncture [10].

The use of low-dose warfarin for prophylaxis against thrombosis in CVADs has been studied in oncology patients. A recent meta-analysis of four studies including a total of 1236 patients concluded that prophylaxis with low-dose warfarin did not significantly decrease the risk of thrombosis [12]. The authors of the meta-analysis recognized that these results are limited by the small number of studies and the treatment variations among them [12]. The concern for bleeding risk is a primary reason patients are not routinely given systemic prophylaxis. Prolonged coagulation times have been documented in patients receiving low-dose anticoagulants for prevention of catheter-related thrombus, indicating that monitoring is necessary [13].

Nonthrombotic catheter occlusions consist of catheter malposition, catheter migration, drug or mineral precipitation, and fat emulsion residue [14]. Immediate assessment of catheter tip location and entire catheter position should be performed using radiographic studies to rule out malposition or migration as the primary cause of the occlusion.

Drug precipitant occlusions can be caused by the administration of incompatible drugs, drugs with a high risk of precipitation or instability, or inadequate flushing of catheters when administering these drugs. These types of occlusions usually require clearance using a solution that changes the pH within the catheter where the occlusion has occurred. The change in pH increases the solubility of the precipitate, thereby enhancing its clearance. The appropriate solution should be carefully chosen, taking into consideration the probable causative precipitate. It is imperative to avoid forceful flushing with any occlusion coexisting with resistance because

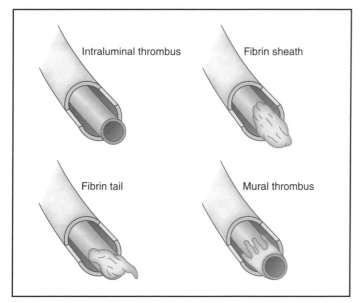

Figure 34-5. Types of thrombotic catheter occlusions. (*From* Herbst *et al.* [35]; with permission.)

forceful flushing into an occluded catheter can result in catheter rupture and catheter emboli. The size of the syringe used for flushing any CVAD should always be greater than 10 mL to prevent excessive pressure on the catheter. Table 34-3 outlines drug precipitate treatment interventions.

INFECTION

CVAD-related infections are highly prevalent and are associated with significant morbidity and mortality. Catheter-related bloodstream infections cost the health care industry $60 to $460 million per year [15]. The rate of catheter-related bloodstream infections varies greatly depending upon patient risk factors, patient location (*eg*, intensive care unit, general care floor, home care), type of infusate (*eg*, parenteral nutrition), and type of VAD. The cost per catheter-related bloodstream infection can reach $25,000, with an associated mortality rate of 12% to 25% [6,16]. Sepsis related to infection from catheters occurs in 1% to 5% of patients with CVADs [17]. The use of CVADs has facilitated the complex management of cancer patients in the 21st century; however, we are challenged with protecting our patients from device-related life-threatening complications. Cancer patients are particularly vulnerable to catheter-related bloodstream infection during their treatment continuum. Infections can be classified as localized, including the exit site, tunnel, or port pocket.

Exit site infections are generally within 2 cm of catheter exit site and exist in the absence of bacteremia. Signs include erythema and tenderness with or without purulence. Tunnel infections occur in tunneled CVADs more than 2 cm from the exit site and extending through the tunnel. Erythema can be seen on the skin and along the tunnel with palpable tenderness. Port pocket infections occur at the subcutaneous pocket and, if severe, can lead to erosion of the port through the skin.

Systemic infections occur from colonization of thrombi or intraluminal or extraluminal colonization of the catheter. Colonization of the hub or catheter exit site by bacteria is the most common source of catheter-related bloodstream infections [15]. Contamination of infusate as a source of infection has decreased over the years and is not a primary source of catheter-related bloodstream infections. Changes in pharmacy mixing processes have contributed to the decline in infusate contaminates.

A nationwide focus on decreasing catheter-related bloodstream infections is under way. Many health care systems have successfully decreased these infections with a variety of evidence-based strategies. In lieu of the associated costs and mortality, many institutions are developing a "zero tolerance" policy for catheter-related bloodstream infections. In one randomized trial that was designed to minimize catheter-related bloodstream infections, a reduction of 50% was realized [18]. Most interventions focused on maximum sterile barrier insertion techniques using large sterile drapes, masks, caps, sterile gloves, gowns, aseptic technique, and chlorhexidine in a 2% aqueous solution as the skin preparatory agent. Chlorhexidine is considered the superior skin preparatory agent for catheter insertion and maintenance [6,19,20].

The practice of routinely replacing or rewiring central venous catheters is no longer recommended due to increased risks of infection and insertion complications. Other known risk factors for catheter-related bloodstream infections include the use of an antimicrobial ointment at the catheter insertion site, the use of multilumen catheters, and placement of a catheter in the jugular or femoral vein [6,21]. Table 34-4 outlines various strategies to reduce catheter-related bloodstream infections.

Catheter-related bloodstream infection rates appear to be the highest in traditional nontunneled, noncuffed, central venous catheters. An average rate of 2.7% per 1000 catheter-days has been documented but can vary in other catheter types depending upon host factors and specific catheter characteristics. PICCs have traditionally been associated with lower infection rates when compared with other CVADs. Lower colony-forming units of bacteria exist on the arm as opposed to the chest or neck insertion sites, creating a more favorable placement location. However, it must be noted that the increased use of PICCs in critically ill and immunocompromised patients may increase the risk of infection. A prospective study of 251 PICCs placed in high-risk hospitalized patients demonstrated catheter-related bloodstream infections comparable with other lines traditionally

placed in this population, suggesting that the host risk factors may be more predictive of infection than the type of line utilized [22]. This comparison requires further study in the oncology patient population, with special focus on hematologic malignancy patients.

Another well-known risk factor for catheter-related bloodstream infections is the administration of parenteral nutrition. Parenteral nutrition is a hyperosmolar solution that contains large amounts of dextrose and amino acids. The use of parenteral nutrition should include stringent standards of care to minimize or prevent catheter-related bloodstream infections. Some proven practice standards include dedication of a catheter lumen if feasible, avoidance of opening or accessing the dedicated line, and strict aseptic technique in catheter and line maintenance. The Centers for Disease Control and Prevention (CDC) recommends changing IV tubing containing lipids or parenteral nutrition/lipid admixtures every 24 hours due to the high propensity for infection [6].

The materials used in catheter manufacturing also impact infection rates. Polyvinyl chloride and polyethylene materials are less able to resist adherence of microorganisms on their surface and therefore are not recommended for use. Newer catheter materials, such as polyurethane, have emerged to combat this adherence problem. Antimicrobial-coated catheters are now a viable option for reducing catheter-related bloodstream infections and, despite their cost, have proven successful in various studies [23]. Catheters coated with antiseptic and silver-impregnated catheters have also been described for infection reduction and need further study to determine benefit. Cuffs are used by some central-line catheter manufacturers to combat infection and/or for catheter securement (Fig. 34-6).

Table 34-3. Drug Precipitates*

Precipitate	Clearing agent
Lipid residue	70% ethanol or sodium hydroxide
Low-pH drug (pH 1–5)	Hydrochloric acid (0.1% N)
High pH-drug (pH 9–12)	Sodium bicarbonate ($NaHCO_3$)
Calcium phosphate	Hydrochloric acid (0.15% N)
	Cysteine hydrochloride

*For volume and concentration, refer to manufacturer's guidelines.
(*Adapted from* Infusion Nurses Society [14] and Rabinowitz and Olsen [34].)

Table 34-4. Catheter-Related Bloodstream Infection Prevention Strategies

Trained and competent health care providers

Minimize lumens when choosing a central venous access device

Central-line insertions checklist and written standard of care

Avoidance of femoral insertion

Hand hygiene

Skin antisepsis with chlorhexidine (superior to povidone-iodine)

Central-line supply cart or bundle

Maximum sterile barrier drape

Sterile gown, gloves, mask, and face shield for provider

Avoidance of topical antimicrobial ointments (increased risk of *Candida* infection)

Strict aseptic technique to prevent colonization of hub of catheter

Avoidance of guidewire exchange to replace catheters suspected of being infected

Cover catheter and catheter connections during showering

Change dressing whenever site is soiled, loose, or wet

Eliminate scheduled catheter rewires unless mechanical problems exist

(*Adapted from* CDC [6], Heaton *et al.* [13], Pronovost *et al.* [32], and O'Grady *et al.* [33].)

Dressings and dressing components have also been an area of considerable investigation. Impregnated sponges, such as chlorhexidine-saturated types, are round discs placed at the catheter exit site to reduce catheter colonization. In a recent meta-analysis, seven randomized clinical trials of the chlorhexidine sponge were reviewed. The author concluded that the use of a chlorhexidine-impregnated sponge appeared to be associated with a lower infection rate than placebo [24].

The type of dressing used to cover CVADs has been largely debated. The two most common dressing types are gauze and transparent dressings. Transparent dressings are advantageous because they facilitate the securement of the external portion of the catheter, allow visualization of the site, and are changed less frequently. They also may allow moisture to escape from the catheter insertion site. The frequency of dressing changes and the ideal dressing for central venous catheters remains an area of investigation. Dressing choices should be based upon specific patient needs, such as skin integrity, sensitivities, and preference. The Infusion Nurses Society recommends gauze dressing changes every 48 hours and transparent, semipermeable dressing changes at least every 7 days [14]. The catheter and catheter connections should be covered during showering to prevent water-borne infections [6]. All dressing types should be changed immediately if found loose, soiled, or wet. Diaphoretic patients may need more frequent dressing changes.

Historically, organisms most commonly implicated in catheter-related infections of cancer patients included coagulase-negative staphylococci and *Staphylococcus aureus* [6]. Currently, coagulase-negative staphylococci (37%), *S. aureus* (13%), *Enterococci* (13%), and gram-negative rods (14%) have emerged as the most common cause of catheter-related bloodstream infections [6].

Organisms present in catheter-related bloodstream infections and the treatment of these organisms are specific to host-related factors and geographical areas. In general, 80% of coagulase-negative staphylococci infections can be treated with antimicrobial therapy without having to remove the catheter [25]. In contrast, removal of infected CVADs improves treatment response in patients with *S. aureus* infections and should be considered [25]. The presence of a catheter-related bloodstream infections related to gram-negative rods necessitates catheter removal because these infections are associated with significant sepsis. Successful treatment of the infection requires removal of the catheter and the immediate initiation of antimicrobial therapy [25]. *Candida* species are less common causes of catheter-related bloodstream infections; however, they can lead to increased mortality and should be a consideration in the immunocompromised host.

The CDC and Joint Commission on Accreditation of Health Care Organizations state that catheter-related bloodstream infections are expressed per 1000 CVAD-days or catheter-days [6,26]. Challenges with determination of catheter-related bloodstream infections exist when varying surveillance definitions and techniques are used. Most surveillance definitions include all bloodstream infections in patients with CVADs, whereas other sites have been excluded. Ideally this definition should be combined with a thoughtful review of the clinical data to ensure that undocumented sources and other clinical symptoms are not present. The presence of other infectious sources and/or clinical symptoms in the patient would preclude confirmation of a catheter-related bloodstream infection [6].

The Infectious Diseases Society of America recommends obtaining simultaneous quantitative blood cultures from the suspected catheter and a peripheral blood source to assist in accurate identification of a catheter-related bloodstream infection [27]. In 2005, a meta-analysis of this method was found to have sensitivity rates of 93% and specificity rates of 100% in long-term catheters [28]. The use of CVAD blood cultures alone can be used to identify an infection; however, they may not be highly sensitive for a catheter-related bloodstream infection, especially in immunocompromised patients [25].

Treatment of catheter-related bloodstream infections must be approached in an evidence-based manner to prevent unnecessary removal of a central venous catheter. The catheter may be able to remain in place while antimicrobial treatment is initiated. The decision to "treat the catheter" through the infection is dependent upon the specific organism and the host's defense status. Some organisms are particularly virulent and difficulty clearing them from the catheter surface and bloodstream necessitates prompt catheter removal. Additionally, if bacteremia persists despite antimicrobial therapy, a thrombus should be considered and catheter removal is indicated. Strong indications for catheter removal include fungemia related to the catheter, hemodynamic instability, and patient complaints of chills or rigors when flushing the catheter. A full discussion of the specific antimicrobial treatments for catheter-related bloodstream infections is beyond the scope of this chapter.

OTHER

Other complications associated with CVADs include phlebitis, air emboli, catheter emboli, brachial plexus injury, subclavian artery damage, cardiac tamponade, pneumothorax, and catheter pinch-off syndrome (Table 34-5). Air embolus is caused when a significant amount of air is inadvertently allowed to enter the venous system. The air travels to the right side of the heart and into the pulmonary circulation, which causes vasoconstriction of the pulmonary circulation, resulting in an acute onset of hypoxia, hypotension, neurologic symptoms, and even death. Immediate treatment of an air embolus includes positioning of the patient on the left lateral decubitus with the head down. Prevention of air emboli includes placing the patient in Trendelenburg position during central venous catheter placement and removal, asking the patient to undergo a Valsalva test during insertion and removal, and avoiding accidental air insertion through syringes or IV tubing. The Trendelenburg procedure is believed to increase pressure in the larger veins to above atmospheric pressure, thereby reducing the risk of air aspiration into the venous system. After removal of a central venous catheter, an occlusive dressing should be applied over the site [29]. Additionally, care must be taken to clamp open-ended central-line catheters prior to accessing the hub of the catheter. The use of Luer-Lok (Becton Dickinson, Franklin Lanes, NJ) connections on catheter hubs and extension tubing is recommended to prevent accidental hub exposure [14].

Pinch-off syndrome is a rare but serious condition that occurs with catheters placed in the subclavian vein between the clavicle and the first rib. A complete occlusion may be noted; however, when the patient lifts his or her arm in the air or turns the head to the opposite side of the catheter, the catheter may resume function. Repositioning is a temporary solution and pinch-off syndrome should be ruled out. Continued compression of the catheter by the clavicle can shear the catheter and cause it to be severed in part or full [30] (Fig. 34-7).

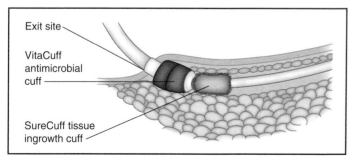

Figure 34-6. Central venous access device cuffs. VitaCuff antimicrobial cuff and SureCuff ingrowth cuff (Bard Access Systems, Salt Lake City, UT).

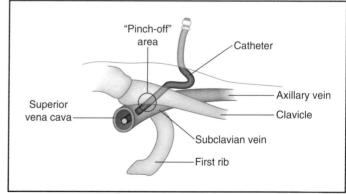

Figure 34-7. Catheter pinch-off.

Table 34-5. Select Venous Access Device Complications

Complication	Description
Phlebitis	Most common with PICCs. Characterized by redness, warmth, tenderness, and presence of a palpable "cord" along the vein. Risk factors include catheter material and size, vein in which the catheter is placed, and administration of irritating fluids. Mechanical phlebitis occurs ~ 4–7 d postinsertion; treat with warm compresses; usually resolves spontaneously. Chemical phlebitis can be avoided or minimized by ensuring catheter tip is in the SVC/RA juncture
Pinch-off syndrome	Caused by placement at the subclavian vein between the clavicle and first rib. Shearing of the catheter can result in catheter emboli
Catheter embolism	Catheter fragment(s), which can travel to the pulmonary artery. Caused by breakdown of catheter material, patient movement, pinch-off syndrome, or laceration of catheter during insertion. Sequelae can include sepsis, thrombus, perforation, or pulmonary emboli
Air embolism	Air travels to the right side of the heart and into the pulmonary circulation, causing vasoconstriction that results in an acute onset of hypoxia, tachypnea, chest pain, cyanosis, hypotension, neurologic symptoms, and even death
Cardiac tamponade	Catheter tip location and infusion of fluids with high osmolarity are risk factors. Catheter tip can erode through the heart wall. Symptoms include dyspnea, chest pain, tachycardia, hypotension, and pulsus paradoxus. Stop infusions immediately and aspirate from the catheter. Confirm tip location with radiography prior to use
Pneumothorax	More common with subclavian vein cannulation than internal jugular vein. Risk increases with frequent needle sticks and in emergency situations
Brachial plexus injury	Most common with jugular or subclavian insertion location. Loss of sensation, muscle weakness, paralysis of shoulder and upper limb muscles. Can result from a hematoma caused during insertion that caused brachial plexus compression. Transiently caused by anesthetic. Can be decreased with ultrasound use during insertion
Cardiac arrhythmias	Can be caused during guidewire insertion with chest lines. Avoid inserting the wire too deep during insertion. Catheter tip location is a significant cause. Ensure catheter tip is in lower SVC at the juncture of the RA. Catheter placed deep in the RA increases the risk of arrhythmias. Cardiac perforation can occur with catheters in the RA

PICC—peripherally inserted central-line catheter; RA—right atrium; SVC—superior vena cava.

REFERENCES

1. Barton AJ, Danek G, Johns P, Coons M: Improving patient outcomes through CQI: vascular access planning. *J Nurs Care Qual* 1998, 13:77–85.
2. Slaughter SE: Intravascular catheter-related infections: strategies for combating this common foe. *Postgrad Med* 2004, 116:59–66.
3. Moureau N, Poole S, Murdock MA, *et al.*: Central venous catheters in home infusion care: outcomes analysis in 50,470 patients. *J Vasc Interv Radiol* 2002, 13:1009–1016.
4. Crnich CJ, Maki DG: Infections caused by intravascular devices: epidemiology, pathogenesis, diagnosis, prevention, and treatment. In *APIC Text of Infection Control and Epidemiology*, edn 2. Washington, DC: Association for Professionals in Infection Control and Epidemiology; 2005:24.21–24.26.
5. Stephens LC, Haire WD, Kotulak GD: Are clinical signs accurate indicators of the cause of central venous catheter occlusion? *JPEN J Parenter Enteral Nutr* 1995, 19:75–79.
6. Centers for Disease Control and Prevention: Guidelines for the prevention of intravascular catheter-related infections. *MMWR Morb Mortal Wkly Rep* 2002, 51(RR-10):1–36.
7. Rosovsky RP, Kuter DJ: Catheter-related thrombosis in cancer patients: pathophysiology, diagnosis, and management. *Hematol Oncol Clin North Am* 2005, 19:183–202, vii.
8. Wilkin TD, Kraus MA, Lane KA, Trerotola SO: Internal jugular vein thrombosis associated with hemodialysis catheters. *Radiology* 2003, 228:697–700.
9. Bern MM, Lokich JJ, Wallach SR, *et al.*: Very low doses of warfarin can prevent thrombosis in central venous catheters. A randomized prospective trial. *Ann Intern Med* 1990, 112:423–428.
10. Ong B, Gibbs H, Catchpole I, *et al.*: Peripherally inserted central catheters and upper extremity deep vein thrombosis. *Australas Radiol* 2006, 50:451–454.
11. Lee AY, Levine MN, Butler G, *et al.*: Incidence, risk factors, and outcomes of catheter-related thrombosis in adult patients with cancer. *J Clin Oncol* 2006, 24:1404–1408.
12. Rawson KM, Newburn-Cook CV: The use of low-dose warfarin as prophylaxis for central venous catheter thrombosis in patients with cancer: a meta-analysis. *Oncol Nurs Forum* 2007, 34:1037–1043.
13. Heaton DC, Han DY, Inder A: Minidose (1 mg) warfarin as prophylaxis for central vein catheter thrombosis. *Intern Med J* 2002, 32:84–88.
14. Infusion Nurses Society: *Policies and Procedures for Infusion Nursing*, edn 3. Norwood, MA: Infusion Nurses Society; 2006.
15. Mermel LA: Prevention of intravascular catheter-related infections. *Ann Intern Med* 2000, 132:391–402.
16. Pittet D, Tarara D, Wenzel RP: Nosocomial bloodstream infection in critically ill patients: excess length of stay, extra costs, and attributable mortality. *JAMA* 1994, 271:1598–1601.
17. Theaker C: Infection control issues in central venous catheter care. *Intensive Crit Care Nurs* 2005, 21:99–109.
18. Render ML, Brungs S, Kotagal U, *et al.*: Evidence-based practice to reduce central line infections. *Jt Comm J Qual Patient Saf* 2006, 32:253–260.
19. Maki DG, Ringer M, Alvarado CJ: Prospective randomised trial of povidone-iodine, alcohol, and chlorhexidine for prevention of infection associated with central venous and arterial catheters. *Lancet* 1991, 338:339–343.
20. Mimoz O, Pieroni L, Lawrence C, *et al.*: Prospective, randomized trial of two antiseptic solutions for prevention of central venous or arterial catheter colonization and infection in intensive care unit patients. *Crit Care Med* 1996, 24:1818–1823.
21. O'Grady NP, Dezfulian C: The femoral site as first choice for central venous access? Not so fast. *Crit Care Med* 2005, 33:234–235.
22. Safdar N, Maki DG: Use of vancomycin-containing lock or flush solutions for prevention of bloodstream infection associated with central venous access devices: a meta-analysis of prospective, randomized trials. *Clin Infect Dis* 2006, 43:474–484.
23. Borschel DM, Chenoweth CE, Kaufman SR, *et al.*: Are antiseptic-coated central venous catheters effective in a real-world setting? *Am J Infect Control* 2006, 34:388–393.
24. Ho KM, Litton E: Use of chlorhexidine-impregnated dressing to prevent vascular and epidural catheter colonization and infection: a meta-analysis. *J Antimicrob Chemother* 2006, 58:281–287.

25. Raad I, Hanna H, Maki D: Intravascular catheter-related infections: advances in diagnosis, prevention, and management. *Lancet* 2007, 7:645–657.

26. Maki DG, Kluger DM, Crnich CJ: The risk of bloodstream infection in adults with different intravascular devices: a systematic review of 200 published prospective studies. *Mayo Clin Proc* 2006, 81:1159–1171.

27. Mermel LA, Farr BM, Sherertz RJ, *et al.*: Guidelines for the management of intravascular catheter-related infections. *J Intraven Nurs* 2001, 24:180–205.

28. Safdar N, Fine JP, Maki DG: Meta-analysis: methods for diagnosing intravascular device-related bloodstream infection. *Ann Intern Med* 2005, 142:451–466.

29. Ingram P, Sinclair L, Edwards T: The safe removal of central venous catheters. *Nurs Stand* 2006, 20:42–46.

30. Aitken DR, Minton JP: The "pinch-off sign": a warning of impending problems with permanent subclavian catheters. *Am J Surg* 1984, 148:633–636.

31. Bagnall-Reeb H: Evidence for the use of the antibiotic lock technique. *J Infus Nurs* 2004, 27:118–126.

32. Pronovost P, Needham D, Berenholtz S, *et al.*: An intervention to decrease catheter-related bloodstream infections in the ICU. *N Engl J Med* 2006, 355:2725–2732.

33. O'Grady NP, Alexander M, Dellinger EP, *et al.*: Guidelines for the prevention of intravascular catheter-related infections. Centers for Disease Control and Prevention. *MMWR Recomm Rep* 2002, 51(RR-10):1–29.

34. Rabinowitz N, Olsen M: Venous access devices. *Manual of Cancer Nursing*, edn 2. Philadelphia: Lippincott Williams & Wilkins; 2004:484–497.

35. Herbst SL, Kaplan LK, McKinnon BT: Vascular access devices: managing occlusions and related complications in home infusion. *Infusion* 1998, 4(Suppl):S1–S32.

36. The Johns Hopkins Hospital: Adult vascular access device (VAD) policy: Appendix B: catheter choice. *Interdisciplinary Clinical Practice Manual.* Available at http://www.hopkinsmedicine.org/heic/policies/pdf/IFC035_VAD_B.pdf. Accessed May 12, 2008.

Page numbers followed by *f* indicate figures; page numbers followed by *t* indicate tables.